Pediatric Ophthalmology

Pediatric Ophthalmology

DAVID TAYLOR FRCS FRCP
Consultant Paediatric Ophthalmologist,
The Hospital for Sick Children,
Great Ormond Street, London

WITH

EDUARD AVETISOV

MICHAEL BARAITSER

JOHN BRAZIER

NICHOLAS CAVANAGH

SUSAN DAY

JOHN ELSTON

WILLIAM GOOD

CREIG HOYT

SCOTT LAMBERT

ANTHONY MOORE

ELIZABETH THOMPSON

FOREWORD BY
MARSHALL M. PARKS
Washington DC

BLACKWELL SCIENTIFIC PUBLICATIONS

BOSTON OXFORD

LONDON EDINBURGH MELBOURNE

© 1990 by
Blackwell Scientific Publications, Inc.
Editorial Offices:
3 Cambridge Center, Suite 208
  Cambridge, Massachusetts 02142, USA
Osney Mead, Oxford OX2 0EL, England
25 John Street, London WC1N 2BL, England
23 Ainslie Place, Edinburgh EH3 6AJ, Scotland
54 University Street, Carlton
  Victoria 3053, Australia

First published 1990

Set by Setrite Typesetters,
Hong Kong; printed and
bound by Printek s.a., Bilbao, Spain

90   91   92   93   5   4   3   2   1

DISTRIBUTORS
USA and Canada
  Mosby-Year Book, Inc.
  200 North LaSalle Street
  Chicago, Illinois 60601
  (*Orders*: Tel: 1 800 621-9262)

Australia
  Blackwell Scientific Publications
  (Australia) Pty Ltd
  54 University Street
  Carlton, Victoria 3053
  (*Orders*: Tel: 03 347-0300)

Outside North America and Australia
  Marston Book Services Ltd
  PO Box 87
  Oxford 0X2 ODT
  (*Orders*: Tel: 0865 791155
         FAX: 0865 791927
         Telex: 837515)

Library of Congress
Cataloging-in-Publication Data

Pediatric ophthalmology/[edited by] David Taylor; with Eduard
  Avetisov ... [et al.]: foreword by Marshall M. Parks.
       p   cm.
    Includes bibliographical references.
    ISBN 0-86542-117-X
    1. Pediatric ophthalmology. I. Taylor, David, 1942—
  II. Avetisov, E. S. (Eduard Sergeevich)
    [DNLM: 1. Eye Diseases — in infancy & childhood.
  WW 600 P3713]
  RE48.2. C5P432 1990
  618.92'0977 — dc20

British Library
Cataloguing in Publication Data

Taylor, David
  Pediatric Ophtalmology.
  1. Children. Eyes. Diseases
  I. Title
  618.92'0977

ISBN 0-86542-117-X

Contents

List of Contributors

Eduard S Avetisov *Moscow Helmholtz Research Institute of Ophthalmology, 103064 Moscow, USSR*

Michael Baraitser FRCP, *Consultant Clinical Geneticist, Hospital for Sick Children, Great Ormond Street, London WC1*

John Brazier, FRCS, *Consultant Ophthalmologist, University College Hospital, Gower Street, London WC1*

Nicholas Cavanagh MD, FRCP, *Consultant Paediatric Neurologist, Westminster Children's Hospital, Vincent Square, London WC1; Charing Cross Hospital, Fulham Palace Road, London W6; and Cheyne Centre for Spastic Children, 61 Cheyne Walk, London SW3*

Susan Day MD, *Pacific Presbyterian Medical Center, 2100 Webster Street, Suite 214, San Francisco, California 94115, USA*

John S Elston BSc, MD, FRCS, *Consultant Ophthalmologist, Radcliffe Infirmary, Woodstock Rd., Oxford*

William V Good MD, *Assistant Professor of Ophthalmology, Department of Ophthalmology K301, University of California, San Francisco, California 94143, USA*

Creig S Hoyt MD, *Professor and Director of Pediatric Ophthalmology, University of California, Suite 751, 400 Parnassus Avenue, San Francisco, California 94143, USA*

Scott R Lambert MD, *Assistant Professor and Chief of Pediatric Ophthalmology, Emory University School of Medicine, Atlanta, Georgia 30322, USA*

Anthony Moore MA, FRCS, *Consultant Ophthalmologist, Addenbrookes Hospital, Hills Road, Cambridge CB2 2QQ*

David Taylor FRCS, FRCP, *Consultant Paediatric Ophthalmologist, Hospital for Sick Children, Great Ormond Street, London WC1*

Elizabeth Thompson MB, FRACP, *Consultant Clinical Geneticist, Kennedy-Galton Centre, Northwick Park Hospital, Harrow, Middlesex HA1 3UJ*

Foreword

Many years ago my 6-year-old son and his classmates attended their first performance of the Washington Symphony Orchestra; an extracurricular activity intended to introduce children to classical music. That evening in response to my inquiry about his day's unique experience he locked at me with sadness in his eyes and replied, 'But dad, they play such long songs.' Were this lad asked to comment about this text authored by Taylor and colleagues I suspect a similar response would be evoked perhaps — 'it is such a long story.'

Nearly all specialties in medicine and surgery share a natural division of their discipline into pediatric and geriatric portions. Ophthalmology is no exception to this generalization since the bulk of its pathology occurs either in pediatric or geriatric patients. Moreover, each age group has special ophthalmic care delivery needs with a special type of support from the physician and technical personnel in the specialties surrounding ophthalmology and unique facilities to render appropriate diagnostic and therapeutic methods. Also texts written for one group must differ from texts written for the other in order to include the relevant material and exclude the irrelevant. But the range and volume of material to be included in a text written either for pediatric ophthalmology or geriatric ophthalmology are comparable. A relatively complete text in either by necessity must be a long story.

The first text I recall written exclusively for pediatric ophthalmology was thirty years ago (Doggart 1959). Since then, as the subspecialties became established, the pace of new pediatric ophthalmology texts appearing on the market has broken into full stride. This is good, for the ultimate beneficiaries of this trend are our patients. This trend provides maximal opportunity to us who must learn or constantly review the multitude of details required for delivering quality care. We are fortunate to be surrounded by such a plethora of excellent minds with so many motivated physicians willing to collect and organize all the material for us.

The contrast is striking between Doggart's text (1959) and Taylor et al.'s (1990) text on pediatric ophthalmology. One is thin, the other is thick. The quantity of information imparted in the thick one is amazing. Is this difference in thickness between the two texts due solely to the amount of new knowledge that has been revealed during the past thirty years? I am afraid the answer is yes. At the time of my entry into pediatric ophthalmology in 1947, the total knowledge developed in this subspecialty was even less than that contained in Doggart's thin text. Prior to 1950 only a very few ophthalmologists had any idea that the subspecialty was needed and none appreciated the importance of the role it was destined to play in relationship to the flowering of the multiple subspecialties in either pediatrics or ophthalmology.

During the century prior to 1950 every advanced nation evolved special care facilities and health care delivery systems for their children. Eventually ophthalmology would certainly become a part of this scheme. The start of ophthalmology's involvement was slow, but by 1959 the pace had quickened; training in the subspecialty had become structured and was sought. A text was needed and Doggart, an Englishman, delivered it.

The task of producing a text today which provides the reader with the entire knowledge relevent to our field has become almost insurmountable. The array of diseases that affect the visual system and the anatomy surrounding the eye is enormous. Add to this the advent of the rapidly advancing field of genetics, its annual revelations of new basic facts and newly categorized diseases and now one can sense the magnitude of the onrushing front of new knowledge that has to be cataloged and disseminated. From such a crowded knowledge base, the first decision an editor of a comprehensive text in our subspecialty must face is what to include and exclude. It would be much easier to continue the trend of publishing theme texts which focus on only one facet, such as genetics, strabismus, pediatric ocular oncology, pediatric glaucoma, etc. Such limited texts serve a purpose, but there is always the need for a comprehensive text covering the entire breadth of our specialty. To accomplish this mission in 1990 requires a thick book. Taylor and his associate authors have succeeded in this mission by bringing us their monumental treatise on pediatric ophthalmology.

The text is divided into seven parts using 84 chapters to record this long list of subjects. Almost every statement is backed up by a total of 3688 references spotted throughout this book and the comprehensive coverage of this broad subspecialty deserves a note of gratitude from each reader to each of the authors. It is a thick book with the melodious appeal of a symphony. It is a long song.

Marshall M. Parks MD

Reference

Doggart JH. *Diseases of Children's Eyes.* The CV Mosby Co., St Louis, 1959

Preface

We have aimed to make this book a combination of a useful referenced text for referral and a practical clinical guide to pediatric ophthalmology.

Pediatric ophthalmology has changed greatly in ten years and this book aims to reflect the change. The thrust of the change has been due to the greater interest that ophthalmologists have developed in the care of the whole child and in medical as well as surgical care. In my experience this worldwide change has been spurred by demand from pediatricians with sick children with eye problems and where eye signs form vital diagnostic clues. The ophthalmologist has responded by arming himself with not only vital knowledge about strabismus, cataracts and other eminently treatable eye conditions but also with the wider fields of medicine which have expanded so much in the decade. This has the dual benefit to the pediatric ophthalmologist that he has become highly specialized in the care of a tiny, but vital, organ and he is one of the few ophthalmologists who can justify being a real generalist dealing with conditions as widely diverse as orbital disease and metabolic disease, strabismus and neuro-ophthalmology. We also have to thank our pediatrician colleagues for showing us how to approach the child and his problems. I believe that the child has benefited from these changes.

We have achieved an international flavour by close Anglo-American and Russian collaboration. This has been very rewarding and reflects the nature of post-graduate education that was achieved by the imagination and effort of the contributors, not by government sponsorship — long may we be able to continue to help each others' apprentices for the widening and deepening of their training!

We have tried to avoid overlap of subjects by careful planning, editing and indexing but some overlap is inevitable and deliberate to avoid the need to jump around the book too much. Individual subjects have not been treated in excessive depth in most areas, but references have been provided for the reader with greater curiosity.

The problems in the appendix have been included to help the clinician to find a way through the process of diagnosis. Most of the sections provide only guidelines and their use should be supplemented by reading appropriate areas of the main text.

Sexism creeps into any publication and we have not done much to avoid it other than by using a liberal mix of him and her when referring to babies. We were unable to stomach the use of generic pronouns (shem, shim, thon, na, per, hir, himorher, himmer) although we endorse Burkhart's (1987) principles of non-sexist writing!

The spelling of the title of this book is a pragmatic response to a majority view; we expect that anyone who has been so meticulous as to read the Preface as far as this will judge the work more on its content than its packing!

The photographs have come mainly from my own collection with occasional ones lent by kind colleagues who are acknowledged in the legends. The purpose has been to illustrate pertinent points in the text rather than to form an all-encompassing collection, on the one hand, or to initiate the beginner in the basics of pediatric ophthalmology, on the other hand.

Surgery is not learnt from books and we have confined ourselves to surgical principles and indications. The best place to learn surgery is in the operating room or theatre guided by surgical texts and papers.

Aspects of genetics have been dealt with in a general section by Baraitser and Thompson and some details are given in each relevant section. In genetics lies not only the future of so much pediatric ophthalmology but it is also a fascinating and rewarding area for study with enormous benefits to families.

I would like to express my personal gratitude to my friends and mentors, particularly to Bill Hoyt, Kenneth Wybar, Marshall Parks, Otto Wolf and Stephen Miller who have enriched and enlarged my view of ophthalmology.

David Taylor

Reference

Burkhart S. Sexism in medical writing. *Br Med J* 1987; **295**: 1585

Acknowledgements

No book like this can be published without the help of an enormous number of people who do a lot but receive little credit. This is one of those books that has been helped by very many more people than the number of authors, some of whom are mentioned below:

Mr Chris Lyons, Dr Mike Levine, Jeremy Squire and Dr John Pritchard helped with either proof reading or with editorial suggestions, and one of our authors, Dr Nicholas Cavanagh, helped with very many chapters by removing ophthalmological jargon, making the chapters readable by the non-ophthalmologist.

Josephine Lace, Yvonne Robinson, Gill Alger and Anna Taylor all helped with the manuscript but most of all I owe a debt of gratitude to Mrs Linda White who prepared the final text in an amazingly short time with considerable accuracy.

Clair Bourhiz organized the slide library from which the illustrations have been drawn. The photographers at Great Ormond Street — in particular, Carol Reeves, Ray Lunnon and Simon Brown — took most of the photographs and Karen Abadee acted as the subject for many of the illustrations in Chapter 33.

My heartfelt thanks go to all of these kind and hard working people. If there has been any pleasure in producing this book it has largely been due to them!

Finally, I would like to express my gratitude to the staff at Blackwell Scientific Publications — in particular, Rebecca Huxley, Edward Wates and Peter Saugman for their prompt and meticulous handling of this book, and unfailing good humour.

Section 1
Epidemiology, Growth and Development

1 Epidemiology of Visual Handicap in Childhood

JOHN ELSTON

Visually handicapped children are a complex and heterogenous group. Although there is a large amount of information potentially available about them, it is scattered throughout the paediatric and ophthalmological literature. The subject is, however, an important one, for several reasons: for the individual child, the early recognition of visual handicap may allow effective treatment, for example of congenital cataract. Recognition is important also because, even as an isolated defect, visual handicap may have serious implications for many developmental functions (Reynell 1978). Finally, an understanding of the epidemiology of childhood visual handicap may enable us to reduce its occurrence in future generations.

The problem

Establishing the current causes of childhood visual handicap in the UK is a daunting task. The definition of the condition is not agreed, and although there can be no argument that the completely blind child is visually handicapped, there are considerable difficulties in evaluating and measuring visual function between light perception and normality (Robinson 1977). It may be done by using clinical methods, preferential looking techniques, or electrodiagnostic studies. It may be carried out by an ophthalmologist, orthoptist, developmental paediatrician, or neurologist. Visual function may be documented on the blind registration (BD8) form, where childhood blindness is defined in educational terms, or according to some other concept of the effect of visual handicap. The age at which the evaluation takes place is very variable but obviously important. The cause of the visual handicap may be given anatomically (e.g. corneal opacity), descriptively (e.g. optic atrophy) or on the basis of the presumed underlying disorder (e.g. rubella syndrome).

Most available surveys therefore have serious epidemiological deficiencies. It is difficult to eliminate bias in the selection of the patients studied since the spectrum of affected children stretches from those with an isolated visual problem to the multiply handicapped (Bleeker-Wagemakers 1981) child whose poor vision may be thought relatively unimportant, and who is not, therefore, on the blind register (Robinson 1977). For example, of 7700 retarded children examined by Warburg et al. (1975), 200 were already on the blind register, but a further 369 were found to have a serious, unrecognized, visual handicap. The reported prevalence of associated mental handicap may vary from 2% when children in schools for the blind are examined (Fraser & Friedman 1967), to 57% of the total population of visually handicapped children (Bryars & Archer 1977). Ascertainment in the surveys of visually handicapped children is at best 80% (Bryars & Archer 1977). Since visual handicap may be classified in a number of different ways, the diagnostic criteria are open to different interpretations and regional variations are apparent (Brennan & Knox 1973). These may be due to the policies and awareness of individual ophthalmologists and developmental paediatricians. Since the primary purpose of blind and partially sighted registration in children is identification of individuals requiring educational assistance, surveys may rely on these statistics, but registration is often not obligatory. Because diagnostic evaluation is variable and may rely either on clinical signs alone or include extensive electrodiagnostic and radiological investigation, up to 25% of visually handicapped children may not have an established diagnosis (Hatfield 1972; Schappert-Kimmijser et al. 1975). All the studies are retrospective and it is important to know the date of birth of the patients and be aware of neonatal treatment policies at that time in order to comment sensibly on the contribution of, for example, retinopathy of prematurity.

3

Current causes

Estimates of prevalance (disease frequency in the community) in the developed world are often difficult to assess due to demographic and educational trends and in Europe the prevalence of blindness may be less accurate than in some developing countries (Johnson and Minassian 1989). In an attempt to give an overview of the current causes in Western Europe, North America and Australia, the findings in eight surveys from these areas from 1965 onwards have been analysed together (Fraser & Friedmann 1967; Fraser 1968; Hatfield 1972; Lindstedt 1972; Schappert-Kimmijser *et al.* 1975; Bryars & Archer 1977; Robinson 1977; Bleeker-Wagemakers 1981). Because of differences of population and method, they are not strictly comparable. For the purpose of this analysis, therefore, the causes have been classified as either prenatal, perinatal or postnatal (Table 1.1).

1 Prenatal causes are either genetic, e.g. albinism, tapetoretinal degeneration or cataracts, or other, e.g. infection or structural maldevelopment of the eye.

2 Perinatal factors include prematurity, the complications of labour (especially neonatal asphyxia), and neonatal infections such as meningitis and ophthalmia neonatorum.

3 Postnatal causes are trauma, including non-accidental injury, infection, raised intracranial pressure and tumours.

Considering the eight studies together, agreement on several important points emerges (Table 1.2). It is

Table 1.1 Analysis of childhood visual handicap.

Aetiological factor	Clinical example
Prenatal	
Genetic	Cataract
	Albinism
	Tapeto-retinal degeneration
Other	Infection
	Pre-eclampsia
Perinatal	Prematurity
	Neonatal asphyxia
	Infection
Postnatal	Trauma
	Infection
	Tumour

clear that genetic defects are the single most important cause of visual handicap in childhood, accounting for between 34 and 51% of cases. Taken together with the other prenatal influences, between a half and two thirds of all cases are accounted for. This has not always been the case. Serial studies of registered blind schoolchildren in the USA indicate that in the early years of this century, postnatal causes (particularly infection) were more important (Hatfield 1963). In 1906/7 for example, ophthalmia neonatorum accounted

Table 1.2 Aetiology of visual handicap in childhood: data assembled from eight recent surveys.

Reference	Country	Aetiology (% of total)				
		Prenatal				
		Genetic	Other	Perinatal	Postnatal	Not established
Hatfield (1963)	USA	68		9	5	18
Fraser & Friedman (1967)	England and Wales	50	6	33	11	—
Fraser (1968)	Australia	34	20	16	14	16
Lindstedt (1972)	Sweden	58		17	12	13
Robinson (1977)	Canada	41	10	20	10	19
Schappert-Kimmijser (1975) *et al.*	W. Europe	45	6	8	16	25
Bryars & Archer (1977)	N. Ireland	51	11	11	5	22
Bleeker-Wagemakers (1981)	Netherlands (mentally retarded patients)	40	11	36	5	8

for 28% of cases, and in so far as the studies allow us to make the comparison, rural African populations still suffer in this way. Keratitis accounted for 21% of childhood blindness in one study from Nigeria (Olurin 1970) and infections, including meningitis, 32% in another from Malawi (Benezra & Chirambo 1977). The prophylaxis and management of pre and postnatal infections in developed countries has radically altered the picture so that by 1972 only 10% of cases of childhood blindness in the USA were due to an infection, and 75% of these were prenatal (congenital rubella) (Hatfield 1972). The prevalence of the other major blinding prenatal infection in the USA, syphilis, fell by 91% between 1933 and 1958 (Hatfield 1963).

Perinatal influences are next in importance in developed countries. Again, continuing improvements in the management of pregnancy and labour in recent years are tending to improve these figures. The picture is not entirely straightforward, however, and the problem is illustrated by retinopathy of prematurity. The population which was at risk from this condition in the 1940s and 1950s is now protected by routine precautions in oxygen administration. The prevalence fell from 7.9 per 100 000 in 1950 to 1.8 per 100 000 in 1965 (Hatfield 1972). The disease is now, however, reappearing since its occurrence is inversely related to the birth weight of the baby, and current neonatal expertise allows the survival of very low birth weight babies, who even 10 years ago would have died (Ashton 1984). Seventy one per cent of children born at between 500 and 750 g, for example, show acute proliferative retinopathy of prematurity, despite assiduous oxygen monitoring (Flynn et al. 1979). Although the majority of cases will resolve spontaneously, no consensus has yet emerged on effective prophylaxis or treatment. Similarly, contemporary medical and surgical treatments and policies allow the survival of children with severe structural abnormalities of the central nervous system. These children usually have multiple handicaps, with visual difficulties as only a part of their problem (Robinson 1977). For these reasons, although the incidence of visual handicap in childhood is stable, the prevalence of the condition is rising (Hatfield 1963; Robinson 1977).

Control of environmental factors in Western Europe has had an important impact on the postnatal development of visual handicap. Ocular trauma, for example, still represents a major problem in developing countries (Merin et al. 1972; Baghdassarian & Tabbara 1975), but is now numerically of little importance in the USA and the UK. Cataract associated with congenital rubella is still important in countries

without a rubella vaccination programme (Moriarty 1988). Technical developments in the treatment of, for example, infantile glaucoma and congenital cataracts have meant that the extent of the visual disability in these conditions has been reduced. Congenital cataract, however, is now the commonest single anatomical diagnosis in childhood visual handicap in the UK. It may be that the survival of low birth weight, especially dysmature, neonates with a tendency to hypoglycaemia, may be partly responsible (Merin & Crawford 1971). The importance of developments in neonatal medicine, alluded to above, are thereby emphasized. A recent study (Robinson et al. 1987) has emphasized the changes taking place in British Columbia over a 40-year period; there has been an increase in children born with optic nerve lesions, a decrease followed by a re-emergence of retinopathy of prematurity, and a decrease in lens diseases reflecting the decrease in rubella. Overall there was a decrease in registered blindness and those registered had fewer handicaps.

The future

The trend in childhood visual handicap is away from identifiable environmental causes that may be preventable, towards pre and perinatal influences, often ill understood, over which we have much less control. Genetic causes now predominate, but there are over 50 different conditions with Mendelian inheritance involved, polygenic inheritance accounts for others and there is also the possibility of a new mutation of a dominant gene (Phillips et al. 1975; Baraitser 1981). There is, however, a real possibility of prevention in this field. Primary prevention is by genetic counselling. The ophthalmologist has an important role here, since the geneticist relies on the diagnosis established in one child to give the parents advice about the possibility of a similar defect occurring in others. It may not be possible to establish the diagnosis precisely on the basis of one clinic visit, and it is, therefore, extremely important that both the ophthalmologist and the parents of a visually handicapped child appreciate this before advice about subsequent pregnancies is given.

Secondary control of genetically determined disease is now possible by abortion of a fetus with a recognized defect. The recognition of the gene locus for conditions such as X-linked retinitis pigmentosa (Bhattacharya et al. 1984) and retinoblastoma (Sparkes et al. 1983) may enable prenatal diagnosis to control these conditions.

It is clear that genetic studies, both in the population

to establish inheritance, and in the laboratory to define gene loci, are of prime importance in the future control of childhood visual handicap. The difficulty of introducing effective, preventive measures to control the other major contributor to the problem, perinatal environmental factors, is illustrated by the dilemma with regard to retinopathy of prematurity. The increasingly effective treatment of conditions such as congenital cataracts lessens the impact of visual handicap on development as a whole, but preventive measures are clearly more important.

Most recent studies of the current causes suffer from serious objections as to bias, low ascertainment and diagnostic imprecision. However, previously unrecognized factors have emerged in the aetiology of specific diseases such as congenital cataracts. An epidemiologically adequate study of childhood visual handicap in England and Wales would be a major advance in further defining, and therefore combatting, the problem.

References

Ashton N. Retrolental fibroplasia, now retinopathy of prematurity. *Br J Ophthalmol* 1984; **68**: 689

Baghdassarian SA, Tabbara KF. Childhood blindness in Lebanon. *Am J Ophthalmol* 1975; **79**: 827–30

Baraitser M. The genetics of blindness. *Hospital Update* 1981; **23**: 516–27

Benezra D, Chirambo MC. Incidence and causes of blindness among the under 5 age group in Malawi. *Br J Ophthalmol* 1977; **61**: 154–7

Bhattacharya SS, Wright AF, Clayton JF, *et al.* Close genetic linkage between x-linked retinitis pigmentosa and a restriction fragment length polymorphisin identified by recombitant DNA probe L1.28. *Nature* 1984; **309**: 253–5

Bleeker-Wagemakers EM. *On the Causes of Blindness in the Mentally Retarded.* Bartimeus Foundation, The Nederlands 1981

Brennen ME, Knox EG. An investigation into the purposes, accuracy and effective uses of The Blind Register in England. *Br J Prev Soc Med* 1973; **27**: 154–9

Bryars JH, Archer DB. Aetiological survey of visually handicapped children in Northern Ireland. *Trans Ophthalmol Soc UK* 1977; **97**: 26–30

Flynn JT, Cassady J, Essner D, *et al.* Fluorescein angiography in retrolental fibroplasia: experience from 1969–1979. *Ophthalmology* 1979; **86**: 1700–23

Fraser GR. The causes of severe visual handicap among school children in South Australia. *Med J Aust* 1968; **1**: 615–20

Fraser GR, Friedman AI. The causes of blindness in childhood: a study of 776 children with severe visual handicaps. Johns Hopkins, Baltimore 1967

Hatfield EM. Causes of blindness in school children. *Sight Saving Review* 1963; **33**: 218–33

Hatfield EM. Blindness in infants and young children. *Sight Saving Review* 1972; **42**: 69–89

Johnson GJ, Minassian DC. Prevalence of blindness and eye disease. *J R Soc Med* 1989; **82**: 351–4

Lindstedt E. Severe visual impairment in Swedish children. *Doc Ophthalmol* 1972; **31**: 173–204

Merin S, Crawford JS. Hypoglycaemia and infantile cataract. *Arch Ophthalmol* 1971; **86**: 495–8

Merin S, Lapithis AG, Horovitz D, Michaelson IC. Childhood blindness in Cyprus. *Am J Ophthalmol* 1972; **74**: 538–42

Moriarty BJ. Childhood blindness in Jamaica. *Br J Ophthalmol* 1988; **72**: 65–8

Olurin O. Aetiology of blindness of Nigerian children. *Am J Ophthalmol* 1970; **70**: 533–40

Phillips CF, Stokoe NL, Hughes HE. An ophthalmic genetic clinic. *Trans Ophthalmol Soc UK* 1975; **95**: 472–6

Reynell J. Developmental patterns of visually handicapped children. *Child Care Health Dev* 1978; **4**: 291–304

Robinson GC. Causes, ocular disorders, associated handicaps and incidence and prevalence of blindness in children. In Jan JE, Freeman RD, Scott EP (eds). *Visual Impairment in Children and Adolescents.* Grune & Stratton, New York 1977; pp 27–47

Robinson GC, Jan JE, Kinnis C. Congenital Ocular blindness in children 1945–84. *Am J Dis Child* 1987; **141**: 1321–4

Schappert-Kimmijser J, Hansen E, Haustrate-Gosset MF, Lindstedt E, Skeydgaard H, Warburg M. Causes of severe visual impairment in children and their prevention. *Doc Ophthalmol* 1975; **39**: 213–41

Sparkes RS, Murphree AL, Lingua RW, *et al.* Gene for hereditary retinoblastoma assigned to human chromosome 13 by linkage to esterase-D. *Science* 1983; **219**: 971–3

Warburg M, Frederiksen P. Blindness among 7700 mentally retarded children in Denmark. In Smith B, Kein J (eds). *Visual Handicap in Children.* W. Heinemann, London 1977.

2 Normal and Abnormal Visual Development

SUSAN DAY

The development of vision in infants is a difficult area to study since the process of seeing, as well as the evaluation of this process, encompasses ocular, central nervous system, and behavioural development. A baby's eyesight nevertheless represents the most important source of information about his new environment and is of vital developmental significance. Indeed, general development may be severely affected when visual perception is impaired.

Neonatal vision

The visual system is relatively mature at birth. The first year of life represents a very dynamic period in vision development, and any pathology which impairs visual development has a longstanding impact. The visual system remains malleable at least for the first decade, and thus attention to this visual plasticity is paramount in the management of childhood eye problems.

When directly questioned, parents are indeed aware of their baby's visual development. Although traditional teaching suggests that the fixation and following reflexes are present at the age of 6 weeks, many parents will report their baby sees at a much younger age. Parents will also observe a baby's fascination with brightly coloured objects, such as mobiles, rapidly moving objects such as fans, and fascination simply with the human face. In the event that their baby has poor vision, many parents are almost intuitive in their ability to discern it.

Various anatomical and physiological factors influence the developing vision of an infant. Not only the eye's maturation, but also the central nervous system's growth and maturation must be considered.

Anatomical aspects

Prenatal development of the eye and brain occurs relatively early in comparison to other systems. By 6 weeks of gestation, the ocular structures and differentiation of the brain are fairly well developed. Teratogenic factors occurring within the first trimester commonly result in ocular defects. At birth, the anteroposterior diameter of the infant's eye is 70% that of an adult, measuring approximately 17 mm. The volume of the infant's eye in contrast, is only 50% that of an adult's eye. Thus, differential growth of the eye occurs after birth. The anterior structures consisting of cornea, lens and iris are in general more completely developed than the posterior segment of the eye (Swan & Wilkins 1984).

7

Periorbital tissue also is relatively well developed at birth although some growth does occur after birth. The muscle insertions and their relationships to the limbus and equator change dramatically within the first year of life; such knowledge must be considered with regards to timing of strabismus surgery. It has been recommended that strabismus surgery not be performed prior to the age of 6 months because of the changing relative anatomic relationships (Swan & Wilkins 1984).

The inner layers of the eye also undergo further growth and differentiation after birth. Although human studies are relatively few, examination of neonatal monkeys has shown that differentiation of the fovea occurs relatively late in comparison to other regions of the retina (Hendrickson & Kupfer 1976) and may be incomplete until 4 months after birth (Hendrickson & Kupfer 1976; Abramov et al. 1982; Hendrickson & Yuodelis 1984). Clinically, one often sees a relatively dull foveal reflex which gains an added sense of dimension presumably due to thickening and the development of the internal limiting membrane within the first few months. The peripheral temporal retina does not achieve complete vascularization until 44 weeks gestation. Due to the greater length between the optic nerve and temporal ora serrata compared to the nasal ora serrata, there is a predilection for abnormal vascularization in the temporal retina as in retinopathy of prematurity.

The optic nerve head itself is relatively full size at birth although there may be minimal postnatal growth. Clinical evidence of severe optic nerve hypoplasia implies a severe early insult occurring at 6–10 weeks gestational age; such a hypoplastic nerve has no potential of postnatal growth to any significant degree. Minor degrees of optic nerve hypoplasia may result from later prenatal influences.

In addition to the growth of the eye postnatally, the central nervous system is also maturing. The myelination of visual pathways, for instance, is not complete until 2 years of age (Magoon & Robb 1981). Control of eye movements may also be influenced by the development of supranuclear eye movement systems involving the cerebellar, brain stem, and vestibular input.

Physiological aspects

The development of normal function of the visual system, both sensory and motion, in large part parallels anatomic development. It is not surprising, for instance, that visual evoked potential (VEP) and forced preferential looking (FPL) data show rapid improvement of grating resolution in the first months of life when we recognize that foveal differentiation is incomplete at birth (Banks et al. 1988). The variation of binocular alignment (Nixon et al. 1985) during the first months of life may reflect orbital growth, ocular growth, and maturation of supranuclear eye movement control as well as improved acuity and binocular function. To isolate one particular system and study its role in changing functions becomes a very difficult task.

One approach toward understanding normal physiology is to study the ramifications physiologically of abnormal function, such as with amblyopia. Then, single cell recordings and other direct studies of function can be made. A detailed consideration of such abnormal functions will follow later in this chapter.

Extrageniculostriate vision

One recent report (Dubowitz et al. 1986) suggests that in early neonatal vision, subcortical regions may play a significant factor in vision behaviour. Premature infants were assessed behaviourally by their ability to track a red yarn ball as well as with visual evoked responses and a version of preferential looking. Infants were also assessed neurologically, and cranial ultrasounds and CT scans were also performed. Curiously, some infants with ultrasound or radiological evidence of occipital cortex abnormality had good initial visual function behaviourally as well as the presence of a visual evoked response (VER). In fact, one infant appeared to see initially despite postmortem documentation of an absent occipital cortex.

Normal visual development

The development of visual acuity in infants has been measured in various ways. The standard clinical techniques of 'fix and follow' response and the CSM (centrally, steadily and maintain fixation) classification, each rely upon interpretation of motor responses. Early attempts to quantify visual acuity were made with optokinetic nystagmus testing in which stripes of varying size were passed in front of an infant's eye (Gorman et al. 1957; Dayton et al. 1964). The presence of induced optokinetic nystagmus implied the infant's ability to see the stripes. More recent efforts to quantify infant vision fall into two basic categories — psychophysical testing and electrophysiologic techniques.

Psychophysical measurement

The most common psychophysical test is some variant of preferential looking (PL); it is often described as forced preferential looking, or FPL. With psychophysical testing, interpretation of a child's ability to see is dependent upon a child's motor response. A child is given a choice of looking at a homogenous target or at a target with gratings. When the child appears to see a large grating, subsequent test samples are performed with progressively finer grating size.

Measurements with this technique have suggested that an ability to resolve 20/100 equivalent gratings is present by the age of 1 year (Fig. 2.1) and 20/20 equivalent gratings by the age of 3 years (Teller *et al.* 1986) (Fig. 2.2). FPL techniques have been applied clinically to patients with strabismus, amblyopia, and aphakia (Catalano *et al.* 1987). The 1–2-year age group appears to be most easily tested with this technique, but one must remember that the responses to the FPL test are always dependent on a movement, and may be defective for motor as well as visual

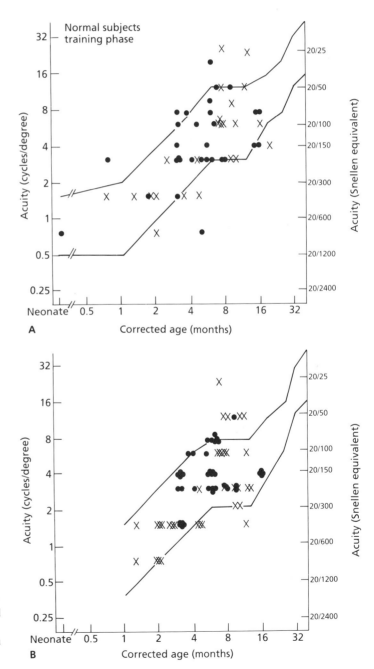

Fig. 2.1 Estimates of binocular (A) and monocular (B) acuity of normal children 1–32 months old. Acuity card acuity norms are within the solid lines. Data from experienced testers are represented by ● and data from inexperienced testers by x. From Sebris *et al.* (1987).

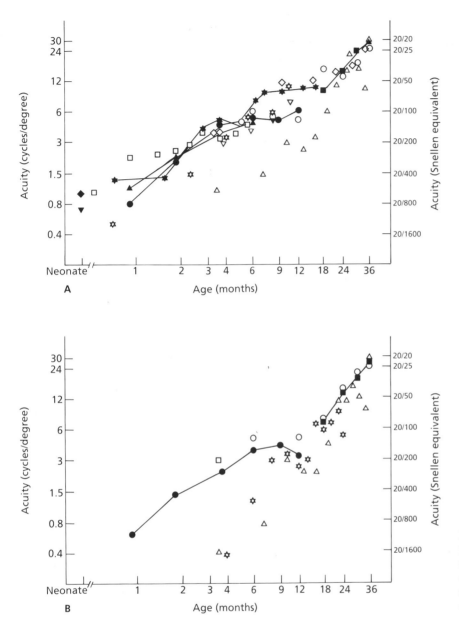

Fig. 2.2 Pooled data from normal 0–3-year-olds with acuity cards (filled symbols) and PL or operant procedures (open symbols). Upper figure, binocular acuities, lower monocular. From Teller *et al.* (1986).

reasons. Strictly speaking, there is no direct equivalence between Snellen acuity and FPL gratings which are measured in cycles per degree.

Electrophysiological measurement

The second method of measurement, electrophysiologic testing, records infants' visual evoked potentials to projected gratings of various sizes; it is not dependent on eye movements. Both checker board and stripe gratings have been used. The techniques of acuity estimation vary, and include reliance upon a signal generated by a series of quickly projected samples (Sokol 1978). Extrapolation of visual acuity

on the basis of the visual evoked response to a rapidly changing grating size known as the 'sweep' technique (Tyler *et al.* 1979) and direct measurement in which acuity is estimated on the basis of responses (Eizenman *et al.* 1987). The quantified visual acuity with this technique implies the ability to resolve 20/20 gratings by the age of 6–8 months.

The apparent difference in visual acuities between VEP and FPL quantification arises from the basic differences between electrophysiologic and psychophysical testing. Application of both the FPL and the visual evoked response in infants has been helpful in establishing normal vision development. Application of either of these techniques to pathological conditions is far more difficult; the limitations are greatest in the very children in which we need this information.

Other research techniques have been used to measure maturity of the visual system in infants, including vernier visual acuity (Shimojo & Held 1987) and contrast sensitivity (Norcia *et al.* 1987). It should be emphasized that each of these techniques is measuring a very precise function. Attempts to directly correlate acuities obtained with these techniques to Snellen acuities are *not* appropriate. Thus, a mother who is told that her baby is seeing 20/80 by any given technique should not be led to believe that this will necessarily be the level obtained when her child is 15 years old. Rather than providing us with the precise number, these techniques have been helpful in research settings in documenting differences between the two eyes, improvement or worsening of vision, and an estimate of severe versus mild visual loss in comparison to other age-matched controls.

Clinical assessment

Establishing normal levels of visual function is, despite research efforts to quantify them, still primarily one of observation of behaviour. Guidebooks for new parents will rightly tell them the baby should steadily fix on an object (such as their faces) by 6 weeks. In fact, many parents will volunteer that their babies were able to fix steadily within the first few days.

Specific guidelines for the neonatal examination have been made to help assessment of a baby's development. Although some tests are directly intended to assess a baby's vision, others designed to assess motor development are in fact vision-dependent, highlighting the key role that vision plays in the normal general development of a child. By 2 months, a following response should be present, and the baby should smile responsively to a parent. At 4 months, a child should reach for an object. At 6 months, a child plays with an object in his or her hand. Shortly after 1 year of age, a child begins to scribble with a crayon and point to desired objects (Swaiman & Wright 1975).

Assessment of vision in toddlers (McDonald 1986) becomes easier due to the child's ability to communicate. Although many clinicians rely too simply on fix-follow or CSM criteria (see Chapter 7) vision can be quantified without research techniques. One must remember, however, the shortness of the attention span and the tendency to become quickly bored by anything that does not resemble a game.

Acuity tests designed for the toddler can be regarded as to the task which must be performed by the child.

Detection acuity tasks are commonly used by developmental paediatricians, especially the Stycar graded balls vision test (Sheridan 1973). The examiner observes a child's response to moving white balls of progressively smaller size. The Catford drum (Catford & Oliver 1973) and the dot visual acuity test (Kirschen *et al.* 1983) are also detection tests and do not measure acuity. The recognition acuity tasks include: (a) direction-orientated tasks such as the illiterate E and Landolt C; (b) letter charts; (c) picture charts; and (d) Bailey–Hall cereal test. Of these, the illiterate E test enjoys the greatest popularity, although the limitation placed by a child's orientational skill make this a difficult test to rely upon before the age of 3 years. Letter charts may be used at this age and are best adapted into a matching format where the child holds a key card. Picture charts including the lighthouse test (Grier 1973) and the Allen picture cards (Allen 1957) each have some limitation as a consequence of cultural and social differences among children. The Bailey Hall cereal test uses breakfast cereal-like objects to entice a child's response (Bailey 1983).

Visual acuity norms in the 18-month to 3-year-old child have been highly variable, depending not only on the type of testing (detection vs recognition vs resolution) but also on the particular research centre. Regardless of the type of test, there is a variation of one octave, that is a halving or doubling of spatial frequency, such as from 10′ arc to 5 or 20′ of arc: comparable to the difference between 20/20 and 20/40 and 20/80 vision (McDonald 1986). To the busy clinician, it appears that the best advice regarding norms in this age group is to gain familiarity with one or two of the available tests, gather one's own sense of what is normal, and pursue equivocal results with further testing and careful follow-up. Above all, any specific number obtained for a toddler's vision must be matched with the clinical story to give an interpretation of testing results.

Visual acuity norms in children age 3–6 years have received considerable attention from Simons (1983). He recommends the use of a single optotype test (such as Landolt C or HOTV) with a constant surround which is non-memorizable. Particular attention must be paid to the child's difficulty lateralizing, i.e. distinguishing between right and left, if an E optotype is used. A further recommendation is made to perform distance testing at 3 rather than 6 m. Specific visual acuity norms are largely dependent upon the type of optotype used (Simons 1983).

At age 4, most researchers have found 'normal' vision to be between 20/20 and 20/40 (Slataper 1950;

Simons 1983; Romano *et al.* 1975). A visual acuity of 20/20 is reached by more than 70% of those tested not until the age of 7 years (Simons 1983). The National Society to Prevent Blindness (1976) has established the following criteria for referral: 3–4-year-olds — 20/50 or less in either or both eyes by isolated symbols; 5–6-year-olds — 20/40 or less in either or both eyes and/or an interocular acuity difference of one line on isolated symbols or two lines on linear presentations. Further guidelines for ophthalmologic assessment as well as a review of current screening practices are reviewed by Ehrlich *et al.* (1983).

Abnormal visual development

Critical period

Historically, an understanding of the critical time period for visual development has been gained only through observation of abnormal circumstances, be they experimental or clinical observation. Weisel and Hubel (1963a, 1963b, 1965) documented the parallel between visual behaviour created by unilateral eye closure and visual physiology in which cortical cells from the deprived eye functioned abnormally. One of their major contributions was to confirm the significance of an abnormal visual experience during a critical time period.

That a critical period exists for normal visual development is demonstrated clinically by studies of the child born with cataract and operated upon at several years of age. Despite clearing of the media, and even with proper optical correction, such a child has a permanent profound visual deficit.

The critical time period for development of normal infant vision when the insult is binocular appears to be within the first 3 months of life, i.e. with failure of a focussed image such as with complete congenital cataracts. Clearing of the media and optical correction should be in place within the first few months of life in order to ensure vision which will allow a relatively normal life (Vaegan & Taylor 1979). From a practical standpoint, however, the clinician is rarely completely assured of what an infant's past visual experience has been. The benefit of the doubt must be given to the infant presenting with this clinical circumstance and treatment rendered as promptly as is possible.

In the most severe example of deprivation, a child with unilateral congenital cataract, it appears that the 'window of opportunity' for successful treatment may be as short as from birth to 6 weeks. In long-term follow-up of children with congenital cataracts, acuity

better than 20/40 is rarely obtained when surgery and optical correction is delayed beyond 2 months (Vaegan & Taylor 1979), although other reports have been far more encouraging (Beller et al. 1981; Robb *et al.* 1987).

Plasticity of the visual system

The infant with his or her 'window' of critical vision development is replaced by an individual with a more mature visual system. Its fragility, however, remains, and any new insult has the potential for impairing good vision (Von Noorden 1985). The plasticity of the visual system extends up to 12 years after birth. Any acquired abnormality such as strabismus or a traumatic cataract can result in altered visual development. Most clinicians have established a cut-off at 10–12 years in terms of any possible responses to treatment aimed at recovering vision.

Abnormal visual development occurs whenever a clearly focussed image on the retina is not maintained during the first months to years of life. The type of 'insult', be it poor focus (ametropia), poor 'aim' (strabismus), or media opacity does not seem to be nearly as important as other critical factors: the age of onset, the severity of the insult, the age of initiation of treatment, compliance with treatment, and the health of the fellow eye.

In general, the younger the onset, the more severely damaging is the insulting factor. This is especially true if the insult occurs within the first few months of life during the critical time period. For instance, a child with bilateral congenital cataracts must receive attention within the first few months of life if vision better than 20/40 to 20/60 is likely to be achieved. Clinically, the most difficult feature in this regard is determining the age of onset: parental observation, the position of the cataract, and the degree to which the media are opaque are indicators of a true congenital onset of the visual defect, whilst if there has been a postnatal assessment of a red reflex or in some instances the presence of a microphthalmic eye (suggesting persistent hyperplastic primary vitreous) are stronger indicators of an early onset visual defect. A congenital cataract, though present at birth, is not necessarily associated with a significant visual defect from birth (such as a small anterior polar cataract) or at least not at all stages of its development; it is the onset of the visual defect that is the important factor and the most difficult to determine.

The severity of the insult also contributes to the prognosis. Significance is in part related to the location of the abnormality. An anterior polar cataract, far away from the nodal point of the eye, is unlikely to result in any significant visual disturbance whilst an opacity of similar size which is posteriorly placed may impair vision significantly.

The earlier the initiation of appropriate treatment, the better the prognosis; compliance with treatment, such as with occlusion therapy, also is important. Finally, the status of the fellow eye appears to be a significant feature relating to permanent visual loss. Large differences between the two eyes appears to evoke a more extensive visual loss in the poorer eye. Some clinicians have argued that in conditions which are essentially unilateral such as monocular congenital cataract, treatment should include *bilateral* occlusion prior to completion of surgery and optical correction of the pathologic eye so that asymmetric development of vision does not occur (Cynader *et al.* 1976).

Amblyopia

DEFINITION

When significant interruption of normal visual development occurs, then amblyopia is the term used to describe this loss of vision. Amblyopia, derived from the Greek word for 'dullness of vision', can be unilateral or bilateral and always implies a deprivation during the early months or years of life. Amblyopia is significant in that it is a potentially reversible condition. Although classic definitions stress that amblyopia is visual loss 'with no associated organic defect', in fact there is always an abnormality, be it strabismus, anisometric amblyopia, isoametropia, or media opacity, which predisposes the eye or eyes to amblyopia.

CLASSIFICATION

Amblyopia is usually classified as to the type of associated pathology: most commonly the pathology occurs in one eye only. The most common type of unilateral amblyopia is strabismic amblyopia. Strabismic amblyopia is most commonly associated with esotropia although it can occasionally occur with exotropia as well. The amount of deviation cannot be correlated with the degree of amblyopia. The second most common form of unilateral amblyopia is anisometropic amblyopia, in which a difference in refractive error in the two eyes results in poor visual development in one eye. Hypermetropic anisometropic amblyopia may occur when a difference of greater than one dioptre is present. Myopic anisometropia must be considered as a potential amblyogenic factor if a difference in excess of -3 dioptres is present. Astigmatic amblyopia, far less common, should be considered in terms of the sphere-equivalent of the two eyes. The resultant amblyopia may be meridional, i.e. at only one axis. Deprivational amblyopia occurs monocularly whenever any inbalance in media clarity occurs between the two eyes, such as cataract, ptosis, corneal opacity, hyphaema, vitreous haze, occlusion amblyopia, or even the prolonged use of atropine.

Bilateral amblyopia occurs occasionally. Deprivational amblyopia is the classic example, as in the infant with bilateral congenital cataracts. Isoametropic amblyopia occurs with bilateral refractive errors which are so severe as to prevent any clear image from forming on the developing retina. Hypermetropic isoametropia is of concern whenever the refractive error exceeds 4 dioptres, but is usually clinically relevant with refractive errors of 6 dioptres or greater (Schoenleber & Crouch 1987). Myopic isoametropic amblyopia may occur with refractive errors exceeding $8-10$ dioptres.

The classification of amblyopia may in the future be regarded not on the basis of underlying predisposing factor but rather on a functional basis. Psychophysical research has highlighted differences in contrast sensitivity function between predominantly strabismic and predominantly anisometropic amblyopia (Bradley & Freeman 1985; Hess & Pointer 1985). Ocular motility research has shown abnormalities of fixation (Schor & Flom 1975), saccades and pursuits (Schor 1975), and optokinetic nystagmus (Schor & Levi 1980). Further research will be required to more fully understand the sensory and motor abnormalities associated with amblyopia, as well as an attempt to understand whether these associated abnormalities are a cause of or an effect of the amblyopia. With better understanding of these mechanisms better treatment of amblyopia could be rendered.

INCIDENCE

Amblyopia affects between 2 and 5% of the general population. The vast majority of amblyopia occurs in one eye only. Strabismus is by far the most common cause of amblyopia, followed by anisoametropia and media opacities such as congenital cataract.

Anisometropic amblyopia can be a difficult condition to detect in the absence of strabismus. The better seeing eye provides vision which allows the child to function normally. Routine primary care physician screening tests do not in general include an examination for refractive errors although assessment of the Brückner reflex (Tongue & Cibis 1981) or photophorefraction has been advocated to assess for amblyogenic factors including anisometropic amblyopia (Atkinson *et al.* 1983; Day & Norcia 1986). The degree of anisometropia which is sufficient to induce amblyopia seems to vary greatly from individual to individual. Nevertheless, any child with a difference of 1 dioptre of hyperopia or 3 dioptres of myopia must be carefully followed to exclude the possibility of amblyopia. The optical correction of anisometropic amblyopia at times warrants a monocular contact lens to eliminate concerns about aniseikonia.

Media opacities of various types can also cause unilateral amblyopia. Some conditions are obvious such as a near complete ptosis of one eye. Others, such as a posterior capsular cataract, can only be detected with careful screening. Teaching primary care physicians to use the direct ophthalmoscope to screen for this condition at birth, 6 weeks and 6 months is essential.

SIGNIFICANCE

Although an adult with unilateral amblyopia usually has no significant limitations of day-to-day life, prevention of amblyopia is in large part warranted to guard the devastating effect of loss of the good eye at an age where amblyopia can no longer be treated. One study cites the risk of blindness as being greater when amblyopia is present (Tommila & Tarkkanen 1981). Although some authors have claimed that in adulthood the use of an amblyopic eye can improve in the event of loss of the good eye (Rabin 1984), most clinicians have observed that profound amblyopia is not reversible during adulthood.

Strabismic amblyopia occurs when in association with strabismus, a strong fixation preference for one eye is made. Although the visual loss often follows the onset of strabismus, the strabismus can be a consequence of poor vision in one eye. The presence of amblyopia does not appear to have any correlation with the angle of deviation although amblyopia is far more commonly associated with esotropia than exotropia. In the management of strabismus, one must first reverse the amblyopia as best as possible before proceeding with strabismus surgery.

BILATERAL AMBLYOPIA

Bilateral amblyopia is a far less common condition, although its effects on any individual are far more serious than unilateral amblyopia. The most severe type of bilateral amblyopia occurs in instances where the management of media opacities has been delayed. In many children with bilateral severe congenital cataracts who have had surgery at the age of 1 year, despite the clearing of the media the best visual acuity may be in the 20/400 range. A similar visual level also results if the child has had surgery at 1 month but did not receive optical correction of the resultant hyperopia until the age of 1 year. It must also be appreciated that the ultimate vision achieved in these cases is not simply dependent on timing or on anatomical factors. There are still several cases in which, despite 'perfect' management and no complications, the visual results are still poor. Although it is probably not correct to ascribe all of the deficit to amblyopia, it is likely that bilateral amblyopia plays a significant role in these cases.

More mild forms of bilateral amblyopia occur when refractive errors prevent a clearly focussed image on both retinas at all times. This condition, isoametropic amblyopia, most commonly occurs with hyperopia. No specific refractive error can be regarded as the exact cut-off for susceptibility to this condition, although most clinicians feel that any refractive error in excess of 4 dioptres of hyperopia, 8 dioptres of myopia or 2 dioptres of astigmatism potentially creates a condition which could lead to bilateral amblyopia. The majority of people with isoametropic amblyopia have hyperopia in excess of 6 dioptres. Detection of this condition may often not be made until visual acuity tests are performed at school. When the refractive error is symmetrical in the two eyes, strabismus may not develop, since additional accommodative effort still results in a blurred image and accommodative convergence is not used because it does not result in clearing of the image.

Any patient who has hyperopic isoametropia must be regarded as possibly having other pathology. Retinal dystrophies especially Leber's congenital amaurosis may have a high incidence of hyperopia.

The proper management of hyperopic isoametropia includes either spectacles or contact lenses. Contact lenses provide a greater derive to peripheral fusion since the peripheral visual field is enhanced with lens wear. The ability of young children to wear lenses is highly variable, and the child's motivation as well as parental support must be excellent.

Bilateral myopic isoametropic amblyopia is far less common since bilateral myopia still allows for a focussed image to develop at near; thus, bilateral amblyopia is unlikely unless the myopia exceeds 8 dioptres. High degrees of myopia in a child warrant concern about systemic health (see Chapter 6).

TREATMENT

The treatment of abnormal visual development rests on simple principles. Firstly, attention must be directed to the amblyogenic factor. If significant refractive error exists, then optical correction must be made. If significant media opacities are present, then these must be dealt with, usually surgically. If strabismus is present, then amblyopia must first be reversed with occlusion therapy prior to any surgical treatment. Occlusion therapy itself is not innocuous. In general, total full time occlusion should not be prescribed in excess of 1 week of occlusion per year of age. A 2-year-old child, for instance, should be given 2 weeks of occlusion therapy with a follow-up appointment 2 weeks. A 6-month-old baby, on the other hand, can only be occluded safely for a few *days* before repeat assessment is indicated. To ensure the best possible compliance, it is best to initially recheck vision after 3 weeks of patching, with longer gaps in older children. Also, occlusion appears to work best when a concentrated effort is made so that therapy is nearly full time. Reports of occlusion amblyopia (amblyopia in the eye that is being occluded) have cautioned us in ensuring that any patient who is patched must be followed carefully.

Finally, some debate has been raised as to the 'healthiness' of the good eye in conditions of amblyopia; confusingly both 'supernormal' function (Bradley & Freeman 1981; Rentschler & Hitz 1985) and 'subnormal' function (Kandel *et al.* 1986) have been found in research settings.

NEUROPHYSIOLOGY AND NEUROANATOMY

Wiesel and Hubel (1963a) from single-unit recordings of kitten striate cortex found abnormal cortical cells firing when driven by the deprived eye; this abnormal recording was accompanied by behaviourally poor vision. These abnormal recordings could not be reproduced when deprivation was imposed upon an adult cat. They concluded that the affected pathways had been normal at birth but were then influenced by the deprivation. Von Noorden *et al.* (1970a, 1970b; Von Noorden 1973) produced experimental esotropia in infant monkeys and created deprivation amblyopia with lid suturing. Both behavioural studies (Von Noorden *et al.* 1970a, 1970b; Von Noorden 1973) and neurophysiological recordings (Baker *et al.* 1974)

demonstrated findings similar to the previous animal experiments: deprivation resulted in abnormal responsiveness in cortical cells driven either by the amblyopic eye or in cells which required binocular input.

A search for the histopathological correlate, seemingly a simple task given the prevalence of this condition, has yielded sparse findings. Weisel and Hubel (1963a) demonstrated shrinkage in regions of the lateral geniculate body in kittens with one sutured eye. A single report of similar lateral geniculate nucleus (LGN) pathology in one human with anisometropic amblyopia has been made (Von Noorden *et al.* 1983). Ikeda and Tremain (1979), because of changes they found in ganglion cells, have argued that a site for amblyopia is within the retina on the basis of studies of kittens with strabismus. Von Noorden contests the clinical relevance of this research by arguing that with strabismic amblyopia (as opposed to deprivation amblyopia), the fovea of the deviating eye does in fact receive a clear image but that the brain is unable to process the conflicting information from the two eyes (Von Noorden 1985).

The search for the neuroanatomical location of the amblyopic locus has in part been guided by the pupillary responses. In general, relative afferent pupillary defects, or Marcus Gunn's pupils, are not clinically apparent in patients with amblyopia. However, clinical observation (Greenwald & Folk 1983) and more sophisticated testing have pointed to more subtle pupillary abnormalities in some of these patients, supporting the possibility for a very anteriorly located abnormality in these patients (Ikeda 1980).

FUTURE DIRECTIONS

Considering that Hippocrates in 400 BC defined amblyopia as 'when the doctor and the patient see nothing', and that the grandfather of Charles Darwin was one of the first to advocate occlusion therapy, our understanding of the complexities of amblyopia may have improved, but our understanding of the effective management has not changed significantly. Several avenues of investigation have suggested a potential next step to be in the neurobiochemical direction. Experimentally, amblyopia has been reversed with bicuculline in animals, as evidenced by neurophysiological recordings (Duffy *et al.* 1985). Unfortunately, a constant side effect of seizures accompanies the 'cure', and thus human studies have not been performed. A second avenue of research centers on a better understanding of the plasticity of the central nervous system. It has been postulated that certain biochemicals may prolong plasticity so that the effective window for treatment of amblyopia might be prolonged.

Colour vision

Normal development

When does a baby develop colour vision? As with visual acuity testing, quantification is an awesome task. Simple observation was used by Charles Darwin who reported that his newborn son could see a candle at 9 days but could not appreciate colour until 48 days (Darwin 1877). Parents often decorate infants' rooms with brightly coloured, highly colour saturated toys, mobiles, and furniture. Tutors of poorly sighted infants suggest the use of brightly coloured objects to encourage vision development.

Scientific understanding of infant colour vision has relied initially on behavioural tests, in ways analogous to preferential visual acuity testing. One aspect of colour vision testing was to determine which colours were most interesting to children. Using preferential grabbing as an indicator, several observers found yellow to be the most appealing colour (Valentine 1914; Shirley 1933). An ability to match colours is present by 2 years (Cook 1931). More recent studies have isolated different aspects of colour vision development into spectral sensitivity and brightness determinators, and chromatic vision discriminations (Bornstein 1978). Although one such study showed relatively depressed blue sensitivity (Trincken 1955) in infants 3 months and younger, other behavioural tests show spectral sensitivity identical to adults (Peeples & Teller 1978). Electrophysiological recordings have shown better sensitivity in wave lengths shorter than 550 nm. A similar study performed longitudinally agreed that infants do have such developmental differences when compared to adult spectral sensitivity (Moskowitz-Cook 1979). These differences have been explained on the basis of differing absorption characteristics of the infant lens and macular pigment (Dobson 1976) and on developmental factors involving the infant's rods and cones (Moskowitz-Cook 1979) in the parafoveal and foveal regions.

The routine testing of children for colour vision is included in many screening systems for children's eyes (Ehrlich et al. 1983).

Abnormal colour vision

Abnormal colour vision is a common condition which has an impact on individuals and society (Fletcher & Voke 1985). Defective colour vision can be defined as congenital or acquired on the basis of response to colour vision testing.

Congenital colour vision abnormalities affect approximately 5–6% of males in Western Europe and North America (Waardenberg et al. 1963) due to its X-linked inheritance pattern. Their classification is based on the presence of three colour classes of cones: red-, green-, and blue-sensitive systems. A person is termed trichromatic if all systems are present, dichromatic if one is absent, and monochromatic if two are absent. The abnormal system is indicated by the terms protanomaly (red defect), deuteranomaly (green defect), and tritanomaly (blue defect). If function is completely absent (as opposed to defective) the suffix '-anopia' is used (hence: protanopia, deuteranopia, tritanopia).

Deuteranomaly represents the most common inherited abnormality; other X-linked inherited abnormalities are deuteranopia and protanopia. Tritanomaly and tritanopia are inherited as autosomal dominant conditions but affect only 0.005% of the population (Verriest 1974). The impact of inherited colour vision, referred to loosely as colour blindness and sometimes in the UK as Daltonism, has been studied extensively. From an educational standpoint, children with congenital defects do not appear to have any difficulty during elementary school (Lampe et al. 1973). Children themselves may report limits in appreciation of colour television or food appearance, or difficulty seeing car rear lights (Voke 1984). The greatest impact of defective colour vision appears to be on career choice. Although understandably difficult to compile, a list of vocations in which colour vision defects are possible handicaps or career limitations is available (Voke 1980). Strict requirements limiting military careers, particularly with regards to flying airplanes, still exist.

Acquired colour vision defects imply an entirely different set of underlying conditions. Testing for these defects centers not on one of defining a particular spectral sensitivity which is defective, but rather in defining loss of brilliance, or desaturation of colours. Such colour vision loss is often termed dyschromatopsia.

Acquired colour vision defects can occur with media opacity, optic nerve or retinal disorder with central nervous system pathology. Amblyopia typically does not cause a colour vision deficit although subtle abnormalities may be present (Marre & Marre 1978; Bradley *et al.* 1986). A review of the specific defect in these abnormalities indicates defects predominantly in the blue–yellow distribution (Fletcher & Voke 1985).

Binocular vision and stereo-acuity

The phenomenon of stereopsis is one particularly important to a baby, where his or her world is all relatively at near and in which monocular clues of relative size have not yet been experienced. The normal development of stereopsis has been presumed as a consequence of observation of a baby's convergence to a near target (Hoyt *et al.* 1982). Braddick and Atkinson (1983) have assessed stereo-acuity development by VEP and OKN techniques (optokinetic nystagmus) and found existence of this function by 3 months of age; even earlier binocular development has been found by Eizenmann *et al.* (1988). The proliferation of more purely basic science research on stereo-acuity has been great over the past 25 years in part as a consequence largely of computer technology (Julesz 1986).

The neurophysiologic basis for binocular vision has evolved from an understanding of the endothial striate cortex cell's abilities to be stimulated by either eye (Hubel & Wiesel 1959) to a definition of columned cortical cell layers which contribute to stereopsis (Maunsell & Van Essen 1983).

That much remains unknown in the realm of binocular vision, not only on the basis of neurophysiology, but also in psychophysical and theoretical modelling roles, has been outlined by Bishop and Pettigrew (1986). One major problem in this research relates to differences in the animal model which invalidate transposition of data to the human model.

The zone of single binocular vision, or Panum's space, encompasses a physiologically defined horopter, a curved plane on which each point falls on corresponding retinal points in each eye. Beyond Panum's space, objects cannot be fused, and physiologic diplopia results. Although physiologic diplopia can be recognized if a concentrated effort is made, these doubled images in our day-to-day function are either suppressed or ignored.

Clinically, binocular vision is regarded as an ability to fuse as well as an ability to perceive depth, or stereopsis. Fusion is regarded as motor and sensory; although an artificial division, these terms have aided the clinician in assessing his patient.

Abnormal binocular vision is a common partner of strabismus and amblyopia, and conventional clinical testing include tests of fusion and stereopsis (see Chapter 7). The adaptation of the patient depends in large part on his age. In an adult with recently acquired strabismus, diplopia will result; in a young child, diplopia is not expected, but rather suppression is present. Many regard this phenomenon as an unconscious effort to avoid diplopia (the image falling on a nonfoveal region in one eye) or confusion (two separate objects in space projected onto corresponding areas in the two eyes). Suppression may be further classified as 'central' versus 'peripheral', 'monocular' versus 'alternating', and 'facultative' versus 'obligatory'. The status of binocular vision function is regarded as an important parameter in predicting the outcome of strabismus surgery, and the desire to enhance normal binocular vision development is cited as an indicator to perform surgery before the age of 2 years in children with infantile esotropia.

Impact of abnormal vision on general child development

Abnormal visual development begets abnormal child development. Vision is the most important sense for general development and education (Jan *et al.* 1977). A baby learns by imitating, by becoming aware of his own hands and feet through vision, and by eye contact from parents providing clues about his performance. The blind or partially sighted baby is deprived, in varying degrees, of these ingredients to normal development.

Blindness has a profound effect on motor development, and developmental milestones are delayed. Sighted babies will raise their heads and look about at 12 weeks of age; blind babies are unhappy in this position, and prefer to be on their backs (Jan *et al.* 1977) which causes a delay in control of the head and trunk. The ability to grasp an object, usually present at 5–6 months, is often delayed until 1 year. Walking readiness, on the other hand, is not retarded, whereas crawling is more difficult. The physiotherapist can play an important role in helping the parents pace the motor development of the blind child and in developing postural position which will enhance mobility (Siegal & Murphy 1970).

In contrast to motor development, speech development commences at about the same age — 8 weeks — in sighted and unsighted children. However, lack of visual input slows progress, as words are less meaningfull without the corresponding visual symbol.

Typically, blind children repeat words (echolalia) much more commonly than sighted children (Fay 1973). Finally, non-verbal communication, such as a smile in response to others is understandably delayed.

Does blindness enhance the other senses, such as hearing or touch? Although this notion is much talked about, infant research has disproved this theory. Rather, educational efforts are enhanced in other disciplines such as tactile sense. The limitations in playing certain sports may, for instance, result in opportunities to have music lessons at an earlier age (Jan *et al.* 1977).

Some physiologic functions of the blind child are, however, influenced by blindness. These changes exist even when other congenital abnormalities are not present. Electroencephalograms show altered recordings, such as an absence of rapid eye movement (REM) recordings (Berger *et al.* 1962). The response to caloric testing of the vestibular system is reduced (Forssman 1964). Altered growth patterns, circadian rhythms and sleep patterns also occur in blind children (Jan *et al.* 1977).

As the child grows older, mobility skills and educational needs become increasingly important. Mobility is greatly enhanced by the slightest of remaining vision, not only in getting about but also in awareness of his or her own body parts. Mobility education of such children must be individualized due to the multiple factors involved with this skill (Garry & Ascarelli 1960). Schools for the blind concentrate teaching resources dealing with issues such as maximum use of remaining vision, special technology providing education means (such as magnifying book print) and practical vocational counselling. A major effort is made to allow contact with sighted individuals and encourage incorporation of the blind child into the sighted society (Lowenfeld 1973).

Undoubtedly the blind child's general development is heavily influenced by other congenital limitations. Mental retardation is present in 25–80% of blind children, depending on one's definition of blindness and mental retardation (Graham 1968). Cerebral palsy, present in 6–15% of blind children, represents a particular impact on the blind child when the hands are spastic (Jan *et al.* 1977). Varied degrees of hearing loss are found in 10% of blind children (Robinson 1974), the combination of deafness and blindness necessitates particularly creative efforts in education and socialization (Van Dijk 1971).

Finally, the responsibility of the blind child's general development and incorporation rests not only with the blind child and the family, but also with the attitudes of the sighted toward the child (ophthalmologists included!). Helen Keller reflected that 'not blindness, but the attitude of the seeing to the blind is the hardest burden to bear' (Jan *et al.* 1977).

References

Abramov I, Garden J, Hendrickson A *et al.* The retina of the newborn infant. *Science* 1982; **217**: 265–7

Allen H. A new picture series for preschool vision testing. *Am J Ophthalmol* 1957; **44**: 38–41

Atkinson J, Braddick O. The use of isotropic photorefraction for vision screening in infants. *Acta Ophthalmol (Copenh)* (Suppl.) 1983; **157**: 36–45

Bailey I. *Bailey–Hall Cereal Test.* University of California, Berkeley, CA 1983

Baker F, Griggs P, Von Noorden G. Effects of visual deprivation and strabismus on the response of neurons in the visual cortex of the monkey, including studies on the striate and prestriate cortex in the normal animal. *Brain Res* 1974; **66**: 185

Banks MS, Bennett PJ, Schefrin B. Inefficient cones limit infants' spatial and chromatic vision. *Invest Ophthalmol Vis Sci* 1988; **29**: 59

Beller R, Hoyt CS, Marg E. *et al.* Good visual function after neonatal surgery for congenital monocular cataracts. *Am J Ophthalmol* 1981; **91**: 559–65

Berger R, Olley P, Oswald I. The EEG, eye movements, and dreams of the blind. *Q J Exp Psychol* 1962; **14**: 183–6

Bishop P, Pettigrew J. Neural mechanisms of binocular vision. *Vision Res* 1986; **26**: 1587–600

Bornstein M. Chromatic vision in infancy. In: *Advances in Child Development and Behaviour*, vol. 12. Reese H, Lipsett L, Eds. Academic Press, New York 1978; 117–82

Braddick O, Atkinson J. The development of binocular function in infancy. *Ophthalmology* 1983; **157**: 27–35

Bradley A, Dahlman C, Switkes E, De Valois K. A comparison of colour and luminance discrimination in amblyopia. *Invest Ophthalmol Vis Sci* 1986; **27**: 1404–9

Bradley A, Freeman RD. Contrast sensitivity in anisometropic amblyopia. *Invest Ophthalmol Vis Sci* 1981; **24**: 467–76

Bradley A, Freeman RD. Temporal sensitivity in amblyopia: an explanation of conflicting reports. *Vision Res* 1985; **25**: 39–46

Catalano RA, Simon JW, Jenkins PL, Kandel GL. Preferential looking as a guide for amblyopia therapy in monocular infantile cataracts. *J Pediatr Ophthalmol Strabismus* 1987; **24**: 56–63

Catford G, Oliver A. Development of visual acuity. *Arch Dis Child* 1973; **48**: 47–50

Cook W. Ability of children in colour discrimination. *Child Dev* 1931; **2**: 303–20

Cynader M, Berman N, Hein A. Recovery of function in cat visual cortex following prolonged deprivation. *Exp Brain Res* 1976; **25**: 139–56

Darwin C. A biographical sketch of an infant. *Mind* 1877; **2**: 285–94

Day SH, Norcia AM. Photographic detection of amblyogenic factors. *Ophthalmology* 1986; **93**: 25–8

Dayton G, Jones M, Ain P. *et al.* Developmental study of coordinated eye movements in the human infant. I. Visual acuity in the newborn human: a study based on induced optokinetic nystagmus recorded by electro-oculography. *Arch Ophthalmol* 1964; **71**: 865−70

Dobson V. Spectral sensitivity of the 2 month infant as measured by the visual evoked cortical potential. *Vision Res* 1976; **16**: 367−74

Dubowitz L, de Vries L, Mushin J, Arden G. Visual function in the newborn infant: is it cortically mediated? *Lancet* 1986; **i**: 1139−41

Duffy FH, Burchfiel JL, Maver GD, Joy RM, Snodgrass SR. Comparative pharmacological effects on visual cortical neurones in monocullary deprived cats. *Brain Res* 1985; **339**: 257−64

Ehrlich M, Reinecke R, Simons K. Preschool vision screening for amblyopia, strabismus. Programs, methods, guidelines. *Surv Ophthalmol* 1983; **28**: 145−63

Eizenman M, Schneck M, Skarf B. Optimum estimation of acuity using visual evoked potentials. *Invest Ophthalmol Vis Sci* (Suppl.) 1987; **28**: 00−00

Eizenman M, Skarf B, McCulloch D. Detection of early development of binocular fusion in infant. *Invest Ophthalmol Vis Sci* 1988; **29**: 25

Fay W. On the echolalia of the blind and the autistic child. *J. Speech Hear Disorder* 1973; **38**: 478−89

Fletcher R, Voke J. *Defective Colour Vision. Fundamentals, Diagnosis and Management.* Adam Hilger, Bristol 1985

Forssman B. Vestibular reactivity in cases of congenital nystagmus. *Otolaryngol* 1964; **57**: 539−55

Garry R, Ascarelli A. Teaching typographical orientation and spatial orientation to congenitally blind children. *J Education* 1960; **143**: 1−49

Gorman J, Cogan D, Gellis S. An apparatus for grading the visual acuity of infants on the basis of optokinetic nystagmus. *Pediatrics* 1957; **19**: 1088−92

Graham M. *Multiply Impaired Blind Children: A National Problem.* New York, American Foundation for the Blind 1968

Greenwald MJ, Folk ER. Afferent pupillary defect in amblyopia. *J. Pediatr Ophthalmol Strabismus* 1983; **20**: 63−7

Grier T. Visual acuity development and evaluation in the preschool child. *Optometric Weekly* 1973; **64**: 370−4

Hendrickson A, Kupfer C. The histiogenesis of the fovea in the Macaque monkey. *Invest Ophthalmol Vis Sci* 1976; **15**: 746−56

Hendrickson AE, Yuodelis C. The morphological development of the human fovea. *Ophthalmology* 1984; **91**: 603−12

Hess RF, Pointer JS. Differences in the neural basis of human amblyopia: the distribution of the anomaly across the visual field. *Vision Res* 1985; **25**: 1577−94

Hoyt C, Nickel B, Billson F. Ophthalmological examination of the infant. *Surv Ophthalmol* 1982; **26**: 177−89

Hubel D, Wiesel T. Receptive fields of single neurones in the cat's striate cortex. *J Physiol London* 1959; **148**: 574−91

Hubel D, Wiesel T. Binocular interaction in striate cortex of kittens reared with artificial squint. *J Neurophysiol* 1965; **28**: 1041−59

Ikeda H. Visual acuity, its development and amblyopia. *J. Royal Soc Med* 1980; **73**: 546

Ikeda H, Tremain K. Amblyopia occurs in retinal ganglion cells in cats reared with convergent squint without alternating fixation. *Exp Br Res* 1979; **35**: 559

Jampolsky A. Unequal visual inputs and strabismus management: a comparison of human and animal strabismus. In: *Symposium on Strabismus.* Transactions of the New Orleans Academy of Ophthalmology. CV Mosby 1978; St Louis 358

Jan J, Freeman R, Scott E. *Visual Impairment in Children and Adolescents.* New York, Grune & Stratton 1977

Julesz B. Stereoscopic vision. *Vision Res* 1986; **26**: 1601−12

Kandel GL, Simon JW, Drylewski A. Acuities of dominant eyes of infant amblyopes are subnormal before treatment. *Invest Ophthalmol Vis Sci* 1986; **27**: 2

Kirschen D, Rosenbaum A, Ballard C. The dot visual acuity test − a new acuity test for children. *J Am Optom Assoc* 1983; **54**: 1055−9

Lampe J, Doster M, Beal B. Summary of a three year study of academic and school achievement between colour defective and normal primary age pupils. *J Sch Health* 1973; **43**: 309−11

Lowenfeld B (ed). *The Visually Handicapped Child in School.* John Day, New York 1973

Magoon EH, Robb RM. Development of myelin in human optic nerve and tract, a light and electron-microscopic study. *Arch Ophthalmol* 1981; **99**: 655−9

Marre M, Marre E. Colour vision in squint amblyopia. *Mod Probl Ophthalmol* 1978; **19**: 308

Maunsell J, Van Essen D. Functional properties of neurons in middle temporal visual area of macaque monkey. II. Binocular interactions and sensitivity to binocular disparity. *J Neurophysiol* 1983; **50**: 1148−67

McDonald M. Assessment of visual acuity in toddlers. *Surv Ophthalmol* 1986; **31**: 189−210

Moskowitz-Cook A. The development of spectral sensitivity in human infants. *Vision Res* 1979; **19**: 1133−42

National Society to Prevent Blindness. *A Guide for Eye Inspection and Testing Visual Acuity of Preschool Children − a Screening Process.* New York, NY 1976

Nixon RB, Helveston EM, Miller K. *et al.* Incidence of strabismus in neonates. *Am J Ophthalmol* 1985; **100**: 798−801

Norcia AM, Tyler CW, Hamer RD. Development of contrast sensitivity in human infants. *Invest Ophthalmol Vis Sci* 1987; **28**: 5

Peeples D, Teller D. White-adapted photopic spectral sensitivity in human infants. *Vision Res* 1978; **18**: 49−53

Rabin J. Visual improvement in amblyopia after visual loss in the dominant eye. *Am J Optom Physiol Optics* 1984; **61**: 334−7

Rentschler I, Hitz R. Amblyopia processing of positional information. Part 1: vernier acuity. *Exp Brain Research* 1985; **60**: 270−78

Robb RM, Mayer DL, Moore BD. Results of early treatment of unilateral congenital cataracts. *J Pediatr Ophthalmol Strabismus* 1987; **24**: 178−81

Robinson G. *Epidemiological Studies of Congenital and Acquired Blindness in Blind Children Born in British Columbia − 1944−1973.* First National Multi-Disciplinary Conference on Blind Children, Canadian Medical Association, Vancouver, Canada. 1974 p 1−21

Romano P, Romano J, Puklin J. Stereoacuity development in children with normal binocular single vision. *Am J Ophthalmol* 1975; **79**: 966−71

Schoenleber DB, Crouch ER. Bilateral hypermetropic amblyopia. *J. Pediatr Ophthalmol Strabismus* 1987; **75**: 77−79

Schor CM. A directional impairment of eye movement control in strabismic amblyopia. *Invest Ophthalmol Vis Sci* 1975; **14**:

692−97

Schor CM, Flom MC. Eye position control and visual acuity in strabismus amblyopia. In *Basic mechanisms of Ocular Motility and their Clinical Implications*. Pergamon Press, Oxford 1975; 555−69

Schor CM, Levi D. Disturbances of small field horizontal and vertical optokinetic nystagmus in amblyopia. *Invest Ophthalmol* 1980; **19**: 668−683

Sebris SL, Dobson V, McDonald MA, Teller DV. Acuity cards for visual acuity assessment of infants and children in clinical settings. *Clin Vis Sci* 1987; **2**: 45−58

Sheridan M. The stycar graded balls vision test. *Dev Med Child Neurol* 1973; **15**: 423−32

Shimojo S, Held R. Vernier acuity is less than granting acuity in 2- and 3-months olds. *Vision Res* 1987; **27**: 77−86

Shirley M. *The First Two Years. Intellectual Development.* Minneapolis: University of Minnesta Press 1933

Siegel I, Murphy T. *Postural Determinants in the Blind.* Final Project Report, Grant RD-3512, SB-700C2. Division of Research and Demonstration Grants, Social Rehabilitation Service, DHEW, Washington DC 1970

Simons K. Visual acuity norms in young children. *Surv Ophthalmol* 1983; **28(2)**: 84−92

Slataper F. Age norms of refraction and vision. *Arch Ophthalmol* 1950; **43**: 466−79

Sokol S. Measurement of infant visual acuity from pattern reversal evoked potentials. *Vision Res* 1978; **18**: 33−9

Swaiman K, Wright F. The neurologic examination in children. In: *The Practice of Pediatric Neurology.* CV Mosby, St Louis 1975; p. 50

Swan KC, Wilkins JH. Extraocular muscle surgery in early infancy − anatomical factors. *J Pediatric Ophthalmol Strabismus* 1984; **21**: 44−9

Teller D, McDonald M, Preston K, Sebris S, Dobson V. Assessment of visual acuity in infants and children: the acuity card procedure. *Dev Med Child Neurol* 1986; **28**: 779−90

Tommila V, Tarkkanen A. Incidence of loss of vision in the healthy eye in amblyopia. *Br J Ophthalmol* 1981; **65**: 575−7

Tongue AC, Cibis GW. Bruckner test. *Ophthalmology* 1981; **88**: 1041−4

Trincken D. Die ontogenetische entwicklung des helligkeits- und forbensehens bein menschen. I. Die entwicklung des helligketissehens. Albrecht v. *Graefes Arch Clin Exp Ophthalmol* 1955; **156**: 519−43

Tyler C, Apkarian P, Levi D, Nakayama K. Rapid assessment of visual function: an electronic sweep technique for the pattern visual evoked potential. *Invest Ophthalmol Vis Sci* 1979; **18**: 703−13

Vaegan, Taylor D. Critical period for deprivation amblyopia in children. *Trans Ophthalmol Soc UK* 1979; **99**: 432−7

Valentine C. The colour perception and colour preference of an infant during its fourth and eighth months. *Br J Psychol* 1914; **6**: 363−86

Van Dijk J. Educational approaches to abnormal development. In: *Deaf−Blind Children and Their Education.* Proceedings of the 1970 International Conference on the Education of Deaf−Blind Children. Rotterdam University Press, Rotterdam 1971

Verriest M. Recent progress in the study of acquired deficiencies of colour vision. *Bull Soc Ophthalmol Fr* 1974; **74**: 595−620

Voke J. *Colour Vision Testing in Specific Industries and Professions.* Keeler, London 1980

Voke J. But spinach is black. *The Optician* 1984; **187**: 35−6

Von Noorden G. Experimental amblyopia monkeys. Further behavioural observation and clinical correlations. *Invest Ophthalmol* 1973; **12**: 721

Von Noorden G. Amblyopia: a multi-disciplinary approach (Proctor Lecture). *Invest Ophthalmol Vis Sci* 1985; **26**: 1704−16

Von Noorden G, Crawford M, Levery R. The lateral geniculate nucleus in human amnisometropia amblyopia. *Invest Ophthalmol* 1983; **24**: 788−90

Von Noorden G, Dowling J, Ferguson D. Experimental amblyopia in monkeys. II. Behavioural studies in strabismus amblyopia. *Arch Ophthalmol* 1970a; **84**: 215

Von Noorden G, Dowling J, Ferguson D. Experimental amblyopia in monkeys. I. Behavioural studies of stimulus deprivation amblyopia. *Arch Ophthalmol* 1970b; **84**: 206

Waardenberg P, Franceschetti A, Klein D. *Genetics and Ophthalmology.* Thomas Springfield, Illinois 1963

Wiesel T, Hubel D. Effects of visual deprivation of morphology and physiology of cells in the cat's lateral geniculate body. *J Neurophysiol* 1963; **26**: 578−85

Wiesel T, Hubel D. Single cell response in striate cortex of kittens deprived of vision in one eye. *J Neurophysiol* 1963; **26**: 1003−17

Wiesel T, Hubel D. Comparison of the effects of unilateral and bilateral eye closure on cortical unit response in kittens. *J Neurophysiol* 1965; **28**: 1029−40

3 Delayed Visual Maturation

DAVID TAYLOR

When a baby is referred because the parents are worried about its vision, the cause is usually evident on the first examination or at least there is usually a very strong suspicion about the site of the problem. In some babies no cause can be found: their vision just seems worse than their chronological age would indicate, and their estimated or measured visual function is indeed worse but improves with time without specific treatment.

This phenomenon has been recognized for many years, the first report being by Beauvieux (1926, 1947) who noted anomalous appearance of the optic discs which improved with time. Believing this to be due to a defect in myelinization, they coined the terms 'pseudo-atrophie optique', and 'dysgenesie myelinique'. Other terms that have been used are visuo-perceptive blindness, papilla grisea, dissociated visual development, visual development delay, myelogenesis retardata or delayed visual development. It is most frequently known as delayed visual maturation (DVM).

Clinical presentation

Parents and most doctors do not expect the newborn baby to see, so it is only when the child is not fixing and following by 2–4 months that they are referred by the parents themselves, or their advisers, to the ophthalmologist or paediatrician.

The diagnosis of DVM is really retrospective; it is essential that the vision should improve with time, but since DVM can be 'added on' to ocular or systemic disease the eventual vision is not necessarily normal. Delayed vision development, therefore, occurs when a baby shows visual responses that are not consistent with his age (chronological or developmental) in the absence of disease of the visual pathways or brain.

Classification

Patients with DVM can be subclassified usefully into three main groups (Uemura 1979; Fielder *et al.* 1985):
1 Isolated DVM.
2 DVM with systemic disease or mental retardation.
3 DVM with ocular disease.

Group I: Isolated DVM

In these babies, general and neurological development is normal (Illingworth 1961) and the only problem is that the baby appears to see less well than expected for his age. They have normal ocular examination and no systemic abnormalities. Neurophysiological studies are not grossly abnormal — the flash electroretinogram (ERG) is normal though the flash visual evoked potential (VEP) may show some persistence of more juvenile waveforms and some delay in the major positive components (Mellor & Fielder 1980; Harel *et al.* 1983). Pattern onset/offset visual evoked responses (VER) were mildly delayed and noticeably attenuated (Hoyt *et al.* 1983) but Lambert *et al.* (1989) found that their patients in this group had normal pattern VEP's. The EEG must be normal for the child to fall within this group. Most patients in this group present by 3 or 4 months of age and it is very unusual for improvement to be prolonged after 6 months; quite frequently the short delay during the referral process is enough to allow considerable improvements, so that the diagnosis in these cases can only be made retrospectively, by the history. Because measurement of vision in small children is difficult, the determination of whether 'normal' vision has been achieved is largely subjective. However, the eventual outcome should not only be normal for vision but for intellectual and other development. Cole *et al.* (1984), warn that long-term follow-up may not show a completely normal development, but in their group subclassification of cases was not undertaken and neurophysiological studies rarely performed, i.e. they probably included cases from groups II and III.

Finally, this group probably includes the patients described earlier in the 20th century as optic nerve dysmyelination. Although today the presence of optic disc pallor or greyness is not usually noted, the finding of neurophysiological abnormalities might suggest that there is indeed some organic disorder of the visual pathways underlying the phenomenon.

Group II: DVM with systemic disease or mental retardation

Babies who were very premature or had severe intercurrent illness early in their life may show delay in vision development but this usually improves in the same way as it does in group I patients, with residual defects only related to their illness.

Most patients in this group have severe mental retardation; it is most frequently seen in children who have infantile spasms, or other seizure disorders in relation to severe birth asphyxia, hypoglycaemia, hypocalcaemia, tuberous sclerosis, Aicardi's syndrome, etc. In most cases there are diagnostic clues to the underlying cause and the neurophysiological studies are more frequently abnormal, including the EEG. Vision appears to improve with control of the seizures. Children with other causes of mental retardation without seizures, such as hydrocephalus or brain malformations, may also show DVM, often to a lesser degree. Their vision is variable, may be stimulated or excited by sound as well as visual stimuli — i.e. they appear to see better when excited, interested and aroused. In this group the prognosis is less good, there are often residual visual defects or problems with visual perception or hand—eye co-ordination and the recovery of vision also takes longer.

Group III: DVM with ocular disease

Children with early onset ocular disease including nystagmus (with or without albinism), cataract or other cause of a partial visual defect, may have vision that is much worse than would be expected from the primary disease alone and it is a reasonable hypothesis that these patients have DVM in addition to their organic defect. Children in this group improve to their final level more slowly and less fully than in group I but faster and more completely than group II.

Differential diagnosis

The main differential diagnosis is that of the baby with poor vision with no gross ocular or systemic disorder — of course this group includes patients who have, on more detailed examination, discernable disorders but who present to the specialist with no obvious problem (see Problem 1).

Investigation and management

DVM is yet another example of an area where the ophthalmologist and paediatrician or paediatric neurologist can work well together. If the child with suspected DVM is developmentally normal, any associated eye or systemic disease has been ruled out by joint consultation, and the non-invasive neurophysiological studies are normal or not markedly abnormal, then no further investigations need be undertaken, and a good outcome can be expected. These children probably need to be followed rather more carefully than average in their developmental clinic or by their general practitioner after their improvement has been observed by the ophthalmologist.

Where the child has eye disease or systemic problems then these are investigated and managed as is appropriate for the condition.

References

Beauvieux J. La pseudo-atrophie optique des nouveau-nes (dysgénésie myelinique de voies optiques). *Ann d'Occulistique* 1926; **163**: 881−921

Beauvieux M. La cécité apparante chez le nouveau-né la pseudo−atrophie grise du nerf optique. *Arch Ophthalmol (Paris)* 1947; **7**: 241−9

Cole GF, Hungerford J, Jones RB. Delayed visual maturation. *Arch Dis Child* 1984; **59**: 107−10

Fielder AR, Russell-Eggitt IR, Dodd KL, Meller DH. Delayed visual maturation. *Trans Ophthalmol Soc UK* 1985; **104**: 653−61

Harel S, Holtzman M, Feinsod M. Delayed visual maturation. *Arch Dis Child* 1983; **58**: 298−309

Hoyt CS, Jastrebski G, Marg E. Delayed visual maturation in infancy. *Br J Ophthalmol* 1983; **67**: 127−32

Illingworth RS. Delayed visual maturation. *Arch Dis Child* 1961; **36**: 407−9

Lambert SR, Kriss A, Taylor D. Delayed visual maturation, a longitudinal clinical and electrophysiological assessment. *Ophthalmology* 1989; **96**: 524−9

Mellor DH, Fielder AR. Dissociated visual development: electrodiagnostic studies in infants who are 'slow to see'. *Dev Med Child Neurol* 1980; **22**: 327−55

Uemura Y. The assessment of visual ability in children. In François J, Maione M (Eds). *Paediatric Ophthalmology*. Wiley, Chichester 1979; pp. 329−31

4 Normal Child Development

NICHOLAS CAVANAGH

Although child development can only be said to have begun from the time of conception, it is clear that there are many factors before conception that will have an important bearing on the outcome. Not only do these include the genetic material, both nuclear and mitochondrial, and the chromosomal configuration of either gamete, but also the immediate environment of the dividing blastocyst. The taking of the family history, the clinical counterpart of the genetic probe, is the first step in the elucidation of these factors, and the next stage is enquiring about the pregnancy, delivery and neonatal period.

Family history

This should include enquiries about possible consanguinity, and the health of first-degree relatives. Sibling deaths may not be referred to by the parent unless such information is directly (but delicately) sought. Relatives should also be examined when appropriate.

The pregnancy

The answer to a seemingly innocuous question, 'was the pregnancy planned?' may indicate the need for cautious enquiries about attempts to abort, and may also lead on naturally to questions about the mother's health at the time of conception and throughout pregnancy. Whereas the affect of parental inebriation at the moment of conception remains speculative (how many of us owe our origin to such prevailing conditions?), the deleterious effect of maternally ingested alcohol in moderate or large quantities on the developing fetus is now well recognized. Thus, a drug history should include information about alcohol and tobacco, coffee and tea, in addition to other more readily recognized drugs such as anti-convulsants and hormones, or narcotics and glue-sniffing. The relationship of maternal anaemia, state of nutrition, blood pressure, haemorrhage, intercurrent infection and illness, to fetal growth and development is well known, and such information is often volunteered by the mother, but if not should be asked for directly. Other enquiries about the course of the pregnancy should include the strength of fetal movements, particularly if a neuromuscular condition is suspected, and also if any irradiation was given especially at an early stage.

Delivery

Since birth injury continues to be a significant case of physical and mental handicap, the following are some important considerations regarding the delivery: Was it at term, and if not, how much pre or post-term?

Was there evidence of fetal distress as shown by meconium staining of the liquor, irregularities of fetal heart rate on monitoring, intrapartum acidosis, etc? Was the delivery assisted and, if so, why?

Neonatal period

The state of the infant at birth and within the next few days of life is a summation of much that has happened in the previous 40 weeks gestation as well as during the delivery. Important questions include: Did the infant breathe immediately? Was there jaundice requiring specific therapy? Was feeding by breast or bottle and were there any difficulties? Was the baby unduly irritable or quiet? What was the birth weight?

Developmental milestones

It is doubtful whether the answer to questions about stages of development are always reliable. Accuracy of recall is dependant upon a number of factors which include the age of the child (the older the child the more likely the earlier milestones are forgotten), how many siblings there are to confuse with, and whether baby books were kept from which information can be subsequently retrieved. Sometimes no more accurate information can be obtained than whether the development of the child was comparable with his siblings, though most parents are able to remember the age of walking unaided and talking in sentences. The experience of Caputes et al. (1985) is more hopeful in this respect and he reported a percentage of parents recording motor milestones ranging from 72% for sit up alone to 98% pull to stand in children up to the age of 2 years. The figures in Table 4.1 are derived from that paper.

Whereas the recall of dates and acquisition of skills can be an unreliable basis of developmental assessment, direct observation by the doctor, coupled with information from parents of their child's current ability is likely to produce an accurate record of function. What follows is a practical guide to the normal abilities of children of the following ages: 3 months, 6 months, 1 year, 18 months, 2 years, 3 years, 4 years, 5 years and 7 years. No attempt will be made to be fully comprehensive and the information given is intended as a check list which the ophthalmologist may use to help him to decide about his patient. It is presented under the conventional categories of vision and fine movements, hearing and language, posture and gross movements, social and emotional development, and these broad headings are useful *aide-mémoires* for the

Table 4.1 Gross motor milestones which may be recalled by parents of young children. From Caputes *et al.* (1985).

Movement	Mean age	Age range
Roll prone to supine	3.7 months	+/− 1.4 months
Sit alone	6.4 months	+/− 1.3 months
Crawl	7.8 months	+/− 1.7 months
Walk	11.5 months	+/− 1.9 months

doctor to use in framing questions and channelling observations. The data given here is a composite derived from the authors own experience, the incomparable observations of Drs Sheridan (1975) (Table 4.2), Illingworth (1980) and Egan *et al.* (1969) and the revised Denver developmental screening test. Where recent papers have been published giving precise information concerning the range about the mean of the age when skills are acquired, these are sometimes quoted, but at all times it should be appreciated that there is considerable normal variation in human development and that care must be taken in interpreting the significance of apparent aberation (see below).

Table 4.2 is one which doctors, who are not themselves developmental specialists but who need to make rapid assessments, may find useful. What follows is a list of skills grouped under the headings used previously, with approximate dates when they might be expected to be present. Although the data in this form might appear to be more precise, caution is necessary in interpreting variation from the norm.

Vision and fine movements

Follows with eyes with increasing side to side range from birth onward	
Hand regard	3−5 months
Reaches out	3−4 months
Transfer objects from hand to hand	6−8 months
Pincer grasp between thumb and forefinger	9−10 months
Touches objects with forefinger	9−10 months
Looks for the fallen toy	9−10 months
Builds tower of three bricks	18 months
Copies circle	3 years
Knows colours	3 years
Draws a man with head, trunk, arms and legs	4 years

Table 4.2 Normal developmental milestones. Modified from Sheridan (1975).

Age	Vision and fine movements	Hearing and language	Posture and gross movements	Social and emotional development
3 months	Follows adults with eyes Watches own hands before face Fixes still objects briefly	Startled by loud sounds Consoled by comforting sounds Coos	Hands open mostly Lifts head and chest when placed prone	Becomes excited by preparation for happy events, e.g. bath Responds happily to tickle
6 months	Reaches out for small objects he has fixed on Palmar grasp	Uses mostly single syllables, e.g. ah, goo; occasional double sounds, e.g. adah Turns to voices	Grasps own feet Rolls front to back Sits alone very briefly	Takes everything to mouth Beginning to be shy of strangers
1 year	Pincer grasp between forefinger and thumb Looks for toy which has fallen out of sight	Understands several words, e.g. car, spoon Imitates sounds	Has been crawling for several months Beginning to walk holding on or alone	Waves bye-bye Gives on request
18 months	Builds tower with three bricks Enjoys picture books and points	Says 20 or more words	Beginning to run Picks up toys without falling	Drinks well from cup Bowel control Takes off shoes and socks
2 years	Builds tower with six bricks Imitates vertical line Recognizes people in photos	Makes short sentences Can show hands, feet, eyes, etc. on request	Walks up and down Stands alone Can throw a ball	Uses spoon well Bladder control in day Puts on shoes
3 years	Copies a circle Beginning to know colours Cuts with scissors	Knows name, age and sex Asks what, where?	Can stand on one foot Can stand on tip toe	Washes own hands Eats with fork and spoon
4 years	Copies a cross Draws a man with head, trunk and limbs	Asks why? Recounts experiences	Hops	Dresses and undresses and can manage buttons
5 years	Draws a recognizable man and house and copies a square and triangle	Beginning to ask the meaning of abstract words	Can skip on alternate feet	Co-operates with other children and understands the need for rules

Hearing and language

Turns to sounds	3–5 months
Single syllable sounds	Up to 6 months
Double syllable sounds	6–8 months
Imitates clapping hands	9–10 months
Waves bye-bye	9–10 months
Many single words with meaning	18 months
Short sentences	2 years
Identifies parts of body	2 years
Asks 'what'	3 years
Asks 'why'	3–4 years

Posture and gross movements

Lifts head when prone	birth onwards
Lifts head when supine	3 months
Rolls from front to back	4 months
Resting on elbows	5 months
Grasps own feet	5 months
Sits alone	6 months
Crawls	8 months
Walks alone	1 year
Stands on one foot	3 years
Hops	4 years

Social and emotional

Smiles	3–8 weeks
Shy of strangers	6–12 months

FEEDING

Chews	6 months
Drinks from cup	9 months
Uses spoon	18 months

DRESSING

Helps with dressing	9 months
Takes off shoes	15 months
Takes off pants	15–24 months
Dresses	3–4 years
Shoe laces	5–7 years

Interpreting results

There are a number of factors which should be taken into account when interpreting motor developmental milestones, such as racial differences, prematurity, normal variants, etc.

Racial differences

In general black children achieve motor milestones earlier than white. Capute *et al.* (1985) found this to be true for all motor comparisons except rolling prone to supine, but showed such differences to be small, e.g. less than 1 month difference for milestones prior to walking.

Prematurity

Prematurely born children are generally reported to be delayed in locomotor development. Largo *et al.* (1985) showed that this was the case even when correcting the age for the amount of prematurity and even in neurologically normal children. The differences become more marked with increasing age (hence making it unlikely that the difference is due to inaccurate estimation of prematurity), for example:
- Preterm: mean age walking 14.1 months, males.
- Term: mean age walking 13.4 months, males.
- Preterm: mean age walking 14.4 months, females.
- Term: mean age walking 13.5 months, females.

(Although slight sex differences are manifest in the above data and despite the finding of Capute *et al.* (1985) that black/white differences were greater between females than males, comparisons between the sexes in the motor sphere do not show any consistent differences.)

Normal variation

For motor milestones it is important to comment on a normal variant, bottom shuffling. Between 8 and 9% of the normal population show this method of early locomotion in preference to crawling and such children walk independently later than their more conventional colleagues (Robson 1970). Forty eight per cent of idiopathic late walkers were shown by Chaplais and MacFarlane (1984) to be bottom shufflers and for there to be a family history of this in half. Apart from mild hypotonia and joint hyperextensibility, bottom shufflers are usually normal, though Robson and MacKeith (1971) did point out that one child in eight with spastic diplegia shuffles.

Vision impaired children

The medical literature referring to developmental milestones in visually handicapped children is surprisingly limited. Part of the problem is that generalizations cannot be made without reference to the degree of visual impairment and sometimes that is difficult to quantitate, particularly in a young child.

The single most helpful volume on this topic is *Blindness and Early Childhood Development* (Warren, 1984). What follows in this text is a list of highly selective comments and observations which it is hoped will be helpful to the ophthalmologist.
1 Seventy per cent of congenitally visually handicapped babies have additional major handicaps (Robinson 1977).
2 One third of 91 babies were found to be hypotonic (Jan *et al.* 1975).
3 In another series of 100 visually impaired children, 68% were at three quarter level of development or less for their age (Zinkin 1979).

Motor development of vision impaired children

Motor development of the congenitally blind child in the first few months of life is not markedly different from that of a sighted child, and adequate maturation of postural milestones is achieved, e.g. independent sitting and standing (Fraiberg 1977). There are, however, qualitative differences, e.g. the blind baby sits in a frozen attitude (Sonksen 1983). Delay becomes manifest in the acquisition of self-initiated mobility, e.g. extension of arms prone, pulling to stand, crawling (achieved late in the first year). The parachute response is delayed by 6 months in blind babies, occurring at 18 months of age.

The blind baby tends to move his legs more than his arms which may be held flexed at the elbow (Egan 1975). Although he starts to 'look at' his hands by bringing them up to his face at the normal time (16 weeks) reaching out is delayed beyond the 3−4 months norm (Reynell & Zinkin, 1975) and development of his pincer grasp is a year behind normal (Zinkin 1979).

Hearing and language of vision impaired children

Babbling is probably the same in sighted and visually impaired children, but the evidence is mixed as to whether 10−20-word vocabulary is acquired at the same stage (Warren 1984). However, three-word sentences are heard in both groups of children at the same time (Wilson & Halverson 1947). The young blind baby is slow to localize sounds by reaching out to touch them and tends simply to still to the sound.

Social and emotional development of vision impaired children

The blind child smiles at the normal time. He is very slow to localize with his eyes a part of his body which has been touched (this normally occurs around 7 months and in blind babies it may be 2 years or more before he does this; Sonksen 1983). The social competence of blind children and adolescents is not as strong as normal. Tilman (1967) refers to comparison of sighted and blind children on the various parts of the Wechsler Intelligence Scale for Children (WISC).

What do you do if the child seems abnormal?

The developmental scales given earlier are simply a guide to normal development and as Hall and Baird (1986) eloquently indicate, although a below-average performance can be described in terms of age equivalents, i.e. how many months behind, the significance of that delay is uncertain. The best the ophthalmologist can do when a possible delay has been detected is to acknowledge this uncertainty and refer to a paediatrician or to a children's psychologist for more formal psychometric assessment when more specific and rigorously standardized tests can be applied.

References

Capute AJ, Shapiro BK, Palmer FB, Ross A, Wachtel RC. Normal gross motor development: the influences of race, sex and socio-economic status. *Dev Med Child Neurol* 1985; **27**: 635−43

Chaplais J de Z, MacFarlane JA. A review of 404 late walkers. *Arch Dis Child* 1984; **59**: 512−16

Egan D. The early development of visually handicapped children. In: *Visual Handicaps in Children*, Vol. 17 1975; **17**: 139−44 Spastics International Medical Publications

Egan DF, Illingworth RS, MacKeith RC. *Developmental screening 0−5 years.* Clinics in Developmental Medicine 1969; **30**

Fraiberg S. *Insights from the Blind.* Souvenir Press, London 1977

Hall DMB, Baird G. Developmental tests and scales. *Arch Dis Child* 1986; **61**: 213−15

Illingworth RS. *The Development of the Infant and Young Child, Normal and Abnormal*, 9th edition. Churchill Livingstone, Edinburgh 1980

Jan JE, Robinson GC, Scott EP, Kinnis C. Hypotonia in the blind child. *Dev Med Child Neurol* 1975; **17**: 35−40

Largo RH, Molinari L, Weber M, Comenate Pinto L, Duc C. Early development of locomotion: significance of prematurity, central palsy and sex. *Dev Med Child Neurol* 1985; **27**: 183−91

Reynell J & Zinkin P. New perspectives for the developmental assessment of young children with severe visual handicap. *Child Care Health Dev* 1975; **1**: 61−9

Robinson GC *Visual Impairment in Children and Adolescents.* Eds J Jan, R Freeman, E Scott. Grune & Shatton, New York 1977

Robson P. Shuffling, hitching, scooting or sliding − some observations in 30 otherwise normal children. *Dev Med Child Neurol* 1970; **12**: 608−17

Robson P, MacKeith RC. Shufflers with spastic deplegic central palsy: a confusing clinical picture. *Dev Med Child Neurol* 1971; **13**: 651−9

Sheridan M. *The Developmental Process of Infants and Young Children.* HMSO No. 102, 1975

Sonksen P. Vision and early development. In: *Paediatric Ophthalmology*, Eds K Wybar and D Taylor, Dekker, New York, 1983

Tilman MH. Performance of blind and sighted children on the WISC. *Int J Educ Blind* 1967; **16**: 65−74, 106−12

Warren DH. *Blindness and Early Childhood Development*, 2nd revised edition. American Foundation for the Blind, New York 1984

Wilson J, Halverson HM. Development of a young blind child. *J Genet Psychol* 1947; **71**: 155−75

Zinkin P. The effect of visual handicap on early development. In *Visual Handicap in Children*, Vol. **16**: 132−8 Spastics International Medical Publications, London.

5 Postnatal Growth of the Eye

SCOTT LAMBERT AND CREIG HOYT

The premature eye

Premature infants (30–35 gestational weeks) have shorter ocular axial lengths (mean 15.1 +/− 0.9 mm), steeper corneas (53.6 +/− 2.5 dioptres), and higher lenticular refractive powers (43.5 +/− 3.6 dioptres) than full-term infants (Gordon & Donsiz 1985). The pupils are miotic and remnants of the tunica vasculosa lentis are frequently present (Kalina 1979). Bilateral symmetrical lens opacities may occur in premature infants. Initially, they consist of vacuoles along the peripheral edges of the posterior Y suture of the lens, but may progress to a dense opacification of the posterior subcapsular area. Their peak incidence occurs 7–10 days after birth. They usually resolve within 1–2 weeks with no residual abnormalities (McCormick 1968).

Vascularization of the retina is completed nasally during the eighth gestational month and temporally during the ninth month. The peripheral retina has a silver-grey appearance in areas in which vascularization is incomplete (Kalina 1979).

The infant eye

By 40 gestational weeks, the mean axial length of the eye increases to 16.8 +/− 0.6 mm, the cornea flattens to 51.2 +/− 1.1 dioptres, and the lens power decreases to 34.4 +/− 2.3 dioptres (Gordon and Donzis 1985). The peripheral retina is vascularized and the extrafoveal retina functions at nearly adult levels, but the fovea is immature in full-term infants. Neonatal foveolas have both an increased diameter and a lower cone density than adult foveolas. Infants have a rod-free zone or foveola 1000 μm in diameter with a cone density of 18 cones/100 μm, whereas adults have a rod-free zone with a mean diameter of 650–700 μm and a cone density of 42 cones/100 μm. These differences arise secondary to the greater width of the neonatal cone inner segments which decrease from a mean diameter of 7.5 μm at birth to 2.0 μm by adulthood. Conversely, the length of the cone inner segments increases from 10 μm at birth to 25 μm by adulthood. The length of the cone outer segments increase even more dramatically from 3 μm at birth to 60 μm by adulthood (Yuodelis & Hendrickson 1986).

The immaturity of the infant's foveal cones limits their visual acuity in several ways. First, the lower cone density of infants impairs their ability to detect spatial frequency (Hirsch & Hylton 1984). As the cone density of the foveola increases during the first year of life, there is a comparable improvement in the spatial frequency resolving ability (Yuodelis and Hendrickson 1986). Second, the increased length of the cone outer segments which occurs postnatally, probably enhances the efficiency of the cones in detecting light as well as colour. Although the maturation of the visual cortex and other areas of the visual pathway may be of some importance, changes in the morphology and packing density of foveolar cones are primal in mediating the visual maturation of infants.

Growth after infancy

The human eye undergoes rapid growth during the first year of life. During the first 6 weeks of life the cornea flattens from a mean of 51 dioptres to 44 dioptres (Inagaki 1986). The axial length increases from a mean of 17 mm at birth to 20 mm by 1 year of age, the lens power decreases from 34 dioptres at birth to 28 dioptres by 6 months of age (Gordon 1985).

Infants during the first year of life have a mean

refractive error of 1.00−1.25 dioptres of hyperopia and a 15−30% incidence of astigmatism exceeding 1.0 dioptre (Ingram 1979; Fulton *et al.* 1980). Five per cent of infants between 6 and 9 months of age have greater than 3 dioptres of hyperopia and 0.5% have greater than 3 dioptres of myopia (Atkinson *et al.* 1984). Both the prevalence of astigmatism (Abrahamsson 1988) and hyperopia (Mantyjarui 1985) decrease with age. By 3 years of age, the incidence of 1 dioptre or more of astigmatism decreases to 8% (Ingram *et al.* 1979). Premature and full-term infants do not differ in terms of their spherical or astigmatic refractive errors unless retinopathy of prematurity is present when they tend to be myopic (Kushner 1982).

Emmetropization refers to the developmental process in which the growth of the various components of the eye is adjusted so as to achieve emmetropia. Since the corneal curvature assumes its adult dimensions by 8 weeks of age, a decrease in the lens power is believed to compensate for the increase in the axial length of the infant eye during the first year of life (Inagaki 1986).

Aberrant growth

The growth of the infant eye can be altered by visual deprivation and by physical forces. Physical forces which may alter the growth of the infant eye include lid and orbital haemangiomas, an elevation in the intraocular pressure in congenital glaucoma, aberrant innervation of the recti muscles in Duane's syndrome, and the regional gigantism associated with neurofibromatosis. Eyes with congenital glaucoma often develop axial myopia (Costenbader & Kwitko 1967). Eyes with associated capillary haemangiomas frequently develop axial myopia and astigmatism with the axis of plus cylinder parallel to the axis of compression of the globe (Robb 1977). Kirkham (1970) reported a 40% incidence of anisometropia and a 20% incidence of anisometropic amblyopia in patients with Duane's syndrome. He also noted that almost invariably the more ametropic eye was the eye affected by Duane's syndrome and he thought that forces exerted on the globe by co-contraction of the medial and lateral rectus muscles may induce the ametropia. However, other studies have failed to confirm such a high incidence of anisometropia or amblyopia in patients with Duane's syndrome (Tredici & Von Noorden 1985). While patients with neurofibromatosis may have bupthalmic globes secondary to congenital glaucoma, a distinct phenomenon occurs in some patients with regional gigantism in which the globe may assume astronomical dimensions (Hoyt & Billson 1977).

Visual deprivation during infancy may also interfere with the emmetropization process. Using Macaque monkeys, Raviola and Weisel (1985) demonstrated that lid closure or corneal opacification during infancy resulted in axial myopia. The increase in the axial length occurred exclusively in the posterior segment. This phenomenon appeared to be light-dependent, since myopia did not develop when the monkeys were raised in the dark. The process also appeared to be species dependent since transecting the optic nerve or paralysing accommodation with atropine prevented the myopia in some species of monkeys, but not others. Since myopia developed even after surgical ablation of the visual cortices, the process is most likely mediated at the retinal or subcortical level. Defocussing by contact lenses in *Cynomolgus* monkeys produced hyperopia (Crewther *et al.* 1988) so there may be a difference induced by different forms of deprivation. An interesting phenomenon is the lower field myopia which may be due to regional refractive adaptation, i.e. the eye adapts to the proximity of objects in the visual field (Holden *et al.* 1988). Visual deprivation of the nasal or temporal half of the retina of the chick has been shown to result in asymmetrical growth of the posterior portion of the eye (Wallman *et al.* 1987). The eyes of neonatal monkeys which have undergone lensectomy have retarded growth compared to the unoperated eye but this is irrespective of whether they are optically corrected (Wilson *et al.* 1987).

Many reports have documented axial myopia in patients visually deprived during infancy secondary to congenital cataracts (Rabin *et al.* 1981; Johnson *et al.* 1982; Von Noorden & Lewis 1987; Rasooly & BenEzra 1988), corneal opacities (Curtin 1985; Gee & Tabbara 1988), and ptosis (Robb 1977; Hoyt *et al.* 1981; Von Noorden & Lewis 1987), albeit less dramatically than in experimental animals. In addition, chronic cycloplegia has been reported to retard the development of myopia in children, suggesting that accommodation may contribute to its progression (Kelly *et al.* 1975; Brodstein *et al.* 1984). While the refractive state of the eye appears to be programmed genetically, the visual experience during infancy and childhood undoubtedly has an impact on it as well (Richler & Bear 1980).

Similarly the close relationship between myopia and intellectual performance is not in doubt but the nature of this relationship is not yet clear (Rosner & Belkin 1987).

Retinal dystrophies are also commonly associated

with significant degrees of ametropia. Leber's congenital amaurosis is often associated with high hyperopia (Wagner *et al.* 1985; Schroeder *et al.* 1987; Lambert *et al.* 1989), whereas retinitis pigmentosa (Sieving & Fishman 1978) and congenital stationary night-blindness (Merin *et al.* 1970) are commonly associated with high myopia. Albinos are frequently high myopes or hyperopes or have significant astigmatism (Fondal 1962). Patients with retinopathy of prematurity (ROP) are commonly myopic (Rabin *et al.* 1981). Tasman (1979) reported an 80% incidence of 6 dioptres or more of myopia in a series of patients with cicatricial retinopathy of prematurity (ROP). Sixty-seven per cent of these patients had a greater axial length in the more myopic eye. Many patients with regressed ROP also have lenticular myopia (Gordon & Donzis 1986) and astigmatism (Kushner 1982).

References

Abrahamsson M, Fabian G, Sjostrand J. Changes in astigmatism between the ages of 1 and 4 years: a longitudinal study. *Br J Ophthalmol* 1988; **72**: 145–50

Atkinson J, Braddick OJ, Durden K *et al*. Screening for refractive error, in 6–9 month old infants by photorefraction. *Br J Ophthalmol* 1984; **68**: 105–12

Brodstein RS, Brodstein DE, Olson RJ, Hunt SC, Williams RR. The treatment of myopia with atropine and bifocals. *Ophthalmology* 1984; **91**: 1373–9

Costenbader FD, Kwitko ML. Congenital glaucoma. An analysis of seventy-seven consecutive eyes. *J Pediatr Ophthalmol* 1967; **2**: 9–15

Crewther SG, Nathan J, Kiely PM, Brennan NA, Crewther DP. The effect of defocussing contact lenses on refraction in *Cynomolgus* monkeys. *Clin Vis Sci* 1988; **3**: 221–8

Curtin BJ. *The Myopias: Basic Science and Clinical Management*. Harper & Row, Philadelphia 1985

Fondal G. Characteristics and low-vision corrections in albinism. *Arch Ophthalmol* 1962; **68**: 754–61

Fulton AB, Dobson V, Salem D, Mar C, Petersen RA, Hansen RM. Cycloplegic refractions in infants and young children. *Am J Ophthalmol* 1980; **90**: 239–47

Gee S, Tabarra KF. Increase in ocular axial length in patients with corneal opacification. *Ophthalmology* 1988; **95**: 1276–9

Gordon RA, Donzis PB. Refractive development of the human eye. *Arch Ophthalmol* 1986; **103**: 785–9

Gordon RA, Donzis PB. Myopia associated with retinopathy of prematurity. *Ophthalmology* 1986; **93**: 1593–8

Hirsch J, Hylton R. Quality of the primate photoreceptor lattice and limits of spatial vision. *Vision Res* 1984; **24**: 347–55

Holden AL, Hodos W, Hayes BP, Fitzke FW. Myopia: induced, normal and clinical. *Eye* (Suppl.) 1988; **2**: S246–56

Hoyt CS, Billson FA. Bupthalmos in neurofibromatosis: is it an expression of regional giantism? *J Pediatr Ophthalmol Strabismus* 1977; **14**: 228–34

Hoyt CS, Stone RD, Fromer C, Billson FA. Monocular axial myopia associated with neonatal lid closure in human infants. *Am J Ophthalmol* 1981; **91**: 197–200

Inagaki Y. The rapid change of corneal curvature in the neonatal period and infancy. *Arch Ophthalmol* 1986; **104**: 1026–7

Ingram RM. Refraction of 1-year-old children after atropine refraction. *Br J Ophthalmol* 1979; **63**: 343–7

Ingram RM, Traynar MJ, Walker C, Wilson JM. Screening for refractive errors at age 1 year: a pilot study. *Br J Ophthalmol* 1979; **63**: 243–50

Johnson CA, Post RB, Chalupa LM, Lee TJ. Monocular deprivation in humans: A study of identical twins. *Invest Ophthalmol Vis Sci* 1982; **23**: 135–8

Kalina RE. Examination of the premature infant. *Ophthalmology* 1979; **86**: 1690–4

Kelly TS-B, Chatfield C, Tustin G. Clinical assessment of the arrest of myopia. *Br J Ophthalmol* 1975; **59**: 529–38

Kirkham TH. Anisometropia and amblyopia in Duane's syndrome. *Am J Ophthalmol* 1970; **69**: 774–9

Kushner BJ. Strabismus and amblyopia associated with regressed retinopathy of prematurity. *Arch Ophthalmol* 1982; **100**: 256–61

Lambert SR, Kriss A, Taylor D, Coffey R, Pembrey M. Follow-up and diagnostic reappraisal of 75 patients with Leber's congenital amaurosis. *Am J Ophthalmol* 1989; **107**: 624–31

Mantyjarui MI. Changes of refraction in school-children. *Arch Ophthalmol* 1985; **103**: 790–3

McCormick AQ. Transient cataracts in premature infants: a new clinical entity. *Can J Ophthalmol* 1968; **3**: 202–6

Merin S, Rowe H, Auerbach E *et al*. Syndrome of congenital high myopia with nyctalopia: report of findings in 25 families. *Am J Ophthalmol* 1970; **70**: 541–7

Rabin J, Van Sluyters RC, Malach R. Emmetropization: A vision-dependent phenomenon. *Invest Ophthalmol Vis Sci* 1981; **20**: 561–4

Rasooly R, BenEzra D. Congenital and traumatic cataract: the effect on ocular axial length. *Arch Ophthalmol* 1988; **106**: 1066–9

Raviola E, Wiesel TN. An animal model of myopia. *N Engl J Med* 1985; **312**: 1609–15

Richler A, Bear JC. Refraction, near work and education. *Acta Ophthalmol* 1980; **58**: 468–78

Robb RM. Refractive errors associated with haemangiomas on the eyelids and orbit in infancy. *Am J Ophthalmol* 1977; **83**: 52–8

Rosner M, Belkin M. Intelligence, education and myopia in males. *Arch Ophthalmol* 1987; **105**: 1508–12

Schroeder R, Mets MB, Maumenee IH. Leber's congenital amaurosis. Retrospective review of 43 cases and a new fundus finding in two cases. *Arch Ophthalmol* 1987; **1195**: 356–9

Sieving PA, Fishman GA. Refractive errors of retinitis pigmentosa patients. *Br J Ophthalmol* 1978; **62**: 163–7

Tasman W. Late complications of retrolental fibroplasia. *Ophthalmology* 1979; **86**: 1724–40

Tredici TD, Von Noorden GK. Are anisometropia and amblyopia common in Duane's syndrome. *J Pediatr Ophthalmol Strabismus* 1985; **22**: 23–5

Von Noorden GK, Lewis RA. Ocular axial length in unilateral congenital cataracts and blepharoptosis. *Inv Ophthalmol Vis Sci* 1987; **28**: 750–2

Wagner RS, Caputo AR, Nelson LB, Zanoni D. High hyperopia in Leber's congenital amaurosis. *Arch Ophthalmol* 1985; **103**: 1507−9

Wallman J, Gottleib MD, Rajaram V, Fugate Wontzek LA. Local retinal region control eye growth and myopia. *Science* 1987; **237**: 73−7

Wilson JR, Fernandes A, Chandler CV *et al.* Abnormal development of the axial length of aphakic monkey eyes. *Inv Ophthalmol Vis Sci* 1987; **28**: 2086− 99

Yuodelis C, Hendrickson A. A qualitative and quantitative analysis of the human fovea during development. *Vision Res* 1986; **26**: 847−55

6 Myopia in Children

EDUARD AVETISOV

Myopia is important because not only is it a common refractive error but also because it is a significant cause of untreatable visual defect. Although it is the butt of misplaced humour it is a significant disorder which, even in its minor degrees may significantly limit a child's life — for life!

Myopia may be congenital, it may develop in the preschool period but most frequently it is observed in schoolchildren. The number of myopic children increases every school year and the degree of myopia rises also. By the age of majority, some 20% of all students with myopia have already had certain restrictions in their choice of profession. Progressive myopia may lead to irreversible changes in the eye and it may be associated with significant loss of vision.

High, complicated, myopia remains significant among the causes of visual disability, and this condition affects both young and mature people, i.e. those who are at the peak of their creative ability. There are many hypotheses on the origin of myopia, most do not have a scientific background and are based on speculative conclusions, but we would like to consider some interesting speculations as to its natural history.

Traditional theories of causation

According to earlier authors, the vitreous presses on the sclera, if the choroid acting as an elastic capsule does not prevent it. In 'insufficiency' of the ciliary muscle ('intoxication', previous diseases, congenital weakness or stress) it may fail to ensure sufficient tension on the choroidal coat of the eye; as a result, the vitreous body presses more directly upon the sclera, and the latter being weak, gradually stretches making the eyeball longer.

The Swiss ophthalmologist, Steiger (1915), propounded a hereditary–biological theory, in which the ocular elements responsible for the refraction of the eye do not depend on each other but combine in a random fashion. Each of these elements — the refractive power of the media and the axial length of the eyeball — are inherited and predetermined by sex; environment can in no way influence the development of refraction.

Vogt (1924) presumed that the protective coats of the eye correspond to its shape and volume and not the opposite way; therefore a small retina would make the eye hypermetropic, the moderate one —

emmetropic, and when the retina is large the eye would develop myopia.

Sondermann's hypothesis (1950) was based on the observations of Ammon in 1801 who noted protrustion of the sclera at the posterior pole of the eye in 4–7-month embryos. This protrusion was thought to be the result of an imbalance between the intraocular pressure and the ocular coats. By the time of birth, the sclera is already firm at the point, but if this imbalance remains, it may give rise to myopia.

Poos (1950) believed that the final shape and size of the eyeball depends on the active growth of the sclera and the mechanical effect of the ocular muscles. If the muscles complete their growth early, the eyeball remains short; if the muscle stopped growing later in development, the eyeball elongates.

Comberg (1929) felt that the weakness of the sclera was the basis of myopia. Strain on the sclera, weakened under the influence of various unfavourable factors takes place by summation of brief rises of intraocular pressure and the movements of the eyes in reading.

Aetiology

It has become clear there is no single cause of myopia (Curtin 1970, 1985), but Avetisov (1986) has highlighted three factors in its development: (a) near vision efforts—weak accommodation interrelationships; (b) hereditary predisposition; and (c) weak sclera—intraocular pressure interrelationships.

The first two factors are involved to a different extent in the initial period of myopia, the third one in advanced degrees of myopia, causing its further progression. In principle, myopic refraction can also start at the third stage, and all stages are to varying degrees interrelated. Mechanical forces acting on the globe, ocular inflation, and to a lesser extent growth pattern are the important factors in the genesis of myopia (Weale 1988).

In weak accommodation, near vision efforts become a real muscular exertion for the eye. In these cases an eye has to change its optical system so that it can be adapted for near working distances without the strain of accommodation. As a result, during the period of ocular growth and the formation of refraction, the anteroposterior axis of the eye becomes longer. Unfavourable conditions for near vision work induce myopia to the degree to which they hinder accommodation. Such myopia generally does not exceed 3 dioptres.

Weakness of accommodation may be the consequence of congenital morphological defects of the ciliary muscle, its insufficient 'training' or in some systemic diseases. Accommodation may also be weak due to poor blood supply of the ciliary muscle and its reduced activity, in turn, disturbs the haemodynamics of the eye.

Myopia is inherited either as an autosomal dominant or autosomal recessive trait. In autosomal dominant inheritance, myopia develops later in childhood and usually does not reach high degrees. The autosomal recessive type is characteristic of communities with a high percentage of consanguinity but also accounts for many supposedly sporadic cases. A phenotypic polymorphism is common; this myopia is known for its early onset, progressiveness and complications and the association with congenital disease of the eye, and in some instances for a more severe disease process in each successive generation.

When the sclera is weak due to impaired fibrillogenesis (Fig. 6.1), which may be congenital or develop from systemic diseases, there is an inappropriate growth response of the eye and subsequent elongation under the influence of even normal intraocular pressure (Figs. 6.2, 6.3). Intraocular pressure by itself, even when increased, cannot elongate the eye with a normally strong sclera. It is not the static but more the 'dynamic' intraocular pressure which is important, i.e. transient disturbances of the ocular fluids in movements of the body or head. In walking or some activities associated with visual control these movements are mostly performed in the anteroposterior direction. The anterior part of the eye has a barrier (the ciliary body—lens diaphragm), so the disturbance primarily affects the posterior pole of the eye. Once the posterior pole has an increased radius of curvature in accordance with hydrodynamic laws, it becomes the least resistant place.

Excessive elongation of the eye produces an adverse effect on the choroid and retina; these tissues are less plastic and have a physiological limit for their growth. Outside this limit, the choroid and retina develop trophic lesions especially in high degrees of myopia. Decreased haemodynamics of the eye also contributes to the trophic changes.

Congenital myopia has some special pathogenetic features. There are three forms of its origin:

1 Congenital myopia due to poor correlation between anatomical and optical components of refraction, i.e. a combination of a relatively long antero-posterior axis of the eye and a relatively strong refractive power of the optical media (usually the lens). When the sclera is strong, this congenital myopia normally does not progress: elongation of the eye is compensated for

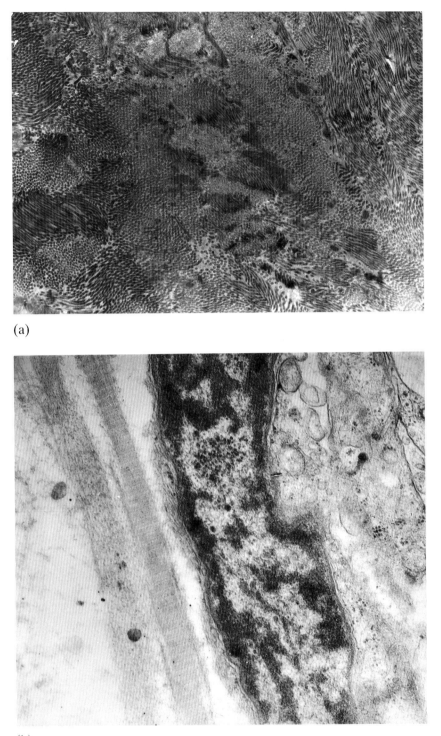

(a)

(b)

Fig. 6.1 (a) Sclera of the posterior ocular segment in emmetropia. Notice dense packing of collagen structures and binding of collagen fibrils in different directions. (b) Posterior sclera in high myopia. Granular destruction of collagen fibrils (original x 30 000).

by a reduction of the refractive power of the lens.

2 Congenital myopia when the sclera is weak and is constantly stretching: it progresses rapidly and the prognosis is poor.

3 Congenital myopia associated with developmental anomalies of the eyeball. This kind of myopia, apart from the poor anatomical and optical correlation, is complicated by other pathology (strabismus, nystagmus, colobomas, subluxation of the lens or its partial opacification, optic nerve atrophy or hypo-

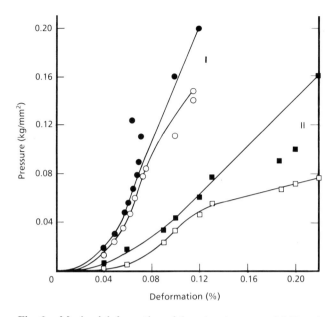

Fig. 6.2 Maximal deformation of the sclera in equatorial (i) and sagittal (ii) directions. Light circles and squares, + approximal data; dark ones, + results of experimental studies.

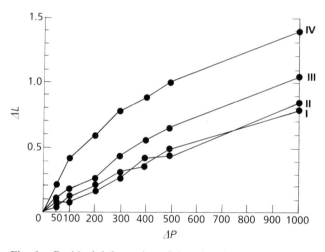

Fig. 6.3 Residual deformation of the sclera in emmetropia (i), low myopia (ii) and high myopia (iii, + near equator; iv, + near posterior pole).

plasia, degenerative changes of the retina, etc.). In combination with a weak sclera this form of myopia can progress.

INTERNATIONAL ASPECTS

The incidence of myopia in the world is different in different places (Borish 1970). In the UK, Ware (1813) found myopia in 1% of schoolchildren and in 25% of university students. Almost the same figures (20%) for students were obtained by Clarke (1924). Accord-

ing to Witte (1923), and Hess and Diederichs (1924) cited from Borish, the myopia rate varied in Germany between 13.8 and 27.8%.

In Austria, 4.5% of the screened population in Vienna were myopic (Von Reuss 1881); in Switzerland, 24% (Franceschetti 1935); in Sweden, 11% (Heinonen 1928); and in Egypt, 18% (Meyerhof 1914). In the USA myopia was diagnosed in 25% of the population, ranging from 24 to 54 years (Sperduto et al. 1983). In the USSR 8.8% of schoolchildren have myopia (Avetisov 1986).

Although reports of its incidence vary, myopia is widely distributed in all developed countries of the world. In some countries it is especially frequent. In Japan, from 15 (Tamura 1932) to 70% (Sato 1957) of students are myopic. In China, this figure varies between 22.1−58% (Rush 1920) and 70% (Rasmussen 1936).

Grading of myopia

Myopia may be of low, moderate and high degrees. The gradation of myopia by its severity varies in different parts of the world: our scheme in the Soviet Union is that low myopia runs up to −3.0 dioptres, moderate from −3.25 to −6.0 dioptres, and high myopia is more than −6.0 dioptres. Low, moderate and high myopia constitue about 82, 12 and 6% respectively of the myopes in the population of the USSR.

Systemic and ocular associations of myopia

Systemic disorders with myopia

1 Down's syndrome.
2 Marfan's syndrome, homocystinuria, and Weill−Marchesani syndrome (see Chapter 24).
3 Ehlers−Danlos syndrome.
4 Stickler's and Kneist's syndromes.
5 Pierre Robin's syndrome.
6 Others:
   (a) Prader−Willi syndrome: hypotonia obesity, small hands and feet, squint (50%) and amblyopia upslanting palpebral fissures, (Hered et al. 1988).
   (b) Cohen's syndrome: hypotonia, mental retardation, obesity, prominent incisors (Cohen et al. 1973).
   (c) Marshall's syndrome: increased growth in length, failure to thrive, shallow orbits, upturned nose, small mandible (Fitch 1980).
   (d) Noonan's syndrome: appearance of Turner's

syndrome — without the XO chromosomal configuration of Turner's syndrome. Epicanthic folds, high myopia, keratoconus and strabismus are frequent (Schartz 1972; Rogers 1975).

(e) Schwartz—Jampel syndrome: short stature, myotonia, rigid joints, blepharophimosis (Schwartz & Jampel 1962). Malignant hyperpyrexia may be associated (Seay & Ziter 1978).

(f) Spranger and Wiedemann's spondyloepiphyseal dysplasia congenita: barrel chest, short trunk, growth deficiency, flat face, malar hypoplasia. High myopia, vitreoretinal degeneration and retinal detachment (Hamidi-Toosi & Maumenee 1982; Murray et al. 1985).

(g) Rubinstein—Taybi syndrome.

Ocular conditions frequently associated with myopia

- Congenital cataract, corneal opacities, ptosis (see Chapter 5).
- Retinal and choroidal dystrophies:
  congenital stationary night-blindness;
  choroideremia;
  gyrate atrophy;
  retinitis pigmentosa;
  cone dystrophy.
- Ectopia lentis
- Myelinated nerve fibres and amblyopia (Fig. 6.4a, 6.4b) (see Chapter 28).
- Wagner's disease (usually a part of Stickler's syndrome).
- Retinopathy of prematurity.
- Albinism.

Presentation and progression

The first sign of myopia is reduced distance acuity which usually corrects with glasses to normal. Myopia, near its onset, may be transient.

Typical complaints of schoolchildren with incipient myopia include fatiguing of the eyes at close working distances, blurring of distant objects or of writing on the blackboard. They prefer to sit at the front of a class and may need to occupy places close to the screen or stage in the cinema or theatre. To improve their vision, myopes often narrow their eyes in order to reduce the size of the pupil and to achieve a sort of pinhole effect.

The far point is nearer than in emmetropia and the near point is also nearer. The amplitude of absolute accommodation remains stable for long periods. The capacity of the ciliary muscle is frequently reduced

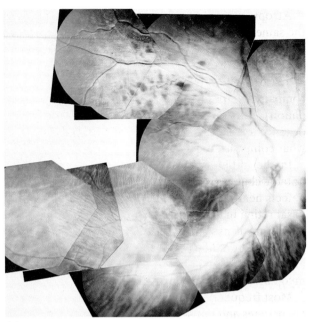

(a)

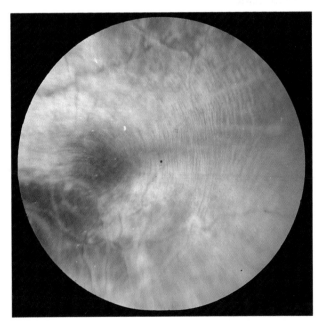

(b)

Fig. 6.4 (a) High myopia with myelinated nerve fibres and amblyopia. (b) The anatomy of the median raphe made outstandingly clear by the visible nerve fibres.

and the amplitude of the positive part (reserve) of relative accommodation is decreased.

Ophthalmoplethisomography and ophthalmorheography often show reduced ocular blood supply, particularly of the ciliary muscle, which becomes more pronounced in advanced stages of myopia.

Atropinization in the initial stages of myopia reveals the same degree of ametropia as in the uncyclopleged state. Sometimes, with cycloplegia, the degree of myopia improves greatly and in rare cases it even increases. The first phenomenon indicates an accompanying pseudomyopia (spasm of accommodation), the second one intensification of the far distance relaxation of accommodation which somewhat compensates the degree of myopia.

In the initial stages of myopia there are not any notable changes in the fundus, except occasional conus defects near the optic disc and in tilted optic discs the nasal retina may be dragged over the optic disc giving one form of pseudopapilloedema (Fig. 6.5). In congenital or hereditary myopia there are fundus alterations but these are more characteristic of severe myopia.

Most frequently, myopia develops to low or moderate degrees and remains static. Commonly, it does not cause reduction in visual functions or pathological transformations in the ocular coats or refractive media. This type of myopia is not a 'disease'. Sometimes the eyeball continues to elongate, simultaneously increasing the degree of myopia. The far point comes closer to the eye, the amplitude of accommodation reduces, weakness of the ciliary muscle increases, and the haemodynamics become poor.

The progression of myopia may give rise to irrevers-

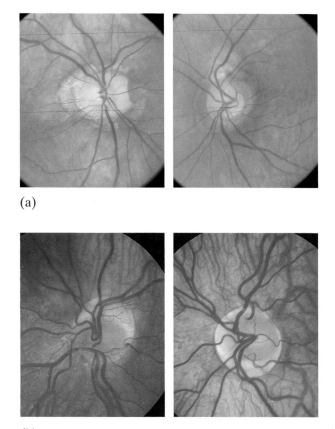

(a)

(b)

Fig. 6.6 Peripapillary myopic degeneration; in (b) conus defects virtually surround the discs.

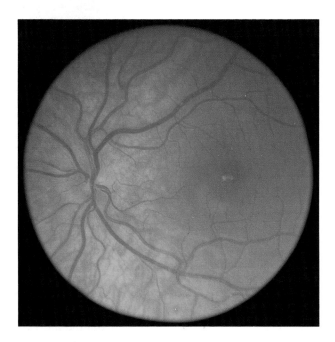

Fig. 6.5 Myopic pseudopapilloedema. This low myope has a mildly 'tilted' optic disc with the nasal retina dragged over the optic disc giving a false appearance of mild papilloedema.

ible ocular changes and visual loss. Spectacles are of little help, dark adaptation may be disturbed, and visual field losses may occur. This elongation of the posterior segment first affects the area of the optic disc. Newly developed conus defects gradually enlarge, embracing the optic disc in the form of an irregular ring (Fig. 6.6). Sometimes the optic disc itself becomes longer, larger and flat, with a greyish tint (Fig. 6.7).

In severe progressive myopia true bulgings (staphylomas) are observed at the posterior pole. They are demarcated by an arc-shaped line located concentrically with the optic disc with the retinal vessels bending over it (Fig. 6.8, 6.9).

With increasing atrophy of choroid and retina the degenerative processes become more pronounced. Whitish-yellow strips appear: these are often multiple and may be criss-crossed but are usually basically horizontal. They are known as lacquer cracks and are thought to be mechanical breaks in Bruch's membrane and the retinal pigment epithelium (Klein & Curtin

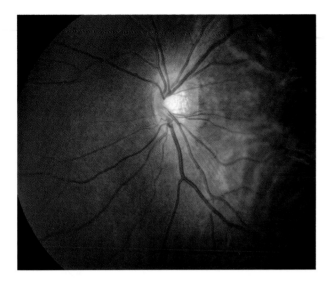

Fig. 6.7 Myopia. The optic disc is vertically oval and has peripapillary degeneration showing around it. There is a posterior staphyloma evidenced by the more visible choroidal vascular pattern.

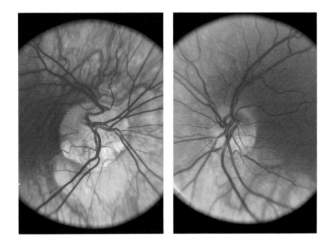

Fig. 6.8 Tilted discs with conus defects. The right eye has a staphyloma above the disc and the left below the disc.

1975). They may presage more serious complications. Later, round or irregular white foci with pigmented margins or inclusions occur. These foci may eventually merge affecting a significant area of the fundus. Depigmentation and disappearance of both small and larger choroidal vessels make the fundus acquire an albinotic appearance with a sparse network of choroidal vessels; in other cases pigmentation of the choroid intensifies and with accumulation of pigment between the vessels a parquet-like appearance of the fundus may be observed.

Decrease in visual acuity is especially great when a yellow spot is involved in the atrophic processes. The macular reflexes are absent, the macular region looks darker and small white atrophic, and some pigmented foci are seen. Degeneration of the peripheral retina with local hyperpigmentation, thinning, cystoid and lattice degeneration, schisis, and small defects and tears associated with vitreous degeneration can induce retinal detachment. Sometimes the integrity of retinal vessels walls is spoiled resulting in retinal haemorrhages which produce a large pigmented focus with a light rim — a so-called Fuch's spot (Fig. 6.9). These haemorrhages may be related to subretinal neovascularization (Hotchkiss & Fine 1981). As a result of haemorrhages and destruction of the vitreous body, the latter develops opacifications which are interpreted by a myope as dark shadows or whispy floaters in the visual field (Fig. 6.10).

When a myope brings an object close to his eyes the medial rectus muscles experience great strain which may lead to fatigue of the muscles and symptoms of asthenopia. If the muscles are not able to perform the convergence efforts, binocular vision is compromised by strabismus. Exophoria or exotropia result from reduced need for accommodation which in turn reduce the stimulus to convergence. If myopia continues to progress, ultrasound biometry shows the elongation of the anteroposterior axis of the eye, which correlates with the degree of myopia and the incidence of complications.

Prognosis

In stabilized low myopia visual prognosis with spectacle correction is favourable. In high severe myopia

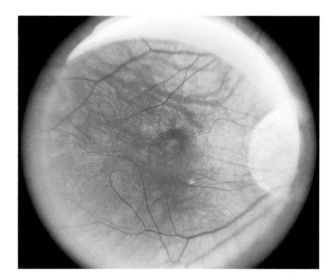

Fig. 6.9 Fuch's spot.

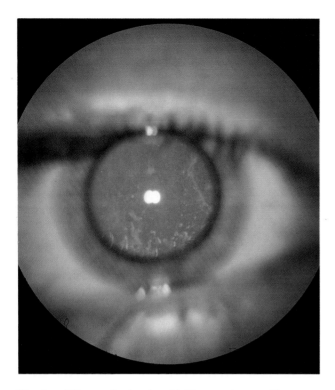

Fig. 6.10 Vitreous floaters in a highly myopic eye with posterior vitreous detachment. The fellow eye had a retinal detachment.

visual acuity often becomes or remains low. In progressive myopia degenerative changes in the retina make the visual prognosis worse particularly where the macular region is affected. In some cases of high myopia without any evidence of significant retinal disease or other pathology of the visual pathways the acuity fails to correct to 100%, this may be due to micropsia from the spectacle correction or an 'organic' myopia from stretching of the retinal elements (Romano 1988).

Diagnosis

Diagnosis of myopia is based on the objective assessment of refraction including, in some cases, the use of cycloplegic drugs.

HISTORY

This should include questions on the time when first signs of visual disturbance were noted, the subjective feelings of the patient, his daily visual work, vocation, general health, whether any glasses were used and any family history of myopia.

GENERAL EXTERNAL EXAMINATION AND COVER TESTS

Heterophorias (usually exophoria) or heterotropias are noted, binocular functions are examined including binocular vision, muscle balance (type and degree of heterophoria for far and near vision), and convergence.

ACUITY TESTING AND REFRACTION

Visual acuity is assessed for each eye individually and both eyes together without correction and with the patient's glasses. If these glasses do not produce normal visual acuity or if the patient has never used spectacles, the doctor should use the minimal minus spherical and astigmatic lenses which give maximal visual acuity. If spherical lenses do not substantially increase visual acuity, amblyopia or organic lesions of the vision should be suspected.

EYE EXAMINATION

Examination of the ocular media and fundi. Apart from ophthalmoscopy, biomicroscopy (with white or red free light) of the vitreous and the posterior segment of the eye are useful. Indirect ophthalmoscopy is especially helpful in examination of the fundi of high myopes, but direct ophthalmoscopy should not be forgotten especially in examination of the optic disc for minor degrees of hypoplasia.

CYCLOPLEGIC REFRACTION

The static refraction of the eye is tested by means of retinoscopy or by automated refractometry in conditions of cycloplegia.

Anisometropia of −2.0 dioptre and more may be important in the spectacle correction of myopia and may be an indication for contact lenses although many children can tolerate higher degrees of anisometropia with a spectacle correction.

EXAMINATION OF ACCOMMODATION

To know the potential of the ciliary muscle, the reserve of relative accommodation should be determined. Data shows the role of accommodation in the origin of one distinct type of myopia and is of value for the choice of management and far/near spectacle correction.

For suspected spasm or paresis of accommodation,

absolute accommodation should be examined; and a determination of far and near point and calculation of the amplitude of accommodation. Cyclopegia should be performed, too.

STARTING SPECTACLES

Spectacles are started after the effect of any cycloplegic agent has worn off.

FURTHER EXAMINATIONS IN SUBOPTIMAL ACUITY

In cases where full optical correction does not produce a high visual acuity or where there are pathological alterations in the ocular fundus, the central visual fuctions are evaluated by the use of perimetry, determination of retinal visual acuity and electrophysiological tests.

Follow-up

Subsequent annual examinations of refraction permit one to judge whether myopia is stationary (steady refraction for 2 years and longer) or progressive and allow judgement of the rate of progression. In cases where astigmatism is present, refraction of each eye is judged by spherical equivalent (the power of the sphere plus half the power of the cylinder).

To estimate the rate of myopia rise, a year's gradient of its progressiveness is calculated from this formula:

$$YG = \frac{SE2 - SE1}{T} \text{ dioptres per year}$$

where YG is a year's gradient, $SE2$ is the spherical equivalent of the eye at the end of follow-up, $SE1$ is the spherical equivalent at the beginning of follow-up, and T is time in years. A year's gradient of less than 1.0 dioptre per year indicates slow progressive myopia, and 1.0 dioptre per year evidences rapidly progressive myopia. Ultrasonic examination of the axial length helps to assess the dynamics of the myopic process.

Prevention

Prevention of myopia lies in the general improvement and physical development of a child or teenager's life and visual environment. Intensification of physical activity and exercise is especially significant for urban schoolchildren. Prophylaxis and treatment of systemic and chronic diseases is also important for prevention of myopia.

Special attention should be paid to using the correct distance when reading or writing: it should be within 30–35 cm. Changes of fixation of vision from near objects to far ones and vice versa during reading with frequent breaks may help to prevent development of myopia. It is important to ensure sufficient lighting of the working place of schoolchildren.

Optical correction

In low or moderate myopia, distance correction ensuring binocular visual acuity of 0.7–0.8 (6/9–6/7.5, 20/30–20/25) is recommended; this correction should not exceed the degree of myopia detected in cycloplegic conditions. In myopia of −1.0 to −2.0 dioptre, spectacles should not be used all the time, but may be used only as required for detailed work in the distance. Optical correction for near vision is determined by the state of accommodation. If it is weak (a reduced reserve of relative accommodation or visual discomfort when reading or writing), a second pair of spectacles is prescribed for near vision or bifocal spectacles for constant use. The upper part of these spectacles corrects myopia almost fully and serves for far vision; the lower part intended for near vision and is weaker by +1.0 to +2.0 dioptres, depending on the subjective feelings of the patient and the degree of myopia. The higher the degree of the myopia the greater the difference in power between the near and distance parts of the bifocal spectacles. If accommodative ability is good (with normal reserve of relative accommodation, absence of discomfort with spectacles), a full or almost full correction is prescribed; in these cases the spectacles promote more active accommodation.

In high myopia the glasses should be constantly worn, the power is determined by tolerance for near and far distance. Where spherical or astigmatic lenses fail to improve visual acuity over 0.4–0.5 (6/12–6/18 or 20/40–20/60), contact lenses may be fitted.

Myopic astigmatism of more than −1.5 dioptres should be corrected. Lesser degrees of astigmatism which reduce visual acuity to a significant extent may also be corrected.

Accommodation treatment

Weak accommodation is treated either with lenses or with home exercises.

LENSES

It is our clinical practise to recommend exercises with lenses. The basis of these exercises lies in the use of

Table 6.1 Clinical classification of myopia.

By degree	By refraction ratio of both eyes	By astigmatism	By period of onset	By course of development	By the stage of complications		Morphological changes	Stage of functional changes (reduction in visual acuity of the best eye with correction)
					By complications	Form		
Low (up to 3.0 D inclusive)	Isometropic	Without astigmatism	Congenital	Stationary	Complicated	Chorioretinal: around disc; macular 'dry' form sand 'exudative' form; peripheric; widespread	*Initial*: cone or ring near optic disc less than ¼ dd. Macular reflex may be absent, small lumps of pigment may appear	1 Visual acuity, 0.8–0.5
Mild (3.25–6.0 D)	Anisometropic*	With astigmatism†	Early acquired (in preschool period)	Slow progressive (less 1.0 D per year)	Non-complicated	Vitreoretinal	*Advanced*: enlargement of cone or ring near optic disc up to 1 dd, change in the form of disc, pigmentation and spottedness of macular region, depigmentation of the fundus	2 Visual acuity, 0.4–0.2
High (more than 6.0 D)			Acquired during school years	Fast progressive (1.0 D per year)		Haemorrhagic	*Far advanced*: further enlargement of cone or ring which frequently merge, forming irregular counter up to 1.5 dd and more, pallor of the disc pronounced depigmentation of the fundus, dense spottedness of macular region, formation of staphylomas	3 Visual acuity, 0.1–0.05
			Acquired in advanced ages			Mixed		4 Visual acuity, 0.04 and lower

* When the difference in refraction of eyes is of 1.0 D and more.
† When astigmatism is of 1.0 D and more.

minus and plus lenses for physiological 'massage' of the ciliary muscle. The effect on the accommodative apparatus is graduated so as not to exceed slightly submaximal accommodative efforts.

First put a book before a patient at a 33 cm distance and determine positive and negative parts of relative accommodation; subtract 0.5−1.0 dioptre from maximal plus and maximal minus lenses. The resultant lenses require submaximal efforts for the ciliary muscle.

After correction of myopia with lenses, commence reading exercises with a minus lens of 0.5 dioptre. Gradually increase the power of the lens by 0.5−1.0 dioptre up to the lens for the submaximal amount of the positive part of relative accommodation. Continue these exercises with every new lens for 3−5 minutes. Then go on with training in the reverse order down to −1.0 dioptre applying each lens for 1 minute. Now use plus lenses. Their power should be gradually increased up to the submaximal amount of the negative part of relative accommodation. Duration of reading with every new lens is 3 minutes.

In the first 3 days of treatment these exercises should be performed once a day, and twice in subsequent days. Every 3 days determine the amount of relative accommodation for specification of submaximal efforts. The course of training consists from 15 to 20 exercises. If the first course of treatment does not stabilize activity of the ciliary muscle, repeat the course after a 1 or 2 month interval. To stabilize the effect of training or where the use of lenses is impossible, home exercises are recommended.

HOME EXERCISES

Ask the child to put on his or her distance glasses and stand at a 30−35 cm distance from the window. Put a round mark 3−5 mm in diameter on the window glass at the level of the patient's eyes. Ask him to choose any object at the far distance the viewing of which requires looking through the mark on the window. He should look alternately at the mark and at the remote object. The exercises are done twice a day for 15−20 days. If the effect of exercises is not evident, he should continue to perform them regularly at 10−15 days interval. Duration of exercises for the first 2 days − 3 minutes, for the 2 subsequent days − 5 minutes, for other days − 7 minutes. Exercises for the ciliary muscle are indicated in low or mild myopia. These are effective mostly in initial myopia.

For normalization of accommodative ability 1% solution of neosinephrine (phenylephrine) can be used. It should be instilled by 1−2 drops at bed time on alternate days. Neosinephrine is also indicated when a myope experiences great visual efforts (e.g. during examination). This technique is not widely practised outside the USSR.

Restrictions to the myope's life

Myopic patients should follow precisely reading instructions. Visual work, other than school lessons, should be reduced within reasonable limits. In progressive myopia, 40−45 minutes of reading require a 5-minute rest. In high myopia, continuous reading should be limited to 30 minutes with a 10-minute break. Patients with myopia higher than −6.0 dioptre (or −4.0 dioptre, if there are changes in the ocular fundus) should avoid lifting of heavy loads, viewing small objects or keeping the body in the bent position with the head being kept downward.

The choice of vocation is very individual; medical considerations are based on the state of visual acuity, the degree of myopia, the stability or progressiveness of the myopia, the presence and type of complications, the visual field (the presence of central or paracentral scotomas). General health and professional conditions should also be considered.

In uncomplicated myopia it is possible and even useful to go in for sports. If the child does not like to wear spectacles during sport they may be taken off. Sports necessitating high acuity without spectacles should not be recommended.

In complicated myopia all sports associated with sharp movements of the body or its shaking are contra-indicated. However, graduated exercises in the gymnasium, walking, rowing and swimming are possible. Recommendations are based on common sense, practicability and must take into account the patients personal philosophy − it is not advisable to wrap the child in cotton wool.

Drug treatment

Some authorities believe that complicated myopia and its progressiveness can be prevented by a number of drugs. These are divided into 5 groups: (a) drugs for reinforcement of the sclera: calcium gluconate, ascorbic acid; (b) for haemodynamics of the eye: nicotinic acid, halidor, nihexinum, trental, etc.; (c) for improvement of metabolism of the retina and choroid: adenosine triphosphoric acid, riboflavin, etc.; (d); haemostatic drugs: rutin, ascorbic acid, dicinon, vicasol, calcium chloride, etc.; and (e) resorption drugs: glucose, sodium iodide. The choice of drug, technique and frequency of application are made on the basis of a variety of indications; they are not widely used outside the USSR (Curtin 1970).

The use of cycloplegic drugs in the arrest of myopic progression has had many advocates over nearly two centuries. The arguments for and against have been many, and although even the best conducted studies (Brodstein *et al.* 1984) may have been cautiously enthusiastic, there is still not clear evidence about the efficacy of this form of treatment.

Keratorefractive surgery

The author and editor do not believe that there is currently a role for keratorefractive surgery in children except in some older cases with substantial astigmatism or anisometropia when the standard optical correction is not tolerated. Excimer laser keratorefractive treatment is still experimental and in children will remain so for many years.

Scleroplasty

Myopia can be significantly arrested by scleroplastic operations. Curtin (1961) suggested strengthening the sclera with an X-shaped graft taken from autologous fascia lata which was put behind the eyeball with a special instrument. Nesterov and Libenson (1967) also used X- and Y-shaped grafts taken from autologous fascia lata.

Belyaev and Iljina (1972, 1975) and Whitwell (1971) used a scleral graft from which a calotte is cut; one end of which is split and placed into the retrobulbar space. Snyder and Thompson (1972) passed a scleral graft vertically around the posterior pole of the eye. Avetisov and Tarutta (1981) also used a scleral graft, but they cut it so that it covers the postero-exterior ocular segment. The authors considered this the most extensible part of the eye in progressive myopia.

Avetisov *et al.* (1986) also suggested a non-surgical method of scleral reinforcement by injecting a special composition under the Tenon's capsule in the postero-external segment of the eye. In 2–3 minutes this composition becomes solid, forming an extra layer on the surface of the sclera. Its slow resorption allows collagen formation and stimulates growth of the connective tissue. This phenomenon improves strength of the sclera making it stretch less.

LENS EXTRACTION

Extraction of the lens to reduce the amount of high myopia is contraindicated in the young due to the high complication rate (Rodriguez *et al.* 1987).

References

Avetisov ES. *Myopia*. Meditsina, Moscow. 1986

Avetisov ES, Tarutta EP. New operation for myopia and its results. *Vestn Oftalmol* 1981; **3**: 21–4

Belayev VS, Ilyina TS. Scleroplasty as a method of surgical treatment in progressive myopia. *Vestn Oftalmol* 1972; **3**: 60–3

Belayev VS, Ilyina TS. Late results of scleroplasty in surgical treatment of progressive myopia. *Eye Ear Nose Throat J* 1975; **54**: 109–13

Borish IM. *Clinical refraction*, 3rd edition. Professional Press, Chicago. 1970

Brodstein RS, Brodstein DE, Olson RJ, Hunt SC, Williams RR. The treatment of myopia with atropine and bifocals. *Ophthalmology 1984*; **91**: 1373–9

Clarke E. *The Errors of Accommodation and Refraction of the Eye and Their Treatment*. 5th ed. Baillière, Tindall & Cox, London. 1924

Cohen MM, Hall BD, Smith DW, Graham CB, Lampert KJ. A new syndrome with hypotonia, obesity, mental deficiency and facial, oral, ocular and limb anomalies. *J. Pediatr 1973*; **83**: 280–6

Comberg W. Anatomic and experimental examinations of the mechanical factors in origin of myopia. *Arch Ophthalmol* 1929; **1**: 286–90

Curtin BJ. Myopia: a review of its etiology, pathogenesis and treatment. *Surv Ophthalmol* 1970; **15**: 1–17

Curtin BJ. *The Myopias: Basic Science and Clinical Management*. Harper & Row, Philadelphia. 1985; 221–5

Curtin, BJ. Scleral support of the posterior sclera. Part II: clinical results. *Am J Ophthalmol* 1961; **52**: 853–62

Fitch N. The syndromes of Marshall and Weaver. *J Med Genet* 1980; **17**: 174–84

Franceschetti A. Zur Refraktionskurve des Neugeboren. *Klin Monatsbl Augenheilkd* 1935; **95**: 98–9

Fuchs E. Der centrale schwarze Fleck bei Myopie. *Z Augenheilkd* 1901; **5**: 171–8

Hamidi-Toosi S, Maumenee IH. Vitroretinal degeneration in Spondyloepiphyseal dysplasia congenita. *Arch Ophthalmol* 1982; **100**: 1104–7

Heinonen O. Etiology of school and occupational myopia. *Acta Ophthalmol (Copenh)* 1928; **6**: 238–50

Hered RW, Rogers S, Zang Y-F, Biglan AW. Ophthalmologic features of Prader–Willi syndrome. *J Pediatr Ophthalmol Strabismus* 1988; **25**: 145–51

Hess C, Diederichs C. Skiaskopische Schuluntersuchungen. *Arch Augenheilkd* 1924; **29**: 1–13

Hotchkiss ML, Fine SL. Pathologic myopia and choroidal neovascularization. *Am J Ophthalmol* 1981; **91**: 177–83

Klein RM, Curtin BJ. Lacquer crack lesions in pathologic myopia. *Am J Ophthalmol* 1975; **79**: 386–92

Meyerhof M. Etude sur la myopie comme maladie de race et

maladie hereditaire chez les Egyptiens. *Ann Oculist* 1914; **151**: 257−73

Murray TG, Green WR, Maumenee IH. Spondyloepiphyseal dysplasia congenita. *Arch Ophthalmol* 1985; **103**: 407−18

Nesterov AP, Libenson NB. Strengthening of the sclera with the broad fascia of the hip in progressive myopia. *Vestn Oftalmol* 1967; **80(1)**: 15−19

Poos F. Kausale Genese der spharischen und aspharischen Refraktionszustande. *Graefes Arch Ophthalmol* 1950; 245−78

Rasmussen OD. Incidence of myopia in China. *Br J Ophthalmol* 1936; **20**: 350−60

Reuss A von. Augen-Untersuchungen an zwei Wiener Volksschulen. *Wien Med Presse* 1881; **22**: 200−2m 234−6

Rodriguez A, Gutierrez E, Alvira G. Complications of clear lens extraction in axial myopia. *Arch Ophthalmol* 1987; **105**: 1522−4

Rogers GL. Noonan's syndrome and autosomal dominant inheritance. *J Pediatr Ophthalmol Strabismus* 1975; **12**: 54−6

Romano PE. The cause of organic amblyopia in high myopia. *Ophthalmology* 1988; **95**: 288.

Rush CC. Treatment of myopia. *China Med J [Engl]* 1920; **34**: 605−7

Sato T. *The Causes and Prevention of Acquired Myopia.* Kanehara Shuppan, Tokyo 1957

Schartz DE. Noonan's syndrome associated with ocular abnormalities. *Am J Ophthalmol* 1972; **73**: 955−60

Schwartz O, Jampel RS. Congenital blepharophimosis associated with a unique generalized myopathy. *Arch Ophthalmol* 1962; **68**: 52−60

Seay AR, Ziter FA. Malignant hyperpyrexia in a patient with Schwartz Jampel syndrome. *J Pediatr* 1978; **93**: 83−4

Snyder AA, Thompson FB. A simplified technique for surgical treatment of degenerative myopia. *Am J Ophthalmol* 1972; **74**: 273−7

Sondermann R. Beitrag zur Frage der Myopiegenese. *Klin Monatsbl Augenheilkd* 1950; **117**: 573−8.

Sperduto RD, Seigel D, Roberts J, Rowland M. Prevalence of myopia in the United States. *Arch Ophthalmol* 1983; **101**: 405−7

Steiger A. Ueber Erbeinheiten am menschlichen Auge. *Z Augenheilkd* 1915; **34**: 1−25

Tamura K. An experimental examination concerning the aetiology of myopia. *Acta Soc Ophthalmol Jap* 1932; **36**: 17−30

Vogt A. Zur Genese der spharischen Refraktionen. *Ber Dtsch Ophthalmol Ges* 1924; **44**: 67−71

Ware J. Observations relative to the near and distant sight of different persons. *Philos Trans R Soc Lond* 1813; **103**: 31−50

Weale RA. Corneal shape and astigmatism: with a note on myopia. *Br J Ophthalmol* 1988; **72**: 696−9

Whitwell J. Scleral reinforcement in degenerative myopia. *Trans Ophthalmol Soc UK* 1971; **91**: 679−86

Witte O. Zur Myopiafrage. *Z Augenheilkd* 1923; **51**: 163−80

Section 2
Management

7 History, Examination and Further Investigation

SUSAN DAY

Taking a history

One initially wonders how detailed a history can be when considering infants' and children's eyes: especially with babies, the vast majority of time seems to be spent sleeping and eating! Many parents do not consciously evaluate how their baby is seeing; yet, when directly questioned about vision, parents often have a very good understanding of how well their baby sees.

The history is of utmost importance in understanding the problem and offering solutions. Although obvious questions about vision will be made, great care must be taken in assessing the child's general health. Perhaps the simplest and most open question to pose is 'Are you, your paediatrician, or doctor, concerned about any aspect of your child's health or development?' Such a question might elicit a response that, for instance, the child has had a special hearing test. As a consequence of this response, one might be alerted to conditions such as retinitis pigmentosa, Waardenberg's syndrome, and Alport's syndrome.

Another key question is to ask about the child's general development. Most of a child's motor development within the first year of life is vision-dependent. What appears to be developmental delay may therefore be a clue that not all is right with the child's vision. Similarly, a child who is not growing properly, or who fails to thrive, may have a combination of developmental abnormalities which results in not only endocrine disturbance but also in hypoplasia of the optic nerves or other vision defect.

A query into the prenatal history is also of utmost importance, especially when congenital infections are suspected. Such questions must be carefully phrased because parents may blame themselves unnecessarily for a congenital defect. Nevertheless, the occurrence of maternal rash, fever, use of medications, and drug abuse must be reviewed.

A review of medications given to the child and taken by the mother during the pregnancy or while breast feeding must be made. Particularly, use of anticonvulsants may influence a child's apparent visual performance. The possibility of allergies to medications must also be covered. Young children, and particularly those with Down's syndrome, may be sensitive to Atropine and other cycloplegic agents.

Once systemic issues have been covered, the baby's vision must be addressed. The most important question to ask the parents is 'How well does your baby see?' Parent and other relatives are keenly perceptive of the baby's vision in an intuitive fashion — they are rarely wrong! Parents often volunteer that they have been concerned about vision for a number of months even though the primary care physician failed to register similar concern. If the child has older siblings, parents also are able to compare the younger child's development to the older child's progress.

Beyond simply intuitive ideas of how good the vision is, the parents should then be questioned about habits which may be directly related to vision or behaviour which implies poor eyesight. A baby with poor vision will often stare at bright lights, have flickering eyelid movements, and may develop nystagmus noticeable to the parents. They may also observe eye poking or rapid hand waving in front of the eyes by such an infant. This infant may fail to smile or seemingly be disinterested in his environment, and hold his head with the chin tucked in when in a sitting position. In contrast, parents of a baby with good sight will volunteer that eye contact is made, or that the baby mimics facial expressions, or that a mobile overlying the crib fascinates the child. The physician must be cautious in considering behaviour as vision-generated whenever the stimulus also makes a noise, such as a music box with a lullaby.

Visual behaviour in an older child often centres around the child's playing habits. A child with poor vision may hold the toy within 1–2 inches (2–5.5 cm) of one or both eyes, inspecting the toy in a way that maximizes his vision. This child too, may be disinterested in television, or insist on moving to within inches of the screen where scanning the entire view is not possible without moving the head. Keep in mind, however, that virtually all children do tend to sit more closely to a TV screen than adults, presumably due to (a) their desire to be immersed in the activity on the screen; and (b) their ability to accommodate more fully and maintain focus at a shorter viewing distance.

Apparent visual difficulty may be present under very specific circumstances, such as in dim illumination or very bright illumination. In the former case, the child may become very irritated when the night light is turned off or have inordinate difficulty in finding his way around in dimly lit situations. Children with poor photopic vision, on the other hand, may hate to go outside or insist on protection from the sun.

With an older child, be sure to include him in the discussion; valuable information is offered, and rapport is established which leads to better co-operation during the examination.

Children who are born with poor vision are not likely to tell you that their vision is poor. Children who acquire poor vision will usually only volunteer that they are unable to see well if the visual loss is bilateral. Unilateral visual loss, either acute or chronic, is usually not noticed by a young child unless or until the other eye becomes involved.

In summary, the taking of the history is the beginning of a good eye examination in infants and children. Much reliability is placed not only on the parents' observations, but also on those of other close relatives, as well as the children themselves. A general development and health history, as well as history of medications and allergies, are elementary aspects of history taking. The importance of taking and documenting a family history is described in the genetics section. A detailed history of vision behaviour may give the ophthalmologist an accurate refinement of where to look for pathology.

Finally, the mood set by taking a history helps to establish rapport with the child which makes examination more fun for the child and more rewarding for the doctor.

Clinical examination

As specialists, ophthalmologists must keep in mind that the child has already been seen, in all likelihood, by another physician who has raised concern about a potential problem with the eyes. Although great variability exists in the quality of screening examinations by primary care physicians, babies in general will receive an initial examination of the eyes for clarity of the media, evidence of conjunctivitis, and any obvious abnormalities such as a squint or congenital defect of the globe. At the baby clinics within the first 4 months, the ability to 'fix and follow' should be documented with each eye, as well as the assessment of oculomotor alignment and analysis of red reflex. Repeated assessment of vision (both subjectively by the parents and objectively by the physician), alignment, and media clarity must be continued on each routine visit within the first 3 years of life. Vision is first routinely quantified by primary care physicians initially between the ages of 3.5 and 7 years.

Once a paediatrician has detected a potential problem, a not insignificant hurdle in the child's care is gaining a prompt appointment. It is absolutely essential that the busy ophthalmologist give specific guidelines to appointment personnel for children as to what represents an urgent problem; leukocoria, for instance, warrants immediate attention to rule out retinoblastoma. A 2-week-old baby with bilateral congenital cataracts represents another urgent matter. Access to the examination is perhaps as important in the practice of paediatric ophthalmology as the examination itself!

The milieu of the examining room is very important. A large examining area is at times almost essential to accommodate the special pushchair, nappy bags, two siblings, two neighbour's children, mum, dad, and the special education teacher! As the initial history is being taken from the parents, the patient may be more comfortable in his own cradle, or playing quietly with a toy on the floor. Fragile examining equipment or dangerous items such as needles or surgical instruments must be out of reach.

The doctor's image portrayed when the child is initially seen must be carefully considered. Many paediatric ophthalmologists prefer to not wear a traditional white laboratory coat. The child is also less frightened if the doctor is at eye level with the child, rather than imposing a 6-foot tall authority-figure on the young child. Talking directly to the older child (rather than to the parents) initially also focuses the attention appropriately on the patient.

The clinical examination by the ophthalmologist starts with observation of the child as the history is being taken. How alert is the child? How does the baby react to sudden changes in the environment, such as a change in lighting or noise or someone coming into the room? Does the head appear to be misshapen, enlarged, or microcephalic? Are there any signs of external bruising which might suggest non-accidental injury? Does there appear to be any asymmetry between the two eyes? Is fixation steady?

Examination for ptosis, blepharophimosis, the external appearance of the lids and adnexae, and skin lesions all must be made.

Early in the visit, an examination of the clarity of the media with a retinoscope provides key information. Examination for factors which lead to amblyopia, including refractive error, strabismus, and media opacities can be made with this simple instrument. The retinoscope seems not to bother infants and children as much as ophthalmoscopes which may have brighter lights or which require touching of the child, but an ophthalmoscope with the rheostat turned down can also be used for most purposes, although not for refraction.

Assessment of visual function is a complex task consisting of numerous components including visual acuity, visual fields, colour vision, and afferent pupillary function. Visual acuity, or the ability to resolve contrasts, develops over the first year of life and there is plasticity in this system up to the age of 12 years. Methods of visual acuity assessment changes as the child grows older.

Fixation and following

In a baby, several techniques of assessing vision on the basis of ocular motor responses are commonly used by paediatric ophthalmologists. Most simply, a baby's ability to fix and follow is noted. Fixation should be steady, and pursuit movements smooth. It must be kept in mind that the ability to follow does not imply any particular Snellen equivalent of visual acuity. Many older children with 20/200 to 20/400 vision demonstrate a good fix and follow response. The fix and follow technique, as well as all of the others mentioned below, should be applied not only binocularly but also monocularly. Occlusion of one eye may result in an unhappy child, and many clinicians rely upon objection to occlusion as an indicator that vision is poor in the unoccluded eye. However, often the occluder itself is enough to upset a child; more subtle occlusion, such as with the examiner's thumb over one eye, may be more successful.

CSM notation

A popular method of notation system is the CSM system. The ability of each eye to fixate Centrally, Steadily, and Maintain fixation is documented. Central fixation implies that the patient's fixation is foveal; that is, that the light reflex is in the centre or paracentral area of the pupil. Steady fixation implies that no nystagmoid movements are imposed on the fixing eye which is regarding a static target. Maintained fixation refers to the ability of one eye to maintain fixation when viewing is converted from a monocular condition to a binocular condition. As an example, a child with a right esotropia is suspected of having an underlying visual problem with the right eye: if the left eye is covered, the right eye takes up fixation which may for the purpose of this illustration be central and steady. Once the occlusion is removed from the left eye, failure of the right eye to move would earn a 'maintained' notation; a shift inward warrants a notation of unmaintained fixation, with implied poor vision in the right eye relative to the left eye.

Quantification of vision

The earliest attempts at visual acuity quantification relied upon an infant's ability to detect stripes on an optokinetic nystagmus drum. The examiner noted the presence or absence of nystagmus by directly observing the baby's eye movements (Gorman *et al.* 1957; Linkz 1973).

Quantification of visual acuity represents a particular challenge in children, due to their communication, developmental, and educational skills. This limitation to testing contrasts with the examiner's need to know just how good the vision is — relative to previous examinations, as in the child undergoing occlusion therapy for amblyopia, one eye relative to the other eye, and relative to vision in age-matched controls. (See Chapter 2 for guidelines for visual acuity in different age groups.)

Standard methods of visual acuity testing can rarely be used before the age of 3 years. Newer tests which rely upon electrophysiological or behavioural end-points have been introduced to broaden our knowledge of vision development in infants and children.

Guidelines for testing of children must adhere to those which we use for adult patients. Whenever possible, distance and near visual acuity measurements must be defined. Testing of each eye separately must be performed, being sure that complete occlusion of one eye is achieved. Establishment of the specific level of best acuity must be refined by the ophthalmologist with repeated testing of targets around the endpoint. Children may often 'quit' prematurely due simply to lack of interest rather than lack of vision.

Techniques for testing, however, must be artfully refined for children. The examination must be more of a game than a test. Reinforcement and reward for positive responses should be somewhat more enthusiastic on the examiner's part than with the middle-aged bank executive! Control of parental coaching must be maintained. The testing will only last as long as the child's attention span, and several tries at different times may be necessary. Extraneous competition for the child's attention by active siblings, ringing telephones, or unnecessary movement, must be kept at a bare minimum.

Despite the above cautions, proper visual acuity estimates can usually be obtained within a matter of minutes once the examiner's skills for performing them have been adapted to children.

Snellen visual acuity and other optotypes

Quantification of visual acuity depends upon a patient's ability to discriminate differences in contrasting colours (traditionally black and white) and upon the examiner's ability to interpret the patient's response. The standard test is the Snellen visual acuity chart, which relies on letter recognition; the smallest subtended angle is defined by gaps in the letter which give identity clues to the patient.

The Snellen visual acuity chart represents one optotype visual acuity chart. An optotype is any symbol whose identification implies visual acuity, or resolution capability, of a particular subtended angle. The shape of the optotype can vary. Although letters appear on the standard Snellen chart, other examples of optotype acuity charts include the Landolt C rings, number charts, schematic picture, and the E (or illiterate E) charts.

All optotype forms of visual acuity testing are psychophysical tests; i.e., interpretation of the test is a subjective one measured by the patient's ability to communicate this subjective recognition to the examiner.

There are many limitations to optotype testing in paediatric ophthalmology. Although some children are able to recognize a few letters by the age of 4 years, the complexities of Snellen visual acuity testing makes it unreliable before the age of 6–8 years. Failure to see a line on the chart must raise the question as to whether the child knows what the letter is.

Many optotype tests have been designed to counter the limitations in letter recognition. The E chart is popularly used not only for the pre-school child, but also for illiterate adults as well as persons from countries whose alphabet is of non Roman figures. With children, the E game has basic limitations. First, a child's co-ordination and left—right discrimination may present apparently inaccurate answers. Some examiners will therefore ignore any miss when left is confused with rightward direction. Second, the test is inherently repetitive, and the child's attention span may fall short of the examiner's needs.

Picture optotypes (Fig. 7.1) may be very helpful in testing a 2–5-year-old child, since recognition of symbolic cars, birthday cakes, and birds can be adapted into a game format more easily. There are cultural limitations which can impair this test's validity; some

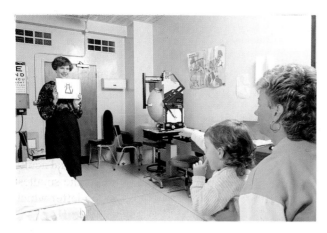

Fig. 7.1 Picture optotypes such as Kay's pictures shown here can be used for acuity measurements but they have cultural limitation due to their being recognition tests.

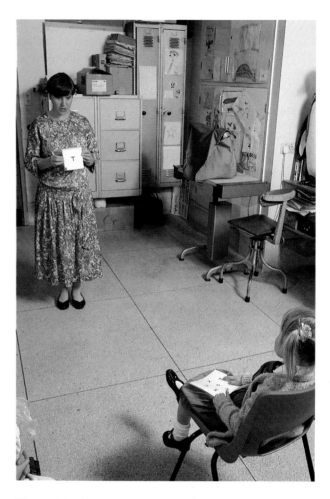

Fig. 7.2 Matching optotypes such as the Sheridan–Gardiner single optotype matching test shown here cannot be used with children as young as the picture optotypes but are nearer to Snellen acuity because recognition is less important.

children may not recognize a telephone because there is none at home, or because the abstracted shape of the telephone on the chart is entirely different from the telephone at home. A second drawback to the picture tests is that the construction of the individual optotypes is less optically accurate than, for instance, the Landolt C ring in which the subtended angle of contrast recognition is very precise. In comparison to the Snellen letter chart, where 26 possible answers are present, the alert child quickly learns that there are usually only five or six possible choices on picture charts.

One final adaptation of optotype visual acuity testing for children is the use of a matching technique. As with the picture chart, the number of possible correct choices is significantly reduced, usually to four or seven possible correct answers. The child need not know the name of a particular optotype but need only pair the examiner's choice of optotype with the patient's available matching optotype which he holds.

The most popular matching optotypes are the HOTV., Sheridan–Gardner (Fig. 7.2) or Sonksen–Silver charts.

VER and FPL

More recently, researchers have introduced two techniques to define vision development in infant and preverbal children. These two methods — preferential looking (PL or FPL) (Fulton *et al.* 1981; Jacobson *et al.* 1982;) Mayer *et al.* 1982) and visual evoked potentials (VEP) (Sokol 1980, Odom *et al.* 1981) — have aided our understanding of both normal and abnormal visual development. Although still used predomi-

nantly in research settings due to time and economic constraints, their impact on clinical ophthalmology is becoming more evident (Ellis *et al.* 1988).

Both the FPL and the VEP provide visual acuity measurements which cannot be directly correlated to Snellen acuity measurements, as their basic principles (behavioural response with FPL and electrophysiologic response with VEP) differ from the optotype tests.

The FPL technique is based on a child's inherent interest in patterned, as opposed to homogenous, targets (Fantz *et al.* 1962; Mayer & Dobson 1978). The patient is presented with two targets positioned in a homogenous background, one of which matches the background, the other of which contains gratings. If the infant responds by turning its eyes or its head toward the striped target as they are simultaneously presented, then this response is interpreted as an ability of the child to see the target. The child is then presented with progressively smaller gratings until the examiner believes the grating targets are no longer eliciting a response different from the homogenous targets. The FPL technique has been refined to help eliminate observer bias and to standardise selection of grating size (Teller *et al.* 1974; Held *et al.* 1979). Commercially available PL cards (McDonald *et al.* 1985; Teller *et al.* 1986) have allowed this technique to enter the clinician's domain (Fig. 7.3).

The PL technique has been helpful in establishing norms for visual acuity development in infants. Their grating acuity estimates that most normal infants reach the ability to resolve 20/20 gratings by the age of 1–3 years (Teller *et al.* 1974; Gwiazda *et al.* 1980; Mayer & Dobson 1982). Abnormal visual development, as occurs with amblyopia, cataract, and strabismus, has been assessed with the PL technique as well (Catalano *et al.* 1987) and correlated when possible with standard Snellen testing (Sokol *et al.* 1983; Birch & Stager 1985; Moskowitz *et al.* 1987) as well as clinical assessment by a paediatric ophthalmologist (Ellis *et al.* 1988). The advantages of the test appear to be a relative ease of administration, a relatively low cost, and rapid answers as long as no pathology is present. With any abnormality, however, testing becomes more time consuming. Its use by paediatric ophthalmologists has remained primarily in centres in which ongoing research is present and in which clinicians work in association with infant vision basic scientists.

The VEP represents a second major area of interest in infant vision research. It's recent evolution is in large part a consequence of computer technology. Its value rests upon the occipital cortex's electrical signal in response to a visual stimulation (Sokol 1976; Regan & Spekreijse 1986). The appearance of the waveform is highly variable as a consequence of different testing circumstances and equipment, and a thorough knowledge of any particular testing situation is required to ensure validity of the test (Sokol 1976).

In general, two types of stimuli, the unpatterned and the patterned, can evoke visual cortical potentials. The quantification of infant vision is limited to patterned stimuli which in general are in either bar gratings or in checkerboard form. Focussing of the image is essential in interpreting its results; thus, knowledge of, and correction of any significant refractive error is essential (Millodot & Riggs 1970).

Two major types of pattern VERs have been developed for the quantification of infant vision. The pattern reversal technique (Sokol & Dobson 1976,) has suggested maturation of 20/20 equivalent grating resolution between the ages of 6 and 12 months. The swept

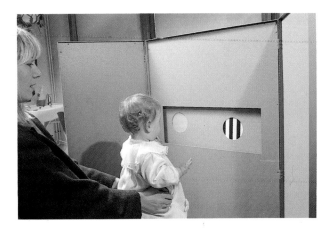

Fig. 7.3 The acuity card procedure. The child sits in front of the screen with as little to distract him or her as possible and cards with varying grating size are placed in the central panel and he is observed through a minute central peep hole as to whether his fixation is drawn to the side with the grating.

VEP technique, which relies upon extrapolation of the VEP signal generated by a 'sweeping' of grating size from large to small in 10 seconds also suggests this tempo of infant vision development (Norcia and Tyler 1985). The difference in these values compared to FPL data has been thought to be due to the superimposed behavioural requirements placed on the infant with the PL technique (Allen *et al.* 1987). The VEP has been applied to clinical circumstances in patients with strabismus (Sokol 1980; Day *et al.* 1988). Its current use remains predominantly in the research laboratory and in circumstances in which clinicians and basic scientists closely collaborate, as the VEP remains a time consuming test in circumstances where there is pathology.

Tests for children with very poor vision

In a child who is obviously poorly sighted, tests must be designed to determine even very low levels of vision. Particularly helpful in the young infant is the spinning or VOR (vestibulo-ocular reflex) test in which the child's fixation reflex is assessed after vestibulo-ocular nystagmus has been induced by spinning, rotating with the child held at arm's length in front of the examiner. With spinning, horizontal nystagmus is induced. After several rotations, the turning is discontinued. The examiner then assesses the baby's eye movements. On cessation of spinning, there are normally only one or two beats of after-nystagmus; in a blind baby, or one with severe cerebellar disease, there will be prolonged after-nystagmus. It is helpful to perform this manoeuvre on normal babies to gain experience in what represents a normal response.

In the most severe cases of poor vision, the examiner simply wishes to know if the child is able to see light at all. A threat response is less helpful in babies than in older individuals because this response may normally not appear for several months. However, a baby's response by blinking to a bright light or camera flash is easy to obtain.

All these tests however, rely on the child's motor responses thus, they must be interpreted cautiously bearing this in mind — if he cannot move his eyes he may appear blind until head control improves and he moves his head to the response instead (See Chapter 43).

Other clues that the vision may be poor may be gained by a child's appearance. The presence of nystagmus, eye poking, and a sunken appearance of the eyes all suggest chronically poor vision.

Other visual functions

Visual fields

Visual field testing is often ignored in infants and children since there is a general concept that this test requires sophisticated equipment and an immense amount of co-operation. Although it is true that Goldmann visual field cannot be performed without co-operation, a useful assessment at any age can be made of significant defects such as haemianopias by simple confrontation techniques. The examiner simply faces the child and attracts the child's attention centrally; then, a toy or light is introduced silently from the far periphery (Fig. 7.4). A child with normal fields will make a very rapid head movement or saccadic eye movement in the direction of the new stimulus. The child may well become bored with repeated attempts, and the availability of several different toys is helpful. Finger counting or detection of which of the examiner's fingers is wiggling may also be useful in older semi-co-operative children (Fig. 7.5). Visual evoked response testing will also reveal significant haemianopias if an array of occipital electrodes is used.

Colour vision

Testing of colour vision also should be attempted. Standard Ishihara colour plates can be used (Fig. 7.6), with adaptation of the usual testing technique so that instead of identification of numbers in the standard way, one can ask a child to trace with his finger the area which is coloured. Ishihara plates test only red—

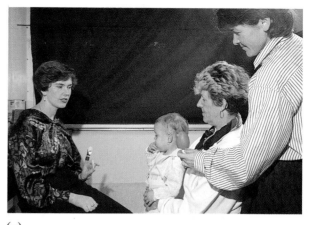

(a)

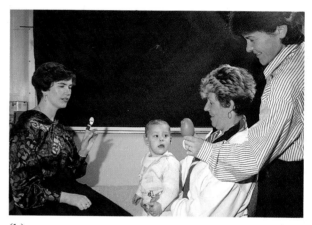

(b)

Fig. 7.4 Infant visual field testing. The first tester on the left, attracts the babies attention (a) while the other brings an object in silently from the side to see if his attention is drawn to it (b). Although crude, if defects are detected by this method they are likely to be functionally significant in the future.

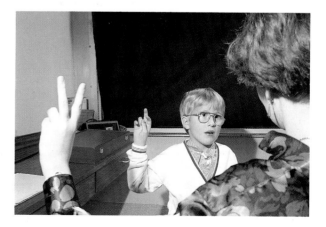

Fig. 7.5 'Finger matching' fields. While the tester watches the fixation, the child tells her when the tester's fingers are wiggling or may match or count the fingers if he is able to.

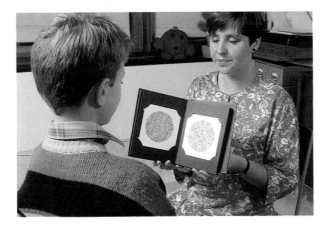

Fig. 7.6 The Ishihara test detects red−green defects only.

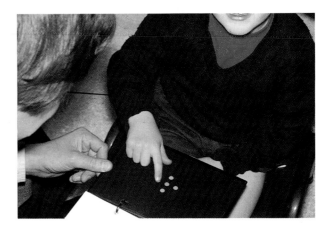

Fig. 7.8 The City University colour test will detect and grade colour defects (see text).

green deficiency but others include blue−yellow testing. The Llantony plates are purely tritan plates (Fig. 7.7). The City University colour vision test also is adaptable to testing children, since the response does not depend on pattern recognition but rather identification of individual dots (Fig. 7.8). The child has to identify which of four different coloured spots is nearer the same colour to a spot around which they are grouped. The HRR plates, currently out of print, provide good testing targets for the 3−5-year-old, as the geometric targets (circle, Xs and triangles) are familiar to them. With tests such as the D-15 test, one can ask that the child match two of three colours which are more similar to each other. One can also keep a group of different coloured socks and ask the child to pick out the two which match. Colour naming may be useful but should be interpreted with caution because many young children with normal colour vision are rather poor at naming colours.

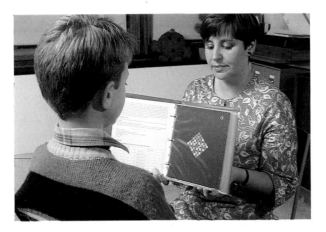

Fig. 7.7 Llantony's tritan plates detect blue−yellow defects.

Pupil inspection

Pupil testing required interpretation of second cranial nerve function (afferent system) as well as third cranial nerve function (efferent system). Simple inspection of pupil size may reveal anisocoria; unless the size difference exceeds 1 mm and/or there is other evidence of III nerve dysfunction such as ptosis or paralytic exotropia, small differences in pupil size are of no consequence. Typically, the neonate's pupil is small (2−3 mm) and minimally reactive to light. The intrinsic iris muscles, the dilator and the sphincter, develop relatively late embryologically. As a consequence, interpretion of pupil size and reactivity must be modified in the infant less than 3 months old.

In the older child, although pupil size is more easily obtained, the light- and near-pupillary reactions may be difficult to judge. A child's fixation must be controlled at a distance fixation target; otherwise, shifts in fixation may result in either falsely positive or negative interpretation of a relative afferent pupil defect (RAPD). Hippus, or physiologic variation in pupil size, also creates difficulty in pupil testing, since this phenomenon is more noticeable in younger individuals. This natural variation in pupil size is particularly noticeable in patients with lightly pigmented irides.

Inevitably, parents are curious about the colour of their child's eyes. 'Can you tell what colour they will be?' and 'When will the eyes turn the final colour?' are foremost in young parents' minds. The evolution of iris pigmentation tends to be complete by 9−12 months; in many circumstances, eye colour can be predicted much earlier on the basis of the colour of the parents' eyes as well as the relative degree of pigmentation of the neonate's eyes. Conditions which result in lightening of the eyes with age are rare; thus it is fairly safe to provide this information to parents.

Tests of binocular vision

Binocularity carries a vast overlap into the field of strabismus where maintenance or improvement of this function influences one's management of the child with strabismus. Several clinical tests have become traditional means of assessing binocularity.

STEREOPSIS

Stereopsis is a binocular function in which a perception of depth is created by either nasal or temporal disparity in the projection of similar retinal images, one from each eye, to the brain. It is not synonymous with 'depth perception' which contains many monocular clues. Although stereopsis implies excellent visual acuity in each eye, poor stereopsis can occur in patients with excellent monocular acuity as well as diminished acuity in one or both eyes (Donzis *et al.* 1983). Although some screening programs have advocated stereopsis tests as helpful in young children it must be remembered that visual acuity and stereopsis are two different functions.

In clinical practice, the Titmus fly stereopsis test (Fig. 7.9) remains the most commonly used form of assessment. A child wearing polarized lenses is asked to point to apparently elevated figures in a book with two superimposed, slightly displaced images creating a 3-dimensional effect. The test is therefore a psychophysical one, and the less refined targets can in fact be seen using monocular clues. The Randot series of

tests uses red/green goggles to create disparate images (Fig. 7.10). Co-operation is required, and in general a fail response is regarded as unreliable in children less than 5 years old. Other stereopsis tests may be used for younger children, in which they point to figures that are elevated or depressed by their position in special plastic cards, such as the Lang or Frisby tests, no special lenses or glasses are required (Fig. 7.11).

In recent years, research has expanded in the field of stereopsis, again largely as a consequence of computer technology. One avenue of study has been to

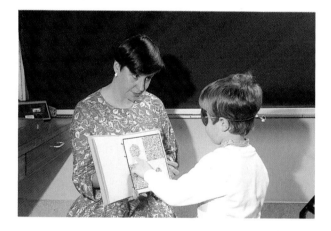

Fig. 7.10 The Randot stereo-acuity test uses a red−green system for creating the disparity between the eyes which allows the child to see shapes on the test card. This child is viewing the demonstration plate.

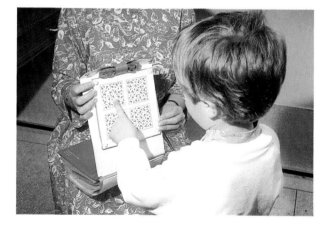

Fig. 7.11 The Frisby test does not require glasses instead the figures in a central panel of one of the test squares are printed on the other side of the perspex sheets so that the child can only see it if he or she has binocular depth perception. In this picture this is demonstrated by the flash gun's shadow cast by the test figure to which the child points. The thickness of the perspex varies, the thicker plates giving greater disparity and therefore are easier to see.

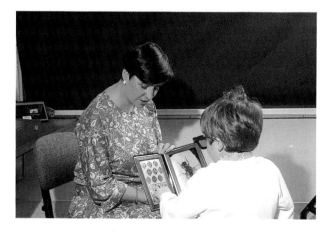

Fig. 7.9 The Titmus stereo-acuity test requires the use of polaroid glasses with the plane of polarization at right angles to each other in the spectaces.

explore stereopsis development, which appears to be most impressive between 3 and 7 months of age (Teller 1986). A second area has explored different forms of testing, especially the random dot stereogram (Julesz 1986). Clinicians have compared the various forms of commercially available stereopsis tests and raised their potential use as screening tests for vision since excellent visual acuity is required in each eye for good stereopsis (Donzis *et al.* 1983). Researchers also have begun to study young infants' stereopsis and the effects of esotropia on stereopsis in an effort to better define the most appropriate time for surgery in children with infantile esotropia (Mohindra *et al.* 1985).

FUSION

The binocular function of fusion includes both sensory and motor fusion. In the former, the visual cortex receives and unifies two images, one from each eye, similar in size and shape. Sensory fusion infers that corresponding retinal points are present in the two eyes which project to one site within the cortex. When fusion is not present, then the abnormal binocular sensory states of diplopia, confusion, or suppression are present (See Chapter 2.) Sensory fusion is most commonly tested with the Worth four-dot test. The child is instructed to wear a pair of glasses in which a red filter is over one eye and a green filter over the other eye. An illuminated target consisting of one red dot, two green dots, and one white dot is held at near (33 cm) and at distance (6 m) and the child is asked the number and colour of the dots. When fusion is present, four dots are seen, with the white dot changing colours due to retinal rivalry. When diplopia is present, five dots are seen. Suppression results in the child's seeing two or three dots, depending on which eye is suppressed. This test is performed at distance and near to assess for central (with the distance testing) and peripheral (with the near testing) fusion as a consequence of the subtended angle covered by the dots at varied distances. Although the Worth four-dot test is widely used to assess pre-operative fusional status in children with strabismus its reliability has been criticised on the basis of the artificiality of an environment interrupted by red and green filters.

Motor fusion refers to vergence movements — either convergence or divergence — evident when an apparent image is 'moved' on the retina, such as holding a prism in front of one eye. Although there is a natural limit to normal fusional amplitudes (von Noorden 1985) the ability of a patient to make this vergence movement implies excellent binocular func-

tion since the impetus for the motor response is unification of the images.

RETINAL CORRESPONDENCE

With orthophoria, binocular vision develops as a consequence of normal retinal correspondence, or a point-to-point coupling of retinal receptor information in the two eyes which is projected to a single cortical region. With early onset malalignment, or strabismus, this coupling is altered, resulting in abnormal input to the visual cortex, or anomalous retinal correspondence. The retinal receptor fields are, in a sense reordered such that under binocular circumstances, there is a shift in the coupling of the projected images from the two eyes that achieves an alteration in binocularity. Tests for normal and anomalous retinal correspondence (ARC) rely upon a subjective interpretation by the patient of two groups of tests. The 'after image' test stimulates the fovea of each eye either with viewing under monocular conditions. A bright flash with a central gap is horizontally viewed first by one eye; this eye is then occluded and the fellow eye views a vertically oriented flash. With both eyes closed, the patient then is asked to describe the orientation of these two relative positions as a cross with one gap (normal correspondence) or as a cross in which the gaps are shifted. The alignment of the eyes must be known as well, since a similar description in an esotropic patient would imply abnormal retinal correspondence, or an apparent reordering of object perception which allows for the basic deviation.

The second form of testing for ARC involves simultaneous viewing of an object which is thus projected onto one foveal and one extrafoveal retinal locus in the patient with strabismus. Since one goal of sensory testing is to create as little interruption to the natural environment as is possible (or, in strabismus jargon, to try to maintain fusion), the Bagolini lenses have gained popularity in this group of testing. The surfaces of plano lenses are 'scratched' in a way that a pinpoint source of light is displayed through the lens in a linear fashion. The orientation of the striations is projected so that the striations in one eye are perpendicular to the fellow eye (Fig. 7.12). The patient's interpretation of the striation's direction as well as the point source of light will then allow the examiner to judge normal and anomalous retinal correspondence as well as the type of ocular deviation when the patient's alignment and fixation are also known.

A second test in which the patient views one target through dissimilar circumstances for the two eyes is

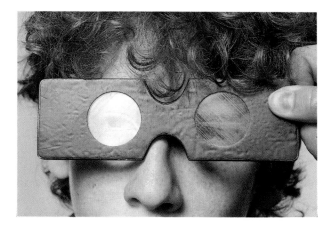

Fig. 7.12 Bagolini's striated glasses. The striations can be clearly seen in the glass in front of the patient's left eye (see text).

the red glass, or diplopia test. A white light is viewed by the patient with a red filter over one eye. A vertical prism will allow separation of the red and white. Interpretation of the patient's responses must be correlated with the patient's alignment at a similar testing distance. The patient responds by assessing the relative position of the red and white lights. By comparing to the alignment of the eye, the examiner can then define whether normal or abnormal retinal correspondence is present.

Contrast sensitivity

Contrast sensitivity testing has been proven to be helpful in patients with subtle visual loss, especially in conditions such as visual pathway gliomas, optic neuritis, and glaucoma. Its value has been that its testing may be abnormal when other standard tests such as visual acuity, colour vision and visual field testing have been normal (Zimmern *et al.* 1979; Regan *et al.* 1980; Stamper *et al.* 1982).

Although contrast sensitivity testing is not routinely performed by paediatric ophthalmologists, researchers have considered its potential role in the management of paediatric problems such as monitoring of amblyopia. Contrast sensitivity function appears to develop rapidly during the first few months of life (Norcia *et al.* 1987).

Eye movements and strabismus

Another important aspect of examination is that of the ocular motor system; strabismus is an extremely common referral diagnosis in children. One must constantly keep in mind the interplay between strabismus and amblyopia. Thus, the examination of the motor system is a reflection of both eye movements and visual function, both monocular and binocular.

As with visual acuity assessment, oculomotor assessment varies in its completeness with the child's age. In infancy, assessment of the corneal light reflex (Hirschberg) is the simplest estimate of ocular alignment. One must keep in mind the tendency for children to have a nasal displacement of the corneal light reflex or 'positive angle kappa'. Additionally, one must be aware that despite apparently straight eyes as judged by corneal light reflex testing, a small tropia may be present with more sophisticated cover test techniques. Nevertheless, corneal light reflex testing is a very important technique to master as a screening technique for strabismus.

In the Krimsky test a prism bar is used to equalize the position of the light reflex in the two eyes — it is particularly useful in non-fixing eyes because it does not need the eye to shift to take up fixation to indicate the magnitude of the deviation.

There are several useful tips about testing for the corneal light reflex: (a) when the corneal light reflex is checked at near, the light source itself must also be held at near, at the same distance as the observer; and (b) the child should fix not on the light source but preferably on a small, accommodative, target, such as a small picture. With this type of stimulus, an accommodative component of the strabismus can more easily be elicited (See Fig. 44.4).

Confirmation of strabismus is made with the alternate cover test and the cover–uncover test (Fig. 7.13). Both of these tests are difficult to perform on the younger child, since control of fixation is mandatory and often children tend to randomly refixate. Also, children tend to object to the presence of a large plastic occluder. The examiner's thumb may be used as an occluder as long as one is careful to hold the thumb close enough so as to truly prevent fixation with the occluded eye.

When a small angle strabismus is present which cannot be detected on traditional cover techniques, the 4 dioptre base-out prism test may reveal information about the patient's alignment and sensory status. With controlled distance fixation (Fig. 7.14), the prism is introduced over one eye, and the examiner assesses for a fixation shift. The test is then repeated with the prism held over the fellow eye. If a difference exists between the two eyes, i.e. a refixation effort is made with the prism over one eye only, a small angle

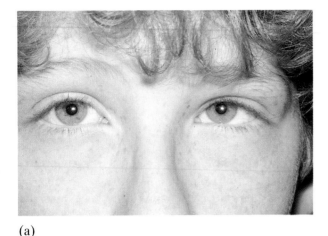

(a)

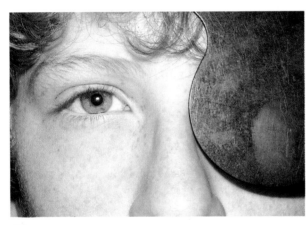

(b)

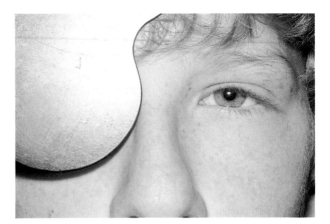

(c)

Fig. 7.13 The cover test. (a) The asymmetrical light reflexes in the pupils can be seen. (b) No shift of the right eye on left eye cover. (c) On the right eye being covered the left eye moves out to take up fixation. Meticulous control over fixation must be maintained (see text).

strabismus with suppression scotoma is suspected (Jampolsky 1964).

The basic deviation is defined as the deviation present at distance with accommodation suspended or controlled. It can be measured with both the Krimsky

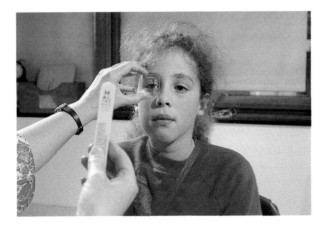

Fig. 7.14 The 4-dioptre base-out prism test. Holding fixation with a target appropriate to the age of the child is vital (see text).

and the cover tests, and is a very important single parameter for assessing alignment. The complete ocular motility exam, however, must be far more comprehensive, however. Measurement of the deviation at near, definition of phoric versus tropic deviations, measurements in the nine positions of gaze, and head tilt measurements are indicated in patients with strabismus and their relevance expanded upon in strabismus section.

Squints may be subtly hidden by an abnormal or preferred head position. Other ocular causes of abnormal head positions are nystagmus with nullpoint, refractive error (usually astigmatism or myopia), a homonymous hemianopia or torticollis caused by muscular, skeletal or neuro-otological defect.

In some circumstances, attention must be given to supranuclear eye movement function including saccades and pursuits, especially when one suspects oculomotor apraxia, progressive external ophthalmoplegia, and other neurological conditions.

In general, the oculomotor examination gives information about the function of cranial nerves III, IV,

VI, as well as the supranuclear control of eye movements. One additional assessment of the cranial nerve III is pupillary shape, size and response to light as well as accommodation.

Slit lamp examination

Slit lamp examination is one vital test which is often overlooked in young children. Examination of the young infant is easy if one merely raises the slit lamp to a comfortable height for the mother to hold the baby in a prone position, steadying the chin with one hand and supporting the body with that arm. The second arm steadies the head posteriorly. The mother is instructed to bring the baby in this prone position up toward the slit lamp until the baby's forehead rests against the forehead strap (Fig. 7.15). Alternatively, hand-held slit lamps may be of particular benefit in other situations, such as inpatient consultations or in the operating room.

Slit lamp examination is particularly important in examining infants with nystagmus, as patients with albinism may clearly show iris transillumination defects on retroillumination. Other specific indications for slit lamp examination include determination of the level of media opacity, examination for foreign bodies and corneal abrasions, determination of corneal abnormalities such as breaks in Descement's membrane from congenital glaucoma, and assessment of the conjunctiva to identify underlying causes of inflammation.

Refraction

See Chapter 8.

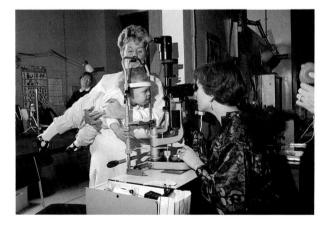

Fig. 7.15 Slit lamp examination can be performed at almost any age in nearly all children but requires a firm but gentle person to hold the child so that his forehead touches the strap.

Photorefraction

New screening devices based on photographic refraction techniques are offered for screening the preverbal child. Using several optical principles (Howland & Howland 1974; Kaakinen 1979) these devices are primarily designed to detect refractive error photographically. In addition to detecting refractive error (Atkinson *et al.* 1987), other amblyogenic factors such as cataract and strabismus have been documented with this technique in infants and preverbal children (Day & Norcia 1986). A commercially available device is used for screening (Morgan 1987), but the technique remains in further evolution prior to widespread use.

Fundoscopy

Fundoscopy in infants and children represents a particular challenge, not only due to limited co-operation, but also due to the different appearance of the fundus in very young children compared to adults. Adequate mydriasis is essential and is best obtained by supplementing the cycloplegic agent (cyclopentolate 1/2 or 1%) with a mydriatic agent such as either tropicamide (Mydriacyl 1%) or phenylephrine 2.5%, especially in an infant with brown irides. Both indirect and direct ophthalmoscopy must be performed. The first instrument to be used should be the indirect ophthalmoscope, as a quick overview of the fundus can lead one to pay particular attention to areas with the direct ophthalmoscope. Although the +20 dioptre lens is frequently used, the +28 to +30 lens can provide a wider field and the +14 lens can provide further details of structures such as the optic nerve. With the tiny infant, it is best to ensure that the baby is quiet and content during the indirect examination. Often this can be achieved by having the baby suck on a bottle or breast. The baby can be cradled in the mother's arms or lying on the mother's lap, whichever allows the baby to be most comfortable. Usually the lids can be held with the examiner's fingers. It is best to first line the lens up and once in place, quickly bring the ophthalmoscope's light into view. Several quick glimpses seem to allow greater cooperation than one attempted prolonged look. As soon as the baby begins to squeeze the lids, the Bell's phenomenon will occur, and the examiner is thwarted!

In the older child, the fundus examination itself can become a game. One technique would be to suggest that by looking in the eyes, the examiner is able to determine what the child has eaten for breakfast (a guess is made based on the current best selling cereal or local favourite!) Another trick is to suggest that there is a particular animal that can be seen, describing the features of the animal until the child is able to identify what the animal is. It is sometimes helpful to demonstrate on either the parents or older siblings what the examination is like, and then the child may ask for his own turn or understand that fundoscopy is not painful.

With children of all ages, it is best to have the room lights dimmed to improve the image of the fundus, but the room should not be completely darkened, as some children may be afraid.

In examining with the direct ophthalmoscope, specific anatomical features must be sought. Examination of the fovea is often easy, as the child will look at the light. If one get the child's attention away from the light by asking him to look at a distance fixation target, then control of the area of examination is easier to obtain. Some children will tolerate the red-free light more easily.

The premature baby

Examination of the premature infant requires special preparation, since the eye evaluation is most commonly in the setting of an intensive care nursery. Co-ordination of the examination must be made with the neonatalogists and charge nurses, as these infants often require other tests or special care throughout the day. A telephone call 30–60 minutes in advance of the examination should be made to ensure adequate mydriasis for the examination. One must use low doses of dilating agents due to the systemic absorption of the medication. A combination drop, such as commercially available Cyclomydril (0.2% cyclopentolate, 0.1% phenylephrine) is best used as one drop to each eye, repeated once in 5–10 minutes. Alternatively, one drop of cyclopentolate 0.5% and phenylephine 2.5% should ensure adequate mydriasis. *Never* allow phenylephrine 10% to be used, as its systemic absorption may result in severe hypertensive crises or death in the premature baby. Equipment must be brought for the examination as well, including an indirect ophthalmoscope, +20 or +30 lens, lid speculum, scleral indentation device, and topical anaesthesia.

The actual examination itself is often performed in the large intensive care nursery room which for consideration of others is brightly lit and hectic! It is necessary to keep in mind the precarious state of health of these infants. At all times during the eye examination, a nurse should be assisting as minor positioning changes can quickly compromise airways or other important lines. The examination must be performed with a lid speculum and scleral indentor since the peripheral retina must be assessed thoroughly due to concerns about retinopathy of prematurity. If pupil dilation is poor, look carefully for synechia formation which may be a clue that significant retinopathy of prematurity is present.

One must keep in mind other features besides retinal status in the premature infant as the examination continues. Slight haziness of the cornea, and vitreous haze in the premature infant, may obscure examination but may be entirely normal.

Additional portable equipment, such as hand-held slit lamps and Perkins applanation tonometers, may be invaluable in the premature infant. Concern about congenital glaucoma, metabolic or infectious disorders, and other particular reasons for ophthalmologic consultation should be known by you prior to your arrival in the neonatal unit. Retinoscopy, too, may be highly desirable in the older premature infant still dependent on life support systems since high refractive errors may be present. Retinoscopy bars (hand-held racks of lenses) can be obtained to aid in this part of the examination.

Until recently, the treatment of retinopathy of prematurity (ROP) has remained highly controversial (Sira *et al.* 1988), and repeated examinations in some centers have mainly served to provide information as to the status of the eyes to be passed to the parents. A multicenter prospective trial has recently demonstrated efficacy in treating these patients with cryotherapy in certain stages of ROP (CRCPG 1988). Thus, the compulsive examination of premature infant has gained even greater significance.

Examination under sedation

Rarely, a standard examination is insufficient to provide all information which is necessary in making the appropriate medical decisions. An oral form of sedation such as chloral hydrate may be considered in such circumstances when general anaesthesia is to be avoided. When chloral hydrate sedation is to be performed, great care must be given that support staff trained in management of sedated infants and children is available, or else the sedation should not be carried out. It should not be carried out without appropriate resuscitation equipment being available. Sedated examinations must be used especially judiciously in infants less than 6 months and in infants who have neurologic abnormalities. An oral dose between 50 and 100 mg/kg of chloral hydrate will usually provide adequate sedation. Patients must be healthy, and their cardiovascular as well as pulmonary status must be ascertained prior to sedation. The infant should have no food or drink for approximately 4 hours beforehand. When chloral hydrate sedation is used, the child must be isolated in a quiet dimly lit room. Adequate sedation will usually allow checking of intra-ocular pressure, use of a portable slit lamp, use of lid speculum, and fundus photography. If any manipulation is to be performed, such as removal of nasolacrimal stents or removal of sutures which will require pulling, chloral hydrate sedation is often not sufficient. Chloral hydrate sedation is most commonly indicated in children who have congenital glaucoma and require repeated follow-up, in children who have unexplained visual loss who cannot co-operate well enough on a routine examination, and in severely retarded children who are unable to co-operate for an examination. Ketamine is a useful alternative, although its use does require the presence of an anaesthetist which in itself implies the use of hospital facilities. Ketamine has gained popularity as an agent for oculinum administration to young children (Magoon 1988).

Examination under anaesthetic

Occasionally, an examination under anaesthesia (EUA) is warranted. The indications include inability to sedate sufficiently with a safe dose of chloral hydrate, need for manipulation such as stent removal or suture removal, re-examination of child with congenital glaucoma who may require further glaucoma surgery immediately after the examination, and examination of children with suspected retinoblastoma who will subsequently undergo enucleation. Additionally, children with known retinoblastoma who require follow-up bone marrow aspirations and lumbar punctures may be co-ordinated under one anesthetic to allow follow-up ophthalmoscopy in addition to the other testing. Finally, an examination under anaesthesia is warranted when detailed electroretinography studies, fluorescein angiography, and combined procedures with other paediatric subspecialities are needed. In most infants, neurophysiological studies do not require anaesthesia. When an examination is scheduled under anaesthesia, then all data possible must be obtained during this golden opportunity. These measurements include corneal diameters, gonioscopy, tonometry, hand-held slit lamp examination, cycloplegic retinoscopy, and microscopic examination of the anterior segment of the eye as well as

posterior segment with special contact lenses when indicated. The consequences of an EUA often require proceeding immediately to surgery such as goniotomy, lensectomy, biopsy or enucleation. Thus, proper counselling of the parents of these possible procedures must be performed prior to the EUA, so that a subsequent anaesthetic can be avoided. If it is known that an EUA will be done, it is appropriate to check if the child requires other elective surgery such as hernia repair, cleft palate repair or even venesection, as simultaneous procedures or sequential procedures may be performed with proper co-ordination.

Other examination and diagnostic testing of infants and children warrants particular co-ordination, including electrophysiology, ultrasonography, photography, and radiology.

The measurement of intraocular pressure in suspected congenital glaucoma is critical to its management. Ketamine sedation, although not universally accepted by anaesthetists, is in widespread use as an agent for producing narcosis. Standard techniques of anaesthesia can be used (Dear *et al.* 1987) providing the pressure is measured before or at least 10 minutes after intubation.

Neurophysiological studies

Electrophysiological studies include electro-oculogram (EOG), electroretinogram (ERG), and visual evoked potential (VEP), and are best perfomed in conjunction with a technician or scientist with special training in these fields, but one who also needs to be good with children and understand their problems, and what questions may or may not be answered by the tests (Fig. 7.16). Electrophysiological studies may clarify one's clinical diagnosis so that appropriate recommendations can be made regarding prognosis and treatment, including possible need for special schooling or genetic counselling. Specific diagnoses are rarely made purely on the basis of electrophysiological studies. Applications of electrophysiological studies in infants and children include the diagnosis of a wide variety of retinal disorders, either with specific findings such as in juvenile X-linked retinoschisis, congenital stationary night-blindness or non specific findings such as retinal detachment or retinal dysplasia in which the amplitude of the ERG is variably reduced. The ERG is particularly helpful in infants who appear blind but in whom fundus changes cannot be distinguished. The diagnosis of Leber's amaurosis for instance, is dependent upon an ERG unless a strongly positive family history with documentation of electro-

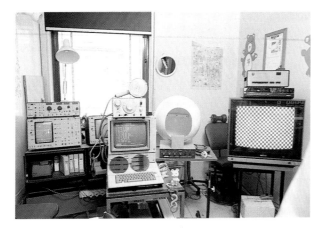

Fig. 7.16 A neurophysiological laboratory for studies of children. The ability of the scientist and technician to get on with children and to thus be able to complete a full examination is extremely important. (Photograph by courtesy of Dr A. Kriss.)

physiological changes in other family members has been made. Children with multi-system disorders require ERG testing as well, since it may be abnormal before other clinical symptoms or signs are evident. Congenital stationary night-blindness and rod monochromatism, represent other retinal abnormalities in which ERG testing may be helpful.

The electro-oculogram is rarely performed in children, since conditions in which it is helpful, such as Best's vitelliform maculopathy and Stargardt's disease, often manifest themselves within the second or third decade of life.

Ultrasound

Ultrasonography has particular applications to infants and children as well. In general, the A- and B-scan ultrasound can be performed on infants and children and has been used to detail the development of the eye (Larsen 1971a, 1971b). With skilled examiners, sedation is rarely required in order to answer specific questions when a baby with opaque media, where details of the vitreous cavity and posterior pole are sought. This is particularly helpful in an infant with a corneal opacity or a cataract when the normality of the posterior segment must be ensured before surgery. Ultrasonography is also helpful before vitrectomy (Restori & McLeod 1977) in cases of ocular trauma in which retinal detachments or retained foreign bodies are suspected. Real-time studies, in which the movements of the intraocular contents can be observed, are particularly helpful (McLeod & Restori 1977). Care must be taken in cases where a ruptured globe is

suspected, however, as inadvertent pressure on the globe may result in further damage to the eye. In cases of retinoblastoma, intralesional calcification may be demonstrable by ultrasonography. The use of A-scan ultrasound is sometimes helpful to determine axial length. Although this may be of aid to an infant who is being fitted with a contact lens, axial lengths may be more of interest in following a child who has high ametropia, and in which the retinoscopic or refractive error appear to have other factors than axial length (Belkin *et al.* 1973). Orbital ultrasound (Restori & Wright 1977) is helpful in some cases, especially if real-time studies are carried out.

Photography

Photography in infants and children can be of particular value, providing documentation to assess changes or to demonstrate pathology to patients, other physicians, or for medicolegal purposes. Photographs of the lens or fundus are especially helpful to the parents when the pathology is not obvious to them as they look at their child. Photography may also be helpful in demonstrating pre and postoperative differences, such as in children with strabismus or ptosis. Children are often most easily photographed with a portable fundus camera since the special positioning of the patient, necessary with formal fundus photography, are difficult. When a child is to receive sedation or a general anaesthetic, it is wise to co-ordinate this with the ophthalmic photographer so that the photographs can be taken at the time of the EUA (Johns 1983; Reeves 1985).

Radiology

Finally, radiology plays a particularly important role in the examination of a child with ocular trauma, suspected non-accidental injury, orbital tumours, and intraretinal masses. Additionally, such studies may be valuable in the assessment of suspected phakomatoses. The CT scan has in large part replaced plain X-rays of the orbits and skull. The CT scan's merits include details of the orbit, oculomotor nerves and muscles, as well as concurrent study of the central nervous system. Calcification of intracranial masses, in particular retinoblastoma, can be well demonstrated with the CT scan. Newer magnetic resonance imaging techniques (MRI) may be less valuable in retinoblastoma cases, since calcification is not so well detected with this technique. Nevertheless, the MRI may be helpful in determining pre-operatively whether optic nerve extension is present since bone artifact is reduced (Schulman *et al.* 1986). However, the MRI is very valuable in assessing posterior fossa abnormalities, suspected demyelinating processes, and in identifying parachiasmal structures. Plain X-rays of the orbits may still have special indications in identifying histiocytosis, defects in association with dermoids, and in fibrous dysplasia and other bony defects. Blow-out or skull fractures may also be better demonstrated by plain X-rays or tomograms of the orbits and skull.

A child who is sedated for a CT scan can easily be assessed for fundus examination if dilating drops have been used ophthalmologist coordinate with the radiology staff an appropriate time for examination.

Summary

The examination of the infant and child entails the same components as that of the adult ophthalmologic examination. The techniques, however, differ due to the different disease processes, differing degrees of co-operation, and the child's personality. Ancillary testing, although not routine, can usually be performed in children as long as the indications for the tests are weighed against their inherent risks. Foremost, the examination of a child must be systematic and complete, and can in fact be great fun if the physician develops the skills necessary to play with children while he is doing a detailed examination.

References

Allen D, Bennett P, Banks M. Effects of luminance on FPL and VEP acuity in human infants. *Invest Ophthalmol Vis Sci Suppl* 1987; **28**: 5

Atkinson J, Braddick O, Wattam-Bell J *et al.* Photorefractive screening of effects of refractive correction. *Invest Ophthalmol Vis Sci* 1987; **28**: 399

Belkin M, Ticho U, Susal A, Levinson A. Ultrasonography in the refraction of aphakic infants. *Br J Ophthalmol* 1973; **57**: 845−8

Birch E, Stager D. Monocular acuity and stereopsis in infantile esotropia. *Invest Ophthalmol Vis Sci* 1985; **26**: 1624−30

Catalano R, Simon J, Jenkins P, Kandel G. Preferential looking as a guide for amblyopia therapy in monocular infantile cataracts. *J Pediatr Ophthalmol Strabismus* 1987; **24**: 56−63

CRCPG (Cryotherapy for Retinopathy of Prematurity Cooperative Group). Multi centre trial of cryotherapy for retinopathy of prematurity. *Arch Ophthalmology* 1988; **106**: 471−9

Day S, Norcia A. Photographic detection of amblyogenic factors. *Ophthalmology* 1986; **93**: 25−8

Day S, Orel-Bixter D, Norcia A. Abnormal grating acuity in infants with esotropia. *Invest Ophthalmol Vis Sci* 1988; **29**: 327−92

Dear G De L, Hammerton M, Hatch DJ, Taylor D. Anaes-

thesia and intraocular pressure in young children. *Anaesthesia* 1987; **42**: 259−65

Donzis P, Rapazzo J, Burde R, Gordon M. Effect of binocular variations of Snellen's visual acuity on Titmus stereoacuity. *Arch Ophthalmol* 1983; **101**: 930−2

Ellis G, Hartmann E, Love A, May J, Morgan K. Teller acuity cards versus clinical judgement in the diagnosis of amblyopia with strabismus. *Ophthalmol* 1988; **95**: 788−91

Fantz RL, Ordy JM, Udele MS. Maturation of pattern vision in infants during the first six months. *J Comp Physiol Psychol* 1962; **55**: 907−17

Fulton AB, Hanson RM, Manning KA. Measuring visual acuity in infants. *Surv Ophthalmol* 1981; **25**: 325−32

Gorman JJ, Cogan DG, Gellis SS. An apparatus for grading the visual acuity of infants on the basis of optokinetic nystagmus. *Pediatrics* 1957; **19**: 1088−92

Gwiazda J, Brill S, Mohindra I, Held R. Preferential looking estimates of visual acuity in infants from 2 to 58 weeks of age. *Am J Optom Physiol Opt* 1980; **57**: 428−32

Held R, Gwiazda J, Brill S *et al.* Infant visual acuity is underestimated because near threshold gratings are not preferentially fixated. *Vision Res* 1979; **19**: 1377−9

Howland H, Howland B. Photorefraction: a technique for study of refractive state at a distance. *J Opt Soc Am* 1974; **64**: 240−9

Jacobson SG, Mohindra I, Held R. Visual acuity of infants with ocular diseases. *Am J. Ophthalmol* 1982; **93**: 198−209

Jampolsky A. The prism test for strabismus screening. *J Pediatr Ophthalmol Strabismus* 1964; **1**: 30−33

Johns M. Fluorescein angiography in the young child. In Wybar K, Taylor D (eds) *Pediatric Ophthalmology Current Aspects.* New York 1983; pp. 77−81

Julesz B. Stereoscopic vision. *Vision Res* 1986; **26 (9)**: 1601−12

Kaakinen K. A simple method for screening of children with strabismus, anisometropia or ametropia by simultaneous photography of the corneal and the fundus reflexes. *Acta Ophtahlmol (Copenh)* 1979; **57**: 161−71

Larsen JS. The sagittal growth of the eye I. Ultrasonic measurement of the depth of the anterior chamber from birth to puberty. *Acta Ophthalmol (Copenh)* 1971a; **49**: 239−62

Larsen JS. The sagittal growth of the eye II. Ultrasonic measurement of the axial diameter of the lens and the anterior segment from birth to puberty. *Acta Ophthalmol (Copenh)* 1971b; **49**: 427−52

Linkz A. Visual acuity in the newborn with notes on some objective methods to determine visual acuity. *Doc Ophthalmol* 1973; **34**: 259−70

Magoon EH. The use of oculinum in children. *Ophthalmology* 1988; (Suppl.) **95**: 142

Mayer D, Dobson V. Visual acuity development in infants and young children, as assessed by apparent preferential looking. *Vision Res* 1978; **18**: 1469

Mayer DL, Fulton AB, Hansen RM. Preferential looking obtained with a staircase procedure in pediatric patients. *Invest Ophthalmol Vis Sci* 1982; **23**: 538−43

McDonald M, Dobson V, Sebris S *et al.* The acuity card procedure: a rapid test of infant acuity. *Invest Ophthalmol Vis Sci* 1985; **26**: 1158−62

McLeod D, Restori M. Real-time B-scanning of the vitreous. *Trans Ophthal Soc UK* 1977; **97**: 547−51

Millodot M, Riggs LA. Refraction determined electrophysiologically: responses to alternation of visual contours. *Arch*

Ophthalmol 1970; **84**: 272−78

Mohindra I, Zwaan J, Held R *et al*. Development of acuity and stereopsis in infants with esotropia. *Ophthalmology* 1985; **92**: 691−7

Morgan K. The evaluation of a commercial off-axis photorefractor. *Ophthalmology* 1987; **94**: 63

Moskowitz A, Sokol S, Hansen V. Rapid assessment of visual function in pediatric patients using pattern VEPs and acuity cards. *Clin Vis Sci* 1987; **2**: 11−20

Norcia A, Tyler C. Spatial frequency sweep VEP: visual acuity during the first year of life. *Vision Res* 1985; **25**: 1399−408

Norcia A, Tyler C, Hamer R. Development of contrast sensitivity in human infants. *Invest Ophthalmol Vis Sci* 1987; **28**(Suppl.): 5

Odom JV, Hoyt CS, Marg E. Effect of natural deprivation and unlateral eye patching, on visual acuity of infants and children; evoked potential measurements. *Arch Ophthalmol* 1981; **99**: 1412−6

Reeves C. *Paediatric ophthalmic photography*. FBIPP Thesis. Institute of Child Health, London 1985; 153 pp

Regan D, Spekreijse H. Evoked potentials in vision research 1961−86. *Vision Res* 1986; **26**: 1461−80

Regan D, Whitlock J, Murray T, Beverly K. Orientation-specific losses of contrast sensitivity in multiple sclerosis. *Invest Ophthalmol Vis Sci* 1980; **19**: 324−8

Restori M, McLeod D. Ultrasound in pre-vitrectomy assessment. *Trans Ophthalmol Soc UK* 1977; **97**: 232−4

Restori M, Wright J. C-scan ultrasonography in orbital diagnosis. *Br J Ophtahlmol* 1977; **61**: 735−40

Schulman J, Peyman G, Mafee M *et al*. The use of magnetic resonance imaging in the evaluation of retinoblastoma. *J Pediatr Ophthalmol Strabismus* 1986; **23**: 144−7

Sira I, Nissenkorn I, Kremer I. Retinopathy of prematurity. *Surv Ophthalmol* 1988; **33**: 1−16

Sokol S. Visually evoked potentials: theory, technique and clinical applications. *Surv Ophthalmol* 1976; **21**: 18−44

Sokol S. Pattern visual evoked potentials: their use in pediatric ophthalmology. *Int Ophthalmol Clin* 1980; **20**: 251−68

Sokol S, Dobson V. Pattern reversal visually evoked potentials in infants. *Invest Ophthalmol Vis Sci* 1976; **15**: 58−62

Sokol S, Hansen V, Moskowitz A, Greenfield P, Towle V. Evoked potentials and preferential looking estimates of visual acuity in pediatric patients. *Ophthalmology* 1983; **90**: 552−62

Stamper R, Hsu-Winges C, Sopher M. Arden contrast sensitivity in glaucoma. *Arch Ophthalmol* 1982; **100**: 947−52

Teller D, McDonald M, Preston K *et al*. Assessment of visual acuity in infants and children: the acuity card procedure. *Dev Med Child Neurol* 1986; **28**: 779−89

Teller DY, Morse R, Borton R, Regal D. Visual acuity for vertical and diagonal gratings in human infants. *Vision Res* 1974; **14**: 1433−9

Teller D, Movshon A. Visual development. *Vision Res* 1986; **26**: 1483−521

von Noorden G K. *Burian−von Noorden's binocular vision and ocular motility: Theory and management of strabismus*. 3rd ed., CV Mosby Co., St. Louis 1985; pp. 205

Zimmern R, Campbell F, Wilkinson I. Subtle disturbances of vision after optic neuritis elicited by studying contrast sensitivity. *J Neurol Neurosurg Psychiatry* 1979; **42**: 407−12

8 Refraction of Infants and Young Children

ANTHONY MOORE

Although ophthalmologists are mainly concerned with children with abnormal refractive errors, it is important to be aware of the normal postnatal development of the eye and the changes in refraction that occur with increasing age before an informed decision can be made about the correction of refractive errors in childhood.

Postnatal development of the eye

At birth the sagittal diameter of the eye is 17–18 mm (Sorsby & Sheridan 1960; Swan & Wilkins 1984) compared with 24 mm of the average emmetropic adult eye. The eyes of premature infants are correspondingly smaller and the axial length is closely related to birth weight (and postconceptual age). Similarly the volume of the adult eye is twice that of the newborn (Swan & Wilkins 1984). Most of the increase in size from newborn to adult values occurs in the first 12–18 months of life (Sorsby & Sheridan 1960; Larsen 1971; Swan & Wilkins 1984) thereafter there is a slow increase in size so that final adult levels are reached by age 13.

The development of the eye can be seen to occur in two distinct phases. During the initial rapid infantile growth phase the axial length of the eye increases from 17 mm to about 23 mm. If the eye is to remain near emmetropic this change in axial length will need to be accompanied by a reduction in refractive power of the eye of approximately 20 dioptres (Sorsby et al. 1961). It is not clear whether most of this compensation is carried out by the lens or the cornea.

Following the rapid changes in growth that occur in infancy there is a slower juvenile growth phase. Cross-sectional studies show that between the ages of 3 and 13 years the axial length of the globe increases by about 1 mm (Sorsby et al. 1961). This small increase would, if there were no compensatory changes, result in a reduction of hypermetropia of about 3 dioptres. The actual change in refraction is less due to flattening of the lens and cornea (Sorsby et al. 1961).

Although the growth of the eye appears to fall into two distinct phases with different growth characteristics, the changes in the various refractive compartments of the eye are co-ordinated in order to ensure that the refraction remains close to emmetropia.

Changes in refraction during childhood

The refraction of young infants has been assessed using cycloplegic retinoscopy (Goldschmidt 1969; Ingram 1979; Fulton et al. 1980), non-cycloplegic retinoscopy (Gwiazda et al. 1984; Mohindra et al. 1978) and photorefraction (Howland et al. 1978; Howland & Sayles 1984).

Spherical refractive errors

Newborn babies have refractive errors which are normally distributed about a mean of about +2.0 dioptres (Banks 1980). The standard deviation is higher than that seen in adult studies which may in part reflect the difficulties of performing retinoscopy in this young age group. The actual hypermetropia may be less than the measured value; Glickstein and Millodot (1970) have produced evidence that the retinoscopy reflex arises anterior to the photoreceptor layer probably from the internal limiting membrane and that retinoscopy therefore overestimates the degree of hypermetropia. This discrepancy is larger the smaller the axial length and is more important in infant eyes.

Similar studies of the refractive errors of premature infants have shown that such infants tend to have refractive errors on the more myopic side (Graham & Gray 1963; Scharf et al. 1975), but that the refractive errors become more emmetropic with increasing age (Banks 1980).

With increasing age there is a gradual decrease in the level of hypermetropia (Sorsby et al. 1961; Banks 1980) so that the refraction becomes more emmetropic; a process which has been termed emmetropisation. This process may be disturbed in certain pathological eye conditions such as Leber's amaurosis and achromatopsia where high refractive errors are common. About 6% of infants still have large refractive errors at the age of 6−9 months (Atkinson et al. 1984); most are hypermetropic and it is this group which may be at highest risk of developing strabismus and amblyopia (Ingram 1977). There is no significant change in normal refraction after the age of 13 (Sorsby et al. 1961).

Astigmatism

It is generally agreed that there is a high prevalence of astigmatism in normal infants (Howland et al. 1978; Mohindra et al. 1978; Ingram 1979; Dobson et al. 1984) and that the degree of astigmatism reduces with increasing age (Mohindra 1978; Ingram & Barr 1979; Howland & Sayles 1984). By the age of 3−5 years the prevalence of astigmatism is similar to that seen in the adult population (Howland & Sayles 1984). The axis of astigmatism also changes; in infants against the rule astigmatism predominates whilst in children over the age of 5 years, with the rule astigmatism is more common (Dobson et al. 1984). Infants who have no astigmatism in the first year of life are unlikely to develop it later (Gwiazda et al. 1984).

Consequences of abnormal refractive errors in infancy

About 6% of 1-year-olds have a significant refractive error (Ingram 1979; Atkinson et al. 1984) and most are hyperopic. Hyperopic infants are at greatly increased risk of developing strabismus and amblyopia (Ingram 1977; Ingram et al. 1986). Uncorrected anisometropia may lead to amblyopia in the more ametropic eye and anisometropia is commonly associated with microstrabismus and defective stereo-acuity. Bilateral high refractive errors which are uncorrected in infancy may lead to bilateral ametropic amblyopia (Abrahamson 1964); patients with bilateral high hyperopia and myopia since infancy may not correct to normal levels of visual acuity in adult life, presumably due to lack of clear retinal image in early childhood. Similarly uncorrected astigmatism in childhood may be associated with a reduced ability to discriminate gratings orientated in the more ametropic meridian, so called meridional amblyopia (Mitchell & Wilkinson 1974). Fulton et al. 1982 have suggested that amongst myopic children those who have uncorrected astigmatism in infancy are more likely to develop progressive myopia.

Assessment of refractive error in children

In older children the refractive error may be assessed objectively and verified subjectively using similar techniques to those used in adults. In infants and in children with mental handicap the refractive error must be estimated from the objective findings alone.

Retinoscopy remains the standard method by which refractive errors are assessed in young children although, photorefraction (Howland et al. 1978; Atkinson et al. 1984), autorefractors (Evans 1984; Helveston et al. 1984) and even techniques using visual evoked potentials (Regan 1973) have also been used.

Retinoscopy

Retinoscopy is carried out either as a static procedure with accommodation relaxed or dynamically with the subject fixed on a near point. Dynamic retinoscopy although useful as a research tool to investigate accommodation in infancy or to evaluate the effectiveness of cycloplegic drugs is rarely used clinically.

Mohindra *et al.* (1978) have described a technique of non-cycloplegic retinoscopy in infancy using near retinoscopy and has claimed a good correlation with cycloplegic refraction. Although this method may be useful as a rapid screening procedure it has yet to gain widespread acceptance in clinical practice, where it is often necessary to perform fundoscopy with pupillary dilatation so that a cycloplegic refraction and fundoscopy can be combined. Relaxation of accommodation in static retinoscopy is achieved either by distance fixation or the use of cycloplegic drugs. In older children the former method can be used and if a 'fogging' technique is used routinely a spurious result can be avoided. Young children, those with mental handicap and all children with strabismus, should have a refraction performed under cycloplegia.

CHOICE OF CYCLOPLEGIC DRUGS

The commonest cycloplegic drugs used in clinical practice are cyclopentolate and atropine. Cyclopentolate is used as a 0.5% solution in the neonate and 1% solution after the age of 3 months. Two drops are instilled into each eye half an hour before retinoscopy; cycloplegia is maximal within 30 minutes and returns to normal with 24 hours (Vale & Cox 1978). It is less effective in darkly pigmented irides. Toxic effects are rare and usually occur if higher doses are given (Praeger & Miller 1964; Bauer *et al.* 1973).

Atropine is used as a 0.5% ointment in young infants and 1% after the age of 3 months. Ointment is preferable to drops as the systemic absorption is thought to be less. The onset of cycloplegia is slower than cyclopentolate taking 3 hours for full effect. Recovery of accommodation starts 2–3 days after the last dose but full amplitude of accommodation may not recover for 10 days. It is more effective than cyclopentolate in pigmented irides.

Traditionally atropine ointment is instilled twice daily for 3 days preceding retinoscopy. Parents should be warned to discontinue the medication if there are signs of local sensitivity or systemic toxicity; very serious toxic reactions may occur after ingestion of as little as 10 mg of atropine; the amount contained in a 10 ml bottle of 1 per cent atropine drops.

Although atropine is a more effective cycloplegic, in most children cyclopentolate gives adequate cycloplegia. Rosenbaum *et al.* (1981) for example showed that in a population of white esotropic children atropine only uncovered a mean of +0.34 dioptres more hyperopia than cyclopentolate although the difference was greater in the more hyperopic eyes. This small difference is unlikely to be clinically significant. Cyclopentolate is preferable for routine cycloplegia in children as it is less toxic and its rapid action means that refraction can be carried out at the initial clinic visit. Furthermore the rapid recovery of normal function is preferable in older children in whom the prolonged pupillary dilatation and cycloplegia associated with atropine use is unacceptable. Atropine may however have a role in selected cases. Children with significant hyperopia or accomodative esotropia, those with darkly pigmented irides and those in whom cyclopentolate appears to give adequate cycloplegia may require a further refraction under atropine cycloplegia. It is also useful in children who are unduly upset by the instillation of drops in the clinic and are thereafter difficult to examine or refract. The parents can instill atropine at home, during sleep if necessary and the child can be seen immediately on arrival in the clinic when a refraction and fundus examination is usually possible.

PRACTICAL ASPECTS

Older children present few problems and after the age of 3 or 4 will readily co-operate with retinoscopy and later subjective refraction. However, retinoscopy may be difficult in infants and young children mainly because of difficulty in obtaining full co-operation and ensuring that refraction takes place along the visual axis. The key to obtaining an accurate refraction is to carry out the procedure when the child (and parent) is relaxed and happy. It is preferable that the mydriatic drops are instilled by a clinic nurse or assistant so that the child does not associate the ophthalmologist with this unpleasant procedure. At the beginning of the examination it is best to obtain as much information as possible using the retinoscope alone before putting lenses in front of the child's eye. It is possible to estimate the approximate degree of the refractive error by the appearance of the retinoscopy reflex. For example in low hyperopia the reflex is very distinct and bright, whereas in moderate and high hyperopia the reflex is duller. It is possible to estimate the degree of myopia by varying the working distance gradually approaching the eye until a null point is reached. Neutralization of the retinoscopy reflex is faster if a lens rack is used rather than individual lenses. In unco-operative infants it is often helpful to give the child a bottle feed at the time of the refraction. It is important to attract the child's attention to the light and in strabismic patients to occlude the preferred eye so that retinoscopy takes place along the optical axis;

off-axis retinoscopy may give rise to false oblique astigmatic refractive errors. Finally it must be realized that refraction in infants and children is difficult and very dependent on the mood and hence co-operation of the child. It is better to accept defeat gracefully and try again another day than to attempt refraction with the child restrained which is normally counterproductive.

It is very rare that an accurate refraction cannot be achieved even in difficult children. In the case of repeated failure, photorefraction is a useful procedure and if this suggests a high refractive error, or if the child has a squint or amblyopia, refraction may very rarely need to be performed under general anaesthesia.

Autorefraction

Modern autorefractors are of two types; objective instruments require only that the patient remains still and fixes the target within the instrument. With subjective autorefractors the patient must in addition be able to appreciate changes in the appearances of the target. Objective autorefractors clearly have more potential for use with children. Objective autorefraction gives comparable values to retinoscopy for cylinder axis and power and spherical power if cycloplegia is used but is unreliable for non-cycloplegic refractions (Evans 1984; Helveston et al. 1984). Helveston et al. (1984) in their study using the Nidek autorefractor found that children as young as 3 years could be refracted successfully.

Autorefractors can be used by non-medical personnel in the clinic and may be used as a basis for subjective refraction in older children. The major limitation is that their use is confined to the very group of children in which retinoscopy is quick and easy to perform. Autorefraction is of no value in infants and retarded children where retinoscopy is most time consuming and least accurate.

Photorefraction

Photorefraction is a technique by which the refractive error of the eye can be assessed by the analysis of flash or video photographs. Although there are several different forms of photorefraction (orthogonal, isotropic and eccentric) the optical principles are similar. The subjects's eye is illuminated by a small flash source and the light returning from the eye captured on the photographic film (or video) of a camera positioned close to the light source. The light will have traversed the eye twice before reaching the film and the refractive error of the eye can be estimated from the pattern of image on the camera film. The detailed optics have been reviewed by Howland et al. (1983). Photorefraction can be used to assess refractive errors and also to study accomodation in infancy (Braddick et al. 1979). Photorefraction is especially well suited to infants and young children. Only brief fixation is necessary and both eyes can be measured simultaneously. The instrument is at a distance from the child's face and no trial lenses need to be held close to the eye so it is easier to obtain the childs co-operation.

The limitation of photorefraction in its present form is that it is not sufficiently accurate over a range of abnormal refractive errors for a spectacle correction to be prescribed on the basis of the measurement. It is, however, excellent for detecting abnormal refractive errors and may have a role to play in infant visual screening (Kaakinen 1979; Atkinson et al. 1984).

Refraction as a method of visual screening

Screening of preschool children for visual abnormalities is traditionally performed between the ages of 3 and 4 years using visual acuity testing, assessment of ocular alignment and stereopsis. Ingram (1977, 1986) has suggested an alternative approach using refraction in infancy as a means of identifying those at risk of developing squint and amblyopia. He has demonstrated that spherical hypermetropia in infancy is significantly associated with the later development of squint and amblyopia. Nearly half of infants with greater than +3.50 dioptres of hypermetropia in any meridian at age 1 year developed amblyopia and strabismus (Ingram et al. 1986).

Widespread refractive screening using retinoscopy would clearly be expensive and impractical but photorefraction which uses relatively inexpensive equipment and can be used by non-medical personnel may be feasible. Atkinson et al. (1984) have demonstrated, in a large population study, that photorefraction can be used to identify the 6% of infants who have abnormal refractive errors and who are at high risk of developing squint and amblyopia. Although early visual screening by refraction is theoretically attractive as it allows early recognition of children at risk of developing amblyopia, there is as yet no evidence that the correction of abnormal refractive errors in infancy is effective in the prevention of later ocular abnormalities (Ingram et al. 1985).

Correction of abnormal refractive errors

In children who are 3 years or older and able to co-operate with visual acuity testing the decision whether to correct a refractive error or not is seldom controversial. Spectacles may be prescribed if an improvement of visual acuity is demonstrated or may be necessary as part of the treatment for strabismus and amblyopia. Spectacles may sometimes be indicated for asthenopic symptoms, but correction of low refractive errors is unlikely to improve non-specific headaches and 'acheing eyes'. There is some evidence that there is a significant degree of over prescribing of spectacles in school age children (Stewart-Brown 1985).

In infants and younger children there is less general agreement about when refractive errors should be corrected. In this section it is hoped to give some general guidelines to treatment.

Bilateral and equal refractive errors

HYPEROPIA

In the esotropic child all the hypermetropia found on retinoscopy is prescribed; a correction is made for the working distance but no reduction should be made for the cycloplegic agent even if atropine is used. There is no good evidence that an adjustment needs to be made for latent hyperopia. The child should be reassessed wearing the spectacle correction and if the angle of strabismus reduces with the glasses they will need to be continued. Children with a near esotropia and a high AC : A ratio may be managed with bifocals; executive bifocals are used with the top of the bifocal segment covering the lower third of the pupil.

Infants who are bilaterally aphakic form another group with hyperopia; contact lenses are the treatment of choice initially but spectacles may be used when the child is older. Initially the child is overcorrected by about +3.0 dioptres so that close objects are in focus but at about the age of 4 or 5 the correct distance prescription is given with a bifocal addition for near work.

There is less general agreement about the management of the infant who is found to be highly hyperopic, either on routine refraction or screening, but is asymptomatic. Although it is clear that such infants are at risk of amblyopia and strabismus (Ingram et al. 1986) there is as yet no evidence that early spectacle correction affects outcome (Ingram et al. 1985). Until more studies have been performed it is probably sensible to correct any bilateral hypermetropia of greater than 4.0 dioptres and to prescribe 1 dioptre less than the full cycloplegic refractive error which will bring the infant to within the normal range.

MYOPIA

The myopic infant is less likely to develop strabismus and amblyopia and low degrees of myopia can be left uncorrected in infancy. In children with exo-deviations the full myopic correction should be prescribed as this may help reduce the angle of strabismus. Myopia greater than −3.0 dioptres should be fully corrected and in school age children lower degrees of myopia are corrected when reduced distance vision interferes with school work or games.

ASTIGMATISM

There is a high prevalence of astigmatism in normal infants which reduces with increasing age. Although low levels of astigmatism may be safely left uncorrected in infancy there is some evidence that more marked astigmatism if left uncorrected may lead to meridional (Mitchell & Wilkinson 1974) or bilateral ametropic amblyopia (Abrahamson 1964). In view of the high prevalence of astigmatism in normal infants it is impossible to give dogmatic advice on when such errors should be corrected.

If spectacles are prescribed for another reason, for example high spherical errors or in the treatment of strabismus and amblyopia it is reasonable to correct all the astigmatic refractive error found at retinoscopy. In infants with bilateral astigmatism with no other indication for refractive correction a short period of observation and repeat refraction is advisable. If the astigmatism does not reduce with time, it should be corrected; errors of less than 1.5 dioptres may probably be safely ignored.

Unequal refractive errors (Anisometropia)

Anisometropia in early infancy is a barrier to the establishment of normal binocular vision; the more ametropic eye may be suppressed and amblyopia may result. Amblyopia is commoner and more profound in hyperopic anisometropia (Jampolsky et al. 1955; Flynn & Cassady 1978) although it may also occur in myopic and astigmatic anisometropia. At what level therefore should anisometropia be corrected? Ingram (1977) has presented evidence that hypermetropic spherical or cylindrical anisometropia greater than 1 dioptre is significantly associated with the later development of amblyopia. Furthermore in most cases of anisometropic amblyopia there are only small differences in the refractive errors between the two eyes (Flynn & Cassady 1978). It would seem sensible therefore in infants whose acuity cannot easily be measured to correct any anisometropia of greater than 1.0 dioptre, especially if both eyes are hyperopic. The need for optical correction can be reviewed when the child is old enough to be formally tested.

References

Abrahamson SV. Bilateral ametropic amblyopia. *J Pediatr Ophthalmol Strabismus* 1964; **1**: 57−61

Atkinson J, Braddick OJ, Durden K, Watson PG, Atkinson S. Screening for refractive errors in 6−9 month infants by photorefraction. *Br J Ophthalmol* 1984; **68**: 105−12

Banks M. Infant refraction and accommodation. *Int Ophthalmol Clin* 1980; **20**: 205−32

Bauer CR, Trottler MCT, Stern L. Systemic cyclopentolate (Cyclogyl) toxicity in the newborn infant. *J Pediatr* 1973; **82**: 501−5

Braddick OJ, Atkinson J, French J, Howland HL. A photorefractive study of infant accomodation. *Vision Res* 1979; **19**: 1319−30

Dobson V, Fulton AB, Lawson Sebris S. Cycloplegic refractions of infants and young children: the axis of astigmatism. *Invest Ophthalmol Vis Sci* 1984; **25**: 83−7

Evans E. Refraction in children using the Rx 1 autorefractor. *Br Orthop J* 1984; **41**: 46−52

Flynn JT, Cassady MS. Current trends in amblyopia therapy. *Ophthalmology* 1978; **85**: 428−50

Fulton AB, Dobson V, Salem D *et al*. Cycloplegic refractions in infants and young children. *Am J Ophthalmol* 1980; **90**: 239−47

Fulton AB, Hansen RM, Peterson RA. The relation of myopia and astigmatism in developing eyes. *Ophthalmology* 1982; **89**: 208−302

Glickstein M, Millodot M. Retinoscopy and eye size. Science 1970; **168**: 605

Goldschmidt E. Refraction in the newborn. *Acta Ophthalmol (Copenh)* 1969; **47**: 570−8

Graham MV, Gray OP. Refraction of premature babies eyes. *Br Med J* 1963; **5**: 1452−4

Gwiazda J, Scheiman M, Mohindra I, Held R. Astigmatism in children: changes in axis and amount from birth to six years. *Invest Ophthalmol Vis Sci* 1984; **25**: 88−92

Helveston EM, Pachtman MA, Caderew W, Ellis FD, Emmerson BS, Weber J. Clinical evaluation of the Nidek AR autorefractor. *J Pediatr Ophthalmol Strabismus* 1984; **21**: 227−30

Howland HC, Atkinson J, Braddick O, French J. Infant astigmatism measured by photorefraction. *Science* 1978; **202**: 331−2

Howland HC, Braddick O, Atkinson J, Howland B. Optics of photorefraction: orthogonal and isotropic methods. *J Opt Soc Am* 1983; **73**: 1701−8

Howland HC, Sayles N. Photorefractive measurements in infants and young children. *Invest Ophthalmol Vis Sci* 1984; **25**: 93−101

Ingram RM. Refraction as a basis for screening children for squint and amblyopia. *Br J Ophthalmol* 1977; **61**: 8−15

Ingram RM, Barr A. Changes in refraction between the ages of 1 and 3½ years. *Br J Ophthalmol* 1979; **63**: 339−42

Ingram RM, Walker C, Wilson JM *et al*. A first attempt to prevent amblyopia and squint by spectacle correction of abnormal refractions from age 1 year. *Br J Ophthalmol* 1985; **69**: 851−3

Ingram RM, Walker C, Wilson JM, Arnold PE, Dally S. Prediction of amblyopia and squint by means of refraction at one year. *Br J Ophthalmol* 1986 **70**: 12−15

Jampolsky A, Flom BL, Weymouth JW, Moses L. Unequal corrected visual acuity as related to anisometropia. *Arch Ophthalmol* 1955; **54**: 893−905

Kaakinen K. A simple method for screening of children with strabismus, anisometropia or ametropia by simultaneous photography of corneal and fundus reflex. *Acta Ophthalmol Kbh* 1979; **57**: 161−71

Larsen JS. The saggital growth of the eye III. Ultrasonic measurements of the posterior segment (axial length of the vitreous) from birth to puberty. *Acta Ophthalmol (Kbh)* 1971; **49**: 441−53

Mitchell D, Wilkinson F. The effect of early astigmatism on the visual resolution of gratings. *J. Physiol (London)* 1974; **243**: 739−56

Mohindra I, Held R, Gwiazda J, Brill S. Astigmatism in infants. *Science* 1978; **202**: 329−30

Praeger DL, Miller SN. Toxic effects of cyclopentolate. *Am J Ophthalmol* 1964; **58**: 1060−1

Regan D. Rapid objective refraction using evoked brain potentials. *Invest Ophthalmol Vis Sci* 1973; **12**: 669−79

Rosenbaum AL, Bateman JB, Bremer DL. Cycloplegic refraction in esotropic children. *Ophthalmology* 1981; **88**: 1031−4

Scharf J, Zonis S, Zeltzer M. Refraction in Israeli premature infants. *J Pediatr Ophthalmol Strabismus* 1975; **12**: 193−6

Sorsby A, Benjamin B, Sheridan M. Refraction and its components during the growth of the eye from the age of 3 years. In Medical Research Council (Gt Britain) Special Report Series No. 301; Medical Research Council London, 1961; pp. 1−67

Sorsby A, Sheridan M. The eye at birth: measurements of the principle diameter in fourty eight cadavers. *J Anat* 1960; **94**: 192−7

Stewart-Brown SL. Spectacle prescribing among 10 year old children. *Br J Ophthalmol* 1985; **69**: 874−80

Swann KC, Wilkins JH. Extraocular muscle surgery in early infancy − anatomical factors. *J Pediatr Ophthalmol Strabismus* 1984; **21**: 44−49

Vale J, Cox B. *Drugs and the eye*. Butterworth, London 1978; p. 21

9 Ophthalmic Genetics

MICHAEL BARAITSER AND ELIZABETH THOMPSON

Most parents after the birth of a child with a malformation of the eye or with a progressive disease leading to visual impairment want to discuss the possibility that the handicap was genetically determined and its prevention during a subsequent pregnancy. This might be handled by the ophthalmologist or at the genetic clinic or perhaps preferably by a combination of the two. The word counselling is a misnomer as few parents would expect 'counsel' but would want to receive all the available information so that they can come to a meaningful decision, given their own individual circumstances.

An approach to counselling

There are two essentials before counselling. One is an accurate three generation family history; something which can usually be achieved even in a busy ophthalmic clinic. Its importance is that the taking of a family history, followed by non-directive counselling, is a potent way of preventing serious malformation. An accurate diagnosis is the other essential prerequisite for counselling. In its absence, a category diagnosis, i.e. an anterior chamber defect or colobomatous microphthalmia is useful. These latter two diagnoses do not describe single entities but at least the geneticists can draw on empirical data to counsel approximate risks.

Counselling in recessively inherited disease

The following general points are relevant:

Affected siblings of both sexes, given unaffected parents in a condition which is totally penetrant and is not frequent in the population, usually indicate autosomal recessive inheritance. This is mostly the situation with oculocutaneous albinism. Confusion might arise because occasionally, a parent (both must be heterozygotes) manifests a degree of translucency of the iris and might have fair hair and skin. Some black people who are carriers have slightly lighter skin and hair colour, but in general, carriers do not show signs. If the condition is such that carriers can be detected then it would be expected that both parents would be found to have the changes. The fact that oculocutaneous albinism might be heterogeneous (tyrosinase positive or negative) does not make any difference as all the subgroups seem to be recessively inherited. That the genes are at separate loci will only affect counselling if there were DNA markers for a specific type of albinism as in that case a prenatal prediction would apply only to one specific category.

Many different loci for albinism would also affect counselling of two albinos who wanted to marry and have children. The prediction would be that all their children would be affected if albinism was always the result of homozygosity at a single locus. If different loci were involved, then all the children would have normal pigmentation of the skin, hair, and iris.

Genetic counselling in autosomal recessive conditions is usually straightforward. The risk of recurrence in subsequent children of the same parents is one in four or 25%; this is known as a high-risk category, as are all risks greater than one in ten, but counselling is non-directive and parents will choose whether the risk is acceptable or not. It is clear that in albinism, the ocular complications are not necessarily severe and some parents are happy to accept this risk.

71

What is needed, given this variability, is that parents should be furnished with information about the proportion of children who will have mild, moderate or severe handicap. In order to understand risks in general, it is always helpful for parents to know the background risk that any couple run every time they have a child. This figure is in the vicinity of one in 50, i.e. about 2% of children are born with a major malformation. From this perspective, a 1–2% risk should be regarded as a reasonable risk. Despite a general acceptance that a one in four risk is high, no couple should be made to feel guilty for taking that risk. Counselling remains essentially advice-giving. Risks should be numerically expressed in the form of odds which should always be put into perspective. Directive counselling should seldom be given and is rarely asked for.

The biggest problem for parents is how to cope with high risks of serious conditions. Leber's amaurosis is a good example. It is often difficult for parents whose first child is diagnosed as having this serious autosomal recessive condition to contemplate another pregnancy especially in the absence of a prenatal diagnosis. Only artificial insemination by donor (AID) or ovum transplantation are ways around the problem but the first option is not acceptable to many people and the latter option is not readily available at present. Nevertheless in each situation, the subject should be raised. The decision whether to accept the risk will also depend on the family structure. If parents already have two other normal children, then they might not want to enlarge the family. The most agonizing choice is for those parents where the affected child is the first in the family. They might be reluctant to accept the genetic implications by suggesting that it 'cannot be genetic because there is no family history' but unfortunately, there is often no family history in those conditions which are inherited as an autosomal recessive. In the face of unpleasant information which the parents will receive, the counsellor will often seek to balance the gloomy news by pointing out that neither their normal or affected children are likely to have affected children themselves unless they marry a close relative, or a visually handicapped person with exactly the same diagnosis. It is also at times difficult for parents who must be carriers for the condition not to feel responsible for the child's handicap; it should therefore be pointed out that on average, everyone in the population is a carrier for at least one potentially harmful recessive gene which in single 'dose' is harmless. The realization that often results from this explanation is that somehow, the parents had been unlucky enough to have chosen from the population at large another gene carrier for a rare condition, say Leber's amaurosis. This may provoke a situation where one partner says to the other with some regret, that they had clearly made a wrong choice and the counsellor should be aware of the tensions that could arise from each statement that is made, in an effort to try to explain the genetic situation.

Genetic counselling must always be dynamic and flexible so that misconceptions or an over emphasis on blame or bad luck must be countered and put into perspective. An interview might take longer than anticipated and ample time should be allowed.

The risks to the offspring of the parents' siblings or the affected child's siblings are likely to be small, even allowing for there being a 50% chance that a parent's sibling is a carrier and a two thirds chance that a normal sibling of the affected child is a carrier. The probability that they would marry another carrier is small, unless they marry a cousin, and cautious reassurance is mostly all that is necessary. A figure quantifying the risk is usually possible to derive. For instance, given that the population frequency for Leber's amaurosis is one in 40 000 then the carrier frequency in the population is only about one in a 100. The chance therefore of a parent's sibling having an affected child is one in two, times one in a 100, times one in four ($1/2 \times 1/100 \times 1/4$). This gives an overall risk of one in 800 which is acceptable to most people.

Counselling in dominantly inherited disease

This follows one of three sequences. If there is a family history of a rare condition stretching over at least two generations and there has been male to male transmission thereby excluding X-linked inheritance, counselling of risks to offspring of those who are affected is simple. The risk is one in two or 50% (a high risk) and if the condition is serious and no prenatal diagnosis is available, then a significant number of people decide that the risk is unacceptable. AID should be discussed if the gene carrier is male. At present, ovum donation is a less practical consideration.

The second common situation is where the condition is known to be dominant, but there is no family history, i.e. a child has uncomplicated aniridia with normal chromosomes and the parents have normal irises. Given that the condition is usually totally penetrant, then it would be reasonable to reassure the parents that the affected child has the condition as a fresh mutation. This concept will nearly always need an explanation and by far the easiest is to indicate that each child inherits half of its genes from each parent and in order to do so, DNA has to replicate itself by a process of copying. It is a miscopy of one of the genes that leads to a fresh mutation. It is comforting for parents to be told that there is nothing wrong with their genes per se, but that the fault lies in the innate difficulty of accurately copying many thousands of genes.

It should also be noted that in some dominantly inherited conditions where for instance a pigmentary retinopathy has been transmitted for many generations that the parents usually have a good understanding of the burden of the condition or the absence thereof and it would be inappropriate for the counsellor to comment in a directive way. Parents will always decide whether or not they could cope although they might want to know whether a particular condition could be more or less severe than their own experience of it.

The third counselling problem in dominantly inherited conditions has to do with variable expression and penetrance. For instance in dominant optic atrophy, it could appear on taking the pedigree that certain members seem to transmit the condition without being affected themselves. However, if they are examined by an experienced ophthalmologist, then pale optic discs will in all probability be found. No parent should therefore be reassured that recurrence risks are small in any condition known to be dominantly inherited with variable expression until they themselves have been examined.

Counselling in X-linked disorders

It might be that a simple appraisal of the pedigree will be sufficient to recognize an X-linked condition. If a mother has an affected son and an affected brother but is herself unaffected or if an affected father produces both normal male and female children but his grandsons through his daughters have the same condition, then this is good evidence for X-linkage. It is more difficult in those situations where a woman has two affected sons as this could be either autosomal recessive or X-linked. If a diagnosis has been made, i.e. of ocular albinism which is mostly X-linked and rarely autosomal recessive, then on balance, counselling should proceed as if the inheritance pattern were X-linked. However, if both males have an unidentifiable condition, then it becomes impossible from the pedigree to distinguish between an X-linked and an autosomal recessive mode of transmission.

When a single male is born with a known X-linked condition, the relevant counselling problem is to know whether mother is a carrier. The affected male could arise in two ways: either as a fresh mutation or because mother is a carrier. Even an absence of a family history does not preclude the possibility that mother is a carrier as she might be a fresh mutation herself or the mutation could have arisen in her own mother. Some female carriers of an X-linked condition show minimal manifestations which should always be looked for. For instance, carriers for Lowe's syndrome might show lens opacities and despite some overlap with the normal population, there are those situations where a slit lamp examination of mother might give a clear cut result; or at least a high probability that mother is a carrier. If there is no way of carrier detection as is the case in Norrie's disease, then there are theoretical reasons for assuming that in X-linked conditions which are so handicapping that boys seldom reproduce, at least two thirds of mothers are carriers. This presumes equal mutation rates in sperm and ova. In this situation, the risk of having an affected male is half of two thirds, i.e. one third which is unfortunately an uncomfortably high risk.

Mitochondrial inheritance

The zygote receives virtually all its cytoplasmic DNA from maternal mitochondria which in man are the only source of extranuclear DNA. Each mitochondrion contains a number of DNA molecules which encode the RNA and protein needed by the mitochondrion.

Some diseases, most notably Leber's optic neuropathy and mitochondrial cytopathy, have characteristics which have led to the belief that they result from mutations in mitochondrial DNA. They have virtually exclusively maternal transmission (as opposed to transmission through affected males via carrier daughters, to grandsons in X-linked disease), a high proportion of offspring are affected or transmit the disease, and some have a proven defect in mitochondrial enzymes (Poulton 1988). Alternative explanations, such as a slow virus or a transplacentally transmitted maternal factor are less attractive alternatives for this pattern of inheritance.

Counselling when no diagnosis is possible

Problems in genetic counselling arise when there is no precise diagnosis. For instance, a girl with normal chromosomes who is mentally handicapped presents with congenital blindness due to a retinal dysplasia.

Experience suggests that the majority of these cases seem to be sporadic although rare recessives have been reported. Parents should be given the complete facts but be told that recurrence risks are still likely to be small in view of the fact that the vast majority of cases have been single events. A risk of 2–3% might be appropriate in this situation and parents should understand that this is a small risk but that in no way could we totally exclude the unusual possibility of a recurrence.

It becomes even more difficult when the affected person is a single male without a specific diagnosis as there is the added problem of X-linked inheritance. An experienced dysmorphologist used to looking at congenital malformations and having experience in the diagnosis of rare malformations will argue that if he or she cannot make a diagnosis, then at least a large proportion of genetic diseases have been excluded. Recurrence risks are therefore reduced to an empirical figure of between 3 and 5% depending on the specific combination of defects. The careful counsellor will also make use of one of the dysmorphology databases which can be easily used in the office on a microcomputer in order to scan the available world literature to make sure that the specific combination has not been described in a possibly obscure paper. Prenatal diagnosis can occasionally be achieved by high resolution ultrasonography. Measurements of the globe in microphthalmia or anophthalmia should be considered, and in these conditions the test could be offered early in a subsequent pregnancy.

Clinical application of DNA technology

DNA analysis can be used to provide information for carrier detection, presymptomatic and prenatal diagnosis of an increasing number of genetic disorders. Frequently, this is accomplished by genetic linkage of DNA markers to the disease locus. The presence of a disease gene itself often cannot be detected before the disease is expressed clinically.

Genetic markers whose presence *can* be detected and which are transmitted with the disease gene, can be used to predict whether or not the disease gene has been inherited. In order to give an accurate prediction, the marker must be physically close (closely linked) to the disease gene to minimise the chance that the two loci will become separated at meiosis, a process called recombination.

In recent years, recombinant DNA technology has provided a rich source of DNA markers called DNA probes which can be used to detect normal variation (polymorphisms) in DNA. Restriction enzymes recognise specific sequences of DNA and cut the DNA at these sites. Normal variations in the presence or absence of cutting sites gives rise to different sized fragments which can be separated by electrophoresis. Such restriction fragment length polymorphisms (RFLP) can be detected by radioactively, or biotin-labelled DNA probes, in a process called Southern blotting. (Emery 1988; Weatherall 1985). RFLPs are inherited in a simple Mendelian fashion, and provided they are close to the disease gene in question, can be used to determine whether an individual has inherited the disease gene without having to know anything about the disease gene itself. A family study is undertaken to track the inheritance of the disease gene using RFLP analysis.

The development of chorion villus sampling, done at 9–10 weeks of pregnancy, has meant that early prenatal diagnosis can be offered if the fetus is at risk of a genetic disorder for which reliable DNA markers have been identified. It is always preferable for the family to have had genetic counselling before a pregnancy so that the gene tracking can be done because, for technical reasons, not all families can be offered a prenatal test (as will be discussed below) and the limitations of the tests need to be fully discussed with the family. Decisions about prenatal diagnosis and termination of affected fetuses need to be fully discussed as well as the risks of the procedures; current risk for a miscarriage after chorion villus sampling is about 3%, but depends upon the operator. The analysis of fetal DNA takes at least 2 weeks, but the advent of new procedures such as the polymerase chain reaction (PCR) will mean that results may be available in 1–2 days in some cases.

Two genetic disorders of the eye, namely Norrie's disease and retinoblastoma are discussed in order to highlight the uses and limitations of DNA technology for carrier detection, presymptomatic and prenatal diagnosis.

Norrie's disease

This X-linked disorder is characterized by early vascular proliferation (pseudoglioma) in both retinas, atrophic irides, corneal clouding and cataracts, progressing to shrinkage of the globes (phthisis bulbi). About, two thirds of cases are moderately or severely mentally retarded (Warburg 1966) and other abnormalities may be present including odd behaviour patterns, seizures, microcephaly, poor muscle bulk, hearing loss, and perhaps a similar facial appearance with a narrow nasal bridge, hypotelorism, flattened nasal area, thin upper lips, and large ears (Donnai *et al.* 1988). The diagnosis is usually made on the ocular findings, but this is sometimes difficult in an isolated case.

About two thirds of mothers who have one affected boy are carriers, and 50% of the male offspring of a known carrier will be affected. Until recently, no method of detection of carriers or prenatal diagnosis was available, and families were counselled on the basis of Bayesian calculation of risks which depends on the number of unaffected male relatives.

However, in 1985, Gal *et al.* reported close linkage of Norrie's disease and the polymorphic X chromosome locus DXS7 defined by the DNA probe L1.28, which localised the Norrie disease gene to the short arm of the X chromosome at band 11.3, that is, at Xp 11.3. This linkage has been confirmed (Gal *et al.* 1985 (b); Kivlin *et al.* 1987) and could be used to provide carrier detection and prenatal diagnosis in suitable families.

For example, in Fig. 9.1 using probe L1.28 to detect DNA polymorphisms, it can be seen that the two X chromosome RFLPs of the mother (an obligate carrier) can be distinguished and can be called A and B. Clearly her affected sons both inherited allele A, so that, in this family, the disease gene is 'tracking' with allele A. The daughter, at 50% risk of being a carrier on pedigree grounds has inherited the A allele from father and the B from mother. Thus, she is predicted not to be a carrier, barring the risk of recombination, estimated at about 5% and her risk of having an affected son is 2.5%. Similarly, the mother herself could be offered a prenatal test. If a male fetus inherited the maternal A or B allele, he would be at 95% or 5% risk of being affected, respectively.

This example highlights three important points. First, the mother must be heterozygous for the markers, to be able to be offered a prenatal test. This is called being 'informative' for the test. If the mother were homozygous, i.e. AA, her two alleles could not be distinguished and a prenatal test would not be possible. However, as new markers are identified, it becomes increasingly likely that a given female will become informative for the test. The second point is that the risk of a wrong prediction due to recombination must be explained to the woman and her partner; some couples would not be prepared to take this risk and might prefer to opt for fetal sexing and termination of affected males. The degree of risk a woman is prepared to take often reflects her experience of the disease; a woman who has had two

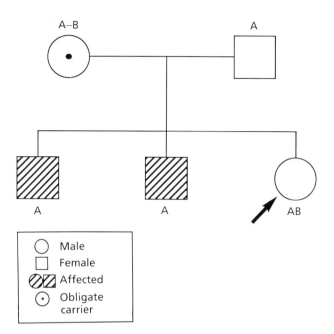

Fig. 9.1 Norrie's disease. The probe L1.28 reveals RFLPs with the enzyme Eco R1. The RFLPs have been designated A and B. The mother (a carrier) has alleles A and B; the affected sons inherited allele A. The maternal allele A is tracking with the Norrie's disease gene. The daughter inherited allele A from father and B from mother, so is predicted not to be a carrier.

affected brothers may be prepared to take less risk than her cousin who has never lived with an affected boy. Thirdly, in the example shown in Fig. 9.1, the accuracy of the prediction that the daughter is unlikely to be a carrier is based on the assumption of correct paternity. If her true father in fact had allele B, then the prediction would be that the girl is likely to be a carrier. Thus a test for paternity should be carried out in situations where a result is dependent on correct paternity.

A factor which can limit the availability of the test is family structure. For example, if the affected boys had died, it would not be possible to 'track' the gene and know which RFLP was travelling with the disease gene in the family. For this reason, it is often important to store a DNA sample from an affected individual, particularly if they are likely to die. It is interesting to note however that all may not be lost if the affected boy has died without a DNA sample being stored. In Fig. 9.2 the healthy brother gives information about the normal allele and would allow the prediction that his sister is not a carrier. Even if the healthy brother were not available and the daughter's risk could not be altered by DNA analysis, she could be offered a prenatal exclusion test in pregnancy. If her male fetus inherited the B allele which she inherited from her

ESTERASE D ACTIVITY

Patients with a constitutional deletion at 13q14 have 50% normal levels of the enzyme esterase D (ESD) in their cells (Cowell *et al.* 1986). Some patients with apparently normal karyotypes may have reduced ESD levels, which suggests that there is a constitutional submicroscopic deletion, (Cowell *et al.* 1986). These patients also have the heritable form of Rb. Junien *et al.* (1982) have shown that it is possible to measure esterase D activity in amniotic fluid. Presumably, this could also be carried out on chorionic villus cells, but this has not yet been done.

Of 200 of Cowell *et al.*'s (1986) Rb patients, 9(4.5%) had low red cell ESD levels and 5 had not previously been diagnosed as deletion carriers. A particular case in point was described by Cowell *et al.* (1987a) of a boy with unilateral Rb and no family history of Rb. The parents were counselled that sibling and offspring risks to their affected child were 2% and 6%, respectively. Although the karyotype was originally reported as normal, the red cell ESD level in the affected child was 50%; the levels in his parents were normal, indicating that a fresh germline mutation causing a deletion had occurred in the affected boy. Re-examination of the karyotype revealed a small 13q14 deletion. The parents were recounselled that the risks to siblings were extremely small but that risks to the offspring of their affected child approached 50%.

It is possible that measurement of ESD levels could miss some deletions in which the Rb but not the ESD locus was involved, but only two such cases have been reported (Cowell *et al.* 1987a).

Finally, it is important to note that *normal* ESD levels do not mean the case is *non*-hereditary. The mutation which disrupts the Rb locus may not necessarily be a deletion. Low ESD levels however, allow a heritable deletion case to be identified.

OTHER METHODS OF PREDICTIVE TESTING

Linkage of electrophoretic variants of ESD to the Rb Gene

ESD occurs in two electrophoretic variants designated type 1 and type 2 (Hopkinson *et al.* 1973). A given individual can be ESD 1–1, ESD 2–2 or ESD 1–2. Because the ESD and Rb loci are closely linked, these variants of ESD can be used to track the Rb gene in families in a linkage study. Fig. 9.3 shows an example of a family which is informative for prenatal or pre-symptomatic screening. Clearly Rb is tracking with

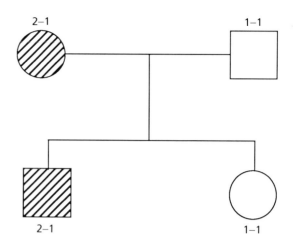

Fig. 9.3 Familial retinoblastoma. Predictive tests using the Esterase D protein polymorphism. The affected mother passed the type 2 allele to her affected son and the father clearly passed the type 1 allele to both children. The sister of the affected boy inherited the type 1 allele from mother, and is predicted to be unaffected with Rb.

the 2-allele in this example. The electrophoretic variants of ESD can be detected in chorion villus samples and cord blood, so that this approach can be used for prenatal diagnosis (Cowell *et al.* 1987b). A limiting factor is that the 2-allele occurs at a frequency of only about 12% in the population, so that the number of heterozygotes will be few. Cowell *et al.* (1987b) found that only about 10–15% of 41 Rb families were informative using this method. Nevertheless, the determination of the ESD polymorphism is easy and quick and the reliability of the test is good; no recombinations between the ESD and Rb loci have yet been observed (Squire *et al.* 1986).

DNA polymorphisms

1 Flanking markers: Predictive tests in informative families have been undertaken using DNA markers which lie outside the Rb gene where two markers flank the gene (Cavenee *et al.* 1986).
2 Intragenic markers: Now that the Rb gene has been localized, DNA polymorphisms *within* the Rb locus have been identified and can be used for predictive tests. The first prenatal diagnoses using intragenic markers were reported by Mitchell *et al.* (1988) and Wiggs *et al.* (1988). An example of a predictive test using intragenic markers is shown in Fig. 9.4. The authors point out that because the marker is within the gene, the risk of recombination between the gene and the marker is small, so that the test is very reliable. There is, however, a very small theoretical

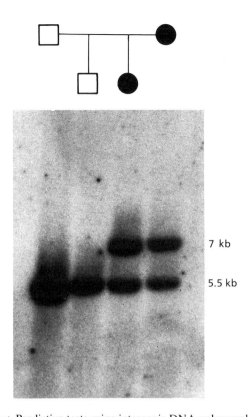

Fig. 9.4 Predictive tests using intragenic DNA polymorphisms. The family has been studied with probe p88PRO.6 using the restriction enzyme Xba1 which reveals a 2 allele polymorphism. The smaller lower band is 5.5 kb (kilobases) in length and the upper band is 7 kb. The affected daughter inherited the 7 kb band from her affected mother. In this family, the retinoblastoma predisposing gene is tracking with the 7 kb band. The father is homozygous for the 5.5 kb band. The son inherited a 5.5 kb band from father and from mother and so is predicted not to be at risk of retinoblastoma. (Father's band looks larger than son's because there is more DNA in the track.) (Photograph by courtesy of Dr. C. Mitchell.)

risk that the actual mutation and the marker could become separated at meiosis (Wiggs *et al.* 1988). Wiggs *et al.* (1988) also reported predictive testing using intragenic markers in 20 kindreds. Predictions could be made in 19 (95%); the other family was complicated by uncertainty about the clinical diagnosis in a key family member. Their conservative estimate (95% confidence interval) of error rate in this method of diagnosis of a predisposition to cancer is less than 12%. As more data accumulates, the error rate is expected to fall. As mentioned above, the results may depend on correct paternity.

3 Direct analysis of the mutation: Horsthemke *et al.* (1987) used direct analysis of the mutation (a very small deletion) in DNA from peripheral blood in three of 11 unrelated patients with familial Rb. A specific DNA sequence detected a heterozygous submicroscopic deletion. They point out that this gives a firm prediction, since the mutation itself is detected, but other authors note that technical difficulties can be encountered (Mitchell *et al.* 1988).

4 Sporadic cases: So far, predictive testing has been limited to familial Rb. It would however, be possible to *exclude* the predisposition to Rb in some siblings of cases with no family history. If the sibling of an affected child shared no Rb gene allele in common with the affected child, then the sibling would be at very low risk of developing the tumour and frequent examinations under anaesthetic could perhaps be avoided (Fig. 9.5).

Similarly, if it could be shown in a sporadic bilateral case whose constitutional karyotype is normal but in whom the tumour itself contained a deletion say in the maternally derived allele, then it might be reasonable to expect that the paternally derived allele is the one which carries a germline mutation. This information could be used to offer a prenatal test to the patient in the future. The same would be true of a familial case in whom the pedigree structure did not allow the abnormal allele to be identified, if for example, an affected parent had died. For this reason, it is important to arrange to store DNA from all Rb tumours and national registers of Rb are useful to help co-ordinate the arrangements (Jay *et al.* 1988).

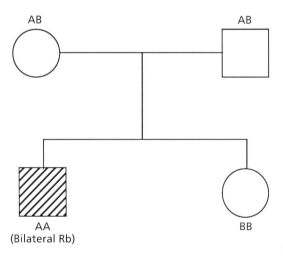

Fig. 9.5 Sporadic retinoblastoma: use of intragenic DNA polymorphisms in a sporadic case to exclude risk to siblings. Since the sibling of the affected boy has no alleles in common with her brother, it is unlikely that she carries the predisposition to Rb, even if one parent has the predisposing gene but has not manifested Rb.

References

Abramson DH, Ellsworth RM, Kitchin FD, Tung G. Second nonocular tumours in retinoblastoma survivors. *Ophthalmology* 1984; **91**: 1351−5

Balaban G, Gilbert F, Nichols W, Meadows AT, Shields J. Abnormalities of chromosome 13 in retinoblastomas from individuals with normal constitutional karyotypes. *Cancer Genet Cytogenet* 1982; **6**: 213−21

Benedict WF, Murphree AL, Banerjee A, Spina CA, Sparkes MC, Sparkes RS. Patients with 13 chromosome deletion: evidence that the retinoblastoma gene is a recessive cancer gene. *Science* 1983; **219**: 973−5

Buchanan JA, Cavanee WK. Review article. Genetic markers for assessment of retinoblastoma predisposition. *Disease Markers* 1987; **5**: 141−52

Carlson EA, Desnick RJ. Mutational mosaicism and genetic counselling in retinoblastoma. *Am J Med Genet* 1979; **4**: 365−81

Cavenee WK, Dryja TP, Phillips RA *et al*. Expression of recessive alleles by chromosomal mechanisms in retinoblastoma. *Nature* 1983; **305**: 779−84

Cavenee WK, Murphree AL, Shull MM, Benedict WF, Sparkes RS, Kock E, Nordenskjold M. Prediction of familial predisposition to retinoblastoma. *N. Engl J Med* 1986; **314**: 1201−7

Cowell JK, Jay M, Rutland P, Hungerford J. An assessment of the usefulness of electrophoretic variants of esterase-D in the antenatal diagnosis of retinoblastoma in the United Kingdom *Br J Cancer* 1987b; **55**: 661−4

Cowell JK, Rutland P, Jay M, Hungerford J. Deletions of the esterase D locus from a survey of 200 retinoblastoma patients. *Hum Genet* 1986; **72**: 164−7

Cowell JK, Thompson E, Rutland P. The need to screen all retinoblastoma patients for esterase D activity: Detection of submicroscopic chromosome deletions. *Arch Dis Child* 1987a; **62**: 8−11

de la Chapelle A, Sankila EM, Lindlof M, Aula P, Norio R. Norrie disease caused by a gene deletion allowing carrier detection and prenatal diagnosis. *Clin Genet* 1985; **28**: 317−20

Donnai D, Mountford RC, Read AP. Norrie disease resulting from a gene deletion: clinical features and DNA studies. *J Med Genet* 1988; **25**: 73−8

Dryja TP, Cavenee W, White R, Rapaport JM, Peterson R, Albert DM, Bruns GAP. Homozygosity of chromosome 13 in retinoblastoma. *N Engl J Med* 1984; **310**: 550−3

Emery AEH. *An Introduction to Recombinant DNA*. John Wiley & Sons, Chichester 1988

Friend SH, Bernards R, Rogelj S, Weinberg RA, Rapaport JM, Albert DM, Dryja TP. A human DNA segment with properties of the gene that predisposes to retinoblastoma and osteosarcoma. *Nature* 1986; **323**: 643−6

Gal A, Stolzenberger C, Wienker TF *et al*. Norrie's disease: close linkage with genetic markers from the proximal short arm of the X chromosome. *Clin Genet* 1985(a); **27**: 282−3

Gal A, Bleeker-Wagemakers L, Wienker TF, Warburg M, Ropers HH. Localisation of the gene for Norrie's disease by linkage to the DXS7 Locus. HGM8. *Cytogenet Cell Genet* 1985(b); **40**: 633

Hopkinson DA, Mestriner MA, Cortner J, Harris H. Esterase D: A new human polymorphism. *Ann J Hum Genet* 1973; **37**: 119−37

Horsthemke B, Barnet HJ, Greger V, Passage E, Hopping W. Early diagnosis in hereditary retinoblastoma by detection of molecular deletions at gene locus. *Lancet* 1987; Feb. **28**: 511−512

Jay M, Cowell J, Hungerford J. Register of retinoblastoma: preliminary results. *Eye* 1988; **2**: 102−105

Junien C, Despoisse S, Turleau C *et al*. Retinoblastoma deletion 13 q 14 and esterase D: Application of gene dosage effect to prenatal diagnosis. *Cancer Genet Cytogenet* 1982; **6**: 281−7

Kivlin JD, Sanborn GE, Wright E, Cannon L, Carey J. Further linkage data on Norrie disease. *Am J Med Genet* 1987; **26**: 733−6

Knudson AG. Mutation and cancer: A statistical study of retinoblastoma. *Proc Natl Acad Sci USA* 1971; **68**: 820−3

Mitchell C, Nicolaides K, Kingston J, Hungerford J, Jay M, Cowell J. Prenatal exclusion of hereditary retinoblastoma. *Lancet* 1988; April **9**: 826

Murphree AL, Benedict WF. Retinoblastoma: Clues to human oncogenesis. *Science* 1984; **223**: 1028−33

Poulton J. Mitochondrial DNA and genetic disease. *Arch Dis Child* 1988; **63**: 883−5

Sparkes RS, Sparkes MC, Wilson MG *et al*. Regional assignment of genes for human esterase D and retinoblastoma to chromosome band 13 q 14. *Science* 1980; **208**: 1042−4

Sparkes RS, Murphree AL, Lingua RW, Sparkes MC, Field LL, Funderbunk SJ, Benedict WF. Gene for hereditary retinoblastoma assigned to human chromosome 13 by linkage to esterase-D. *Science* 1983; **219**: 971−3

Squire J, Dryja TP, Dunn J *et al*. Cloning of the Esterase D Gene: A polymorphic gene probe closely linked to the retinoblastoma locus on chromosome 13. *Proc Natl Acad Sci USA* 1986; **83** 6573−7

Vogel F. Genetics of retinoblastoma. *Hum Genet* 1979; **52**: 1−54

Warburg M. Norrie's disease, a congenital progressive oculo-acoustico-cerebral degeneration. *Acta Ophthalmol* (Suppl.) *Kbh* 1966; **89**: 1−147

Weatherall DJ. *The New Genetics and Clinical Practice*. Oxford University Press, Oxford 1985

Wiggs J, Nordenskjold M, Yandell D, *et al*. Prediction of the risk of hereditary retinoblastoma, using DNA polymorphisms within the retinoblastoma gene. *New Engl J Med* 1988; **318**: 151−7

Yunis JJ, Ramsay N. Retinoblastoma and subband deletion of chromosome 13. *Am J Dis Child* 1978; **132**: 161−3

10 The Visually Handicapped Baby and the Family

DAVID TAYLOR

Although it is preferable to work with, or refer to, a paediatrician or another professional with a special interest in the development of visually handicapped or multiply handicapped children, the ophthalmologist and general paediatrician must learn to understand the needs of the visually impaired baby and his family. By understanding the whole family's needs their shock and pain of having a child with special needs will be eased, and the baby himself will be helped to best overcome his handicap.

The blind child

Effect of visual handicap on the baby

The absence or blunting of sight from birth has effects that stretch far beyond the simple loss of vision because vision is necessary in the development of other primary senses and perceptions and also for normal social integration.

Early in the baby's life, as any parent knows, there is a deep bond that forms aided by visual communication — the mother *knows* that her baby is not just pointing both his eyes at her but actually communicating and their relationship builds on that early interaction. The poverty of facial expression of a blind child may be a problem to the parents unless it is explained that they only show extremes of facial expressions, that the smile may be rather fixed and that their face becomes passive when they are concentrating on speech.

The meaning of things touched such as other parts of the child's body, other people or objects, is enhanced by the use of vision. In a sighted child, the full meaning of an object that is explored by touch may be gained, it is in reference to a visual memory of that object; because a blind baby lacks this visual memory his tactile exploration is less rewarding.

Sight is partly necessary for the learning of speech; the baby mimicks the parent's lip movements and by also using his hearing to modify the sounds he makes, speech is formed. Sightless babies do not turn their head towards a source of sound nearly as accurately, as quickly, or as persistently as sighted babies.

The blind baby is very late in appreciating the disposition of the world around him in three dimensions. Sounds, touch, and other communication reach him as though from anywhere and it is a long time before he builds up a 'map' or frame of reference that is similar to that of a sighted person. The concept of permanence of the surroundings, and perspective are difficult to grasp — perspective in particular is almost impossible for a blind person to understand. Descriptions of brightness and colour are meaningless and names of colours with second meanings (such as blue, yellow, purple) probably mean less as well!

The social interaction of a blind child with other blind or with sighted children is more difficult; their lack of mobility, sometimes odd appearance and delay in other areas of development makes them poor companions for sighted children. Even as toddlers, the blind have greater difficulties in socialising and interacting in their play groups and in infant school. This pattern, set in early life, persists, although at some stage many children over-react against it, and go through a precocious stage that lasts a variable period. Later they often lack drive, initiative and independence, and tend to prefer their own company or that of close relatives.

Blind babies who do not have appropriate help in the early years, especially if they have additional handicaps, are at risk of developing a form of autism the effects of which are lifelong and may be devastating.

There is little doubt that advice and help can enable many parents to help their child to lead a more fulfilling life.

The older visually handicapped children

The advantage of referring a visually handicapped child to an expert in child development is that they can get specific help and preventitive advice, so that it is best to refer them routinely and as early as possible. Every ophthalmologist, and paediatrician involved in the case of visually handicapped children should read about the subject — a book such as that of Jan, Freeman & Scott (Jan *et al.* 1985) may give insight into the problems and how to help them. It is helpful if the advice given is consistent and even offered before a problem arises, so the ophthalmologist and general paediatrician should be conversant with the main problems that confront blind babies. It is important that a strong, early relationship builds up between the doctor, the parents and children and that it is based on mutual trust and respect.

The advice given has to be tailored to each child's needs, so that, for example specific advice regarding schooling in the later years is not usually the province of the primary doctor but of the educators, agencies and local authorities working in concert. Especially if there are multiple handicaps, the doctors will be re-quired to give advice about not only the child's visual capabilities but also how these problems interact with the other handicaps.

Mannerisms and stereotyped behaviour

Blind children develop a wide variety of mannerisms; eye-poking or rubbing, body rocking, head banging, light seeking or sun staring, making repetitive noise, and even, in severe cases usually associated with mental retardation, self mutilation. There is no clear cause for these abnormal forms of behaviour but it may be related to the way in which they are handled in early life. Early intervention by encouraging the parents to handle the baby frequently and to keep him occupied for much of his waking hours may help. Once the mannerisms have become established it is very difficult to stop them. Most doctors involved with visually handicapped children do not recommend psychiatric treatment by adversive therapy, preferring to encourage the parents to intervene when the child is employing the mannerism and substitute it for another one with less risk and that is less socially odd; for instance to change eye-rubbing for thumb-sucking.

Self image, self esteem and cosmetic problems

Cosmetic problems, such as an ugly appearance of the eyes, a squint or roving eye movements need to be considered early because of their potential to alter the way other people may react to the baby. Older children, where reasonably possible, should be reassured that they are nice-looking as this will all help with their confidence and self esteem which is easily shaken and often only rises to levels that would be considered low in sighted people.

Psychological and psychiatric problems

Psychiatric problems are more common in blind children, and especially those with multiple handicaps. Many of these problems, including the autistic behaviour of some blind children may be prevented by appropriate early management but once established require expert help. Behaviour disorders, personality abnormalities, manipulative behaviour are all frequent and require patience and understanding together with pre-emptive counselling as a way of prevention by appropriate handling. Interestingly, depression is probably no more frequent in blind than sighted children.

Sport and mobility

One of the major difficulties in social interaction and the building of self esteem is the immobility of blind children and their inability to take part in games and sport like sighted children. It is only very rare that blind or partially sighted children need to be excluded from sport and activity on the grounds that it might endanger their eyes, so the main reasons why they don't take part are visual. Water sports, even sailing, skiing, walking, running, pottery, woodcarving, sulpture, tandem bicycle riding, gymnastics, and many other activities can be done by blind children, but from very early on the parents need to be encouraged to let their child take part in the rough and tumble of nursery games and to stifle their natural desire to overprotect the child.

The degree to which a visually handicapped child is mobile depends on several factors: intelligence, the amount of vision that he has, how well and how early he was encouraged to be mobile, the type of visual defect, when he became blind and above all his drive and personality. Mobility is essential to achieve independence and it usually requires a very high degree of commitment to training by the child, his parents and the agencies.

The parents and other family members

Impact of the diagnosis on the parents

Most parents react positively to the diagnosis of blindness in their child but may react in a negative and even destructive way. However, even those who have an outwardly calm demeanour will later admit that the realization of the extent of the visual handicap and its awesome implications on their and their children's lives brought with it the most difficult time in their lives.

Parents may react with a mixture of anger, resentment, terror and aggression in varying mixtures which may be destructive and against the best interests of their child. These reactions start early and until they are overcome they only make things worse for the child; they are all made worse by the lack of a cure, the absence of a diagnosis, the making of a diagnosis that is later changed, and the great uncertainty about the future.

The uncertainly is compounded by a changing handicap, uncertainty about the medical diagnosis and prognosis, a failure by the parents to be able to grasp the full impact of the diagnosis and much deeper worries about the educational implications (will it take him away from home?), genetic worries, and rarely discussed but none the less important concerns about the cause (is it a throwback, was it anything that the parents did?).

Early and positive intervention and good consistent advice can help prevent all of these worries.

When and how to talk to the parents

Every doctor will acquire his own way of doing this very rewarding but difficult job but it is generally best to save the definitive discussion until the diagnosis is established, if this is not immediately obvious. A preliminary discussion will be necessary until the diagnosis is established to keep the parents informed of the plan of investigation and how much is known so far.

Repeated interviews are very helpful, as even the most intelligent parents (or their doctor!) can remember only a few items from each interview. It is essential to give them plenty of time for questions and to leave an open invitation to come back at any time. To write with their questions is a helpful invitation but it is surprisingly rarely taken up by the parents.

The way in which the parents questions are answered is vital. A friendly, simple approach using simple diagrams and no jargon, will help the parents to understand the defect and its impact on the life of their baby, and on the rest of the family. It is essential to be honest about how much or how little you know; it is just as important to most parents to know the limits of your knowledge about their child's problem as it is to know how much you know.

The role of the first adviser is by far the most difficult. Very few non-ophthalmologists understand how difficult it is to be the first adviser in the chain of visual handicap experts that the parents of a blind child are helped by. The first ophthalmologist is often blamed by the parents and their later advisers, sometimes with justification, because he has been too blunt, too indirect, too evasive, too insensitive, etc.; perhaps the later adviser should try being the first!

The meaning of visual handicap to a family

'Blindness', 'partial sight', 'visual handicap', 'blunted sight' all have different meanings to different people. Statutory definitions usually involve the ability of the child to be educated by sighted or non-sighted means, or in older people regarding employment. A child may be blind from the educational point of view but able to behave almost normally until the time comes for him to read and write. It is vital to define for the parents what you mean by any of these terms, for instance to define that blindness does not necessarily mean to be stone blind and a child may be able to do numerous things whilst still being registered blind. The commonest mistake is to be too pessimistic which makes things more difficult for the parents. Be accurate as far as you can and build up the value of the residual vision. Even ability to perceive light only is better than no perception of light. Use all the diagnostic aids at your disposal but rely most on clinical judgement as this is still what will give you the best guide. It is probably not an exaggeration to say that the parents should not be told the child is stone blind unless he is anophthalmic!

Other children in the family can be profoundly affected by the blind sibling and show reactions of anger, jealousy because of the attention the child gets, hysterical conversion symptoms, attention-seeking behaviour difficulties, and embarassment because of the appearance of the child. There is no one way to handle these problems, but pre-emptive advice to the parents on not overprotecting the blind baby (or the sibling), being fair in their attentions especially early in the life of the handicapped baby, and being equal in their rewards and punishment, all help to make the normal sibling feel at least equal. The sighted older sibling can be given special responsibilities for the blind baby and often reacts positively to this. It is important to let the children sort out their own interpersonal problems and for the parents to interfere as little as possible.

Second opinion

It is better to suggest a second opinion to the parents. It is more confidence building for the parents if the suggestion comes from the doctor but if the parents or their other advisers suggest it first it is only possible to co-operate whole-heartedly with the suggestion. When the first specialist suggests a second opinion he can usually influence to whom the child is referred to make sure that the best opinion is obtained.

Positive ways of helping

Early and positive intervention

The diagnosis of a severe visual handicap need not be accompanied by negative advice as the parents are often aware of what a blind child cannot do and they need positive advice to help them to help their child (they need to know what he can do). This is not just a way of 'keeping them occupied' but appropriate advice can help the baby to make the best of his life.

Starting the advice early (early 'intervention') is helpful not only to the baby but it can help the parents in the early days to live with the awful shock of the discovery of blindness in their child.

One of the most common reactions of the parents is to feel overawed by their babies problems and to have a rather stand–offish attitude to the child, they treat him like porcelain. It is good to show them that he is like any other baby and can enjoy all the cuddling, playing and the gentle rough and tumble that sighted children get.

Any residual vision, however little, should be encouraged by stimuli appropriate to the visual defect: lights, mirrors, brightly coloured, and coarse patterned toys, especially toys that have interesting and different textures and preferably ones which make a noise.

Helping the child to learn to explore things with his hands can be started from birth. The parents can be encouraged to hold their baby close to them and to hold his hands to their faces to explore them.

The more auditory–tactile stimuli that the blind baby gets the better will he learn to understand and react to new stimuli later.

Physiotherapy

Home physiotherapy and posture-improving exercises are advised by some experts who rightly note that the odd posture and manerisms of blind children may be one of their difficulties in communication with others.

Consistent advice, where possible from the same doctor or other adviser, is very much to be encouraged; as in other areas inconsistently leads to loss of confidence and failure to take any advice. Unfortunately not many state medical systems make this possible.

Other family members

Other children in the family need to be remembered. It is very easy for them to be overlooked by the parents in their desire to do their best for the blind child; they can often be encouraged to help the baby with visual stimulation and just general play, with mutual benefit.

The parents of a blind child are often so involved with the immediate problems that it is very easy for them to overlook the needs of their own parents. The baby's grandparents are often less able to accept his problem than the parents but they can be given help by the parents who should be encouraged to involve the grandparents in any discussion and in getting them to help with the day-to-day life of the baby; not least in baby-sitting while the parents get out by themselves.

The burdens (and the joys) should be shared between all the members of the family. Often the doctor can be helpful if he identifies the 'expert' parent or grandparent; one who takes on all the tasks, reads and knows all about blindness, and tends to exclude other members.

When there is no treatment

Three-quarters of child blindness is totally untreatable. The parents often expect that treatment will be available somewhere or sometime; we have been so bombarded with news reports of medical breakthroughs that many people believe that most conditions are treatable.

A frank discussion, emphasizing that although no formal cure is possible there is still a lot that can be done for the child, and that no cure is available anywhere else (if this is true) will help the parents to accept the situation and look forward positively. In this respect it is often best to broach the subject of eye transplant to the parents and to tell them why no such operation is possible or is likely to be possible in the future. Many parents think that a transplant (of one of their eyes) might help the baby but some are too shy to bring up the question themselves.

Simple support measures

Most support measures are the province of the blind agency workers or others local to the family's home but it is important for all to be aware of the possibility of helping the parents and the rest of the family by simple means.

It may be possible to arrange help with baby sitting, either for evenings or parts of weekends so that the parents can be together and go to do things such as shopping, meeting the bank manager, visiting friends, etc. whilst being confident that the child is safe and happy. Longer-term child care, short-term fostering, or even admission to hospital, nursing home or childrens home for short periods may enable parents to go on holiday together or for the wife to accompany the husband on business or visit her husband who is working away from home.

When the day-to-day management of the child is a major stress factor in a family it may be possible to reduce the burden, and increase the familys positive attitude towards the child by arranging for the child to board at a school or home during the week, coming home at the weekends.

Blindness agency workers may have access to a toy library of suitable toys for visually handicapped children. These workers become very expert at understanding and helping parents and perform a valuable service in the broader management of the child; by intervention, advice, and counselling.

Specific problems for the family

Lack of bonding

The lack of mutual visual communication, together with the shock of the diagnosis and many other factors can give rise to an incomplete bonding or even a source of rejection or distancing in the parents. These feelings probably reflect on the child and affect him too. It is best prevented by early intervention and encouraging bodily contact and baby-game playing together with the other aspects of visual stimulation.

Guilty feelings

Many parents feel a sense of guilt that they have brought a handicapped child into the world; this is most especially so if the cause is thought to be genetic, due to prenatal infection or drug ingestion or postnatal injury. The effect of these feelings can be all-consuming with harmful effects on both parents, the baby and the rest of the family: many are irrational but many are founded on lack of understanding of the condition and its cause, so the best remedy is in the fullest explanation and early intervention.

Family stress

Whilst the birth of a blind baby can result in a deeper and stronger relationship between the parents and other members of the family it very frequently results in enormous stresses within the family. The parents may argue, start to drink alcohol heavily or behave aggressively towards each other or their children, and the marriage may break up especially if there were pre-existing problems. The ophthalmologist is usually in no position to help here; it is usually the paediatrician, health worker or blindness agency worker who is in closer contact and who may be able to help in small but positive ways.

Parents who reject help

Sometimes the reaction of the parents is very strongly against what is seen as the conventional medical wisdom especially if the doctors are seen as failing to provide a cure. They may fail to recognise the handicap and are determined to treat their child as normal until he 'gets better' or they reject any help or counselling. This is quite a common problem, in varying degree, and it can be handled in various ways but it is unlikely to be resolved by forcing or bullying the parents who, providing the physical and mental welfare of the child is being looked after, are usually well within their rights. Usually the best approach is to maintain contact and there are often small problems that the parents can be helped with that may gradually establish a useful relationship again between the parents and the doctor. Again prevention by early and positive advice is the best cure.

Genetic counselling

Unless the cause of the child's blindness is clearly non-genetic, such as in cases of proven (not suspected), congenital infection, the parents should be encouraged to have genetic counselling. Even if the condition is not obviously hereditary, or if the diagnosis is not known there is usually a lot that the geneticist can do to help the parents either in diagnosis by association of ocular and non-ocular conditions, by giving empirical recurrence risks or by newer forms of genetic and chromosomal investigation. Advice is also helpful for older children and young adults who may be concerned about their chances of passing on the defect. Around one half of blind children have an hereditary condition.

Parents groups

In many parts of the world parents meet in self help groups. These may be disease orientated, i.e. rubella or retinitis pigmentosa, or handicap based, i.e. deaf–blind or partially sighted, and the parents meet for discussion of mutual problems, or act as local or nationwide pressure groups. Some of the disease-orientated groups have charity status and raise money for research. Some parents get great comfort and help from these groups but initially it is often best to arrange for a meeting with one parent, on the understanding that the 'new' parent of a blind baby realizes

that no two cases are the same. It is often very reassuring to the new parent to hear how the older child is getting on and managing; often much better than the new parent would have guessed.

Multiple handicaps

Further handicaps do not just add to the visual handicap, they multiply it. One of the biggest problems that faces the parent is that numerous experts become involved. It is therefore most important that there is only one conductor to the medical orchestra (usually it is best if this is a paediatrician with a special interest in handicap) and that he works in close co-operation with, and preferably geographically close to the specialists. Multi-disciplinary teams are one way of getting around this problem although they may be a relatively inefficient use of specialists time. If the care can be confined within one hospital and the number of visits curtailed there is an enormous saving of the parents time, money and stress.

Visual problems are frequent in children with developmental delay and there is a high incidence of other defects in children with poor vision. Vigilance for both is necessary to give the child his best chance in life.

Mental retardation is defined by the World Health Organization as 'incomplete or insufficient general development of mental capacities'. There are many other definitions.

In the UK the term educationally subnormal (ESN) is used, with moderate (M) or severe (S) sub-classifications. ESN(M) children have IQs between 50 and 69, and ESN(S) children have IQs below 50; those below 30 usually being designated profound ESN(S).

In assessing the ability of visually handicapped children special tests are necessary to reduce the effect of the visual handicap on the childs performance (Reynell & Zinkin 1979).

Chromosomal abnormalities (e.g. Down's syndrome) genetic conditions (e.g. the phakomatoses) 'acquired' causes such as congenital infections, ante-partum haemorrhage or toxaemia and intrauterine growth retardation, or prenatal toxic effects (such as drugs and alcohol), are all important prenatal causes. Perinatal anoxia is a large cause of cerebral palsy and many affected children are also mentally retarded. Postnatal damage is a less frequent cause of mental retardation in most developed countries; nonetheless malnutrition, deprived social conditions as well as meningitis, hydrocephalus, hypoglycaemia, encephalitis, and trauma (including non-accidental injury) all play their role. One form of epilepsy in infancy is the so called infantile spasm which is characteristically a generalized seizure with spasm in flexion. Many children who have infantile spasms appear to be blind as their EEG is grossly abnormal and they are constantly fitting and most of these children turn out to be substantially mentally retarded even when the spasms are controlled. They may have structural brain disease, e.g. tuberose sclerosis, or Aicardi's syndrome (in which infantile spasms, agenesis of the corpus collosum, ectopic grey matter and characteristic retinal defects are associated in girls). Neurometabolic disease such as phenylketanuria, Tay Sachs, or Batten's disease are unusual associations of epilepsy with blindness and congenital infections are uncommon but significantly preventable causes.

The apparently poor vision in these children appears to improve as the fits are controlled and mental development occurs.

Cerebral palsy (CP) is a common cause of disability in childhood. It is a motor defect due to non-progressive brain damage in infancy or early childhood. It may be characterised by spasticity, rigidity, athetosis, ataxia, or occasionally tremor or it may be mixed. Various forms occur such as hemiplegia, or doube hemiplegia (tetraplegia) diplegia (bilateral but legs more affected than arms) or athetoid (with involuntary movements being present). From the ophthalmologist's point of view the two commonest problems in CP are optic atrophy and squint. Optic atrophy is common in children with perinatal anoxia as the cause of their CP and its effects are often multiplied by the presence of widespread cerebral damage. Early diagnosis is important so as to institute early intervention. Squints in CP children should be treated in just the same way as in normal children. There is often a temptation to think one is being kind to spare a CP child surgery just for cosmetic reasons. The cosmetic indication is even more important in a CP child, who has already a good enough reason for strangers reacting oddly with him, and in any case some CP children with squints may develop useful binocular vision if treated appropriately. Caution should be exercised with surgery as they often make a larger response than usual to standard amounts of surgery and consecutive squints are frequent.

Education

PLAYGROUPS

Preschool contact with other blind and with sighted children is helpful in improving the blind child's confidence and inquisitiveness. Many ordinary playgroups will accept visually handicapped babies and young children and in some areas there are playgroups attached to schools for older visually handicapped children.

PRESCHOOL TRAINING

It is important to start thinking about education long before the child actually needs to go to school. The availability of special education and extra help with education in a normal school varies enormously from country to country and in different areas within each country. The visual defect needs to be registered so that the education authorities are aware of the further needs of the child and of the needs for special education within a community. The earlier these needs are known the easier it is to arrange for appropriate education. Registration may be delayed, or the categorisation left uncertain if the vision of the child is changing but in general it is still best for the child's handicap to be registered and his needs recognised for the future.

There is a very strong trend towards integration of children into local schools, either in the normal classroom for those with minimal defect or into a local special school for visual handicap, the type of education offered depending on the visual abilities of the child and the presence of any other handicap. Many normal schools have visual handicap units in them, offering specialized extra help in teaching together with special facilities for the partially sighted such as closed circuit TV reading aids.

Special boarding schools are usually available for older children and may have the advantage of being able to offer special facilities and a better environment.

The agency responsible for placement varies from country to country but ultimately it is the parent who has to decide on the best of the alternatives on offer. The school which has the right atmosphere and facilities for the child's combination of defects is often difficult to find near to the parent's home and there has to be a major commitment to travelling throughout the child's education. The parents will need to visit all the schools available and to have discussion with the staff before they can be sure of their choice and time will show a proportion that theirs was not the right choice!

Although integration into the sighted community is the aim, in many countries there can be little doubt that there is still a role for boarding schools for certain categories of children.

The young and some older multiply handicapped children may fare better in a more ordered environment and his family may benefit from a rest from his demands during the week in cases where weekly boarding is possible.

The older child may benefit from the special facilities available, from the training of the staff, and from contact with other children in the same predicament.

Bibliography for parents

Carson S, Arthbertson D, Frobes C. *Off to a good start!* A rescue manual for parents of young blind and visually impaired children (largely for those in Massachusetts, USA, but with ideas for others). Massachusetts International Institute for the Visually Impaired, Newton, Mass., USA

Heart to heart. Parents of blind and partially sighted children talk about their feelings. Blind Children's Center, 4120 Marathan Street, PO Box 29159, Los Angeles, California 90029, USA

Scott EP, Jan JE, Freeman RD. *Can't Your Child See?*, 2nd edn. Pro-Ed 5341 Industrial Oaks Bvd, Austin, Texas 78735, USA 1985

References

Brett EM. *Paediatric Neurology.* Churchill Livingston, London 1983

Fraiberg S. *Insights from the blind: Comparative Studies of Blind and Sighted Infants.* Basie Books, New York 1977

Jan JE, Freeman RD, Scott EP. *Visual impairment in children and adolescents.* Grune & Stratton, New York, London 1977

Reynell J, Zinkin P. Developmental aids for young visually handicapped children. *Child Care Health Dev* 1: 1979; 61−9

Wybar KC, Taylor DSI. (Eds.) The visually handicapped child. In *Paediatric ophthalmology − current aspects.* Marcel Dekker, New York & Basel 1983, pp. 85−141

Section 3
Infectious, Allergic and External Eye Disorders

hepatosplenomegaly, thrombocytopenic purpura, microcephaly, osteopathy, lymphadenopathy, diabetes, a retinal pigmentary disturbance, glaucoma, and keratitis (Alfano 1966; Wolff 1972). They also have abnormal dermaglyphics (Purvis Smith 1969) with an increased frequency of fingertip whorl pattern. CT scanning shows low-density areas and flecks of calcification of the white matter, and calcification in the basal ganglia (Ishikawa *et al.* 1982).

The prevalence of these abnormalities correlates closely with the gestational stage during which the rubella infection occurs. Intrauterine infections during the first 3 months of pregnancy result in a 50% incidence of the rubella embryopathy (Hanshaw *et al.* 1985), whereas infections after the fourth gestational month rarely result in the full rubella syndrome (Manson *et al.* 1960).

Cataracts are present in 20% of children with the congenital rubella syndrome (Hertzberg 1968). They are bilateral 75% of the time and conform closely to Greg's original description (Fig. 11.1). The rubella virus has been cultured from the cataractous lenses of children with the congenital rubella syndrome up to 4 years of age and is probably responsible for the intense inflammatory response that may occur after cataract surgery (Cotlier 1966).

The most common ocular abnormality of the congenital rubella syndrome is a pigmentary retinopathy (Marks 1946). It is usually bilateral and is present in 40% of affected patients. The retinopathy is characterized by mottled pigmentary changes throughout the fundi most marked at the posterior pole (Fig. 11.2). Although progression of the pigmentary changes may occur, the vision typically remains 6/12 or better (Hertzberg 1968; Collis 1970). Rarely subretinal neovascularization may occur with a precipitous fall in the visual acuity (Fig. 11.3). The electrooculogram is usually normal, suggesting the function of the retinal pigment epithelium is not affected by the pigment mottling (Krill, 1967). Electroretinograms may show subtle abnormalities. A pigment disturbance of the iris is common (Fig. 11.4).

The corneas of infants with the rubella syndrome may be hazy either secondary to a keratitis or less commonly to an elevation in the intraocular pressure (Fig. 11.5). The intraocular pressure is usually normal when the cornea is hazy from keratitis. The keratitis typically clears in weeks or a few months. Glaucoma is found most frequently in microphthalmic eyes (Fig. 11.6) and is usually bilateral (Wolff 1972). It has been estimated to occur in 10% of children with the congenital rubella syndrome (Sears 1967).

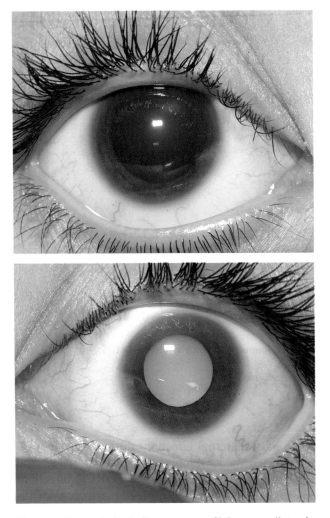

Fig. 11.1 Congenital rubella cataract. 25% have a unilateral cataract associated with microphthalmos. Virus can be grown from the lens up to 4 years of age.

The development of an attenuated rubella virus vaccine and its subsequent widespread usage beginning in 1969 has dramatically decreased the incidence of the congenital rubella syndrome (Meyer *et al.* 1966; Krugman 1969). Whereas 30 000 children were estimated to have been born with the congenital rubella syndrome during the rubella epidemic of 1964 in the USA, only four were born with the syndrome in 1983 (Krugman *et al.* 1985).

Toxoplasmosis

Intrauterine toxoplasmosis was first recognized as a cause of chorioretinitis and intracranial calcification in 1939 (Wolf *et al.* 1939). Chorioretinitis is the most frequently recognized feature of the congenital toxoplasmosis syndrome. Other less common findings

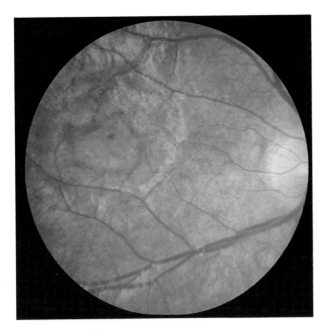

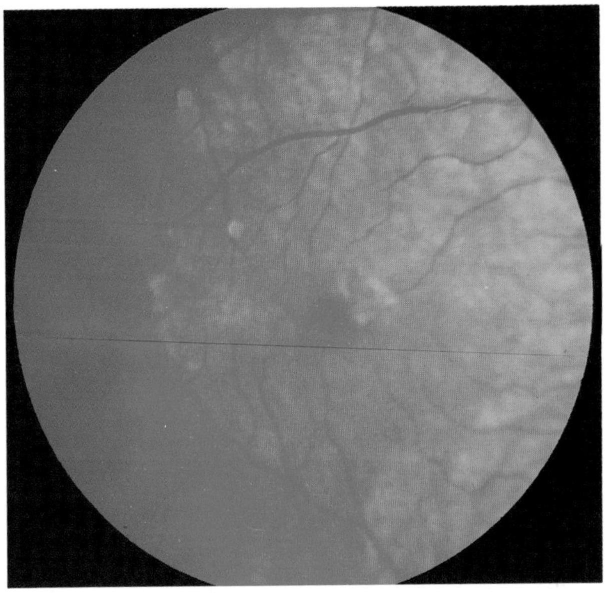

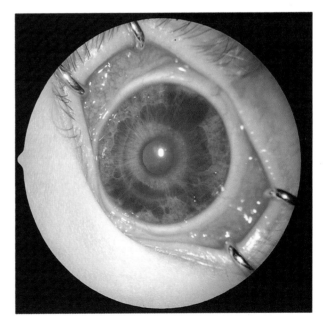

Fig. 11.3b Same patient. The right eye has a mild retinal pigment epithelial disturbance and 6/6 acuity.

Fig. 11.2 Congenital rubella retinopathy. There are diffuse retinal pigment epithelial changes most marked at the posterior pole. The acuity is 6/12.

include intracranial calcification, seizures, hydrocephalus, microcephaly, hepatosplenomegaly, jaundice, anemia, and fever (Eichenwald 1957). The incidence of intrauterine toxoplasmosis infections in the USA ranges from 1:1000 to 1:8000 live births

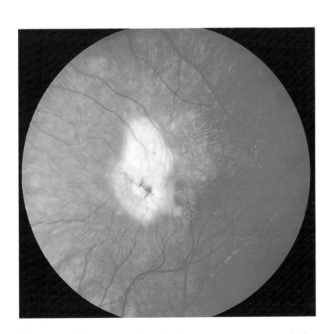

Fig. 11.3a Left eye showing disciform scarring in congenital rubella. The patient aged 9 years has an acuity secondary to subretinal neovascularization in this eye of 5/60.

Fig. 11.4 Congenital rubella. Iris pigment disturbance.

(McCabe & Remington 1988). Only 10–15% of the offspring of women with toxoplasmosis during the first trimester demonstrate serological evidence of intrauterine disease, however these children typically have the most severe manifestations of the syndrome. A higher percentage of foetuses infected during later

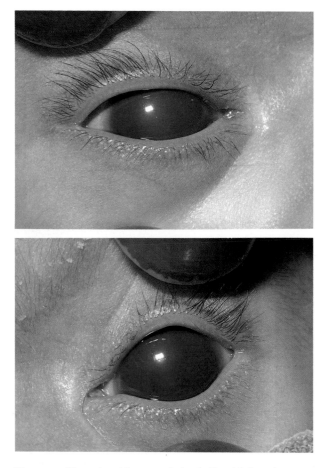

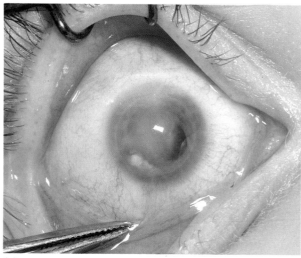

(a)

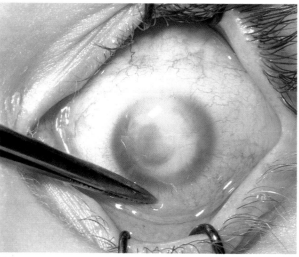

(b)

Fig. 11.5a Neonate with congenital rubella with hazy large appearing corneas. The intraocular pressure was normal.

Fig. 11.6a, 11.6b Congenital rubella with microphthalmos cataract, iris damage glaucoma, and corneal scarring. The right eye (a) had had a partially successful graft and had navigation vision.

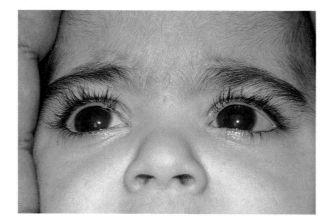

Fig. 11.5b Same patient aged 3. The intraocular pressure has not been raised at any of the subsequent examinations. The corneas had cleared by 3 months of age.

stages of gestation are seropositive to toxoplasmosis, but usually have minimal if any abnormalities (Desmonts & Couvreur 1974). It has been increasingly recognized that some infected neonates who are apparently normal on initial examination may develop chorioretinitis, blindness, hydrocephalus, mental retardation, and deafness even years later (Koppe *et al.* 1986; Remington & Wilson 1987).

Toxoplasmosis is acquired from eating undercooked meat or exposure to cat faeces. Marked regional differences occur in the prevalence of seropositivity to toxoplasmosis presumably due to differing dietary and living customs. For example, 84% of pregnant women in Paris were seropositive to toxoplasmosis (Desmonts & Couvreur 1974) in contrast to 22% of pregnant women in London (Ruoss 1972). Women of child-bearing years emigrating from an area of low immunity to a region of high immunity are at the greatest risk of contracting toxoplasmosis.

Ocular manifestations of congenital toxoplasmosis include chorio-retinitis (Fig. 11.7, 11.8, 11.9), microphthalmos, cataracts, panuveitis, and optic atrophy. The chorioretinal scarring is usually heavily pigmented and associated with areas of chorioretinal atrophy (Noble & Carr 1982). It is commonly bilateral and frequently involves the macula. Toxoplasmosis acquired after birth rarely results in chorioretinitis (Perkins 1973). Children with congenital toxoplasmosis may have quiescent chorioretinal scars, or active chorioretinitis with an accompanying vitritis and anterior uveitis. While only primary maternal toxoplasmosis infections have conclusively been shown to result in the congenital toxoplasmosis syndrome, multiple siblings have been reported to develop toxoplasmosis chorioretinitis on rare occasions. In most instances of multiply affected siblings the chorioretinitis is secondary to an acquired toxoplasmosis infection (Asbell et al. 1982; Lou et al. 1978).

All neonates with serological evidence of an intrauterine toxoplasmosis infection, whether or not they

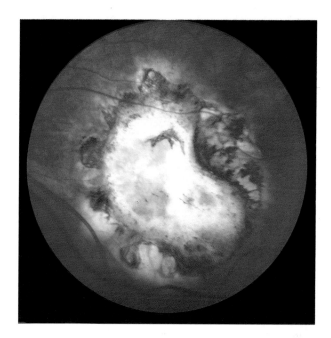

Fig. 11.8 Raised toxoplasmosis macular scar.

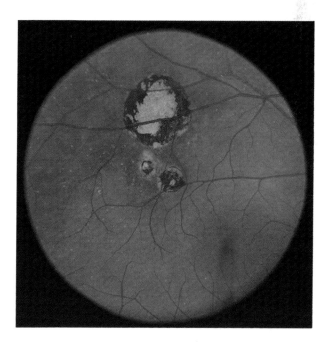

Fig. 11.9 Paramacular toxoplasmosis scar.

have signs of active infection, should be treated with a 21-day course of pyrimethamine and sulfonamides (either sulfadiazine or the triple combination of sulfapyrazine, sulfamethazine, and sulfamerazine). Folinic acid should be administered concurrently to reduce the haematoxicity of pyrimethamine. A 4–6-week course of spiramycin should then be given. Alternating

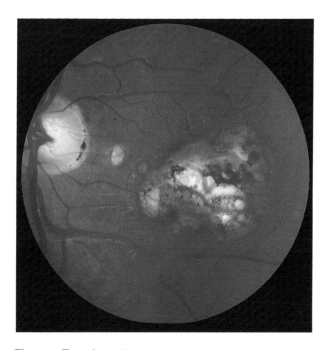

Fig. 11.7 Toxoplasmosis macular retinal pigment epithelial disturbance.

courses of these antibiotics are recommended for a total of 6 months (Feldman Remington 1987). Congenital toxoplasmosis can be diagnosed in utero by serology and ultrasound examinations. Pregnant women with a primary toxoplasmosis infection treated with spiramycin have offspring with less severe manifestations of congenital toxoplasmosis (Daffos 1988).

Women seronegative to toxoplasmosis should not eat undercooked meat and should minimize their exposure to cats during pregnancy. Fruits and vegetables, which might be contaminated with toxoplasmosis oocytes, should be washed carefully before being eaten.

Cytomegalovirus

Congenital cytomegalovirus infections are the most common intrauterine infection; they occur in 0.5–2.5% of all newborns (Stagno *et al.* 1986). Most children with congenital cytomegalovirus infections develop normally, but 10–20% have congenital abnormalities (Hanshaw 1971; Pass *et al.* 1980).

Intrauterine cytomegalovirus infections damage the foetus as a consequence of tissue necrosis rather than interference with organogenesis. Infections early in gestation are probably more embryopathic, although it is often times difficult to determine the gestational age at which the infection occurred since 95% of primary cytomegalovirus infections are asymptomatic (Stagno *et al.* 1986). Primary maternal cytomegalovirus infections are much more embryopathic than recurrent infections (Stagno *et al.* 1982). Abnormalities associated with congenital cytomegalovirus infections include jaundice, hepatosplenomegaly, microcephaly, psychomotor retardation, cerebral calcifications, a petechial rash, optic atrophy, and chorioretinitis (Weller 1971).

Ocular manifestations of congenital cytomegalovirus are uncommon, but include chorioretinitis (Fig. 11.10), microphthalmos, cataracts, keratitis (Fig. 11.11), and optic atrophy (Tarrkanen *et al.* 1972). Congenital cytomegalovirus chorioretinitis is rarely seen as an acute retinitis; typically it consists of discrete areas of chorioretinal pigmentation and atrophy resembling a toxoplasmosis chorioretinal scar (Lonn 1972).

The diagnosis of congenital cytomegalovirus should be suspected in neonates with hepatosplenomegally, jaundice, petechiae or thrombocytopenia, cerebral calcification, chorioretinitis and microcephaly. As the clinical features of congenital CMV may also develop with other congenital infections the diagnosis must be

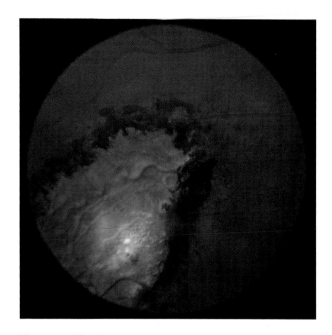

Fig. 11.10 Chorioretinal lesion in a child with proven CMV infection without serological evidence of toxoplasmosis.

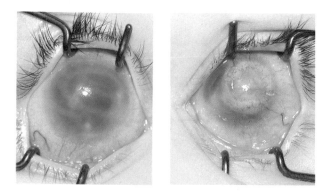

Fig. 11.11 Congenital CMV with bilateral keratopathy and glaucoma.

confirmed by viral isolation and serological tests. The virus can usually be cultured from the urine, stool, and throat of congenitally infected neonates for many months; cytomegalovirus specific IgM antibody titres are also elevated. People working with children excreting cytomegalovirus are not at increased risk of acquiring cytomegalovirus (Divorsky *et al.* 1983) In contradistinction, seronegative mothers of young children attending day-care centres are at great risk of acquiring the infection (Pass *et al.* 1987). It is probably necessary to have intimate contact with a person excreting cytomegalovirus in order to acquire the infection.

Herpes simplex

Herpes simplex infections most commonly occur in neonates delivered to mothers with active genital herpes simplex vesicles. The risk of neonatal infection is considerably greater from primary genital herpes infection than from recurrent lesions (Nahmias *et al.* 1971). Premature rupture of the amnionic membranes may allow infection to occur via an ascending route. The herpes simplex type 2 strain is responsible for most neonatal infections.

Neonatal herpes simplex is often first detected as a cutaneous vesicular eruption which progresses to a disseminated systemic infection in 50% of infants, resulting in hepatitis, pneumonia, and disseminated intravascular coagulation. Central nervous system infections are most commonly manifested as an encephalitis. Seventy per cent of neonates with disseminated infections have involvement of both the viscera and the central nervous system. The eye is rarely the only organ affected by a neonatal herpes simplex infection (Nahmias & Hagler 1972).

Ocular involvement most commonly consists of blepharoconjunctivitis with vesicles on the eyelids and injection of the conjunctiva. A keratitis may occur initially as an epithelial dendrite, but progress to stromal involvement if left untreated. In rare instances, chorioretinitis with an accompanying vitritis may occur, particularly in infants with central nervous system involvement. Cataracts may form secondary to the accompanying uveitis.

A disseminated neonatal herpes simplex infection is associated with a 70% mortality rate. A high percentage of children surviving herpes simplex encephalitis are neurologically handicapped (Whitley *et al.* 1980). Because of the risk of dissemination, all neonates less than 1 month of age with a herpes simplex infection, even if initially limited to cutaneous or ocular involvement, should be treated with systemic antiviral therapy. Most children born by vaginal delivery to women with recurrent genital herpes simplex infections, do not acquire the infection, so treatment should only be initiated in neonates if symptoms of a herpes simplex infection develop (Prober *et al.* 1987). Intravenous acyclovir, an agent which specifically inhibits viral DNA production, is the agent currently recommended for the treatment of neonatal herpes simplex infections. Herpetic keratitis should be treated with either acyclovir ointment or triflurothymidine solution topically. Herpes simplex blepharoconjunctivitis should also be treated with topical antiviral therapy as prophylaxis against the development of keratitis.

The diagnosis of a herpes simplex infection should be considered in infants with progressive icterus, fevers, hepatosplenomegaly, and cutaneous vesicular lesions. The isolation of herpes simplex from fresh vesicles or from corneal scrapings confirms the diagnosis. The presence of multinucleated giant cells on scraping from vesicles or from the cornea are suggestive of a herpes simplex infection, but are not diagnostic since they may occur with several other viral infections.

Women with active genital herpes infections should have caesarean sections to reduce the risk of a disseminated infection in their offspring.

Syphilis

Congenital syphilis only occurs in fetuses exposed to *Treponema pallidum* after the 16th gestational week. Virtually all of the offspring of women with primary syphilis acquired after the 16th gestational week have congenital syphilis, whereas the incidence decreases to 90% with secondary syphilis and 30% with latent syphilis. Syphilis infections acquired at an earlier gestational age frequently result in foetal death.

Congenital syphilis may result in early manifestations occurring in infancy secondary to an active infection or late manifestations occurring later in childhood secondary to ongoing inflammation or a hypersensitivity reaction. Early manifestations include skeletal abnormalities, rhinitis, a maculopapular rash, fissures around the lips, nares and anus, hepatosplenomegaly, anemia, and uveitis. Late manifestations include sensorineural hearing loss, bone changes, dental abnormalities, and interstitial keratitis (Fiumara & Lessell 1983). The finding of interstitial keratitis, deafness, and malformed incisors are known as Hutchinson's triad which suggests congenital syphilis.

Ocular manifestations of congenital syphilis include chorioretinitis (Fig. 11.2), interstitial keratitis, anterior uveitis, and optic atrophy. Interstitial keratitis occurs in 10−40% of children with untreated congenital syphilis. It most commonly occurs in children 5−20 years of age. It is characterized by either sectorial or diffuse corneal oedema infiltrated by interstitial vessels. Visual loss occurs secondary to corneal scarring and residual ghost vessels. It is bilateral in 80% of affected children and usually accompanied by an iridocyclitis and iris atrophy. It occurs secondary to a hypersensitivity reaction and responds best to topical corticosteroids. The chorioretinitis occurring with congenital syphilis most commonly results in periph-

the time of vaginal delivery to mothers with recurrent genital herpes simplex virus infections. *N Engl J Med* 1987; **316**: 240−4

Purvis Smith S. Dermatoglyphic defects and rubella teratogenesis. *JAMA* 1969; **00**: 1865−8

Remington JA, Wilson CB. Toxoplasmosis. In Fergin RD, Cherry JD (eds) *Pediatric Infectious Diseases*, 2nd edn. WB Saunders, Philadelphia, London 1987, pp. 2067−78

Rothenberg R, Woelfel M, Stoneburner R *et al*. Survival with the acquired immunodeficiency syndrome. Experience with 5833 cases in New York City. *N Engl J Med* 1987; **317**: 1297−302

Rouss CF, Bourne GL. Toxoplasmosis in pregnancy. *J Obstet Bynaecol Br Commonw* 1972; **779**: 1115−8

Ryan SJ, Hardy PH, Hardy JM *et al*. Persistence of a virulent *Treponema pallidum* despite penicillin therapy in congenital syphilis. *Am J Ophthalmol* 1972; **73**: 258−61

Savage MO, Moosa A, Gordon RR. Maternal varicella infection as a cause of fetal malformations. *Lancet* 1973; **1**: 352−4

Scott GB, Fischl MA, Klimas N *et al*. Mothers of infants with the acquired immunodeficiency syndrome. Evidence for both symptomatic and asymptomatic carriers. *JAMA* 1985; **253**: 363−8

Sears ML. Congenital glaucoma in neonatal rubella. *Br J Ophthalmol* 1967; **51**: 744−8

Siegel M. Congenital malformations following chicken pox, measles, mumps, and hepatitis. Results of a cohort study. *JAMA* 1973; **226**: 1521−4

Stagno S, Pass RF, Coud G *et al*. Primary cytomegalovirus infection in pregnancy: incidence, transmission to foetus, and clinical outcome. *JAMA* 1986; **256**: 1904−8

Stagno S, Pass RF, Dworsky ME *et al*. Congenital cytomegalovirus infection: the relative importance of primary and recurrent maternal infection. *N Engl J Med* 1982; 306: 945−9

Stagno S, Reynolds DW, Hurry E. Congenital CMV infection: occurrence in immune population. *N Eng J Med* 1977; **296**: 1254−8

Tarkkanen A, Merenmias L, Holmstron T. Ocular involvement in congenital cytomegalic inclusion disease. *J Pediatr Ophthalmol* 1972; **9**: 82−6

Thiry L, Spricher-Goldberger S, Jonckheer T *et al*. Isolation of AIDS virus from cell-free breast milk of three healthy virus carriers. *Lancet* 1985; **2**: 891−2

Weibel RE, Neff BJ, Kater BJ *et al*. Live attenuated varaicella virus vaccine. Efficacy trial in healthy children. *N Engl J Med*. 1984; **310**: 1409−15

Weller TH. The cytomegaloviruses: ubiquitous agents with protean clinical manifestations. *N Engl J Med* 1971; **285**: 203−14

Weller TH. Varicella and herpes zoster. Changing concepts of the natural history, control, and importance of not-so-benign virus. *N Engl J Med* 1983; **309**: 1362−8, 1434−40

Whitley RJ, Nahmias AJ, Visentine AM, *et al*. The natural history of herpes simplex virus infection of mother and new born. *Pediatrics* 1980; **66**: 489−94

Wolf A, Cowen D, Paige BH. Toxoplasmis encephalomyelitis. III. A new case of granulomatous encephalomyelitis due to a protozoon. *Am J Path* 1939; **15**: 657−94

Wolff SM. The ocular manifestations of congenital rubella. *Trans Am Ophthalmol Soc* 1972; **70**: 577−614

12 Ophthalmia Neonatorum

SCOTT LAMBERT AND CREIG HOYT

A purulent conjunctivitis is one of the most common infections occurring during the first month of life (Sandstrom *et al.* 1984). Although its incidence has been reported to be as low as 1.6% of newborns in the USA (Armstrong *et al.* 1976), in certain parts of the world it occurs in 7−12% of all neonates (Pierce *et al.* 1982; Fransen *et al.* 1986; Laga *et al.* 1988).

Infants with ophthalmia neonatorium typically develop a purulent discharge associated with lid oedema, conjunctival hyperemia and occasionally pre-auricular adenopathy.

The period of time after birth until the onset of neonatal conjunctivitis is quite variable and may be helpful in dignosing the causative agent. Conjunctivitis during the first few days of life commonly occurs as a toxic effect of topically administered silver nitrate at the time of birth. Gonococcal conjunctivitis usually develops during the first week of life. Chlamydial conjunctivitis may also develop during the first week of life, but is frequently delayed in its onset. Prophylactic treatment with erythromycin may prolong the interval before chlamydial conjunctivitis is detected. Bell *et al.* (1987) reported that chlamydial conjunctivitis was not detected in infants who had received erythromycin prophylaxis until 9−45 days after birth, whereas infants who received silver nitrate prophylaxis presented with chlamydial conjunctivitis 6−26 days after birth.

The pathogen responsible for neonatal conjunctivitis varies between different geographic areas due to differences in the prevalence of maternal infections and the use of prophylactic antibiotics or silver nitrate. In a large hospital in Nairobi, Kenya where 6% of all pregnant women had cervical gonococcal infections, 3% of all newborns had gonococcal ophthalmia neonatorium (Laga 1986). In contrast, gonococcal ophthalmia neonatorium is rare in the USA where women are routinely cultured for Neisseria gonorrhoeae during pregnancy. Neonatal conjunctivitis is most commonly caused by Chlamydia trachomatis in the USA (Rapoza *et al.* 1986). A variety of other pathogens including *Haemophilis influenzae, Staphylococcus aureus, Streptococcus viridans, Strep. pneumoniae* and enterocococci may also be cultured from neonates with conjunctivitis (Rapoza *et al.* 1986, Sandstrom 1987).

Laboratory studies

Because of the difficulty in distinguishing between the various types of neonatal conjunctivitis by clinical characteristics alone, laboratory studies are paramount in establishing the correct diagnosis and selecting the best treatment. A Gram stain should be performed on a conjunctival scraping from the palpebral conjunctiva of all infants with early infantile conjunctivitis (Winceslaus *et al.* 1987). If Gram-negative diplococci are present in polymorphonuclear leukocytes, the child should be treated for presumed gonococcal conjunctivitis. Sandstrom *et al.* (1984) reported that while the identification of Gram-negative coccobacili on a gram stain of the conjunctiva correlated with the isolation of *Haemophilus* species, the presence of Gram-positive cocci did not correlate with positive cultures of *Staphylococcus aureus*, enterococci or *Streptococcus pneumoniae*. White blood cells are also present more frequently on the Gram stain of infants with conjunctivitis than controls (Sandstrom et al. 1984).

A Giemsa stain is also helpful in identifying intracytoplasmic inclusion bodies in infants with chlamydial conjunctivitis. Unlike adults with chlamydial conjunctivitis, intracytoplasmic inclusion bodies may be seen in 60–80% of all infants with chlamydial conjunctivitis. In addition, cultures for chlamydia may be obtained or a rapid diagnosis may be made with direct immunofluorescent monoclonal antibody staining of conjunctival scrapings (Rapoza et al. 1986). Cultures for other bacterial pathogens should also be obtained before antibiotic therapy is initiated.

Gonococcal conjunctivitis

Gonococcal ophthalmia neonatorium is still common in certain parts of the world, but is rare in the USA (Laga et al. 1986). However, because of its propensity to produce a severe keratitis, a gonococcal infection should be excluded in all children with neonatal conjunctivitis by Gram staining and culturing a conjunctival scraping. Neisseria gonorrhoeae isolates are resistant to penicillin in many urban areas in the USA and many other parts of the world (50–60% in certain areas of Africa) (Laga et al. 1986). While systemic penicillin was the recommended treatment for gonococcal ophthalmia neonatorium as recently as 1985, systemic administration of a third generation cephalosporin (ceftriaxone 28–50 mg/kg/day) is now advised in areas where penicillinase-producing N. gonorrhoeae is endemic (1% or more of isolates) (Lepage et al. 1988). Irrigation of the eyes with saline may also be helpful as adjuvant therapy. A concurrent infection with Chlamydia trachomatis should be considered in neonates who do not respond to systemic ceftriaxone.

Chlamydial conjunctivitis

Chlamydia trachomatis is one of the most commonly isolated pathogens in infants with neonatal conjunctivitis in the USA with a prevalence of three to four per 1000 live births (Pierce et al. 1982, Schachter 1978). Because chlamydial conjunctivitis may also be associated with a neonatal pneumonitis, it is important that the correct diagnosis be promptly established (Schachter et al. 1975; Beem & Saxon 1977; Harrison et al. 1978). The pneumonitis generally develops during the first 6 weeks of life and is characterized by a nasal discharge, cough, and tachypnoea. The recommended treatment for infants with chlamydial conjunctivitis is a 14-day course of oral erythromycin

syrup (50 mg/kg/day) in four divided doses (Heggie et al. 1985). Oral erythromycin not only treats chlamydial pneumonitis and eradicates nasopharyngeal carriage of Chlamydia, but it is also more effective than topical erythromycin in preventing a relapse of chlamydial conjunctivitis (Patamasucan et al. 1982). However, chlamydial conjunctivitis may recur even after a course of oral erythromycin possibly due to poor compliance with antibiotic therapy, an inadequate dose of antibiotics or a reinfection (Rees et al. 1981). A second course of oral erythromycin should be given when a recurrence occurs. Adjuvant therapy with topical erythromycin or tetracycline may also be beneficial. In addition, parents of infected children should be treated with oral tetracycline or erythromycin for 2 weeks. Untreated chlamydial conjunctivitis usually resolves spontaneously after 8–12 months but may result in the formation of a micropannus and scarring of the tarsal conjunctiva (Mordhorst & Dawson 1971). In addition, children with untreated chlamydial conjunctivitis are at increased risk of developing a pneumonitis or otitis (Beem et al. 1977, Harrison et al. 1978).

Non-gonococcal, non-chlamydial conjunctivitis

The most common pathogens isolated from neonates with conjunctivitis aside from Neissera gonorrhoeae and Conjunctivitis trachomatis are Haemophilus species, Staphylococcus aureus, Streptococcus pneumoniae and enterococci (Sandstrom et al. 1984). Broad-spectrum antibiotics should be administered to infants with severe conjunctivitis until culture results have identified the pathogen and its antibiotic sensitivity. Infants with mild to moderate conjunctivitis may be treated with lid hygiene alone until a microbe has been isolated. Conjunctival cultures are sterile in 20–60% of neonates with conjunctivitis (Pierce et al. 1982; Sandstrom et al. 1984; Sandstrom 1987). Lid hygiene alone may be a sufficient treatment for these infants (Sandstrom 1987).

Congenital dacrostenosis

A congenital nasolacrimal duct obstruction is also frequently associated with neonatal conjunctivitis. Dacrostenosis should be suspected in children with unilateral conjunctivitis and epiphora who have a reflux of mucopurulent material from the lacrimal punctae after massaging the lacrimal sac. Dacrocystitis in infants with congenital dacrostenosis is usually caused by *Haemophilus* species and *S. pneumoniae* (Sandstrom *et al.* 1984). Congenital dacrostenosis should be treated initially with topical antibiotics and massage of the lacrimal sac using the Crigler technique to increase the hydrostatic pressure in the lacrimal sac (Crigler 1923). If the dacrostenosis fails to resolve spontaneously by 6–12 months of age, probing of the nasolacrimal system is generally advised (Kushner 1982). Dacrocystitis secondary to congenital dacrostenosis may on occasion progress to periorbital cellulitis (Kushner 1982; Katowitz & Welsh 1987). Periorbital cellulitis should be treated with the appropriate systemic antibiotics. Infants with congenital dacrostenosis and a persistent dacrocystitis which fails to respond to topical antibiotics and massaging should have their nasolacrimal system probed at an earlier age (Katowitz & Welsh 1987).

Viral

Non-chlamydial viral conjunctivitis also occurs in neonates, but less frequently. Herpes simplex conjunctivitis usually occurs in neonates exposed to a maternal herpes infection at the time of birth. Vesicles may be present on the eyelids or on other parts of the body. Herpetic keratitis may also develop. The diagnosis can be confirmed by culturing the fluid in a vesicle. Neonates with a suspected herpes simplex infection should be treated with systemic acyclovir to reduce the risk of a disseminated infection developing.

Prophylaxis for ophthalmia neonatorum

Crede (1881), introduced 2% silver nitrate as a prophylactic treatment for ophthalmia neonatorum in Leipzig in 1881. After its introduction the incidence of ophthalmia neonatorum fell from 13.6% to zero in Leipzig, with the only adverse effect being a slight hyperemia, with now and then an increase in conjunctival secretions during the first 24 hours (Créde 1881; Forbes and Forbes 1971). The widespread use of silver nitrate prophylaxis was subsequently associated with a dramatic decline in the incidence of ophthalmia neonatorum in Europe and the USA (Barsam 1966). With the advent of modern antibiotics, the use of prophylactic silver nitrate has waned because of the chemical conjunctivitis it frequently produces. All but eleven States now permit topical erythromycin or tetracycline to be substituted for 1% silver nitrate as prophylaxis against ophthalmia neonatorum (Dillon 1986). The position of the American Academy of Pediatrics in 1986 was that 1% silver nitrate, 0.5%

erythromycin ointment and 1% tetracycline are equally acceptable for the prevention of gonococcal ophthalmia neonatorum (Peter 1986).

The best form of prophylactic treatment for children exposed to chlamydia or penicillinase producing strains of *Neissera gonorrhoeae* at birth is still controversial. In a retrospective study of 120 women with a *Chlamydia trachomatis* infection of the cervix, chlamydial conjunctivitis developed in 25% of their offspring even after prophylactic silver nitrate or topical erythromycin (Bell *et al.* 1987). Laga *et al.* (Laga 1988), reported that 10.1% of infants exposed to a maternal chlamydial infection at birth developed chlamydial conjunctivitis after silver nitrate prophylaxis, compared to 7.2% of neonates receiving tetracycline prophylaxis. Topical tetracycline was also a more effective prophylaxis against *N. gonorrhoeae* conjunctivitis. In their study only 3% of infants exposed to *N. gonorrhoeae* at birth developed gonococcal conjunctivitis after tetracycline prophylaxis compared to 7.0% of the infants after silver nitrate prophylaxis (Laga *et al.* 1988). Hammerschlag *et al.* (1989) reported a lower incidence of chlamydial conjunctivitis in the offspring of women with chlamydial cervicitis treated with 0.5% erythromycin (14%) or 1% tetracycline (11%), than with 1% silver nitrate (20%), but the difference was not statistically significant. Gonoccocal conjunctivitis only developed in seven infants (0.6%). Six of the mothers had not received any prenatal care. The most effective prophylaxis for gonococcal and chlamydial conjuctivitis is prenatal screening and treatment of maternal infections (Schachter *et al.* 1986).

Because the incidence of gonococcal ophthalmia neonatorum is extremely low in Europe, several countries including England and Belgium no longer require prophylaxis against ophthalmia neonatorum. Children born by caesarean section within 3 hours of the time the amniotic membranes ruptures, have a particularly low risk of developing ophthalmia neonatorum (Isenberg *et al.* 1988). Children born to women with poor prenatal care have the highest risk of developing gonococcal conjunctivitis.

References

Armstrong JH, Zacarias F, Rein MF. Ophthalmia neonatorum: a chart review. *Pediatrics* 1976; **57**: 884–92

Barsam PC. Specific prophylaxis of gonorrheal ophthalmia neonatorum: a review. *N Engl J Med* 1966; **274**: 731–4

Beem MO, Saxon EM. Respiratory-tract colonization and a distinctive pneumonia syndrome in infants with *Chlamydia trachomatis*. *N Engl J Med* 1977; **296**; 306–10

Bell TA, Sandstrom KI, Gravett MG *et al*. Comparison of ophthalmic silver nitrate solution and erythromycin ointment for prevention of natally acquired *Chlamydia trachomatis*. *Sex Transm Dis* 1987; **14**: 195−200

Crédé CSF. Reports from the obstetrical clinic in Leipzig: prevention of eye inflammation in the newborn. *Arch Gynecol* 1881; **71**: 50−3

Crigler LW. The treatment of congenital dacrocysticis. *JAMA* 1923; **81**: 23−4

Dillon HC. Prevention of gonococcal ophthalmia neonatorum. *N Engl J Med* 1986; **22**: 1414−15

Forbes GB, Forbes GM. Silver nitrate and the eyes of the newborn: Crede's contribution to preventive medicine. *Am J Dis Child* 1971; **121**: 1−4

Fransen L, Nsanze H, Klauss V, Stuyft P, D'Costa L, Brunham RC, Piot P. Ophthalmia neonatorum in Nairobi, Kenya: the roles of *Neisseria gonorrhoeae* and *Chlamydia trachomatis*. *J Infect Dis* 1986; **5**: 862−9

Hammerschlag MR, Cummings C, Roblin PM, Williams TH, Delke L. Efficacy of neonatal ocular prophylaxis for the prevention of chlamydial and gonococcal conjunctivitis. *N Engl J Med* 1989; **320**: 769−72

Harrison HR, Phil D, English MG, Lee CK, Alexander ER. *Chlamydia trachomatis* infant pneumonitis. *N Engl J Med* 1978; **13**: 702−8

Heggie AD, Jaffe AC, Stuart LA *et al*. Topical sulfacetamide vs oral erythromycin for neonatal chlamydial conjunctivitis. *Amer J Dis Child* 1985; **139**: 564−6

Isenberg SJ, Apt L, Yoshimor R *et al*. Source of the conjunctival bacterial flora at birth and implications for ophthalmia neonatorum prophylaxis. *Am J Ophthalmol* 1988; **106**: 458−62

Katowitz IA, Welsh MG. Timing of initial probing and irrigation in congenital nasolacrimal duct obstruction. *Ophthalmology* 1987; **94**: 698−705

Kushner BJ. Congenital nasolacrimal system obstruction. *Arch Ophthalmol* 1982; **100**: 597−600

Laga M, Naamara W, Brunham RC *et al*. Single-dose therapy of gonococcal ophthalmia neonatorum with ceftriaxone. *N Engl J Med* 1986; 1382−5

Laga M, Plummer FA, Piot P *et al*. Prophylaxis of gonococcal and chlamydial ophthalmia neonatorum. *N Engl J Med* 1988; **11**: 653−7

Lepage P, Bogaerts J, Kestelyn P, Meheus A. Single-dose cefotaxime intramuscularly cures gonococcal ophthalmia neonatorum. *Br J Ophthalmol* 1988; **72**: 518−20

Mordhorst CH, Dawson C. Sequelae of neonatal conjunctivitis and associated diseases in parents. *Am J Ophthalmol* 1971; **71**: 861−7

Patamasucan P, Rettig PJ, Faust KL, Kusmiesz HT, Nelson JD. Oral v topical erythomycin therapies for chlamydial conjunctivitis. *Am J Dis Child* 1982; **136**: 817−21

Peter G. *1986 Red Book: Report of the Committee on Infectious Diseases*, 20th edn. American Academy of Pediatrics, Elk Grove, Illinois 1986

Pierce JM, Ward ME, Seal DV. Ophthalmia neonatorum in the 1980s: incidence, aetiology and treatment. *Br J Ophthalmol* 1982; **66**: 728−31

Rapoza PA, Quinn TC, Kiessling LA, Green R, Taylor HR. Assessment of neonatal conjunctivitis with a direct immunofluorescent monoclonal antibody stain for *Chlamydia*. *JAMA*, 1986; **24**: 3369−73

Rees E, Tait A, Hobson D, Karayiannis P, Lee N. Persistence of chlamydial infection after treatment for neonatal conjunctivitis. *Arch Dis Child* 1981; **56**: 193−8

Sandstrom I. Treatment of neonatal conjunctivitis. *Arch Ophthalmol* 1987; **105**: 925−8

Sandstrom KI, Bell TA, Chandler JW *et al*. Microbial causes of neonatal conjunctivitis. *J Pediatr* 1984; **5**: 706−11

Schachter J. Chlamydial infections. *N Engl J Med* 1978; **298**: 540−9

Schachter J, Lun L, Gooding CA, Ostler B. Pneumonitis following inclusion blennorrhea. *J Paediatr* 1975; **87**: 779−80

Schachter J, Sweet RL, Grossman M *et al*. Experience with the routine use of erythromycin for chlamydial infections in pregnancy. *N Engl J Med* 1986; **314**: 276−9

Winceslaus J, Goh BT, Dunlop EM, Mantell J, Woodland RM, Forsey T, Treharne JD. Diagnosis of ophthalmia neonatorum. *Br Med J* 1987; **295**: 1377−9

13 Preseptal and Orbital Cellulitis

ANTHONY MOORE

Periorbital infections, particularly sinusitis, may cause infection or a severe inflammatory reaction of the orbital tissues leading to preseptal or orbital cellulitis. The proximity of the paranasal sinuses to the orbital walls, and the interconnection between the venous system of the orbit and the face allow infection to spread from the sinuses to the orbit either directly or via the blood stream. The orbital venous system is devoid of valves and two-way communication is permitted with the venous system of the nose, face and pterygoid fossa. The superior and inferior ophthalmic veins which drain the orbit empty into the cavernous sinus, hence orbital and facial infections may lead to the serious complication of cavernous sinus thrombosis.

Certain anatomical structures help to limit the direct spread of infection. The orbital periosteum acts as a barrier to spread from infected sinuses, but may become stripped from the orbital wall by a collection of pus which forms a subperiosteal abscess. The orbital septum limits the spread of infection from the preseptal space to the orbit.

Orbital infections and their complications can be classified into five types (Chandler 1970) (Table 13.1).

Preseptal cellulitis

Aetiology

Preseptal cellulitis is much more common than orbital cellulitis and may have a variety of causes including eyelid trauma, extraocular infections and upper respiratory tract infections (Barkin 1978; Weiss 1983). Children with this condition can be divided into three main groups (Jones 1983). The first group includes those who have developed periorbital oedema from an associated lid infection such as impetigo, herpes simplex or varicella, or have a local cause for the oedema such as infected chalazion, or dacrocystitis (Fig. 13.1). Secondly, suppurative cellulitis may develop from lid trauma (Fig. 13.2), in which case the causative organism is usually *Staphlococcus aureus* or a beta-haemolytic streptococcus. Thirdly, in preseptal cellulitis associated with an upper respiratory tract infection (Fig. 13.3), *Haemophilus influenzae* and *Streptococcus* are the usual organisms involved (Weiss 1983; Smith 1978). In this last group of children there, is often an associated sinusitis (Barkin 1978; Weiss 1983). *Haemophilus influenzae* infection is commoner in young children (Weiss 1983; Smith 1978); for example in the series of Smith *et al.* (1978) 12 out of 15 children with proven haemophilus preseptal cellulitis were less than 3 years of age.

Table 13.1 Classification of orbital infections. Modified from Chandler (1970).

Preseptal cellulitis
Orbital cellulitis
Subperiosteal abscess
Orbital abscess
Cavernous sinus thrombosis

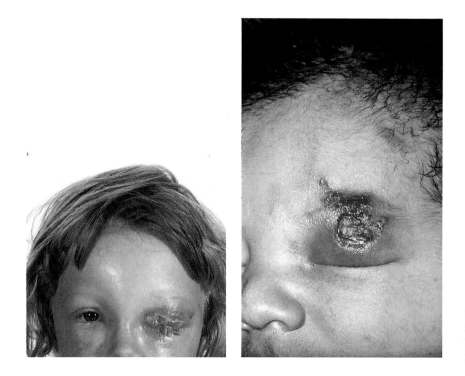

Fig. 13.1 Preseptal cellulitis caused by spread from a stye in a patient with leukaemia (left).

Fig. 13.2 Preseptal cellulitis caused by infection of a necrotic ulcer caused by a forceps injury (right) (Dr S. Day's patient).

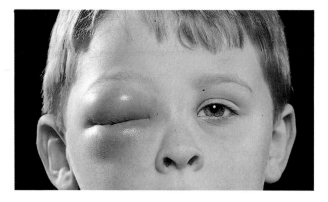

Fig. 13.3 Preseptal cellulitis associated with sinus infection in an otherwise healthy child.

Clinical manifestations

The usual clinical presentation is unilateral periorbital oedema in a child with recent eyelid trauma or upper respiratory tract infection. Bilateral involvement is rare (Barkin 1978). In contrast with orbital cellulitis vision is usually normal and there is no proptosis or limitation of ocular motility. The child is often generally unwell with a raised temperature and a full blood count will usually show a leucocytosis. Local causes for the lid swelling such as chalazion or dacryocystitis are easily excluded on clinical examination. In the neonate it is important to exclude inclusion conjunctivitis; osteomyelitis of the maxilla (Cavenagh 1960), and Caffey's disease (infantile cortical hyperostosis).

The clinical picture may vary with the different organisms involved. In staphylococcal infections there is a purulent discharge, whilst haemophilus infection leads to a non-purulent cellulitis with a characteristic bluish-purple discoloration of the eyelid. In streptococcal infection there is usually a sharply demarcated red area of induration (Jones 1983).

Rarely meningitis may complicate preseptal cellulitis (Weiss *et al.* 1983).

Management

Children with a local cause for the periorbital oedema, such as dacryocystitis need specific treatment for the underlying condition and rarely need further investigation. In suppurative cellulitis following lid trauma it is sufficient to culture the wound discharge as there is rarely any bacteremia and blood cultures are usually negative (Weiss *et al.* 1983). In children who develop

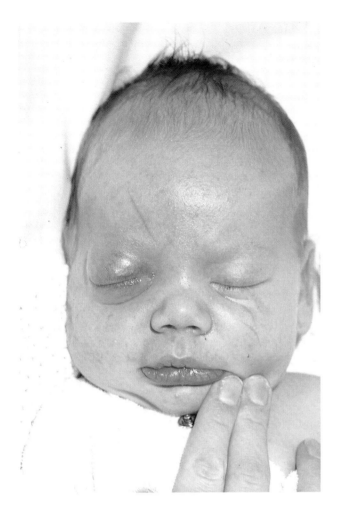

Fig. 13.4a Orbital cellulitis.

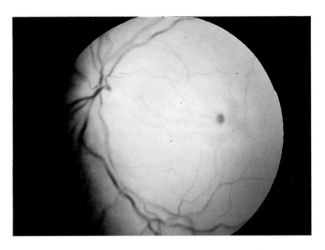

Fig. 13.5 Central retinal artery occlusion in orbital cellulitis (Dr S. Day's patient).

periorbital cellulitis following an upper respiratory tract infection, cultures should be taken from nose, throat, conjunctiva and from aspirates of the periorbital oedema. Blood cultures should also be taken and sinus X-rays performed, although the latter may be difficult to interpret in children under the age of 2 years due to the lack of development of the sinuses (Weiss *et al.* 1983). A CT scan to exclude orbital involvement is indicated when marked lid swelling prevents an adequate examination of the globe (Goldberg 1978). (Fig. 13.6.)

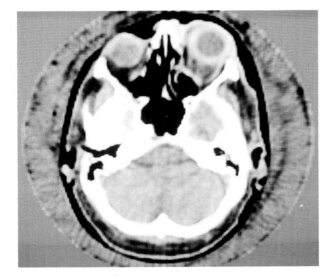

Fig. 13.4b Scan of a patient with orbital cellulitis with axial proptosis. The child was ill and pyrexial with pneumococcal septicaemia. (Same patient as 13.4a.)

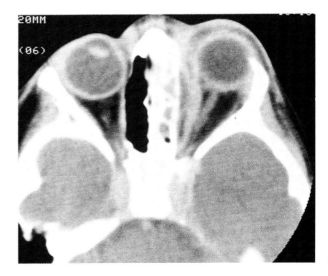

Fig. 13.6 CT scan showing left ethmoid sinusitis and subperiosteal abscess.

Older children with a suppurative cellulitis following lid trauma who are not generally unwell, can be managed as an out patient using oral antibiotics. The initial choice of antibiotic is based upon the Gram stain of the discharge and can be reviewed when culture and sensitivity results are available. If the Gram stain is negative a broad-spectrum penicillin such as ampicillin combined with a penicillinase-resistant penicillin such as cloxacillin should be given initially.

In young children and infants overall management is best undertaken by a paediatrician in consultation with the ophthalmologist and ENT surgeon. Unless there is a clearly positive Gram stain result, initial antibiotic treatment should be intravenous chloramphenicol combined with a penicillinase-resistant penicillin such as cloxacillin or a cephalosporin. Chloramphenicol or the newer cephalosporins are preferred to ampicillin because of the prevalence of ampicillin resistant strains of *Haemophilus influenzae* (Lerman *et al.* 1980). This initial treatment may be modified once culture and sensitivity results are available. The lid swelling and temperature usually subside within 2 to 3 days when oral treatment may replace intravenous antibiotics.

An excellent guide to the antibiotic treatment of bacterial preseptal and orbital cellulitis has been published by Jones (1982).

Surgical treatment is seldom necessary; about 10% of children will require surgical drainage of a lid abscess or paranasal sinus (Weiss 1983).

Orbital cellulitis

Orbital cellulitis is an uncommon but important condition which may give rise to a variety of serious systemic and ocular complications (Table 13.2). In the pre-antibiotic era one fifth of patients died from septic intracranial complications and one third of the sur-

Table 13.2 Complications of orbital cellulitis.

Optic neuritis
Optic atrophy
Exposure keratitis
Central retinal artery occlusion (Jarret 1969)
Retinal and choroidal ischaemia (Sherry 1973)
Subperiosteal and orbital abscess (Schramm 1978; Krohel 1980)
Cavernous sinus thrombosis (Clune 1963)
Meningitis (Weiss *et al.* 1983)
Brain abscess
Septicaemia (Krohel 1980)

vivors had visual loss in the affected eye (Duke-Elder 1974). This poor outlook has been dramatically altered by the introduction of effective antibiotics but prompt diagnosis and treatment are essential if such complications are to be avoided.

Aetiology

In contrast to preseptal cellulitis, orbital cellulitis is more frequent in children older than 5 years and in over 90% of cases occurs secondary to sinusitis (Watters 1976; Weiss 1983) especially of the ethmoid. When it does occur in infants it is usually due to infection with type B *Haemophilus influenzae* (Londer 1974). Other less common causes are penetrating orbital trauma, especially when there is a retained foreign body, dental infections (Flood 1982), extraocular and retinal surgery (Von Noorden 1972) and haematogenous spread during a systemic infectious illness. Rarely a necrotic retinoblastoma (Rozanksy 1964) or Coats' disease (Judisch 1980) may cause severe panophthalmitis and secondary orbital cellulitis.

The common bacterial pathogens are *Staphylococcus aureus*, *Streptococcus pyogenes*, *Strep pneumoniae* and *Haemophilus influenzae*. Other Gram-negative organisms such as *Escherichia coli* and anaerobic bacteria which may form gas within the orbit (Sevel 1973), may occasionally be implicated. Atypical mycobacteria have also been reported to cause orbital cellulitis in young children (Levine 1969). Fungal infections are rare but should be excluded when orbital cellulitis occurs in an immunosuppressed or diabetic child (Schwartz 1977) (see page 00).

Clinical manifestations

The usual presentation is with a painful red eye and increasing lid oedema in a child who has had a recent upper respiratory tract infection. The child is usually pyrexial and generally unwell. There is usually conjunctival chemosis and injection, axial proptosis and limitation of eye movements (Fig. 13.4). Visual loss when it occurs is usually due to an associated optic neuritis but may also be caused by exposure keratitis or even a retinal vascular occlusion (Jarret 1969; Sherry 1973; Schramm 1978) (Fig. 13.5).

The acute onset, pain, fever and systemic illness help to differentiate orbital cellulitis from other causes of unilateral proptosis. Occasionally orbital cellulitis may cause proptosis and limitation of ocular motility without marked inflammatory signs and may be confused clinically with a rapidly growing orbital tumour or inflammatory pseudotumour. In such cases the distinction is made on plain films and CT scan of the orbit.

In young infants under 3 months of age osteomyelitis of the superior maxilla (Cavenagh 1960) which gives a similar clinical picture should be excluded.

Management

Children with orbital cellulitis should be admitted to hospital immediately for investigation and treatment. Initial investigations should include blood cultures and cultures from nose, throat and conjunctivae. These are often negative, but a positive result is helpful in planning antibiotic treatment. Sinus X-rays and a dental examination should be performed and an ENT consultation obtained. In the absence of any local cause for the orbital cellulitis a careful search should be made for any septic focus elsewhere in the body. If there are signs of meningism lumbar puncture is indicated.

It is preferable to obtain a CT scan in all cases of orbital cellulitis as CT scan has been shown to detect subperiosteal and orbital abscesses which are not apparent clinically or on plain films (Goldberg 1978; Schramm 1978). Orbital ultrasound may also detect orbital abscess but is less reliable (Schramm 1978; Krohel 1980).

The initial treatment of orbital cellulitis in infants should be with high dose intravenous chloramphenicol combined with a penicillinase resistant penicillin, or a cephalosporin (Guttman 1977). In older children in whom haemophilus infection is less likely ampicillin can be used instead of chloramphenicol. The initial regime may be modified in the light of later culture results. About 60% of children will be cured by antibiotics alone but the remainder will require surgical drainage of an infected sinus or orbital abscess (Weiss 1983). With prompt treatment complications (Table 13.2) are fortunately rare.

Subperiosteal and orbital abscess

The incidence of subperiosteal and orbital abscess complicating orbital cellulitis varies in different series but is probably about 10% (Hornblass 1984). The vast majority of such cases have associated sinus infection. In subperiosteal abscess, a purulent infection within a sinus breaks through the orbital bony wall and lies beneath the periosteum which is stripped from the bone. Orbital abscess occurs either when a subperiosteal abscess breaches the periorbita or when a collection of pus forms within the orbit in a child with orbital cellulitis. The usual causative organism is *Staphylococcus* but *Streptococcus* and *Haemophilus* may also be responsible. Unless there is non-axial proptosis or a palpable fluctuant swelling at the orbital rim, it is difficult to distinguish orbital abscess from uncomplicated orbital cellulitis clinically. It should be suspected whenever there is marked systemic toxicity and severe orbital signs, or when orbital cellulitis is slow to respond to adequate doses of intravenous antibiotics. Initial CT scanning of all new cases of orbital cellulitis will allow early detection of orbital and subperiosteal abscess, and serial orbital ultrasound may be used to follow the course of the abscess once treatment has been started.

The management of orbital or subperiosteal abscess is by surgical drainage including the involved sinus and high-dose intravenous antibiotics.

Osteomyelitis of the superior maxilla

This condition which usually presents in the first few months of life with fever, general malaise and marked periorbital oedema, may be confused with orbital cellulitis, or subperiosteal abscess (Cavenagh 1960). There may be conjunctival chemosis and mild proptosis and early central abscess formation in the superior maxilla with pointing at the inner or outer canthus. The diagnosis should be suspected if there is pus in the nostril and oedema of the alveolus and palate on the affected side. A fistula may be present in the area of the first deciduous molar.

Staphylococcus aureus is the usual infecting organism but the mode of infection is uncertain; it may result from haematogenous spread to the dental sac of the first deciduous molar which has a rich blood supply or may develop secondary to mastitis in the mother.

Treatment is with high-dose intravenous cloxacillin and surgical drainage of the abscess preferably via the nose. Cavenagh (1960) has reviewed the literature on this condition and reported a series of 24 infants she has personally treated with excellent results.

Cavernous sinus thrombosis

Since the introduction of antibiotics this dreaded complication of orbital cellulitis is rare. In the pre-antibiotic era the mortality rate was almost 100% (Grove 1936). Antibiotics have reduced the mortality of this complication of orbital cellulitis to 25% (Clune 1963) from 100% (Grove 1936). In its early stages cavernous sinus thrombosis may be difficult to distinguish clinically from orbital cellulitis. In the former there is more severe pain and a marked systemic illness, proptosis develops rapidly and there may be IIIrd, IVth, and VIth cranial nerve palsies compared with the purely mechanical limitation seen in orbital cellulitis. Hyperalgesia in the distribution of the Vth cranial nerve is common. The presence of retinal venous dilatation and optic disc swelling, especially if bilateral, is very suggestive of cavernous sinus thrombosis. In the later stages, bilateral involvement in cavernous sinus thrombosis makes the clinical distinction from orbital cellulitis easier.

The management of cavernous sinus thrombosis is best undertaken by a paediatric neurologist or neurosurgeon and involves treatment with high-dose intravenous antibiotics with anticoagulants and systemic steroids in selected cases.

Fungal orbital cellulitis

Fungal orbital cellulitis is rare in childhood but fungi of the class phycomycetes, may cause orbital infection in children who are acidotic, diabetic, or immunosuppressed.

Orbital phycomycosis

In adults this infection is seen mainly in diabetics in ketoacidosis but may occur in mild diabetes (Schwartz 1977) and in patients who are immunosuppressed. The main predisposing condition in childhood is metabolic acidosis associated with gastroenteritis (Hale 1971) although less commonly it may occur in children who are diabetic or immunosuppressed (Schwartz 1977). Blodi et al. have reported two cases occurring in otherwise healthy children (Blodi 1969). Untreated, it is rapidly fatal so that prompt diagnosis is essential.

The condition begins with colonization of the sinuses by Phycomycetes followed by direct or haematogenous spread to the orbit. Orbital involvement is heralded by periorbital pain, marked lid oedema, conjunctival chemosis and proptosis. Later spread to the orbital apex will result in IIIrd, IVth, and VIth cranial nerve palsies and optic neuropathy. Central retinal artery occlusion may occur. Sinus X-rays will normally show ethmoid or maxillary sinusitis. Phycomycetes have a tendency to invade arteries and cause thrombosis and subsequent tissue necrosis; involvement of the facial arteries causes gangrene of the nose, palate and facial tissues. Once spread to the cavernous sinus and intracranial vessels has occurred, the prognosis is very poor.

Orbital phycomycosis should therefore be suspected in any diabetic, acidotic or immunosuppressed child who develops a rapidly progressive orbital cellulitis, especially if accompanied by necrosis of skin or nasal mucosa. To confirm the diagnosis, scrapings from infected tissues should be cultured and Gram and Giemsa stained. Larger tissue biopsies should be fixed in 10% formalin and processed for histological examination. These fungi have an affinity for haematoxylin and are therefore easily recognized in haematoxylin and eosin sections. A positive culture result should be interpreted with caution as phycomycetes are common contaminants in most microbiology laboratories. The presence of the typical non-septate branching hyphae in scrapings or histological sections of involved tissues is necessary to make a definite diagnosis.

The management of this condition consists of specific antifungal therapy, correction of the underlying metabolic or immunological abnormality and surgical debridement of necrotic tissues. The specific treatment of choice is amphotericin B which should be given intravenously and may also be used locally to irrigate infected sinuses. It is nephrotoxic so renal function should be carefully monitored. Any metabolic abnormality should be corrected and immunosuppressive drugs especially steroids should be withdrawn if possible. Surgical debridement of necrotic tissues should be performed when the patient's general condition allows.

References

Barkin, RM, Todd JK, Amer J. Periorbital cellulitis in children *Pediatrics* 1978; **62**: 390−2

Blodi FC, Hannah FT, Wadsworth JAC. Lethal orbitocerebral phycomycosis in otherwise healthy children. *Am J Ophthalmol* 1969; **67**: 698−704

Cavenagh F. Osteomyelitis of the superior maxilla in infants. *Br Med J* 1960; **1**: 468−72

Chandler JR, Langenbrunner DJ, Stevens ER. The pathogenesis of orbital complications of acute sinusitis. *Laryngoscope* 1970; **80**: 1414−28

Clune JP. Septic thrombosis within the cavernous sinus. *Am J Ophthalmol* 1963; **56**: 33−9

Duke-Elder S, MacFaul PA. In: Duke Elder S (Ed.) *Ocular Adnexae: Lacrimal Orbital and Para-orbital Diseases. System of Ophthalmology*, vol. XIII, part 2. CV Mosby Co, St Louis 1974; pp. 859−89

Flood TP, Braude LS, Jampol LM, Herzog S. Computed tomography in the management of orbital infections associated with dental disease. *Br J Ophthalmol* 1982; **66**: 269−74

Goldberg F. Berne AS, Oski FA. Differentiation of orbital cellulitis from preseptal cellulitis by computed tomography. *Paediatrics* 1978; **62**: 1000−9

Grove WE. Septic and aseptic types of thrombosis of the

cavernous sinus. *Arch Otolaryngol* 1936; **24**: 29−50

Guttmann L. Appropriate antibiotics in orbital cellulitis. *Arch Ophthalmol* 1977; **95**: 170−6

Hale LM. Orbito-cerebral phycomycosis. *Arch Ophthalmol* 1971; **86**: 39−43

Hornblass A, Herschorn BJ, Stern K, Grimes C. Orbital abscess. *Surv Ophthalmol* 1984; **29**: 169−78

Jarrett W, Gutman F. Ocular complications of infection in the paranasal sinuses. *Arch Ophthalmol* **1969**; **81**: 683−8

Jones DB. Microbial pre-septal and orbital cellulitis. In: Duane TD, Jaeger AJ (Eds.) *Clinical Ophthalmology*, Vol. 4. Harper and Row, London 1982; pp. 1−19

Jones DB. Discussion on paper by Weiss *et al.* Bacterial periorbital cellulitis and orbital cellulitis in childhood. *Ophthalmology* 1983; **90**: 201−3

Judisch F. Orbital cellulitis secondary to Coats disease. *Arch Ophthalmol* 1980; **98**: 2004−6

Krohel GB, Krauss HR, Christensen RE, Minckler D. Orbital abscess. *Arch Ophthalmol* 1980; **98**: 274−6

Lerman SJ, Brunken JM, Bollinger M. Prevalence of ampicillin resistant strains of *Haemophilus influenzae* causing systemic infection. *Antimicrob Agents Chemother* 1980; **18**: 474−5

Levine RA. Infection of the orbit by an atypical mycobacterium. *Arch Ophthalmol* 1969; **82**: 608−10

Londer L, Nelson DL. Orbital cellulitis due to *Haemophilus influenzae*. *Arch Ophthalmol* 1974; **91**: 89−98

Rozansky NM. A necrotic retinoblastoma simulating panophthalmitis. *Surv Ophthalmol* 1964; **9**: 381−3

Schramm VL, Myers EN, Kennerdell J. Orbital complications of acute sinusitis. Evaluation management and outcome. *Otolaryngol* 1978; **86**: 221−30

Schwartz JN, Donnelly EH, Klintworth GK. Ocular and orbital phtycomycosis. *Surv Ophthalmol* 1977; **22**: 3−28

Sevel D, Tobias B, Sellars SL, *et al.* Gas in the orbit associated with orbital cellulitis and paranasal sinusitis. *Br J Ophthalmol* 1973; **57**: 133−7

Sherry T. Acute infarction of the choroid and retina *Br J Ophthalmol* 1973; **57**: 204−5

Smith TF, O'Day D, Wright PF. Clinical implications of preseptal (periorbital) cellulitis in childhood. *Pediatrics* 1978; **62**: 1006−9

Von Noorden GK. Orbital cellulitis following extraocular muscle surgery. *Am J Ophthalmol* 1972; **74**: 627−9

Watters E, Waller H, Hiles D, Michaels RH. Acute orbital cellulitis *Arch Ophthalmol* 1976; **94**: 785−8

Weiss A, Friendly D, Eglin K, Chang M, Cold B. Bacterial periorbital and orbital cellulitis in childhood. *Ophthalmology* 1983; **90**: 195−203

14 Endophthalmitis

ANTHONY MOORE

Intraocular infections may be caused by bacteria, fungi or parasites; organisms may enter the eye directly (exogenous endophthalmitis) or may be blood-borne from a distant source of infection (endogenous endophthalmitis). Bacterial infections which usually present acutely and progress rapidly will be considered separately from fungal and parasitic endophthalmitis.

Bacterial endophthalmitis

Bacterial endophthalmitis is rare in childhood but prompt recognition and early treatment is essential if blindness and destruction of the globe is to be avoided. A high 'index of suspicion' is necessary to diagnose this rare condition early and a systematic approach to diagnosis and management should be followed for optimum results.

Exogenous bacterial endophthalmitis

AETIOLOGY

Pathogenic bacteria may enter the eye by a variety of routes; direct infection may occur during intraocular surgery or follow penetrating trauma or inadvertent performation of the globe during extraocular surgical procedures such as strabismus and retinal surgery (McMeel *et al.* 1978; Salamon 1982). Endophthalmitis may also develop secondary to an infected glaucoma drainage bleb, suppurative keratitis (Fig. 14.1) or even orbital cellulitis.

In adults most bacterial infections develop following intraocular surgery but this complication is fortunately rare (for example the incidence of post operative endophthalmitis following cataract surgery is about 0.1%) (Allen & Mangiaracine 1964, 1973). The patient is the usual source of infection although contaminated instruments or solutions or less commonly the surgeon may be the cause. In children, in whom intraocular surgery is rarely performed, trauma is a more important predisposing factor (Weinstein *et al.* 1979).

PATHOGENIC ORGANISMS

The common organisms causing bacterial endophthalmitis are *Staphylococcus epidermidis*, *Staph. aureus*, *Streptococcus* spp., *Proteus* spp. and *Pseudomonas* spp. (Forster *et al.* 1976; Forster 1978; Olson 1983). A single organism is usually responsible although in post-traumatic endophthalmitis mixed infections are common. Postoperative infections are most commonly due to Gram-positive organisms (Olson 1983) and staphylococcal infections are responsible in about 50% of cases. Late glaucoma drainage bleb infections are due to streptococci in a high proportion of cases. Most studies of the bacteriology of endophthalmitis have been concerned with the adult population but in Weinstein's study of children with endophthalmitis the results were very similar with 75% of culture-positive cases being caused by Gram-positive organisms (Weinstein 1979).

CLINICAL PRESENTATION

The clinical presentation of bacterial endophthalmitis depends on the route of infection and the virulence of

114

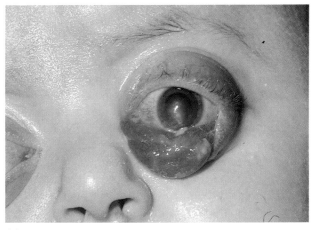

(a)

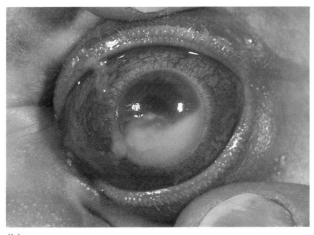

(b)

Fig. 14.1 (a)Exposure keratitis with conjunctival chemosis in a child with subluxation of the globe caused by shallow orbits in Crouzon's disease. (b)Same patient with endophthalmitis and hypopyon following exposure keratitis. Although the eye was saved by prompt antibiotic treatment the acuity 5 years later was very poor due to amblyopia. Occlusion of the other eye was made difficult by the craniofacial deformity.

the organism. Postoperative endophthalmitis typically presents 1 to 3 days after surgery with pain and blurring of vision. There is usually lid swelling, conjunctival injection and chemosis, a severe uveitis, hypopyon and vitreous haze. With less virulent organisms such as *Staph. epidermidis* the onset of symptoms and signs may be delayed for several weeks after surgery. In endophthalmitis following penetrating trauma there is a persistent severe uveitis and vitreous haze often with infiltration of the wound edges. Retinal periphlebitis may be an early sign of bacterial endophthalmitis in those cases in which a fundus examination is possible. Endophthalmitis should always be suspected after intraocular surgery or trau-

matic perforation whenever the degree of inflammation is greater than expected.

The main differential diagnosis is from fungal endophthalmitis and severe uveitis. Rarely retinoblastoma or metastatic tumour may present with uveitis and hypopyon (Table 14.1).

BACTERIOLOGICAL INVESTIGATION

Culture specimens from aqueous, vitreous and any other obviously infected site should always be taken before starting therapy. Children with suspected endophthalmitis often need a general anaesthetic to allow a thorough examination and bacteriological specimens to be taken. The microbiologist should be informed so that fresh culture media are available in the operating room and that immediate Gram and Giemsa stains can be performed.

We recommend the protocol suggested by Forster *et al.* (1980). Aqueous and vitreous specimens are plated out on blood agar, chocolate agar and thioglycollate and incubated at 37°C for bacterial isolation; further specimens are incubated at 25°C on Sabauraud's medium and blood agar for fungal growth. In addition, both aqueous and vitreous should be placed on glass slides and stained with Gram and Giemsa stains. Once all the specimens have been taken, intravitreal and subconjunctival antibiotic injections can be given during the same anaesthetic.

MANAGEMENT

There are few published reports on the management of endophthalmitis in childhood and as it seems that similar organisms are responsible for childhood and adult infections, antimicrobial therapy should be guided by experience in treating adult endophthalmitis (Forster 1980; Ramsey 1983; Olson *et al.* 1983) Young children present special problems in management and frequent sedation or general anaesthetics may need to be given to allow the progress of treatment to be monitored and subconjunctival injections given. Be-

Table 14.1 Causes of hypopyon in childhood.

Endophthalmitis
Severe uveitis
Retinoblastoma
Leukemia
Lymphoma
Neuroblastoma
Langerhans cell histiocytosis (LCH)

fore starting treatment, the Gram and Giemsa stains of aqueous and vitreous should be reviewed; if there is no evidence of fungal infection treatment should be started with broad spectrum antibiotics (Gram-stain results are not sufficiently reliable to allow specific antibacterial treatment to be given at this stage). Gentamicin and cephalazolin are given intravitreally, subconjunctivally and systematically as detailed in Table 14.2. Special care should be taken in preparing the intravitreal antibiotics because of the risk of retinal toxicity if higher doses are inadvertently given (Jeglum 1981). Renal function and intravenous drug levels should be monitored while gentamicin is being used. Antibiotic therapy is reviewed in the light of culture and sensitivity results. Once a causative organism has been isolated and there is improvement on specific antibacterial therapy local and systemic steroids should be given to reduce intraocular inflammation. (Steroids are however contraindicated if a co-existant fungal infection is suspected.)

The role of vitrectomy in the early management of bacterial endophthalmitis is not established. Although it offers the theoretical advantage of allowing removal of bacterial toxins from the eye and facilitating the spread of intraocular antibiotics it is technically difficult in infected eyes and complications such as retinal detachment may occur (Olson 1983); in children especially the lens may have to be sacrificed to allow a complete vitrectomy to be performed.

In cases where medical treatment is not successful in controlling the infection and vision is lost evisceration should be performed.

Table 14.2 Initial treatment* of bacterial endophthalmitis.

1. *Intravitreal*
    Gentamicin 0.1 mg (in 0.1 ml)
    Cephazolin 2.25 mg (in 0.1 ml)
2. Subconjunctival
    Gentamicin 40 mg (10–20 mg in infants)
    Cephazolin 125 mg (or cefuroxime 125 mg)
3. Systemic
    Gentamicin 2 mg/kg i.v. or i.m./8 hourly
    Cefuroxime 60 mg/kg/day in divided i.v. or i.m. doses 6–8 hourly (or ceftazidime 60 mg/kg/day in divided doses 8 hourly)
    Monitor serum levels and adjust doses accordingly
4. Topical
    Atropine 1% b.d. (0.5% b.d. in infants)
    Genticin hourly
    Cephazolin 5% (or cefuroxine 5%) hourly

* Review therapy when culture results available.

PREVENTION

In postoperative endophthalmitis the patient is the usual source of infection; children with extraocular infection such as blepharitis or conjunctivitis or with impaired nasolacrimal drainage should have ocular surgery deferred until these conditions are remedied. We routinely use topical chloramphenical for 24 hours pre-operatively and give a subconjunctival injection of gentamicin or a cephalosporin at the end of intraocular surgery. In addition, meticulous attention should be paid to a sterile non-touch operative technique. In penetrating trauma it is important to remove any intraocular foreign body or devitalized tissue and to commence local and systemic antimicrobials immediately after wound repair. Aphakic infants wearing contact lenses are at risk of developing suppurative keratitis and endophthalmitis; the parents should be warned to remove the contact lens immediately and seek advice if there is conjunctival injection, corneal haze, purulent discharge, photophobia or pain.

Endogenous bacterial endophthalmitis

Metastatic endophthalmitis results from haematogenous spread of infection from a distant focus of infection such as meningitis (Hedges 1956; Jenson & Naidof 1973) bacterial endocarditis, skin infections, abdominal sepsis and otitis media (Gammel & Allansmith 1974). Bilateral involvement occurs in about 50% of cases (Gammel & Allensmith 1974). Streptococci. staphylococci and meningococci (Fig. 14.2, 14.3) are the organisms most commonly involved.

The usual presentation is with insidious onset of blurred vision, often bilaterally (Jensen & Naidoff 1973) and photophobia. Initially the clinical picture may be confused with a chronic uveitis (Gammel & Allansmith 1974) and the diagnosis delayed until there are signs of a severe vitritis or hypopyon. The presence of significant vitreous inflammation and posterior segment changes such as vasculitis and localized choroidal or retinal infiltration suggest an infective aetiology.

Metastatic endophthalmitis should be managed in the same way as post-operative infection. Aqueous and vitreous specimens should be obtained for culture before starting treatment with broad spectrum antibiotics. In children who are too sick to undergo a general anaesthetic, antibiotic therapy can be guided by the results of blood culture.

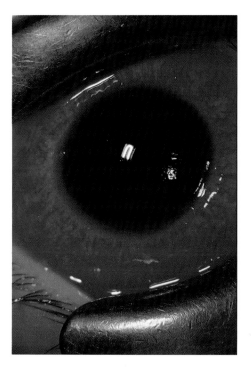

Fig. 14.2 Panophthalmitis in meningococcal septicaemia. Fifty per cent of such cases are bilateral.

Fungal endophthalmitis

Fungal endophthalmitis is fortunately rare in child-hood and is usually seen as a complication of fungal septicaemia in sick children with compromised im-munity. Rarely fungal infection may complicate pen-etrating trauma especially when there is retained foreign material (Meyer & Hood 1977).

Endogenous fungal endophthalmitis

Candida albicans is the organism most commonly implicated in endogenous fungal endophthalmitis although other fungal pathogens are occasionally res-ponsible. It usually develops in sick children with candidal septicaemia; risk factors include immuno-suppression, intravenous feeding (Parke *et al*. 1982), haemodialysis (Parke *et al*. 1982), prematurity (Baley *et al*. 1981) and broad-spectrum antibiotic use (Baley *et al*. 1981) Endophthalmitis is seen clinically in about 40% of patients with candidal septicaemia Baley *et al*. 1981; Parke *et al*. 1982) although postmortem studies (Edwards *et al*. 1974) have shown histopathological evidence of intraocular infection in 85% of cases.

The typical appearance of intraocular candida in-fection is of discrete fluffy white chorio-retinal lesions sometimes with an associated retinal haemorrhage.

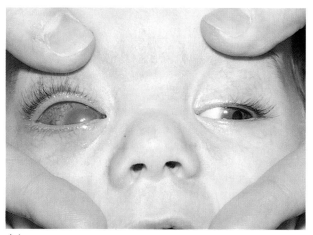

(a)

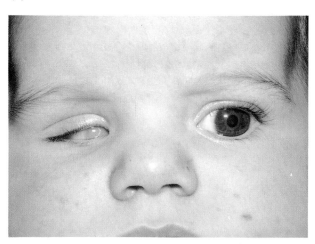

(b)

Fig. 14.3 Meningococcal endophthalmitis (a) leading to phthisis bulbi (b).

There is usually overlying vitreous inflammation, and as the condition evolves the retinal lesions enlarge and white 'snowballs' may appear in the vitreous (Edwards *et al*. 1974). In most cases, when the ocular lesions are small and *candida* has been isolated from blood cul-tures treatment can be started without the need for culture of aqueous and vitreous. Diagnostic vitrectomy is indicated when the diagnosis is in doubt or when there is a large vitreous abscess. Until recently the treatment of choice has been amphotericin B (despite its toxicity) which may be used in combination with flucytosine, although resistance may develop to the latter (Edwards 1978). Ketoconazole, an antifungal agent, which is less toxic than amphotericin B has been successfully used in *Candida endophthalmitis* (Salmon *et al*. 1983) and may eventually replace amphotericin B although experience is at present limited. The overall management of these children should be undertaken by a paediatrician with a special interest in infectious disease.

Exogenous fungal endophthalmitis

This may rarely complicate penetrating trauma in children, especially if there is a retained wooden foreign body. Symptoms and signs of intraocular infection may develop weeks or months after the injury following which there is a slow progression, with uveitis, vitritis and later hypopyon and vitreous abscess.

In suspected fungal endophthalmitis aqueous and vitreous specimens should be aspirated and cultured as for bacterial endophthalmitis. Gram and Geimsa stains will often show fungal hyphae and allow a prompt diagnosis to be made. If fungi are seen on microscopic examination amphoteracin B (5µg) is injected intravitreally and broad spectrum antifungal treatment given locally and systemically. Steroids should not be used. The detailed treatment of fungal endophthalmitis has been reviewed by Jones (1978) and Smolin et al. (1984).

Parasitic endophthalmitis

Toxocara

See Chapter 23.

Toxoplasmosis

See Chapter 11.

Immune-mediated ophthalmitis

Mahdi et al. (1988) proposed an immune-mediated mechanism for endophthalmitis in a 7-month-old with meningococcal septicaemia whose panophthalmitis failed to respond to systemic antibiotic therapy but which responded to topical steroids and mydriatics.

References

Allen HF, Mangiaracine AB. Bacterial endophthalmitis after cataract extraction: a study of 22 infections in 20,000 operations. *Arch Ophthalmol* 1964; **72**: 454–62

Allen HF, Mangiaracine AB. Bacterial endophthalmitis after cataract extraction: II Incidence in 36000 consecutive operations with special reference to pre-operative antibiotics. *Trans Am Acad Ophthalmol Otolarygol* 1973; **77**: 581–8

Baley J, Annable WL, Kliegmann RM. *Candida endophthalmitis* in the premature infant. *J Pediatr* 1981; **98**: 458–61

Edwards JE. Severe candidal infections, clinical perspectives, immune defense mechanisms and current concepts of therapy. *Ann Intern Med* 1978; **89**: 91–106

Edwards J, Foos R, Montgomerie J, Gaze L. Ocular manifestations of Candida Septicaemia. Review of 76 cases of haematogenous *Candida endophthalmitis*. *Medicine* 1974; **53**: 47–5

Forster RK, Etiology and diagnosis of bacterial post operative endophthalmitis. *Ophthalmology* 1978; **85**: 320–6

Forster RK, Abbot RL, Gelender H. Management of infectious endophthalmitis. *Ophthalmology* 1980; **87**: 313–19

Forster RK, Zacchary I, Cottingham A, Norton E. Further observations on the diagnosis, cause and treatment of endophthalmitis. *Am J Ophthalmol* 1976; **81**: 52–6

Gammel J, Allansmith M. Metastatic staphylococcal endophthalmitis presenting as chronic iridocyclitis. *Am J Ophthalmol* 1974; **77**: 454–8

Hedges TR, McAllister R, Coriell LL *et al*. Metastatic endophthalmitis as a complication of meningococcic meningitis. *Arch Ophthalmol* 1956; **55**: 503–05

Jeglum EL, Rosenberg SB, Benson WE. Preparation of intravitreal drug doses. *Ophthalmic Surg* 1981; **12**: 355–9

Jensen AD, Naidoff MA. Bilateral meningococcal endophthalmitis. *Arch Ophthalmol* 1973; **90**: 396–8

Jones DB. Therapy of post surgical fungal endophthalmitis. *Ophthalmology* 1978; **85**: 357–70

Mahdi G, Tulton M, Evans-Jones G. Ophthalmitis in meningococcal disease. *Arch Dis Child* 1988; **63**: 550–1

McMeel JW, Naegele DF, Badrinath SS, Murphy PL. Acute and subacute infections following scleral buckling operations. *Ophthalmology* 1978; **85**: 341–9

Meyer R, Hood I. Fungus implantation with wooden intraocular foreign bodies. *Ann Ophthalmol* 1977; **9**: 271–8

Olson JC, Flynn HW, Forster RK, Clubertson WW. Results in the treatment of post operative endophthalmitis. *Ophthalmology* 1983; **90**: 692–9

Parke D, Jones D, Gentry L. Endogenous endophthalmitis among patients with candidemia. *Ophthalmology* 1982; **89**: 789–96

Ramsey JJ, Newsom DL, Sexton DJ, Harms WK. Endophthalmitis current approaches. Ophthalmology 1982; **89**: 1055–65

Salamon S, Friborg T, Lukenberg M. Endophthalmitis after strabismus surgery. *Am J Ophthalmol* 1982; **93**: 39–41

Salmon JF, Partridge B, Spalton DJ. *Candida endophthalmitis* in a heroin addict: a case report. *Br J Ophthalmol* 1983; **67**: 306–9

Smolin G, Tabbara K, Whitaker J. *Infectious Diseases of the Eye*. Williams & Wilkins, Baltimore 1984; pp. 161–71

Weinstein GS, Mondino BJ, Weinberg RJ, Biglan AW. Endophthalmitis in a pediatric population. *Ann Ophthalmol* 1979; **11**: 935–43

15 External Eye Diseases

DAVID TAYLOR

Infections of the external eye

Epidemiology

Corneal disease is the commonest cause of blindness in many parts of the world today (Foster 1988). In pre-antibiotic days infective keratitis was the major cause of child blindness and that situation still applies to the developing world especially in areas where there is chronic malnutrition, endemic trachoma and unhygenic living conditions.

In developed countries external eye infections comprise one of the commonest referrals to casualty clinics (Chiapella & Rosenthal 1985), and keratitis is a small but significant cause of blindness especially amongst children whose health is already compromised.

The normal flora of the conjunctiva is different to that of adults with children having fewer anaerobic bacteria and more *Streptococcus* species (Singer *et al.* 1988).

The 'soil and the seed'

Normally the eye has a very strong resistance to the damaging effects of even the most virulent of micro-organisms. That resistance is based on a number of factors:

1 A normal volume tear production, and the ability to produce more when needed.
2 Normal tear constituents, including lysozyme and other antibacterial substances, immunoglobulins, cells and interferon.
3 A stable tear film that covers the whole cornea evenly and does not break down between blinks.
4 Normal tear spreading by blinking.
5 Corneal sensation and the ability to detect and react to corneal foreign bodies.
6 An intact epithelium with properties of resistance to penetration by micro-organisms, rapid repair, and a continued turnover of cells.

Should there be a breakdown in any one of those mechanisms the cornea and the eye itself are at threat from infection. In the developed world measles (rubella) gives rise to a keratoconjunctivitis with photophobia, grittiness and redness of the eyes that lasts a few days, clearing without residua. In the malnourished child, low in vitamin A, it results in a liquefactive keratitis and blindness. The soil is as important as the seed. Other common examples are the severity of herpes simplex keratitis in leukaemic children, the severity of fungal ulcers on the immuno-suppressed, the devastating rapidity of deterioration of corneal ulcers in children with a combination of 5th and VIIth nerve palsy, and the almost exclusive occurrence of *Candida* keratitis in the immune compromised, i.e. in mucocutaneous candidiasis (Wagman *et al.* 1987).

Symptoms and signs

The classic symptom of conjunctivitis is discharge giving rise to an eye that is stuck in the morning and has a greenish or yellowish discharge during the day. The eye is also red from blood vessel dilatation and haemorrhages may occur from endothelial damage and dilatation. Swelling of the conjunctiva is due to oedema and to follicles which are nests of lymphoid tissue within the conjunctiva which quickly swell during infections and to other antigenic stimuli; they have blood vessels around their margins whereas the papillae seen in chronic conjunctivitis are solid blocks of cellular aggregations around a central vascular core. Acute conjunctivitis causes the eye to feel hot and sometimes to itch a little. Vision is unaffected except by the strands of mucous floating around which can be blinked away to clear the vision.

Keratitis results in discomfort (except in anaesthetic eyes) and a foreign body sensation or grittiness; fresh ulcers may be frankly painful. The vision is unaffected until the corneal transparency is impaired, especially in the axial area. Eyes with keratitis almost invariably have a degree of conjunctivitis. Examination with magnification, preferably the slit lamp, is mandatory and fluorescein is helpful, painless and safe in demonstrating breaks in corneal and conjunctival epithelium.

Laboratory diagnosis

Although there is no necessity for culture of the discharge in every case seen in a general practice, the ophthalmologist must have access to good microbiology services if he is to make the correct diagnosis and institute the best treatment. Collaboration with a microbiologist colleague is the way in which most ophthalmologists achieve their goal. The pace of change in antibiotic therapy and microbiological diagnosis is so great that few ophthalmologist have adequate expertise in this area.

Bacterial culture is rarely necessary in acute conjunctivitis but is the counsel of perfection. In keratitis, the ulcer that fails to respond to antibiotics may need to have all treatment stopped for 48 hours before re-culturing. Scrapings are useful for culture and direct examination for fungi and bacteria when stained. Viral isolation is important in the neonate and also in herpes simplex keratitis.

Acute catarrhal conjunctivitis

Acute conjunctivitis without specific features in childhood results from infection with a vast array of organisms probably the commonest are the influenza virus, infectious mononucleosis, and with exanthemata such as measles.

Gigliotti *et al.* (1981) identified an organism in 72% of children with acute conjunctivitis. *Haemophilus influenza* accounted for 42% of those, adenovirus for 20% and *Streptococcus pneumoniae* for 12%. *H influenza* was more common in the winter, adenovirus in the late summer. If the children had pharyngitis then adenovirus was the most common organism. It was interesting that *Moraxella* and *Chlamydia* were not isolated in the group of children up to 18 years of age. *Moraxella* species usually cause a subacute conjunctivitis.

Acute follicular keratoconjunctivitis

Acute follicular conjunctivitis is usually bilateral, affecting one eye then the other, within a few days, and there is usually a history of contact with someone with similar symptoms. After the first few days the conjunctival follicles are enlarged and 'juicy' and there is often a systemic upset.

Epidemic keratoconjunctivitis (EKC)

EKC is often caused by adenovirus type 8 or 19 but other adenoviruses have been implicated. It is highly infectious. The incubation period is 1 week and the follicular conjunctivitis is associated with a keratitis with multiple small round, raised, white epithelial and subepithelial lesions which cause considerable discomfort. The symptoms may last some weeks and small white stromal lesions which represent an immune reaction may remain for months. A systemic illness occurs in nearly half the patients (Darougar *et al.*

1983). The disease spreads rapidly and is notorious for infecting patients and staff in an ophthalmology department.

Persistent lacrimation may be caused by a multifocal nasolacrimal duct and canalicular obstruction which may require probing, corticosteroid irrigation and intubation if dacryocystorrhinostomy is to be avoided (Hyde & Berger 1988).

Treatment is not usually helpful but dilute steroids may improve the symptoms and chloramphenicol may be used to prevent secondary bacterial infection.

Pharyngoconjunctival fever (PCF)

PCF is highly infectious and is due to the adenovirus type 3 or other subtypes. The patient has a fever, pharyngitis and a keratoconjunctivitis similar to EKC. No treatment alters the cause of the disease which lasts up to 2 weeks.

Herpes simplex keratoconjunctivitis

Darougar et al. (1985) studied primary herpes virus infections in 108 patients: 69% were over 15 years and 7% were under the age of 5 years. Upper respiratory tract infections were found in 35% and other systemic disturbance including fever, malaise and aching in 31%. Symptoms included redness, watering, discharge and itching lids. The major signs were lid vesicles and ulcers, papillary conjunctivitis mainly in the upper lid conjunctiva and follicles in the lower lid conjunctiva. Punctate epithelial keratitis was common but dendritic ulcers occurred in 15% and disciform keratitis in 2%. Seven per cent of patients presented with a keratoconjunctivitis without any clinical clues as to the diagnosis and a chronic blepharoconjunctivitis developed in 15% of patients.

The conjunctivitis may be severe with a pseudomembrane obscuring the conjunctiva but it is self-limiting in most patients. Special precautions need to be taken for the immunocompromised patient who should be treated with topical antiviral agents in conjunction with an infectious diseases specialist.

One of the most interesting things about the ubiquitous herpes simplex virus is why in some individuals the normally amicable relationship between the virus and host is disturbed (Monnikendam 1988). Most patients resolve spontaneously (Simon et al. 1986) only the minority developing keratitis.

Haemorrhagic keratoconjunctivitis

This occurs in epidemics and is due to various picornavirus types (enterovirus type 70). The epithelial keratitis is painful and the presence of multiple subconjunctival haemorrhages and the short duration (often only a few days) are characteristic. Coxsackie virus type A24 has also been implicated (Yin-Murphy et al. 1986).

Chlamydia

Chlamydia trachomatis strains cause neonatal inclusion conjunctivitis but Chlamydia strains cause acute trachoma and TRIC (oculogenital disease). The oculogenital types are not common in nonsexually active persons but acute trachoma occurs in children and young adults as a more or less subacute keratoconjunctivitis which is characterized by follicles prominent on the upper tarsal plate and a marginal keratitis. The changes which make it such a prominent cause of blindness relate to subconjunctival scarring with consequent dry eyes entropion and trichiasis. The clinical picture and progression vary with the health of the population in which trachoma is endemic and the area of the world. Treatment is with tetracycline ointment for 2 months and systemic erythromycin.

Other micro-organisms

Molluscum contagiosum infections (Fig. 15.1), mononucleosis, psittacosis and occasionally bacteria and fungi may cause a follicular conjunctivitis.

Subacute and chronic follicular conjunctivitis

Normal childhood folliculosis

It is normal in childhood to have prominent follicles especially in the fornices, in the lower lid especially and without much evidence of inflammation. It seems to be analogous to the normal lymphoid hyperplasia that occurs in tonsils, lymph nodes, etc.

Moraxella conjunctivitis

The bacteria Moraxella lacunata causes 'external angular conjunctivitis' — so called because it tends to affect the external angle most particularly with bulbar injection and involvement of the lids. It is a subacute infection which may give rise to marginal infiltrates.

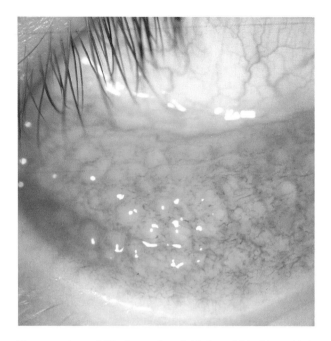

Fig. 15.1 Acute follicular conjunctivitis in a child with multiple molluscum cantagiosum lesions.

Other micro-organisms

Molluscum contagiosum and some bacterial or fungal conjunctivitis especially if partially treated may give rise to a chronic follicular conjunctivitis.

Drugs

Various drugs including idoxuridine, eserine and adrenaline can cause a subacute or chronic follicular conjunctivitis.

Keratitis

The most common forms of keratitis are those associated with acute virus infections but these are almost invariably self-limiting except in sick children. Herpes simplex keratitis forms a small but important group of older children with chronic disease who may lose vision as a result of the disease and amblyopia combined.

Bacterial keratitis

Microbial keratitis in children is a small cause of blindness (Coster *et al.* 1981), but one in which predisposing factors are vitally important (Ormerod *et al.* 1986); these include overwhelming systemic infections,

immunodeficiency, orbital malignancies, exposure, trauma, or dry eye.

Pseudomonas species (Ormerod *et al.* 1986) and *Streptococcus viridans* (Seal *et al.* 1982) are the most common bacteria isolated in early life. Mixed infections are common (Jones 1981). Older children are most commonly infected with *Strep pneumoniae* (Okumoto & Smolin 1974) and males are most frequently affected (Klein 1981; Ormerod *et al.* 1986). Beta-haemolytic streptococci, *Staphylococcus, Haemophilus* species, *Moraxella* species, *Coliform*, and *Shigella* (Schmeidt & Cimma 1983) are less frequent pathogens.

PREVENTION

Prevention is an important factor in the management of microbial keratitis. Paediatricians need to understand the relevance of corneal exposure, trichiasis and dry eyes and orbital neoplasms may require special attention due to the combination of exposure, dryness, immune deficiency, radiation keratitis, and corneotoxicity of chemotherapeutic drugs (Ormerod *et al.* 1986). Correct and careful nursing techniques may prevent many severe nosocomial corneal infections in children in intensive care units (Hilton *et al.* 1983).

TREATMENT

Treatment relies heavily on skilled paediatric management, and skilled and kind nursing so that frequently repeated eye drops can be instilled and subconjunctival doses of antibiotics given using oral or intravenous sedation or anaesthesia if necessary. Delivering the treatment is the most difficult part of the management but delivering the right treatment is also vital and usually requires collaboration with the microbiology team. Culture of the discharge and scraping are the most important prelude to treatment which should not be withheld awaiting the culture and antibiotic sensitivity results, but started immediately. Chloramphenicol remains the most effective topical treatment and tetracycline is also useful (Seal *et al.* 1982). Gentamycin is the most effective against *Pseudomonas* species (Dart & Seal 1988). Hourly drops are usually best given in a form without preservative because irritation by most preservatives can cause slow healing.

Intravenous antibiotics based on the sensitivity of the cultured organism should be given in the immunocompromized or septicaemic child.

Later treatment such as tectonic grafts, debridement, conjunctival flap, and penetrating keratoplasty all have their place but the visual prognosis is often poor due to the scarring from the disease and amblyopia in younger children.

Specific features of various forms of bacterial keratitis

PSEUDOMONAS AERUGINOSA

Pseudomonas ulcers most frequently affect young children (Fig. 15.2). It is a virulent organism that is mobile and produces collagenase which gives rise to a rapidly spreading liquefactive ulcer with hypopyon. Gentamycin remains the most frequently used antibiotic against *Pseudomonas*, and most other Gramnegative bacteria, but medical adjunctive therapy (i.e. cycloplegics, steroids, and protease inhibitors) and surgical treatment may help in some cases (Dart & Seal 1988).

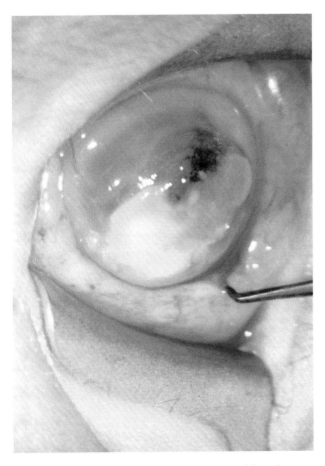

Fig. 15.2 Pseudomonas keratitis in a neonate with no known predisposing factors.

MORAXELLA

Moraxella species are diplococci which give rise to external angular keratitis and indolent corneal ulcers that are oval in shape with undermined edges.

STAPHYLOCOCCUS

Staphylococcal ulcers tend to be limited or with sattelite lesions and rather round in shape. *Staph aureus* is more virulent and *Staph epidermidis*, though much more common, only causes infection when the corneal resistance is compromised.

STREPTOCOCCUS

Streptococcus pneumoniae is a common organism that may invade corneas compromised by disease or contact lens wear. The ulcers may be very rapid in onset and spread with an undermined edge and hypopyon is frequent. *S pyogenes* usually causes marginal ulcers in an eye with blepharoconjunctivitis or dacryocystitis.

Streptococcus viridans is the usual cause of infectious crystalline keratopathy. The majority of hosts have had corneal surgery, trauma, herpes simplex or *Acanthamoeba* keratitis. The characteristic appearance is of a white, feathery crystalline deposit in the anterior stroma without much inflammation. Previous steroid treatment is frequent. The diagnosis is usually made by microscopy of corneal donor buttons but culture of a corneal scrape or swab may be possible (Watson *et al.* 1988).

GONOCOCCI

Gonococcal keratitis leads to a very rapidly spreading ulcer especially dangerous in the neonate. Perforation occurs rapidly if untreated. Meningococci give rise to similar ulcers.

ENTEROBACTERIA

Escherichia coli, Aerobacter, Proteus and *Klebsiella* species usually affect debilitated children.

Interstitial keratitis (IK)

Interstitial keratitis is a non-ulcerative stromal keratitis with vascularization which affects a variable proportion of the cornea.

Classically IK was caused by congenital syphilis early in the course of the disease, more frequently in

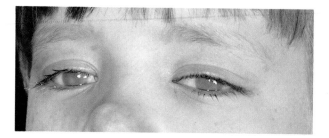

Fig. 15.3 Interstitial keratitis of unknown cause.

girls. Pain, photophobia, and limbal vascular engorgement occur, and the cornea becomes cloudy, usually diffusely and bilaterally (Fig. 15.3), a uveitis accompanies the corneal changes. Heavy vascularization extends from the limbus giving the orangey-red 'salmon patch'. Clearing proceeds from the periphery leaving a central hazy cornea and ghost vessels.

Diagnosis depends on clinical suspicion of the disease and the finding of a positive FTA-ABS test. Treatment consists of the treatment of the underlying disease and topical steroids. Syphilitic IK may represent an allergic mechanism.

Interstitial keratitis also occurs with onchocerciasis, leprosy and TB which give rise to localized disease whilst viral IK is usually discoid or more or less diffuse, causes including mumps, measles and herpes simplex.

Cogan's syndrome

Cogan's syndrome is an unusual condition in which there is a bilateral painful IK with deep stromal involvement and vascularization associated with orbital inflammatory signs and a progressive deafness. The keratitis, but not the deafness responds to corticosteroids. Vasculitis (Cheson *et al.* 1976) or an immunological mechanism has been proposed (Char *et al.* 1975).

Nummular keratitis

Nummular keratitis is a localized form of keratitis with often multiple round corneal lesions with minimal conjunctivitis. The corneal lesion may be faceted but not ulcerated. They are mostly caused by viruses including adenovirus, herpes simplex and zoster, EB (Epstrein−Barr) virus but it also occurs with sarcoid, onchocerciasis, and TB. The lesions often respond to topical steroids which must be used with care when herpes simplex is a possibility.

Fungal keratitis

Fungi are unusual causes of keratitis and occur in children predisposed by severe systemic disease (Wagman *et al.* 1987), trauma with dirty wounds (Hirst *et al.* 1979) topical and systemic steroid (Ralph *et al.* 1976). Prior administration of steroids remains a significant problem in weakening resistance to the infection and although they may have a role in the treatment of some infective keratitis when combined with antibiotics, they should be withheld where possible.

The commonest causitive organisms are Actinomycetaceae (*Actinomyces* and *Nocardia* in particular and *Candida*. *Candida* produces marginal infiltration or elevated multiple chronic white anterior stromal and epithelial defects with later penetration of the stroma (Fig. 15.4a, b), liquefaction and endophthalmitis. *Nocardia* are aerobic and produce penetrating single corneal ulcers with a slow onset but later they may have a severe keratitis, with hypopyon that may be resistant to antibiotic treatment and may require debridement and a conjunctival flap (Hirst *et al.* 1979).

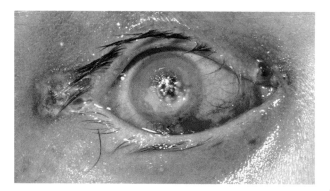

(a)

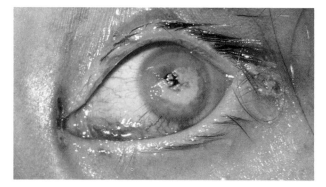

(b)

Fig. 15.4 Bilateral *Candida* keratitis in a severely immunocompromised child.

Small sattelite lesions around the main ulcer occur and coalesce with each other. They may respond to treatment with sulphonamides and co-trimoxazole.

Filamentous fungi such as *Fusarium* species, *Mucor*, *Penicillium* and *Aspergillus* also cause keratitis in dirty wounds and in compromised hosts.

Protozoal keratitis

Acanthamoeba species are ubiquitous protozoa that exist in soil and water. Acanthamoeba keratitis occurs in people exposed to the organism by swimming in brackish and standing water, in chlorinated swimming pools or hot tubs and by using contact lenses that are inadequately sterilized.

The ulcers are chronic and indolent, but are associated with few inflammatory signs. Infection often follows minor trauma, exposure to soil, standing water etc. and pain is a prominent symptom. The lesions are stromal infiltrates, often ring-shaped with variable anterior uveitis (Mannis *et al.* 1986). Diagnosis is made by Giemsa stains or fluorescent antibody techniques from corneal scrapes or keratoplasty buttons (Epstein *et al.* 1986).

It may be that the use of corticosteroids should be only instituted with caution because of the occurence of an additional bacterial keratitis, i.e. with *streptococcus viridans* causing infectious crystalline keratopathy (Ficker 1988) or *Pseudomonas* (Davis *et al.* 1987).

treatment with 0.1% propamidine isesthionate 0.15% dibromopropamidine, neomycin or miconazole has been successful (Wright *et al.* 1985), but the infection is often resistant to treatment and results in stromal keratitis which may require keratoplastly often with recurrence in the graft.

Heat sterilizing contact lenses is important in prevention together with the once only use of contact lens solution or sterilizing solutions that are discarded weekly (Ficker 1988). Contact lens cases should also be sterilized regularly.

Non-infective external eye disease

Phlyctenular disease

Phlyctenular conjunctivitis occurs in all parts of the world, often in undernourished children.

There is a single localized inflammatory lesion with a white centre that is raised and later ulcerates. The lesions are usually transient, lasting up to 2 weeks before disappearing without trace, only to reappear elsewhere. There are few symptoms. The cornea may be involved with a marginal infiltrate and an ulcer that is painful. Most cases are associated with staphylococcal lid disease by some form of immunological mechanism. No direct infective agent has been proved but it seems to be associated with systemic infections including tuberculosis, fungal and worm infections.

Ligneous conjunctivitis

Ligneous conjunctivitis is a disorder of children which presents with redness and watering, sometimes following acute conjunctivitis. There are thickened nodular masses composed of amorphous fibrous hyalinized material.

It has been reported in siblings (Bateman *et al.* 1986) and an autosomal recessive inheritance is suggested. Infective causes have never been proven. Other mucus membranes may be involved.

Treatment has been with excision, steroids, chromoglycate and with anti-fibrin agents with varying success. Excision by itself is followed by rapid recurrence (Hidayat & Riddle 1987). Spontaneous resolution occurs and cases in Hidayat and Riddle's series of 17 had the disease for 4 months to 44 years.

Chronic papillary conjunctivitis

Papillae form as a chronic response to a variety of stimulants. They are characterized by the presence of loops of vessels surrounded by variable cellular aggregations so that the papillae measure from 0.5 to 5 mm. The cells are inflammatory and later there is organization of the whole mosaic-like mass which is best seen on the tarsal plates of the upper lids.

CHRONIC ATOPIC CONJUNCTIVITIS

The prime symptom of this condition is itching, with redness, burning, watering, and stickiness also being present. It can be very troublesome but on examination there are very few signs — usually these are limited to the finding of numerous small pale tarsal papillae. There is often a personal or family history of atopy and conjunctival swabs show eosinophils in the mucous discharge. The serum IgE levels are raised. Although many cases are, like the eczema from which many of them suffer, self-limited, some go on to form a troublesome chronic keratoconjunctivitis (Jay 1981) and some develop keratoconus possibly related to eye rubbing.

Treatment is best kept to the minimum required for

the symptoms. Decongestants and antihistamine drops may be useful and many patients feel better with simple lubricants. Sodium cromoglycate is often helpful but needs to be used prophylactically if there is a seasonal element, and started well before the onset of symptoms. Steroids are best avoided, only being used in short courses under strict supervision.

PHYSICAL AND CHEMICAL IRRITANTS

Atropine, skin irritants, eye drop preservatives, oily vehicules and atmospheric and industrial chemicals may give rise to a chronic papillary conjunctivitis. Physical irritants include contact lenses, artificial eyes, eye sutures; lacrimal concretions with fungal infection may also cause a similar picture.

Certain 'soft' contact lenses and artificial eyes are associated with a giant papillary conjunctivitis almost identical to vernal disease. It starts after months or years of successful wear and develops gradually. It seems to be related to mechanical disturbance of the conjunctival epithelium.

VERNAL DISEASE

Vernal disease is a chronic conjunctivitis with an onset in childhood that is more frequent in boys than girls. It is seasonally exacerbated and occurs in all parts of the world although its incidence and manifestations vary greatly from area to area.

The onset is rarely before 4 years and many patients have a personal or family history of atopy (Frankland & Easty 1971) and there is often other evidence of hypersensitivity including high IgE levels in blood and tears and an eosinophilia.

Pollen-specific IgE and IgG have been found in tears and blood (Ballow & Mendelson 1980; Ballow *et al.* 1983) indicating that various forms of immune reactions may be involved.

The main symptom is itching with redness, watering, lid swelling, a mucus discharge being usual. The itching is invariable and matches the severity of the disease. There are two forms, palpebral and limbal with a mixed form.

The palpebral form is characterized by a generally more severe course with characteristic flat topped giant papillae in the upper tarsal conjunctiva which are red at first (Fig. 15.5), become whiter with ageing and in remission (Fig. 15.6). The papillae may be mucus laden and become very hypertrophic and when actively inflamed they may be indirectly associated with keratopathy but probably don't cause it.

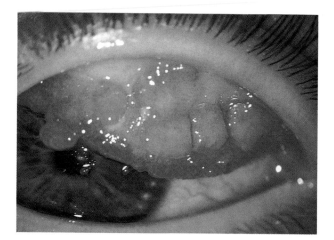

Fig. 15.5 Giant papillae in active vernal disease.

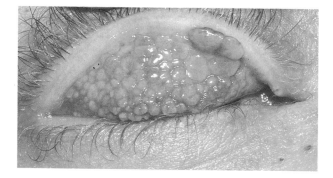

Fig. 15.6 Large papillae and residual giant papillae in chronic vernal disease on treatment.

Limbal vernal disease starts as a swelling and opacification at the limbus, often nodular (Fig. 15.7). The nodules are papillae with a central vascular tuft; they may become cystic or have white deposits in them known as Trantas Spots. The cornea becomes vascularised in the affected area of the limbus and arcus-like changes occur (Fig. 15.8).

Vernal keratopathy starts usually in the upper third of the cornea as epithelial opacities which coalesce and extend to form a punctate fluorescein-staining area which may shed to form a 'macro-erosion' (Buckley 1981). These erosions are very indolent with a slightly raised margin and a base which becomes filled with mucus and cellular debris known as vernal plaque. Sub-epithelial scarring and arcus lipoides (Fig. 15.8) occur related to the affected areas.

Treatment has been greatly aided by two drugs. The first, soluble steroids, can be used with great effect in acute and severe disease, usually being started

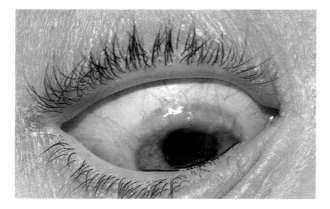

Fig. 15.7 Limbal vernal.

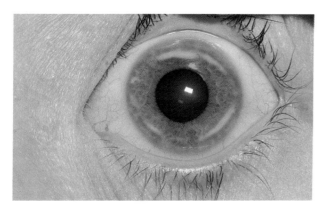

Fig. 15.8 Arcus lipoides in longstanding vernal disease currently in remission.

in high dose and rapidly tailed off, but chronic usage is often necessary. Therein lies the greatest problem because up to 10% may be susceptable to steroid-induced glaucoma. Since these children often pose great difficulty in examination, if tonometry is not possible they may require periodic anaesthetics in order to be sure that glaucoma has not supervened. The practise of prescribing acetazolamide routinely with steroids to 'prevent' glaucoma cannot be justified in view of the side effects of acetazolamide and the low risk of anaesthetic. The second drug is disodium cromoglycate which seems to lack side effects and to be at least moderately effective (Foster 1988). The drops sting especially in an already inflamed eye and they seem to take some time to become effective; it is often best to start them before an exacerbation if it is predictable or to cover the start of their use by increasing the steroid dose. Some cases can be controlled by disodium cromoglycate alone.

Vernal keratitis usually responds to the above medical treatment. There is no benefit to the cornea from removing the lid papillae however large and vicious looking, but corneal plaque may simply be excised (Buckley 1981).

Hay fever conjunctivitis

These children have recurrent, often seasonal red eyes and running nose in response to a variety of more or less well defined allergens, the commonest being pollen, moulds, horse dander and cat fur. The onset is rapid with itching and pale, baggy swelling of the lids and conjunctiva. They water and become red with time with mucoid discharge.

Treatment may be by desensitization, topical (rarely systemic) steroids, or antihistamines by drop or systemically. In principal treatment is usually started with antihistamines or decongestants being used depending on response.

Staphylococcal hypersensitivity

A form of hypersensitivity to staphylococcal exotoxins is used to explain a variety of external eye disease including some forms of blepharoconjunctivitis, meibomitis, and acute keratitis as in toxic epidermal necrolysis.

Episcleritis

Episcleritis occurs in self-limiting attacks lasting up to a month and recurring after an interval of months. The eye becomes red in a circumscribed area deep to the conjunctiva which may be swollen ('nodular') and irritable. No cause is found in children but in adults there is a definite association with gout. Treatment with a short course of topical steroids usually shortens the attack and oral non-steroidal anti-inflammatory agents may help.

References

Ballow M, Danshik PC, Mendelson L, Rapacz P, Sparks K. IgG specific antibodies to rye grass and ragweed pollen antigens in the tear secretions of patients with vernal conjunctivitis. *Am J Ophthalmol* 1983; **95**: 161−8

Ballow M, Mendelson L. Specific immunoglobulin E antibodies in tear secretions of patients with vernal conjunctivitis. *J Allergy Clin Immunol* 1980; **66**: 112−8

Bateman JB, Isenberg SJ, Pettit TH, Simons KB. Ligneous conjunctivitis: an autosomal recessive disorder. *J Pediatr Ophthalmol Strabismus* 1986; **23**: 137−40

Buckley RJ. Vernal keratopathy and its management. *Trans Ophthalmol Soc UK* 1981; **101**: 234−8

Char DM, Cogan DG, Sullivan WR. Immunologic study of

non-syphilitic interstitial keratitis with vestibuloauditory symptoms. *Am J Ophthalmol* 1975; **80**: 491−7

Cheson BD, Bluming AZ, Alroy J. Cogan's syndrome: a systemic vasculitis. *Am J Med* 1976; **60**: 549−51

Chiapella AP, Rosenthal AJR. One year in an eye casualty clinic. *Br J Ophthalmol* 1985; **69**: 865−70

Coster DJ, Wilhelmus K, Jones BR. Suppurative keratitis in London. In: Trevor-Roper PD (Ed.) *The Cornea in Health and Disease.* Academic Press, London 1981; pp. 395−8

Darougar S, Grey RHB, Thaker U, McSwiggan DA. Clinical and epidemiological features of adenovirus keratoconjunctivitis in London. *Br J Ophthalmol* 1983; **67**: 1−7

Darougar S, Wishart MS, Viswalingham ND. Epidemiological and clinical features of primary herpes simplex virus ocular infection. *Br J Ophthalmol* 1985; **69**: 2−6

Dart JK, Seal DV. Pathogenesis and therapy of *Pseudomonas aeruginosa* keratitis. *Eye* (Suppl.) 1988; **2**: 546−55

Davis RM, Schroeder RJP, Rowsey JJ, Jensen HG, Tripathi R. Acanthamoeba keratitis and infectious crystalline keratopathy. *Arch Ophthalmol* 1987; **105**: 1524−7

Epstein RJ, Wilson LA, Visvesvara GS, Plourde EG. Rapid diagnosis of acanthamoeba keratitis from corneal scraping using indirect fluorescent antibody staining. *Arch Ophthalmol* 1986; **104**: 1318−21

Ficker L. Acanthamoeba keratitis. The quest for a better prognosis. *Eye* (Suppl.) 1988; **2**: 537−45

Foster A. Childhood blindness. *Eye*(Suppl.) 1988; **2**: 527−36

Foster CS, The Cromolyn Sodium Collaborative Study Group. Evaluation of topical cromolyn sodium in the treatment of vernal keratoconjunctivitis. *Ophthalmology* 1988; **95**: 194−202

Frankland AW, Easty DL. Vernal keratoconjunctivitis, an atopic disease. *Trans Ophthalmol Soc UK* 1971; **91**: 479−82

Gigliotti F, Williams WT, Hayden FG, Hendley JO. Etiology of acute conjunctivitis in children. *J Pediatr* 1981; **98**: 531−6

Hidayat AA, Riddle PJ. Ligneous conjunctivitis. *Ophthalmology* 1987; **94**: 949−59

Hilton E, Uliss A, Samuels S, Adams AA, Leser, ML, Lowy FD. Nosocomial bacterial eye infections in intensive care units. *Lancet* 1983; i: issue 8337, 1318−20

Hirst LW, Harrison, GK, Merz WG, Stark WJ. *Nocardia asteroides* keratitis. *Br J Ophthalmol* 1979; **63**: 449−54

Hyde KJ, Berger ST. Epidemic keratoconjunctivitis and lacrimal excretory system obstruction. *Ophthalmology* 1988; **95**: 1447−9

Jay JL. Clinical features and diagnosis of adult atopic keratoconjunctivitis and the effect of treatment with sodium cromoglycate. *Br J Ophthalmol* 1981; **65**: 335−40

Jones DB. Polymicrobial keratitis. *Trans Am Ophthalmol Soc* 1981; **79**: 153−67

Klein JO. The epidemiology of pneumococcal disease in infants and children. *Rev Infect Dis* 1981; **3**: 246−53

Mannis MJ, Tamaru R, Roth AM *et al.* Acanthamoeba sclerokeratitis: determining diagnostic criteria. *Arch Ophthalmol* 1986; **104**: 1313−17

Monnickendam MA. Herpes simplex ophthalmia. *Eye* (Suppl.) 1988; **2**: 556−69

Okumoto M, Smolin G. Pneumococcal infections of the eye. *Am J Ophthalmol* 1974; **77**: 346−52

Ormerod LD, Murphree AL, Gomez DS, Schanzlin DJ, Smith RE. Microbial keratitis in children. *Ophthalmology* 1986; **93**: 449−55

Ralph RA, Lemp MA, Liss G. Nocardia keratitis: a case report. *Br J Ophthalmol* 1976; **60**: 104−6

Schmiedt R, Cimma R. Shigella corneal ulceration. *Clin Pediatr* 1983; **24**: 460−1

Seal DV, Barrett SP, McGill JI. Aetiology and treatment of acute bacterial infection of the external eye. *Br J Ophthalmol* 1982; **66**: 357−60

Simon JW, Lango F, Smith RS. Spontaneous resolution of herpes simplex blepharoconjunctivitis in children. *Am J Ophthalmol* 1986: **102**: 598−600

Singer TR, Isenberg SJ, Apt L. Conjunctival anaerobic and aerobic bacterial flora in paediatric versus adult subjects. *Br J Ophthalmol* 1988; **72**: 448−52

Wagman RD, Kazdan JJ, Kooh SW, Fraser D. Keratitis associated with the multiple endocrine deficiency, autoimmune disease, and candidiasis syndrome. *Am J Ophthalmol* 1987; **103**: 569−75

Watson AP, Tullo AB, Kerr-Muir MG, Ridgway ACA, Lucas DR. Arborescent bacterial keratopathy (infectious crystalline keratopathy). *Eye* (Suppl.) 1988; **2**: 517−22

Wright P, Warhurst D, Jones BR. *Acanthamoeba* keratitis successfully treated medically. *Br J Ophthalmol* 1985; **69**: 778−82

Yin-Murphy M, Baharuddin-Ishak, Phoon MC, Chow UTK. A recent epidemic of Coxsackie virus type A24 acute haemorrhagic conjunctivitis in Singapore. *Br J Ophthalmol* 1986; **70**: 869−73

16 Erythema Multiforme (Stevens–Johnson Syndrome)

ANTHONY MOORE

Erythema multiforme is an acute systemic disorder with variable skin and mucus membrane involvement. In its mildest form it is characterized by a localized or generalized skin eruption often with typical 'target' or 'iris' lesions. In the more severe form, often termed the Stevens–Johnson syndrome (Stevens & Johnson 1922), there is an extensive bullous form of erythema multiforme with involvement of mucus membrane and conjunctiva.

Although the exact aetiology is unknown, the disorder is thought to be due to an acute hypersensitivity reaction and may follow bacterial, protozoal, fungal, viral or mycoplasmal infection or be related to food or drug sensitivity (Gottschalk & Stone 1976; Hurwitz 1981;). In many cases the cause is unknown. Histological and immunohistochemical studies suggest that the skin and mucus membrane abnormalities are caused by an immune complex mediated vasculitis (Kazmierowski *et al.* 1979; Wuepper *et al.* 1980; Foster *et al.* 1988). In children most cases follow infection. Although the acute disorder is self limiting it can produce serious longterm ocular abnormalities (Wright & Collin 1983). Recurrent disease of the skin, eyes, and mucus membranes may occur in a minority of patients (Bean & Quezada 1983; Foster *et al.* 1988).

Clinical features

The clinical features of this disorder are extremely variable; in some cases there is a mild self-limiting skin rash with no mucus membrane involvement, whereas in others there is widespread skin and mucus membrane disease. Conjunctival involvement is similarly variable and tends to parallel the severity of the skin involvement.

In most cases the onset of the skin eruption is preceded by a prodromal period with mild fever, malaise and joint and muscle pains. The skin lesions are symmetrical, and may involve any part of the surface including palms and soles of the feet. The appearance is variable and includes patchy erythema, bullae or the typical target lesions (Hurwitz 1981). Oral lesions are common and are seen as swelling and blistering of the lips and erosions of the oral mucosa and tongue. Conjunctival involvement varies from mild injection to severe disease with membrane formation and symblepharon (Fig. 16.1, 16.2).

The most severe involvement occurs in the Stevens–Johnson syndrome. In this variant there is usually a prodromal period of general malaise, fever, gastrointestinal upset and arthralgia followed by acute onset of an extrusive bullous skin eruption with severe involvement of ocular, oral, anal and genital mucosa with later scarring (Fig. 16.3).

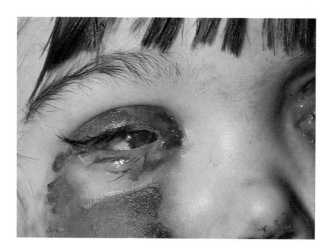

Fig. 16.1 Stevens–Johnson syndrome; early stage with acute keratoconjunctivitis and skin lesions.

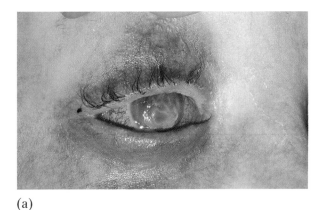

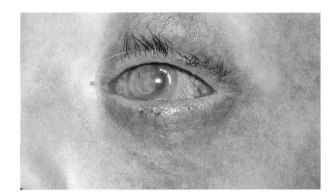

(a)

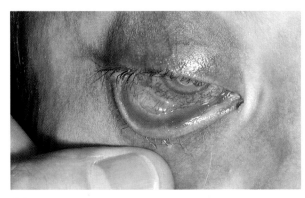

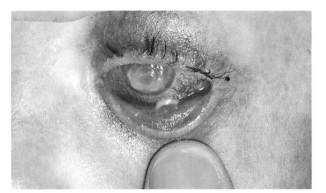

(b)

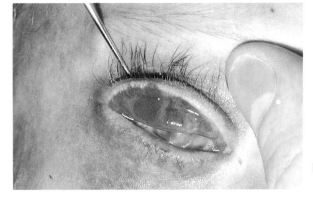

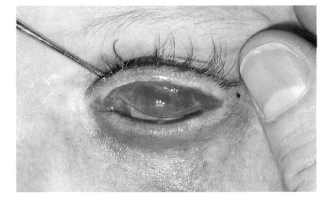

(c)

Fig. 16.2a, b, c Stevens–Johnson syndrome; bilateral desquamative conjunctivitis with areas of necrosis. There is a severe keratitis which resulted in chronic scarring worsened by the later occurrence of a dry eye.

Ocular involvement

In the acute phase there is usually a mucopurulent conjunctivitis (Fig. 16.1) with a marked papillary re-action of the subtarsal conjunctiva. In more severe cases there is infarction of the conjunctiva (Fig. 16.2) with membrane formation and adhesions may form between the lid and bulbar conjunctiva (Wright & Collin 1983). Secondary infection may occur if topical antibiotics are not used.

Although the initial conjunctival changes are self-limiting, late scarring and secondary epithelial changes may give rise to serious ocular problems. Lid margin deformities, punctal occlusion, metaplastic lashes, and trichiasis are common. Keratinization of the tarsal conjunctiva (Fig. 16.4) may lead to chronic irritation (Wright & Collins 1983). Some patients develop the

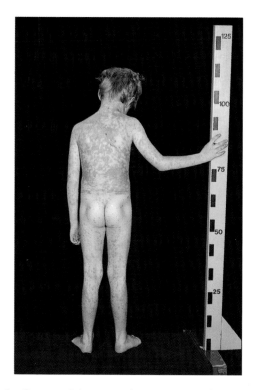

Fig. 16.3 Stevens–Johnson syndrome; same patient as in Fig. 16.2. There is extensive scarring and pigmentation of the skin.

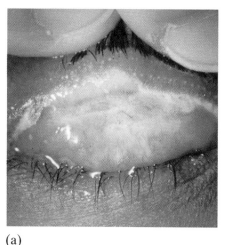

(a)

(b)

Fig. 16.4 Stevens–Johnson syndrome; late stage with subconjunctival scarring and squamous metaplasia of the lid margins.

dry eye syndrome due to extensive mucosal scarring. Corneal changes such as punctate epithelial keratitis and neovascularization may be seen and are usually secondary to conjunctival and lid margin abnormalities.

Management

Most children with the Stevens–Johnson syndrome require hospital admission and systemic steroids are usually prescribed to control the widespread vasculitis (Rasmussen 1976). The acute eye management includes frequent topical steroids (without preservatives), often given half hourly, and less frequent topical antibiotics to prevent any secondary infection. The nursing management is vital because these miserable sick children are almost always reluctant to accept the treatment that is so vital; help with the nursing by the mother is often necessary. If adhesions start to form between the bulbar conjunctiva and lid these may be separated with a glass rod or divided with scissors under local anaesthesia. This may need to be carried out daily to prevent permanent adhesions. The acute conjunctival changes settle on treatment

with steroids but the late complications may present long term problems in management. Dry eyes may require frequent treatment with artificial tear drops and a simple ointment lubricant at night. Squamous metaplasia and keratinization of the conjunctiva may respond to topical retinoid therapy (Kaz Soong et al. 1988). Trichiasis is best treated with cryotherapy although if there is a true cicatricial entropion a lid everting procedure such as a Trabut's operation may be necessary (Wright & Collins 1983). If there is extensive scarring and shortening of the tarsus a mucus membrane graft may be required in addition. Children with this disorder should be followed carefully in the eye department and any lid margin deformity or trichiasis corrected early to prevent permanent corneal damage.

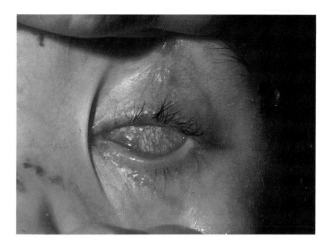

Fig. 16.5 Toxic epidermal necrolysis with conjunctivitis in a 3-year-old girl.

Toxic epidermal necrolysis (TEN)

This disease is similar in many ways to the Stevens–Johnson syndrome. It appears to be a hypersensitivity phenomenon and it is characterized by the occurrence of widespread erythema and a bullous reaction. The epidermis may separate when gently stroked (the Nikolsky sign). Mucus membrane and conjunctival involvement is common (Fig. 16.5).

Lyell's disease is the form of TEN that occurs in response to many of the same factors that cause erythema multiforme. The blisters form at the dermal–epidermal junction and may represent the most severe form of erythema multiforme.

Ritter's disease is a form of TEN that occurs in response to a bacterial exotoxin produced by group 2 phage type *Staphlococcus aureus*. The Nikolsky sign is positive but the cleavage plane is intraepidermal with resultant early healing. Conjunctive involvement may occur in both disorders.

References

Bean SF, Quezada RK. Recurrent oral erythema multiforme. Clinical experience with 11 patients. *JAMA* 1983; **249**: 2810–12

Foster CS, Fong LP, Azar D, Kenyon KR. Episodic conjunctival inflammation after Stevens–Johnson syndrome. *Ophthalmology* 1988; **95**: 453–62

Gottschalk HR, Stone OJ, Stevens–Johnson syndrome from ophthalmic sulphonamide. *Arch Dermatol* 1976; **112**: 513–14

Hurwitz S. Hypersensitivity syndromes. In: Hurwitz S (Ed.) *Clinical Pediatric Dermatology*. WB Saunders, London 1981; pp. 392–4

Kazmierowski JA, Wuepper KD. Erythema multiforme: immune complex vasculitis of the superficial cutaneous microvasculature. *J Invest Dermatol* 1978; **71**: 366–9

Kaz Soong H, Martin NF, Wagener MD. Topical retinoid therapy for squamous metaplasia of various ocular surface disorders. *Ophthalmology* 1988; **95**: 1142–6

Rasmussen JE. Erythema multiforme in children — response to treatment with systemic steroids. *Br J Dermatol* 1976; **95**: 181–5

Stevens AM, Johnson FC. A new eruptive fever associated with stomatitis and ophthalmia: a report of two cases in children. *Am J Dis Child* 1922; **24**: 526–33

Wuepper KD, Watson PA, Kazmierowski JA. Immune complexes in erythema multiforme and the Stevens–Johnson syndrome. *J Invest Dermatol* 1980; **74**: 368–71

Wright P, Collin JRO. Ocular complications of erythema multiforme and their management. *Trans Ophthalmol Soc UK* 1988; **10**: 338–41

Section 4
Systemic Paediatric Ophthalmology

17 Disorders of the Eye as a Whole

SUSAN DAY

Influence of the eye on the development of the orbit

Although the absence of a developing eye in itself does not affect the initial development of a bony orbit (Mann 1937), the growth of the orbit is highly influenced by the presence or absence of an eye. At birth, the normal eye occupies a higher percentage of the orbital volume; growth of the orbital volume increases dramatically during the first year of life (Peyton 1940).

How does absence of an eye, either congenitally or surgically at an early age, influence the growth of the bony orbit? Although orbital volume cannot be assessed with X-rays, the horizontal and vertical measurement of the orbital rim can be taken easily. Kennedy (1965) has shown that these parameters are reduced by 15% in adults who had anophthalmos or had the eye removed within the first year of life. He has also shown that in humans, cats, and rabbits this retardation of orbital growth is approximately halved when an orbital implant is used and that the severity of the overall reduction in volume diminishes if the insult occurs at a later date. Orbital growth appears to be complete by age 15 years, so that subsequent enucleation will not result in any appreciable size difference.

Determination of the influence of an eye on orbital volume cannot be detected radiologically, but measurements of skulls have shown a 60% reduction in volume (Kennedy 1973).

Orbital growth may be secondarily influenced by radiotherapy as well (Guyuron et al. 1983). This consideration as well as intracranial radiotherapy's effects becomes important clinically in the management of children with retinoblastoma, rhabodomyosarcoma, and other radiosensitive neoplasms involving the orbit (Starceski et al. 1987).

Anophthalmos

Anophthalmos is the term used when the eye is nonexistent as a true eye or more commonly a tiny cystic remnant of the eye is present when the term cryptophthalmos is preferred. Variable abnormalities of the orbit occur. Orbital growth is retarded to some extent (Pfeiffer 1945; Kennedy 1965). Extraocular muscles may be absent, and optic foramen size decreased (Pico & Townsend 1979). The conjunctival sac may be very small in size, and its growth must be stimulated with insertion of a prosthesis within the first few years of life, these prostheses require periodic enlargement to continue growth stimulation.

Anophthalmos represents either a complete failure of budding of the optic vesicle or early arrest of its development. To differentiate between anophthalmos and extreme microphthalmos, the examiner can touch the lids to feel for any movements representing rudimentary extraocular muscle function. CT scans may demonstrate buried residual soft tissue mass in cases of extreme microphthalmos, but histological sectioning alone can clarify the presence of neural ectoderm derivatives cells or microphthalmos or their absence in true anophthalmos (Pearce et al. 1974; Brownstein et al. 1977; Sassani Yanoff 1977; Guyer & Green 1984; Brunquell et al. 1984; Pe'er & BenEzra 1986). Unilateral anophthalmos is often associated with anomalies of the other eye (O'Keefe et al. 1987).

Many underlying causes have been proposed for

anophthalmos. Its bilaterality implies an early generalized teratogenic event. Most are sporadic (Warburg 1981A) although case reports involving siblings do exist (Zeiter 1963). Chromosomal abnormalities (Zimmerman & Font 1966; Warburg 1981b) include many syndromes in which extreme microphthalmos is one of many congenital defects. Prenatal infections, X-rays, chemical agents such as LSD (Bogdanoff et al. 1972) and other environmental agents may all play a role in the anophthalmos–microphthalmos spectrum of disorders (Guyer & Green 1984). Some families have shown a dominant gene for coloboma with variable expression with extreme microphthalmos or cryptophthalmos at one end of the spectrum and coloboma, sometimes quite trivial at the other.

The ophthalmologist's management of true anophthalmos is the same as that of extreme microphthalmos — to stimulate growth of the adnexal structures and orbit (Kennedy 1973; Soll 1982). We must additionally play a sensitive role in parental support of such a child. When bilateral, blindness is inevitable and networking with the appropriate agencies will provide great support. A search for possible causes in conjunction with primary care physician may help ease guilt, and genetic counselling will aid the parents in understanding risks of future children being involved. When unilateral, emphasis must be placed on the integrity of the fellow eye if this is the case, and on the relatively normal life that can be expected in a monocular child. Safety glasses must be considered at an early age to protect the good eye.

Cryptophthalmos syndromes

The cryptophthalmos syndrome describes the concurrence of microphthalmos with a varying degree of skin covering the eyeball and lids being variably attached to the cornea.

François (1969) described three subgroups:
1 Complete cryptophthalmos. The lids are replaced by a layer of skin without lashes or glands, and the skin is fused with the microphthalmic eye without a conjunctival sac.
2 Incomplete cryptophthalmos. The lids are rudimentary and there is a small conjunctival sac. The exposed cornea is often opaque.
3 Abortive form. In this form the upper lid is partly fused with the upper cornea and conjunctiva. The globe is small.

The systemic associations include nose deformities, cleft lip, and palate, syndactyly and many others (François 1941; Ide & Wollschlaeger 1969; Brazier et al. 1986). Surgical treatment is usually unsatisfactory and mainly indicated to protect an eye at risk from further deterioration of corneal clarity.

Microphthalmos

The spectrum of anophthalmos merges with microphthalmos. The net volume of a microphthalmic eye is reduced. Often, clinical suspicion is created on the basis of cornea size. Although microphthalmos is usually associated with a small cornea, there may be microphthalmos with a normal cornea (Bateman 1984) and microcornea without microphthalmos (Judisch et al. 1979). Ultrasonographic determination of an axial length less than 20 mm substantiates a diagnosis of microphthalmos (François & Goes 1977). Microphthalmos is a relatively rare condition, with an incidence of 0.25% (Heimonen et al. 1977) and its prevalence accounting for approximately 10% of blind children in one study (Fujiki et al. 1982).

The defect of vision depends on the severity of the microphthalmos and whether it is bilateral.

Microphthalmos can be further divided into colobomatous (Fig. 17.1) and non-colobomotous categories (Bateman 1984) on the basis of associated uveal abnormalities. The association between the processes. of eye growth and closure of the fetal fissure are interlinked and important since closure of the cleft is completed early in development (Mann 1964).

Many causal associations of microphthalmos have been suggested, and possible causes must be kept in mind while considering the child's overall health. Bateman (1984) carefully classifies according to heredity, environmental causes, chromosomal aberrations and unknown causes which have additional systemic abnormalities. Of particular interest is the cat's eye syndrome characterized by uveal coloboma, renal malformations, and imperforate anus as a consequence of an abnormal chromosome 22 (Schachenmann et al. 1965; Schinzel et al. 1981) and the CHARGE syndrome in which ocular coloboma with microphthalmos are associated with heart defects, choanal atresia, retarded growth, genital anomalies, and ear anomalies (Hall 1979; Pagon et al. 1981). Warburg and Friedrich (1987) have reviewed the association of coloboma or microphthalmos with mental retardation and found that multiple chromosomal aberrations can lead to these findings. The Lenz microphthalmos syndrome includes developmental delay, 'bat' ears, ptosis, dental, digital, and other skeletal, urogenital and clefting anomalies (Traboulsi et al. 1988).

Ophthalmic intervention, *per se*, is limited to prescribing glasses to offset amblyogenic refractive errors, supervising oculiarist's role in fitting cosmetic shells or contact lenses in non-seeing eyes, and diagnosing and treating glaucoma. Microphthalmic eyes with corneal opacities may be successfully treated by corneal grafting (Feldman *et al.* 1987).

Microphthalmos with cyst

One unusual form of microphthalmos can present with progressive swelling from birth. The eye often cannot be seen, and the uninitiated ophthalmologist often fears a rapidly growing neoplasm at first. This condition is a colobomatous microphthalmos where cyst formation occurs on the course of the optic nerve, often with free communication with the intraocular contents (Dollfus 1968; Makley & Battles 1969; Waring *et al.* 1976; Helveston *et al.* 1970). Presentation may be as a massive orbital mass distending the lids and hiding the eye or as proptosis in which a microphthalmic eye is visible. Ultrasonography (Fisher 1978) and CT scanning (Weiss *et al.* 1985) aid in its diagnosis. Although management is usually conservative, extremely large cysts must be handled either with repeated aspiration (Weiss *et al.* 1985) or surgical removal of the cyst (Makley & Battles 1969; Waring *et al.* 1976), although because of the communication with the eye, the removal of the eye may necessarily deflate the microphthalmic eye which may need to be removed.

Nanophthalmos

Nanophthalmos (Fig. 17.2) is a rare disease characterized by a small eye, eye hypermetropia, weak but thick sclera, and a tendency to angle closure glaucoma (O'Grady 1971; Calhoun 1975) and uveal effusion (Brockhurst 1974). There is an increased fibronectin level in nanophthalmic sclera and cells (Yue *et al.* 1988). Fibronectin is a glycoprotein involved with cellular adhesion and healing.

Any surgery, but especially intraocular surgery and even laser trabeculoplasty (Good & Stern 1988) may be complicated by severe uveal effusion and should be avoided where possible. Some cases may be autosomal recessive. MacKay *et al.* (1987) described a consanguineous family with seven affected offspring, with a pigmentary retinopathy, cystic macular degeneration, high hypermetropia, nanophthalmos and angle closure glaucoma.

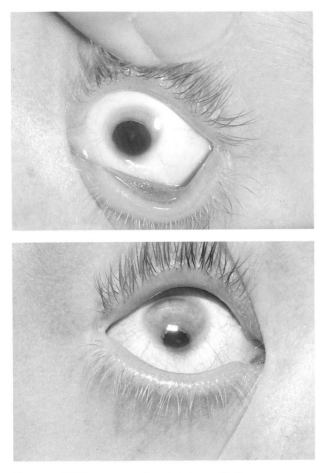

Fig. 17.1 Colobomatous microphthalmos. Both eyes are generally small with an inferior coloboma in the fundus. Although vision was limited to an acuity of 2/60 in each eye, he had a useful visual field and navigated without problems.

Thus, the ophthamologist faced with a new patient with microphthalmos must carefully address several questions:
- What is the level of visual function?
- What is the refractive error; if it is asymmetrical is amblyopia present in addition?
- Are any colobomas present?
- Is there evidence of glaucoma or uveal effusion?

Additionally, the ophthalmologist in conjunction with the primary care physician must answer these critical questions:
- Are there any contributing factors to its presence; congenital infection, chromosomal abnormality, environmental factors?
- Is there a risk of involvement in future children?
- Are there life-threatening associations (such as cardiac defect) or factors which may alter parental expectations of the child (such as mental retardation or deafness)?

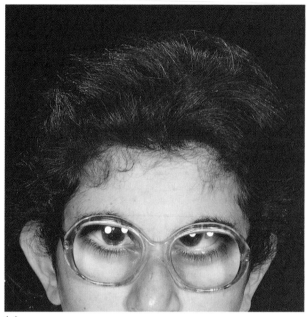

(a)

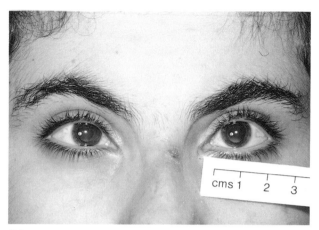

(b)

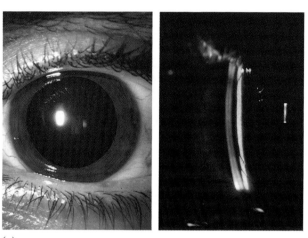

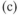
(c)

Fig. 17.2 (a) Nanophthalmos showing the high hypermetropia. The phakic corretion was +10 right, +11 left. (b) Nanophthalmos showing the small eyes and abnormal red reflex. (c) Nanophthalmos showing the shallow anterior chamber. The eyes are prone to angle closure glaucoma. (d) Nanophthalmos showing the crowded optic disc and prominent yellow foveal pigment. Nanophthalmic eyes are very prone to choroidal effusions in response to intraocular surgery.

Cyclopia and synophthalmos

Complete (cyclopic) or partial (synophthalmos) fusion of the two eyes is a very rare birth defect. The brain also fails to develop two hemispheres, and the orbit has gross deformities. The defects are incompatible with life except in very rare circumstances (Panum 1878).

These conditions result from inadequate embryonic neural tissue anteriorly, with subsequent maldevelopment of midline mesodermal structures (Torczynski *et al.* 1977). Because of the close parallel of eye and central nervous system embryological development, the brain is almost always malformed as well (Leech & Shuman 1986) the telencephalon fails to divide, and a large dorsal cyst develops (Mettler 1947). Midline structures such as the corpus callosum, septum pellucidum, and olfactory lobes are often not present (Jellinger *et al.* 1981) and anomalies may extend to the mesencephalic region with thalamic abnormalities.

The orbits are markedly affected as a consequence of the abnormal development of midline mesodermal structures. The normal nasal cavity is replaced by the

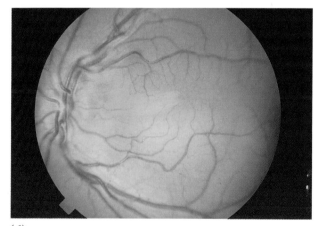

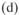
(d)

'pseudo-orbit' (Duke-Elder 1964), and the bones show multiple malformations, especially in midline structures. The defects additionally involve the skull, with absence of the sella turcica and clinoids.

The eyes are more commonly partly fused than completely fused. One optic nerve is present, and no chiasm is recognizable. Structures are best developed laterally, such as the muscles innervated by cranial nerves IV and VI in comparison to those innervated by cranial nerve III (Gartner 1947). Other intraocular abnormalities may exist such as persistent hyperplastic primary vitreous, cataract, coloboma, and microcornea (Spencer 1985).

Chromosomal aberrations are commonly present (Batts *et al.* 1972; Fujimoto *et al.* 1973; Howard 1977). Familial occurrences and association with consanguinous marriages have also been noted (Howard 1977).

Other aetiological considerations include maternal health (Stabile *et al.* 1985) and toxic factors, based on a high incidence in animals who grazed on an alkaloid-containing substance (Bryden *et al.* 1971).

The importance of cyclopia and synophthalmos is primarily one of academic embryological interest; the overwhelming systemic abnormalities place management of this condition in the hands of perinatologists and geneticists.

References

Bateman JB. Microphthalmos. *Int Ophthalmol Clin* 1984; **24**: 87−107

Batts JA, Punnett HH, Valdes-Dapena M, Coles JW, Green WR. A case of cyclopia. *Am J Obstet Gynecol* 1972; **112**: 657−61

Bogdanoff B, Rorke LB, Yanoff M, Warren WS. Brain and eye abnormalities: possible sequelae to prenatal use of multiple drugs including LSD. *Am J Dis Child* 1972; **123**: 145−8

Brazier DJ, Hardman-Lea SJ, Collin JRO. Cryptophthalmos: surgical treatment of the congenital symblepharon variant. *Br J Ophthalmol* 1986; **70**: 391−5

Brockhurst RJ. Nanophthalmos with uveal effusion: a new clinical entity. *Trans Am Ophthalmol Soc* 1974; **72**: 371−403

Brownstein S, Bright M, Kirkham TH, Carpenter S. Anophthalmos. Report of two cases. *Can J Ophthalmol* 1977; **12**: 143−6

Brunquell PJ, Papale JH, Horton JC, Williams RS, Zgrabik MJ, Albert DM, Hedley-Whyte ET. Sex-linked hereditary bilateral anophthalmos, pathologic and radiologic correlation. *Arch Ophthalmol* 1984; **102**: 108−13

Bryden MM, Evans HE, Keeler RF. Cyclopia in sheep caused by plant teratogens. *J Anat* 1971; **110**: 507

Calhoun FP. The management of glaucoma in nanophthalmos. *Trans Am Ophthalmol Soc* 1975; **73**: 97−122

Dollfus MA, Marx P, Langlois J, Clement JC, Forthomme J. Congenital cystic eyeball. *Am J Ophthalmol* 1968; **66**: 504−9

Duke-Elder S. Anomalies in the size of the eye. In *Normal and Abnormal Development. System of Ophthalmology* vol. III, part 2. Kimpton, London, 1964; pp. 429−51, 488−90

Feldman ST, Frucht-Pery J, Brown SI. Corneal transplantation in microphthalmic eyes. *Am J Ophthalmol* 1987; **104**: 164−7

Fisher YL. Microphthalmos with ocular communicating cyst-ultrasonic diagnosis. *Ophthalmology* 1978; **85**: 1208−11

François J. Syndrome malformatif avec cryptophtalmie. *Acta Genet Med Gemellol (Roma)* 1969; **18**: 18−50

François J, Goes F. Ultrasonographic study of 100 emmetropic eyes. *Ophthalmologica* 1977; **175**: 321−7

Fujiki K, Nakajima A, Yasuda N *et al.* Genetic analysis of microphthalmos. *Ophthalmic Paediatr Genet* 1982; **1**: 139−49

Fujimoto A, Ebbin AJ, Towner JW, Wilson MG. Trisomy 13 in two infants with cyclops. *J Med Genet* 1973; **10**: 294−6

Gartner S. Cyclopia. *Arch Ophthalmol* 1947; **37**: 220−31

Good WV, Stern WH. Recurrent nanophthalmic uveal effusion syndrome following laser trabeculoplasty. *Am J Ophthalmol* 1988; **106**: 234−5

Guyer DR, Green WR. Bilateral extreme microphthalmos. *Ophthalmic Paediatr Genet* 1984; **4**: 81−90

Guyuron B, Dagys AP, Munro IR, Ross RB. Effect of irradiation on facial growth: a 7- to 25-year followup. *Ann Plast Surg* 1983; **11**: 423−7

Hall BD. Choanal atresia and associated multiple anomalies. *J Pediatr* 1979; **95**: 395−8

Helveston EM, Malone E, Lashmet MH. Congenital cystic eye. *Arch Ophthalmol* 1970; **84**: 622−4

Heinonen OP, Shapiro S, Slone D. *Birth Defects and Drugs in Pregnancy*. Publishing Sciences Group, Littleton, Massachusetts 1977

Howard RO. Chromosomal abnormalities associated with cyclopia and synophthalmia. *Trans Am Ophthalmol Soc* 1977; **75**: 505−38

Ide CH, Wollschlaeger PB. Multiple congenital abnormalities associated with cryptophthalmia. *Arch Ophthalmol* 1969; **81**: 640−4

Jellinger K, Gross H, Kaltenback E, Grisold W. Holoprosencephaly and agenesis of the corpus callosum: frequency of associated malformations. *Acta Neuropathol (Berl)* 1981; **55**: 1−10

Judisch GF, Martin-Casals A, Hanson JW, Olin WH. Oculodentodigital dysplasia. Four new reports and a literature review. *Arch Ophthalmol* 1979; **97**: 878−84

Kennedy RE. The effect of early enucleation on the orbit in animals and humans. *Am J Ophthalmol* 1965; **60**: 277−306

Kennedy RE. Growth retardation and volume determination of the anophthalmic orbit. *Am J Ophthalmol* 1973; **76**: 294−302

Leech RW, Shuman RM. Holoprosencephaly and related midline cerebral anomalies: a review. *J Child Neurol* 1986; **1**: 3−18

Llorca FO. Le cerveau et l'oeil de deux embryons humains cyclopes de 37 et 45 jours. *Acta Anat (Basel)* 1955; **23**: 379−85

MacKay CJ, Shek MS, Carr RE, Yanuzzi LA, Gouras P. Retinal degeneration with nanophthalmos, cystic macular degeneration, and angle closure glaucoma. A new recessive syndrome. *Arch Ophthalmol* 1987; **105**: 366−71

Makley TA, Battles M. Microphthalmos with cyst. Report of two cases in the same family *Surv Ophthalmol* 1969; **13**: 200−6

Mann I. *Developmental abnormalities of the Eye*. Cambridge University Press, London 1937; pp. 46−64

Mann I. *The Development of the Human Eye* 3rd ed. British Medical Association, London 1964; p. 277–00

Marin-Padilla M. Study of the sphenoid bone in human cranioschisis and craniorhachischisis. *Virchows Arch Path Anat Physiol* 1965; **339**: 245–53

Mettler FA. Congenital malformation of the brain. Critical review. *J Neuropathol Exp Neurol* 1947; **6**: 98–110

O'Grady RB. Nanophthalmos. *Am J Ophthalmol* 1971; **71**: 1251–3

O'Keefe M, Webb M, Pashby RC, Wagman RD. Clinical anophthalmos. *Br J Ophthalmol* 1987; **71**: 635–8

Pagon RA, Graham JM, Zonana J, Young S–L. Coloboma, Congenital heart disease, and choanal atresia with multiple anomalies: CHARGE association *J Pediatr* 1981; **99**: 223–7

Panum PL. Beitrage zur Kenntniss der physiologischen Bedeutung der argebornen Missbildungen. *Virchows Arch Path Anat* 1878; **72**: 289–324

Pearce WG, Nigam S, Rootman J. Primary anophthalmos histological and genetic features. *Can J Ophthalmol* 1974; **9**: 141–5

Pe'er J, BenEzra D. Heterotopic smooth muscle in the choroid of two patients with cryptophthalmos. *Arch Ophthalmol* 1986; **104**: 1665–70

Peyton WT. A topographic study of the orbit and bulbus oculi during a part of the growth period. *Anat Rec* 1940; **76**: 343–55

Pfeiffer RL. The effect of enucleation on the orbit. *Trans Am Acad Ophthalmol Otolaryngol* 1945; **49**: 236–9

Pico G, Townsend W. Congenital and developmental anomalies of the orbit. In Jones IS, Jakobiec FA (eds.) *Diseases of the Orbit*. Harper Hagerstown & Row 1979; pp. 123–33

Sassani JW, Yanoff M. Anophthalmos in an infant with multiple congenital anomalies. *Am J Ophthalmol* 1977; **83**: 43–8

Schachenmann G, Schmid W, Fraccaro M, Mannini A, Tiepolo L, Perona GP, Sartori E. Chromosomes in coloboma and anal atresia. *Lancet* 1965; **2**: 290

Schinzel A, Schmid W, Fraccaro M *et al*. The cat-eye syndrome: dicentric small marker chromosome probably derived from a No. 22 (tetrasomy 22 pter -q11) associated with a characteristic phenotype: report of 11 patients and delineation of the clinical picture. *Hum Genet* 1981; **57**: 148–58

Soll DB. The anophthalmic socket. *Ophthalmology* 1982; **89**: 407–23

Spencer WH. Abnormalities of scleral thickness and congenital anomalies. In Spencer WH (ed.) *Ophthalmic Pathology. An Atlas and Textbook*, 3rd ed. vol. 1. WB Saunders, Philadelphia 1985; pp. 394–5

Stabile M, Bianco A, Iannuzzi S, Buonocore MC, Ventruto V. A case of suspected keratogenic holoprosencephaly. *J Med Genet* 1985; **22**: 147–9

Starceski PJ, Lee PA, Blatt J, Finegold D, Brown D. Comparable effects of 1800- and 2400- rad (18- and 24- cGy) cranial irradiation on height and weight in children treated for acute lymphocytic leukemia. *Am J Dis Child* 1987; **141**: 550–2

Torczynski E, Jacobiec FA, Johnston MC, Font RL, Madewell JA. Synophthalmia and cyclopia: a histopathologic, radiographic, and organogenetic analysis. *Doc Ophthalmol* 1977; **44**: 311–78

Traboulsi EI, Lenz W, Gonzales-Ramas M, Siegel J, Macrae WG, Maumenee IH. The Lenz microphthalmia syndrome. *Am J Ophthalmol* 1988; **105**: 40– 5

Warburg M. Genetics of microphthalmos. *Int Ophthalmol* 1981(a); **4**: 45–65

Warburg M. Diagnostic precision in microphthalmos and coloboma of heterogenous origin. *Ophthalmic Paediatr Genet* 1981(b); **1**: 37–42

Warburg M, Friedrich U. Coloboma and microphthalmos in chromosomal aberrations. Chromosomal aberrations and neural crest cell developmental field. *Ophthalmic Paediatr Genet* 1987; **8**: 105–18

Waring GO, Roth AM, Rodrigues MM. Clinicopathologic correlation of microphthalmos with cyst. *Am J Ophthalmol* 1976; **82**: 714–21

Weiss A, Martinez C, Greenwald M. Microphthalmos with cyst: clinical presentations and computed tomographic findings. *J Pediatr Ophthalmol Strabismus* 1985; **22**: 6–12

Yue BYJT, Kurosawa A, Duvall J, Goldberg MF, Tso MOM, Sugar J. Nanophthalmic sclera. Fibronectin studies. *Ophthalmology* 1988; **95**: 56–60

Zeiter HJ. Congenital microphthalmos. A pedigree of four affected siblings and an additional report of forty-four sporadic cases. *Am J Ophthalmol* 1963; **55**: 910–22

Zimmerman LE, Font RL. Congenital malformations of the eye. Some recent advances in knowledge of the pathogenesis and histopathological characteristics. *J Am Med Assn* 1966; **196**: 684–92

18 Lids

CREIG HOYT AND SCOTT LAMBERT

Embryology and anatomy

During the first month of embryonic development, the optic vesicle is covered by a thin layer of surface ectoderm. During the second month, active cellular proliferation of the adjacent mesoderm results in the formation of a circular fold of mesoderm lined on both sides by ectoderm. This fold constitutes the rudiments of the eyelid which gradually elongates over the eye. The mesodermal portion of the upper lid arises from the fronto-nasal process, the lower lid from the maxillary process. The covering layer of ectoderm becomes skin on the outside and conjunctiva on the inside. The tarsal plate, connective and muscular tissues of the eyelids are derived from the mesodermal core. The process of fusion of the eyelids by an epithelial seal begins at the two extremities at the 3.1 mm stage and is complete at the 3.5 mm stage. The eyelids remain adherent until approximately the end of the fifth month. Separation begins on the nasal side, a process which is usually completed during the sixth or seventh month of development. Very rarely this process is incomplete at birth in a full term infant. The specialised structures in the lids develop between 8 weeks to 7 months and by term the lid is fully developed with functioning muscles, lashes and meibomian glands (Sevel 1988).

The eyelids have several characteristic folds. The most conspicuous is a well demarcated superior palpebral sulcus 3–4 mm above the lid margin which flattens out on depression of the upper eyelid and becomes deeply recessed when the upper lid is elevated. It divides each eyelid into an orbital and tarsal portion. The orbital portion lies between the margins of the orbit and the globe, and the tarsal portion lies in direct relationship to the globe. The palpebral fissure, the opening between the upper and lower lids, is the entrance into the conjunctival sac bounded by the margins of the eyelids. This aperture forms an asymmetric ellipse that is approximately 22–30 mm long and 12–15 mm high when the lids are open (Feingold & Bossert 1974).

When the eyelids are opened in a newborn infant, the upper eyelid rises well above the cornea while the lower eyelid crosses the inferior margin of the cornea. However, by adulthood the upper eyelid covers the upper 1–2 mm of the cornea while the lower lid lies slightly below its inferior margin (Feingold & Bossert 1974).

The principle muscle involved in opening the upper lid and in maintaining normal lid position is the levator palpebri superioris. Müller's muscle and the frontalis muscle play an accessory role.

The levator palpebri superioris arises as a short tendon blended with the underlying origin of the superior rectus from the under surface of the lesser wing of the sphenoid bone. Its flat muscle belly passes forward below the orbital roof and just superior to the superior rectus muscle until it is about 1 cm behind the orbital septum where it ends in a membranous expansion or aponeurosis. The aponeurosis of the levator spreads out in a fan-shaped manner across the length of the eyelid, inserting primarily into the septum that separates the bundles of the orbicularis oculae muscle in the lower half of the eyelid. Some of the fibres of the aponeurosis also attach to the anterior surface of the tarsal plate. The lateral and medial extensions of the aponeurosis are referred to as its horns. The lateral horn is attached to the orbital tubercle and to the upper aspect of the lateral palpebral ligament. The medial horn is attached to the medial palpebral ligament. The levator palpebri superioris is innervated by branches from the superior division of the oculomotor nerve.

Müller's muscle is composed of a thin band of smooth muscle fibres about 10 mm in width that arise on the inferior surface of the levator palpebri superioris. The muscle courses anteriorly directly between the levator tendon and the conjunctiva of the upper eyelid to insert into the superior margin of the tarsus. Branches of the ocular sympathetic pathway innervate the fibres of Müller's muscle.

The eyelid is indirectly elevated by attachment of the frontalis muscle into the superior orbital portions of the orbicularis oculae muscle. The frontalis muscle is innervated by the temporal branch of the facial nerve. A tarsal plate composed of dense connective tissue is found in both the upper and lower eyelids. The upper lid tarsal plate has a marginal length of 29 mm and is 10–12 mm wide. The lower lid tarsal plate is 5 mm wide.

Lid retraction in infancy

Occasionally infants may present with a history of one or both eyelids appearing to be retracted. There are several conditions which can give rise to this appearance.

1 A false appearance of lid retraction may be given by ipsilateral proptosis or a contralateral ptosis when the child is trying to elevate the ptosed lid; and with inferior rectus fibrosis or Brown's syndrome which restricts upward movement of the eye, not the lid.
2 Bilateral lid elevation with an upgaze palsy is the classic 'setting sun' sign in hydrocephalus of any cause and also in dorsal midbrain disease.
3 Lid retraction, unilateral or bilateral, occurs with the Marcus Gunn jaw winking phenomenon. Sometimes there is no ptosis — the lid just elevates.
4 Neonatal Grave's disease (Shield's et al. 1988).
5 A sequel to third nerve palsy with aberrant regeneration.
6 Myasthenic patients may have transient lid retraction particularly after looking down for a period.
7 Lid lag is a defective relaxation of the lids which occurs in hyperthyroidism, myopathic disease, a congenitally short levater tendon (Zak 1984) or occasionally in myasthenia, after looking up for a few seconds.

Congenital abnormalities

Cryptophthalmos

Cryptophthalmos (Fig. 18.1) is a rare condition in which there is complete failure of development of the eyelid folds. As a result, the epithelium that is normally differentiated into cornea and conjunctiva becomes part of the skin that passes continuously from the forehead to the cheek (Gupta & Saxena 1963) (see Chapter 17).

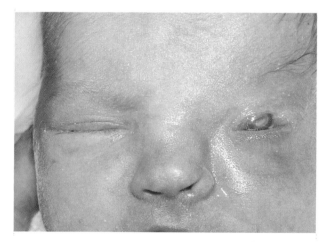

Fig. 18.1 Cryptophthalmos (Fraser's) syndrome. This child with a unilateral form has a fused eye and lid. The upper lid is also defective. The nares are notched on the left. Other features include partial syndactyly, ear anomalies and anomalous genitalia (Gupta & Saxena 1963).

Coloboma

Congenital colobomas are clefts of varying configurations found throughout the visual system. Eyelid colobomas (Fig. 18.2) may be found in all areas of the eyelids but are most commonly found in the nasal half of the upper lid (Roper-Hall 1969). More than one lid may be involved in the same patient, or there may be multiple colobomas in the same lid. They may also occur as isolated anomalies, but are sometimes seen in patients with other congenital lesions, most commonly dermoids and dermolipomas. Eyelid colobomas result from anomalous development of the visual system, between the 15 and 32 mm embryonic stage. A predominant aetiologic theory incriminates the mechanical action of amniotic bands. Heredity does not usually play a significant role in the aetiology of most lid colobomas (Smith & Chrubini 1970). An exception is the lower lid coloboma associated with mandibulo-facial dysostosis (Treacher–Collins syndrome) which appears to be an autosomal dominant trait of varying penetrance and expressivity.

Epiblepharon

Epiblepharon (Fig. 18.3) is a condition characterized by the presence of a horizontal fold of skin across either the upper or lower eyelid which forces the lashes against the cornea. There is often a familial tendency towards this condition and it occurs more frequently in chubby-cheeked infants and in orientals. It usually corrects itself as a result of differential growth of the facial bones. It is seldom associated with keratitis. Surgical intervention is, therefore, rarely indicated but when needed because of persistence of symptoms or corneal compromise may consist simply

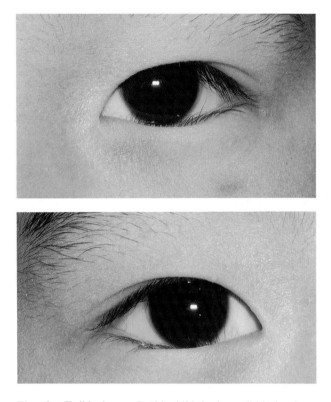

Fig. 18.3 Epiblepharon. In this child the lower lid lashes have turned in from birth, but the cornea has remained undamaged. Spontaneous improvement usually occurs.

of excision of an ellipse of skin and subcutaneous fat near to the lash margins.

Entropion

Congenital entropion (Fig. 18.4), the turning inward of the lid margin, rarely occurs as an isolated anomaly. When it does present as an isolated defect, it usually involves the lower lid, although involvement of the upper lid has been documented. Entropion in infants and children is most often part of a condition secondary to epicanthus or epiblepharon of the lower lid. It is frequently associated with microphthalmos and enophthalmos as the result of lack of support of the posterior border of the eyelid. Isolated primary entropion results from an absence of the tarsal plate or from a hypertrophy of the marginal portion of the orbicularis muscle. Congenital absence of the tarsal plate is the most common cause of congenital entropion of the upper lid (Tse 1983). When hypertrophy of the marginal portions of the orbicularis muscle is responsible, the resulting entropion is referred to as the spastic type. Entropion in children is often familial with more than one instance occurring in the same

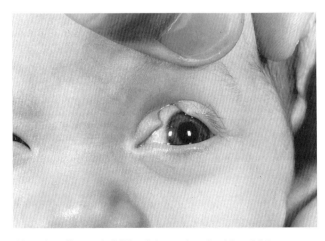

Fig. 18.2 Congenital lid coloboma in a healthy child.

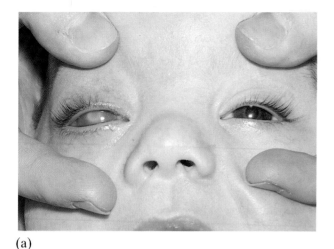

(a)

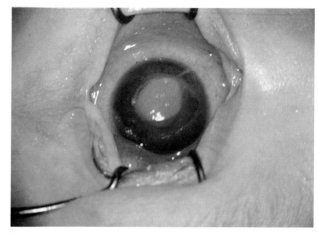

(b)

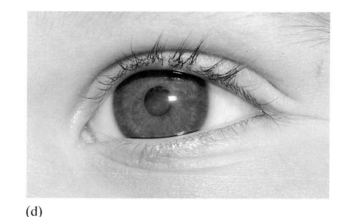

(c)

(d)

Fig. 18.4 (a) Congenital entropion. Shortly after birth this child's eye was found to be swollen, at EUA there was right upper lid entropion. (b) The corneal abrasion caused by the entropion. (c) After taping the lids the entropion resolved and ultimately there was only minimal subepithelial opacity. (d) The normal left eyelids.

sibship. Congenital entropion can be treated conservatively by lid suture or taping but sometimes it may be necessary to excise an ellipse of skin and orbicularis muscle with attachment of the excised margins to the tarsal plate.

Tarsal kink

Congenital horizontal kinking of the tarsus causes entropion which can be corrected by a simple surgical procedure (Price & Collin 1987).

Ectropion

Congenital ectropion rarely occurs as an isolated anomaly. Eversion of lid margins usually occur in conjunction with congenital ptosis, epicanthus inversus, and blepharophimosis (Callahan 1973). It may also occur in association with microphthalmos, buphthalmos and orbital cysts.

Eversion

Congenital eversion (Fig. 18.5) of the lids (Bentsi-Enchill 1981), which occurs most frequently in children with Down's syndrome, or those who have had a difficult delivery or with skin disorders, may be treated simply by reparting of the lids and taping (Moanie *et al.* 1982). More severe cases are best treated by the insertion of a skin graft in the eyelids.

Epitarsus

Primary epitarsus is an apron-like fold of conjunctiva attached to the inner surface of the upper lid, it occurs secondary to conjunctivitis, amniotic bands or as a congenital anomaly (Khurana *et al.* 1986).

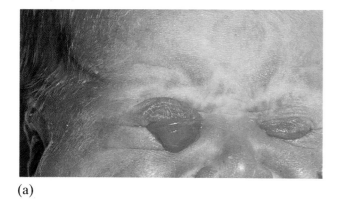

(a)

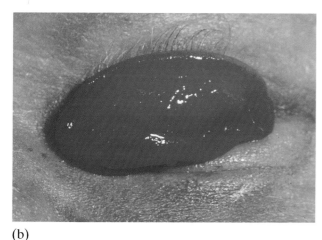

(b)

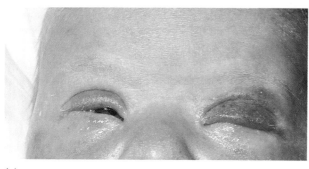

(c)

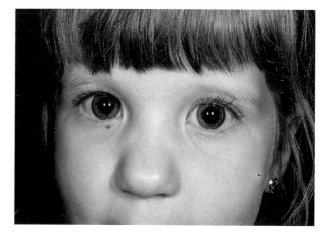

Fig. 18.6 Epicanthic folds.

Fig. 18.5 (a) This neonate with Down's syndrome developed lid eversion when crying that rapidly became permanently present. The birth history was unremarkable. (b) The lid eversion was maintained by the very marked chemosis. (c) After taping the lids for 4 days the swelling resolved leaving bruising, indicating that haemorrhage may play a causative role.

Epicanthus

Epicanthal folds (Fig. 18.6) are found as a racial characteristic in a large portion of the world's population. In races in which epicanthus is not typical of the normal face, it may be found either as congenital or as an acquired abnormality. Congenital epicanthus may occur as an isolated anomaly or it may be associated with other conditions, such as ptosis, telecanthus (in which the medial canthi are displaced in the lateral direction), or with abnormally small eyelids as well as with ptosis and telecanthus in the condition known as the blepharophimosis syndrome (Mustardé 1963, 1971).

Telecanthus

Telecanthus refers to an increased width between the medial canthi with a normal interpupillary distance. This may occur as an isolated condition or in association with other abnormalities such as epicanthus and blepharophimosis. It also occurs in Aarskog's facial−digital−genital syndrome (Berry *et al.* 1980). Hypertelorism refers to an increased 'interpupillary distance caused by an increased interorbital width. The normal intercanthal distance is 20 +/− 2 mm (1SD) at birth increasing to 26 +/− 1.5 mm by 2 years of age. The normal interpupillary distance is 39 +/− 3 mm at birth increasing to 48 +/− 2 mm by 2 years of age (Feingold 1974).

Blepharophimosis

A more complicated clinical picture is seen in patients with blepharophimosis (Fig. 18.7), a condition in which there is not only a considerable degree of telecanthus and small inverted epicanthal folds, but also ptosis and flattening of the supraorbital ridges (Callahan 1973). The palpebral aperture is reduced in width, and the eyelids are decreased in size (McCord 1980). Strabismus and nystagmus may also be associ-

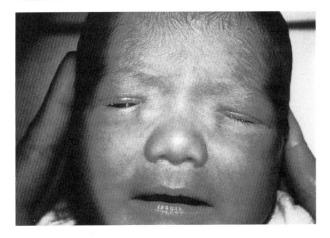

Fig. 18.7 Blepharophimosis.

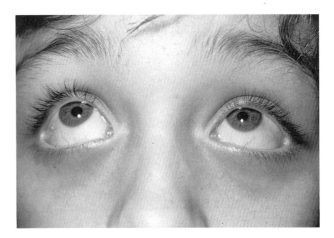

Fig. 18.8 Euryblepharon.

ated with this abnormality. Chromosomal studies are usually normal in these patients, but duplication of 6p and 10q chromosomes has been reported. There may be an association with female infertility (Jones & Collin 1984).

Ankyloblepharon

Ankyloblepharon exists when the eyelid margins are partially or completely fused together, thus producing shortening of the palpebral fissure. This condition may be subdivided into external ankyloblepharon in which the inner canthus is fused. External ankyloblepharon is the most common type. This abnormality, which was described by Van Hasner in 1881, may be inherited as an autosomal dominant trait, sometimes in association with ectodermal defects, cleft lip and palate (Ehlers & Jensen 1970; Hay & Wells 1976; Akkerman & Stern 1979). Ankyloblepharon filiforme adnatum is a similar condition in which a small tag, or a few small tags, of skin jam the two lids, they may be divided simply. They are usually isolated but have been described with systemic abnormalities including meningomyelocoele and hydrocephalus (Kazarian & Goldstein 1977) or in trisomy 18 (Clarke & Patterson 1985).

Euryblepharon

Euryblepharon (Fig. 18.8) is a condition in which generalized enlargement of the palpebral aperture occurs, usually greatest in the lateral aspect (Keipert 1975). As a result, localized outward displacement of the lateral canthus occurs. The lateral canthus is displaced inferiorly with a resulting downward displace-

ment of the lateral half of the lower lid. This may superficially mimic the appearance of congenital ectropion. It may occur as an isolated anomaly, inherited as an autosomal dominant trait, or may be associated with craniofacial dysostoses.

Distichiasis

Distichiasis refers to a congenital abnormality in which a secondary row of lashes occurs (White 1975). This usually involves the lower eyelid only. It may occur as an isolated anomaly, or be inherited as an autosomal dominant trait. It may also be associated with chronic lymphedema of the lower extremities, the Falls–Kertsz syndrome (Anderson & Harvey 1981). If patients are symptomatic it may be treated by cryotherapy of the lashes of the lower lid, in the upper lid by lid splitting and cryotherapy to the posterior lamella, or by excision of individual follicles (Wolfley 1987). Ectopic lashes occurring either singly or in bunches in the lids are rare anomalies (Fig. 18.9).

Ptosis

Congenital ptosis

Ptosis may be produced by damage to the motor system controlling eyelid elevation and position at any level of the pathways, from the cerebral cortex to the levator muscle itself or to the tissues surrounding the muscle (Beard 1981, 1989). Topical diagnosis of ptosis depends upon the character of the deficiency and on evidence of associated neuropathic, neuromuscular or myopathic disease. Lowering of the upper eyelid position may occur without a true ptosis. This may occur

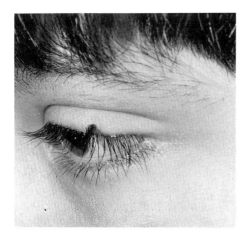

Fig. 18.9 Ectopic lashes.

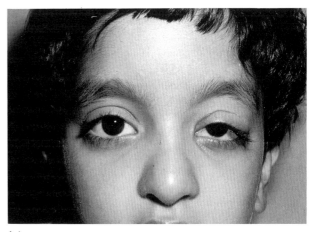

(a)

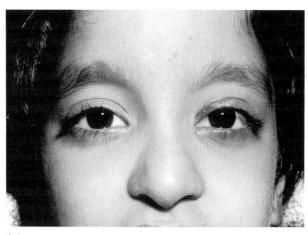

(b)

Fig. 18.10 (a) 5-year-old child with a 3.5 mm left congenital ptosis and poor levator function. The patient had an unsuccessful 24 mm levator resection 1 year earlier. (b) Six months post-operatively after a 6 mm left full-thickness lid resection. Photographs by courtesy of Man Kim MD.

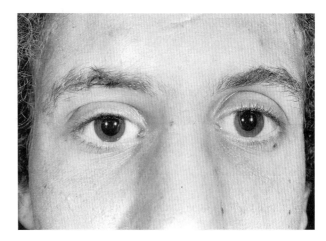

Fig. 18.11 Teenage patient with mild ptosis in both eyes. He was diagnosed to have progressive external ophthalmoplegia 2 years later.

as the result of reduced orbital volume, for example, in association with microphthalmos or enophthalmos. A pseudoptotic appearance commonly accompanies ipsilateral hypotropia and should not be mistaken for a true ptosis. 'Congenital' ptosis is the most common anomaly of the eyelids. The term congenital ptosis is usually used by most authorities to designate a group of cases in which the ptosis is due to a developmental dystrophy of the levator muscle or its tendon, and is not associated with any innervational abnormalities (Berke & Wadsworth 1955). Thus, infants born with a third nerve palsy or Horner's syndrome are not usually referred to as a congenital ptosis (Frueh 1978). Congenital ptosis may be unilateral or bilateral, and of varying severity. A significant proportion of patients with congenital ptosis show weakness of the ipsilateral superior rectus muscle (Fig. 18.10) (Isaksson 1960). The association is best explained by the close embryologic development of the two muscles (Anderson & Baumgartner 1980b). The other muscles supplied by the third cranial nerve are not affected. Most cases of congenital ptosis are not familial, but sometimes there may be ptosis in the immediate or distant family. Congenital ptosis may be an isolated abnormality or it may be associated with other defects including epicanthus, abnormalities of the puncti, congenital cataracts, anisometropia, and amblyopia. Non-ocular defects including those of the skeletal muscles, (Fig. 18.11, 18.12, 18.13) or hearing, also occur.

The severity of congenital ptosis varies widely. The ptosis may be so mild as to be hardly noticeable or so severe that vision is only possible by tilting the head backward (Fig. 18.14, 18.15). Patients with severe ptosis often wrinkle their forehead and contract the frontalis muscle in an effort to pull the eyelid upward.

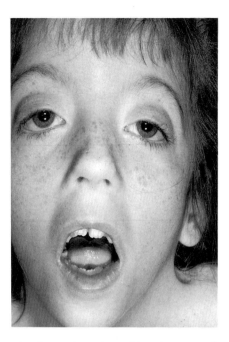

Fig. 18.12 Ptosis seen in patient with arthyrogryposis.

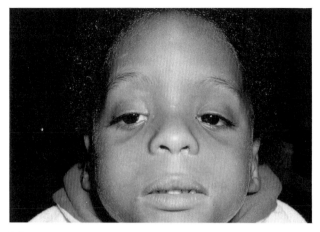

(a)

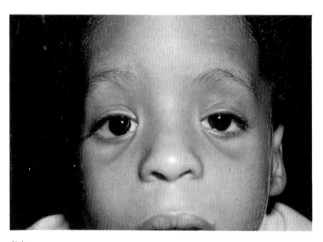

(b)

Fig. 18.13 (a) Three-year-old child with the fetal alcohol syndrome and bilateral congenital ptosis. There was 2 mm of levator function bilaterally. (b) Six months post-operatively after silicone rod suspensions, bilaterally.

In these cases, inactivation of the frontalis muscle with the examiner's hand is necessary in order to ascertain the full extent of the ptosis. Congenital ptosis persists throughout life and generally does not improve and may in fact worsen with age.

While amblyopia rarely occurs secondary to occlusion of the visual axis with ptosis, anisometropic and strabismic amblyopia frequently co-exist (Anderson & Baumgartner 1980b). Careful evaluation of the fixation reflexes of a ptotic eye and refraction are, therefore, essential to exclude amblyopia. In all cases treatment of the amblyopia should precede any attempt at surgical correction of the ptosis unless the ptotic eye completely occludes the pupil.

In general, a congenital ptosis should be repaired when accurate measurements can be obtained on repeated examinations. This is rarely possible before the age of 1, and in most situations surgical correction is best deferred until a child is between 2 and 4 years of age (Beard 1981). In deciding what surgical procedure to use in correcting congenital ptosis, it is important to evaluate both the amount of ptosis as well as the degree of levator function. Congenital ptosis of up to 1.5 mm with more than 8 mm of levator function may be corrected using the Fasanella–Servat procedure. If the patient has more than 4 mm of levator function a levator resection may be performed. In patients with 3 mm or less of levator function, a frontalis suspension procedure is usually

recommended. This may utilize autogenous or banked fascia, or banked sclera as material for the suspension. Careful attention must be paid to not overcorrect patients with severe ptosis, especially when Bell's phenomenon is absent, since exposure keratopathy may ensue as the result of incomplete eyelid closure.

Marcus Gunn phenomenon

Four to 6% of congenital ptosis cases are associated with the jaw-winking phenomenon of Marcus Gunn (Beard 1981). This syndrome is characterized by paradoxical ptosis in that it is reduced or overcompensated for when the patient makes chewing or swallowing movements (Fig. 18.16). This may be demonstrated by having the patient open and close the mouth or

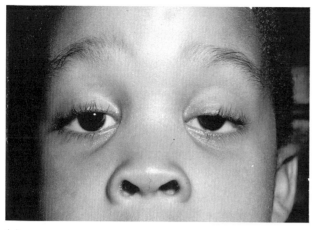

(a)

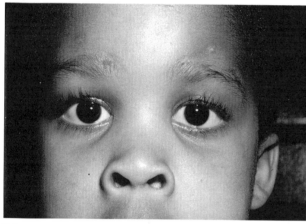

(b)

Fig. 18.14 (a) Six-year-old child with bilateral congenital ptosis. There was only 4 mm of levator function bilaterally. The child has adopted a chin-up head posture. (b) Two months post-operatively after a bilateral frontalis suspension using autogenous fascia lata. Photographs by courtesy of Man Kim MD.

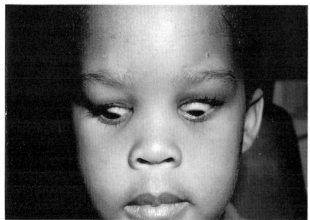

Fig. 18.15 Lagophthalmos postoperatively on downgaze. (Same patient as Fig. 14a, b.) Photograph by courtesy of Man Kim MD.

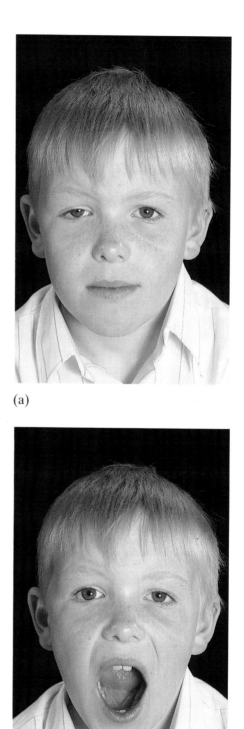

(a)

(b)

Fig. 18.16 (a) Moderate right ptosis (Marcus Gunn). (b) With jaw open the right upper lid elevates.

move the jaw from side to side. With each appropriate movement, the ptotic eyelid elevates, often to a level higher than the normal position. Usually the lid elevates when the patient opens the mouth and moves the mandible to the side opposite to the involved eye. Occasionally the ptosis increases when the mouth opens, and is overcompensated for when the jaws are forcibly closed. Marcus Gunn jaw-winking ptosis is almost always unilateral and more frequently involves the left side than the right. It varies from minimal to an exaggerated and cosmetically intolerable ptosis. It would appear that Marcus Gunn jaw-winking ptosis arises as the result of congenitally misdirected fibres from the Vth cranial nerve innervating the levator muscle which should be ordinarily innervated by the IIIrd cranial nerve. As a result, stimulation of the jaw moving mechanism results in an excess of impulses being sent to the poorly innervated levator muscle, which momentarily raises the eyelid (Sano 1959). This syndrome is associated with weakness of the superior rectus muscle on the affected side in about 75% of cases. This condition is usually sporadic, but familial cases have been reported. Some authorities believe that jaw-winking ptosis improves with age, while others are adamant that the anomaly persists (Beard 1981).

The inverse Marcus Gunn phenomena is a rare condition in which the ipsilateral eyelid closes as the external pterygoid muscle moves the jaw to the opposite side. Patients with this condition invariably have a mild degree of ptosis of the involved eyelid when the eyes are in a primary position and the mouth is closed. Electromyographic studies have demonstrated that downward movement of the lower jaw is associated with total inhibition of the levator and unassociated with any activity of the orbiculus oculae muscle (Lubkin 1978). This syndrome is truly the inverse of the Marcus Gunn jaw-winking phenomena, since the upper eyelid is not actively closing. There is a synkinesis between the oculomotor and trigeminal nerves.

Surgical correction of Marcus Gunn jaw-winking is difficult (Collin 1988). If the primary abnormality is the ptosis with very little synkinetic movement of the eyelid, standard ptosis surgery may be all that is appropriate. If the synkinetic movements are most cosmetically troublesome, these may be eliminated by disinserting the levator from its tarsal insertion and performing a frontalis sling. Regrettably, since most patients with the Marcus Gunn jaw-winking phenomenon have a unilateral disorder, this surgical correction is not ideal. Beard has recommended that in severe cases, a bilateral frontalis sling be performed even in the presence of a normal functioning contralateral lid (Beard 1965).

Ptosis in brain disease

Most patients with neuropathic ptosis have involvement of the IIIrd cranial nerve or the sympathetic pathway. However, unilateral or bilateral cerebral or cortical ptosis may rarely occur. Cortical ptosis is uncommon and usually occurs contralateral to the cortical lesion (Caplan 1974); the ptosis is usually mild and easily overlooked. The subnucleus that subserves levator function is a midline structure that is located at the caudal end of the third nerve nuclear complex (Warwick 1963). Lesions that affect this region will thus produce bilateral ptosis. Mesencephalic ptosis may be congenital, occurring as a consequence of dysplasia or aplasia of the IIIrd nerve nuclear complex. It is much more commonly seen as an acquired disorder secondary to ischemic, inflammatory, infiltrative, compressive or traumatic lesions.

Third nerve palsy and ptosis

Ptosis from involvement of the IIIrd nerve fascicle is usually unilateral and is commonly associated with weakness of one or more extraocular muscle innervated by this nerve. Pupil involvement is common but is not invariably present. Rarely ptosis will occur prior to the development of other evidence of a third nerve lesion. In some patients with mild involvement of the levator muscle from an early IIIrd nerve lesion, eyelid position during gaze straight ahead and in the vertical plane may appear to be normal, but when the patient performs a series of rapid blinks, slow and incomplete eyelid opening is immediately evident on the affected side. Paresis of the IIIrd cranial nerve in infants or children usually occurs as the result of trauma or congenital abnormality. Although ptosis is usually associated with these pareses, some patients with congenital IIIrd nerve palsies show little or no ptosis. The frequent association of contralateral monoparesis or hemiparesis patients with congenital IIIrd nerve palsies suggest that the site of the pathology is within the mid-brain (Balkan & Hoyt 1984). Paresis of the IIIrd cranial nerve rarely occurs in children as a result of compression of the intracranial portion of this nerve. Severe amblyopia is often associated with congenital IIIrd nerve palsies.

Horner's syndrome

Lesions of the sympathetic pathway may produce a mild unilateral ptosis as part of the Horner's syndrome. The ptosis seen in Horner's syndrome is usually mild, variable, and associated with ipsilateral miosis. Strabismus is not an associated finding in children with Horner's syndrome. Hypochromia of the affected iris commonly occurs in association with the congenital Horner's syndrome (Hyodo & Kase 1983). Injury to the brachial plexus at birth appears to be responsible for many of these cases although cases have been reported in association with congenital tumours and intrauterine infections (Spieglblatt *et al.* 1976). Congenital Horner's syndrome has been reported in association with other congenital defects, including facial hemiatrophy and cervical vertebral anomalies but it most often occurs without associated defects.

Myopathic ptosis

Ptosis that occurs from direct involvement of the levator or its tendon may occur as a congenital or an acquired phenomena. Acquired myopathic ptosis occurs in a number of mitochondrial cytopathies that are characterized by chronic progressive external ophthalmoplegia. In some patients, however, the ptosis is the presenting sign and may persist as an isolated phenomena for months or years. Ptosis of this type is usually bilateral, symmetrical and very slowly progressive. Bilateral partial ptosis contributes to the characteristic facies of patients with myotonic dystrophy and may also occur in various forms of familial periodic paralysis. Ptosis may be the initial and only sign of the various forms of infantile myasthenia gravis. Recent reports have emphasized that the prevalence of myasthenia gravis in infancy is probably much greater than previously recognized.

Trauma

Ptosis may occur following various types of ocular surgery, including cataract extraction and enucleation. This almost certainly occurs as the result of traumatic disinsertion of the levator tendon (Paris & Quickert 1976). Acquired ptosis in children who wear contact lenses should arouse the suspicion that the contact lens is embedded in the soft tissues of the superior fornix.

Blepharochalasis

Blepharochalasis is a rather uncommon condition first described by Fuchs in 1896. It is limited to the upper lids in which a myogenic ptosis occurs. This disorder initially manifests itself in childhood with recurrent attacks of severe oedema of the eyelids. Each succeeding attack leaves some residual damage to the tissues. Eventually the levator aponeurosis becomes thin and stretched. At surgery it may be even difficult to identify it. The orbital septum breaks down and orbital fat and even the orbital lobe of the lacrimal gland may prolapse into the eyelid, all of which cause the eyelid to droop. The aetiology of this syndrome is unknown, although it is frequently familial. In some children a mild ptosis, usually unilateral, may be associated with a high levator insertion with unequal lid creases, the condition may be familial, it rarely requires treatment. When treatment is required it may consist of a combination of levator aponeurosis tuck, blepharoplasty lateral canthoplasty and dermis fat graft in atrophic cases (Bergin *et al.* 1988).

Tumours

The most common congenital tumours affecting the lids are naevi, angiomas, and neurofibromas; rhabdomyosarcoma may also start in the lids. Melanocytic naevi are flat lesions and usually small, becoming larger and darker with age. Divided naevi (Fig. 18.17) are a form of congenital melanocytic naevus which involves the upper and lower lids (McDonnell & Mayou 1988). Haemangiomas (Fig. 18.18, 18.19) have a propensity for rapid growth in early life but usually resolve spontaneously, injection with depot corti-

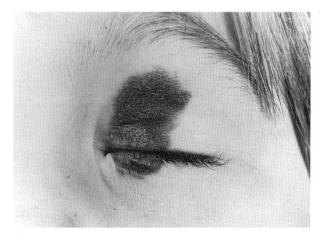

Fig. 18.17 Congenital divided naevus.

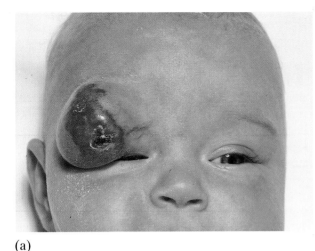

(a)

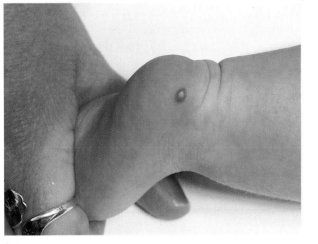

(b)

Fig. 18.18 (a) Large haemangioma with surface ulceration, which is almost certain to cause amblyopia; if the left eye is occluded the amblyopia could be avoided because the eye can just see below the lid. (b) The same child has other haemangiomas — a useful diagnostic guide.

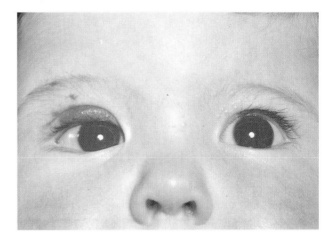

(a)

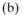

(b)

Fig. 18.19 (a) Three month old baby with right upper lid haemangioma. (b) Same child at 5 months after corticosteroid injection.

costeroid preparations may help (Fig. 18.19). The main concern is the development of amblyopia associated with the covering of the lid and with astigmatism, typically the astigmatism is hypermetropic with the axis at right angles to the centre of the haemangioma (Robb 1977).

Because of the position of the haemangioma it causes an understandably high degree of worry by the parents and this is often associated with pressure for treatment. Small lesions do not require treatment apart from occlusion of the fellow eye to counter amblyopia. Larger lesions may improve with injected depot steroids (Kushner 1982) or occasionally a short course of systemic steroids. Both depot and systemic steroids may result in adrenal suppression (Weiss 1989). Other treatments, including surgery, radiotherapy or injections of sclerosing agents leave permanent scars or carry unjustifiable risks so for larger lesions it is probably best to try steroids. If they do not work it is important to reassure the parents that the lesions always improve with time and that surgery can be carried out to improve any residual defect.

Dermoid cysts may occur in the lids, but these are usually primary tumours of the orbit and orbital margin and involve the lid secondarily (see Chapter 22). Molluscum contagiosum (Fig. 18.20, 18.21) and warts of viral origin also frequently occur on the eyelids. Molluscum lesions may require curettage and diathermy of their core. Juvenile xanthogranuloma lesions occasionally occur in the lids (Mansour *et al*. 1985).

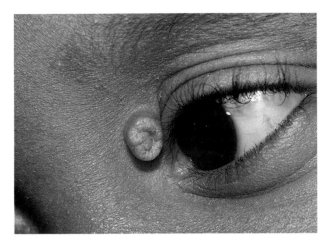

Fig. 18.20 Large molluscum contagiosum lesion (Dr S. Day's patient).

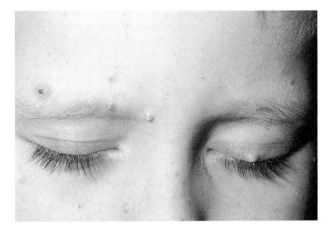

Fig. 18.21 Multiple molluscum contagiosum lesions.

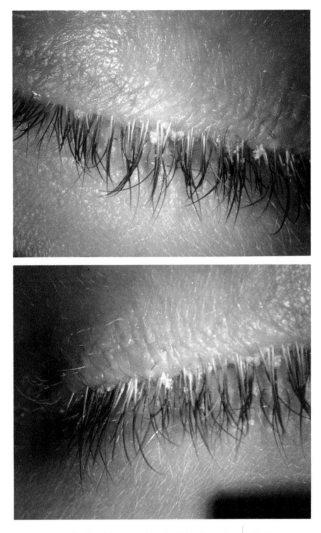

Fig. 18.22 Blepharitis associated with chronic staphylococcus infection.

Chalazia

A chalazion is a lipogranuloma of the meibomian gland that results from obstruction of the gland duct and is usually located in the midportion of the tarsus, away from the lid border, sometimes they may occur well away from the lid margin (Gonnering 1988). It may occur on the lid margin if the opening of the duct is involved. A secondary infection of the surrounding tissues may develop with swelling of the entire lid. Chalazia can cause pressure on the globe thereby altering the refractive error. Small chalazia may resolve spontaneously. If they are large, however, or secondarily infected, treatment is usually required. This usually involves the use of warm compresses with topical antibiotic therapy. Incision of the conjunctival wall of the lesion and curettage is sometimes necess-

ary, although this is avoided whenever possible in young children since it usually necessitates a general anaesthetic. Chronic meibomitis and blepharitis (Fig. 18.22), which may predispose to recurrent chalazion formation, should be treated by lid cleaning with isotonic solution on a cotton wool ball together with antibiotic/hydrocortisone ointment for a circumscribed period before resorting to curettage (Fig. 18.23) which usually requires general anaesthesia. Chronic chalazia should be treated with suspicion as rhabdomyosarcoma may present in this guise.

Acute blepharitis

Acute blepharitis presents with ulceration of the lid margins and is usually caused by *Staphylococcus aureus*, other organisms and viruses, including

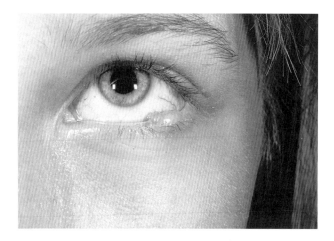

Fig. 18.23 Chronic chalazion that failed to respond to simple medical treatment of lid toilet and antibiotic cream.

Moraxella species, herpes simplex, and various fungi in immunosuppressed patients. Staphylococcal and *Moraxella* blepharitis usually respond well to antibiotic cream and lid toilet, and fungi or herpes simplex usually respond to appropriate chemotherapy.

Chronic blepharitis

Chronic blepharitis is much more common than acute form. It presents as irritable eyelids that are red, scaly and sometimes rather swollen. The anterior lid margin is usually most affected but occasionally the posterior lid margin is more red and swollen when the meibonium glands are affected (chronic meibomitis). Infection plays a role with *Staphylococcus aureus*, *Propionibacterium acnes* or coagulase-negative staphyloccal species being important (Dougherty & McCully 1984). The role of yeasts like *Pityrosporum ovale* is uncertain but it seems clearer that the mite *Demodex folliculorum* plays a role, perhaps as a vector for bacteria and yeasts. Lice, *Phthirus palpebrarum* or *P. pubis*, may be found on slit lamp examination of the lash bases or their eggs ('nits') may be found attached to the lashes.

Most cases of chronic blepharitis have a seborrhoeic element with greasy, scaly lids associated in some cases with seborrhoeic dermatitis of the scalp (dandruff) or elsewhere.

Treatment is by regular lid cleaning with isotonic solutions on a cotton wool ball or bud, with particular attention to the lid margins. Expression of greasy meibomian secretion by firm pressure may also help the symptoms of burning and irritation. This simple treatment should be carried out long after the symp-toms have improved. Reinfected or severe cases, in some of which there may be an associated kerato-conjunctivitis, may be treated in addition by a short course of a steroid-antibiotic combination ointment.

Trichiasis

Trichiasis is an acquired condition of the lid margin in which the cilia are misdirected, usually backward, causing corneal and conjunctival irritation. It differs from entropion in that the lid margin itself is in normal position, but because of fibrosis or cicatrization, the ciliae are misplaced. Historically, the most common cause of this condition has been trachoma. In most developed countries, however, more common causes of trichiasis include the Stevens−Johnson syndrome, severe burns, and pemphigus. The treatment of trichiasis is not usually simple and many techniques have been suggested for its cure. Although the clinical distinctions between trichiasis and mild cicatrical entropion is not always easy, it is of tremendous importance in the surgical treatment of these two conditions; if the lid borders turn in, then none of the procedures described for trichiasis alone are effective. Trichiasis may be treated by epilation, electrolysis, or various resection techniques.

References

Akkerman CH, Stern LM. Ankyloblepharon filiforme adnatum. *Brit J Ophthalmol* 1979; **63**: 129−31

Anderson L, Baumgartner A. Amblyopia in ptosis. *Arch Ophthalmol* 1980a; **98**: 1068−9

Anderson L, Baumgartner A. Strabismus in ptosis. *Arch Ophthalmol* 1980b; **98**: 1062−7

Anderson RL, Harvey JT. Lid splitting in posterior lamellar cryosurgery for congenital and acquired distichiasis. *Arch Ophthalmol* 1981; **99**: 631−41

Balkan R, Hoyt CS. Associated neurologic abnormalities in congenital third nerve palsies. *Am J Ophthalmol* 1984; **97**: 315−19

Beard C. A new treatment for severe unilateral ptosis and for ptosis with jaw-winking. *Am J Ophthalmol* 1965; **59**: 252−7

Beard C. *Ptosis*. CV Mosby, St Louis 1981; pp. 32−84

Beard C. A new classification of blepharoptosis. *Int Ophthalmol Clin* 1989; **29**: 214−16

Bentsi-Enihill KO. Congenital total eversion of the upper eyelids. *Br J Ophthalmol* 1981; **65**: 209−13

Bergin DJ, McCord CD, Berger T, Friedberg H, Waterhouse W. Blepharochalasis. *Br J Ophthalmol* 1988; **72**: 863−7

Berke RN, Wadsworth JAC. Histology of levator muscle in congenital and acquired ptosis. *Arch Ophthalmol* 1955; **53**: 413−6

Berry C, Cree J, Mann T. Aarskog's syndrome. *Arch Dis Child* 1980; **55**: 706−11

Callahan AC. Surgical correction of blepharophimosis syndromes. *Trans Am Acad Ophthalmol Otolaryngol* 1973; **77**: 687—95

Caplan LR. Ptosis. *J Neurol Neurosurg Psychiatry* 1974; **34**: 1—7

Clarke DI, Patterson A. Ankyloblepharon filiforme adnatum in trisomy 18 (Edward's syndrome). *Br J Ophthalmol* 1985; **69**: 471—3

Collin JRO. New concepts in the management of ptosis. *Eye* 1988; **2**: 185—9

Dougherty JM, McCully JP. Comparative bacteriology of chronic blepharitis. *Br J Ophthalmol* 1984; **68**: 524—9

Ehlers N, Jensen IK. Ankyloblepharon filiforme congenitum: associated with harelip and cleft palate. *Acta Ophthalmol* 1970; **48**: 465—7

Feingold M, Bossert WH. Normal values for selected physical parameters: an aid to syndrome delineation. *Birth Defects* 1974; **10**: 13

Frueh BR. The mechanistic classification of ptosis. *Ophthamology* 1978; **98**: 1019—21

Gonnering RS. Extratarsal chalazia. *Br J Ophthalmol* 1988; **72**: 202—6

Gupta SP, Saxena RC. Cryptophthalmos. *Brit J Ophthalmol* 1963; **46**: 629—31

Hay RJ, Wells RS. The syndrome of ankyloblepharon, ectodermal defects and cleft lip and palate: an autosomal dominant condition. *Br J Dermatology* 1976; **94**: 277—89

Isaksson I. A study of congenital blepharoptosis. *Trans Ophthalmol Soc UK* 1960; **80**: 231—8

Jones CA, Collin JRO. Blepharophimosis and its association with female infertility. *Br J Ophthalmol* 1984; **68**: 533—4

Kazarian EL, Goldstein P. Ankyloblepharon filiforme adnatum with hydrocephalus, meningomyelocele and imperforate anus. *Am J Ophthalmol* 1977; **84**: 355—7

Keipert JA. Euryblepharon. *Br J Ophthalmol* 1975; **59**: 57—8

Khurana A, Ahluwalia B, Mehtani V. Primary epitarsus: a case report. *Br J Ophthalmol* 1986; **70**: 931—2

Kushner BJ. Intralesional corticosteroid injection for infantile Adnexal hemangioma. *Am J Ophthalmol* 1982; **93**: 496—506

Lubkin V. The inverse Marcus Gunn phenomena: electomyographic contribution. *Arch Neurol* 1978; **35**: 249—54

Mansour AM, Traboulsi E, Frangieh G. Multiple recurrences of juvenile xanthogranuloma of the eyelid. *J Pediatr Ophthalmol and Strabismus* 1985; **22**: 156—7

McCord CD. The correction of telecanthus and epicanthal folds. *Ophthalmic Surg* 1980; **11**: 446—56

McDonnell PJ, Mayou BJ. Congenital divided naevus of the eyelids. *Br J Ophthalmol* 1988; **72**: 198—202

Moanie R, Kopelowitz N, Rosenfeld W, Jhaderi R. Congenital eversion of the eyelids. *J Pediatr Ophthalmol and Strabismus* 1982; **19**: 326—7

Mustardé JC. Epicanthal folds and the problem of telecanthus. *Trans Ophthalmol Soc UK* 1963; **83**: 397—411

Mustardé JC. *Plastic Surgery in Infancy and Childhood*. Longman, London 1971, pp. 251—60

Paris GL, Quickert MH. Disinsertion of the aponeurosis of the levator palpebri superioris muscle after cataract extraction. *Am J Ophthalmol* 1976; **81**: 337—40

Price NC, Collin JR. Congenital horizontal tarsal kink: a simple surgical correction. *Br J Ophthalmol* 1987; **71**: 204—7

Robb RM. Refractive errors associated with hemangiomas of the eye lids in infancy. *Am J Ophthalmol* 1977; **83**: 52—8

Roper-Hall MJ. Congenital colobomata of the lids. *Trans Ophthalmol Soc UK* 1969; **88**: 556—7

Sano K. Trigemino-oculomotor synkinesis. *Neurolgia* 1959; **1**: 29—51

Sevel D. A reappraisal of the development of the eyelids. *Eye* 1988; **2**: 123—9

Shields LC, Nelson LB, Carpenter GC, Shields JA. Neonatal Grave's disease. *Br J Ophthalmol* 1988; **72**: 424—8

Smith B, Chrubini T. *Occuloplastic Surgery*. CV Mosby. St Louis 1970, pp. 9—12, 18—20

Speilgelblatt L, Benoit T, Jacob JL. Neuroblastoma with heterochromia and Horner's syndrome. *J Pediatr* 1976; **88**: 1067—8

Tse DP, Anderson RL, Fratkin JD. Aponeurosis disinsertion in congenital entropion. *Arch Ophthalmol* 1983; **101**: 436—40

Warwick R. Representation of the extraocular muscles in the oculomotor nuclei of the monkey. *J Comp Neurol* 1963; **98**: 449—503

Weiss AH. Adrenal suppression after corticosteroid injection of periocular hemangiomas. *Am J Ophthalmol* 1989; **107**: 518—22

White JH. Correction of distichiasis by tarsal resection and mucous membrane grafting. *An J Ophthalmol* 1975; **80**: 507—8

Wolfley D. Excision of individual follicles for the management of congenital distichiasis and localised trichiasis. *J Pediatr Ophthalmol Strabismus* 1987; **24**: 22—6

Von Hasner. Ankyloblepharon filiforme adnatum. *Z Heilkd* Prague 1881; **2**: 429

Zak TA. Congenital primary upper eyelid entropian. *J Ped Ophthalmol Strabismus* 1984; **21**: 69—73

19 Conjunctiva and Subconjunctival Tissue

DAVID TAYLOR

Structure, function, and embryology

The conjunctiva is derived from a band of mesenchyme around the limbus which also forms the sclera, episclera, and Tenon's capsule. In childhood the conjunctiva is thicker than in old age and the epithelial cells are more square in shape and they are more numerous than in mid-life. In childhood Tenon's capsule is thick and the blood vessels are fewer, less tortuous, smaller and less prominent than they are in old age. As every strabismus surgeon knows, the conjunctiva of a child is a much tougher tissue than the underlying Tenon's 'capsule'; it holds sutures well. The subconjunctival tissues do not develop the fatty infiltrates that occur especially in the exposed areas in an adult, this being one of the factors behind the 'bright eyes' of youth. The conjunctiva contains goblet cells which produce mucus, vital to the normal structure of the tear layer and, therefore, vital to the protection of the eye. The growth of the conjunctival fornix, orbital margin, and palpebral fissure correlates with weight and gestational age of term and premature neonates (Isenberg et al. 1987).

Vascular abnormalities

Haemangioma and lymphohaemangioma

Usually occuring predominantly as a haemangioma composed of blood vessels, these are usually associated with lid and orbital haemangiomas (Fig. 19.1) and sometimes with intracranial haemangiomas but may be isolated (Fig. 19.2). They appear as bright red masses which blanch on pressure and which not infrequently haemorrhage spontaneously or with trivial trauma. Treatment may be difficult because removal is often followed by recurrence (Fig. 19.1). Radiotherapy may play some role in their treatment (Fig. 19.1).

Lymphohaemangiomas (Fig. 19.3) are usually more widespread with the whole of one side of the face being affected and the abnormality appearing in other

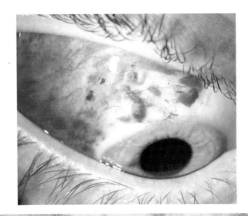

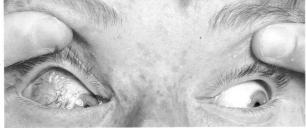

Fig. 19.1 Conjunctival haemangioma. As a baby this 17 year old girl had an orbital and lid haemangioma. The subconjunctival vascular abnormality had bled repeatedly and did not respond to surgical excision of the subconjunctival vessels. The conjunctival haemangiomata became devascularized with low-dose radiotherapy (same patient).

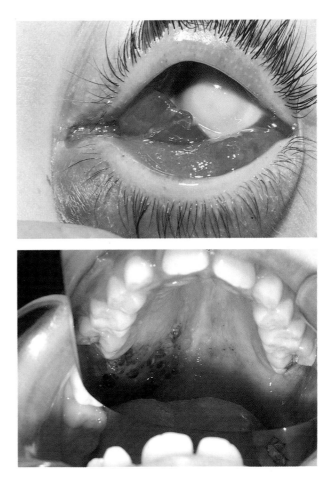

Fig. 19.3 This 2-year-old child had an anomalous left eye from birth; at 18 months of age the lids became swollen due to a lymphohaemangioma which also involved the orbit and maxilla. Palatal clear and blood-filled cysts typical of lymphohaemangioma (same patient).

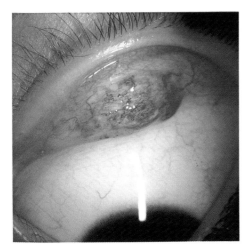

Fig. 19.2 An isolated conjunctival haemangioma in a 2-year-old child that disappeared by the age of 6 years.

parts of the face, in the nose causing nose bleeds or on the palate causing bleeding when eating. Lympho-haemangiomas are less prone to the cessation of growth which many of the pure haemangiomas show by the time the child is a few years of age, but nonetheless some do show resolution and, therefore,

surgery should be restricted only to those cases where relentless growth has occurred, where the cosmetic appearance is extremely poor, or where there appears to be no cessation of growth. Clinically they may be distinguished by the appearance of clear fluid filled cystic areas amongst the blood filled haemangioma tissue.

Sturge—Weber syndrome

Naevus flammeus, the flat form of facial haemangi-oma, may sometimes be associated with congenital glaucoma, intracranial calcification and fits when it is known as the Sturge—Weber syndrome. The conjunc-tiva may be involved showing only a faint blush on the normal whiteness of the conjunctiva or it may be more extensive (Fig. 19.4). It may be limited to sectors of the conjunctiva and may cause difficulty because of

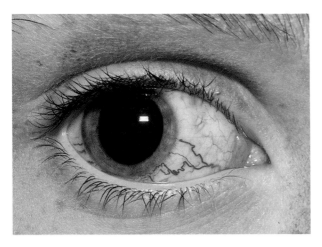

Fig. 19.4 Sturge–Weber syndrome. Conjunctival capillary haemangioma with dilated larger vessels associated with glaucoma.

bleeding at the time of surgery for glaucoma associated with Sturge–Weber syndrome (Chapter 25). The vessels consist of a very fine network of capillary sized vessels.

Klippel–Trenaunay–Weber syndrome

This syndrome which consists of a widespread vascular anomaly causing limb hypertrophy and bluish vascular anomalies of the skin may also have conjunctival angiomas.

Orbital, cerebral, and ocular vascular malformation

A variety of intracranial abnormalities may be associated with orbital and conjunctival varices. The best known of the ocular abnormalities is in the Wyburn–Mason syndrome, in which huge racemose angiomatous malformation of the retina, sometimes with remarkably well preserved vision is associated with intracranial, orbital, and sometimes conjunctival vascular malformations (Theron, *et al.* 1974).

Ataxia telangiectasia (Louis–Bar syndrome)

This disease is autosomal recessively inherited and usually presents with a cerebellar ataxia after a normal early development. Limb and truncal ataxia occur in the first decade and is slowly progressive. Later dysarthria and other movement disorders including extrapyramidal disorders are seen. Usually the child becomes severely handicapped by 12 years of age. Mental retardation is frequent, as is dementia, and growth

retardation occurs especially in those who have recurrent infections. These infections are due to an immunological defect with reduced synthesis of IgA and to a certain extent of IgG. They are also susceptable to a variety of neoplasms and abnormal carbohydrate metabolism (McFarlan & Strober 1972). The characteristic ocular feature is the presence of extremely tortuous and telangiectatic conjunctival vessels which usually occur in the exposed areas (Fig. 19.5). Sometimes they may be quite gross, but they are usually subtle. The bulbar conjunctiva is affected first (Harley *et al.* 1967) and they consist of a post-capillary venular link with vessels of non-uniform calibre with slow flow of red blood cells (Kulikov, 1974).

Another characteristic finding is an eye movement defect consisting of nystagmus and a form of saccade palsy or oculomotor apraxia (Smith and Cogan 1959; Baloh et al. 1978).

Carotid-cavernous fistula

Children who develop a red eye following head trauma by a few days, but occasionally some weeks, should be suspected of having a carotid-cavernous fistula. Although relatively rare in childhood it is sometimes severe and may be associated with raised intraocular pressure. The diagnosis needs to be established promptly for the appropriate treatment to be undertaken.

Sickle cell disease

Although not symptomatic, the conjunctiva is a useful site for observing the vascular changes by slit lamp

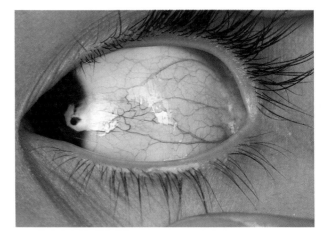

Fig. 19.5 Ataxia telangiectasia. There is a group of telangiectatic and tortuous vessels in the exposed area of the conjunctiva especially temporally.

microscopy. Coma-shaped conjunctiva capillaries and slow flow may be seen.

Hyperviscosity

In blood hyperviscosity states the conjunctiva appears suffused, the capillaries dilated and tortuous with slow flow seen on slit lamp microscopy.

Conjunctival haemorrhage

Most frequently this occurs after minor trauma and it occurs when there has been a rise in central venous pressure such as after a seizure, immediately after birth or any activity involving Valsalva type procedures. They usually improve spontaneously within 2 weeks and do not require treatment.

Spontaneous conjunctival haemorrhages are not infrequent in childhood and are the subject of some mythology as to causation, but they are generally not known to be associated with any serious abnormality. Sometimes they occur repeatedly in one area and slit lamp examination may reveal an anomalous vessel which occasionally needs treatment by cautery to prevent recurrence.

Subconjunctival haemorrhages occur in thrombocytopenic states, for instance in leukaemia. Various forms of conjunctivitis may be associated with subconjunctival haemorrhage.

Fabry's disease

Small conjunctival aneurysms occur in Fabry's disease.

Conjunctival lymphangiectasia

Conjunctival lymphangiectasia may be associated with generalized lymphoedema (Milroy–Meige disease). It has been described with Turner's syndrome (Perry & Cossari 1986) and dilated subconjunctival lymph vessels may be seen and adjacent to plexiform neuromas (Fig. 19.6)

Linear scleroderma (morphoea en coup de sabre)

A perilimbal dilated vascular network (Fig. 19.7) is a not uncommon finding in morphoea en coup de sabre (Taylor & Talbot 1985). Morphoea appears as a linear groove in the scalp or forehead skin and may spread to the lids orbit and eye. Ipsilateral glaucoma may occur (Perrot et al. 1977).

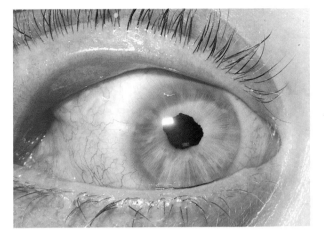

Fig. 19.6 Neurofibromatosis with orbital plexiform neuroma adjacent to which there are dilated lymph vessels — note the ectropion pupillae.

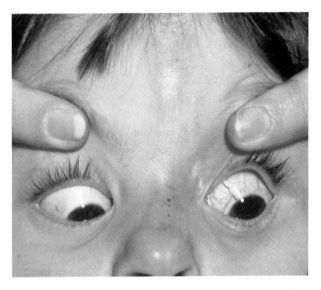

Fig. 19.7 Morphoea en coup de sabre. This child had a left frontal linear scleroderma which can be seen to affect the side of the nose together with conjunctival telangiectasia and glaucoma.

Pigmented lesions

Oculodermal melanosis (naevus of ota)

This shows as a variable slatey blue scleral, conjunctival and subconjunctival pigmentation associated with skin and mucus membrane hyperpigmentation (Fig. 19.8) usually on the same side (Charlin 1973). It is usually noticed in the first year or two of life, but sometimes does not present until later. It may get worse initially and then again later at puberty. There

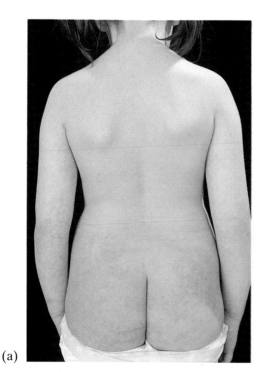

(a)

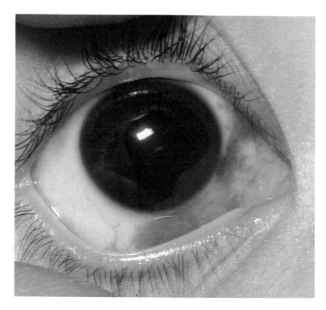

Fig. 19.9 Ocular Melanosis. Congenital slate-blue episcleral pigmentation.

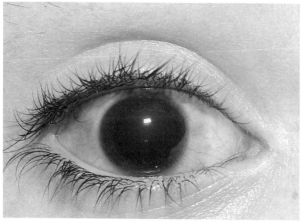

(b)

Fig. 19.8 (a) Oculo-dermal Melanosis with widespread skin and mucous membrane pigmentation. (b) Sub-conjunctival melanosis (same patient).

is said to be an increased risk in this condition of the child later developing uveal or other malignant melanomas (Jay 1965b; Yamomato 1969; Singh *et al.* 1988). Intracranial vascular malformations may also be associated (Orr *et al.* 1978; Massey *et al.* 1979).

Ocular melanosis

This is a usually unilateral slatey blue episcleral pigmentation (Fig. 19.9) sometimes associated with an increase in iris and other uveal pigment. It is present

from birth, but may not present until the first year or two of life and it may become more prominent at puberty. There is some evidence of an increased risk of developing uveal melanomas. Children with this condition should be reviewed periodically because of a risk of pigmentary glaucoma and the risk of melanoma (Roldan *et al.* 1987).

Naevi

These do not usually become obvious until after the first few years of life (Jay 1965a), often after 10 years or even later. They are composed of melanocytic naevus cells sometimes located only within the epithelial layer of the conjunctiva when they are known as junctional naevi. When subepithelial and epithelial naevus cells are present it is known as a compound naevus and sometimes only subepithelial cells are found. They usually occur near the limbus and are well circumscribed and usually flat, although compound naevi are sometimes slightly elevated and may be cystic (Fig. 19.10). Occasionally they are only very lightly pigmented or even non-pigmented. They are the most common childhood epibulbar tumour.

There is little evidence for the progression of naevi into melanomas. Melanomas of the conjunctiva are extremely rare in childhood (McDonnell *et al.* 1989) and are characterized by being somewhat more raised, vascular and fleshy than naevi.

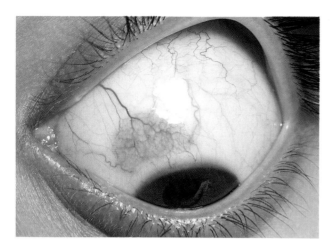

Fig. 19.10 A cystic compound naevus of the conjunctiva in a 14-year-old

Gaucher's disease

Pingueculae and conjunctival pigmentation occur in the chronic forms of Gaucher's disease (see Chapter 36).

Alkaptonuria

Episcleral and conjunctival pigmentation occur in the area of the horizontal rectus muscle insertions. These children, whose urine turns black on standing, have bone disease with arthritis and valvular and atherosclerotic heart disease.

Kartagener's syndrome

In this recessively inherited syndrome children may be born with dextrocardia and they develop bronchiectasis, bronchitis and respiratory tract infections. They are sometimes myopic and may develop glaucoma. They characteristically have marked conjunctival melanosis and hypertrophy of the plica semilunaris (Segal *et al.* 1963).

Peutz—Jegher syndrome

This is a dominantly inherited syndrome with polyposis of the gastrointestinal tract, especially the small bowel. The polyps may bleed and may become malignant. Freckles are seen around the orifices, on the lids and conjunctiva; scleral and corneal pigmented spots have been described.

Tumours and infiltrates

The most common epibulbar tumours are naevi, dermoids inclusion cysts and papillomas (Cunha *et al.* 1987).

Epibulbar dermoid

These are choristomas which contain a combination of fat, hair follicles and sebaceous glands. They may occur at the limbus or even on the cornea alone. Corneal and limbal dermoids appear as yellow white, usually rounded elevations sometimes with pigmentation and hair at the apex (Fig. 19.11, 19.12) and sometimes associated with intraocular abnormalities (Fig. 19.13). The more posterior dermoids known as dermolipomas may be associated with a larger amount of fatty tissue without hairs and they extend posteriorly for some considerable distance and cannot safely be

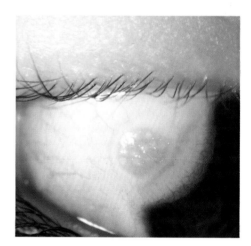

Fig. 19.11 A hairy limbal dermoid.

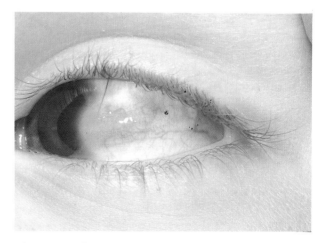

Fig. 19.12 A limbal dermoid encroaching on the cornea, but extending back to the temporal fornix.

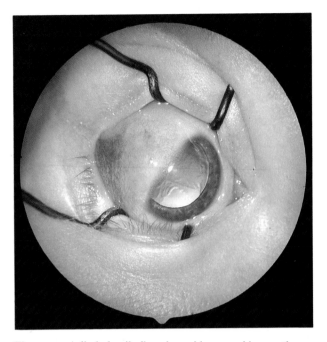

Fig. 19.13 A limbal epibulbar dermoid encroaching on the lateral third of the eye. Although removed leaving minimal scarring, the eye had profound amblyopia due to astigmatism.

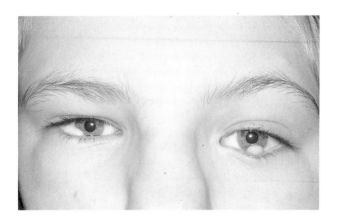

Fig. 19.14 Bilateral limbal dermoids with attachments to the lid and malar hypoplasia in Goldenhaar's syndrome.

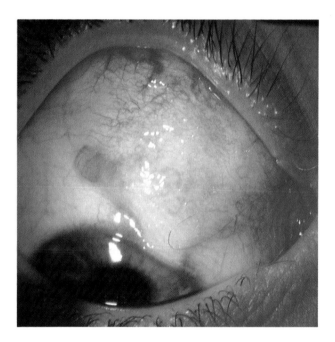

Fig. 19.15 Epibulbar oseous choristoma overlying ectopic lacrimal gland.

removed as a whole. They may be closely related to eye muscles.

Either type of dermoid may be associated with Goldenhaar's syndrome (Fig. 19.14) in which often bilateral epibulbar dermoids occur with a lid coloboma and with pre-auricular skin tags or appendages; and a variety of first branchial arch abnormalities; and occasionally a neuroparalytic keratitis (Romano 1978).

Epibulbar osseous (Fig. 19.15) choristomas are flatter bony and fatty abnormalities which may overly ectopic lacrimal gland which lie in the temporal or superotemporal region under the conjunctiva (Hered & Hiles 1987; Pokorny *et al.* 1987).

Most dermoids can be simply excised for cosmetic reasons; when the cornea is involved a lamellar keratectomy has to be carried out and the results are often only moderately good with an improvement in that the elevated mass is removed, but the remaining cornea is sometimes opalescent or may even become opaque. Freehand corneal lamellar grafting may improve the appearance in refractory cases but the results are sometimes not very satisfactory.

Clear cysts

Occasionally small clear fluid-filled cysts appear in the conjunctiva in older children. These are of no significance and usually disappear spontaneously.

Secondary tumours

The conjunctiva may be invaded by other tumours including rhabdomyosarcoma (Fig. 19.16) and retinoblastoma; rarely retinoblastoma may present as a conjunctival or subconjunctival swelling. Histiocytosis-X occasionally involves the conjunctiva as does juvenile xanthogranuloma. Conjunctival infiltrates occur in childhood leukaemia and neurofibromas, usually associated with a plexiform neuroma of the orbit, may present with a whitish or clear cystic knotted mass in the subconjunctival tissue.

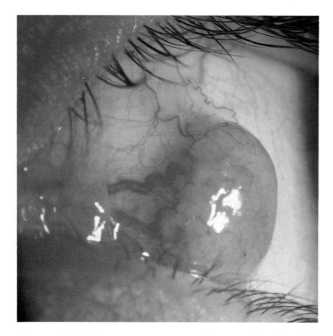

Fig. 19.16 Rhabdomyosarcoma presenting as a subconjunctival nodule.

Xeroderma pigmentosa

This is a rare autosomal recessive disease of infancy and childhood in which the skin is excessively sensitive to light resulting in pigmentation, telangiectasis, keratosis, and the development of basal cell and squamous cell carcinomas, malignant melanomas, and a variety of other tumours. These may include squamous cell carcinomas of the conjunctiva (Fig. 19.17) (Bellows *et al.* 1974) and the syndrome is sometimes associated with neurological abnormalities including deafness, ataxia, mental retardation and cerebellar atrophy when it is known as the De Sanctis–Cacchione syndrome (Handa *et al.* 1978).

Benign hereditary epithelial dyskeratosis

This dominantly inherited condition consists of the presence of elevated whitish plaques of hyperkeratotic and vascular tissue in the exposed areas of the conjunctiva and it may be associated with dyskeratosis of the buccal mucosa (Yanoff 1968). It is rare and has been described in a small group of North American patients.

Papilloma

Conjunctival papillomas are not uncommon in childhood. They present as elevated, sometimes pedunculated lesions that are usually white or yellowish, but

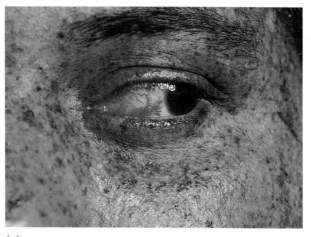

(a)

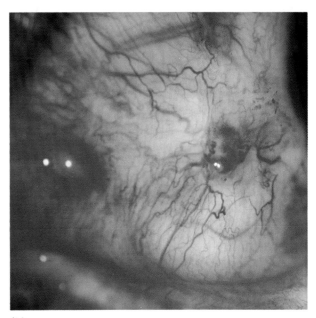

(b)

Fig. 19.17 (a) Xeroderma Pigmentosa. The widespread skin pigmentation can be seen in this girl of Indian origin. (b) The conjunctiva was affected by multifocal recurrent squamous cell carcinoma.

may be quite heavily pigmented or pink in colour (Fig. 19.18). On lamp examination they can be seen to consist of translucent 'flesh' with small red spots which represent the vessels in the core of the papillomatous tissue. They may be multiple and may occur in more than one member of the family. In young children they are usually associated with a virus infection and they often disappear spontaneously (Wilson & Ostler 1974), but if they do not disappear after a few months or if they are causing considerable trouble cryotherapy, surgical excision or diathermy may be indicated.

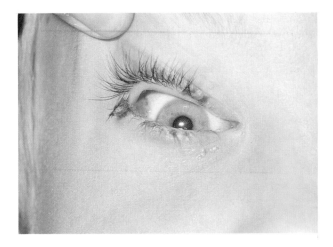

Fig. 19.18 Conjunctival papilloma of the temporal bulbar conjunctiva associated with lid papillomas.

Sarcoidosis

The conjunctiva was once thought to be frequently involved in sarcoidosis and it was not infrequent for 'blind' biopsies of the conjunctiva to be carried out in order to diagnose sarcoidosis. The histological diagnosis must be carefully considered because meibomian cysts have a similar appearance. Conjunctival biopsy is indicated in suspected sarcoidosis (Hoover *et al.* 1986) especially if a discreet elevated lesion is seen. Conjunctival sarcoidosis does not usually cause any symptoms and in itself requires no treatment.

Avitaminosis

Malnutrition is one of the commonest causes of blindness in the world today. Although it warrants deeper study only the conjunctival aspects will be referred to here.

Xerophthalmia, the term applied to the external eye manifestations of blinding malnutrition, usually occurs in the setting of a more widespread protein/calorie malnutrition and is often associated with infection (Brown *et al.* 1979), usually following a period of night-blindness, which is often the first sign but only discovered on direct questioning, a dry appearance or dullness of the eyes appears with the conjunctiva appearing wrinkled, reddened, dull and sometimes pigmented. Bitot's spots are flaky, elevated patches usually in exposed areas of the conjunctiva and most significant if present on both sides of the cornea (Sommer *et al.* 1980). Most of these cases are associated with vitamin A deficiency as well as a more generalized malnutrition and infection of the conjunc-

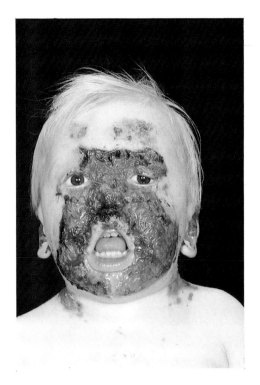

Fig. 19.19 Dystrophic epidermolysis bullosa. Most of the facial skin has debrided. Surprisingly the conjunctival and corneal epithelium had only been mildly affected.

tiva and cornea, already weakened by dryness and vitamin A deficiency plays a major role.

Pingueculum and pterygium

Pingueculae and pterygia are rare in childhood but can occur occasionally in children who come from hot and dry countries. It is unusual for them to give rise to substantial problems in childhood. Pseudopterygia, on the other hand, are not uncommon following inflammatory corneal disease or excision of a corneal lesion, for instance, an epibulbar dermoid. If cosmetically unsightly they may be excised with a wide conjunctival margin and a superficial keratectomy but occasionally a mucous membrane graft may be required.

Conjunctival thinning

Conjunctival thinning occurs in Dego's disease, the scalded baby syndrome, epidermolysis bullosa and in ectodermal dysplasia.

Dego's disease is a rare, multiple organ system disease characterized by a papular eruption on the trunk and extremities with atrophic white centres lesions surrounded by a telangiectatic border. A variety of ocular manifestations may occur including an abnormal retinal vascular pattern (Lee *et al.* 1984), ophthalmoplegia, papilloedema and optic atrophy, together with atrophic telangiectatic conjunctival lesions.

In Dystrophic epidermolysis bullosa eye changes are common including symblepharon, broadening of the limbus, corneal opacities and recurrent erosions (Fig. 19.19) (McDonnell *et al.* 1989).

Conjunctival thickening

Conjunctival thickening occurs in conjunctival scarring, pemphigus, and the Richner–Hanhart syndrome (tyrosinaemia type 2). In the Richner–Hanhart syn-

drome, also known as tyrosinosis, there are hyperkeratotic lesions of the palm, soles and elbows and occasionally mental retardation. It is associated with an increase in serum and urine tyrosine. It is transmitted as an autosomal recessive trait. Children with this condition are photophobic and have watering eyes with thickened conjunctiva and hypertrophy of the tarsal conjunctiva. There are epithelial and subepithelial opacities of the cornea and corneal ulceration which appears dendritic at times. The lesions on the cornea tend to heal spontaneously but may take some time. When they first appear dendritiform and they are often bilateral. The corneal lesions may be treated with corticosteroids and by the appropriate diet (Michalski *et al.* 1988).

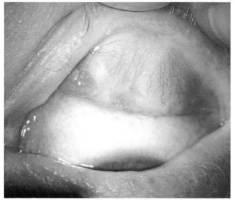

(a)

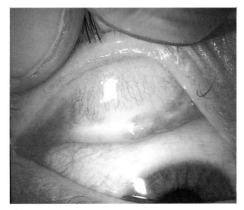

(b)

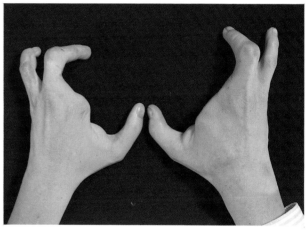

(c)

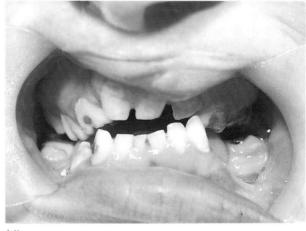

(d)

Fig. 19.20 EEC syndrome. This child had conjunctival thinning especially affecting the tarsal plates (a, b). Marked ectrodactyly (c). Ectodermal dysplasia and other ectodermal defects including teeth (d) and hair abnormalities (see Chapter 20.1).

In ectodermal dysplasia there is conjunctival and corneal thinning which may lead to spontaneous perforation. The EEC syndrome (Fig. 19.20) is an autosomal dominant syndrome with variable expression which has prominent eye complications (McNab *et al.* 1989; Wilson *et al.* 1973).

Conjunctival scarring

Scarring can be caused by the following.
1 Burns:
  (a) Thermal.
  (b) Chemical, including non-accidental injury.
2 Traumatic, including surgery, e.g. squint surgery and surgery to remove dermoids, etc.
3 Infection:
  (a) Trachoma.
  (b) Severe and prolonged bacterial infections or adenovirus.
4 Avitaminosis.
5 Inflammatory disease:
  (a) Stevens—Johnson syndrome.
  (b) Richner—Hanhart syndrome.
  (c) Chronic vernal conjunctivitis.
  (d) Erythema Multiforme.
  (e) Toxic epidermal necrolysis.
6 Dry-eye.
7 Ectodermal dysplasia.

References

Baloh RW, Yee RD, Boder E Eye movements in ataxia telangiectasia. *Neurology* 1978; **28**: 1099–104

Bellows RA, Lahour M, Lepreau FJ, Albert DM. Ocular manifestations of xeroderma pigmentosa in a black family. *Arch Ophthalmol* 1974; **92**: 113–9

Brown KH, Gaffar A, Alamgir SM Xerophthalmia, protein-calorie malnutrition and infections in children. *J Pediatr* 1979; **95**: 651–6

Charlin C. Oculo-dermo-mucous melanosis. Naevus of ota (in French). *Arch Ophthalmol (Paris)* 1973; **33**: 19–28

Cunha RP, Cunha MC, Shields JA. Epibulbar tumours in children: a survey of 282 biopsies. *J Pediatr Ophthalmol Strabismus* 1987; **24**: 249–55

Handa J, Nakano Y, Akiguchi I Cranial computed tomography findings in xeroderma pigmentosum with neurologic manifestations (De Sanctis—Cacchione syndrome). *J Comp Ass Tom* 1978; **2**: 456–9

Harley RD, Baird, HW, Craven Ataxia-telangiectasia. *Arch ophthalmol (Chic)* 1967; **77**: 582–92

Hered RW, Hiles DA. Epibulbar osseous choristoma and ectopic lacrimal gland underlying a dermolipoma. *J Pediatr Ophthalmol Strabismus* 1987; **24**: 255–9

Hoover DL, Khan JA, Giangiacomo J. Review. Pediatric ocular sarcoidosis *Surv Ophthalmology* 1986; **30**: 215–29

Isenberg SJ, McCarty JW, Rich R. Growth of the conjunctival fornix and orbital margin in term and premature infants. *Ophthalmology* 1987; **94**: 1276–81

Jay B. Naevi and melanomata of the conjunctiva. *Br J Ophthalmol* 1965a; **49**: 169–83

Jay B. Malignant melanoma of the orbit in a case of oculodermal melanosis (naevus of ota). *Br J Ophthalmol* 1965b; **49**: 359–63

Kulikov VV. Changes in the microvascular bed of the eye conjunctiva in ataxia-telangiectasis (syndrome of D Louis-Bar). *Arch Patologi (Moscow)* 1974; **36**: 30–8

Lee DA, Su D, Liesegang TJ. Systemic ophthalmology. Ophthalmic changes of Dego's disease (malignant atrophic papulosis). *Ophthalmology* 1984; **91**: 295–9

McNab A, Potts MJ, Welham RAN. The EEC syndrome and its ocular manifestations. *BJ Ophthalmol* 1989; **73**: 261–5

Massey EW, Brannon WL, Morland M. Neavus of ota and intracranial arteriovenous malformation. *Neurology* 1979; **29**: 1625–7

McDonnell JM, Carpenter JD, Jacobs P, Wan L, Gilmore JE. Conjunctival melanocytic lesions in children. *Ophthalmology* 1989; **96**: 986–93

McDonnell PJ, Schofield OMV, Spalton DJ, Mayon BJ, Eady RAJ. The eye in dystrophic epidermolysis bullosa. *Eye* 1989; **3**: 79–84

McDonnell PJ, Spalton DJ. The ocular signs and complications of epidermolysis bullosa. *JR Soc Med* 1988; **81**: 576–8

McFarlan DE, Strober W Ataxia telangiectasia. *Medicine* 1972; **51**: 281–314

Michalski, A, Leonard JV, Taylor DSI. The eye in inherited metabolic disease. *JR Soc Med* 1988; **81**: 286–90

Orr LS, Osher RH, Savino PJ The syndrome of facial nevi, anomalous cerebral venous return, and hydrocephalus. *Ann Neurol* 1978; **3**: 316–8

Perry HD, Cossari AJ. Chronic lympangiectasis in Turner's syndrome. *B J Ophthalmology* 1986; **70**: 396–9

Perrot H, Durand L, Thivolet J, Millon M, Ortonne JP. Sclerodermi en coup de sabre et glaucome chronique homolateral. *Ann Dermatol Venereol* 1977; **104**: 381–386

Pokorny KS, Hyman BM, Jakobiec FA, Perry HD, Caputo AR, Iwamoto T Epibulbar choristomas containing lacrimal tissue: clinical distinction from dermoids and histologic evidence of an origin from the palpebral lobe. *J Am Acad Ophthalmol* 1987; **94**: 1249–58

Roldan M, Llanes F, Negrete O, Valverde F. Malignant melanoma of the choroid associated with melanosis oculi in a child. *Am J Ophthalmol* 1987; **104**: 662–3

Romano P. Neuroparalytic keratitis in Goldenhaar syndrome. *Am J Ophthalmol* 1978; **85**: 111–3

Segal P, Kikela M, Mrzyglod S, Keromska-Zbierska I. Kartagener's syndrome with familial eye changes. *Am J Ophthalmol* 1963; **55**: 1043–9

Singh M, Kaur B, Annwar NM. Malignant melanoma of the choroid is a naevus of ota. *Br J Ophthalmol* 1988; **72**: 131–4

Smith JL, Cogan DG. Ataxia telangiectasia. *Arch Ophthalmol (Chic)* 1959; **62**: 364–9

Sommer A, Emran N, Tjakrasudjatma S. Clinical characteristics of vitamin A responsive and nonresponsive Bitot's spots. *AJO* 1980; **90**: 160–71

Taylor P, Talbot EM. Perilimbal vascular anomaly associated with ipsilateral en coup de sabre morphoea. *Br J Ophthalmol* 1985; **69**: pp. 60–62

Theron J, Newton TH, Hoyt WF. Unilateral retino-cephalic

vascular malformations. *Neuroradiology* 1974; **7**: 185−96

Wilson FM, Grayson M, Pieroni D. Corneal changes in ectodermal dysplasia. *Am J Ophthalmol* 1973; **75**: 17−27

Wilson FM, Ostler HB. Conjunctival papillomas in sibliges. *Am J Ophthalmol* 1974; **77**: 103−10

Yamamoto T. Malignant melanoma of the choroid in the nevus of ota. *Ophthalmologica* 1969; **159**: 1−10

Yanoff M. Hereditary benign intra opithelial dyskeratosis. *Arch Ophthalmol* 1968; **79**: 291−5

20.1 Developmental Abnormalities of the Cornea and Iris

JOHN ELSTON

The prenatal development of the cornea, trabecular meshwork and iris takes place in a co-ordinated, integrated fashion (Mann 1957a). Different structures in the anterior segment are subject to common influences, so that developmental abnormalities of one component are often accompanied by abnormalities of others. Clinically, these disorders are therefore usually bilateral, but often asymmetric, and present as corneal opacity, glaucoma and iris abnormalities, or combinations of these.

Embryology

By the sixth week of intra-uterine life, the surface ectoderm has been restored after the separation of the lens vesicle, and therefore constitutes the future anterior epithelium of the cornea. Mesenchymal tissue accumulates between the surface ectoderm and the anterior lens capsule (O'Rahilly 1975). There is experimental evidence that the mesenchyme is derived, at least in part, from neural crest cells (Kupfer & Kaiser-Kupfer 1979). These are cells formed from the dorsal margin of the neural tube at about the time of it's closure, and are therefore of neuro-ectodermal origin. They are pluripotent, and appear to have an important role in the migration and terminal induction of tissues in many sites (Beauchamp & Knepper 1984). The mesenchyme involved in anterior segment development shows three distinct phases of increased activity from the sixth week onwards.

The first phase (primary mesenchymal development) involves cell multiplication and migration deep to the surface ectoderm (O'Rahilly 1975; Kenyon 1975). A solid disc of tissue, two cells thick by the eighth week, is formed and is the future corneal endothelium (Wulle 1972). The central corneal endothelial cell density diminishes rapidly from the 16th week onwards as the cornea grows, creating a monolayer of cells by the 18th week. The evidence suggests that there is little endothelial cell division after the second trimester (Murphy *et al.* 1984b). Descemet's membrane is secreted by the endothelial cells and from the eighth week onwards they show evidence of high metabolic activity, with plentiful endoplasmic reticulum, mitochondria, Golgi bodies and nucleoli and the deposition of a basement membrane (Wulle 1972). The membrane is regularly thickened by the addition of further lamellae, approximately 30 being present at term. The lamellae are bound by short cross-linking bridges (Murphy *et al.* 1984(a)). The prenatally developed striated Descemet's membrane is 3.0 μm thick. Postnatally it is thickened by the addition of amorphous material. Schwalbe's ring marks the posterior limit of Descemet's membrane and is developmentally part of the trabecular meshwork (see below). Histological examination for the presence of striations in Descemet's membrane in developmental abnormalities of the anterior segment can therefore indicate whether there has been a primary or secondary failure of endothelial cell function.

The second phase of mesenchymal activity results in the migration and multiplication of cells between the developing Descemet's membrane and the surface ectoderm; these cells become keratocytes, and produce the corneal stroma (Mann 1957b). The third phase of cell migration is accompanied by blood vessels and occurs superficial to the lens, thereby creating the anterior chamber between itself and the first phase. Until the 28th week this chamber is lined by a continuous sheet of mesothelium (O'Rahilly 1975).

The trabecular meshwork develops from a circumferential mass of mesenchyme situated at the periphery of the developing cornea, adjacent to the sclera. The anterior border of this mesenchyme develops into Schwalbe's ring; posterior to this, the trabeculae are formed. The angle between the developing cornea and iris progressively extends further posteriorly during intra-uterine life. The developing canal of Schlemm, initially posterior to the anterior chamber and separated from it by a layer of mesenchyme, thereby comes to lie superficial to the trabecular meshwork. Similarly, the extension of the anterior chamber angle posteriorly means that Schwalbe's ring becomes separated from the iris stroma (Hansson & Jerndal 1971).

The process of intra-uterine anterior chamber angle extension was originally ascribed to tissue atrophy or resorption. In 1955, a new hypothesis, based on examinations of fetal eyes and measurement of the relative positions of the angle, ciliary body and corneoscleral junction, was put forward (Allen *et al.* 1955). It was suggested that the angle extended by cleavage of tissue, the splitting force being the relatively high rate of growth and increase in curvature of the cornea. Failure of proper cleavage of the angle could result in the various types of anterior segment maldevelopment, for this reason called 'anterior segment cleavage syndromes' (Allen *et al.* 1955; Reese & Ellsworth 1966, Waring *et al.* 1975).

Subsequent histological studies have produced no support for the theory of tissue cleavage, which is probably an artefact related to the post-fixation detachment of the ciliary body from the overlying sclera (Kupfer 1969; Kupfer & Ross 1971). The angle appears to form by a process of differential growth, altering micro-anatomical relations, and the term anterior segment cleavage syndrome should therefore be abandoned.

The discontinuity in the monolayer of polyhedral endothelial cells lining the trabecular meshwork that develops around the 28th week is reflected in an increase in outflow facility (Kupfer & Ross 1971). Again, the process involved is probably differential cell growth.

At full term birth, the cornea is less than 10 mm in horizontal and vertical diameter (9.3 mm; Murphy *et al.* 1984b), and Descemet's membrane is 3.0 μ m thick. The cornea continues to grow relatively quickly in infancy, reaching adult size (11.7 mm diameter) by 24 months, during which period the endothelial cell density also falls relatively rapidly since cell division is minimal (Speedwell *et al.* 1988). The outflow facility through the trabecular meshwork has usually reached postnatal values by the 32nd week of intra-uterine life (Kupfer & Ross 1971).

Patterns of anterior segment maldevelopment

Anterior segment dysgenesis may be considered to affect primarily either the cornea, the trabecular meshwork or the iris. Recognisable patterns of clinical presentation, physical signs, natural history and systemic associations are seen, but there is considerable overlap. Some conditions are genetically determined and in some, prenatal environmental conditions may be important. Conditions that look the same are not necessarily the same pathological entity, and the best approach is therefore descriptive. Generic terms with aetiological implications that are either wrong ('anterior segment cleavage syndromes') or speculative ('neural crestopathies') are best avoided.

Primary corneal abnormalities

Whole cornea

MEGALOCORNEA

If the cornea is adult size at birth, or 13 mm diameter by 2 years (Fig. 20.1), and provided buphthalmos has been excluded, megalocornea is diagnosed. The condition is non-progressive, bilateral, symmetrical and congenital. The corneal diameter may be as much as 18 mm (Kraft *et al.* 1984) but the thickness is normal, as is endothelial cell density, indicating a process of total corneal hypertrophy (Skuta *et al.* 1983). Other features are astigmatism, atrophy of the iris stroma, meiosis, and iridodonesis due to lens subluxation. X-linked inheritance is usual, but autosomal dominant and recessive, as well as sporadic cases are also described. Ultrasound shows that the posterior segments are of normal size (Kraft *et al.* 1984), and visual development is usually good.

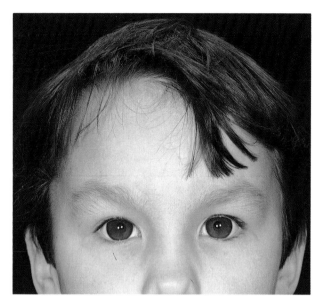

Fig. 20.1.1 Megalocornea — corrected acuities were normal.

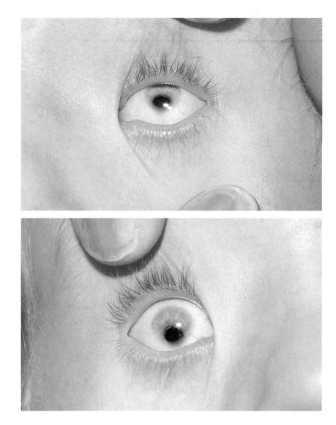

Fig. 20.1.2 Colobomatous microphthalmos, microcornea and cornea plana.

MICROCORNEA

Microcornea is diagnosed when the diameter is less than 9 mm. It may occur in nanophthalmos in which case the eye is grossly normal but small, or microphthalmos, when the eye is small and also otherwise obviously abnormal. Microcornea is a frequent finding as part of other anterior segment developmental anomalies.

CORNEA PLANA

Cornea plana is an abnormality of curvature of the cornea, which is relatively flattened. It may be found as a component of microphthalmos, coloboma or sclerocornea (Fig. 20.1), and is not an isolated condition.

Peripheral

SCLEROCORNEA

Sclerocornea is congenital bilateral, often asymmetric predominantly peripheral corneal opacification with vascularization (Fig. 20.1.3). It may be isolated, or more usually, associated with abnormal corneal size (microcornea) or curvature (cornea plana). With time a relatively clear mid-corneal zone may develop (Fig. 20.1.4). Other ocular associations are raised intra-ocular pressure due to an associated angle dysgenesis, strabismus in asymmetric cases, and nystagmus if the

opacity extends to the central cornea (Goldstein & Cogan 1962; Elliott *et al.* 1985).

Rarely, there are systemic abnormalities, e.g. mental retardation, and abnormal facies. Sclerocornea has also been described in a number of unrelated conditions involving multiple congenital abnormalities. The condition may be inherited as an autosomal dominant characteristic (Elliott *et al.* 1985) or sporadic. Minor degrees of sclerocornea are common in dysgenesis of other anterior segment structures. Histology shows variable collagen fibre diameters, vascularization and a poorly developed or absent Descemet's membrane (Howard & Abrahams 1971).

Management

Glaucoma should be excluded, at an examination under anaesthetic (EUA) which is usually necessary to make the diagnosis. If present, it should be treated medically if possible. An accurate refraction and appropriate correction will also be required. Repeated EUAs may be necessary. If there is a family history of

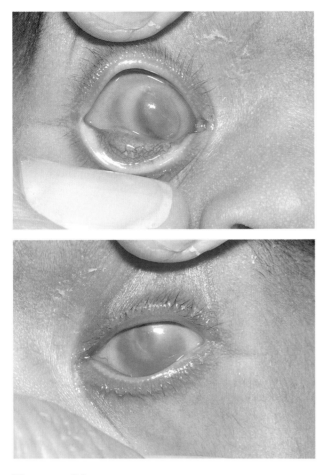

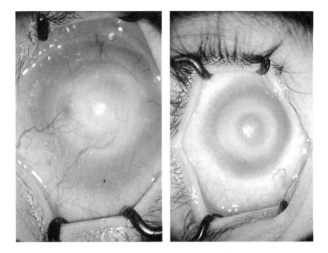

Fig. 20.1.4 Sclerocornea. With time a relatively clear zone may develop between the opaque centre and the periphery.

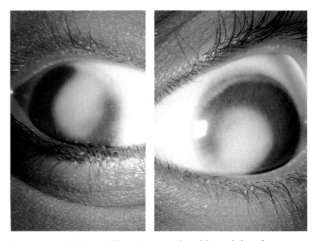

Fig. 20.1.5 Bilateral Peters' anomaly with peripheral scleralization.

Fig. 20.1.3 Sclerocornea.

similar disorders, the parents should be offered genetic counselling.

Central

PETERS' ANOMALY

This consists of a congenital central corneal opacity: 80% of cases are bilateral, and the peripheral cornea is usually clear although scleralization of the limbus is common (Fig. 20.1.5). Over half the cases have glaucoma, and other ocular associations including microcornea, microphthalmos, cornea plana, coloboma, cataract (Fig. 20.1.6), and mesenchymal dysgenesis of the iris (Kenyon 1975). Congenital perforation of the cornea has also been described (Heckenlively & Kielar 1979). Systemic associations are unusual (Kresca & Goldberg 1978). The condition is usually sporadic, although both autosomal dominant and recessive inheritance have been suggested (Stone *et al.* 1976). Peters' anomaly has also been described in association

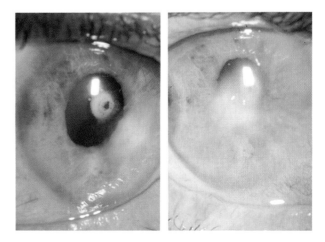

Fig. 20.1.6 Peters' anomaly with cataract underlying the corneal opacity. The iris defect to the left of both pictures is surgical.

with the ring 21 chromosomal abnormality (Cibis *et al.* 1985) and partial deletion of the long arm of chromosome 11 (Bateman *et al.* 1984).

The histopathological hallmark of Peters' anomaly is absence of the central corneal endothelium and Descemet's membrane. The lens is normal ultrastructurally, but may be adherent to the central corneal opacity. The endothelial defect is the primary abnormality (with secondary failure of secretion of Descemet's membrane), but it can be the result of several different pathogenetic mechanisms. These include primary dysgenesis and secondary disruption, e.g. in rubella embryopathy (Stone *et al.* 1976). Secondary keratolenticular contact from a variety of causes in utero may produce the clinical and histopathological features of Peters' anomaly (Townsend *et al.* 1974).

Management

An examination under anaesthetic and microscopy will usually be required to establish the diagnosis. If the condition is predominantly unilateral, with normal pressure and no axial corneal opacity in the less involved eye, no treatment will be required. The intraocular pressure should be measured regularly, and treated, if possible medically, if raised. If there are dense bilateral corneal opacities, then surgical treatment may be offered. An ultrasound will be needed to exclude keratolenticular contact and retinal detachment (Townsend *et al.* 1974). An 'open sky' lensectomy, anterior vitrectomy, and corneal graft will usually be required, although rarely, only the corneal graft is necessary. The visual prognosis in these cases is extremely guarded.

Posterior keratoconus

In posterior keratoconus the anterior corneal curvature is normal, but there is a circumscribed area of stromal thinning on the posterior surface, usually axial, associated with increased curvature. The condition is bilateral, congenital, non-progressive, and very rare (Wolter & Haney 1963). Familial cases are described associated with short stature and a thick neck (Haney & Falls 1961).

Management

These children have myopic astigmatism which should be treated with the appropriate spectacle correction.

Primary angle abnormalities

Schwalbe's ring, developmentally part of the angle, marks the posterior limit of Descemet's membrane. The anterior border is visible as a narrow grey-white line on the inner surface of the cornea, known as posterior embryotoxon.

Posterior embryotoxon

Posterior embryotoxon is a common variant of normality, and may be visible in up to 32% of eyes (Forsius *et al.* 1964). It is more prominent temporally than nasally, and as an isolated finding has no pathological significance. Developmental abnormalities of the anterior segment are, however, frequently accompanied by posterior embryotoxon (Forsius & Eriksson 1964).

Axenfeld's anomaly

Axenfeld's anomaly consists of posterior embryotoxon with, in addition, bridges of iris tissue crossing the angle to Schwalbe's ring (Fig. 20.1.7). It indicates significant angle dysgenesis, and is associated with glaucoma in 50% of patients (Waring *et al.* 1975). It may occur sporadically, or show autosomal dominant inheritance. The glaucoma may be manifest at birth as buphthalmos, or develop in later life, so that regular monitoring of the intraocular pressure is mandatory.

Congenital glaucoma

Primary congenital glaucoma (buphthalmos) is a form of angle dysgenesis due to a failure of development of

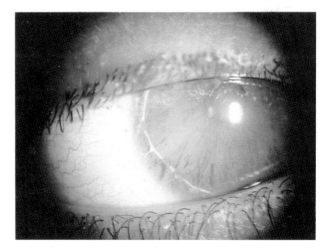

Fig. 20.1.7 Axenfeld's anomaly — marked posterior embryotoxon to which is attached strands of iris.

the normal discontinuity of cells lining the angle (Kupfer & Ross 1971; Kupfer & Kaiser-Kupfer 1979).

Secondary congenital glaucoma is seen in eyes with additional developmental abnormalities, for example of the iris, e.g. Rieger's anomaly, or aniridia. It may also occur in conditions such as von Recklinghausen's disease and rubella embryopathy where the angle may be developmentally or functionally defective.

Primary iris abnormalities

Rieger's anomaly

Rieger's anomaly consists of hypoplasia of the anterior iris stroma, which gives the iris a flat featureless appearance, accompanied by irido-trabecular bridges to Schwalbe's line, and posterior embryotoxon (Fig. 20.1.8, 20.1.9, 20.1.10). The pupil may have an abnormal shape, size or position, or rarely, there may be more than one pupil (Fig. 20.1.11). Ectropion uveae is common (Henkind *et al.* 1965) and coloboma of the iris has been described (Pearce & Kerr 1965). Glaucoma occurs in 60% of cases, but its occurrence and severity do not correspond to the extent of the iris changes (Henkind *et al.* 1965).

Because of the embryology of the anterior segment, other developmental abnormalities such as sclero-

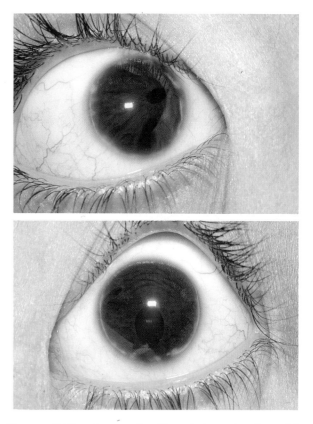

Fig. 20.1.8 Rieger's anomaly with posterior embryotoxon iris adhesions polycoria and glaucoma.

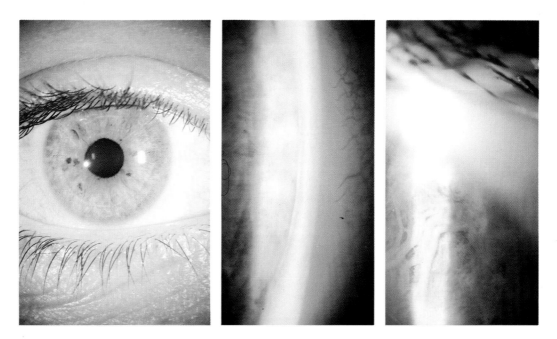

Fig. 20.1.9 Rieger's anomaly with focal iris hypoplasia.

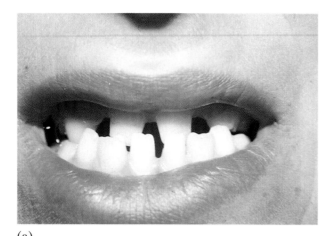

(a)

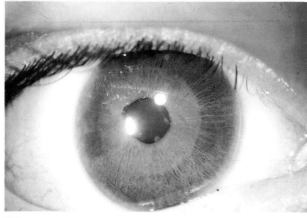

(b)

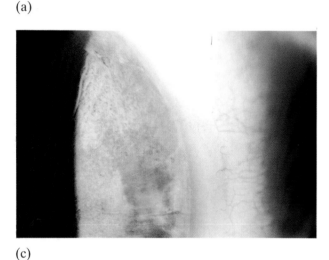

(c)

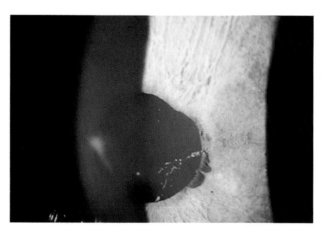

(d)

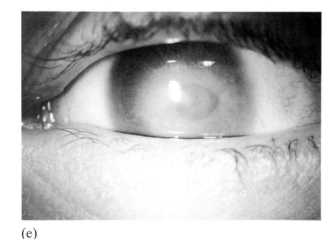

(e)

Fig. 20.1.10 Rieger's Syndrome; the illustrated features are (a) cone shaped teeth, (b) segment of iris hypoplasia, (c) posterior embryotoxon in area related to the iris hypoplasia, (d) ectropion uveæ and a strand of iris which was attached to the cornea, (e) central corneal opacity similar to Peter's anomaly.

cornea may be seen in Rieger's anomaly. In addition, there are consistent corneal endothelial abnormalities. Large, heterogeneous cells, visible on specular microscopy (Fig. 20.1.12) indicate that both the first and third phase of mesenchymal activity in anterior segment development is defective (Hittner *et al*. 1982).

Corneal opacities are common but are usually small and peripheral, at the level of Descemet's membrane. Rarely, however, Rieger's anomaly may present as a central corneal opacity (Hittner *et al*. 1982). Posterior keratoconus has also been described as an association (Mullaney 1968).

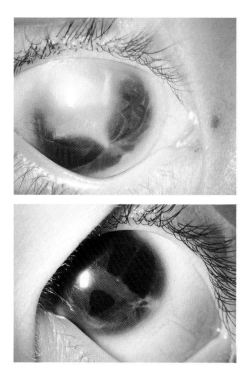

Fig. 20.1.11 Rieger's syndrome — brother of patient in Fig. 20.1.10 with features of Rieger's and Peters' syndromes.

Lens changes are another consistent finding; they consist of small localized cortical opacities (Hittner *et al.* 1982) or epicapsular stars (Henkind *et al.* 1964; Chisholm & Chudley 1983) and are not usually visually significant. Other ocular associations include optic disc anomalies (e.g. tilting, myelination) and high myopia (Tabbara *et al.* 1973).

Rieger's anomaly is inherited as an autosomal dominant characteristic with variable expressivity; some 30% of cases appear to be either sporadic or new mutations (Henkind *et al.* 1965).

Rieger's syndrome

Rieger's syndrome consists of the anomaly with somatic features. Most prominent are the facial abnormalities; maxillary hypoplasia and short philtrum, and dental abnormalities which affect both primary and secondary dentition, and consist of small, widely spaced cone shaped teeth, or even partial anodontia (Wesley *et al.* 1978). Other features of Rieger's syndrome are umbilical and inguinal hernias and hypospadias. Isolated growth hormone deficiency is recognized as an inconstant feature (Sadeghi-Nejad & Sencot 1974; Heinemann *et al.* 1979). Abnormalities of chromosome 6 have been described (Tabbara *et al.*

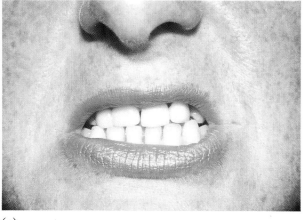

(a)

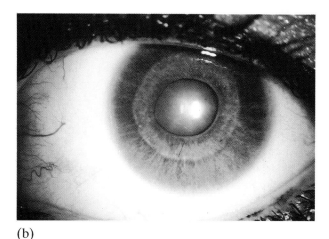

(b)

(c)

Fig. 20.1.12 Rieger's syndrome — mother of patients in Fig. 20.1.10, 20.1.11. (a) With typical teeth (capped). (b) Iris hypoplasia (same patient). (c) Corneal endothelium. Photographs by courtesy of Mr J. Dart.

1973; Heinemann *et al.* 1979) as has deletion of chromosome 13 (Stathacopoulos *et al.* 1987).

Rieger's syndrome is an autosomal dominant condition; some members of a pedigree may have the somatic manifestations without ocular signs (Chisholm & Chudley 1983). Glaucoma occurs in 25–50% of affected individuals.

Management

Cases may present as buphthalmos, corneal opacity, or abnormal-appearing irises or eyes. The diagnosis may require an examination under anaesthetic. Somatic features should be sought and the relatives will need examination, on the slit lamp as a prelude to genetic counselling.

Glaucoma should be treated if possible medically, since it may resolve spontaneously. If uncontrolled a trabeculectomy may be required.

Life-long monitoring of intraocular pressure is required, since the intraocular pressure may become elevated in later life. Genetic counselling should be offered to the parents of affected children.

A newly described primary iris developmental abnormality consists of the association of dysgenesis of the angle with a persistent pupillary membrane attached to the lens (Cibis *et al.* 1986).

References

Allen L, Burian HM, Braley AE. A new concept of the development of the anterior chamber angle. *Arch Ophthalmol* 1955; **53**: 783–98

Bateman JB, Maumenee IH, Sparkes RS. Peters' anomaly associated with partial deletion of the long arm of chromosome 11. *Am J Ophthalmol* 1984; **97**: 11–15

Beauchamp GR, Knepper PA. Role of the neural crest in anterior segment development and disease. *J Pediatr Ophthalmol Strabismus* 1984; **21**: 209–14

Chisholm IA, Chudley AE. Autosomal dominant iridogonio-dysgenesis with associated somatic anomalies: four generation family with Rieger's syndrome. *Br J Ophthalmol* 1983; **67**: 529–34

Cibis GW, Waeltermann J, Harris DJ. Peters' anomaly in association with Ring 21 chromosomal abnormality. *Am J Ophthalmol* 1985; **100**: 733–4

Cibis GW, Waeltermann JM, Hurst E, Tripathi RC, Richardson W. Congenital pupillary-iris-lens membrane with gonio-dysgenesis. *Ophthalmology* 1986; **93**: 847–53

Elliott JH, Feman SS, O'Day DM, Garber M. Hereditary sclerocornea. *Arch Ophthalmol* 1985; **103**; 676–9

Forsius H. Eriksson A. Embryotoxon corneae posterius in a family with slit pupil and in cases with other anomalies of the iris. Acta *Ophthalmology* 1964; **42**: 68–77

Forsius H, Eriksson A, Fellman J. Embryotoxon corneae posterius in an isolated population. *Acta Ophthalmologica* 1964; **42**: 42–9

Goldstein JE, Cogan DG. Sclerocornea and associated congenital anomalies. *Arch Ophthalmol* 1962; **67**: 760–8

Haney WP, Falls HF. The occurence of congential keratoconus posticus circumscriptus. *Am J Ophthalmol* 1961; **52**: 53–5

Hansson HA, Jerndal T. Scanning electron microscopic studies on the development of the iridocorneal angle in human eyes. *Invest Ophthalmol* 1971; **10**: 252–65

Heckenlively J, Kielar R. Congenital perforated cornea in Peters' anomaly. *Am J Ophthalmol* 1979; **88**: 63–5

Heinemann M-H, Breg R, Cotlier E. Rieger's syndrome with pericentric inversion of chromosome 6. *Br J Ophthalmol* 1979; **63**: 40–4

Henkind P, Siegel IM, Carr RE. Mesodermal dysgenesis of the anterior segment: Rieger's anomaly. *Arch Ophthalmol* 1965; **73**: 810–17

Hittner HM, Kretzer FL, Antoszyk JM, Ferrell RE, Mehta RS. Variable expressivity of autosomal dominant anterior segment mesenchymal dysgenesis in six generations. *Am J Ophthalmol* 1982; **93**: 57–70

Howard RO, Abrahams IW. Sclerocornea. *Am J Ophthalmol* 1971; **71**: 1254–60

Kenyon KR. Mesenchymal dysgenesis in Peters' anomaly, sclerocornea and congenital endothelial dystrophy. *Exp Eye Res* 1975; **21**: 125–142

Kraft SP, Judisch GF, Grayson DM. Megalocornea: a clinical and echographic study of an autosomal dominant pedigree. *J Pediatr Ophthalmol Strabismus* 1984; **21**: 190–4

Kresca LJ, Goldberg MF. Peters' anomaly: dominant inheritance in one pedigree, and detrocardia in another. *J Pediatr Ophthalmol Strabismus* 1978; **15**: 141–6

Kupfer C. A note on the development of the anterior chamber angle. *Invest Ophthalmol* 1969; **8**: 69–74

Kupfer C, Kaiser-Kupfer MF. Observations on the development of the anterior chamber angle with reference to the pathogenesis of congenital glaucomas. *Am J Ophthalmol* 1979; **88**: 424–6

Kupfer C, Ross K. The development of outflow facility in human eyes. *Invest Ophthalmol* 1971; **10**: 513–7

Mann I. *Developmental Abnormalities of the Eye.* British Medical Association, London 1957a; 224

Mann I. *Developmental Abnormalities of the Eye.* British Medical Association, London 1957b; 342–64

Mullaney J. The anterior chamber cleavage syndrome. *Trans Ophthalmol Soc UK* 1968; **88**: 757–66

Murphy C. Alvarado J, Juster R. Prenatal and post natal growth of human Desçemet's membrane. *Invest Ophthalmol Vis Sci* 1984a; **25**: 1402–15

Murphy C, Alvarado J, Juster R, Maglio M. Prenatal and postnatal cellularity of the human corneal endothelium. *Invest Ophthalmol Vis Sci* 1984b; **25**: 312–22

O'Rahilly R. The prenatal development of the human eye. *Exp Eye Res* 1975; **21**: 93–112

Pearce WG, Kerr CB. Inherited variation in Rieger's malformation. *Br J Ophthalmol* 1965; **49**: 503–37

Reese AB, Ellsworth RM. The anterior chamber cleavage syndrome. *Arch Ophthalmol* 1966; **75**: 307–318

Sadeghi-Nejad A, Sencot B. Autosomal dominant transmission of isolated growth hormone deficiency in iris–dental dysplasia (Rieger's syndrome). *J Pediatr* 1974; **85**: 644–48

Skuta GL, Sugar J, Ericson ES. Corneal endothelial cell measurements in megalocornea. *Arch Ophthalmol* 1983; **101**: 51−3

Speedwell L, Novakovic P. Sherrard GS, Taylor DSI. The infant corneal endothelium. *Arch Ophthalmol* 1988; **106**: 771−5

Stathacopoulos RA, Bateman JB, Sparkes RS, Hepler RS. The Rieger's syndrome and chromosome 13 deletion. *J Pediatr Ophthalmol Strabismus* 1987; **24**: 198−203

Stone DL, Kenyon KR, Green R, Ryan SJ. Congenital central corneal leukoma, (Peters' anomaly). *Am J Ophthalmol* 1976; **81**: 174−193

Tabbara KF, Knouri FP, Derkaloustian VM. Rieger's syndrome with chromosome anomaly. *Can J Ophthalmol* 1973; **8**: 488−91

Townsend WM, Font RL, Zimmerman LE. Congenital corneal leukomas. *Am J Ophthalmol* 1974; **77**: 192−206

Waring GO, Rodrigues MM, Laibson PR. Anterior chamber cleavage syndrome: a stepladder classification. *Surv Ophthalmol* 1975; **20**: 3−27

Wesley RK, Baker JD, Golnick AL. Rieger's syndrome. *J Pediatr Ophthalmol Strabismus* 1978; **15**: 67−70

Wolter JR, Haney WP. Histopathology of keratoconus posticus circumscriptus. *Arch Ophthalmol* 1963; **69**: 357−62

Wulle KG. Electron microscopy of the fetal development of the corneal endothelium and Descemet's membrane of the human eye. *Invest Ophthalmol* 1972; **11**: 897−904

20.2 Corneal Abnormalities in Childhood

WILLIAM GOOD AND CREIG HOYT

Corneal disease is still the most common cause of blindness in the world today. It is not surgery but the combination of better nutrition, public and private health measures, and antibiotics that have made corneal disease an unusual cause of blindness in the Western World. Nonetheless corneal diseases are a small but significant cause of disability from visual defect, glare or pain and corneal abnormalities may form important clues to the nature of systemic diseases.

Trisomy 18 and trisomy 18 mosaic

In trisomy 18, although the usual eye abnormalities in this syndrome involve the lids, the eye most frequently is colobomatous. The cornea may be diffusely opaque at birth. Discrete corneal opacities caused by breakdown of the corneal epithelium occasionally occur. In trisomy 18 mosaic syndrome (Fig. 20.2.1), geographic corneal opacities are characteristic (Frangoulis & Taylor 1983; Stark *et al.* 1987).

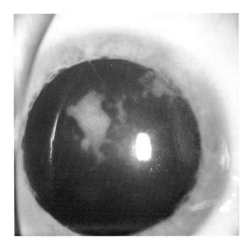

Fig. 20.2.1 Trisomy 18 mosaic syndrome with characteristic geographical corneal opacity.

Dermoids (choristomas)

Dermoids are choristomas that consist of masses of skin, hair follicles, hair, and sebaceous glands in an abnormal location (Mansour *et al.* 1989). These masses were originally destined to become skin but were displaced onto the eye. They usually are found at the corneoscleral junction, in the inferotemporal quadrant. Dermoids can involve the entire thickness of the cornea and sclera. They reduce vision by blocking light (if they occur across the cornea) or by distorting the contour of the cornea giving astigmatism and amblyopia (Fig. 20.2.2). Dermoids may sometimes cover the cornea and some are inherited in an autosomal dominant fashion; X-linked recessive inheritance has also been described (Topilow *et al.* 1981). Dermoids also occur in Goldenhaar's syndrome, congenital generalized fibromatosis (Vangsted and Limpaphayom 1983), and the linear nevus sebaceous syndrome of Fuerstein and Mimms. Corneal dermoids may just involve the cornea and epibulbar tissues. In some sporadic cases there is a much more widespread affection of the eyeball, with the dermoid (more properly described as a dermis-like choristoma since many dermis features are not present) overlying a microphthalmic, disorganized or anterior staphylomotous eye (Fig. 20.2.3) (Bernuy *et al.* 1981).

Treatment is usually necessary on cosmetic grounds alone but must be preceded by a full ocular examination to include gonioscopy to assess the extent of the mass. Lamellar keratectomy is sufficient in most cases and improves the appearance by not only removing the white-yellow appearance but also the elevation. Many cases re-opacify but the appearance is often

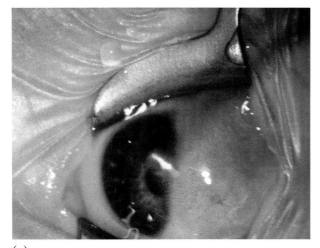

(a)

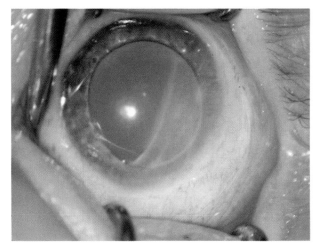

(b)

Fig. 20.2.2 (a) Limbal dermoid which covered half of the cornea and extended posteriorly in the fornix. (b) Same patient, 1 year following lamellar keratectomy which was carried out at 2 months of age. Although, the cosmetic appearance was satisfatory and remained so for 5 years after this photograph the eye was densely amblyopic due to high astigmatism and the corneal opacity.

adequate post operatively and freehand grafting is not usually required. Full thickness dermoids may be treated by excision and corneal (not scleral) grafting (Fig. 20.2.4) but the prognosis should be guarded.

Corneal staphyloma

In congenital corneal staphyloma the cornea is enlarged, ectatic, and opaque (Fig. 20.2.5); the Descemet membrane is missing (Schanzlin *et al.* 1983). The posterior segment of the eye is usually normal (Leff *et al.* 1986), but glaucoma occurs and may cause

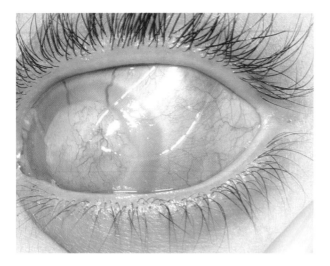

Fig. 20.2.3 Dermis-like choristoma overlying an anomalous eye that has become buphthalmic.

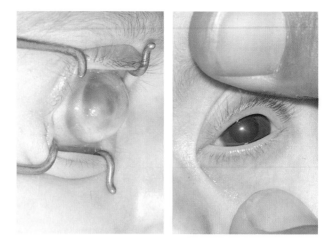

Fig. 20.2.5 Congenital corneal staphyloma of the right eye. The left eye was normal.

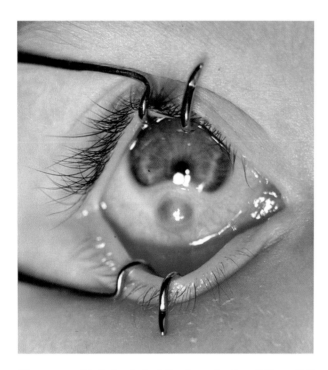

Fig. 20.2.4 Limbal ectasia following scleral graft for a full-thickness limbal dermoid. This had been repeated on three occasions, but the graft repeatedly dissolved and the area became ectatic. It was successfully treated with a corneal graft which lasted permanently.

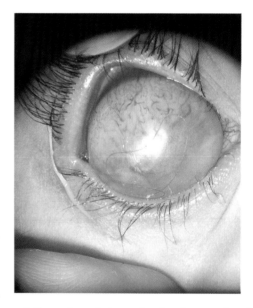

Fig. 20.2.6 Corneal staphyloma that has become keratinized and the cornea thickened.

Amniotic bands

Amniotic bands may be associated with congenital corneal leukomas (Miller *et al.* 1987) or with exposure keratitis from lid defects (Benezra *et al.* 1982).

Treatment of the congenitally opaque cornea

Treatment for these conditions is often hopeless, so unilateral cases are treated as cosmetic problems and the eye is covered with a cosmetic shell or contact lens. The eye is enucleated if painful or excessively

buphthalmus. Corneal metaplasia is a similar condition; both this, sclerocornea and staphyloma may be caused by a neural crest cell migration defect. Intra ocular defects sometimes co-exist (Klauss & Riedel 1983) and the cornea may become opaque and keratinized with time (Fig. 20.2.6).

large. Bilateral cases are best left alone if there is any possibility of vision in one eye. If the infant is blind corneal grafting is indicated, with occasional good results (Zaidman *et al.* 1982). Grafting is probably best performed either early in infancy when the baby can be examined more easily on the slit lamp or later in childhood when he is more co-operative. Corneal grafting in children is less successful in the long term than the same procedure in adults (Mackenson 1977; Khöbel & Demeler 1978; Brown & Salmon 1983).

Keratitis

Allergic

See Section 3.

Infection

See Section 3.

Exposure keratitis

Exposure keratitis is a disorder of the ocular surface due to failure to maintain adequate lubrication and protection for the corneal epithelium, which results in its break down. The cornea will lose its lustre, and this may be followed by punctate loss of corneal epithelium. Larger areas of epithelial loss are followed by thinning of the corneal stroma. In severe cases, corneal perforation can occur. Usually these cases are associated with a bacterial infection which occurs because of the loss of protection afforded by the normal spread of tears.

Eyelid abnormalities may cause exposure keratitis (Miller *et al.* 1987). An ectropion, for example, can result in poor eyelid apposition; the cornea, then, is relatively unprotected. Disorders of the lacrimal gland (e.g. tumors, congenital malfunctions, CNS disease, radiation necrosis (Fig. 20.2.7) result in poor lubrication of the corneal surface. Exopthalmos from orbit disease results in poor lid closure. Seventh nerve palsies affect closure of the eyelids. Fifth nerve palsies also result in keratitis and combined Vth and VIIth cranial nerve palsies cause the most serious problems especially if the eye is also dry (Fig. 20.2.8). Sensory innervation of the cornea may play an important role in maintaining its integrity (Schimmelpfennig & Beurman 1979). Blinking is also influenced by sensory input.

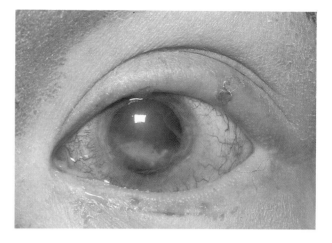

Fig. 20.2.7 Keratitis resulting from a combination of exposure, drying and the direct effects of irradiation for orbital rhabdomyosarcoma.

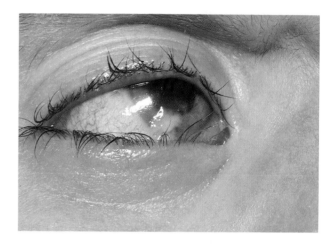

Fig. 20.2.8 Dry and exposed eye giving rise to keratitis in a patient with VIIth nerve palsy associated with the CHARGE association.

Non-accidental injury

A spectrum of corneal injuries can occur in child abuse. The corneal epithelium may be abraded, producing a characteristic stain when fluorescein is placed on the eye. Deeper injuries are produced when the object striking the eye is sharp. Corneal perforation with flattening of the anterior chamber occurs rarely. The presence of lid ecchymoses accompanying the corneal injury should arouse suspicion of abuse. A careful history and physical exam should be conducted, searching for other unexplained injuries. Forceps injuries cause ruptures of Descemet's membrane usually in a vertical direction and are associated with high astigmatism in the axis of the ruptures, myopia, and deep amblyopia (Angell *et al.* 1981). Chemical injuries, sometimes repeated, may be due to non-accidental injury by the parents (Taylor & Bentovim 1976) (Fig. 20.2.9).

Cogan's syndrome

Cogan's syndrome consists of interstitial keratitis and audiovestibular disease (Cogan 1945). The cornea shows bilateral patchy stromal infiltrates, with vascularization and uveitis. Eventually, vascularization of the cornea occurs. The VIIIth nerve impairment may precede or follow corneal involvement. An association of this syndrome with polyarteritis nodosa has been described (Gilbert & Talbot 1969), and there are many case reports of this and other systemic associations (Bicknell & Holland 1978). The cause is unknown although immunological (Char *et al.* 1975) and viral (Darougar *et al.* 1978) agents have been implicated.

Vitamin A deficiency and measles

Deficiency of vitamin A damages the cornea. The surface loses its normal lustre, even though the eye is not always excessively dry. The tears show abnormal electrophoretic responses to measles infections, especially in malnourished children (Kogbe & Listet 1987). Corneal vascularization, keratinization, and oedema can occur. When vitamin deficiency is accompanied by malnourishment and protein deficiency, an acute liquefactive necrosis of the cornea can occur.

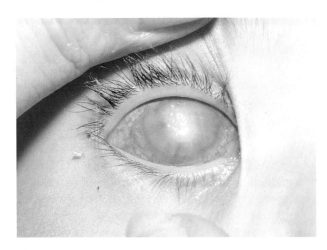

Fig. 20.2.9 Non-accidental chemical injury to the cornea. This child suddenly developed a profoundly severe keratitis in one eye on the day that his mother's boyfriend left the home. Although never proven the situation was highly suggestive.

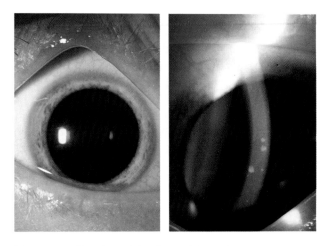

Fig. 20.2.10 Ectodermal dysplasia with small superficial corneal opacities.

This is particularly marked when associated with measles infection, herpes simplex, or the use of traditional eye medicines (Foster & Sommer 1987). If diagnosed early some of these problems are reversible with vitamin A replacement and may be prevented by dietary measures, vitamin A replacement and measles vaccination (Monnickendam & Darougar 1987). The Bitot spot is a triangular foamy appearing lesion that occurs over the conjunctiva in vitamin A deficiency; its presence on the temporal side of the eye suggests active deficiency (Sommer 1978). Vitamin A deficiency also causes night-blindness.

Ectodermal dysplasia

The congenital absence of ectodermal structures (sweat glands, hair follicles and hair) is called ectodermal dysplasia. Occasionally, corneal changes occur (Wilson *et al.* 1973). Epithelial corneal cysts and opacities that are best seen with a slit lamp develop (Fig. 20.2.10). Pannus, the abnormal growth of superficial blood vessels onto the cornea, occurs. A dry-eye state may result from deficient tear production. A more severe keratopathy (Fig. 20.2.11) with severe visual consequences occurs in some cases, it may be due to the combination of the underlying dysplasia, tear film abnormalities and infection (Mawhorter *et al.* 1986).

Epidermolysis bullosa

Corneal abnormalities are surprisingly infrequent in epidermolysis bullosa, but changes include limbal broadening, corneal reticular opacities at the level of

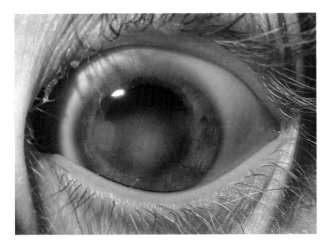

Fig. 20.2.11 Ectodermal dysplasia with an axial keratopathy which resulted in poor vision.

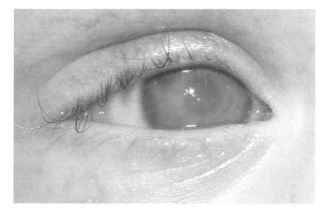

Fig. 20.2.12 Epidermolysis bullosa. Although many cases of epidermolysis bullosa do not have corneal changes some, like this patient, develop acute epithelial erosions as a result of minor trauma.

Bowman's and symblepharon (McDonnell & Spalton 1988). Although the lesions are usually small and anterior (Aurora *et al.* 1975) they may develop widespread corneal epithelial erosion (Fig. 20.2.12).

Ichthyosis

The ichthyosiform dermatoses are a group of disorders characterized by scaling. 'Harlequin baby' and 'collodian baby' (Orth *et al.* 1974) are extreme congenital forms which may have congenital ectropion. They frequently succumb to skin infections in the neonatal period. Ichthyosis vulgaris is the commonest form, inherited as an autosomal dominant trait, with scaling of the extensor surfaces and back. No eye problems occur. X-linked ichthyosis is congenital with

scaling of the scalp, face and neck, abdomen and limbs; palms and soles are spared. Corneal nerves may be thickened and band keratopathy occurs as an isolated abnormality (Jay *et al.* 1968). Superficial corneal lesions, which stain with fluorescein, occur; they are transient but recur and eventually cause superficial scarring (Fig. 20.2.13).

Lamellar ichthyosis (Katowitz *et al.* 1974) and ichthiosis linearis circumflexa are severe autosomal recessive disorders that give rise to ectropion and keratoconjunctivitis mainly due to exposure. Epidermolytic hyperkeratosis and erythrokeratoderma variabilis are two autosomal dominant varieties. Ichthyosis also occurs in the Sjögren Larssen syndrome (see Chapter 27), Netherton syndrome (ichthyosis, sparse hair, eyebrows and eyelashes, and atopic diathesis), Refsum disease (see Chapter 34), and chondrodysplasia punctata (Conradi's disease and rhizomelic dwarfism).

Corneal anaesthesia and hypoaesthesia

Defective corneal sensation may give rise to a keratitis that is chronic, recurrent and often severe. Although termed 'neurotropic', implying that the lack of some nerve factor is important, it is most likely that the main aetiological factors are drying, reduced blinking and repeated trivial trauma. Defective corneal sensation may arise from any cause of fifth nerve damage. As in adults, it occurs with trauma, herpes zoster ophthalmicus, developmental or acquired brainstem lesions, and tumours, in particular cerebello-pontine angle or pontine tumours. It may occur with herpes simplex keratitis or after carbon disulphide (McDonald 1938) or hydrogen sulphide (Sjogren 1939) poisoning.

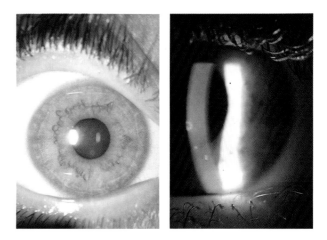

Fig. 20.2.13 Ichthyosis with superficial corneal lesions.

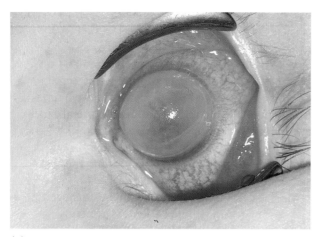

(a)

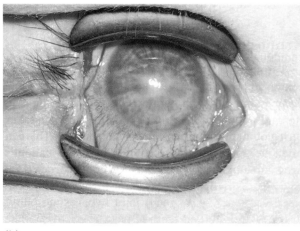

(b)

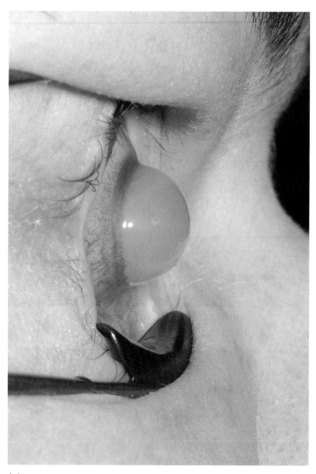

(c)

Fig. 20.2.18 (a) Acute hydrops in a child with Down's syndrome and keratoconus. (b) Same patient. Side view showing extreme keratoglobus. (c) After using elbow restraints to stop her rubbing her eyes, bilateral tarsorrhapies and padding of the eye the keratoglobus resolved and became asymptomatic, but vision was reduced by axial scarring.

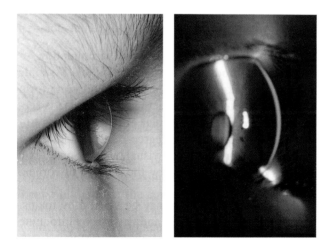

Fig. 20.2.19 X-linked keratoglobus. On the left it is possible to see into the angle between the cornea and the iris by looking laterally at the eye without using a gonioscope.

Wilson's disease is an inherited disorder of copper metabolism. Low levels of the copper transporting protein, cerruloplasmin, accompany low serum, and high tissue levels of copper. Wilson's disease usually presents in the second decade of life. Four organ systems are involved. Central nervous system (CNS) involvement leads to basal ganglia degeneration with tremor, choreoathetosis, and neuropsychiatric changes. Renal tubular staining causes aminoaciduria. The liver is affected by nodular cirrhosis. The cornea often develops staining of the peripheral Descemet's membrane most marked in the 12 and 6 o'clock positions (Fig. 20.2.21) (Kayser–Fleischer ring). The stain which is due to copper deposition is brown-green and is best seen at the slit lamp. Gonioscopy may be

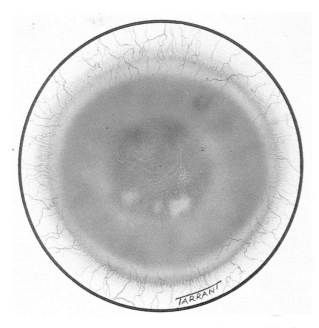

Fig. 20.2.20 Amiodarone keratopathy. It is unusual for these cases to cause visual defect; the most common abnormality is a mild whirl-like opacity as seen in the centre of this painting.

necessary for visualization in some cases. The ring is not absolutely pathognomonic of Wilson's disease; other causes of liver failure, carotenaemia, and multiple myeloma may lead to a similar ring (Fleming 1977). In Wilson's disease a rare but characteristic abnormality is the 'sunflower' subcapsular cataract.

Acrodermatitis enteropathica is associated with radial, subepithelial lines in the superior portion of the cornea (Matta *et al.* 1975). The lines are whorl-like and pass from the corneoscleral junction toward the centre of the cornea. Keratomalacia may be associated (Feldberg *et al.* 1981). This rare dermatitis is characterized by an assymetrical rash that begins in infancy. The nails are dystrophic. A gastrointestinal disturbance causes diarrhoea and poor growth; it is treated successfully with zinc dietary supplements.

In cystinosis a defect in lysosomal transport leads to accumulation of cystine in lysosomes. Growth retardation, renal failure, decreased skin and hair pigmentation, and corneal crystalline deposits occur (Fig. 20.2.22). Infantile cystinosis causes renal failure and early death. Corneal cystals are detected as early as 2 months of life. They start anteriorly, progressing posteriorly (Melles *et al.* 1987). A pigmentary retinopathy also develops. An adult form of cystinosis (non-nephronopathic) causes corneal deposits but no systemic manifestations. The adolescent form resemble the infantile form, with the absence of growth retardation and skin hypopigmentation.

Although corneal crystals in cystinosis are mainly in the anterior stroma, they occur in all tissues. They seldom reduce visual acuity, but photophobia is frequent (Katz *et al.* 1987 (a)). The glare disability may be profound. Patients may also have an abnormal contrast sensitivity (Katz *et al.* 1987 (b)) and reduced corneal sensitivity (Katz *et al.* 1987 (c)). The crystals have different morphologies depending on the site (Frazier & Wong 1968) and can be studied by specular microscopy (Dale *et al.* 1981). Cysteamine treatment has recently been shown to have beneficial effects on

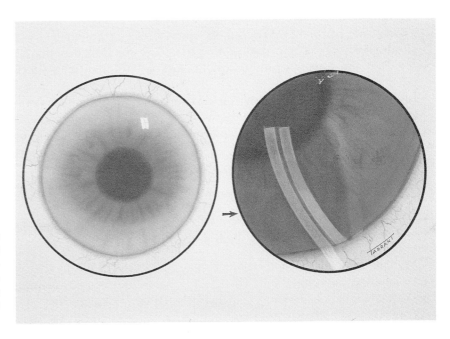

Fig. 20.2.21 Wilson's disease. The brown deposits are most prominent in the 6 and 12 o'clock position and consist of deposition of brown-green copper containing substance in the peripheral parts of Descemet's membrane. Gonioscopy may be necessary for visualization.

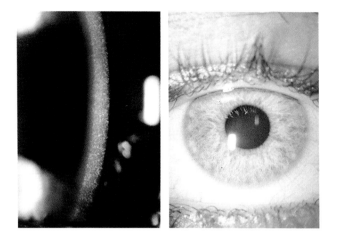

Fig. 20.2.22 Cystinosis. Corneal crystals can be seen by slit-lamp microscopy. The children are often blond, fair-skinned, and very photophobic.

the photophobia (Kaiser-Kupfer *et al.* 1987). Corneal grafts may remain clear at least in the medium term (Kaiser-Kupfer *et al.* 1986). Glaucoma may occur due to crystal accumulation in intraocular tissues (Wan *et al.* 1986).

Corneal crystals

Crystalline corneal deposits or crystal-like deposits occur in the following conditions:

1 Cystinosis.
2 Crystalline corneal dystrophy (Schnyder's dystrophy):
  (a) May present in infancy.
  (b) There are anterior central corneal ring like aggregation of stromal crystals that may be yellowish and hard are composed of cholestorol (Rodriguez *et al.* 1987; Brooks *et al.* 1988).
  (c) They are usually asymptomatic, it does not affect the epithelium.
  (d) It may be autosomal dominant (Rodriguez *et al.*1987).
  (e) It may be accompanied by an arcus lipoides and white limbus girdle.
  (f) There are not usually systemic associations (Lisch *et al.* 1986).
3 LCAT disease.
4 Uric acid crystals (brownish coloured).
5 Granular dystrophy and Bietti's marginal dystrophy (Wilson *et al.* 1989).
6 Multiple myeloma (Knapp *et al.* 1987).
7 Calcium deposition.
8 Dieffenbachia plant keratoconjunctivitis (Ellis *et al.* 1973).

9 A syndrome of corneal crystals, myopathy and nephropathy (Arnold *et al.* 1987).
10 Tyrosinaemia type II — the Richner Hanhart syndrome:
  (a) Plaque-like pseudo-dendritic figures occur with crystalline edges.
  (b) They are intra- and subepithelial, raised, bilateral.
  (c) Ulceration occurs.
  (d) Treatment with steroids and also tyrosine and phenylalanine.
  (e) Diet may prevent the symptoms (Grayson 1983).
  (f) Mental and physical retardation, palmar keratosis, and conjunctival thickening also occur (Beinfang *et al.* 1976).

Band keratopathy

Band keratopathy is the result of ocular inflammation or systemic disease. The band occurs in the region between the eyelids (interpalpebral region), usually with a clear region between the band and the corneoscleral limbus. Bowman's membrane is infiltrated with calcium. Eventually, Bowman's membrane will be destroyed. The deposits of calcium take on a 'Swiss-cheese' appearance, which helps distinguish this condition from simple corneal calcific degeneration. This latter condition is the end product of phthisis bulbi or a necrotic ocular tumour and may involve all corneal layers.

Any condition causing systemic hypercalcaemia can cause band keratopathy. Thus, sarcoidosis, parathyroid disease, and multiple myeloma, are occasionally associated with a band. Chronic ocular inflammation also causes band keratopathy. This is most characteristic in Still's disease (juvenile chronic arthritis) in its pauci-articular form (Fig. 22.2.23). Prolonged corneal oedema and glaucoma rarely lead to band formation. Toxic mercury vapors or eye drops and gout are uncommonly associated with band keratopathy. Gouty band kerotopathy differs from other causes by being brown. Band keratopathy may occur with some forms of ichthyosis (Jay *et al.* 1968).

LCAT deficiency

Lecithin cholesterol acyltransferase deficiency (LCAT) is a rare autosomal recessive condition that causes a central corneal haze in homozygotes. Premature arcus senilus develops in heterozygotes (Vrabec 1988). LCAT esterifies free cholesterol for use in

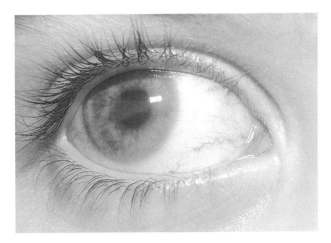

Fig. 20.2.23 Band keratopathy in Still's disease.

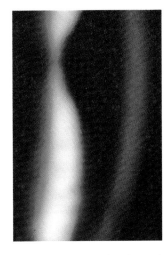

Fig. 20.2.24 Map dot and finger print dystrophy (Mr J. Dart's patient).

synthesis of cell membranes. Its absence causes proteinuria, renal failure, anemia, and hyperlipidemia.

Corneal dystrophies

Corneal dystrophies are bilateral corneal diseases with the following characteristics: they are usually congenital, hereditary, avascular, involve the central cornea, and are progressive. Dystrophies are not associated with systemic disease. They are often classified according to the layer of the cornea involved.

Dystrophies should be distinguished from corneal degenerations (Friedlander and Smolin 1979). Degenerations are secondary processes, resulting from aging, previous corneal inflammation, or systemic disease. This section will focus on the most common dystrophies, according to the affected layer of the cornea.

Epithelial dystrophies

MAP, DOT, AND FINGERPRINT DYSTROPHY

Map, dot, and fingerprint corneal dystrophy (Fig. 22.2.24) affects the corneal epithelium. The inheritance is usually autosomal dominant, with so-called fingerprint lines, map lines, and microcysts forming in the surface lining of the cornea. These anatomical changes are impossible to see without the slit lamp. However, the condition should be suspected when a patient develops recurrent, spontaneous corneal erosions. Treatment is aimed at preventing these recurrent epithelial erosion. Patching and ocular lubricants are the mainstay of treatment. Vision is seldom affected.

MEESMAN'S DYSTROPHY

Meesman's dystrophy is an autosomal dominant epithelial dystrophy. The corneal epithelium and its basement membrane thicken with formation of tiny vesicles best appreciated at the slit lamp in the palpebral fissure. This condition presents in childhood with symptoms of eye irritation or photophobia due to recurrent erosions, despite a reduction in corneal sensation.

RECURRENT EROSIONS

Recurrent erosions may be a dystrophy. The condition is sometimes bilateral with an autosomal dominant inheritance but corneal trauma seems to precipitate it. It is due to faulty adherence of epithelium to its basement membrane. The children present with recurrent painful keratitis often with an onset at night which has led to the suggestion that it may be the nocturnal lagophthalmos and drying that are important aetiological factors. Treatment consists of allowing the epithelium to regenerate, and hopefully to reattach to the basement membrane. Patching, the use of 5% sodium chloride drops, epithelial debridement and soft contact lens use may all help in more severe cases. Prevention of nocturnal drying by the use of simple eye ointment is a useful preventative measure.

Bowman's layer dystrophies affecting children

BOWMAN'S LAYER DYSGENESIS

This is a bilateral progressive congenital corneal clouding with poor prognosis thought to be due to a proliferation of the cells which give rise to Bowman's layer (Apple *et al.* 1984).

REIS BUCKLER'S DYSTROPHY

This autosomal dominant bilateral disease presents in infancy or early childhood with recurrent attacks of photophobia, pain, redness and watering which last days or weeks. The corneal surface is irregular with microscopic epithelial protrusions which eventually become more numerous and opaque with a geographic or honeycomb appearance, worse in the mid peripheral zone. Corneal sensation is reduced. Vision is reduced by infiltration of the Bowman's layer and its replacement by scar tissue by the mid twenties (Rice *et al.* 1968) at which time it becomes less symptomatic.

Treatment of the acute attacks is similar to that of the recurrent erosions; kerotaplasty may be followed by recurrence in the graft (Olson & Kaufmann 1978).

Stromal dystrophies

Granular, macular, and lattice dystrophy all will reduce vision, and may be noticed in the first or second decade of life, but vision only deteriorates later (Waring 1978).

GRANULAR DYSTROPHY

Granular dystrophy (Groenow type I) is an autosomal dominant anterior stromal dystrophy (Fig. 22.2.25). It is distinguished by discrete, granular appearing corneal opacities. Histologically, these consist of hyaline deposits.

Corneal transplant is indicated when vision has

been reduced to an unacceptable level. The dystrophy may recur in the graft.

LATTICE DYSTROPHY

Lattice dystrophy is also autosomal dominant. The deposition of amyloid in the corneal stroma and subepithelial space leads to a characteristic clinical picture of dots interconnected with lattice lines. The central cornea can become hazy. Recurrent corneal erosions occur, and vision deteriorates slowly. Corneal transplant will clear the cornea, but recurrence in the graft is most likely in this condition.

MACULAR DYSTROPHY

Macular dystrophy (Groenow type II) is an autosomal recessive stromal dystrophy (Fig. 22.2.26). Deposits of mucopolysaccharides in corneal stroma, Desçemet's membrane, and corneal endothelium lead to confluent, ill-defined central and peripheral corneal opacification. Visual deterioration is most likely in this stromal dystrophy. It too, may be accompanied by recurrent erosions. Corneal transplant may be followed in several years by recurrence in the graft.

OTHER STROMAL DYSTROPHIES

Schnyder's dystrophy and Bietti's marginal corneal crystalline dystrophy do not usually cause visual disability.

The autosomal dominant central cloudy dystrophy of Francois is an asymptomatic disorder in which there is formation of cloud-like opacities in the central cornea.

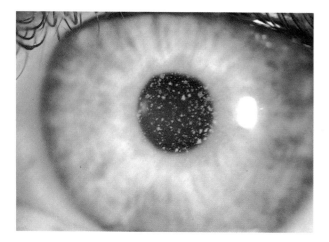

Fig. 20.2.25 Granular dystrophy (Mr J. Dart's patient).

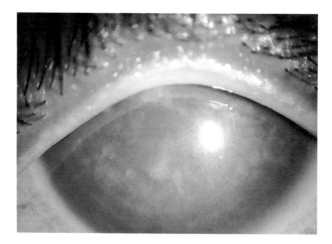

Fig. 20.2.26 Macular dystrophy (Mr J. Dart's patient).

Congenital hereditary stromal dystrophy presents at birth with a ground-glass or flaky white cornea without vessels and with a normal thickness cornea. It is autosomal dominant and not progressive. Histologically the corneal stroma is uniformly abnormal with loose lamellae related to keratocytes (Witschel *et al.* 1978). Treatment by corneal grafting carries a good prognosis.

Endothelial dystrophies

FUCH'S DYSTROPHY

Fuch's endothelial corneal dystrophy is a common dystrophy that presents later in life and only rarely in childhood. Although autosomal dominant inheritance is usual, most patients are women. Bilateral involvement is the rule with rare cases occurring unilaterally. The hallmark of this condition is corneal oedema. Endothelial failure is first represented by central corneal endothelial bumps on slit lamp examination. Histologically, the bumps are thickened areas of Descemet's membrane, caused by abnormal collagen production by sick endothelial cells. Later, the posterior layer of the cornea takes on a bronze appearance. Corneal decompensation occurs, resulting in diminished vision secondary to oedema. At this point, treatment consists of corneal transplant.

CONGENITAL HEREDITARY ENDOTHELIAL DYSTROPHY (CHED)

This important but rare corneal dystrophy was clearly described by Maumenee (1960). It may be due to abnormal final differentiation of neural crest cells (Bahn *et al.* 1984).

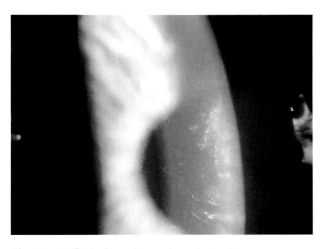

Fig. 20.2.27 Posterior polymorphous dystrophy.

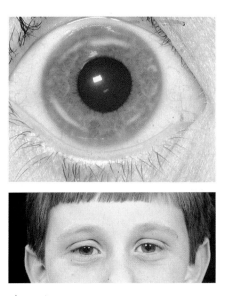

Fig. 20.2.28 Corneal arcus remaining in a child who had severe vernal catarrh.

Usually the presentation is at birth with a variable diffuse avascular haziness of the cornea with photophobia. The cornea is much thicker than normal. The opacification may clear in the first few weeks of life but a significant proportion remain opaque, or become opaque enough to warrant corneal grafting, which carries a relatively good prognosis (Kirkness *et al.* 1987). Autosomal dominant and probable recessive inheritance patterns have been described. The key to the clinical differentiation from congenital hereditary stromal dystrophy is the increased corneal thickness, progressiveness, and pathological changes in Descemet's membrane, all seen in CHED.

POSTERIOR POLYMORPHOUS DYSTROPHY

This is also a bilateral autosomal dominant corneal dystrophy present at birth (Fig. 22.2.30). It is asymmetrical and slowly progressive. The symptoms are often mild and most patients do not require corneal grafting (McCartney & Kirkness 1988). Slit lamp appearances show vesicles, nodules, and vacuoles in the Descemet's membrane area best seen on retroillumination. It seems to have some features of anterior chamber cleavage abnormalities with a prominent Schwalbe's line and irido-corneal adhesions, glaucoma and corectopia (Grayson 1974).

Corneal arcus

Arcus lipoides is due to a deposition of a variety of phospholipids, low density lipoproteins and triglycer-

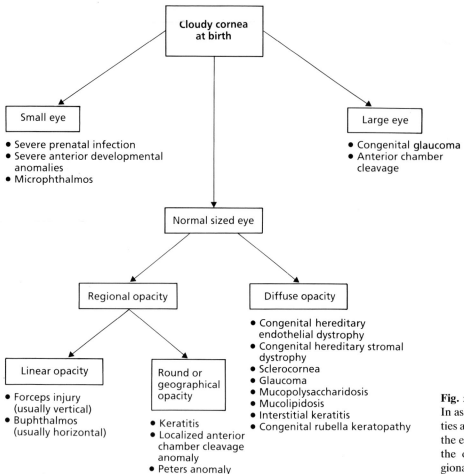

Fig. 20.2.29 The cloudy cornea at birth. In assessing the child with corneal opacities at birth it is important to see whether the eye is small, large or normal sized. Is the opacity diffuse or regional? If regional is it linear or geographical?

ides in the stroma of the peripheral cornea. Unlike xanthomas, corneal arcus is not invariably associated with hyperlipidaemia, but when corneal arcus appears in youth it is highly suggestive of raised plasma low density lipoproteins (LDL). Arcus is not correlated with plasma high density lipoprotein (HDL) or very low density lipoprotein (VLDL). Arcus appears in youth in familial hypercholesterolaemia (Fredrickson's type II) and in familial hyperlipoproteinaemia (type III).

Arcus lipoides may also occur in children adjacent to areas of corneal disease including vernal keratopathy (Fig. 22.2.28), herpes simplex, and limbal dermoid.

Disorders of HDL metabolism tend to cause diffuse corneal clouding; these include LCAT disease, Tangier disease, fish eye disease, and apoprotein AI absence; occasionally however an arcus-like peripheral condensation occurs.

Primary lipoidal degeneration of the cornea is an arcus that occurs in a healthy cornea in a person with normal plasma lipids.

White cornea at birth

The white cornea at birth poses an important differential diagnosis (Fig. 22.2.29). The first consideration is that the newborn suffers congenital glaucoma. The corneal diameter will be large (due to expansion of the globe from increased pressure). Ruptures in Descemet's membrane that are limbus parallel may be present. Intraocular pressure is elevated. The optic nerves will show increased cupping. Urgent intervention in the form of surgery is usually indicated, if vision is to be preserved.

The next possibility is a forceps injury. Forceps marks may be visible on the lids or cheek. A linear, usually vertical, rupture of Descemet's membrane will be present. This causes corneal oedema. Oedema always resolves, leaving varying degrees of astigmatism. Late corneal decompensation is possible.

Certain metabolic conditions are in the differential diagnosis. Cystinosis rarely causes a cloudy cornea at birth. Mucopolysaccharidoses occasionally present as congenital cloudy cornea.

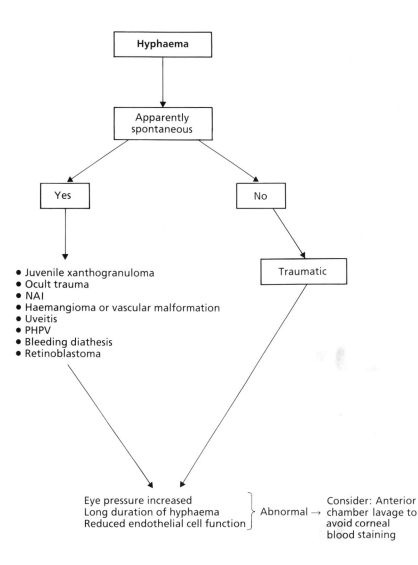

Fig. 20.2.30 Management of corneal blood staining secondary to hyphaema. Hyphaema without obvious cause leads the ophthalmologist to think of certain specific abnormalities.

Hyphaema

↓

Apparently spontaneous

Yes   No

↓   ↓

• Juvenile xanthogranuloma
• Ocult trauma
• NAI
• Haemangioma or vascular malformation
• Uveitis
• PHPV
• Bleeding diathesis
• Retinoblastoma

Traumatic

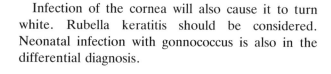

Eye pressure increased
Long duration of hyphaema } Abnormal → Consider: Anterior chamber lavage to avoid corneal blood staining
Reduced endothelial cell function

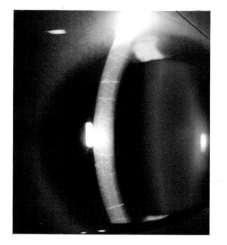

Fig. 20.2.31 Multiple endocrine neoplasia type 2B. Thickened corneal nerves can be seen crossing even the axial area of the cornea.

Infection of the cornea will also cause it to turn white. Rubella keratitis should be considered. Neonatal infection with gonnococcus is also in the differential diagnosis.

Blue sclerae

Hereditary conditions that cause a defect in mesodermal structures will produce a blue appearing sclera. The characteristic blue discoloration is probably related to thinning of the sclera. Blue sclera is a consistent finding in osteogenesis imperfecta. This condition is associated with brittle bones and a conductive hearing loss. Blue sclera occurs in the Ehlers–Danlos and Marfan's syndromes. Rarely, it may occur in association with brittle corneas (Stein 1968) or ectodermal dysplasia (Wilson 1973). In infancy many normal children have blue-ish corneas and some myopic children also have the same appearance.

Hyphaema and corneal blood staining

Blood staining of the cornea is an important and devastating complication of hyphaema (Fig. 20.2.30). Generally, duration of hyphaema, degree of elevation of intraocular pressure, the integrity of corneal endothelium and the occurrence of secondary haemorrhages are the factors associated with staining. The doctor should observe the patient with hyphaema at least daily, give him non-aspirin-containing analgesics and acetazolamide if the intraocular pressure is raised, and when he suspects that staining of the cornea is possible, he may recommend an anterior chamber lavage; the efficacy of antifibrinolytic drugs is not established (Kraft *et al.* 1987). Corneal blood staining may occur within 3 days if the intraocular pressure is high.

The incidence in one series (Agapitos *et al.* 1987) was 17 per 100,000 paediatric population per year. Rebleeds occurred in 7.6% but did not correlate with age, the use of cycloplegics or steroids. Ninety-one per cent of this series achieved acuity of 20/30 or better. Amblyopia occurred in the two children who required cataract extraction of the 316 in the series.

Corneal nerves

Corneal nerves are visible in the periphery of the cornea in normal persons but they may be more visible in certain conditions (Menscher 1974), including the following:

1 Dystrophies: Fuchs, keratoconus.
2 Buphthalmos.
3 Inflammatory disease:-leprosy; after corneal grafts; corneal trauma.
4 Refsum's disease.
5 Ichthyosis.
6 Multiple endocrine neoplasia type IIb.
7 Neurofibromatosis (described but may have been cases of Men IIb).

Multiple endocrine neoplasia (MEN)

There are three main syndromes in which tumours occur in a variety of endocrine organs at a young age. For the ophthalmologist the most prominent of these is MEN IIb. Patients show a marfanoid habitus, full and fleshy lips, nodular neuromas on the tip and edges of the tongue and eyelids, pes cavus, constipation, and peroneal muscular atrophy due to neuroma formation (Dyck *et al.* 1979). It is autosomal dominantly inherited. Prominent corneal nerves within an otherwise

normal cornea (Spector *et al.* 1981) are an important diagnostic feature (Fig. 22.2.31). They are a mixture of myelinated and unmyelinated fibres and are also present in the ciliary body and iris. Because of a very high incidence of thyroid medullary carcinoma in MEN IIb, prophylactic thyroidectomy may be recommended in childhood. Phaeochromocytoma also occur.

References

Agapitos PJ, Noel L-P, Clarke WN. Traumatic hyphaema in children. *Ophthalmology* 1987; **94**: 1238–42

Angell LK, Rovv RM, Berson FG. Visual prognosis in patients with ruptures in Descemet's membrane due to forceps injuries. *Arch Ophthalmol* 1981; **99**: 2137–40

Anseth A. Congenital bilateral corneal anaesthesia. *Acta Ophthalmol* 1968; **46**: 909–11

Appenzeller O. Kornfield M. Snyder R. Acromutilating paralysing neuropathy with corneal ulceration in Navajo children. *Arch Neurol* 1976; **33**: 733–8

Apple DJ, Olson RJ, Jones GR, Carey JC, Van Norman DK, Ohrlaff C, Philippart M. *Am J Ophthalmol* 1984; **98**: 320–8

Arnold RW, Stickler G, Bourne W. Corneal crystals, myopathy and nephropathy: a new syndrome. *J Pediatr Ophthalmol Strabismus* 1987; **24**: 151–5

Aurora AL, Madhaven M, Rao S. Epidermolysis bullosa lethalis. *Am J Ophthalmol* 1975; **79**: 464–70

Bachynski BN, Andreu R. Flynn JR. Spontaneous corneal perforation and extrusion of intraocular contents in premature infants. *J Pediatr Ophthalmol Strabismus* 1986; **23**: 25–8

Bahn CF, Falls HF, Varley GA, Meyer RF, Edelhauser HF, Bourne WM. Classification of corneal endothelial disorders based on neural crest origin. *Ophthalmol* 1984; **91**: 558–63

Beinfang D, Kuwabara T, Puesctel S. The Richner Hanhart syndrome. *Arch Ophthalmol* 1976; **94**: 1133–8

BenEzra D, Frucht Y, Paez JH, Zelikovitch A. Amniotic band syndrome and strabismus. *J Pediatr Ophthalmol Strabismus* 1982; **19**: 33–6

Bernuy A, Contreras F, Maumenee AE, O'Donnell FE. Bilateral, congenital, dermis-like choristomas overlying corneal staphylomas. *Arch Ophthalmol* 1981; **99**: 1995–8

Bicknell JM, Holland JV. Neurologic manifestations of Cogan syndrome. *Neurology* 1978; **28**: 218–33

Biglan AW, Brown SI, Johnson BL. Keratoglobus and blue sclerae *Am J Ophthalmol* 1977; **83**: 225–33

Birndorf LA, Ginsberg SP. Hereditary fleck dystrophy associated with decreased corneal sensitivity. *Am J Ophthalmol* 1973; **73**: 670

Boger WP, Petersen, Robb RM. Keratoconus and acute hydrops in mentally retarded patients with congenital rubella syndrome. *Am J Ophthalmol* 1981; **91**: 231–3

Bowen DI. Clinical aspects of oculoauriculo vertebral dysplasia. *Br J Ophthalmol* 1971; **55**: 145–54

Brooks AMV, Grant G, Gillies WE. Determination of the nature of corneal crystals by specular microscopy. *J Am Acad Ophthalmol* 1988; **95**: 448–53

Brown SI, Salamon SM. Wound healing of grafts in congenitally opaque infant corneas. *Am J Ophthalmol* 1983; **95**: 641–4

Carpel EF. Congenital corneal anaesthesia. *Am J Ophthalmol* 1978; **85**: 357–9

Char DH, Cogan DG, Sullivan WR. Immunologic study of nonsyphilitic interstitial keratitis with vestibulo auditory symptoms. *Am J Ophthalmol* 1975; **80**: 491–5

Cogan DG. Syndrome of non-syphilitic interstitial keratitis and vestibulo auditory symptoms. *Arch Ophthalmol* 1945; **33**: 144–9

Dale RT, Rao GN, Aquavella JV, Metz HS. Adolescent cystinosis: a clinical and specular microscopic study of an unusual sibship. *Br J Ophthalmol* 1981; **65**: 828–32

Darougar S, John AC, Viswalingham M, Cornell L, Jones BR. Isolation of chlamydia psittaci from a patient with interstitial keratitis and uveitis associated with otological and cardiovascular lesions. *Br J Ophthalmol* 1978; **62**: 709–13

Dyck PJ, Carney JA, Sizemore GW, Okazaki H, Brimijoin WS, Lambert EH. Multiple endocrine neoplasia, Type 2b; phenotype recognition, neurological features and their pathological basis. *Ann Neurol* 1979; **6**: 302–14

Ellis W, Barfort P, Mastman GJ. Keratoconjunctivitis with corneal crystals caused by the dieffenbachia plant. *Am J Ophthalmol* 1973; **76**: 143–5

Esakowitz L, Yates JRW. Congenital corneal anaesthesia and the MURCs association: a case report. *Br J Ophthalmol* 1988; **72**: 236–9

Feldberg R, Yassur Y, Ben-sira I, Vasano I, Zelikovitz I. Keratomalacia in acrodermatitis enteropathica. *Metab Pediatr Syst Ophthalmol* 1981; **5**: 207–12

Fleming CR, Dickson ER, Wahner HW, Hollenhorst RW, McCall JT. Pigmented rings in non-Wilsonian liver disease. *Ann Intern Med* 1977; **86**: 285

Ford FR, Wilkins L. Congenital universal: insensitiveness to pain. *Bull Johns Hopkins Hosp* 1938; **62**: 448–66

Foster A, Sommer A. Corneal ulceration, measles and childhood blindness in Tanzania. *Br J Ophthalmol* 1987; **71**: 331–43

Frangoulis M, Taylor D. Corneal opacities — a diagnostic feature of the trisomy 8 mosaic syndrome. *Br J Ophthalmol* 1983; **67**: 619–22

Frazier P, Wong VG. Cystinosis, histologic and crystallographic examination of crystals in eye tissues. *Arch Ophthalmol* 1968; **80**: 93

Friedlander MH, Smolin G. Corneal degenerations. *Ann Ophthalmol* 1979; **11**: 1485–95

Gilbert WS, Talbot FJ. Cogan's syndrome. Signs of periarteritis nodosa and cerebral venous sinus thrombosis. *Arch Ophthalmol* 1969; **82**: 633–000

Grayson M. The nature of hereditary deep posterior polymorphous dystrophy of the cornea. *Trans Am Ophthalmol Soc* 1974; **72**: 516–25

Grayson M. *Diseases of the Cornea*. CV Mosby Co., St Louis 1983, pp. 222–6

Hewson GE. Congenital trigeminal anaesthesia. *Br J Ophthalmol* 1963; **47**: 308–11

Hyams S, Dar H, Neumann E. Blue sclerae and keratoglobus. Ocular signs of a systemic connective tissue disorder. *Br J Ophthalmol* 1969; **53**: 53–8

Jay B, Black RK, Wells RS. Ocular manifestations of ichthyosis. *Br J Ophthalmol* 1968; **56**: 45–52

Kaiser-Kupfer MI, Caruso RC, Minkler DS, Gahl WA. Long-term ocular manifestations in nephropathic cystinosis. *Arch Ophthalmol* 1986; **104**: 706–11

Kaiser-Kupfer MI, Fujikawa L, Kuwabara T, Jain S, Gahl WA. Removal of corneal crystals by topical cysteamine in nephropathic cystinosis. *N Engl J Med* 1987; **316**: 775–9

Katowitz JA, Yolles E, Yanoff M. Ichthyosis congenita. *Arch Ophthalmol* 1974; **91**: 208–10

Katz B, Melles RB, Schneider JA. Glare disability in nephropathic cystinosis. *Arch Ophthalmol* 1987a; **105**: 1670–1

Katz B, Melles RB, Schneider JA. Contrast sensitivity function in nephropathic cystinosis. *Arch Ophthalmol* 1987b; **105**: 1667–70

Katz B, Melles RB, Schneider JA. Corneal sensitivity in nephropathic cystinosis. *Am J Ophthalmol* 1987c; **104**: 413–17

Kirkness C, McCartney A, Rice N, Garner A, Steele A McG. Congenital hereditary corneal oedema of Maumenee: itsclinical features, management and pathology. *Br J Ophthalmol* 1987; **71**: 130–45

Klauss V, Reidel K. Bilateral and unilateral mesodermal corneal metaplasia. *Br J Ophthalmol* 1983; **67**: 320–3

Knapp AJ, Gartner S, Henkind P. Multiple myeloma and its ocular manifestations. *Surv Ophthalmol* 1987; **31**: 343–51

Knobel H, Demeler U. Keratoplastik bei kindern und jugendlichen. *Ophthalmologica (Basel)* 1978; **177**: 146–51

Kogbe O, Listet S. Tear electrophoretic changes in Nigerian children after measles. *Br J Ophthalmol* 1987; **71**: 326–30

Kraft SP, Christianson MD, Crawford JS, Wagman RD, Antoszy KJH. Traumatic Hyphema in children: Treatment with Epsilon-Aminocaproic Acid. *Ophthalmology* 1987; **94**: 1232–8

Lawford JB. Bilateral (?Congenital) anaesthesia of conjunctiva and cornea; neuroparolytic keratitis. Trans Ophthalmol Soc UK 1907; **27**: 80–000

Leff SR, Shields JA, Augsburger JJ, Sakowski AD Jr, Blair CJ. Congenital corneal staphyloma: clinical, radiological and pathological correlation. *Br J Ophthalmol* 1986; **70**: 427–30

Lisch W, Weidle EG, Lisch C *et al.* Schnyder's dystrophy: Progression and metabolism. *Ophthalmol Pediatr Genet* 1986; **7**: 45–50

Mackensen *et al.* (Freiburg). Keratoplasty in childhood. *Klin Monatsbl Augenheilk* 1977; **171**: 199–209

Macnab A. Opacity of the cornea in three members of one family. *Trans Ophthalmol Soc UK* 1907; **27**: 81–2

Manfredi M, Bini G, Cruccu G, Accornero N, Berardelli A, Medolago L. Congenital absence of pain. *Arch Neurol* 1981; **38**: 507–12

Mansour AM, Barber JC, Reinecke RD, Wang FM. Ocular choristomas. *Surv Ophthalmol* 1989; **33**: 339–59

Maumenee AE. Congenital hereditary corneal dystrophy. *Am J Ophthalmol*. 1960; **50**: 1114–8

Matta CS, Felker GV, Ide CH. Eye manifestations in acrodermatitis enteropathica. *Arch Ophthalmol* 1975; **93**: 140–4

Mawhorter LG, Ruttum MS, Koenig SR. Keratopathy in a family with the ectrodactyly-ectodermal dysplasia clefting syndrome. *Ophthalmology* 1985; **92**: 1427–32

McCartney ACE, Kirkness CM. Comparison between posterior polymorphous dystrophy and congenital hereditary endothelial dystrophy of the cornea. *Eye* 1988; **2**: 63–71

McDonald R. Carbon disulfide poisoning. *Arch Ophthalmol* 1938; **20**: 839

McDonnell PJ, Spalton DJ. The ocular signs and complications of Epidermolysis Bullosa. *JR Soc Med* 1988; **81**: 576–8

Melles RB, Schneider JA, Narsing AR, Katz B. Spatial and

temporal sequence of corneal crystal deposition in nephropathic cystinosis. *Am J Ophthalmol* 1987; **104**: 598−605

Menscher JH. Corneal nerves. *Surv Ophthalmol* 1974; **19**: 1−14

Miller MT, Deutsch TA, Cronin C, Keys CL. Amniotic bands as a cause of ocular anomalies. *Am J Ophthalmol* 1987; **104**: 270−85

Mohandessan MM, Romano PE. Neuroparalytic keratitis in Goldenhar-Gorlin syndrome. *Am J Ophthalmol* 1978; **85**: 111−3

Monnickendam M, Darougar S. Editorial: Postmeasles blindness. *Br J Ophthalmol* 1987; **71**: 325

Olson RJ, Kaufman HE. Recurrence of Reis-Bucklers corneal dystrophy in a graft. *Am J Ophthalmol* 1978; **85**: 349−52

Orth DH, Fretzin DF, Abramson V. Collodian baby with transient bilateral upper lid ectropion. Review of ocular manifestations in ichthyosis. *Arch Ophthalmol* 1974; **91**: 206−7

Purcell JJ, Krachmer JH. Familial corneal hypesthesia. *Arch Ophthalmol* 1979; **97**: 872−4

Purcell JJ, Krachmer JH, Thompson HS. Corneal sensation in Adie's pupil. *Am J Ophthalmol* 1977; **84**: 496−500

Purcell JJ, Krachmer JH, Weingeist TD. Fleck corneal dystrophy. *Arch Ophthalmol* 1972; **73**: 670

Rahi A, Davies PD, Ruben M, Lobascher D, Menon J. Keratoconus and coexisting atopic disease. *Br J Ophthalmol* 1977; **61**: 761−4

Rice NSC, Ashton N, Jay B, Black RK. Reis Buckler's dystrophy. *Br J Ophthalmol* 1968; **52**: 577−82

Riley FC, Robertson DM. Ocular histopathology in multiple endocrine neoplasia type 2b. *Am J Ophthalmol* 1981; **91**: 57−64

Rodrigues MM, Kruth HS, Krachner JH, Willis R. Unesterified cholesterol in Schnyder's corneal crystalline dystrophy. *Am J Ophthalmol* 1987; **104**: 157−63

Schanzlin DJ, Robin JB, Erickson G, Lingra R, Minckler D, Pickford M. Histopathologic and ultrastructural analysis of congenital corneal staphyloma. *Am J Ophthalmol* 1983; **95**: 506−14

Schimmelpfennig B, Beurman RW. Evidence for neurotropism in the cornea (abstract) *Invest Ophthalmol Vis Sci* 1979; **18**: 125

Shenk Van H. Hornhautbefunde bei idiopathischer anasthesie der hornhaut. *Klin Monatsbl Augenheilkd* 1958; **133**: 506−18

Shields JA, Waring GO, Monte LG. Ocular findings in leprosy. *Am J Ophthalmol* 1974; **77**: 880−90

Sjogren H. A contribution to our knowledge of the ocular changes induced by sulphuretted hydrogen. *Acta Ophthalmologica* 1939; **17**: 166−71

Smiddy WE, Hamburg TR, Kracher GP, Stark WJ. Keratoconus: contact lens or keratoplasty? *Ophthalmology* 1988; **95**: 487−93

Sommer A. Renewed interest in the ancient scourge xerophthalmia (editorial). *Am J Ophthalmol* 1978; **86**: 284

Spector B, Klintworth GK, Wells SA. Histologic study of the ocular lesions in multiple endocrine neoplasia syndrome type 11B. *Am J Ophthalmol* 1981; **91**: 201−14

Spencer WH, Fisher JJ. The association of keratoconus with atopic dermatitis. *Am J Ophthalmol* 1959; **47**: 332−4

Stark DJ, Gilmore D, Vance J, Pearn J. A corneal abnormality associated with trisomy 8 mosaicism syndrome. *Br Ophthalmol* 1987; **71**: 29−32

Stein RM, Cohen EJ, Calhoun JH, Fendick M, Reinecke RD. Corneal birth trauma managed with a contact lens. *Am J Ophthalmol* 1987; **103**: 596−7

Stein R, Lazer M, Adam A. Brittle cornea, a familial trait associated with blue sclera. *Am J Ophthalmol* 1968; **66**: 67−9

Stewart HL, Wind CA, Kaufman HE. Unilateral congenital corneal anesthesia. *Am J Ophthalmol* 1972; **74**: 334−5

Taylor D, Bentovim A. Recurrent non-accidentally inflicted chemical eye injuries to siblings. *J Pediatr Ophthalmol Strabismus* 1976; **13**: 238−42

Topilow HW, Cykiert RC, Goldman K, Palme E, Henkind P. Bilateral corneal dermis-like choristoma. *Arch Ophthalmol* 1981; **99**: 1387−91

Trope GE, Jay JL, Dudgeon J, Woodruff G. Self-inflicted corneal injuries in children with congenital anaesthesia. *Br J Ophthalmol* 1985; **69**: 551−5

Vangsted P, Limpaphayom P. Dermoid of the cornea. *Acta Ophthalmologica* **61**, fasc 5, 1983; 927−33

Vrabec MB, Shapiro MB, Koller E, Wilbe DA, Henricks J, Albers JJ. Ophthalmic observations in lecithin choline acyltransferase deficiency. *Arch Ophthalmol* 1988; **106**: 225−9

Wan WL, Minckler DS, Rao NA. Pupillary-block glaucoma associated with childhood cystinosis. *Am J Ophthalmol* 1986; **101**: 700−6

Waring GO III, Rodriguez MM, Laibson PR. Corneal dystrophies *Surv Ophthalmol* 1978; **23**: 97−9

Waring GO III, Roth AM, Rodrigues MM. Clinicopathologic correlation of microphthalmos with cyst. *Am J Ophthalmol* 1976; **82**: 714−21

Wilson DJ, Weleber RG, Klein M, Welch RB, Green WR. Bietti's crystalline dystrophy: a clinico-pathologic correlative study. *Arch Ophthalmol* 1989; **107**: 213−22

Wilson FM, Grayson M, Pieroni D. Corneal changes in ectodermal dysplasia: Case report, histopathology and differential diagnosis. *Am J Ophthalmol* 1973; **75**: 17−27

Wilson FM, Schmitt TE, Grayson M. Amiodorone induced corneal verticillata. *Ann Ophthalmol* 1980; **12**: 657

Witschel H, Fine BS, Grutzner P, McTigue JW. Congenital hereditary stromal dystrophy of the cornea. *Arch Ophthalmol* 1978; **96**: 1043−51

Woodward EG. Keratoconus; maternal age and social class. *Br J Ophthalmol* 1981; **65**: 104−7

Zaidman GW, Johnson B, Brown SI. Corneal transplantation in an infant with corneal dermoid. *AJO* 1982; **93**: 78−83

21 Lacrimal System

SUSAN DAY

The lacrimal system consists of a secretory portion, lacrimal and accessory lacrimal glands, meibomian glands, and goblet cells; and an excretory portion, punctae, canaliculus, lacrimal sac, and nasolacrimal duct. Its function is to produce and remove tears. Tears themselves serve in multiple ways to protect the eyes, including lubrication, provision of oxygen, and an antibacterial role; when the tears drain away, irritating substances as well as cellular debris is similarly removed (Lemp & Blackman 1983; Werb 1983). Epiphora represents one of the most common indications for referral in a paediatric ophthalmology practice. Other rare conditions in infants and children warrant a thorough knowledge of its pathology.

Lacrimal gland

Anatomy

The lacrimal gland occupies the lacrimal gland fossa in the supero-temporal aspect of the orbit. It is divided into the orbital and palpebral lobes by the levator aponeurosis. The palpebral lobe can normally be directly prolapsed into the superotemporal cul-de-sac and with abnormal enlargement of the lacrimal gland, direct visualization or direct biopsy of the lacrimal gland can usually be made.

Embryology

The lacrimal gland commences differentiation from the nasal cells by the conjunctiva at 40–45 days of gestation. By the fifth month, lobules are relatively well formed. The lacrimal gland continues to grow up to 3–4 years of age after birth. Reflex tearing, however, begins in infants anywhere from a few weeks to several months (Duke–Elder & Cook 1963; Sevel 1981). The accessory lacrimal glands have common origins but remain within the lids rather than migrating with the remainder of the lacrimal gland precursors.

Congenital abnormalities

Congenital absence of the lacrimal gland is rare. This is usually associated with conditions in which congenital absence of at least part of the conjunctiva is present, such as anophthalmos and cryptophthalmos.

Congenital alacrima or hyposecretion of tears is relatively more common; the lacrimal gland may be present despite the absence of tears. Because tear production, especially reflex tear production, is often small until 6 months after birth, investigation of these patients is not usually indicated unless other systemic disorders seem apparent (Riley et al. 1949; Riley 1952; Riley & Moore 1966). Patrick (1974) has shown that neonates do produce tears and suspected that the apparent absence of tearing was accounted for by an efficient tear pump created by the lids and lacrimal system. Children with familial dysautonomia, or Riley–Day syndrome can develop severe keratopathy as a consequence of the dry-eyes and the corneal hypesthesia (Goldberg et al. 1968). (See Appendix, Problem 7.)

Other congenital abnormalities include ectopic lacrimal gland tissue in which tissue is embryologically misplaced deeper in the orbit. Since no drainage system exists, an apparent enlarging orbital mass may develop (Green & Zimmerman 1967; Jacobs *et al.* 1977). Neoplasms have been reported in association with ectopic tissue; thus its diagnosis is significant (Mindlin *et al.* 1977; Mueller & Borit 1979).

Since the embryology of the lacrimal gland is closely linked to the conjunctival epithelium, the common position of some forms of dermoid cysts supero-temporally can be understood. Dermoid cysts must be distinguished from dacryops, or ectasia of the lacrimal gland ducts, in certain circumstances (Rush & Leone 1981; Brownstein *et al.* 1984). Congenital fistulae may be present in the region of the lateral canthus (Duke−Elder & Cook 1963; Blanksma & Pol 1980) and preauricular region (Mukherji & Mukhopadhay 1972). Crocodile tears (Chorobski 1951) in which tearing is elicited by chewing or sucking, occur as a consequence of congenital aberrant innervation between the Vth cranial nerve (innervating the lacrimal gland) and the gustatory fibres of the VIIth cranial nerve. This has been found in instances of aberrant innervation including the Marcus−Gunn jaw winking phenomenon and Duane's syndrome (Ramsey & Taylor 1980).

Dacryoadenitis

This may occur either unilaterally or more typically bilaterally in children. Often the child is systemically ill. Mumps may result in lacrimal gland as well as parotid gland swelling (Riffenburgh 1961). Other causes include mononucleosis, zoster, histoplasmosis and gonoccocal infection (Duke−Elder & MacFaul 1974). The diagnosis of dacryoadenitis is aided by assessment of the 'S-sign' in which there is a drooping of the lateral aspect of the upper lid. Direct inspection of the palpebral lobe of the gland may confirm evidence of inflammation. CT scans can confirm presence of enlargement but also aid in ruling out lacrimal or other orbital masses if signs and symptoms of dacryoadenitis do not resolve.

Lacrimal gland infarcts

This occurs rarely in children with sickle cell disease. The rapid onset can mimic and must be differentiated from orbital cellulitis, but its treatment consists of reversal of the sickle cell crisis. A bone scan may be particularly helpful in defining the lacrimal infarct.

Lacrimal gland tumours and pseudotumour

With the exception of a dermoid involving the lacrimal gland, tumours are extremely rare in childhood (Duke−Elder & Cook 1963). Pseudotumour is rare in childhood but may affect the lacrimal gland in young people (Chavis *et al.* 1978, Mottow & Jakobiec 1978). Malignant epithelial tumours including mixed cell, adenocystic and other carcinomas (Dagher *et al.* 1980) are also rare but recorded in childhood (Wright *et al.* 1979; Wright 1982).

Lacrimal duct cysts

These appear to be rare in childhood (Smith & Rootman 1986) but occur as translucent swellings under the conjunctiva or lacrimal gland swelling.

Lacrimal drainage system

Embryology

The development of the lacrimal drainage system includes an epithelial lined ectodermal component as well as mesodermal components. The ectodermal precursors of the canaliculi and ducts are in place at the 28−30 mm stage of the embryo. Growth continues with gradual formation of a lumen, and patency is established to the lids. The most distal region of the nasolacrimal duct remains nonpatent, consisting of mesodermal components of the nasolacrimal duct and the mucosa of the inferior nasal meatus. At birth, a substantial number of infants still do not have patency of this terminal region. Muruko-del-Castillo (1983) probed 181 full-term infants and found bilateral patency in 131, unilateral patency in 46, and bilateral blockage in four, concluding a 15% nonpatency of 362 passages. Other anatomical studies have revealed between 35% and 73% nonpatency in full-term infants (Schwarz 1935; Cassady 1952). The bones related to the lacrimal excretory passage are incompletely developed at birth; chondrification and ossification commences 6 weeks after birth and may cause significant difficulty with probing by 18 months.

Congenital abnormalities

CONGENITAL PUNCTAL ABNORMALITIES

These abnormalities, including imperforate punctae and absent punctae, can involve both the upper and lower punctae. A thin gray membrane is often present and additional punctae or slit-like fistulae may be present. Nonpatency of the punctae may be suspected when epiphora is present in the absence of any significant discharge, since stagnation within the nasolacrimal sac is not present.

Treatment

Isolated absence of the upper punctum requires no treatment, but absence of the lower or both upper and lower punctum requires treatment only if there are significant symptoms. Treatment requires microdissection or retrograde cannulation with intubation for at least 6 weeks postoperatively. If that fails a conjunctivo-dacryocysto-rhinostomy with Lester Jones tubes is the only, albeit usually unsatisfactory, treatment.

FISTULAS OF THE NASOLACRIMAL SYSTEM

Fistulas may occur due to false passage formation after incision of a lacrimal sac abscess but more frequently they are sometimes bilateral developmental abnormalities. They are usually asymptomatic unless there is an associated nasolacrimal duct obstruction when they may leak tears or pus. Typically they appear just below the medial canthus (Fig. 21.1), they can be multiple. If they cause symptoms they can be excised after careful delineation of the canaliculi.

CONGENITAL NASOLACRIMAL DUCT OBSTRUCTION

This is more frequent and involves failure of the distal system to establish patency to the nasal mucosa. It is usually an isolated defect but may be associated with the EEC syndrome (electrodactyly ectodermal dysplasia clefting) (Fig. 21.2). The infant characteristically develops epiphora at 2–6 weeks; recurrent conjunctivitis, discharge, or dacryocystitis may also be associated. The condition is bilateral in approximately one third of children (Crawford & Pashby 1984). The symptoms may be aggravated by wind or dust, but photophobia is absent. Diagnosis can be supported by applying gentle pressure to express discharge through the punctae. Alternatively, agents such as fluorescein can be instilled and assessment made within the oropharynx of its drainage with the cobalt blue light — not easy in an infant!

The management of the infant with nasolacrimal duct obstruction depends largely on the age of the infant and severity of symptoms. In general, primary care physicians assume this responsibility until the

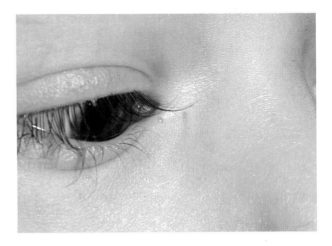

Fig. 21.1 Congenital fistula of the nasolacrimal system. The fistula can be seen as a tiny mark below the medial canthus.

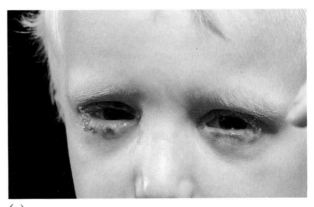

(a)

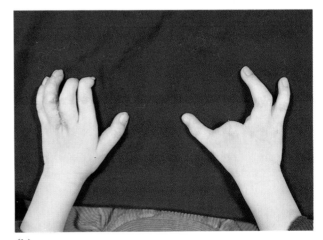

(b)

Fig. 21.2 (a) EEC syndrome with nasolacrimal duct obstruction. **Fig. 21.2** (b) EEC syndrome — clawed deformity of the hands.

child is 6 months old unless the symptoms are particularly prominent or the parents are particularly worried. Many paediatricians will instruct the parents to massage the nasolacrimal sac region in an effort to hasten resolution (Kushner 1982). The most appropriate motion for this manoeuvre is to initially milk any discharge from the sac by gently stroking in an upward motion. Once cleaned, the nasolacrimal system should be firmly massaged with downward pressure. This technique forces any remaining fluid to press against the (presumably) remaining thin mucous membrane between the nasolacrimal duct and the nose. The number of strokes should be three to four and repeated frequently throughout the day. It may be helpful to recommend that every nappy change would be an appropriate time to perform this manoeuvre.

The use of topical antibiotics is rather widespread amongst the primary care physicians in infants with epiphora. This author's practice is to reserve antibiotics until there is evidence of conjunctivitis or purulent characteristics to the expressed discharge.

On the first visit, a complete ophthalmological assessment is indicated. One would be remiss not to diagnose other problems deserving attention. Congenital glaucoma must be excluded as an underlying cause for the epiphora. Diagrams should be drawn for the parents so that they can understand the proposed treatment. Topical antibiotics, usually sulphacetamide, can be prescribed if evidence of infection is present. Proper massage technique should be encouraged.

The decision to proceed with nasolacrimal probing is based primarily on severity, age, parental concern, and is tempered by the general health and the standard practice within the community. Most nasolacrimal probings are performed between 9 and 12 months of age. By waiting until this age, a chance of allowing spontaneous resolution is given (Kushner 1982).

The choice of office probing or hospital probing depends in large part on the ophthalmologists' training but is also influenced by medical economics and parental requests as well. The office probing procedure avoids a general anaesthetic and the expenses of a hospital stay, and many parents will choose this option. The hospital probing in a controlled environment is undoubtedly less nerve-wracking for the ophthalmologist. With current medical economics, a hospital probing may cost 50–100 times as much as an office probing. Probing under chloral hydrate sedation cannot be performed since manipulation is required. An office probing requires a flat surface with overhead illumination, a restraint (or 'papoose') board, sterile

nasolacrimal probing set, standard topical anaesthetic drops, 4% xylocaine topical anaesthetic, applicators, a syringe with irrigating needle, and steady hands (earplugs for the ophthalmologist are optional!). Some ophthalmologists prefer that the parents be with their baby: others will ask them to wait elsewhere. A detailed discussion of the procedure will be necessary if they are to observe, especially emphasizing that the procedure (a) is entirely outside of the globe itself; (b) during the actual probing, the instrument will be rotated such that it appears almost like an acupuncture needle; and (c) the major side effect is a bloody nose or regurgitation of blood into the conjunctival sac. Inevitably, the parents will ask if the procedure 'hurts'; there must be discomfort, but much of the crying is a consequence of being restrained in a foreign setting. The trauma to the baby is probably analogous to the discomfort when an intravenous line is placed in a baby. Virtually all report that their baby sleeps afterward, presumably from being stressed by the procedure. Very few say their child acts differently; the worst reaction that parents have told this author is a baby's anxiety over being placed in a supine position for a day or two. Parents rarely say that, if given the choice again, they would prefer hospitalization, but some paediatricians feel that as the risk of anaesthetic is negligible the psychological trauma is unwarranted.

Hospital probing is undoubtedly a more controlled procedure and is in many ways simple for the physician since the child is under anaesthesia and the familiar operating room mileau is present. The same instrumentation is required, and the same steps are taken with the exception of instillation of anaesthetic drops and holding an applicator moistened with 4% xylocaine over the punctum. One initially dilates the punctum both either superiorly or inferiorly. A small gauge probe is then introduced at the superior punctum, perpendicular to the lid margin, for a short distance (approx 1 mm). The probe is then rotated and advanced to follow the canalicular system in a horizontal and then inferoposterior direction. The probe should pass without much force so that false passages are not created. At the distal extreme, a resistance will be felt from the mucous membrane. A slight pop should be felt as this is broken with the probe. The feel is similar to popping a balloon with a blunt needle. The 000 probe is removed and a larger gauge 00 or 0 probe inserted to provide further dilation. The now-patent system should be irrigated with 1 ml of balanced salt solution.

Probing of the opposite side may be performed at the same time if the baby has tolerated the procedure well. Probing should not be performed if there is evidence of acute dacryocystitis.

Postoperatively, a topical antibiotic drop four times daily for 2 days may be used as well as a nasal decongestant for the same time period (such as 1/4 or 1/8% phenlyephine) or 1/2% ephedrine; do not use this for prolonged periods of time, as it may induce hypertension.

The success of office probing approaches 80% on the initial probing. Patency can usually be judged within days after the procedure. Most physicians prefer a repeat simple probing to tube placement unless the child is older or symptoms are severe. Tube insertion must be considered if two failed probings have occurred or in cases of trauma involving the nasolacrimal system. They may also be used in conjunction with dacryocystorhinostomy.

Silicone tubes are used in which a metal probe is wedged or glued onto each end. Crawford tubes include a probed with a bullous enlargement at the tip; Guibor tubes have a larger bore probe attached on either end. Under general anaesthesia, the superior and inferior systems are probed and irrigated to ensure that patency is present. The inferior system is then probed with one end of the tubing until the probe reaches the nasal cavity. Retrieval of the probe is then obtained either with a special hook-shaped instrument (Crawford 1977) or with a straight clamp. Although direct visualization of the metal probe can be attempted with appropriate nasal speculae, the young child's anatomy with large inferior turbinates often makes this difficult.

The contact of the hook with the probe can be difficult to feel and is improved by connecting the probe and the hook to different levels of an electrical circuit (low ampèrage) in which there is a light bulb and when contact is made, it lights up (Fig. 21.3). One gains skill in prompt location of the probe by visualizing the angle formed between the inserted probe and the retrieving instrument. In comparison to adults, the probe is far more anteriorly located. Once the inferior system has its portion of tubing in place, the superior system is then canalized, leaving a loop of tubing which extends from superior to inferior punctum and two metal probes coming out of the nose. The loose ends are then securely tied to each other with multiple (6–8) squared knots and the tubing then cut 1 cm from the knot. Future retrieval of the knotted end can be ensured by securing a 4.0 silk suture around the knot and cutting its end long. Tubings are usually left in place 3–6 months so that patency may be established (Crawford & Pashby

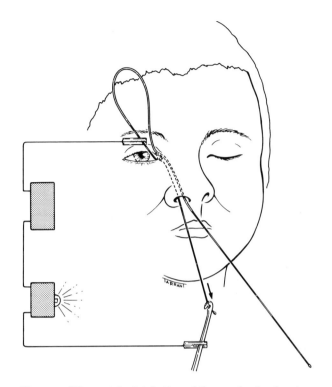

Fig. 21.3 Silicone tube intubation of the nasolacrimal system can be facilitated by location of the Crawford's probe under the turbinate by the use of a low ampèrage electrical circuit.

1984). Removal in the young child usually requires general anesthetic unless the portion of tubing or silk suture can easily be seen in the nasal cavity. The loop is bisected, and tubing is then pulled through the nose.

Rarely, a dacryocystorhinostomy (DCR) must be performed in children. Indications include recurrent epiphora despite prior silicone intubation, inability to establish patency with simple probings and intubation, and trauma (Billson *et al.* 1978) involving the nasolacrimal sac. Although ophthalmologists have traditionally avoided its use in children, its success is comparable to adult DCRs when particular attention is given to paediatric anatomy (Nowinski *et al.* 1985).

Congenital dacryocystocoele (amniotocele, mucocele)

An unusual presentation of nonpatent nasolacrimal system(s) may occur in the neonate when fluid has become trapped within the nasolacrimal sac and distends it. Various terms have been suggested for this condition; 'amniotocele' has been used since, in part, the fluid within the sac was derived from amniotic fluid (Levy 1979), and 'mucocele' to coincide with the appearance of the fluid obtained from the mass

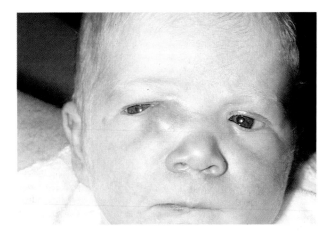

Fig. 21.4 Congenital dacryocystocele

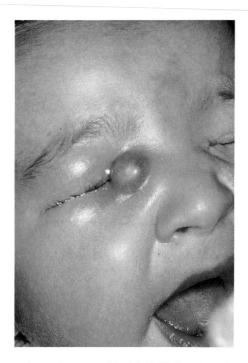

Fig. 21.5 Acute dacryocystitis. Mr R Welham's patient.

(Jackson & Lambert 1963; Scott *et al*. 1979). 'Dacryocystocele' has been suggested (Harris & DiClementi 1982) as an attempt to anatomically describe the condition without implying specific content of the swelling.

The baby has a bluish appearing mass, (Fig. 21.4) often 10–12 mm in diameter, in the region of the nasolacrimal sac. Appropriate management of the swelling has shifted from immediate probing for this condition (Scott *et al*. 1979) to more conservative massage, topical antibiotics, and systemic antibiotics if evidence of dacryocystitis develops (Levy 1979; Harris & DiClementi 1982).

Although meningocele must be considered in the differential diagnosis, the appearance is so classic that further investigation is unnecessary unless the condition is not resolved within a week or unless clinical findings progress. One helpful differentiating feature is the presence of pulsations with a meningocele on palpation.

Acute dacryocystitis

Acute dacryocystitis (Fig. 21.5) frequently accompanies nonpatent nasolacrimal systems since a stagnant system is present. Congenital acute dacryocystitis is very rare; the swelling usually represents a dacryocystocele. Infantile acute dacryocytitis requires systemic antibiotics, often systemic, in much the same way as preseptal cellulitis. Cultures should be taken if discharge can be expressed through the punctum. Probing should *not* be performed, since false passages can lead to orbital cellulitis. Similarly, incision should preferably not be made in the acute phase since fistularization can occur even though much of the inflammation takes place around rather than in the lacrimal sac. If a fluctuant mass remains after resolution of the acute phase, evacuation can be performed with a 19 gauge needle into the lower pole of the sac, lessening the chances of fistularization, and placing the potential fistula trait in the region where a dacryocystorhinostomy incision would be performed anyway. Once all signs of infection have been resolved, probing to establish patency should be performed.

Chronic dacryocystitis

Chronic dacryocystitis (Fig. 21.6) is more common. The nasolacrimal sac is enlarged but the child is comfortable. Rarely purulent discharge can be obtained. These patients require establishment of patency with a probing after attempted irrigation. If a spontaneous fistula has occurred, probing should be hastened to encourage the fistula to spontaneously close.

Canaliculitis

Canaliculitis in children is uncommon. Treatment involves cultures and antibiotics. Probing in the active phase is to be avoided.

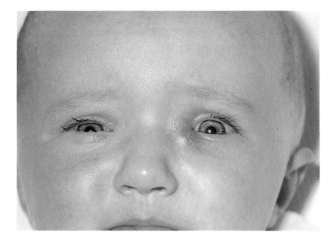

Fig. 21.6 Chronic recurrent dacryocystitis associated with nasolacrimal duct obstruction.

AIDS virus

Recent concern about the presence of AIDS (acquired immune deficiency syndrome) virus in bodily fluids including tears warrants mention since the incidence of neonatal AIDS is increasing. Babies can contract AIDS via maternal transmission as well as through breast milk. Documentation of AIDS transmission to a caretaker of a child has been made, presumably as a consequence of continual exposure to bodily secretions. Although it is highly unlikely that tears were the transmitting vector, it is sensible for the ophthalmologist to wash hands between cases and to be particularly cautious when examining a baby with AIDS (Fujikawa *et al.* 1986). One might also take special precautions such as gloving in procedures such as the examination of a neonate that is failing to thrive.

References

Billson FA, Taylor HR, Hoyt CS. Trauma to the lacrimal system in children. *Am J Ophthalmol* 1978; **86**: 828−33

Blanksma LJ, Pol BAE. Congenital fistulae of the lacrimal gland. *Br J Ophthalmol* 1980; **64**: 515−17

Brownstein S, Belin MW, Krohel GB, Smith RS, Condon G, Codere F. Orbital dacryops. *Ophthalmology* 1984; **91**: 1424−9

Cassady JV. Developmental anatomy of the nasolacrimal duct. *Arch Ophthalmology* 1952; **47**: 141−58

Chavis RM, Garner A, Wright JE. Inflammatory orbital pseudotumour. *Arch Ophthalmol* 1978; **96**: 1817−22

Chorobski J. Syndrome of crocodile tears. *Arch Neurol Psychiatr* 1951; **65**: 299−318

Crawford JA. Intubation of obstructions in the lacrimal system. *Can J Ophthalmol* 1977; **12**: 289−93

Crawford JA, Pashby RC. Lacrimal system disorders. *Int Ophthalmol Clin* 1984; **24**: 39−53

Dagher G, Anderson RL, Ossoinig KC, Baker JD. Adenoid cystic carcinoma of the lacrimal gland in a child. *Arch Ophthalmol* 1980; **98**: 1098−100

Duke−Elder S, Cook C. The lacrimal gland. In: Duke−Elder S (Ed.) *System of Ophthalmology*, Vol. III, part 1. Kimpton, London 1963; pp. 239−41

Duke−Elder S, MacFaul PA. The ocular adnexa. In: Duke−Elder S (Ed.) *System of Ophthalmology*, Vol. VIII, part 1. CV Mosby Co., St Louis 1974; pp. 605−10

Fujikawa L, Salahuddin S, Ablashi D *et al.* HTLV III in the tears of AIDS patients. *Ophthalmology* 1986; **93**: 1479−81

Goldberg MF, Payne JW, Brunt PW. Ophthalmologic studies of familial dysautonomia; the Riley-Day syndrome. *Arch Ophthalmol* 1968; **80**: 732−46

Green WR, Zimmerman LE. Ectopic lacrimal gland tissue: report of 8 cases with orbital involvement. *Arch Ophthalmol* 1967; **78**: 318−27

Harris GJ, DiClementi D. Congenital dacryocystocele. *Arch Ophthalmol* 1982; **100**: 1763−65

Jackson H, Lambert TD. Congenital mucocele of the lacrimal sac. *Br J Ophthalmol* 1963; **47**: 690−1

Jacobs L, Sirkin S, Kinkel W. Ectopic lacrimal gland in the orbit identified by computerized axial transverse tomography. *Ann Ophthalmol* 1977; **9**: 591−3

Kushner B. Congenital nasolacrimal system obstruction. *Arch Ophthalmol* 1982; **100**: 597−600

Lemp M, Blackman H. Physiology of tears. In: Milder B, Weil B (Eds.) *The Lacrimal System*. Appleton-Century-Crofts, Norwalk, Connecticut: 1983; pp. 49−62

Levy NS. Conservative management of congenital amniotocele of the nasolacrimal sac. *J Pediatr Ophthalmol Strabismus* 1979; **16**: 254−6

Mindin A, Lamberts D, Barsky D. Mixed lacrimal gland tumors arising from ectopic lacrimal gland tissue in the orbit. *J Pediatr Ophthalmol* 1977; **14**: 44−6

Mottow LS, Jakobiec FA. Idiopathic inflammatory orbital pseudotumour in childhood I Clinical characteristics. *Arch Ophthalmol* 1978; **96**: 1410−7

Mueller EC, Borit A. Aberrant lacrimal gland and pleomorphic adenoma within the muscle cone. *Ann Ophthalmol* 1979; **11**: 661−3

Mukherji R, Mukhopadhay SD. Congenital bilateral lacrimal and pre-auricular fistulas. *Am J Ophthalmol* 1972; **73**: 595−6

Muruko-del-Castillo J. Development of the lacrimal apparatus. In Milden B, Weil B (Eds.) *The Lacrimal System*. Appleton-Century-Crofts, Norwalk, Connecticut 1983; pp. 9−22

Nowinski TS, Flanagan JC, Mauriello J. Pediatric dacryocystorhinostomy. *Arch Ophthalmol* 1985; **103**: 1226−8

Patrick RK. Lacrimal secretions in full-term and premature babies. *Trans Ophthalmol Soc UK* 1974; **94**: 283−90

Ramsay J, Taylor D. Congenital crocodile tears: a key to the aetiology of Duane's syndrome. *Br J Ophthalmol* 1980; **64**: 518−22

Riffenburgh RS. Ocular manifestations of mumps. *Arch Ophthalmol* 1961; **66**: 739−43

Riley CM. Familial autonomic dysfunction. *J Am Med Assoc* 1952; **149**: 1532−5

Riley CM, Day RL, Greeley D, Langford WS. Central

autonomic dysfunction with defective lacrimation: I. Report of five cases. *Pediatrics* 1949; **3**: 468−78

Riley CM, Moore RH. Familial dysautonomia differentiated from related disorders. *Pediatrics* 1966; **37**: 435−46

Rush JA, Leone CR Jr. Ectopic lacrimal gland cyst of the orbit. *Am J Ophthalmol* 1981; **92**: 198−201

Schwarz M. Congenital atresia of the nasolacrimal canal. *Arch Ophthalmol* 1935; **13**: 301−2

Scott WE, Fabre JA, Ossoinig KC. Congenital mucocele of the lacrimal sac. *Arch Ophthalmol* 1979; **97**: 1656−8

Sevel D. Development and congenital abnormalities of the nasolacrimal apparatus. *J Pediatr Ophthalmol Strabismus* 1981; **18**: 13−19

Smith S, Rootman J. Clinical pathological review lacrimal ductal cysts. Presentation and management. *Surv Ophthalmol* 1986; **30**: 245−51

Werb A. The anatomy of the lacrimal system. In Milder B, Weil B (Eds.) *The Lacrimal System.* Appleton-Century-Crofts, Norwalk, Connecticut 1983; pp. 23−32

Wright JE. Factors affecting the survival of patients with lacrimal gland tumours. *Can J Ophthalmol* 1982; **17**: 3−9

Wright JE, William B, Krohel GB. Clinical presentation and management of lacrimal gland tumours. *Br J Ophthalmol* 1979; **63**: 600−6

22 Orbit

JOHN BRAZIER AND ANTHONY MOORE

22.1 Orbital Disease in Children

ANTHONY MOORE AND JOHN BRAZIER

Table 22.1.1 Proptosis in the neonate.

Unilateral	Bilateral
Encephalocele	Craniofacial dysostoses
Congenital cystic eye	Neuroblastoma
Microphthalmos with cyst	
Dermoid cyst	
Haemangioma	
Lymphangioma	
Juvenile xanthogranuloma	
Teratoma	
Optic nerve glioma	
Neurofibroma	
Rhabdomyosarcoma	
Neuroblastoma	

Abnormalities of the orbit in childhood occur either as a developmental defect or are acquired as a result of orbital disease. Developmental abnormalities may be confined to the orbit or may be part of a more widespread craniofacial malformation; the orbit may be smaller than normal, may be shallow (resulting in proptosis) or the relationship between the two orbits may be disturbed. In hypertelorism the orbits are widely separated whilst in the opposite condition (hypotelorism) they are closely set. Part of the orbital walls may be deficient at birth allowing intracranial tissue to prolapse into the orbit resulting in pulsating exophthalmos. The orbit continues to develop throughout childhood but radiotherapy, for example in the treatment of orbital rhabdomyosarcoma, or enucleation of the globe may result in a failure of the orbit to grow normally on the affected side.

Rarely proptosis may be present at birth or in the early neonatal period; the main causes of orbital disease in this young age group are set out in Table 22.1.1.

Acquired orbital disease usually presents with proptosis, reduced vision, restriction of ocular movements or a combination of all three. Less commonly enophthalmos may develop following orbital trauma. Proptosis is the commonest presenting sign and is due to the presence of abnormal material, tumour, blood, or inflammatory tissue within the orbit, or may be due to oedema or infiltration of the extraocular muscles as in dysthyroid eye disease.

Aetiology

The relative frequencies of the conditions causing proptosis in childhood vary in different series (Porterfield 1962; MacCarty & Brown 1964; Youseffi 1969; Templeton 1971; Eldrup Jorgannsenn & Fledelius 1975; Crawford 1983; Shields et al. 1986) mainly due to differences in the source of the material. Series from eye hospitals (Youseffi 1969) show significant differences from those from neurosurgical (MacCarty 1964) or paediatric units (Crawford 1983). Geographical factors are also important; the major causes of proptosis in African children (Templeton 1971) for example are quite different from those seen in Europe and North America (Youseffi 1969; Crawford 1983). Some series (Porterfield 1962; Edrup Jorgannsenn & Fledelius 1975; Shields 1986) have relied solely on histopathological examination of biopsy specimens. Although such series give a clear indication of the commonest lesions encountered surgically they are not representative of the aetiology of the child who presents clinically with proptosis. Histopathological studies will tend to underestimate conditions such as dysthyroid eye disease, orbital cellulitis, and capillary haemangioma where the diagnosis is made clinically and in which conservative treatment is possible. Also orbital biopsies are often not performed in metastatic or multifocal disease such as neuroblastoma or Langerhans' cell histiocytosis where it is often more convenient to biopsy another peripheral site.

The most extensive and representative series is that of Crawford (Crawford 1983) who reviewed 585 cases of proptosis seen at a large children's hospital (Table 21.1.2). It is clear from this series that orbital tumours are an uncommon cause of proptosis; representing only 16% of the total number of cases in this study. Surprisingly this is also true of histopathologic studies; for example in the study by Shields (1986) only 6% of all specimens were primary malignant tumours of the orbit (Table 21.1.3). The study of Youseffi (1969) gives a representative breakdown of the relative frequencies of benign and malignant orbital tumours encountered surgically in childhood (Table 21.1.4).

Table 22.1.2 Diagnosis in 585 cases of proptosis. Reproduced with permission from Crawford (1983).

Developmental	50
Inflammatory	237
Metabolic disorders and general disease	133
Hyperthyroidism	107
Histiocytosis X	20
Fibrous dysplasia	4
Caffey's disease	1
Osteopetrosis	1
Neoplastic	98
Benign	40
Malignant	
Primary	16
Secondary	40
Vascular	53
Miscellaneous	1
Unknown	13

Table 22.1.3 Types of lesion seen in 250 orbital biopsies in children. From Shields *et al.* (1986).

Cystic	52.0%
Inflammatory	16.4%
Adipose containing	6.8%
Vascular	6.8%
Rhabdomyosarcoma	4.0%
Retinoblastoma	3.6%
Lacrimal Gland	2.4%
Lymphoid/leukaemias	2.4%
Optic nerve/meningeal	2.4%
Peripheral nerve tumours	1.6%
Osseous/cartilaginous	1.2%
Histiocytic	0.4%

Table 22.1.4 Incidence of orbital tumours in 62 children. From Youseffi (1969).

Dermoid cyst	46.7%
Haemangioma	14.5%
Neuroblastoma	9.6%
Rhabdomyosarcoma	3.2%
Sebaceous cyst	3.2%
Dermolipoma	3.2%
Pseudotumour	3.2%
Optic nerve glioma	1.6%
Meningioma	1.6%
Fibrous dysplasia	1.6%
Others	11.6%

Clinical assessment

In the assessment of the child with proptosis it is important to take a careful history and carry out a full examination before investigations can be logically planned. The age of onset, whether unilateral or bilateral and the rate at which the proptosis developed are very important. Bilateral proptosis in early infancy is likely to be due to shallow orbits associated with a craniofacial malformation. Unilateral proptosis in childhood is almost invariably due to the globe being pushed forward by a mass within the orbit. Benign tumours such as haemangioma or dermoid cyst grow very slowly whereas rapid onset of proptosis suggests a metastatic deposit or a rapidly growing tumour such as rhabdomyosarcoma. Rapid growth is often associated with tumour necrosis resulting in periorbital ecchymosis and when this sign is present bilaterally it usually indicates orbital deposits in neuroblastoma. Rapid onset of proptosis is also seen in orbital cellulitis but there is usually associated pain and marked limitation of ocular motility in a child who is generally ill and febrile.

The site of any orbital mass may be indicated by the direction in which the eye is pushed forward. A posterior tumour will generally result in axial proptosis whereas a more anteriorly placed tumour may displace the eye vertically or laterally. For example, in fibrous dysplasia of the orbit which typically affects the frontal bone, the globe is usually displaced downwards and forwards. Proptosis which increases on straining or coughing suggests a vascular tumour, whereas pulsating exophthalmos may be associated with defects of the orbital wall or encephalocele. Refraction is essential because astigmatism associated with orbital tumour is an important cause of amblyopia (Bogan *et al.* 1987).

In the examination of the child with proptosis it is important to assess the visual acuity and in infants, where formal visual assessment is not possible, to look for any differences in fixation between the two eyes. Assessment of the pupillary reactions may provide additional information; the presence of a relative afferent pupil defect may be an early sign of optic nerve compression. The degree of proptosis should be measured using an exophthalmometer and any vertical or lateral displacement assessed using a transparent ruler. A cover test should be performed to ensure that any apparent non-axial proptosis is not due to an associated strabismus. Ocular movements should be carefully assessed and the presence of any lid retraction or lid lag, which may indicate dysthyroid eye disease, noted. Limitation of ocular motility may be due to mechanical restriction by tumour, muscle infiltration, oedema or entrapment or to involvement of the III, IV, or VIth cranial nerves within the orbit. Fundus examination may show optic disc swelling or atrophy in cases of optic nerve compression and in the case of a mass close behind the globe, choroidal folds may be evident.

A systemic evaluation may give useful clues to the diagnosis. Café au lait spots may suggest a diagnosis of neurofibromatosis and similar skin pigmentation may also be seen in fibrous dysplasia. Skin lesions may also be present in Langerhans' cell histiocytosis and juvenile xanthogranuloma and in capillary haemangioma of the orbit there are often other haemangioma elsewhere on the skin. In suspected metastatic disease there may be other involved sites such as an abdominal mass in neuroblastoma or skin, scalp or bony lesions in Langerhans' cell histiocytosis.

In dysthyroid eye disease there will often be other systemic signs which help suggest the diagnosis. In the child with unexplained proptosis it is helpful to obtain opinions from other specialities, in particular from general paediatricians and ENT specialists who may be able to help with confirming the diagnosis.

Investigation

Investigation of the child with proptosis should be guided by the history and clinical findings so that the approach is tailored to each individual case, a similar blanket investigation of all cases should be avoided. In some children where there are other abnormalities, for example the craniofacial malformations, the cause of the proptosis is apparent without the need for extensive investigations. In others further tests will be necessary to confirm the suspected diagnosis or to judge the extent of orbital involvement. In planning the investigation of such children, especially those that may need systemic chemotherapy or sinus or intracranial procedures, it is essential to work closely with other specialists such as paediatricians, ENT surgeons and neurosurgeons from the outset.

Radiological investigations

PLAIN X-RAYS

Although CT scan is the initial radiological investigation in most cases of proptosis, the findings on plain X-ray may allow a definitive diagnosis to be made or may suggest the appropriate next investigation. The finding of a large orbit on the affected side for example suggests that the proptosis is due to a longstanding slow growing benign tumour. In suspected orbital cellulitis the presence of an opaque ethmoid sinus will help confirm the diagnosis. Some of the helpful radiological signs seen on plain X-ray of the orbit are detailed in Table 21.1.5. Plain X-rays are also of value in the evaluation of orbital trauma, including orbital fractures and suspected intraorbital foreign bodies.

Plain X-rays of the orbit are readily obtained and still indicated to evaluate bone quality (Table 21.1.5) (density, erosion, absence) and orbital size. However, the diagnostic yield per unit of radiation exposure is much lower than with CT (Weiss 1984). Optic nerve size is better evaluated directedly by CT than indirectly by plain optic foramen views.

CT AND MRI SCANNING

Diagnostic imaging of orbital structures was revolutionized by the development of computerized tomography (CT) in the early 1970s (Ambrose et al. 1974; Gawler et al. 1974). CT is at present the investigation of choice in the majority of cases because of a proven ability to demonstrate and distinguish causes of proptosis with accuracy and relatively low risk (Lloyd 1977). CT will provide information about intracranial as well as orbital structures and is relatively non-invasive when intravenous contrast is not used. Differential diagnostic yield is increased by use of contrast in selected cases (Moseley & Sanders 1982). Children may require sedation or general anaesthesia to allow CT to be performed without loss of image quality due to movement artefact.

A further advance in the level of anatomical detail in orbital images is offered by the development of magnetic resonance imaging (MRI) (Moseley et al. 1983; Savino 1987), particularly with use of higher

Table 22.1.5 Abnormalities on plain X-ray.

Small orbit
Enucleation in early childhood
Radiotherapy
Anophthalmos
Microphthalmos

Large orbit
Haemangioma
Lymphangioma
Orbital varices
Neurofibromatosis
Meningoencephalocele

Small optic canal
Fibrous dysplasia
Osteopetrosis

Large optic canal
Optic nerve glioma
Neurofibromatosis

Opaque sinus
Orbital cellulitis
Sinus mucocele

Lytic lesion of orbital wall
Langerhans' cell histiocytosis
Leukaemia
Neuroblastoma
Ewing's sarcoma
Fibrous dysplasia

Orbital calcification
Orbital varices
Haemangioma
Dermoid cyst
Retinoblastoma

magnetic fields (1.5 tesla) and surface coils for recording (Bilaniuk *et al.* 1985; Zimmerman *et al.* 1985; Savino 1988). Present problems with MRI include long scanning time (with consequent relative increase in movement artefact) and lack of the ability possesed by CT to reformat images acquired in one plane into another plane. A more specific problem of MRI for orbital work is the relative inability to image bone and calcification (Leib & Kates 1988). A great advantage is the absence of ionising radiation, sometimes a limiting factor when serial or repeated CT scans are required (Moseley 1983). In children, a disadvantage of MRI scanning is that, because of the need to use ferrous materials, a general anaesthetic is difficult to administer.

ULTRASONOGRAPHY

Ultrasonography is a useful adjunct to CT scan in the investigation of soft tissue abnormalities of the orbit. It is relatively inexpensive, painless and has no side effects. It can be used in both A-scan and B-scan modes, and real-time studies may also be helpful.

The usefulness of ultrasound in orbital diagnosis is limited by poor imaging of the orbital apex and lesions involving bone (Char & Norman 1982). It is, however, non-invasive so it retains a role in some centres in investigation of anterior and mid-orbital disease.

References

Ambrose JAE, Lloyd GAS, Wright JE. A preliminary evaluation of fine matrix computerized axial tomography (EMI-scan) in the diagnosis of orbital space-occupying lesions. *Br J Radiol* 1974; **47**: 747−51

Bilaniuk LT, Schenk JF, Zimmerman RA *et al.* Ocular and orbital lesions: surface coil MR imaging. *Radiology* 1985; **156**: 669−74

Bogan S, Simon JW, Krohel GB, Nelson LB. Astigmatism associated with adnexal masses in infancy. *Arch Ophthalmol* 1987; **105**: 1368−70

Char DH, Norman D. The use of computed tomography and ultrasonography in the evaluation of orbital masses. *Surv Ophthalmol* 1982; **27**: 49−63

Crawford JS. In: Crawford JS, Morin JD (Eds.) Diseases of the Orbit. In: *The Eye in Childhood*. Grune & Stratton, New York 1983; pp. 361−94

Edrup−Jorgensen P, Feidelius H. Orbital tumours in infancy: an analysis of Danish cases from 1943−1962. *Acta Ophthalmol* 1975; **53**: 887−96

Gawler J, Sanders MD, Bull JWD, de Boulay G, Marshall J. Computer assisted tomography in orbital disease. *Br J Ophthalmol* 1974; **58**: 571−87

Leib ML, Kates MR. Orbital computer-assisted tomography. In: Lessel S, Van Dalen JTW (Eds.) *Current Neuro-ophthalmology*, Vol. 1. Year Book Medical Publishers, Chicago 1988; Chapter 20

Lloyd GAS. The impact of CT scanning and ultrasonography on orbital diagnosis. *Clin Radiol* 1977; **28**: 583

MacCarty CS, Brown DN. Orbital tumours in children. *Clin Neurosurg* 1964; **11**: 76−84

Moseley I, Brant−Zadawski M, Mills C. Nuclear magnetic resonance imaging of the orbit. *Br J Ophthalmol* 1983; **67**: 333−42

Moseley IF, Sanders MD. *Computerized Tomography in Neuro-ophthalmology*. Chapman & Hall, London 1982.

Porterfield JF. Orbital tumours in children: a report on 214 cases. *Int Ophthalmol Clin* 1962; **2**: 319−26

Savino PJ. The present role of magnetic resonance imaging in neuro-ophthalmology. *Can J Ophthalmol* 1987; **22**: 4−12

Savino PJ. The orbit. In: Lessell S, Van Dalen JTW (eds.) *Current Neuro-ophthalmology*, Vol. 1. Year Book Medical Publishers, Chicago 1988

Shields JA, Bakewell B, Augsburger JJ, Donso L, Bernardino

V. Space occupying orbital masses in children. A review of 250 consecutive biopsies. *Ophthalmology* 1986; **93**: 379–84

Templeton AC. Orbital tumours in African children. *Br J Ophthalmol* 1971; **55**: 254–61

Weiss RA, Haik BG, Smith ME. Introduction to diagnostic imaging techniques in ophthalmology. *Int Ophthalmol Clin* 1986; **26** (Fall): 1–24

Youseffi B. Orbital tumours in children: a clinical study of 62 cases. *J Pediatr Ophthalmol Strabismus* 1969; **6**: 177–81

Zimmerman RA, Bilaniuk LT, Yanoff M *et al*. Orbital magnetic resonance imaging. *Am J Ophthalmol* 1985; **100**: 312–7

22.2 Craniofacial Abnormalities

JOHN BRAZIER

Congenital anomalies of the skull and face require a co-ordinated management approach from paediatrician, ophthalmologist, plastic surgeon, and neurosurgeon to best help the visual, intellectual, and cosmetic problems of affected children. Disorders considered in this section fall into two main groups; the craniosynostosis syndromes, including Crouzon's and Apert's diseases, and the mandibulofacial dysostoses, including Treacher-Collins' and Goldenhar's syndromes.

Craniosynostosis syndromes

Pathogenesis

These congenital disorders affect predominantly the bony development of the cranium and upper face. The common anomaly in these linked conditions is a failure in development of the primitive mesoderm from which the skull bones develop (Duke–Elder 1964). In addition to abnormalities of the bones themselves there is premature closure of one or more sutures which limits skull growth in the direction perpendicular to the suture. When skull growth in certain directions is arrested in this way, compensatory growth occurs in the unrestricted direction(s) to minimize the compressive effect on the growing brain. When brain growth exceeds growth of the skull, intracranial hypertension results. Affected children may have symptoms of headache and vomiting with evidence of papilloedema.

Classification

A variety of deformities occur, depending on the sutures involved (Fig. 22.2.1) and extent of involvement. Classification is difficult as most terms are descriptions of the head shape resulting from deformity. Some terms are used interchangeably. Classification of craniosynostosis was reviewed by Howell (1954), Blodi (1957), Duke–Elder (1964), and, more recently, Marchac and Renier (1982). The classification offered here combines elements from these reports.

In normal development, the skull expands during growth in vertical, anteroposterior and lateral directions. Reduction of growth in one or more directions produces a typical skull shape.

Growth restricted in anteroposterior and lateral directions

This gives rise to a vertically elongated head, a deformity usually called oxycephaly (pointed head). The forehead slopes back in continuity with the dorsum of the nose. This deformity may only become evident in childhood, usually after the age of three years. When the anteroposterior shortening is more marked the term acrocephaly (peaked head) may be applied.

Growth restricted in anteroposterior direction

This causes shortening of the skull and base in the anteroposterior dimension and is called brachycephaly (short head). The most striking cases of anteropos-

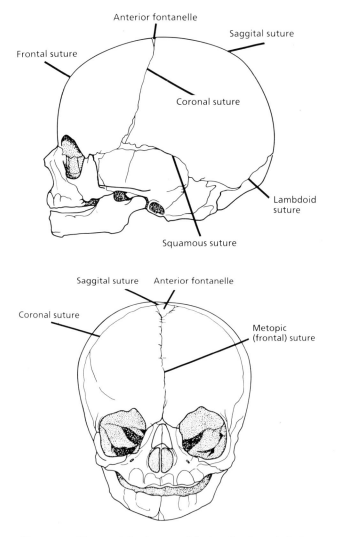

Fig. 22.2.1 The cranial sutures and fontanelles in an infant skull.

terior shortening are those associated with Crouzon's and Apert's diseases. The superior forehead tends to bulge in the newborn and infant, becoming vertical later. The skull is excessively wide to compensate for lack of anteroposterior growth resulting from premature fusion of the coronal suture. When the skull is excessively high as well as short the term turricephaly (turret head) can be applied.

Growth restricted in lateral direction

This causes the skull to become long and narrow — scaphocephaly (boat head).

In addition to these three broad groups, two further types warrant mention to complete the classification.

Trigonocephaly (triangular head)

These are distinguished by a triangular shaped forehead and result from premature closure of the metopic suture.

Plagiocephaly (slanting head)

An asymmetrical deformity due to premature closure of the coronal suture on one side. The forehead is flattened on the affected side and associated with asymmetry of the skull and face.

Common ophthalmic features in craniosynostosis syndromes

In the description of conditions which follows, it will be observed that a number of ophthalmic problems are shared by the different diagnostic groups. These common ophthalmic features, visual failure, proptosis, strabismus, and hypertelorism, are considered in this section.

Visual failure

Visual failure due to optic atrophy is a relatively common finding. Views differ on the pathogenesis of optic nerve damage and it seems that different factors may be involved. Undoubtedly many cases have optic atrophy secondary to raised intracranial pressure and papilloedema (Howell 1954; Tessier 1971; Archer *et al.* 1974; Marchac & Renier 1982; Renier *et al.* 1982). These cases are potentially salvageable by timely intervention to allow skull expansion with consequent reduction of intracranial pressure (Archer 1974). Kinking and stretching of the optic nerves due to abnormal skull and brain development may be responsible for primary optic atrophy in some cases (Howell 1954; Blodi 1957; Duke−Elder 1964), whilst narrow optic canals have been blamed in other cases (Howell 1954; Blodi 1957; Tessier 1971).

In a series of 244 patients with craniosynostosis syndromes, Dufier *et al.* (1986) observed that the incidence of optic nerve involvement varied with the type of deformity. Optic discs were considered either pale or atrophic in 50% of Crouzon's disease, 34% oxycephaly and 24% Apert's disease. Disc swelling was observed at some stage in assessment in 31% Crouzon's disease, 23% oxycephaly and 9.5% Apert's disease.

Proptosis

The proptosed appearance in these patients is due to two factors; shallow orbits and maxillary hypoplasia (especially in Crouzon's disease) with a lowered and relatively posterior origin of the lower lid making sclera visible between the inferior limbus and lid in the primary position. In their review, Dufier *et al.* (1986) carefully call this appearance pseudoexophthalmos, arguing that the proptosis is due to retrusion of the face rather than increased volume of orbital contents. Measurements of exophthalmos in these patients did not exceed a mean of 20 mm with the Hertel exophthalmometer in any patient group, indicating that the proptosis is apparent rather than real.

The shallow orbit and lid position make lagophthalmos, and consequent corneal exposure, a problem in some patients. Rarely, the globe is liable to spontaneously subluxate outside the lids (Blodi 1957; Duke–Elder 1964).

Strabismus

Dufier *et al.* (1986) reviewed 200 patients in seven craniofacial groups who had been examined for squint; and of these, 36.5% had squints. Convergent deviation is more likely in Apert's disease; divergence in Crouzon's disease, and about equal convergent/divergent deviations in isolated oxycephaly. Out of 21 patients suffering from Apert's disease, 24% also had vertical deviations. In unilateral coronal suture stenosis (plagiocephaly) there is often an associated superior oblique palsy on the affected side possibly related to shortening of the orbital roof (Bagolini *et al.* 1982.)

A number of explanations for the strabismus are offered, (Dufier *et al.* 1986) including divergent line of the orbital axes, short anteroposterior orbital dimensions, and hypertelorism. All these factors were considered to favour development of exodeviations. Treatment of the squints is made more difficult by presence of optic atrophy or amblyopia. In addition there may be anomalies of the extraocular muscles, explaining in part the motility problems but making squint surgery more difficult (Wienstock & Hardesty 1965; Dufier 1986 *et al.*).

Hypertelorism

This is a discriptive term applied to the craniofacial deformity characterized by wide separation of the orbits. Hypertelorism occurred in 45% of the patients reviewed by Dufier *et al.* (1986). Normal ranges for interorbital distances were taken from Johr (1953). Hypotelorism (abnormal proximity of the orbit) was a common feature of trigonocephaly but none of the other groups reported.

Description of conditions

Ophthalmic complications are likely in oxycephaly, Crouzon's and Apert's diseases; these conditions are outlined in this section. Pfeiffer's syndrome, a condition similar to Apert's disease, is also mentioned. Hypertelorism is also described.

OXYCEPHALY (Fig. 22.2.2)

Clinically this condition is characterized by high, narrow, pointed, or dome-shaped configuration of skull; the anteroposterior and lateral measurements being decreased and the vertical increased (Mann 1957). The forehead is high, the eyes wide apart and apparently proptosed (orbits being shallow), the superciliary ridges poorly developed. There is superior prognathism (François 1975) and the palatal arch is high and narrow. The deformity results from premature synostosis of all the skull sutures, particularly the coronal suture.

Shallowing of the orbits is the result of medial and forward displacement of the great wing of the sphenoid and to a lesser extent the vertical orientation of the orbital plate of the frontal bone. The orbital roof is thus almost vertical, continuing the line of the forehead (Duke–Elder 1964).

Intracranial hypertension is frequent in oxycephaly (Marchac & Renier 1982) and the troubles resulting from it (visual failure, headache and vomiting) may lead to clinical presentation. Skull X-ray may show marked digital impression reflecting chronically elevated intracranial pressure. Mental ability of patients is related to the intracranial pressure, being poorer when the pressure is highest (Renier *et al.* 1982). Occasionally there is a history of convulsions in infancy (Mann 1957) and the EEG may be abnormal (Blodi 1957).

Ocular problems are secondary to the bony deformity. They tend to become evident in the 2 to 5-year-old age group. Ophthalmic features include visual failure, proptosis, strabismus, restricted eye movements, and nystagmus.

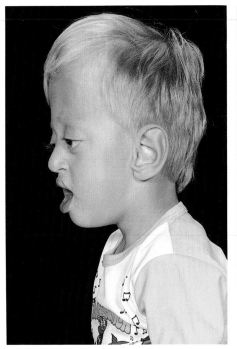

(a)

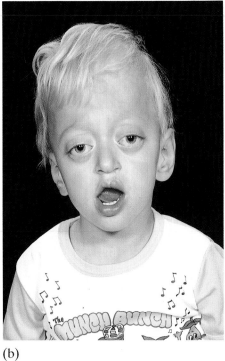

(b)

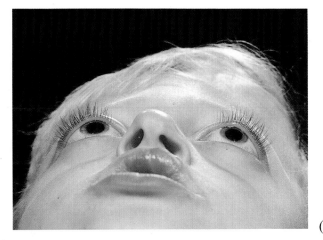

(c)

Fig. 22.2.2 (a–c) Oxycephaly showing the high narrow skull with increased height of the skull, shallow orbits, superior prognathism, and poorly developed superciliary ridges. (d,e) Oxycephaly. Showing papilloedema secondary to craniosynostosis. Marked papilloedema may be an indication for early craniectomy. (Same patients as a–c.)

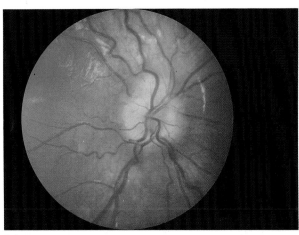

(d)

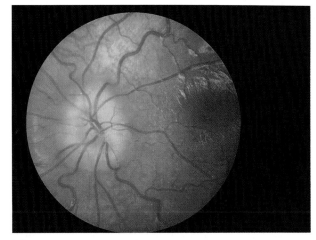

(e)

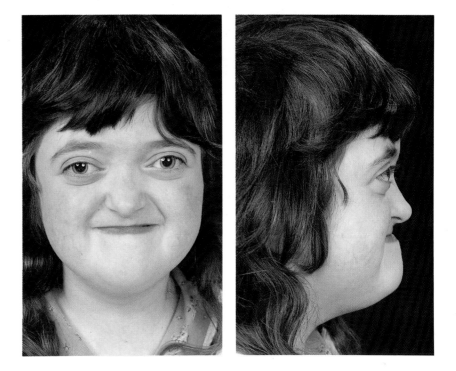

Fig. 22.2.3 Crouzon's disease. This girl has the features of inferior prognathism, maxillary hypoplasia, and a prominent forehead, her nose is quite straight — it often is more 'hooked' in this condition.

CROUZON'S DISEASE (Fig. 22.2.3)

This developmental cranial deformity was described by Crouzon (1912) and has special characteristics. Premature fusion of the cranial sutures gives rise to acrocephaly or scaphocephaly, but there is also a marked abnormality of the face. The forehead is prominent, maxillae hypoplastic and the nose hooked, resembling a parrot's beak (Duke−Elder 1964). Atresia of the nostrils may occur. There is inferior prognathism with an arched palate and the mouth characteristically held half open (François 1975). Again, the orbits are shallow, causing a proptosed appearance, and widely spaced. Other findings include corneal exposure, divergent squint and nystagmus where visual failure occurs early. Other associations include iris coloboma, aniridia, corectopia, micro or megalocornea, cataract, ectopia lentis, blue sclera and glaucoma.

Associated abnormalities include deafness, epilepsy and delayed mental development. Inheritance is autosomal dominant with high penetrance and variable expressivity.

ACROCEPHALOSYNDACTYLY

The association of acrocephaly (brachycephaly) with syndactyly occurs in a group of disorders known as acrocephalosyndactyly. Of the five recognized types (Tentamy & McKusick 1969) Apert's disease (type I) and Pfeiffer's syndrome (type V) are the most common.

Apert's disease (Fig. 22.2.4, 22.2.5)

This condition is closely allied to Crouzon's disease and is characterized by craniosynostosis and syndactyly of hands and feet involving the second to fifth digits. Involvement of the skull sutures is variable but the coronal suture is usually involved. The facial appearance is fairly typical with hypoplasia of the middle third of the face and protusion of the lower jaw. The palate is high arched and the mouth held half open.

Ophthalmic features usually include proptosis, antimongoloid slant of the palpebral fissures, hypertelorism and usually strabismus.

There may be optic atrophy, keratoconus, ectopia lentis, congenital glaucoma, lack of pigment in the fundus, and subluxation of the globes (Collin 1983). Transmission is by autosomal dominant inheritance most cases arising from a fresh mutation made more likely by increased paternal age.

Pfeiffer's syndrome (Fig. 22.2.6)

This disorder is characterized by acrocephaly, mild syndactyly, and characteristic broad short thumbs

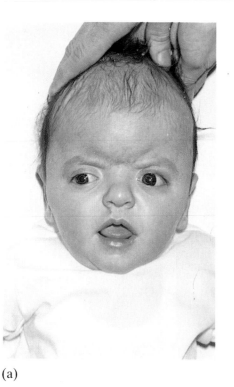

(a)

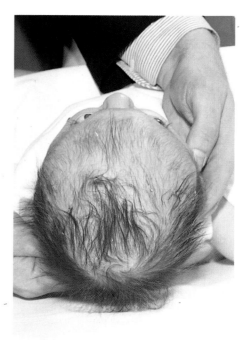

(b)

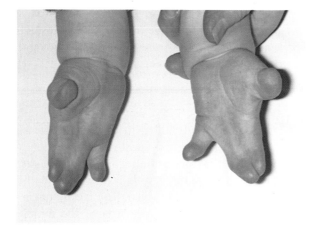

(c)

Fig. 22.2.4 (a,b) Apert's syndrome showing the shallow orbits, strabismus, open mouth with maxillary hypoplasia. (c) Apert's syndrome. The syndactyly usually affects the second to fifth digits of hands and feet.

and great toes. Other characteristics are similar to Apert's disease. Transmission is autosomal dominant with complete penetrance but variable expressivity (Goodman 1977).

HYPERTELORISM

This is a descriptive term introduced by Greig to designate a condition in which the two eyes and orbits are widely separated. It may be difficult to distinguish the point at which wide orbital separation ceases to be a normal variant (morphogenetic hypertelorism) and

becomes a condition determined by anomalous development of the face and head, as described by Greig (embryonic hypertelorism). The latter condition involves characteristic broadening of the nasal bridge with a prominent forehead. The orbits are widely displaced with frequently divergent squint. Visual function is usually good. François (1975) considered transmission to be either dominant (mild form) or recessive (pronounced form).

Assessment of hypertelorism should not overlook the possibility that the orbital displacement reflects some other disorder such as meningocele, encepha-

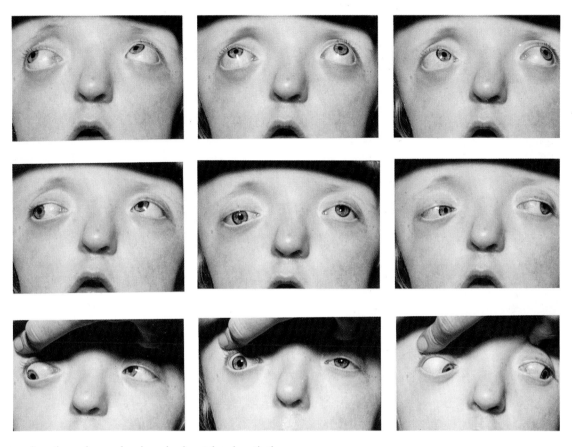

Fig. 22.2.5 Apert's syndrome showing a horizontal and vertical squint which may be associated with anomalies or absence of vertical muscles. A 'V' esotropia is most common in Apert's syndrome (Dufier *et al.* 1986).

locele, or previous trauma. Hypertelorism may be associated with facial cleft (Tessier 1971; Collin 1983).

CLOVERLEAF SKULL (Fig. 22.2.7)

There is a great deal of variation in the expression of the dominant genes of Crouzon's, Carpenter's, and Pfeiffer's syndromes and at their most marked these may present as Cloverleaf skull syndrome (Kleeblattschaedel) (Cohen 1973). It may also occur sporadically and a variety of minor forms occur.

The skull has a flat, trilobed appearance given by synostosis of the coronal and lambdoid sutures (Fig. 22.2.1) — hence the term cloverleaf. Hydrocephalus may be associated and the life expectancy is limited. The orbits are extremely shallow and proptosis with globe subluxation and repeated corneal damage may occur (Walters *et al.* 1973). The definitive treatment of the subluxation is by frontal bone advancement but reposition of the globes followed by a medial

and lateral tarsorraphy may be necessary urgently together with treatment of the corneal ulceration.

Treatment

As mentioned earlier, a multidisciplinary approach to treatment is required. Aims of treatment are to allow brain growth by enlarging the intracranial space (this may be required urgently if the ophthalmologist detects increasing disc swelling), improvement of cosmesis and ophthalmic treatment for complications such as corneal exposure and strabismus.

Surgical approaches to the skull include decompressive osteotomy when intracranial pressure is raised early in life and, later, combined craniofacial techniques as described by Tessier (1971) involving advancement of the forehead, orbital margins, nose and maxillae. This approach may allow alleviation of restricted intracranial space and cosmetic aspects in a single procedure. Squint surgery is best delayed until after craniofacial surgery as alteration of the orbital axes may have a beneficial effect, reducing the degree of extraocular muscle surgery required.

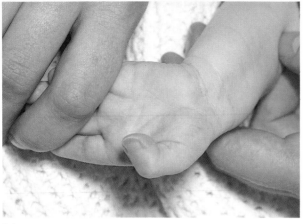

(a)

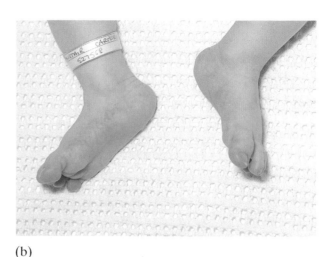

(b)

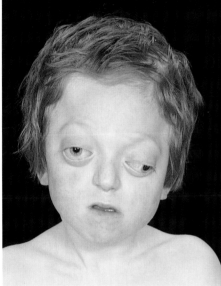

(c)

Fig. 22.2.6 (a,b) Pfeiffer's syndrome showing broad thumb and great toes. (c) Pfeiffer's syndrome showing acrocephaly and hypertelorism (same patient as a,b).

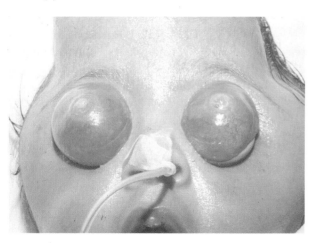

Fig. 22.2.7 Cloverleaf skull with trilobed flattened skull appearance, subluxated globes, exposure keratitis, and chemotic conjunctiva.

Mandibulofacial dysostoses

This term was used by François (1975) to group together a number of congenital disorders of the face due primarily to retarded differentiation of mesoderm derived from the first branchial arch. The two syndromes most frequently encountered are those of Treacher—Collins and Goldenhar.

Treacher—Collins' syndrome

This syndrome was described by Treacher—Collins in 1900 but is also associated with the names of Franceschetti and Zwahlen who made a detailed description in 1944. Transmission is by autosomal

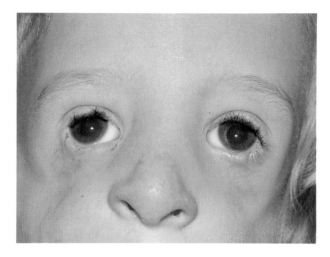

Fig. 22.2.8 Treacher—Collins' syndrome. These patients may have marked malar hypoplasia, an anti-mongoloid slant to the palpebral fissures, and lower lid colobomata together with mandibular hypoplasia and macrostomia. Ear malformations occur and middle and inner ear anomalies may impair hearing.

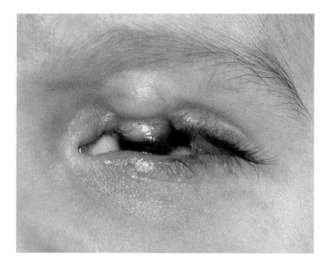

Fig. 22.2.9 Goldenhar's syndrome. This child had preauricular appendages, cardiac disease and hydrocephalus. The left eye has multiple subconjunctival and corneal dermoids and a lid coloboma with a dermoid in the upper lid. The dermoids were excised by lamellar keratectomy, but the residual astigmatism and amblyopia resulted in poor acuity. The right eye had a small limbal dermoid and good acuity.

dominant inheritance with complete penetrance but variable expressivity.

Malformations of the upper face include malar hypoplasia, often with absence of the zygomatic arch, antimongoloid slant of the palpebral fissures and coloboma of the outer third of the lower lid. Absence

of the nasofrontal angle gives a bird or fish-like profile. Malformations of the lower face include hypoplasia of the lower jaw with macrostomia and abnormal dentition. The external ear is malformed and there may be associated middle or inner ear abnormalities. There are often accessory auricular appendages and blind fistulae between the angles of the mouth and ears.

Treatment involves plastic repair of the lid colobomata and, where considered appropriate, surgery to correct the underdevelopment of the zygoma, maxillae and mandible by bone or cartilage grafts (Tulasne & Tessier 1986). Hearing problems also require attention.

Goldenhar's syndrome

The oculoauricular dysostosis of Goldenhar is characterized by epibulbar dermoids or lipodermoids (conjunctiva or cornea) and by preauricular appendages, usually anterior to the tragus, with or without fistulae to the ear. Vertebral anomalies are often associated, and cardiac or pulmonary abnormalities are common. The mode of inheritance is not clearly defined.

Other ophthalmic findings may include microphthalmos, ocular colobomata and coloboma of the eyelid, usually the middle third of the upper lid.

The syndrome shares a number of features with the Treacher—Collins' syndrome, and combinations of the two syndromes have been reported (Goldenhar 1952; François 1975).

References

Archer DB, Gordon DS, Maguire CJF, Glendhill CA. Ophthalmic aspects of craniosynostosis. *Trans Ophthalmol Soc UK* 1974; **94**: 172—96

Bagolini B, Campos E, Chiesi C. Plagiocephaly causing superior oblique deficiency and ocular torticollis. *Arch Ophthalmol* 1982; **100**: 1093—6

Blodi FC. Developmental abnormalities of the skull affecting the eye. *Arch Ophthalmol* 1957; **57**: 593—610

Cohen MM. An etiologic and nosologic overview of the craniosynostosis syndromes. *Birth Defects*, Original Articles Series 1973; **11**: 137—89

Collin R. The craniofacial dysostoses. In: Wybar K, Taylor D (Eds.) *Pediatric Ophthalmology Current Aspects.* Marcel Dekker, New York 1983

Crouzon MO. Dysostose cranio-faciale héréditaire. *Bull Soc Méd Hôp Paris* 1912; **33**: 545—55

Dufier JL, Vinurel MC, Renier D, Marchac D. Les complications ophthalmologiques des crâniofaciosténoses. A propos de 244 observations. *J Fr Ophtalmol* 1986; **9**: 273—80

Duke—Elder S. Normal and abnormal development. Congenital deformities. In: Duke–Elder S (Ed.) *System of Ophthalmology*, Vol. III. Part 2. Henry Kimpton, London 1964; pp. 1037–57

François J. Heredity of the craniofacial dysostoses. *Mod Probl Ophthalmol* 1975; **14**: 5–48

Goldenhar M. Associations malformatives de l'oeil et de l'oreille; en particulier le syndrome dermöide epibulbaire — appendices auriculaires — fistula auris congenita et ses relations avec la dysostose mandibulo — faciale. *J Genet Hum* 1953; **1**: 243

Goodman RM. *Atlas of the Eye in Genetic Disorders*. CV Mosby Co, St Louis 1977; 182

Howell SC. The craniostenoses. *Am J Ophthalmol* 1954; **37**: 359–79

Johr P. Valeurs moyennes et limites normales en fonction de l'âge, de quelques mesures de la tête et de a région orbitaire. *J Genet Hum* 1953; **2**: 247–82

Mann I. *Developmental Abnormalities of the Eye*. British Medical Association, London, 1957

Marchac D, Renier D. *Craniofacial Surgery for Craniosynostosis*. Little, Brown & Co, Boston 1982

Renier D, Sainte–Rose C, Marchac D, Hirsch J-F. Intracranial pressure in craniostenosis. *J Neurosurg* 1982; **57**: 370–37

Temtamy S, McKusick V. Synopsis of hand malformations with particular emphasis on genetic factors. *Birth Defects* 1969; **5**: 125–85

Tessier P. The definitive plastic surgical treatment of the severe facial deformities of craniofacial dysostosis. *Plast Reconstr Surg* 1971; **48**: 419–42

Tulasne JF, Tessier PL. Results of the Tessier integral procedure for correction of Treacher–Collins' syndrome. *Cleft Palate J* (Suppl. 1) 1986; **23**: 40–9

Walters EC, Hiles DA, Johnson BL. Cloverleaf skull syndrome. *Am J Ophthalmol* 1973; **76**: 716–26

Wienstock FJ, Hardesty HH. Absence of superior recti in craniofacial dysostoses. *Arch Ophthalmol* 1965; **74**: 152–3

22.3 Cystic, Vascular, and Primary Bone Disorders

ANTHONY MOORE

Cystic lesions of the orbit

Cystic lesions of the orbit in childhood include dermoid cysts, sinus mucocoeles, microphthalmos with cyst, encephalocele, congenital cystic eyeball, and teratoma. In some parts of the world parasitic cysts such as echinococcus and shistosoma are common, but these are rare in Europe and North America (Jacobiec & Jones 1985). Haemorrhage within orbital lymphangiomas may give rise to the so called 'chocolate' cysts and cystic lesions of the orbital wall may be seen in fibrous dysplasia, ossifying fibroma and aneurysmal bone cyst.

Dermoid cyst

Dermoid cysts of the orbit and periorbital region are common in childhood (Youseffi 1969; Crawford 1983). They are developmental choristomas which are thought to arise from ectodermal rests trapped at the suture line during orbital development. They are found most commonly at the upper outer quadrant (Fig. 22.3.1) (Pfeiffer & Nichol 1948). Histologically, the cysts are found to be lined by epithelium and contain keratin and cholesterol; outside the epithelium is a layer of dermal appendages including sebaceous glands and hair follicles. Leakage from, or rupture of, a cyst usually excites a chronic granulomatous reaction.

In their commonest form, dermoids appear as an isolated superficial cystic mass at the orbital margin, which gives rise to few clinical problems (Sherman *et al.* 1984), although, rarely, larger cysts at the superior

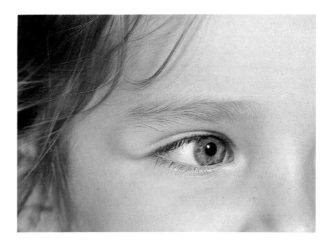

Fig. 22.3.1 External angular dermoid.

orbital margin may cause ptosis or vertical muscle imbalance (Sherman *et al.* 1984). Such superficial dermoids may have a characteristic radiological appearance; on plain X-rays there is indentation of the orbital wall with an inner area of radiolucency and outer rim of incranial bone density (Pfeiffer & Nichol 1984). Occasionally, however, there are deficits of the orbital wall in the region of the dermoid which may indicate that there is a deep component of the cyst within the orbit, temporal fossa, or intracranial cavity (Pfeiffer & Nichol 1948; Sherman *et al.* 1984). All patients with superficial dermoid cysts should have plain X-rays of the area before planning excision. If the posterior extent of the cyst cannot be ascertained on clinical examination, or if a bony defect is identified radiologically, it is wise to arrange an orbital CT scan to assess the extent of the tumour before undertaking surgery. Superficial dermoids can be easily excised through the brow and rarely recur if removed completely. Rupture of the cyst during excision may be followed by a chronic inflammatory reaction.

Less commonly dermoid cysts arise deep within the orbit (Fig. 22.3.2); these tend to be extensive, may be associated with marked proptosis and are difficult to manage (Pfeiffer & Nichol 1948; Sherman *et al.* 1984; Lane *et al.* 1987). An anterior component can often be palpated at the orbital margin. Deep orbital dermoids present in later childhood, adolescence, or early adult life (Lane *et al.* 1987). The management is total surgical excision (Sherman *et al.* 1984; Lane *et al.* 1987) but a careful preoperative clinical and radiological assessment is necessary so that the correct surgical approach to the orbit is used. In children where the orbital cyst is so extensive that a lateral orbitotomy is necessary surgery should be delayed until bone growth has ceased (Lane *et al.* 1987).

Orbital encephalocele

Encephaloceles, where part of the intracranial contents herniate through a congenital bony defect of the skull, may present to the ophthalmologist in two ways. Encephaloceles of the base of the skull may be associated with an optic disc anomaly (Pollock 1968) and this diagnosis should always be considered in a child with such an optic nerve anomaly especially if there is a midline facial anomaly with hypertelorism and a broad root to the nose. A second rare presentation is with proptosis due to an orbital encephalocele.

Orbital encephaloceles are uncommon and are of two main types (Duke–Elder 1964); in anterior orbital encephalocele there is herniation of the intracranial

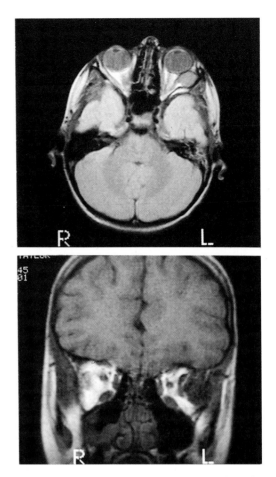

Fig. 22.3.2 Orbital dermoid. MRI scan showing lateral retro-ocular lesion on the left side.

contents in the region of the sutures dividing the frontal, ethmoid, lacrimal and maxillary bones whilst in the posterior type the encephalocoele enters the orbit via the optic foramen, orbital fissures or via a posterior bony defect. Posterior orbital encephaloceles may be associated with neurofibromatosis.

Anterior orbital encephalocele presents in early childhood as a slowly progressive proptosis with the eye being pushed forwards and laterally, or as a cystic swelling at the medial aspect of the orbit extending onto the face. The cyst may be pulsatile and increases on straining or crying (Mortada & E-Toraei 1960; Duke–Elder 1964; Consul 1965; Leone & Marlowe 1970). Plain X-rays will normally show a bony defect and CT scan will demonstrate communication with the intracranial cavity. Prompt neurosurgical referral is advised.

Posterior encephaloceles are rare and present with slowly progressive proptosis which may be pulsatile; the eye is displaced forwards and downwards (Duke–Elder 1964) and the proptosis increases on straining or crying. Plain X-rays will demonstrate abnormally enlarged foraminae or bony defect of the posterior orbit, and CT scan will delineate the extent of the lesion. They occur particularly in neurofibromatosis where the whole sphenoid may be dysplastic.

Sinus mucocele

A mucocele is a cystic swelling of the frontal or ethmoidal sinus which contains mucous secretions; typically the mucocele slowly expands resulting in thinning of the bony walls of the sinus. This results in displacement of the orbital contents causing proptosis. Most mucoceles arise from the frontal sinus so it is not surprising that it is a very rare cause of proptosis in childhood as the frontal sinus is not fully developed until later. The ethmoid sinus, however, is well developed and ethmoidal sinus mucoceles may present in childhood (Alberti *et al.* 1968; Robertson 1969) when they are usually associated with cystic fibrosis.

The usual presentation is with gradual onset of proptosis; the eye is usually pushed forwards laterally and upwards. A firm cystic non-compressible swelling may be palpable at the medial side of the orbit; inflammatory signs are absent. Plain X-rays will show a markedly enlarged sinus on the affected side and on CT scan a cystic lesion of the medial wall of the orbit arising from the ethnoid sinus is seen. Referral to an ENT surgeon is appropriate and the management is primarily surgical.

Other cystic lesions arising in the sinuses may cause proptosis, i.e. dentigerous cysts (Fig. 22.3.3).

Microphthalmos with cyst

Incomplete closure of the foetal fissure in early development (between 7 mm and 14 mm stage) may result in a variety of colobomatous defects of the eye (Pagon 1981). Eyes with severe colobomata are often microphthalmic and proliferation of neuro-ectoderm at the lips of the persistent foetal fissure may result in the formation of an orbital cyst which communicates with the eye. Arrest of development before the 7 mm stage of foetal development results in a congenital cystic eye or 'anophthalmos with cyst' (Dollfus 1968; Helveston *et al.* 1970). In this latter condition no recognizable globe is present within the orbit.

CLINICAL PRESENTATION

The usual presentation is with a bluish cystic lesion in the lower fornix which displaces a severely micro-

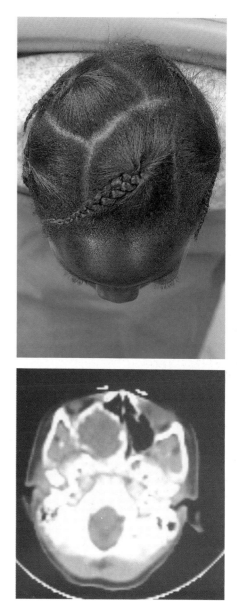

Fig. 22.3.3 Dentigerous cyst. This girl presented with chronic proptosis secondary to a large dentigerous cyst involving the orbit and maxillary sinus.

phthalmic eye up under the upper lid (Fig. 22.3.4) (Waring *et al.* 1976; Weiss *et al.* 1985). Rarely the cyst may be present in the upper lid (Fig. 22.3.5) and the eye is deviated downwards (Nicholson & Green 1981). The cyst communicates with the eye via a narrow stalk. The microphthalmic eye usually has extremely poor vision and associated optic nerve and retinal coloboma. The other eye may be normal or also have optic nerve or retinal coloboma (Waring *et al.* 1976; Weiss *et al.* 1985). Ocular coloboma may be associated

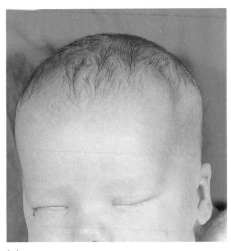

(a)

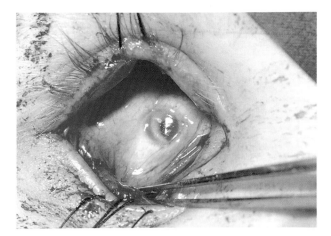

(b)

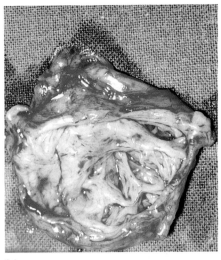

(c)

Fig. 22.3.4 (a) Bilateral microphthalmos with cyst in the lower lid of the right orbit. (b) At surgery the cyst was removed resulting in temporary collapse of the globe due to the connection between the cyst and the eye. (c) The cyst after removal showing trabeculations.

with a variety of systemic malformations (Waring *et al.* 1976; Pagon 1981).

The extent of the cystic component is best delineated by CT scan, although it may also be identified on ultrasound B scan. When the cyst is small it may be asymptomatic and be found incidentally on CT scan.

MANAGEMENT

In most cases no active intervention is needed (Weiss 1985). If the cyst enlarges resulting in an unsightly appearance it is best managed by aspiration. The cyst frequently recurs and repeated aspiration may be necessary. When there is recurrence of the cyst after multiple aspirations surgery may be indicated, although it may be difficult to excise the cyst without sacrificing the globe.

Congenital cystic eyeball (anophthalmos with cyst)

Cystic eyeball can be distinguished from microphthalmos with cyst by complete absence of any rudimentary globe. It presents at birth as a large cystic swelling within the affected orbit which in contrast to microphthalmos with cyst predominantly distends the upper lid (Dollfus 1968; Helvenston *et al.* 1970). Histological examination shows multiple cavities filled with proliferating glial tissue (Dollfus 1968).

Orbital teratoma

Teratomas arise from primitive germ cells and all three germ cell layers are represented; they are classified as choristomas rather than true neoplasms. Malignant change has only rarely been reported in the orbit (Soares *et al.* 1983).

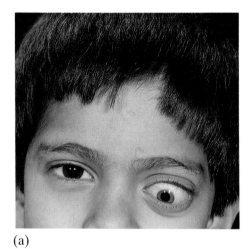

(a)

Fig. 22.3.5 Superior orbital cyst causing proptosis with downwards displacement of the microphthalmic eye.

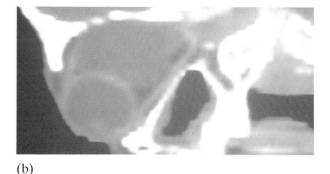

(b)

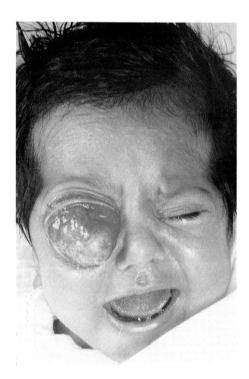

(c)

The usual presentation is with unilateral often massive proptosis in a newborn child (Hoyt & Joe 1962; Barber *et al.* 1974; Chang *et al.* 1980; Levin *et al.* 1986). The eye is usually displaced upwards by a large cystic mass which transilluminates. Plain X-rays will show an enlarged orbit on the affected side and the extent of the lesion is easily delineated on CT scan. Typically there is rapid growth after birth leading to extensive destruction within the orbit and exposure keratitis (Fig. 22.3.6). Less commonly there is slow growth over a number of years (Levin *et al.* 1986).

The treatment of choice is early surgical excision with preservation of the globe (Hoyt & Joe 1962; Barber *et al.* 1974; Chang *et al.* 1980; Levin *et al.* 1986), although aspiration of fluid from the cystic mass may be performed as a temporary measure, to allow surgery to be postponed until the infant is more able to withstand excision (Barber *et al.* 1974). Late malignant transformation is a rare occurrence (Garden & McManus 1986).

Parasitic cysts

Hydatid cysts occur in areas where they are endemic (Morales *et al.* 1988).

Vascular disorders of the orbit

Vascular tumours of the orbit comprise capillary and cavernous haemangiomas, haemangiopericytomas, orbital varices, and lymphangiomas. Capillary haemangiomas are common, usually present in early childhood and characteristically undergo spontaneous

regression (Margileth & Museles 1965; Haik *et al.* 1979). Cavernous haemangiomas and pericytomas are predominantly seen in adults although may rarely cause proptosis in childhood. Lymphangiomas, like

Fig. 22.3.6 Congenital orbital teratoma.

capillary haemangiomas, present in early childhood, but unlike the latter do not undergo spontaneous regression and are often complicated by orbital haemorrhage or infection (Jones 1959; Iliff 1979). Wright (1974) believes that most lesions described in the literature as lymphangiomas (Jones 1959; Iliff 1979) are really congenital orbital varices but this view has yet to gain widespread acceptance.

Capillary haemangioma

Capillary haemangioma is one of the commonest orbital tumours of childhood. It occurs more frequently in females than males (Stigmar *et al.* 1978; Haik *et al.* 1979; Deady & Willshaw 1986) and usually presents at birth or during the first few months of life (Haik *et al.* 1979). The natural history is one of initial increase in size followed by slow spontaneous regression (Margileth & Museles 1964; Haik *et al.* 1979). Histopathologically the haemangioma is a vascular hamartoma consisting of proliferating endothelial cells and pericytes which infiltrate the orbital structures. During periods of active growth mitotic figures may be seen.

CLINICAL FEATURES

Most cases present at birth or early infancy. The lids and superior orbit are most frequently involved, and in most children with an orbital haemangioma causing proptosis there is an anterior component or lid lesion which aids diagnosis (Haik *et al.* 1979). Eversion of the lid may show a bluish cystic lesion representing the vascular anomaly. About 30% of patients will have typical cutaneous 'strawberry' haemangiomatous lesions at other sites (Haik *et al.* 1979). Other findings suggestive of orbital haemangioma are increase in tumour size on crying (Fig. 22.3.7) and the presence of a dark blue 'vascular' hue to the periorbital subcutaneous tissues.

Capillary haemangiomas only rarely cause optic nerve dysfunction (Stigmar *et al.* 1978; Haik *et al.* 1979) but visual loss may result from amblyopia (Robb 1977; Stigmar *et al.* 1978; Haik *et al.* 1979; Deady 1986). This is especially common with anteriorly placed tumours and when there is extensive lid involvement (Fig. 22.3.8, 22.3.9). The amblyopia may be due to stimulus deprivation, when a large lid lesion covers the pupil, anisometropia or strabismus. Anteriorly placed tumours may cause anisometropia and in particular tend to cause astigmatism with the induced minus cylinder perpendicular to the axis of

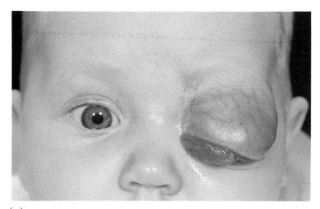

(a)

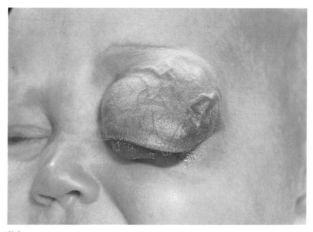

(b)

Fig. 22.3.7 (a) Capillary haemangioma of the anterior orbit and lid. (b) Same patient when crying showing engorgement and mild increase in size.

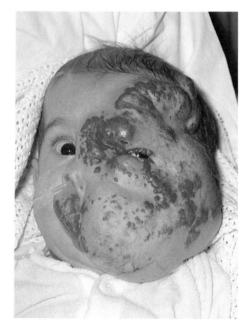

Fig. 22.3.8 Massive facial and orbital haemangioma.

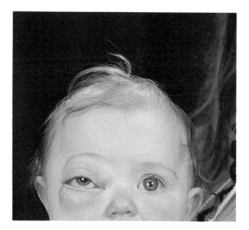

Fig. 22.3.9 Orbital haemangioma. As sometimes happens the mother of this child, on several occasions, was accused of having injured her child.

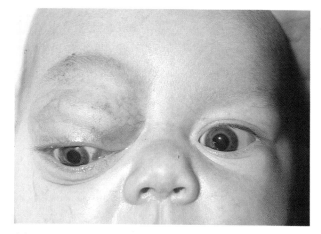

(a)

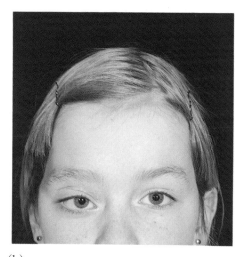

(b)

Fig. 22.3.10 (a) Orbital haemangioma in a child aged 2 months. (b) Same patient aged 9 years after some spontaneous resolution and surgery. Surgery is usually not necessary and best avoided where possible.

compression of the globe by tumour (Robb 1977). The astigmatism may persist even when the haemangioma regresses (Robb 1977). Strabismus may develop in the absence of anisometropia (Stigmar *et al.* 1978).

A rare complication of extensive haemangiomata is thrombocytopenia due to the entrapment of platelets within the vascular hamartoma (Kasabach & Merritt 1940).

INVESTIGATION

In the majority of children presenting with proptosis the presence of lid involvement or other cutaneous haemangiomas allow a clinical diagnosis to be made. Plain X-rays of the orbit will often show an enlarged orbit on the affected side and the extent of the lesion can be judged from CT scan which will show a diffusely infiltrative lesion without a definite capsule. Rarely lesions confined to the posterior orbit, especially during a period of growth, may be mistaken for a malignant tumour such as rhabdomyosarcoma and biopsy may then be necessary.

MANAGEMENT

Most capillary haemangiomas undergo spontaneous regression (Fig. 22.3.10, 22.3.11); in the series of Margileth and Museles (1964) 30% of lesions completely regressed by the age of 3, 60% by age 4 and 76% by age 7. Treatment should initially be confined to the management of any amblyopia with correction of refractive errors and occlusion, while awaiting spontaneous regression. Active treatment to reduce the size of the tumour mass is only indicated when the pupil is totally covered or where a posterior lesion results in progressive proptosis during the initial growth phase. Many different methods of treatment have been advocated including surgical excisions, radiotherapy, injection of sclerosing agents, and local or systemic steroids (Hiles & Pilchard 1971). Kushner (1982) has reported good results with injection of local steroid into the haemangioma. We have similarly obtained good results in anteriorly placed tumours with this technique and recommend the injection of a combination of methylprednisolone 40 mg and triamcinolone 40 mg into the haemangioma. This may be

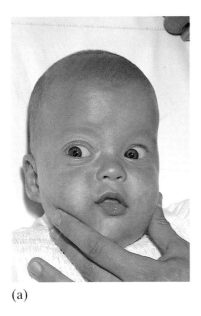
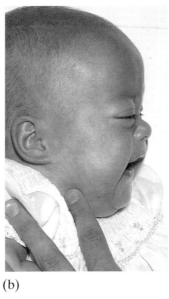
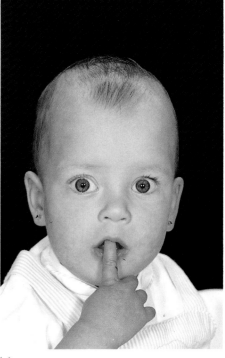

(a)   (b)

(c)

Fig. 22.3.11 (a, b) Right orbital haemangioma in a child aged 5 months. (c) Spontaneous resolution by 15 months (same patient).

repeated if necessary. For posterior orbital lesions, systemic steroids are preferred because of the risk of orbital haemorrhage associated with local injection.

Radiotherapy and sclerosing agents should no longer be used and surgical excision should be deferred until the child is 6 or 7 years when any residual cosmetic defect may be corrected.

Haemangiopericytoma

This tumour which is derived from the pericyte, is predominantly seen in adults although a few cases have been reported in children (Kapoor *et al.* 1978; Croxatto & Font 1982). In children it presents with gradual onset of proptosis, and on CT scan is seen as a well circumscribed lesion that shows marked enhancement with contrast. It is a locally invasive tumour that can undergo distant metastasis and it is best treated by complete local excision attempting to preserve the capsule. Local recurrences are common so that if complete excision is not possible more extensive surgery should be performed.

Lymphangioma

Lymphangiomas may affect the conjunctiva, lids and orbit and may be associated with similar lesions of the face, sinuses and oropharynx (Fig. 22.3.12). The lid and orbital lesions present at birth or early childhood, are slowly progressive and, in contrast to haemangioma, do not undergo spontaneous resolution. The orbit does not contain lymphatics so it is likely that these tumours arise from primitive vascular elements within the orbit. Wright (1974) however, on the basis of venous contrast studies, believes these lesions to be congenital vascular abnormalities rather than true lymphangiomas.

Histopathologically, lymphangioma of the orbit is a diffusely infiltrative lesion composed of endothelial lined channels indistinguishable from lymphatics. Lymphoid follicles are often seen in the fibrous stroma separating the endothelial channels and haemorrhage into the tumour is common giving rise to the so called chocolate cyst.

Orbital lymphangiomas present in infancy or early childhood with progressive proptosis. In Jones' (1959) series of 29 patients with orbital lymphangioma only three cases occurred in adults, the average age of

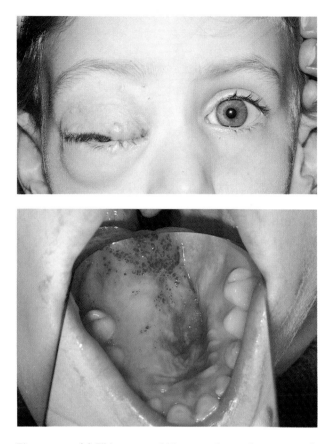

Fig. 22.3.12 (a) This 4-year-old boy was born after a 32-week gestation. Right proptosis developed by 4 weeks and was progressive despite orbital surgery, until age 3. It has been static since then. The diagnosis was a lymphohaemangioma. (b) Same patient showing clear and blood-filled cystic lesions on the palate.

onset was 6.2 years and ten patients had the lesions present since birth. In contrast to haemangiomas the proptosis is variable; exacerbations of the proptosis may occur in association with upper respiratory tract infections and orbital haemorrhage resulting in rapidly increasing proptosis and subconjunctival haemorrhage (Jones 1959). About one third of patients have extension of the lesion to involve the lid or the conjunctiva. Strabismus is common but ptosis and optic nerve compression are rare (Jones 1959).

Examination of the nasal and palatal mucosa may reveal characteristic mixed clear fluid and blood filled blebs (Fig. 22.3.12b). Plain X-rays of the orbit usually show enlargement of the orbit on the affected side, and CT scan will outline the extent of the tumour, which in contrast to haemangioma usually shows a significant cystic component. When active treatment is required because of progression the treatment of choice is surgical excision; as much of the lesion as possible is excised without causing damage to the intra-orbital structures (Jones 1959; Iliff & Green 1979). Radiotherapy is of uncertain value.

Congenital orbital varices

Wright (1974) believes on the basis of venography studies that most cases of lymphangiomas described in the literature are congenital orbital varices. The clinical presentation and management of these two conditions is identical and since CT scan has now replaced venography as the routine radiological investigation of such cases, the distinction is academic. Orbital varices grow slowly during childhood and rarely give rise to visual problems. Plain X-rays show enlargement of the orbit on the affected side and phleboliths are often seen. Surgical excision when indicated for cosmetic reasons should be confined to the anterior varices as attempts to excise deep orbital varicosities may result in optic nerve or other cranial nerve damage (Wright 1974). Repeated and sometimes severe haemorrhage into the lesion may occur (Kremer et al. 1987). Some orbital varices may be associated with extensive intracranial varicosities (Fig. 22.3.13).

Rare vascular lesions of the orbit

STURGE–WEBER SYNDROME

The typical Sturge–Weber syndrome consists of a facial naevus flammeus (port-wine stain) and leptomeningeal angiomatosis. The facial lesion is typically unilateral often involving the distribution of the ophthalmic branch of the trigeminal nerve and may be associated with angiomatosis of a variety of tissues including the eye, respiratory tract, gastrointestinal tract, ovary and pancreas. Cerebral involvement may give rise to seizures, hemiplegia and intellectual retardation. Not all patients however have the complete syndrome and there is wide variability in expression.

The ophthalmic manifestations include unilateral congenital glaucoma, episcleral and conjunctival vascular anomalies and diffuse choroidal haemangiomatosis. The latter may be complicated by serous retinal detachment. Orbital involvement is rare; Hofeldt et al. (1979) described two patients with ipsilateral naevus flammeus and a unilateral orbital vascular malformation causing proptosis. In each case there was no evidence of any intracranial lesion.

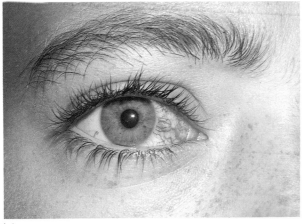

(a)

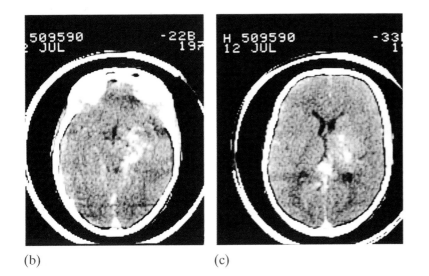

(b)   (c)

Fig. 22.3.13 (a) Subconjunctival varicocities in a patient with an orbital and intracranial haemangioma. (b) Contrast-enhanced CT scans showing the intracranial lesion (same patient).

KLIPPEL–TRENAUNAY–WEBER SYNDROME

This rare syndrome comprises multiple cutaneous naevi associated with various angiomas of one or more limbs which may show hypertrophy of the soft tissues. Rathbun *et al.* (1970) described a 15-year-old girl with the classical features of the syndrome who developed intermittent proptosis secondary to an orbital varix.

BLUE RUBBER BLEB NAEVUS SYNDROME

In this rare syndrome which usually presents in childhood, multiple bluish coloured cutaneous vascular malformations are seen in association with angiomatosis affecting other tissues including the gastrointestinal tract, lung, heart, and CNS. Most cases are sporadic but autosomal dominant inheritance has been reported in several families. Angiomas may involve the conjunctiva, iris, and retina (Crompton & Taylor 1981). Rennie *et al.* (1982) have reported an adult with the syndrome who developed unilateral proptosis secondary to an orbital vascular malformation.

Primary disorders of bone

Fibrous dysplasia of the orbit

Fibrous dysplasia is an uncommon disorder of unknown aetiology characterized by the replacement of normal bone by a cellular fibrous stroma containing islands of woven bone. It usually presents in childhood although lesions may remain asymptomatic until adult life. The condition, although histologically benign, is usually progressive in childhood but growth is often self-limiting; it behaves as a hamartoma rather than a true neoplasm. Rarely malignant transformation can occur, either spontaneously or following radiotherapy (Schwartz *et al.* 1964; Gross & Montgomery 1967; Huvos *et al.* 1972; Feintuch 1973).

Fibrous dysplasia may involve multiple bony sites (polyostotic form) or be confined to a single site (monostotic form). Polyostotic fibrous dysplasia may coexist with cutaneous pigmentation, and endocrine abnormalities. This is known as Albright's syndrome (Albright *et al.* 1937).

CLINICAL FEATURES

Most patients with orbital fibrous dysplasia have the monostotic form of the disease; several contiguous skull bones may be involved and the disease usually remains unilateral. The clinical features depend on which of the orbital walls are predominantly affected. The orbital roof is most commonly involved giving rise to proptosis and downward displacement of the globe and orbit (Gass 1965; Moore 1969; Moore *et al.* 1985). Involvement of the maxilla may displace the eye upwards and if the bony nasolacrimal duct is involved there is persistant epiphora (Moore 1969;

Moore *et al.* 1985). When the sphenoid is involved optic atrophy may develop from narrowing of the optic canal (Fig. 22.3.14) (Sassin & Rosenberg 1968; Moore *et al.* 1985) or optic nerve compression by an associated sphenoidal sinus mucocele (Liakos *et al.* 1979). Rarely involvement of the sella turcica may result in chiasmal compression and bilateral visual failure (Weyand *et al.* 1952). Other uncommon neuro-ophthalmic complications include cranial nerve palsies (Finney & Roberts 1976; Fernandez *et al.* 1980), trigeminal neuralgia (Finney & Roberts 1976) and raised intracranial pressure and papilloedema (Moore 1969; Ameli *et al.* 1981). Extensive orbitocranial involvement may also give rise to severe cosmetic deformity.

Three types of radiological appearance are seen; the lesions may be lytic, sclerotic or show a mixed picture (Fries 1957; Leeds & Seaman 1962). Occasionally, large cystic lesions of the orbital wall may be seen (Moore *et al.* 1985). Fortunately most cases involving the orbit are of the sclerotic type and there is little diagnostic difficulty (Moore 1969). The extent of cranial and orbital involvement is best assessed using

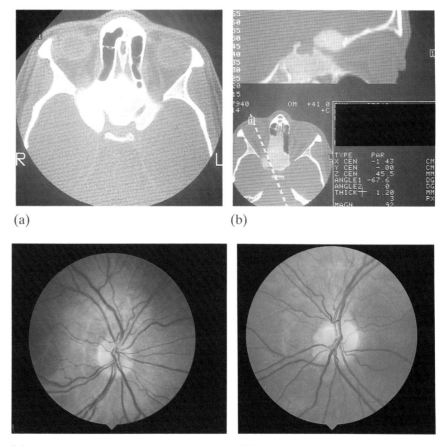

(a)   (b)

Fig. 22.3.14 (a, b) Fibrous dysplasia. CT scan showing sphenoid involvement. The optic canals are narrowed. (c, d) with chronic compressive optic neuropathy with atrophy on the left. The presenting symptoms were at 12 years and she showed no deterioration after 14 years with minimal residual signs or symptoms (same patient).

(c)   (d)

CT scan and careful attention should be given to assessment of the optic canal and chiasmal region.

MANAGEMENT

Fibrous dysplasia is a benign condition which although may be progressive in childhood its growth is self-limiting. However the rate of growth and time of arrest is unpredictable. The aim of treatment is to minimize complications whilst waiting for spontaneous arrest to occur.

In children in whom orbital X-rays show a typical sclerotic appearance, where there is little doubt about the diagnosis an initial period of observation and repeat radiological assessment is advisable. Where there is a lytic or cystic lesion of the orbital wall biopsy is usually necessary to confirm the diagnosis. Surgery is indicated when there is marked cosmetic deformity or optic nerve compression. Radical excision of all diseased bone is advisable, with facial and orbital reconstruction using bone grafts. This is best carried out in a specialised craniofacial unit when good cosmetic and functional results may be obtained (Moore et al. 1985).

Aneurysmal bone cyst

Aneurysmal bone cyst, first described by Jaffe and Lichtenstein (1942) in 1942 is a benign cystic lesion of bone filled with blood and lined by multinucleate giant cells and fibroblasts. They are solitary and typically involve the long bones, small bones of the hands and feet, pelvis or vertebral column (Biesecker et al. 1970). Involvement of the skull and orbit is rare. They usually present in childhood, occasionally later.

Aneurysmal bone cysts of the orbit have been reviewed by Powell and Glaser (1975) and Ronner and Jones (1983). Most cases involve the orbital roof and there is usually a history of gradual onset of unilateral proptosis (Johnson et al. 1988). Large cysts with intracranial extension may give rise to papilloedema (Constantini 1966) and rarely optic nerve compression may occur (Yee et al. 1977). The extent of the lesion is easily identified on CT scan and the treatment of choice is surgical excision with craniofacial reconstruction where necessary (Powell & Glaser 1975; Ronner & Jones 1983).

Juvenile ossifying fibroma of the orbit

This is an uncommon disorder which arises in the bony wall of the orbit and gives rise to slowly pro-

gressive proptosis. Although there are clinical and pathological similarities to fibrous dysplasia it probably represents a distinct entity (Margo et al. 1985).

It usually presents in children and young adults with slowly progressive painless proptosis; it most commonly involves the orbital roof or ethmoid (Blodi 1976; Margo et al. 1985) although rarely maxillary involvement may cause upward displacement of the globe (Shields et al. 1985). CT Scan shows cystic lesion of the orbital wall of variable density. Histopathologically the predominant feature is multiple round mineralized collagenous foci (psammomatoid ossicles) lying within a benign fibrous stroma (Margo et al. 1985). The treatment of choice is surgical excision but recurrence is common (Margo et al. 1985).

Benign osteoblastoma of the orbit

This benign tumour only rarely involves the orbit. Lowder et al. (Lowder et al. 1986) described a 5-year-old boy who developed a firm mass in the left supero-orbital region. CT scan revealed a sclerotic cystic lesion of the orbital roof which was excised and histology revealed a benign osteoblastoma.

Post-irradiation osteosarcoma of the orbit

Survivors of the genetic form of retinoblastoma are at greater risk of developing a second tumour (Strong & Knudson 1973; Abrahamson et al. 1984). Most of these tumours are osteosarcoma (Abrahamson et al. 1984) which may occur within the field of radiation given to treat the retinoblastoma, or at a distant site. In Abrahamson's series (Abrahamson et al. 1984) of 693 patients with bilateral retinoblastoma 89 developed second tumours; 58 within the radiation field and 31 out of the field. The latent period from completion of radiotherapy to development of the second tumour ranged from 10 months to 23 years (mean 10.4 years). The prognosis of osteosarcoma of the orbit is extremely poor; most patients die within a year of diagnosis.

Infantile cortical hyperostosis (Caffey's disease)

This is an uncommon disorder of unknown aetiology which affects infants in the first few months of life. It is characterized by sudden onset of fever, irritability and soft tissue swelling in a young infant. The soft tissue over the involved bone is swollen and tender and plain X-rays show subperiosteal new bone formation and cortical thickening. There is usually a leucocytosis and raised ESR. The mandible is the commonest bone to be involved in which case the infants have a characteristic facial appearance with swollen cheeks. The condition is in general self-limiting and the radiological appearance reverts to normal within a few months.

Involvement of the facial and skull bones may lead to periorbital oedema and even proptosis (Minton & Elliot 1967; Iliff & Ossofsky 1962). The management is generally conservative with an initial period of observation and follow up radiological examination of the involved bones. Systemic steroids may be used for persistant disease, or to hasten remission when there is gross swelling.

Osteopetrosis

This rare disorder of bone is characterized by an increase in thickness and density of bone which may result in narrowing of the marrow cavity and also the bony foraminae of the skull. The bony changes result in an increased susceptibility to fracture. It occurs in a severe (autosomal recessive) form and a more benign form which is usually inherited as an autosomal dominant trait. The mild form is often discovered incidentally on routine X-ray; ophthalmic complications are confined to the severe disease.

The severe form presents in infancy with failure to thrive, anaemia and thrombocytopenia; extramedullary haemopoeisis results in hepatosplenomegaly and lymphadenopathy. Ophthalmic complications occur as a result of changes in the skull leading to narrowing of the bony foraminae. The commonest and most severe complication is optic atrophy (Riser 1941; Ellis & Jackson 1962; Klintworth 1963; Hill & Charlton 1965; Aasved 1970) and usually follows narrowing of the optic canal and optic nerve compression (Fig. 22.2.15). Early decompression of the canal may preserve some vision (Hill & Charlton 1965; Ellis & Jackson 1962). Keith (1968) has described one infant with optic atrophy who had no evidence of optic canal narrowing and in whom there was evidence of rod and cone degeneration at post-mortem; he has suggested that the optic atrophy in some cases may be due to an associated retinal dystrophy.

Other ophthalmic complications include exophthalmos (Ellis & Jackson 1962) nystagmus (secondary to bilateral visual loss) and cranial nerve palsies (Klintworth 1963).

Recently there has been some success in treating these children with bone marrow transplantation (Ballet *et al.* 1977; Sorrel *et al.* 1981).

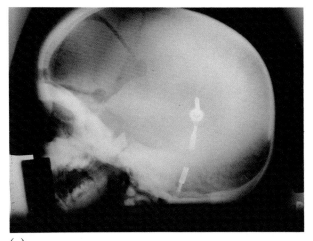

(a)

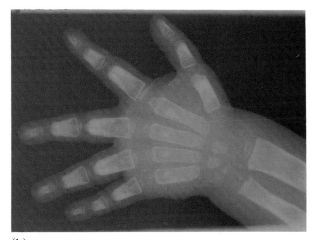

(b)

Fig. 22.3.15 (a) Osteopetrosis. This infant had a bilateral compressive optic neuropathy which failed to respond to surgery. He also has a shunt in situ. Bone marrow transplantation has been successful in some cases. (b) X-ray of hands showing increased density of distal ends of the phalanges (same patient).

Enophthalmos

Congenital enophthalmos is usually due to bone dysplasias, as occurs in sphenoid dysplasia in neurofibromatosis, and in developmental orbital disorders. Acquired enophthalmos is usually due to blow-out fractures or other trauma and rarely to tumours that have become fibrosed or otherwise contracted (Fig. 22.3.16). It also occurs with hemifacial atrophy, the Parry–Romberg syndrome and morphoea en 'coup de sabre' (linear scleroderma).

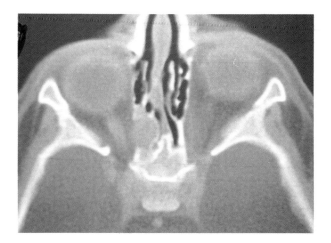

Fig. 22.3.16 Acquired enophthalmos caused by an astroglial tumour involving the paranasal sinuses.

References

Aasved H. Osteopetrosis from the ophthalmological point of view. A report of two cases. *Acta Ophthalmol* 1970; **48**: 771−7

Abrahamson DH, Ellsworth RM, Kitchin D, Tung G. Second non-ocular tumours in retinoblastoma survivors. *Ophthalmology* 1984; **91**: 1351−5

Alberti PWRM, Marshall HF, Munro-Black JI. Frontal-ethmoidal mucocoele as a cause of unilateral proptosis. *Br J Ophthalmol* 1968; **52**: 833−8

Albright F, Butler AM, Hampton AO, Smith P. Syndrome characterised by osteitis fibrosa disseminata, areas of pigmentation and endocrine dysfunction, with precocious puberty in females; report of five cases. *N Engl J Med* 1937; **216**: 727−46

Ameli NO, Rahmat H, Abbassioun K. Monostotic fibrous dysplasia of the cranial bones: report of fourteen cases. *Neurosurg Rev* 1981; **4**(2): 71−7

Ballet JJ, Griscelly C, Coutris C, Milhaud G, Maroteaus P. Bone marrow transplantation in osteopetrosis. *Lancet* 1977; **2**: 1137

Barber JC, Barber LF, Guerry D, Geeraets WJ. Congenital orbital teratoma. *Arch Ophthalmol* 1974; **91**: 45−8

Biesecker JL, Marcove RC, Huvos AG, Mike V. Aneurysmal bone cysts. A clinicopathologic study of 66 cases. *Cancer* 1970; **26**: 615−25

Blodi F. Pathology of orbital bones: Edward Jackson Memorial Lecture. *Am J Ophthalmol* 1976; **81**: 1−26

Chang DF, Dallow RL, Walton DS. Congenital orbital teratoma: report of a case with visual preservation. *J Pediatr Ophthalmol Strabismus* 1980; **17**: 88−95

Constantini F. Aneurysmal bone cyst as an intracranial space occupying lesion: a case report. *J Neurosurg* 1966; **25**: 205−7

Consul BN, Kulshrestha OP. Orbital meningocoele. *Br J Ophthalmol* 1965; **49**: 374−6

Crawford JS. Diseases of the orbit. In: *The Eye in Childhood*. Crawford JS, Morin JD, (Eds.) Grune & Stratton, New York 1983; 361−94

Crompton JL, Taylor D. Ocular lesions in the blue rubber naevus syndrome. *Br J Ophthalmol* 1981; **65**: 133−7

Croxatto JO, Font RL. Haemangiopericytoma of the orbit: a clinicopathological study of 30 cases. *Hum Pathol* 1982; **13**: 210−8

Deady JP, Willshaw HE. Vascular hamartomas in childhood. *Trans Ophthalmol Soc UK* 1986; **105**: 712−6

Dollfus MA, Langlois J, Clement JC, Forthomme J. Congenital cystic eyeball. *Am J Ophthalmol* 1968; **66**: 504−09

Duke-Elder S. Congenital Deformities of the Orbit. In: Duke-Elder S (Ed.) *System of Ophthalmology*, Vol 3, Kimpton, London 1964; pp. 949−56

Ellis P, Jackson WE. Osteopetrosis a clinical study of optic nerve involvement. *Am J Ophthalmol* 1962; **53**: 943−53

Feintuch TA. Chondrosarcoma arising in a cartilaginous area of previously irradiated fibrous dysplasia. *Cancer* 1973; **31**: 877−81

Fernandez E, Colavita N, Moschini M, Fileni A. 'Fibrous dysplasia' of the skull with complete unilateral cranial nerve involvement; case report. *J Neurosurg* 1980; **52**: 404−6

Finney HL, Roberts TS. Fibrous dysplasia of the skull with progressive cranial nerve involvement. *Surg Neurol* 1976; **6**: 341−3

Fries JW. The roentgen features of fibrous dysplasia of the skull and facial bones; a critical analysis of thirty-nine pathologically proved cases. *Am J Roentgenol Radium Ther Nucl Med* 1957; **77**: 71−88

Garden JW, McManus J. Congenital orbital−intracranial teratoma with subsequent malignancy. *Br J Ophthalmol* 1986; **70**: 111−4

Gass JDM. Orbital and ocular involvement in fibrous dysplasia. *South Med J* 1965; **58**: 324−9

Gross CW, Montgomery WW. Fibrous dysplasia and malignant degeneration. *Arch Otolaryngol* 1967; **85**: 653−7

Haik BG, Jakobiek FA, Ellsworth RM, Jones IL. Capillary haemangioma of the lids and orbit: an analysis of the clinical features and therapeutic results in 101 cases. *Ophthalmology* 1979; **86**: 760−89

Helveston EM, Malone E, Lashmet MH. Congenital cystic eye. *Arch Ophthalmol* 1970; **84**: 622−4

Hiles D, Pilchard WA. Corticosteroid control of neonatal haemangiomas of orbit and ocular adnexae. *Am J Ophthalmol* 1971; **71**: 1003−8

Hill BG, Charlton WS. Albers−Schonberg disease. *Med J Aust* 1965; **2**: 365−7

Hofeldt AJ, Zaret CR, Jakobiec FA, Behrens MM, Jones IS. Orbitofacial angiomatosis. *Arch Ophthalmol* 1979; **97**: 484−8

Hoyt WF, Joe S. Congenital teratoid cyst. *Arch Opthalmol* 1962; **68**: 197−201

Huvos AG, Higinbotham NL, Miller TR. Bone sarcomas arising in fibrous dysplasia. *J Bone Joint Surg (Am)* 1972; **54**: 1047−56

Iliff C, Ossofsky H. Infantile cortical hyperostosis: an unusual case of proptosis. *Am J Ophthalmol* 1962; **53**: 976−80

Iliff WJ, Green WR. Orbital lymphangiomas. *Ophthalmology* 1979; **86**: 914−29

Jacobiec FA, Jones IS. Orbital inflammations. In: Duane TD (Ed.) *Clinical Ophthalmology*. Harper & Row, Philadelphia 1985; pp. 60−5

Jaffe WL, Lichtenstein L. Solitary unilateral bone cyst with emphasis on the roentgen picture, the pathological appearance and the pathogenesis. *Arch Surg* 1942; **44**: 1004−25

Johnson TE, Bergin DJ, McCord CD. Aneurysmal bone cyst of

the orbit. *Opthalmology* 1988; **95**: 86−90

Jones IS. Lymphangiomas of ocular adnexae: an analysis of 62 cases. *Trans Am Ophthalmol Soc* 1959; **57**: 602−65

Kapoor S, Kapoor MS, Aurora AL, Sood GC. Orbital haemangiopericytoma: a report of a 3-year-old child. *J Pediatr Ophthalmol Strabismus* 1978; **15**: 40−2

Kasabach HH, Merritt KK. Capillary haemangioma with extensive purpura. *Am J Dis Child* 1940; **59**: 1063−70

Keith CG. Retinal atrophy in osteopetrosis. *Arch Ophthalmol* 1968; **79**: 234−41

Klintworth GK. The Neurologic Manifestations of Osteopetrosis (Albers−Schonbergs Disease). *Neurology* 1963; **13**: 512−00

Kremer I, Nissenkorn I, Feuerman P, Ben−Sira I. Congenital orbital vascular malformation complicated by massive retrobulbar haemorrhage. *J Pediatr Ophthalmol Strabismus* 1987; **24**: 190−3

Kushner BJ. Intralesional steroid for infantile adnexal haemangioma. *Am J Ophthalmol* 1982; **93**: 496−506

Lane CM, Erlich WW, Wright JE. Orbital dermoid cyst. *Eye* 1987; **1**: 504−11

Leeds N, Seaman WB. Fibrous dysplasia of the skull and its differential diagnosis; a critical analysis of thirty-one pathologically proved cases. *Radiology* 1962; **78**: 570−82

Leone CR, Marlowe JF. Orbital presentation of an ethmoida encephalocoele. *Arch Ophthalmol* 1970; **83**: 445−7.

Levin M, Leone CR, Kincaid MC. Congenital orbital teratoma. *Am J Ophthalmol* 1986; **102**: 476−81

Liakos GM, Walker CB, Carruth JAS. Ocular complications in craniofacial fibrous dysplasia. *Br J Ophthalmol* 1979; **63**: 611−6.

Lowder CY, Berlin AJ, Cox W, Hahhn JF. Benign Osteoblastoma of the Orbit. *Ophthalmology* 1986; **93**: 1351−4

Margileth AM, Museles M. Cutaneous haemangiomas in children. Diagnosis and conservative management. *J Am Med Assoc* 1964; **194**: 135−8

Margo CE, Ragsdale BD, Perman K, Zimmerman LE, Sweet DE. Psammomatoid ossifying fibroma. *Ophthalmology* 1985; **92**: 150−9

Minton L, Elliot J. Ocular manifestations of cortical hyperostosis. *Am J Ophthalmol* 1967; **64**: 902−7

Moore AT, Buncie JR, Munro I. Fibrous dysplasia of the orbit in childhood. *Ophthalmology* 1985; **92**: 12−20

Moore RT. Fibrous dysplasia of the orbit. *Surv Ophthalmol* 1969; **13**: 321−34

Morales GA, Croxatto JO, Crovetto L, Ebner R. Hydatid cysts of the orbit: A review of 35 cases. *Ophthalmology* 1988; **95**: 1027−33

Mortada A, E-Toraei I. Orbital meningo-encephalocoele and exophthalmos. *Br J Ophthalmol* 1960; **44**: 309−14

Nicholson DH, Green RW. *Microphthalmos with Cyst in Pediatric Ocuar Tumours.* Nicholson DH, Green RW. (Eds.) Year Book Medical Publishers Inc. Chicago 1981; pp. 219−221

Pagon RA. Ocular coloboma. *Survey Ophthalmol* 1981; **25**: 223−36

Pfeiffer RL, Nichol RJ. Dermoid and epidermoid tumours of the orbit. *Arch Ophthalmol* 1948; **40**: 639−64

Pollock JA, Newton TH, Hoyt WF. Trans-Spenoidal and trans-ethmoidal encephalocoeles. *Radiology* 1968; **90**: 442−53

Powell J, Glaser J. Aneurysmal bone cysts of the orbit. *Arch Ophthalmol* 1975; **93**: 340−2.

Rathbun JE, Hoyt WF, Beard C. Surgical management of orbitofrontal varix in Klippel−Trenaunay−Weber syndrome. *Am J Ophthalmol* 1970; **70**: 109−12

Rennie IG, Shortland JR, Mahood JM, Brown BH. Periodic exophthalmos associated with the blue rubber bleb naevus syndrome: a case report. *Br J Ophthalmol* 1982; **66**: 594−9

Riser RO. Marble bones and optic atrophy. *Am J Ophthalmol* 1941; **24**: 874−8.

Robb R. Refractive errors associated with haemangiomas of the eyelids and orbit in infancy. *Am J Ophthalmol* 1977; **83**: 52−7

Robertson DM, Henderson JW. Unilateral proptosis secondary to orbital mucocoele in infancy. *Am J Ophthalmol* 1969; **68**: 845−7

Ronner HJ, Jones IS. Aneurysmal bone Cyst of the Orbit: A Review. *Ann Ophthalmol* 1983; **15**: 626−9

Sassin JF, Rosenberg RN. Neurological complications of fibrous dysplasia of the skull. *Arch Neurol* 1968; **18**: 363−9

Schwartz DT, Alpert M. The malignant transformation of fibrous dysplasia. *Am J Med Sci* 1964; **247**: 1−20

Sherman RP, Rootman J, La Pointe JS. Orbital dermoids: clinical presentation and management. *Br J Ophthalmol* 1984; **68**: 642−52

Sherman RS, Soong KY. Aneurysmal bone cyst: Its roentgen diagnosis. *Radiology* 1957; **68**: 54−64.

Shields JA, Peyster RG, Handler SD, Augsburger JJ, Kapustiak J. Massive juvenile ossifying fibroma of maxillary sinus with orbital involvement. *Br J Ophthalmol* 1985; **69**: 392−5

Soares E, Lopes K, Adrade J, Faleiro L, Alves J. Orbital malignant teratoma. A case report. *Orbit* 1983; **2**: 235−40

Sorrell M, Kapoor N, Kirkpatrick D *et al.* Marrow transplantation for juvenile osteopetrosis. *Am J Med* 1981; **70**: 1280−7

Stigmar G, Crawford JS, Ward CM, Thomson HG. Ophthalmic sequelae of infantile haemangiomas of the eyelids and orbit. *Am J Ophthalmol* 1978; **85**: 806−13

Strong L, Knudson A. Second Cancers in retinoblastoma. *Lancet* 1973; **2**: 1086

Waring GO, Roth AM, Rodrigues M. Clinicopathologic correlation of microphthalmos with cyst. 1976; *Am J Ophthalmol* **82**: 714−21

Weiss A, Martinez C, Greenwald M. Microphthalmos with cyst. Clinical presentation and computed tomographic findings. *J Ped Ophthalmol* 1985; **22**: 6−12

Weyand RD, Craig WM, Rucker CW. Unusual lesions involving the optic chiasm. *Proc Stf Mtg Mayo Clin* 1952; **27**: 505−11

Wright JE. Orbital vascular anomalies. *Trans Am Acad Ophthalmol Otolaryngol* 1974; **78**: 606−16

Yee RD, Cogan DG, Thorp TR, Schut L. Optic Nerve compression due to aneurysmal bone cyst. *Arch Ophthalmol* 1977; **95**: 2176−9

Youseffi B. Orbital tumours in children: A clinical study of 62 cases. *J Paediatr Ophthalmol Strabismus* 1969; **61**: 177−81

22.4 Histiocytic and Haematopoietic Disorders

ANTHONY MOORE AND JOHN BRAZIER

Histiocytic disorders

The histiocytoses are an uncommon group of disorders in which cells derived from the monocyte−phagocyte system proliferate in many different tissues of the body. They are broadly classified into two groups; in Langerhans' cell histiocytosis (histiocytosis X) the abnormal histiocytes are derived from Langerhans' cells and show typical inclusions on electron microscopy. In non-Langerhans' cells histiocytosis the histiocytes have a different origin and lack the Langerhans' inclusion granules.

Three histiocyte disorders, Langerhans' cell histiocytosis, juvenile xanthogranuloma and sinus histiocytosis, which may involve the eye and orbit will be considered here.

Langerhans' cell histiocytosis (histiocytosis X)

Langerhans' cell histiocytosis (LCH) is an uncommon multisystem disorder of unknown aetiology which is characterized by the accumulation of histiocytes in various tissues, giving rise to a varied clinical picture. Lichtenstein (1953) first coined the term histiocytosis X to cover three related disorders: eosinophilic granuloma, Hand−Schuller−Christian disease and Letterer−Siwe disease which he believed were different clinical expressions of a single disease process. Eosinophilic granuloma is used to describe the condition where the histiocytic lesions is confined to bone. Classical Hand−Schuller−Christian disease consisting of the triad of diabetes insipidus, exophthalmos and bony defects of the skull is rare and this eponym is usually used to describe the chronic disseminated form of LCH, where there is widespread bony visceral and soft tissue involvement. Letterer−Siwe disease was a term usually used for more rapid and aggressive visceral disease. Since it is not possible to distinguish between these three groups histopathologically (Risdall et al. 1983) and because there is considerable clinical overlap between the three conditions, the term histiocytosis X was, until recently, used to cover the whole group of disorders. The term Langerhans' cell histiocytosis is now used instead of histiocytosis X in order to differentiate this condition where the abnormal histiocytes are derived from the Langerhans' cell from other histiocytic disorders.

Ophthalmic involvement

The commonest reason for referral to an ophthalmologist in this condition is orbital involvement (Obermann 1968; Moore et al. 1985) but intraocular (Heath 1959; Moziconacci et al. 1966; Rupp & Holloman 1970; Mittleman et al. 1973; Lahav & Albert 1974; Epstein & Grant 1977) and intracerebral involvement, particularly of the chiasm (Ezrin et al. 1963; Smolik et al. 1968; Bernard & Aguilar 1969; Kepes & Kepes 1969; Goodman et al. 1979) may give rise to visual symptoms.

Orbital involvement

Orbital involvement occurs in about 25% of cases of LCH (Obermann 1968; Moore *et al.* 1985) and is usually seen in children with the chronic form of the disease, especially eosinophilic granuloma (Wheeler 1946; Beller & Kornbleuth 1951; Truhlsen 1954; Nirankari *et al.* 1957, Straatsma 1958; Mortada 1966; Chawla & Cullen 1968; Obermann 1968; Heuer 1972; Baghdassarian & Shammas 1977; Moore *et al.* 1985). It is rare in disease confined to the soft tissues (Moore *et al.* 1985) suggesting that the disease usually arises in bone.

CLINICAL FEATURES

The usual presentation is with unilateral or bilateral proptosis in a child with known LCH. Globe subluxation occurs rarely (Wood *et al.* 1988) when there is marked proptosis. Less commonly the presentation is with isolated orbital involvement in a previously healthy child in which case the disease is usually unilateral. An isolated lesion of the superior orbital wall may present with unilateral ptosis. Optic nerve compression and cranial nerve palsies (Fig. 22.4.1) are rare but may be seen with extensive orbital involvement (Beller & Kornbleuth 1951; Moore *et al.* 1985). Skin tethering may occur (Fig. 22.4.2).

Visual loss is uncommon and may be caused by optic nerve compression (Beller & Kornbleuth 1951; Moore *et al.* 1985), optic atrophy following chronically raised intracranial pressure (Moore *et al.* 1985) chiasmal disease (Ezrin *et al.* 1963; Smolik *et al.* 1968; Bernard & Aguilar 1969; Kepes & Kepes 1969; Goodman *et al.* 1979) or intraocular infiltration (Heath 1959, Mozziconacci *et al.* 1966; Rupp & Holman 1970; Lahav & Albert 1974; Epstein & Grant 1977).

INVESTIGATION

In most children with orbital involvement plain X-rays (Fig. 22.4.3, 22.4.4) will demonstrate a lytic lesion of the orbital wall and CT scan will delineate the extent of intraorbital and intracranial involvement (Fig. 22.4.1a). As the disease arises in bone the orbital tumour usually remains extraconal but with time may spread to within the muscle cone. The diagnosis is confirmed by histologic examination of involved tissue. In children with multisystem disease, a more accessible site such as skin or a peripheral bony site should be biopsied but in children with isolated orbital involvement, orbital biopsy is necessary. Children

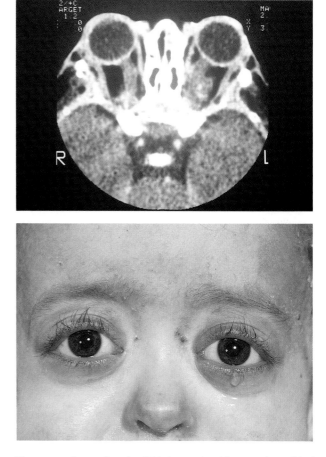

Fig. 22.4.1 Langerhans' cell histiocytosis with extensive orbital involvement on CT scan.

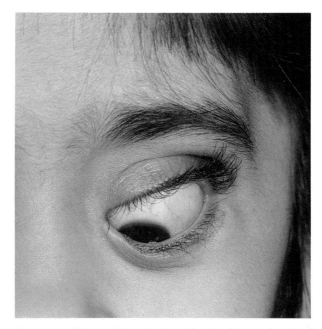

Fig. 22.4.2 Skin and lid tethering with orbital Langerhans' cell histiocytosis.

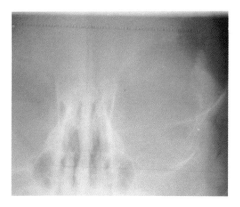

Fig. 22.4.3 Eosinophilic granuloma with punched out skull lesion.

who present initially to the ophthalmologist should be referred to a paediatric oncologist for further investigations including chest X-ray, skeletal survey, lung and liver function tests and early morning specific gravity to define the extent of any systemic involvement.

Light microscopy shows the affected tissues to be infiltrated with histiocytes and multinucleate giant cells together with eosinophils, lymphocytes, plasma cells, and neutrophils. Electron microscopy of the histiocytes demonstrate the presence of typical Langerhans' granules indicating that the proliferating histiocytes are derivatives of the Langerhans' cells, normally present in the epidermis of the skin (Jakobiec & Jones 1983).

MANAGEMENT AND PROGNOSIS

Children with LCH and ophthalmic involvement are best managed by a paediatric oncologist in collaboration with the ophthalmologist. Advice from other specialities such as ENT and orthopaedic surgeons may be needed for specific problems.

The management of orbital involvement depends

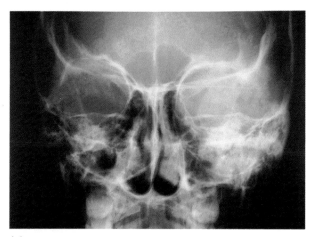

(a)

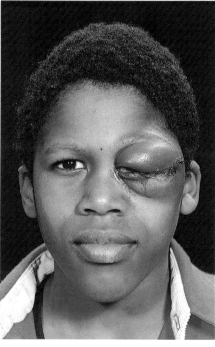

(b)

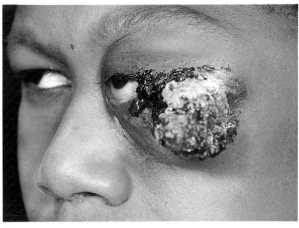

(c)

Fig. 22.4.4 (a) Langerhans' cells histiocytosis extensive bone hypertrophy around a chronic lesion. (b) Same patient with extensive orbital involvement. The vision was unaffected. (c) Same patient with ulcerated skin lesion which ultimately responded to steroid injection and limited surgery.

on whether there is single system for instance skin or bone, or multisystem disease. Children whose disease is confined to a single system, e.g. bone, have a good prognosis (Pritchard 1979) and in cases with a single lesion around the orbit, biopsy, and curettage is often followed by spontaneous resolution (Moore *et al.* 1985). Intralesional steroids may also be used to hasten remission (Moore *et al.* 1985; Wirtschafter *et al.* 1987). Cases with uncomplicated orbital involvement may be managed conservatively, but if there is marked proptosis or evidence of optic nerve compression, a short course of systemic steroids or radiotherapy may be used to induce remission. A radiation dose of 500–600 cGy is usually sufficient and the total dose should not exceed 1000 cGy because of the risk of radiation induced malignancies occurring in later life. Cosmetically disfiguring lesions of the orbital wall may be removed surgically with curettage of the underlying bone.

In patients with generalized LCH orbital involvement will generally respond to systemic chemotherapy but local radiotherapy may be used in addition if there is progressive proptosis or optic nerve compression. The most frequently used systemic agents are prednisolone, vincristine, vinblastine, and VP 16 which are used singularly or in combination (Pritchard 1979; Moore *et al.* 1984). However, because of the tendency for spontaneous regression in this disease an initial period of observation without specific treatment is recommended in uncomplicated disease (Pritchard 1979; Moore *et al.* 1984).

The prognosis in LCH depends upon several factors, the age of the patient, whether single or multisystem disease, and the presence or absence of organ failure. Children with single system disease for example of bone, have a good prognosis (Broadbent 1986). The prognosis is worst in infants and death is rare after the age of 3 years (Lucaya 1971; Lahey 1975). Death is usually due to severe involvement of key organs such as bone marrow, liver, and lungs.

Non-Langerhans' cell histiocytosis

Juvenile xanthogranuloma

Juvenile xanthogranuloma (JXG) is a disorder of unknown aetiology in which there is abnormal proliferation of histiocytes. It is characteristically seen as a benign skin disorders in infants and young children and has a pronounced tendency to undergo spontaneous regression. Rarely the skin lesions (Fig. 22.4.5) may be accompanied by intraocular or orbital

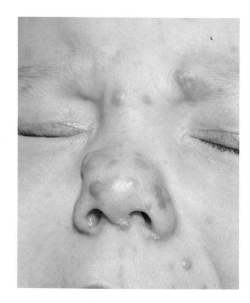

Fig. 22.4.5 Juvenile xanthogranuloma with skin lesion. Both eyes were involved (see Chapter 25).

involvement, but in contrast to Langerhans' cell histiocytosis, visceral, and bony involvement is rare (Zimmerman 1965).

HISTOPATHOLOGY

In JXG the lesion is composed of a mixture of lymphocytes, plasma cells, histiocytes, giant cells, and occasionally eosinophils. The distinctive histological feature however, is the presence of the Touton giant cell, in which a central ring of nuclei enclose an area of eosinophilic cytoplasm. Electron microscopy of the histiocytes fail to show any typical Langerhans' granules seen in histiocytosis X.

OCULAR INVOLVEMENT

JXG is predominantly a disease of infancy; in Zimmerman's series (Zimmerman 1965) 85% of patients with ocular involvement were under the age of 1 year and 64% less than 8 months. Rarely ocular involvement may present in adult life (Zimmerman 1965; Smith & Ingram 1968; Smith *et al.* 1969; Brinkmann *et al.* 1977). Most patients have unilateral disease although a few cases of bilateral involvement have been reported (Smith *et al.* 1969; Hadden 1975).

UVEAL INVOLVEMENT

JXG may involve the iris (Sanders 1960; Gass 1964; Zimmermann 1965; Smith & Ingram 1968; Hadden

1975; Brinkmann *et al.* 1977), ciliary body (Sanders 1960; Zimmermann 1965; Smith *et al.* 1969), or rarely the posterior choroid (Wertz *et al.* 1982). Most cases involve the iris and Zimmermann (1965) has summarized the main presenting signs:

1 An asymptomatic, localized, or diffuse iris tumour. Localized iris tumours may be very vascular and mistaken for a haemangioma (Fig. 22.4.6).

2 Spontaneous hyphaema. The main differential diagnosis of hyphaema in childhood is:

   (a) trauma;
   (b) tumour (retinoblastoma, diktyoma, Langerhans' cell histiocytosis, leukaemia, neuroblastoma);
   (c) rubeosis (secondary to RLF, retinal dysplasia, PHPV);
   (d) A−V malformations of iris.

3 Unilateral glaucoma.

4 Uveitis.

5 Heterochromia iridis.

The diagnosis is usually clear when there is an iris lesion in a child with typical skin lesions; skin biopsy will confirm the diagnosis. When there is doubt about the diagnosis, examination of aqueous obtained at paracentesis may show typical histiocytes; biopsy of the iris lesion is rarely necessary and should be avoided where possible because of the risk of haemorrhage.

Several different methods of treatment have been advocated including topical and systemic steroids, radiotherapy and surgical excision. Conservative treatment is preferred because of the risk of extensive haemorrhage following excision. A reasonable approach is to try a short course of topical (Clements 1966) and systemic steroids to induce remission, combining this with Diamox if the intraocular pressure is raised. If there is no response to steroids, radiotherapy (at a dose not exceeding 500 cGy) should be used.

OPTIC NERVE AND RETINAL INVOLVEMENT

Wertz *et al.* (1982) have reported a 20-month-old infant who presented with heterochromia of the iris and was found on histological examination of the enucleated eye to have massive infiltration of the optic nerve, disc, retina and choroid with histiocytes. Touton giant cells were also present. The overall histological picture was of JXG although there was no evidence of any typical skin lesions.

EPIBULBAR LESIONS

Conjunctival, episcleral, and corneal involvement in JXG is uncommon. The presentation is either with yellowish nodules at the limbus which may grow over the cornea, or as a yellowish or pinkish subconjunctival mass which is similar in appearance to a subconjunctival lymphoma (Zimmerman 1965). If they are progressive they may be treated by systemic steroids or radiotherapy in the same way as uveal involvement.

INVOLVEMENT OF THE OCULAR ADNEXAE

The skin lesions of JXG commonly affect the head and neck so it is not surprising that lid lesions are common. Occasionally a single lid lesion is the only manifestation of JXG and in such cases the diagnosis may not be apparent until histological examination of a biopsy specimen has been performed. The typical skin lesions are orange or yellow-brown papules.

Orbital involvement in JXG is uncommon (Sanders & Miller 1965; Zimmerman 1965; Sanders 1966; Gaynes & Cohen 1967). The usual presentation is with unilateral proptosis in infancy. Most of the cases have presented within the first 6 months of life and there is often involvement of the extraocular muscles, resulting in strabismus and limitation of ocular movement (Zimmerman 1965; Sanders 1966). In contrast to Langerhans' cell histiocytosis in most cases there is no evidence of any bony destruction although the case reported by Gaynes and Cohen (1967), did have a lytic lesion of the orbital wall. If there are no other systemic features it may be difficult to differentiate between JXG and histiocytosis X clinically but light and electron microscopy are diagnostic.

As JXG has a tendency to undergo spontaneous remission, the management of orbital involvement should involve an initial period of observation without specific treatment. If there is progressive proptosis or marked restriction of ocular motility, a short course of systemic steroid should be tried to induce remission (Gaynes & Cohen 1967). In cases unresponsive to steroid, low dose radiotherapy (500 cGy) should be given. The visual and systemic prognosis is usually excellent.

Sinus histiocytosis

Sinus histiocytosis is a disease of unknown aetiology predominantly affecting children and young adults; in the series reported by Foucar (Foucar *et al.* 1979) for

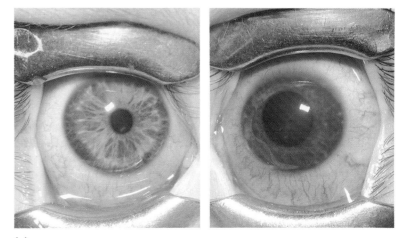

(a)

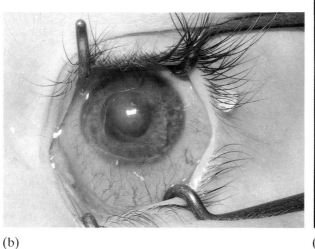

(b)

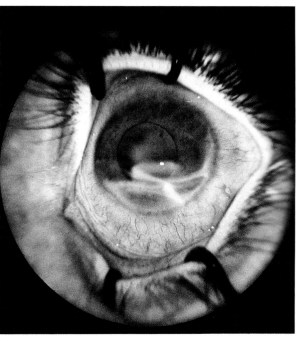

(c)

Fig. 22.4.6 (a–c) Presumed juvenile
xanthogranuloma. The patient had presented
because of recurrent left hyphaema resulting in
glaucoma. There is a vascularized iris which leaked
fluorescein profusely, but no frank mass formation.
(d) One year later. After 350 cGy radiotherapy
there was a very marked improvement and after a
period of occlusion of the right eye the acuity was
6/6. No recurrence occured over 9 years.

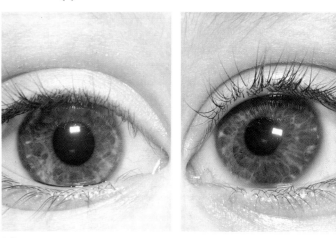

(d)

example, the average age was 8.6 years. There is usually massive painless cervical lymphadenopathy, often with enlargement of other lymph node groups. About 30% of patients have involvement of extranodal sites such as orbit, upper respiratory tract, salivary gland, skin, testes, and bone (Foucar et al. 1979). Laboratory findings include raised erythrocyte sedimentation rate, neutrophil leucocytosis and hypergammaglobulinaemia.

In patients with ophthalmic involvement the usual mode of presentation is with unilateral or bilateral proptosis. The condition affects the soft tissues of the orbit, without bony involvement (Friendly et al. 1977; Foucar et al. 1979; Karcioglu et al. 1988); the tumour mass usually remains extraconal so that optic nerve compression is rare. Less commonly there is an epibulbar mass without proptosis (Karcioglu et al. 1988; Stopak et al. 1988). Progressive proptosis may lead to corneal exposure, ulceration and even endophthalmitis (Friendly et al. 1977; Foucar et al. 1979). Involvement of the lids is common and rarely there may be intraocular involvement with infiltration of the uveal tract with histiocytes (Foucar et al. 1979). The lack of bony and visceral involvement helps to differentiate this condition from Langerhans' cell histiocytosis.

Histopathological examination of orbital biopsy specimens show a dense cellular infiltrate of histiocytes, lymphocytes, and plasma cells surrounded by a coat of connective tissue. The histiocytes often show intracellular phagocytosed lymphocytes and plasma cells. Electron microscopy fails to demonstrate the typical cytoplasmic inclusions of Langerhan cells differentiating this condition from Langerhans' cell histiocytosis.

There is no general agreement in the specific treatment of this disorder; high dose systemic steroids, systemic chemotherapeutic agents such as vinblastine and methotrexate, and radiotherapy have all been used without consistent success. The management of orbital involvement should include frequent assessment of vision and the maintenance of adequate corneal care. Progressive proptosis causing exposure keratitis may require orbital decompression (Friendly et al. 1977; Foucar et al. 1979).

The orbital disease tends to run a chronic course with occasional recurrences, but the overall systemic prognosis is good; there was one death in Foucar's series (Foucar et al. 1979) which may have been related to the use of extensive systemic chemotherapy.

Leukaemia

Orbital involvement in leukaemia was ranked tenth amongst causes of childhood orbital disease by Jones et al. (1983) and accounted for 11% of the 27 cases of unilateral proptosis in children reported by Oakhill et al. (1981). Porterfield (1962) considered leukaemia second only to rhabdomyosarcoma in frequency of childhood malignant orbital disease.

In patients with leukaemia, orbital involvement is more common with acute than chronic forms and more common with lymphoblastic than myelogenous cell types (Jakobiec & Jones 1983). Ridgway et al. (1976) surveyed 657 children with leukaemia and found clinical evidence of orbital involvement in 1%. Kincaid and Green (1983) found postmortem evidence of orbital involvement in 10% of 384 patients.

Clinical features include proptosis, lid oedema, chemosis, and pain (Mortada 1963; Cavdar et al. 1971). One or both orbits may be involved. Proptosis is due either to a mass of leukaemic cells or orbital haemorrhage (Jha & Lamb 1971). When orbital haemorrhage occurs, blood may be evident in the subconjunctival space or cause discolouration of the lids (Rosenthal 1983). Differential diagnosis of rapidly evolving proptosis with chemosis and haemorrhage includes rhabdomyosarcoma, orbital involvement in leukaemia, neuroblastoma, or Ewing's sarcoma and orbital cellulitis (Jha & Lamb 1971; Kincaid & Green 1983). Orbital leukaemic deposits are often associated with meningeal involvement (Ridgway et al. 1976) and are often part of terminal disease (Porterfield 1962; Ridgway et al. 1976), although, in some cases, orbital signs may be the presenting feature of leukaemia and biopsy provides the systemic diagnosis. Orbital disease can involve the lacrimal gland (Zimmerman & Font 1975) or, more rarely, the extraocular muscles (Kincaid & Green 1983). In addition to infiltration with leukaemic cells and haemorrhage, orbital signs in leukaemia may result from opportunistic orbital infection by bacteria or fungi (Rubinfield et al. 1988) or extraocular muscle palsy related to vincristine treatment (Nicholson & Green 1981).

The orbital cell mass consists either of lymphoblastic cells or cells derived from the myeloid series in which case the orbital lesion is called granulocytic sarcoma or chloroma (Fig. 22.4.7). The latter name is derived from green tissue discolouration said to be due to presence of the enzyme myeloperoxidase. Granulocytic sarcoma traditionally carries a poor prognosis; 19 of 32 patients reported by Zimmerman and Font (1975) were dead within 30 months of onset of ophthal-

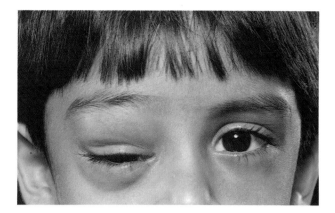

Fig. 22.4.7 Orbital deposit in myeloid leukaemia (chloroma). There was no abnormality in the peripheral blood film. The diagnosis was made by bone marrow aspiration done at the time of orbital biopsy.

mic signs. Granulocytic sarcoma has similar histopathological appearances to reticulum cell sarcoma (histiocytic lymphoma) although the nuclei are more oval, with vesicular nucleoplasm and less well defined nucleoli (Kincaid & Green 1983). Special stains for esterase activity in immature cells may identify differentiation towards myelocytes (Jakobiec & Jones 1983). In young patients diagnosed as having reticulum cell sarcoma it is more likely that they actually have granulocytic sarcoma (Jakobiec & Jones 1983).

Treatment of orbital leukaemia is by systemic chemotherapy and local irradiation, although the dose and effect of the latter (reviewed by Kincaid & Green 1983) are not clearly defined. Intrathecal chemotherapy will not modify orbital disease. Orbital disease in children with acute leukaemia still carries a poor prognosis despite chemotherapy and radiotherapy (Kincaid & Green 1983).

Lymphoma

Knowles et al. (1983) state that they have never seen orbital lymphoma as part of systemic nodal disease in children. Bearing this in mind, the only lymphoma likely to occur in the paediatric orbit is Burkitt's lymphoma.

This condition tends to affect children in tropical Africa. In 60% cases there is a maxillary tumour causing massive proptosis. The tumour responds to chemotherapy with prolonged remission and some patients are reported to show immunological self cure (Jakobiec & Jones 1983). The tumour is linked with the presence of Epstein–Barr virus (Henle 1974).

References

Baghdassarian SA, Shammas HF. Eosinophilic granuloma of orbit. *Ann Ophthalmol* 1977; **9**: 1247–51

Beller AJ, Kornbleuth W. Eosinophilic granuloma of the orbit. *Br J Ophthalmol* 1951; **35**: 220–5

Bernard JD, Aguilar MJ. Localised hypothalamic histiocytosis X: report of a case. *Arch Neurol* 1979; **20**: 368–72

Brinkman RF, Oosterhuis JA, Manschot WA. Recent haemorrhage in the anterior chamber caused by a (juvenile) xanthogranuloma in an adult. *Doc Ophthalmol* 1977; **42**: 329–000

Broadbent V. Favourable prognostic features in histiocytosis X: bone involvement and absence of skin disease. *Arch Dis Child* 1986; **61**: 1219–21

Cavdar AO, Arcasoy A, Gozdaxoglu S et al. Chloroma-like manifestation in Turkish children with acute myelomonocytic leukaemia. *Lancet* 1971; **1**: 680–2

Chawla HB, Cullen JF. Eosinophilic granuloma of the orbit. *J Pediatr Ophthalmol Strabismus* 1968; **5**: 93–5

Clements DB. Juvenile xanthogranuloma treated with local steroids. *Br J Ophthalmol* 1966; **50**: 663–5

Epstein DL, Grant WM. Secondary open angle glaucoma in histiocytosis X. *Am J Ophthalmol* 1977; **84**: 332–6

Ezrin C, Chaikoff R, Hoffman H. Pan-hypopituitarism caused by Hand–Schuller–Christian disease. *Can Med Assoc J* 1963; **89**: 1290–3

Foucar E, Rosai J, Dorfman FR. The ophthalmological manifestations of sinus histiocytosis with massive lymphadenopathy. *Am J Ophthalmol* 1979; **87**: 354–67

Friendly DS, Font RL, Rao NA. Orbital involvement in sinus histiocytosis *Arch Ophthalmol* 1977; **95**: 2006–11

Gass JD. Management of juvenile xanthogranuloma of the iris. *Arch Ophthalmol* 1964; **71**: 344–7

Gaynes PM, Cohen GS. Juvenile xanthogranuloma of the orbit. *Am J Ophthalmol* 1967; **63**: 755–7

Goodman RH, Post KD, Molitch ME, Adelman LS, Altemus LR, Johnston H. Eosinophilic granuloma mimicking a pituitary tumour. *Neurosurg* 1979; **5**: 723–5

Hadden OB. Bilateral juvenile xanthogranuloma of the orbit. *Br J Ophthalmol* 1975; **59**: 699–702

Heath P. The ocular features of a case of acute reticuloendotheliosis (Letterer–Siwe type). *Trans Am Ophthalmol Soc* 1959; **57**: 290–302

Henle W, Henle G. Epstein–Barr virus and human malignancies. *Cancer* 1974; **34**: 1368–74

Heuer HE. Eosinophilic granuloma of the orbit. *Acta Ophthalmol* 1972; **50**: 160–5

Jakobiec FA, Jones IS. Lymphomatous, plasmacytic, histiocytic and haemopoietic tumours. In: Duane TD (Ed.) *Clinical Ophthalmology*, Vol. 2. Harper & Row, Hagerstown 1983

Jha BK, Lamba PA. Proptosis as a manifestation of acute myeloid leukaemia. *Br J Ophthalmol* 1971; **55**: 844–7

Jones IS, Jakobiec FA, Nolan B. Patient examination and introduction to orbital disease. In: Duane TD (Ed.) *Clinical Ophthalmology*, Vol. 2. Harper & Row, Hagerstown 1983

Karcioglu ZA, Allam B, Insler MS. Ocular involvement in sinus histiocytosis with massive lymphadenopathy. *Br J Ophthalmol* 1988; **72**: 793–6

Kepes JJ, Kepes M. Predominantly cerebral forms of histiocytosis X. A reappraisal of 'Gagel's hypothalamic granuloma', 'granuloma infiltrans of the hypothalamus' and 'Ayala's disease' with a report of four cases. *Acta Neuropathol (Berl)* 1969; **14**: 77−98

Kincaid MC, Green WR. Ocular and orbital involvement in leukaemia. *Surv Ophthalmol* 1983; **15**: 211−32

Knowles DM, Jakobiec FA, Jones IS. Rhabdomyosarcoma. In: Duane TD (Ed.) *Clinical Ophthalmology*, Vol. 2. Harper & Row, Hagerstown 1983

Lahav M, Albert DM. Unusual ocular involvement in acute disseminated histiocytosis X. *Arch Ophthalmol* 1974; **91**: 455−8

Lahey ME. Histiocytosis X — an analysis of prognostic factors. *J Pediatr* 1975; **87**: 184−9

Lichtenstein L. Histiocytosis X. Integration of eosinophili granuloma of bone. 'Letterer−Siwe disease' and 'Schueller−Christian disease' as related manifestations of a single nosological entity. *Arch Pathol* 1953; **56**: 84−102

Lucaya JL. Histiocytosis X. *Amer J Dis Child* 1971; **121**: 289−95

Mittelman D, Apple DJ, Goldberg MF. Ocular involvement in Letterer−Siwe disease. *Am J Ophthalmol* 1973; **75**: 261−5

Moore AT, Pritchard J, Taylor D. Histiocytosis X: an ophthalmological review. *Br J Ophthalmol* 1985; **69**: 7−14

Mortada A. Orbital lymphoblastomas and acute leukaemia in children. *Am J Ophthalmol* 1963; **55**: 327−1

Mortada A. Non-lipoid and lipoid reticulo-endotheliosis of orbital bones. *Am J Ophthalmol* 1966; **61**: 558−60

Mozziconacci P, Offret G, Forest A, Attal C, Girard F, Hayem F, Trung FH. Histiocytose X avec lesions oculaires etude anatomique. *Ann Pediatr* 1966; **13**: 348−55

Nicholson DH, Green WR. *Pediatric Ocular Tumours*. Masson, New York, 1981; pp. 257−60

Nirankari MS, Singh M, Manchanda SS, Chitkara NL, Maudgal MC. Eosinophilic granuloma of the orbit. *Arch Ophthalmol* 1957; **58**: 857−61

Oakhill A, Willshaw H, Mann JR. Unilateral proptosis. *Arch Dis Child* 1981; **56**: 549−51

Obermann HA. Idiopathic histiocytosis: a correlative review of eosinophilic granuloma, Hand−Schuller−Christian disease and Letterer−Siwe disease. *J Pediatr Ophthalmol* 1968; **5**: 86−92

Porterfield J. Orbital tumours in children: a report of 214 cases. *Int Ophthalmol Clin* 1962; **2**: 319−35

Pritchard J. Histiocytosis X: natural history and management in childhood. *Clin Exp Dermatol* 1979; **4**: 421−33

Ridgway EW, Jaffe N, Walton DB. Leukaemic ophthalmopathy in children. *Cancer* 1976; **38**: 1744−9

Risdall RJ, Dehner LP, Duray P, Kabrinsky N, Robinson L, Nesbitt ME. Histiocytosis X (Langerhans' cell histiocytosis) — prognostic role of histopathology. *Arch Pathol Lab Med* 1983; **2**: 59−64

Rosenthal AR. Ocular manifestations of leukaemia; a review. *Ophthalmology* 1983; **90**(8): 899−905

Rubinfield RS, Gootenberg JE, Chavis RM, Zimmerman LE. Early onset acute orbital involvement in childhood acute lymphoblastic leukaemia. *Ophthalmology* 1988; **95**(1): 116−20

Rupp RH, Holloman KR. Histiocytosis X affecting the uveal tract. *Arch Ophthalmol* 1970; **84**: 468−70

Sanders TE. Intraocular juvenile xanthogranuloma (nevoxanthogranuloma): a survey of 20 cases. *Trans Am Ophthalmol Soc* 1960; **58**: 59−74

Sanders TE. Infantile xanthogranuloma of the orbit: a report of three cases. *Am J Ophthalmol* 1966; **61**: 1299−1306

Sanders TE, Miller JE. Infantile xanthogranuloma of the orbit. *Trans Am Acad Ophthalmol Otolaryngol* 1965; **69**: 458−64

Smith JLS, Ingram RM. Juvenile oculodermal xanthogranuloma. *Br J Ophthalmol* 1968; **52**: 696−703

Smith ME, Sanders TE, Bresnik GH. Juvenile xanthogranuloma of the ciliary body in an adult. *Arch Ophthalmol* 1969; **81**: 813−814

Smolik EA, Devercerski M, Nelson JS, Smith KR. Histiocytosis X in the optic chiasm of an adult with hypopituitarism: case report. *J Neurosurg* 1968; **29**: 290−295

Stopak SS, Dreizen NG, Zimmerman LE, O'Neill JF. Sinus histiocytosis presenting as an epibulbar mass: a clinicopathologic case report. *Arch Ophthalmol* 1988; **106**: 1426−36

Straatsma BR. Eosinophilic granuloma of bone. *Trans Am Acad Ophthalmol Otolaryngol* 1958; **62**: 771−6

Truhlsen SM. Eosinophilic granuloma involving the orbit. Report of a case. *Am J Ophthalmol* 1954; **37**: 571−5

Wertz FD, Zimmerman LE, McKeown LA *et al*. Juvenile xanthogranuloma of the optic nerve, disc, retina and choroid. *Ophthalmology* 1982; **89**: 1331−5

Wheeler M. Exophthalmos caused by eosinophilic granuloma of bone. *Am J Ophthalmol* 1946; **29**: 980−4

Wirtschafter J, Nesbit M, Anderson P, McClain K. Intralesional methylprednisolone for Langerhan's cell histiocytosis of the orbit and cranium. *J Pediatr Ophthalmol Strabismus* 1987; **24**: 194−7

Wood CM, Pearson ADJ, Craft AW, Howe JW. Globe luxation in histiocytosis. *Br J Ophthalmology* 1988; **72**: 631−4

Zimmerman LE. Ocular lesions of juvenile xanthogranuloma: nevoxanthogranuloma. *Trans Am Acad Ophthalmol Otolaryngol* 1965; **69**: 412−42

Zimmerman LE, Font RC. Ophthalmic manifestations of granulocytic sarcoma/myeloid sarcoma or chloroma. *Am J Ophthalmol* 1975; **80**: 975−90

22.5 Neurofibromatosis and Optic Nerve Tumours

JOHN BRAZIER

Neurofibromatosis

Neurofibromatosis (NF) was described by Von Recklinghausen in 1882 and later included by Van Der Hoeve (1923, 1932), with tuberous sclerosis Von Hippel–Lindau disease and Sturge–Weber syndrome, in a group of disorders known as the phakomatoses. Neurofibromatosis is thought to represent a range of abnormalities resulting from neuroectodermal dystrophy, including cutaneous pigmentary disturbances and a variety of skin and soft tissue tumours arising from cells of the primitive neural crest (Woog et al. 1982). (These tumours include neurofibromas, phaeochromocytomas, meningioma, optic nerve glioma, and medullary carcinoma of the thyroid.) The disease is congenital and inherited as an autosomal dominant trait of variable penetrance and expression. Cases where no family history can be identified are regarded as spontaneous mutations.

Symptoms and signs reflect involvement of multiple systems and organs including orbit, eye, skin, central, and peripheral nervous systems, viscera, and musculoskeletal systems. Signs may be present at birth or appear during infancy. In many patients, initial manifestations do not appear until late childhood or even adult life (Font & Ferry 1972; François 1972).

Orbital involvement consists of bone abnormalities and soft tissue tumours including neurofibroma, schwannoma, optic nerve glioma and nerve sheath meningioma. The pathology of neurofibroma and schwannoma will be described prior to description of the clinical features of neurofibromatosis. Optic nerve glioma and meningioma are described in separate sections.

Pathology

Plexiform neurofibroma is the typical orbital lesion in neurofibromatosis and the most elaborate form of peripheral nerve tumour. Usually presenting during the first decade of life, these tumours consist of interweaving bundles consisting of Schwann cells, axons and endoneural fibroblasts. Each neuromatous unit has a distinct perineural sheath, a finding pathognomonic of neurofibromatosis (Jakobiec & Jones 1983). The hypertrophied nerves are tortuous, forming a plexus, and described on palpation as feeling like a 'bag of worms'. Plexiform neurofibroma dissects through the orbital tissue and is thus extremely difficult to remove surgically. When the lesion involves the lid, the overlying skin may be pigmented and thickened.

Single neurofibromas are not always associated with neurofibromatosis, and tend to occur in adults (Jakobiec & Jones 1983). They are not encapsulated but may be circumscribed and, like plexiform neurofibromas consist of Schwann cells, axons and endoneural fibroblasts. Single neurofibromas are space-occupying in nature and therefore tend to displace other orbital structures. A variation of single neurofibroma, known as diffuse neurofibroma, tends to permeate the orbital structures and is not circumscribed. The cellular elements are again the same, but diffuse neurofibroma is differentiated from plexiform

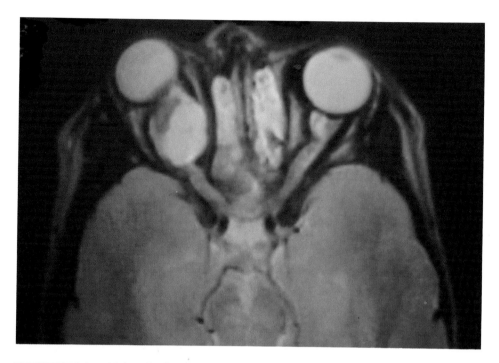

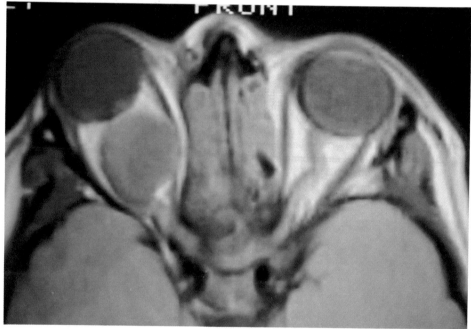

Fig. 22.5.13 Optic nerve glioma with cystic area anteriorly.

enlargement, increased orbital soft tissue shadowing and enlargement of the optic canal where the intra-canalicular optic nerve is involved in the glioma.

MANAGEMENT

Reviewing the literature on optic nerve and chiasmal glioma does not reveal any concensus regarding man-agement. Conservative management, advocated by Hoyt and Baghdassarian (1969), appears very reason-able in many cases where treatment would be of doubtful efficacy and associated with morbidity and expense. Until a large prospective study of conserva-tive management versus the option of surgery and radiotherapy is performed, treatment must be based on retrospective data.

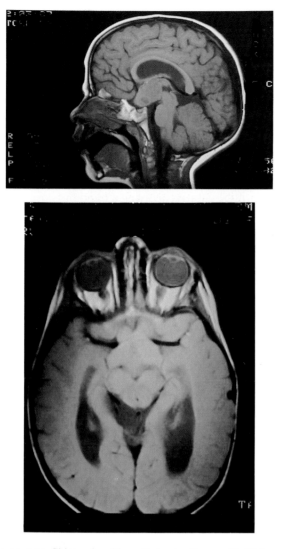

Fig. 22.5.14 Chiasmal and hypothalamic glioma with thickened intracranial optic nerves.

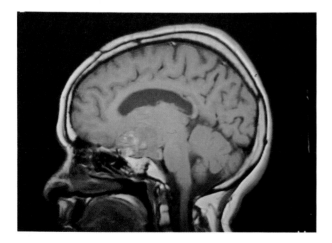

Fig. 22.5.15 Large, vascular, chiasmal and hypothalamic glioma.

Optic nerve glioma

The prognosis in optic nerve glioma is better than chiasmal glioma (Rush *et al.* 1982). Decision to treat depends on the degree of visual loss, proptosis and whether retro-orbital structures are involved. If there is minimum visual loss it is reasonable to keep the child under observation; treatment may not be necessary if the tumour fails to grow or regresses. If there is visual loss without marked proptosis a conservative approach is again indicated. When progressive visual loss occurs radiotherapy may halt the decline (Horwich & Bloom 1985). Biopsy in itself is not usually helpful because the diagnosis can be made with a high degree of certainty on radiological grounds. If the tumour is associated with visual obscurations due to raised pressure in the nerve sheath, biopsy may be combined with decompression of the nerve sheath. If proptosis is marked with a blind eye it is possible to remove the tumour by curettage or via a lateral or subfrontal orbitotomy. Curettage is simple and safe but recurrence possible. Lateral orbitotomy allows access to only the orbital optic nerve, leaves a temporal scar and may interfere with orbital growth. Subfrontal orbitotomy has inherent risks but results in definitive removal of tumour from eye to chiasm though this is not of real benefit when the chiasm is known to be involved.

Chiasmal glioma

As surgical removal of chiasmal glioma is not possible, management options are observation, radiotherapy and, possibly, chemotherapy. Biopsy is rarely necessary because the diagnosis is often clear after radiological studies, but particularly when there is cyst formation or calcium in the tumour biopsy may be indicated. The management plan suggested by Packer *et al.* (1983) and reinforced by Kennerdell and Garrity (1988) seems logical.

In view of remaining uncertainty about the natural history of chiasmal glioma, no treatment is given if the tumour is confined to the chiasm at the time of diagnosis. These patients are reviewed regularly by clinical evaluation of acuity and fields and regular CT (or MRI) scanning.

If the glioma involves the hypothalamus or third ventricle or there is gross enlargement of the optic tract, treatment by radiotherapy is advised. Whilst the effectiveness of radiotherapy for chiasmal glioma is still in doubt (Rush *et al.* 1982; Imes & Hoyt 1986), some authors consider that disease control in up to

50% of patients is possible (Packer *et al.* 1983; Horwich & Bloom 1985). Radiotherapy therefore appears the best treatment option available, especially when visual loss has been rapid and recent. Chemotherapy (Packer *et al.* 1983; Rosenstock *et al.* 1985) may gain acceptance as an alternative to radiotherapy in the future.

Endocrine abnormalities associated with chiasmal glioma require assessment and treatment. Hydrocephalus may require ventricular shunting.

Meningioma

Primary orbital meningiomas are very rare in children. They result from proliferation of meningothelial cells of the arachoroid in the optic nerve sheath and may arise in association with neurofibromatosis. Occasionally, meningiomas in the orbit are unconnected with the nerve sheath (Karp 1974).

Clinical presentation of optic nerve sheath meningioma is with a combination of visual loss and proptosis. More posterior lesions tend to cause predominantly visual loss with little proptosis. A tendency to grow through the dura makes extraocular muscle involvement relatively frequent (Jakobiec & Jones 1983). Compression of the optic nerve results in an afferent pupillary defect and disc swelling or pallor. Optociliary shunt vessels may be present on the disc and are more suggestive of meningioma than the alternative diagnosis of optic nerve glioma (Jakobiec & Jones 1983).

Investigation

CT scanning is the investigation of choice, offering advantages for intraorbital optic nerve imaging over MRI in its present state of development and availability (Holman *et al.* 1985; Leib & Kates 1988). Meningioma usually causes a tubular enlargement of the optic nerve, sometimes with calcification causing a 'tramline' appearance (Jakobiec *et al.* 1984) or excrescent growth through the dura (Rothfus *et al.* 1984). The nerve can usually be identified as a radiolucent region within the tumour on axial and coronal scans (Jakobiec *et al.* 1984; Rothfus *et al.* 1984). The meningioma may show enhancement with intravenous contrast, a feature not seen to a significant extent with optic nerve glioma (Moseley & Sanders 1982). Dutton and Anderson (1985) have drawn attention to the similarity of the perineural variant of orbital pseudotumour and optic nerve sheath meningioma.

Where the differential diagnosis is between meningioma and optic glioma, biopsy may not clarify the situation because of the difficulty in differentiating between meningioma and meningeal hyperplasia (anonymous 1979). Distinctions of these two entities on clinical and radiological grounds is usually possible (Jakobiec *et al.* 1984; Rothfus *et al.* 1984).

Treatment

The main choice lies between observation and surgical excision, although radiotherapy may also be considered (Kennerdell & Garrity 1988). Surgical excision of a lesion not extending backwards through the optic canal will be curative, leaving a blind but cosmetically satisfactory eye (Wolter 1988). Optic nerve sheath meningioma is reported to run a more aggressive course in children than adults so surgical treatment may be favoured (Jakobiec *et al.* 1984). On the other hand, these lesions have no metastatic potential and may grow slowly, so observation to establish the pattern of growth in individual cases appears a reasonable course.

Rare optic nerve tumours in childhood

Leukaemic infiltration of the optic nerve traditionally carries a grave systemic prognosis although with combined radiotherapy and chemotherapy the prognosis is greatly improved. The infiltration may be prelaminar, when the optic disc has a fluffy appearance with oedema and haemorrhage without marked visual loss, or retrolaminar with only moderate disc swelling but profound visual loss (Kincaid & Green 1983; Rosenthal 1983).

Tumours of the optic disc such as melanocytoma, angiomatous malformations, or glial hamartoma (as seen in tuberous sclerosis) may involve the very anterior parts of the optic nerve. Medulloepithelioma, ganglioma, ganglioglioma (Bergin *et al.* 1988), inflammatory lesions, aneuryms, histiocytosis, sarcomas, and other rare entities have also been described (Eggers *et al.* 1976; Brown *et al.* 1985). Margo and Kincaid (1988) found a vascular malformation in the retrolaminar portion of two eyes removed for suspicion of retinoblastoma, one eye had a neuroblastic tumour and the other a form of retina dysplasia.

References

Anonymous. Primary optic nerve meningioma (Editorial). *Br J Ophthalmol* 1979; **63**: 595

Bergin DJ, Johnson TE, Spencer WH, McCord CD. Ganglioglioma of the optic nerve. *Am J Ophthalmol* 1988; **105**: 146–50

Bickler–Bluth ME, Custer PL, Smith ME. Neurilemoma as a

presenting feature of neurofibromatosis. *Arch Ophthalmol* 1988; **106**: 665—9

Binet E, Keiffer SA, Martin SH, Peterson HO. Orbital dysplasia in neurofibromatosis. *Radiology* 1969; **93**: 829—33

Borit A, Richardson EF. The biological and clinical behaviour of pilocytic astrocytomas of the optic pathways. *Brain* 1982; **105**: 161—88

Brown GC, Shields JA. Tumours of the optic nerve head. *Surv Ophthalmol* 1985; **29**: 239—64

Buchanan TAS, Hoyt WF. Optic nerve glioma and neovascular glaucoma; report of a case. *Br J Ophthalmol* 1982; **66**: 96—8

Burrows EH. Bone changes in orbital neurofibromatosis. *Br J Radiol* 1963; **36**: 549—61

Charles NC, Nelson L, Brookner AR *et al*. Pilocytic astrocytoma of the optic nerve with haemorrhage and extreme cystic degeneration. *Am J Ophthalmol* 1981; **92**: 691—5

Charleux J. Les manifestations palpebrale et orbitaires de la neurofibromatose de Recklinghausen. *Ann Oculist (Paris)* 1960; **193**: 930—62

Crowe FW, Schell WJ. Diagnostic importance of café-au-lait spot in neurofibromatosis. *Arch Int Med* 1953; **91**: 758—66

Dutton JJ, Anderson RL. Idiopathic inflammatory perioptic neuritis similating optic nerve sheath meningioma. *Am J Ophthalmol* 1985; **100**: 424—30

Eggers H, Jakobiec FA, Jones IS. Tumours of the optic nerve. *Doc Ophthalmol* 1976; **41**: 43—128

Fletcher WA, Imes RK, Hoyt WF. Chiasmal gliomas: appearance and long-term changes demonstrated by computerized tomography. *J Neurosurg* 1986; **65**: 154—9

Font RL, Ferry AP. Phakomatoses. *Int Ophthalmol Clin* 1972; **12**: 1—50

François J. Ocular aspects of phakomatoses. In: Vinken PJ, Bruyn GW (Eds.) *Handbook of Clinical Neurology*. American Elsevier, New York 1972; pp. 624—39

François J, Katz C. Association homolatérale dehydrophthalmie de névrome plexiforme de la paupière supérerieure et d'hemihypertrophie faciale dans la maladie de Recklinghausen. *Ophthalmologica* 1961; **142**: 549—71

Glaser JS, Hoyt WF, Corbett J. Visual morbidity with chiasmal glioma: long-term studies of visual fields in untreated and irridiated cases. *Arch Ophthalmol* 1971; **85**: 3—12

Grant WM, Walton DS. Distinctive gonioscopic findings in glaucoma due to neurofibromatosis. *Arch Ophthalmol* 1968; **79**: 127—34

Grimson BS, Perry DD. Enlargement of the optic disc in childhood optic nerve tumours. *Am J Ophthalmol* 1984; **97**: 627—31

Haik B, Saint Louis L, Bierly J, Smith M, Abramson D, Ellsworth R, Wall M. Magnetic resonance imaging in the evaluation of optic nerve gliomas. *Ophthalmology* 1987; **94**: 709—718

Harkin J, Reed R. Tumours of the peripheral nervous system. In: *Atlas of Tumour Pathology*, 2nd series, fascicle 3. Armed Forces Institute of Pathology, Washington 1969

Holman RE, Grimson BS, Drayer BP, Buckley EG, Brennan MW. Magnetic resonance imaging of optic gliomas. *Am J Ophthalmol* 1985; **100**: 596—601

Howrich A, Bloom HJG. Optic gliomas: radiation therapy and prognosis. *Int J Radiat Oncol Biol Phys* 1985; **11**: 1067—79

Hoyt CS, Billson FA. Buphthalmos in neurofibromatosis: is it an expression of regional giantism? *J Pediatr Ophthalmol Strabismus* 1977; **14**: 228—34

Hoyt WF, Baghdassarian SA. Optic glioma of childhood. Natural history and rationale for conservative management. *Br J Ophthalmol* 1969; **53**: 793—98

Hoyt WF, Meshel LG, Lessell S *et al*. Malignant optic glioma of adulthood. *Brain* 1973; **96**: 121—32

Huson S, Jones D, Beck L. Ophthalmic manifestations of neurofibromatosis. *Br J Ophthalmol* 1987; **71**: 235—9

Imes RK, Hoyt WF. Childhood chiasmal gliomas: update on the fate of patients in the 1969 San Francisco study. *Br J Ophthalmol* 1986; **70**: 179—82

Jackson IT, Laws ER, Martin RD. The surgical management of orbital neurofibromatosis. *Plast Reconstr Surg* 1983; **71**: 751—8

Jakobiec FA, Depot MJ, Kennerdell J *et al*. Combined clinical and computed tomographic diagnosis of orbital glioma and meningioma. *Ophthalmology* 1984; **91**: 137—55

Jakabiec FA, Jones IS. Neurogenic tumours. In: Duane T (Ed.) *Clinical Ophthalmology*, Vol. 2. Harper & Row; Hagerstown 1983; pp. 1—16

Karp LA. Primary intraorbital meningioma. *Arch Ophthalmol* 1974; **91**: 24

Kennerdell JS, Garrity JA. Tumours of the optic nerve. In: Lessell S, Van Dalen JTW (Eds.) *Current Neuro-ophthalmology*, Vol. 1. Year Book Medical Publishers Inc, Chicago 1988; pp. 25—32

Kincaid MC, Green WR. Ocular and orbital involvement in leukaemia. *Surv Ophthalmol* 1983; **15**: 123—6

Lavery MA, O'Neill JF, Chu FE, Martyn LJ. Acquired nystagmus in early childhood: a presenting sign of intracranial tumour. *Ophthalmology* 1984; **91**: 425—34

Leib ML, Kates MR. Orbital computer-assisted tomography. In: Lessel S, Van Dalen JTW (Eds.) *Current Neuro-ophthalmology*, Vol. 1. Year Book Medical Publishing Inc, Chicago 1988; pp. 323—44

Lewis RA, Gerson LP, Axelson KA *et al*. Von Recklinghausen neurofibromatosis II: Incidence of optic glioma. *Ophthalmology* 1984; **91**: 929—35

Lewis RA, Riccardi VM. Von Recklinghausen Neurofibromatosis. Incidence of iris hamartoma. *Ophthalmology* 1981; **88**: 348—54

Linder B, Campos M, Schafer M. CT and MRI of orbital anomalies in neurofibromatosis and selected craniofacial anomalies. *Radiol Clin North Am* 1987; **25**: 787—802

Lisch K. Ueber beteiligung der Augen, insbesondere das Vorkommen von Iirisknötchen bei der Neurofibromatose (Recklinghausen). *Z Augenheilkd* 1937; **93**: 137—43

Margo CE, Kincaid MC. Angiomatous malformation of the retrolaminar optic nerve. *J Pediatr Ophthalmol Strabismus* 1988; **25**: 37—40

Moseley IF, Sanders MD. *Computerised Tomography in Neuro-ophthalmology*. Chapman & Hall, London 1982

Nicholson DH, Green WR. *Pediatric Ocular Tumours*. Masson, New York 1981

Packer RJ, Savino PJ, Bilaniuk LT *et al*. Chasmatic gliomas of childhood. A reappraisal of natural history and effectiveness of cranial irradiation. *Child's Brain* 1983; **10**: 393—403

Perry HD, Font RL. Iris nodules in Von Recklinghausen's neurofibromatosis. *Arch Ophthalmol* 1982; **100**: 1635—40

Reed D, Robertson WD, Rootman J, Douglas G. Plexiform neurofibromatosis of the orbit. CT evaluation. *Am J Neuroradiol* 1986; **7**: 259—63

Reese AB. *Tumours of the Eye*, 3rd Ed. Harper & Row,

Hagerstown 1976; pp. 156 65

Rosenstock JG, Packer RJ, Bilaniuk L *et al.* Chiasmatic optic glioma treated with chemotherapy. A preliminary report. *J Neurosurg* 1985; **63**: 862−6

Rosenthal AR. Ocular manifestations of leukaemia: a review. *Ophthalmology* 1983; **90**: 899−905

Rothfus WE, Curtin MD, Slamovits TL, Kennerdell JS. Optic nerve/sheath enlargement. *Radiology* 1984; **150**: 409−15

Rush JA, Younge BR, Campbell RJ, MacCarthy CS. Optic glioma: Long-term follow-up of 85 histopathologically verified cases. *Ophthalmology* 1982; **89**: 1213−9

Russell A. A diencephalic syndrome of emaciation in infancy and childhood. *Arch Dis Child* 1951; **26**: 274

Savino PJ. The present role of magnetic resonance imaging in neuro-ophthalmology. *Can J Ophthalmol* 1987; **22**: 4−12

Seiff SR, Brodsky MC, MacDonald G, Berg BD, Howes EL, Hoyt WF. Orbital optic glioma in neurofibromatosis. *Arch Ophthalmol* 1987; **105**: 1689−93

Smith B, English FP. Classical eyelid border sign of neuro-fibromatosis *Br J Ophthalmol* 1970; **54**: 137

Spencer WH. Primary neoplasms of the optic nerve and it's sheaths. *Trans Am Ophthalmol Soc* 1972; **70**: 490−505

Spoor TC, Kennerdell JS, Martinez AJ, Zoras D. Malignant gliomas of the optic pathways. *Am J Ophthalmol* 1980; **89**: 284−92

Taylor D. Congenital tumours of the superior visual system with dysplasia of the optic discs. *Br J Ophthalmol* 1982; **66**: 455−63

Tenzel RR, Royston JR, Miller GE, Buffarn FV. Surgical treatment of eyelid neurofibromas. *Arch Ophthalmol* 1977; **95**: 479

Van der Hoeve J. Eye symptoms in phakomatoses. The Doyne Memorial Lecture. *Trans Ophthalmol Soc UK* 1932; **52**: 380−401

Van der Hoeve T. Eye disease in tuberous sclerosis of the brain and in Recklinghausen's disease. *Trans Ophthalmol Soc UK* 1923; **43**: 534−41

von Recklinghausen FD. Ueber die multiplen Fibrome der Haut und ihre Beziehung zu den multiplen Neuromen. *Festschrift zur Feier des fünfundzwanzigjährigen Bestchens des pathologischen Instituts zu Berlin*; Herrn Rudolf Virchow dargebracht. Hirschwald: Berlin, 1882

Whitehouse D. Diagnostic value of café-au-lait spot in children. *Arch Dis Child* 1966; **44**: 316−19

Wolter JR. Ten years without orbital optic nerve: late clinical results after removal of retrobulbar gliomas with preservation of blind eyes. *J Pediatr Ophthalmol Strabismus* 1988; **25**: 55−60

Wolter JR, Butler RG. Pigment spots of the iris and ectropion uveae with glaucoma in neurofibromatosis. *Am J Ophthalmol* 1963; **56**: 964−73

Woog JJ, Albert DM, Solt LC, Hu DN, Wang WJ. Neuro-fibromatosis of the eyelid and orbit. *Int Ophthalmol Clin* 1982; **22**: 157−87

Wright JE, MacDonald WI, Cal ND. Management of optic nerve gliomas. *Br J Ophthalmol* 1980; **64**: 545−53

22.6 Rhabdomyosarcoma

JOHN BRAZIER

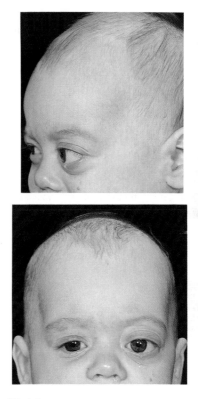

Fig. 22.6.1 Rhabdomyosarcoma. This 3-month-old boy had a 2-week history of left proptosis.

Rhabdomyosarcoma is a tumour of striated muscle cells and the most common primary orbital malignancy in children. Males are slightly more likely to be affected than females (Ashton & Morgan 1965; Jones *et al.* 1965) and most cases present before the age of 10 years, the mean age at onset being 7–8 years (Knowles *et al.* 1983). Over the past two decades treatment has changed from radical surgery to biopsy, radiotherapy and chemotherapy with considerable improvement in disease control and survival rates (Haik *et al.* 1986).

Clinical features

The commonest presenting feature is rapidly progressive proptosis (Frayer & Enterline 1959; Jones *et al.* 1965) (Fig. 22.6.1). There are often quite marked inflammatory signs and in some cases swelling of one or both lids (Fig. 22.6.2) precedes the proptosis (Lederman & Wybar 1976); in others ptosis or a palpable lid mass occurs at onset of the proptosis or shortly after (Knowles *et al.* 1983). Less commonly they present as lid lumps (resembling chalazion), subconjunctival nodules, or periorbital swellings (Fig. 22.6.3).

Clinical appearance is altered by the initial location of the tumour within the orbit. In Jones *et al.*'s (1965) study of 62 cases, the mass was located behind the globe in 50% of cases, in the superior part of the orbit in 25%, inferior in 12%, nasal in 6% and temporal in 6%. Despite frequent location behind the globe, central vision is usually preserved (Frayer & Enterline 1959).

Rhabdomyosarcoma shares the routes of spread of all malignant tumours. Marked local invasiveness tends to be a feature and, whilst direct spread may be confined by the orbital walls, extension into the anterior or middle cranial fossa (parameningeal spread) or nasal cavity occurs. The latter may give rise to nasal stuffiness or nose bleeds. Occasionally a tumour arises within the cranial cavity, giving rise to proptosis when orbital involvement occurs (Shuangshoti & Phonprasert 1976). Although the

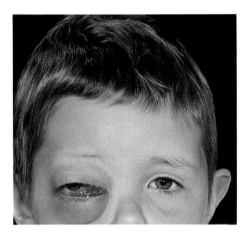

Fig. 22.6.2 Rhabdomyosarcoma. This 6-year-old girl had tumour involving the medial wall of the orbit with chronic proptosis.

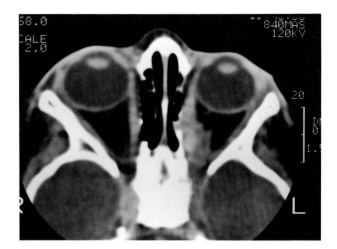

Fig. 22.6.4 Rhabdomyosarcoma. CT scan showing involvement of the left medial rectus and medial wall of the orbit. Transethmoidal biopsy was performed.

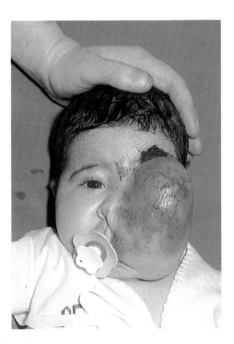

Fig. 22.6.3 Rhabdomyosarcoma. This 15-month-old child had a tumour which had previously been treated as a haemangioma — it involved only the soft tissues of the face.

orbital structures themselves are without lymphatics, deposits may occur in cervical or preauricular lymph nodes. Haematological spread is usually to lung and, occasionally, bone (Knowles *et al.* 1983).

Diagnosis

Rhabdomyosarcoma should be suspected when rapidly progressive proptosis occurs in a child. This clinical situation requires urgent investigation and biopsy if radiological studies identify a neoplasm. CT or MRI scanning will delineate tumour mass and allow the biopsy approach to be planned (Fig. 22.6.4). Plain orbital X-ray may show increased soft tissue density in the orbit or evidence of bone erosion by tumour. Knowles *et al.* (1983) stress the importance of taking a large biopsy to aid identification of diagnostic muscle cell cross-striations. Rhabdomyosarcoma tends to recur along the biopsy tract (Jones *et al.* 1965) so a transcranial biopsy route should be avoided.

Main clinical differential diagnoses are orbital cellulitis, haemangioma, lymphangioma, leukaemia or granulocytic sarcoma, metastatic neuroblastoma, dermoid cyst or retinoblastoma that has spread into the orbit. Most of these can be eliminated by clinical, haematological, and radiological studies, with biopsy where doubt remains.

Pathology

Rhabdomyosarcoma originates in undifferentiated mesenchyme which is either prospective muscle or capable of differentiation into muscle (Harry 1975; Knowles *et al.* 1983). On the basis of their histopathological features orbital rhabdomyosarcomas are classified as embryonal, differentiated or alveolar (Hogan & Zimmerman 1962; Porterfield & Zimmerman 1962; Yannoff & Fine 1976).

Embryonal rhabdomyosarcoma (Ashton & Morgan 1965) is the commonest type. It is composed of malignant embryonal cells (rhabdomyoblasts) in a loose syncitial arrangement. Cells are long and spindle shaped, the majority showing typical cytoplasmic cross-striations. The differentiated type is the least common and associated with a better prognosis (Porterfield & Zimmerman 1962; Charles 1979). Tumour cells are large and, when stained, deeply acidophilic and often granular. Nearly all cells have abundant longitudinal and cross-striations. The alveolar type is more common than the differentiated and carries the worst prognosis (Knowles *et al.* 1983). Cells resemble those of the embryonal type but are divided into alveolar groups by connective tissue trabeculae (Riopelle & Thériault 1956).

Histopathological features of the various types overlap and diagnosis by light microscopy alone may be difficult. Electron microscopy is extremely useful in confirming diagnosis by identification of myofilamentary differentiation (Weichselbaum *et al.* 1980; Ghafoor & Dudgeon 1985). Use of immunohistochemical stains increases the accuracy of diagnosis (Kahn *et al.* 1983; Garrido & Arra 1986).

Treatment

Historical aspects

Orbital rhabdomyosarcoma was treated by surgery alone until the mid 1960s (Jones *et al.* 1965). Frayer and Enterline (1959) reported recurrence requiring orbital exenteration in all five patients treated by local tumour resection in a series of 12 patients. Exenteration remained the treatment of choice, the best published results being those of Jones *et al.* (1965) with 32% 3-year and 29% 5-year survival. Surgical treatment was therefore associated with a poor prognosis.

In 1968 Cassady *et al.* (1968) reported five patients treated by surgery and primary radiotherapy rather than radical surgery. All five patients were alive at follow-up varying from 15 months to 5 years. During the succeeding years there followed reports of improved survival with radiotherapy and benefits of adjuvant chemotherapy (Heyn *et al.* 1974; Abramson 1979).

It is now widely accepted that optimal treatment consists of biopsy, radiotherapy and chemotherapy (Knowles *et al.* 1983; Wybar 1983; Ellsworth 1987).

Present treatment

Clinical and radiological (Vade & Armstrong 1987) diagnosis is confirmed by biopsy, which may be excisional.

Extent of disease within the orbit and surrounding structures is assessed by orbital and head computerized tomography (CT) or magnetic resonance imaging (MRI) scanning. Metastatic disease is identified or excluded by studies including chest X-ray, full blood count, bone scan and marrow studies. When this information is available the disease can be staged. Various staging systems are described; these are reviewed by Weichselbaum *et al.* (1980).

Radiotherapy involves treatment of the orbit and surrounding bony tissues with 3000−6000 cGy in divided doses over 6 weeks (Weichselbaum *et al.* 1979; Knowles *et al.* 1983; Wharam *et al.* 1987). Most patients require in the region of 5000 cGy. Treatment is given with the eye open to reduce the severity of radiation keratoconjunctivitis. Radiotherapy can be expected to control orbital disease in 90% cases (Ellsworth 1987).

Chemotherapy is used as an adjuvent to radiotherapy for orbital and parameningeal disease and to treat metastatic disease. Agents used include vincristine, adriamycin, cyclophosphamide, actinomycin D, and methotrexate (Ghafoor & Dudgeon 1985; Haik *et al.* 1986; Wharam *et al.* 1987). Treatments may need to be continued over 2 years.

Complications of treatment

Complications of treatment by radiotherapy and chemotherapy in 50 patients were reviewed by Heyn *et al.* (1986). Ninety per cent had visual loss of variable degree on the affected eye. Specific eye changes included cataract and keratoconjunctivitis (Fig. 22.6.5, 22.6.6) following treatment of 30−64 cGy to the tumour. Radiological evidence of bone hypoplasia was present in over half the patients with facial asymmetry in many cases. Enophthalmos, lacrimal duct stenosis and dental defects occurred in some patients. Incidental irradiation of the pituitary produced growth reduction in many patients.

Prognosis and future developments

The Intergroup Rhabdomyosarcoma Study (IRS) Committee recently reported 127 patients with rhabdomyosarcoma confined to the orbit and lid treated by subtotal tumour resection or biopsy followed by radiotherapy and chemotherapy (Wharam *et al.* 1987). Excluding diseases from other causes, 3-year survival was 93% indicating a considerable improvement in prognosis over the last 20 years. Eleven of 18 (61%) with parameningeal spread reported by Haik (1986) were alive and well at 6 years. Although late recur-

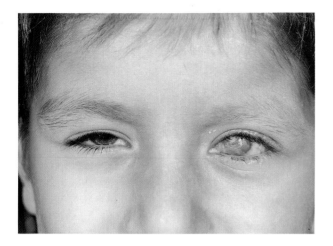

Fig. 22.6.5 Rhabdomyosarcoma. Radiation keratis and dry-eye.

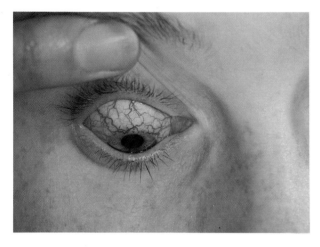

Fig. 22.6.6 Rhabdomyosarcoma. Radiation-induced vascular changes.

rence is unusual, prolonged follow-up is indicated as some cases recur after a long interval (Chestler *et al.* 1988).

Future developments will involve refinement of chemotherapeutic regimes to reduce toxicity of the present drugs (Ghafoor & Dudgeon 1985). The eye can be protected by maintaining orbital irradiation in the 4500–500 cGy range and, in the future, possible use of agents to protect the cornea and lens from radiation damage (Ellsworth 1987).

References

Abramson DH, Ellsworth RM, Tretter P *et al*. The treatment of orbital rhabdomyosarcoma with irradiation and chemotherapy. *Ophthalmology* 1979; **86**: 1330–5

Ashton N, Morgan G. Embryonal sarcoma and embryonal rhabdomyosarcoma of the orbit. *J Clin Pathol* 1965; **18**: 699–714

Cassady JR, Sagerman RH, Tretter P, Ellsworth RM. Radiation therapy for rhabdomyosarcoma. *Radiology* 1968; **91**: 116–20

Charles NC. Pathology and incidence or orbital disorders: an overview. In: Hornblass A (Ed.) *Tumours of the Ocular Adnexa and Orbit*. CV Mosby Co., St Louis 1979; pp. 190–3

Chestler RJ, Dortzbach RK, Kronisch JW. Late recurrence in primary orbital rhabdomyosarcoma (Letter). *Am J Ophthalmol* 1988; **106**: 92–3

Ellsworth RM. Discussion of 'localised orbital rhabdomyosarcoma'. *Ophthalmology* 1987; **94**: 254

Frayer WC, Enterline HT. Embryonal rhabdomyosarcoma of the orbit in children and young adults. *Arch Ophthalmol* 1959; **62**: 203–10

Garrido CM, Arra A. Immunohistochemical study of embryonal rhabdomyosarcomas. *Ophthalmologica* 1986; **193**: 154–9

Ghafoor SY, Dudgeon J. Orbital rhabdomyosarcoma: improved survival with combined pulsed chemotherapy and irradiation. *Br J Ophthalmol* 1985; **69**: 557–61

Haik BG, Jereb B, Smith ME *et al*. Radiation and chemotherapy of parameningeal rhabdomyosarcoma involving the orbit. *Ophthalmology* 1986; **93**: 1001–9

Harry J. Pathology of rhabdomyosarcoma. *Mod Probl Ophthalmol* 1975; **14**: 325–9

Heyn RM, Holland R, Newton WA *et al*. The role of combined chemotherapy in the treatment of rhabdomyosarcoma in children. *Cancer* 1974; **34**: 2128–42

Heyn R, Ragab A, Raney RB Jr *et al*. Late effects of therapy in orbital rhabdomyosarcoma in children. A report from the Intergroup Rhabdomyosarcoma Study. *Cancer* 1986; **57**: 1738–43

Hogan MF, Zimmerman LE. In: *Ophthalmic Pathology: An Atlas and Textbook*, 2nd Edn. WB Saunders & Co., Philadelphia 1962; pp. 746–51

Jones IS, Reese AB, Krout J. Orbital rhabdomyosarcoma: an analysis of 62 cases. *Trans Am Ophthalmol Soc* 1965; **63**: 223–51

Kahn HJ, Yeger H, Kassim O *et al*. Immunohistochemical and electron microscopic assessment of childhood rhabdomyosarcoma. *Cancer* 1983; **51**: 1897–903

Knowles DM, Jakobiec FA, Jones IS. Rhabdomyosarcoma. In: Duane TD (Ed.) *Clinical Ophthalmology*. Harper & Row, Philadelphia 1983

Lederman M, Wybar K. Embryonal sarcoma. *Proc Roy Soc Med* 1976; **69**: 895–903

Porterfield JF, Zimmerman LE. Rhabdomyosarcoma of the orbit. A clinico-pathologic study of 55 cases. *Virchows Arch Path Anat* 1962; **335**: 329–44

Riopelle JL, Theriault JP. A little known form of sarcoma of the soft parts. Alveolar rhabdomyosarcoma. *Ann Anat Path* 1956; **1**: 88–111

Shuangshoti S, Phonprasert C. Primary intracranial rhabdomyosarcoma producing proptosis. *J Neurol Neurosurg Psychiatr* 1976; **39**: 531–35

Vade A, Armstrong D. Orbital rhabdomyosarcoma in childhood. *Radiol Clin North Am* 1987; **25**: 701–14

Weichselbaum RR, Cassady JR, Albert DM, Gonder JR. Multimodality management of orbital rhabdomyosarcoma. *Int Ophthalmol Clin* 1980; **20**: 247−59

Wharam M, Beltangady M, Hays D *et al*. Localized orbital rhabdomyosarcoma. An interim report of the Intergroup Rhabdomyosarcoma Study Committee. *Ophthalmology* 1987;

94: 251−4

Wybar K. Malignant disease. In: Wybar K, Taylor D (Eds.) *Pediatric Ophthalmology* Marcel Dekker, New York 1983; pp. 417−30

Yanoff M, Fine RS. *Ocular pathology: A Text and Atlas*. Harper & Row, New York 1976; pp. 538−40

22.7 Orbital Pseudotumour

JOHN BRAZIER

Definition and introduction

Pseudotumour refers to a space-occupying inflammatory lesion within the orbit that clinically simulates a neoplasm (Blodi & Gass 1968; Jellinek 1969; Mottow & Jakobiec 1978). In this section we use the definition of Jakobiec and Jones (1983a) restricting the term pseudotumour to a category of inflammations without identifiable cause, which may be referred to as idiopathic inflammatory pseudotumour. Lesions due to foreign bodies, bacterial or other infections or related to thyroid dysfunction are excluded.

Whilst orbital pseudotumour is predominantly a disease of adults, it certainly occurs in children (Blodi & Gass 1968; Jakobiec & Jones 1983a, 1983b). Indeed, Jakobiec and Jones (1983b) considered pseudotumour to be the fifth most common cause of orbital disease in children. The condition shows no sex predilection and, in children, symptoms are most likely to commence between 6 and 14 years of age (Mottow & Jakobiec 1978).

Clinical features

Patients typically present with an acute onset of unilateral orbital involvement giving rise to a variety of symptoms and signs. In the cases of 29 children reported by Mottow and Jakobiec (1978), swelling of the lids, particularly in the morning, and pain were the most common symptoms. Ptosis, proptosis, diplopia and an obvious mass were also relatively frequent. Common signs included reduced acuity, conjunctival infection and chemosis, displacement of the globe, a palpable mass, ptosis and anterior uveitis.

Symptoms and signs may vary with the location of the inflammatory mass and a range of disorders can occur. If orbital involvement is diffuse there will be painful ophthalmoplegia and visual loss, if involvement is mainly anterior there will be lid swelling, uveitis and involvement of Tenon's capsule (periscleritis). When the mass is predominantly posterior there may be an orbital apex syndrome (painful ophthalmoplegia with visual loss) or superior orbital fissure syndrome (paralysis of muscles subserved by III, IV and VIth cranial nerves without significant visual loss) (Moseley & Sanders 1982). When the inflammatory response involves the optic nerve (called perineuritis when little inflammation is present elsewhere in the orbit) (Kennerdell & Dresner 1984) disc swelling may be present. Disease may be localized to one or more extraocular muscles (myositis) or the lacrimal gland (dacroadenitis) (Moseley & Sanders 1982; Kennerdell & Dresner 1984).

The acute orbital lesion may be accompanied by systemic symptoms including headache, nausea and vomiting (Mottow & Jakobiec 1978) and malaise (Jellinek 1969). Following presentation, the episode may subside with treatment and never recur, alternatively there are recurrent episodes, affecting one or both orbits over a period of years or the condition becomes chronic, requiring prolonged treatment.

Investigation

Computerized tomographic (CT) scanning of the orbit is the most important investigation although, in the future, magnetic resonance image (MRI) scanning may be preferred because of better diagnostic specificity (Atlas *et al.* 1987). CT findings again depend on the size and severity of inflammation and may vary

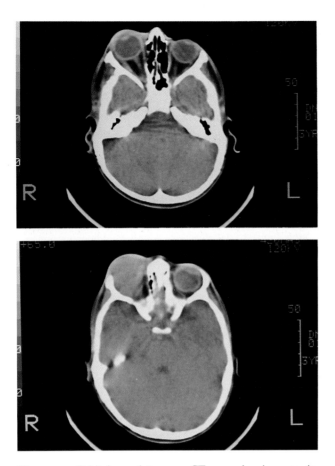

Fig. 22.7.1 Orbital pseudotumour. CT scans showing mass in upper part of the orbit causing proptosis and downward displacement of the eye.

between virtually normal to scans in which virtually no orbital anatomy can be distinguished (Moseley & Sanders 1982). Pseudotumour dacroadenitis must be distinguished from viral dacroadenitis (mumps, infectious mononucleosis) or response to a ruptured dermoid cyst adjacent to the lacrimal gland. Viral causes can usually be distinguished by presence of lymphadenopathy and peripheral blood lymphocytosis (Kennerdell & Dresner 1984). The extraocular muscle enlargement in myositis involves the muscle insertions and this allows differentiation from dysthyroid muscle enlargement where the insertion is spared (Moseley & Sanders 1982). The perineuritis variant may have similar appearances on CT to optic nerve sheath meningioma (Dutton & Anderson 1985). When the mass is located near the orbital fissure, involvement of the cavernous sinus should be excluded.

Other investigations include differential blood count, which may show eosinophilia, and the erythrocyte sedimentation rate (ESR) which is usually raised (Mottow & Jakobiec 1978). ANF titre may be elevated in patients with involvement of the superior orbital fissure.

Biopsy may be indicated under certain circumstances, particularly where response to systemic steroid treatment is poor or the disease recurs after treatment. Mottow and Jakobiec (1978) noted that biopsy was associated with residual deficits in their patients and some cases of biopsy proven pseudotumour have ultimately turned out to be other disorders (Jakobiec & Jones 1983). Biopsy can reasonably be avoided by diagnosis based on typical history, signs and CT appearances, combined with a dramatic response to systemic steroid treatment.

Pathology

A comprehensive account of the pathology of pseudotumour has been provided by Jakobiec and Jones (1983a) and this ground will not be covered again in this account. However, the findings of Mottow-Lippa *et al.* (1981) based on biopsy of orbital pseudotumour in 16 children are of interest and will be summarized.

They found that new lesions showed loose fibrous tissue, widely spaced fibroblasts and scattered inflammatory cells. Progressive disease was associated with increased hyalinization of connective tissue. Cellular infiltration was mainly lymphocytes and plasma cells with no evidence of true immunogenic granuloma formation. Presence of eosinophilic infiltration in biopsy specimens correlated with blood eosinophilia. Late sequelae of inflammation were the consequence of collagen deposition within orbital structures (particularly relevant to residual motility problems).

Treatment

Treatment is with oral corticosteroids. Initial dosage of 1–1.5 mg/kg/day prednisolone should produce a dramatic reduction of pain in 1–2 days (Mottow & Jakobiec 1978). Steroids are tapered gradually depending on symptoms and signs. In recurrent or chronic cases maintenance steroids may be required. Radiotherapy remains an option in chronic disease (Kennerdell & Dresner 1984) but may be ineffective in children (Mottow & Jakobiec 1978) in whom long-term effects of radiotherapy on orbital development must be borne in mind.

Prognosis

Some comments on prognosis were also made by

Mottow & Jakobiec (1978). As judged by residual loss of acuity, ocular motility disturbance and proptosis, prognosis was best after a single unilateral episode and worst in bilateral recurrent disease. Recurrent unilateral attacks formed an intermediate group.

References

Atlas FW, Grossman RI, Savino PJ *et al*. Surface coil MR of orbital pseudotumour. *AJNR* 1987; **8**: 141−6

Blodi FC, Gass DJM. Inflammatory pseudotumour of the orbit. *Br J Ophthalmol* 1968; **52**: 79−93

Dutton JJ, Anderson RC. Idiopathic inflammation perioptic neuritis simulating optic nerve sheath meningioma. *Am J Ophthalmol* 1985; **100**: 424−30

Jakobiec FA, Jones IS. Orbital inflammation. In: Duane T (Ed.) *Clinical Ophthalmology*, Vol. 2. Harper & Row, Hagerstown 1983a

Jakobiec FA, Jones IS. Patient examination and introduction to orbital disease. In: Duane T (Ed.) Vol. 2. *Clinical Ophthalmology*. Harper & Row, Hagerstown 1983b

Jellinek EH. The orbital pseudotumour syndrome and its differentiation from endocrine exophthalmos. *Brain* 1969; **92**: 35−58

Kennerdell JS, Dresner SC. The non-specific orbital inflammatory syndromes. *Surv Ophthalmol* 1984; **29**: 93−103

Moseley IF, Sanders MD. *Computerised Tomography in Neuro-ophthalmology*. Chapman & Hall, London 1982

Mottow LS, Jakobiec FA. Idiopathic inflammatory orbital pseudotumour in childhood. I Clinical characteristics. *Arch Ophthalmol* 1978; **96**: 1410−7

Mottow-Lippa L, Jakobiec FA, Smith M. Idiopathic inflammatory orbital pseudotumour in childhood. II Results of diagnostic tests and biopsies. *Ophthalmology* 1981; **88**: 565−74

22.8 Lacrimal Gland, Metastatic, and Secondary Orbital Tumours

JOHN BRAZIER

Neuroblastoma and Ewing's sarcoma are responsible for the majority of childhood orbital metastatic disease (Albert *et al*. 1967). Other tumours can rarely give rise to orbital metastases including Wilms' tumour (Apple 1968), testicular embryonal sarcoma, ovarian sarcoma and renal embryonal sarcoma (Nicholson & Green 1981).

Jakobiec and Jones (1983) are careful to differentiate between blood borne deposits of a malignant tumour (metastatic disease) and extension of a tumour into the orbital tissues from an adjacent structure (secondary disease). Retinoblastoma extending into the optic nerve or orbital structures is the most important source of secondary orbital disease in children.

Neuroblastoma

Neuroblastoma is the most common cause of orbital metastases in childhood, accounting for 41 of 46 cases of orbital metastatic disease reported by Albert *et al*. (1967). The primary tumour had been diagnosed prior to presentation with orbital disease in 93% of cases. Presentation with orbital neuroblastoma before the primary is detected is therefore relatively unusual, accounting for 8% of the cases reported by Musarella *et al*. (1984). Despite being the most common metastatic orbital tumour in children, neuroblastoma accounted for only 1.5% of 214 orbital tumours reported

by Porterfield (1962) and 3% of 307 orbital tumours in children quoted by Nicholson and Green (1981).

Neuroblastoma is a malignant neoplasm derived from embryonic neuroblastic tissue anywhere within the sympathetic nervous system. It is second only to central nervous system (CNS) tumours and leukaemia as a cause of childhood malignancy, accounting for 10–15% of the total (De Lorimer 1969; Jakobiec & Jones 1983). Primary sites include the adrenals (more than 50% of cases), other retroperitoneal structures, cervical sympathetic chain, mediastinium, and pelvis (Gross *et al*. 1959; De Lorimer 1969). There is a single report of primary orbital neuroblastoma (Levy 1957). Age of onset varies between birth and late teens, the majority of patients being under 4 years.

The systemic diagnosis is often not made until late in the disease when the patient has widespread metastases (Anon 1975; Musarella 1984). Ninety per cent of patients have abnormally high levels of vanilylmandelic acid (VMA) in their urine reflecting secretion of catecholamines by the tumour. This urinary VMA can be used both in diagnosing the condition and monitoring treatment.

Ophthalmic features

Orbital metastases commonly present as unilateral (Fig. 22.8.1) or bilateral proptosis associated with spontaneous orbital ecchymosis in 25% of cases (Mortada 1967; Alfano 1968; Musarella *et al*. 1984). The lesion may be in the orbital soft tissues, zygoma or frontal bone. Bony lesions give rise to swelling of overlying tissues so periobital swelling and ptosis may be present. Musarella *et al*. (1984) drew attention to the association of Horner's syndrome with cervical and thoracic neuroblastoma and opsoclonus–myoclonus with occult, localized neuroblastoma.

Treatment

The primary lesion is removed where possible. Prognosis is improved by age (under 1 year is favourable),

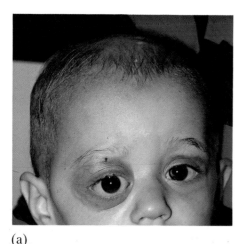

(a)

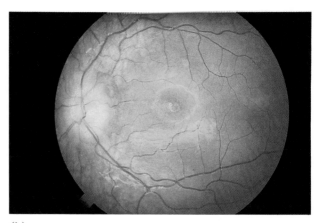

(b)

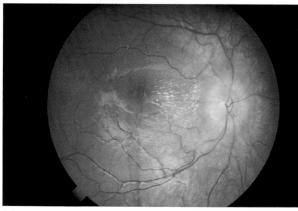

(c)

Fig. 22.8.1 (a) Neuroblastoma. This child presented with bilateral orbital bruising and right proptosis. Dr S. Day's patient. (b, c) Neuroblastoma. This patient had widespread orbital and cranial boney involvement with raised intracranial pressure and papilloedema.

primary site (thoracic lesions better than abdominal) and by absence of widespread metastatic disease at the time of diagnosis. Orbital lesions are treated with radiotherapy and chemotherapy and these treatments used in conjunction with surgery for systemic disease (Green *et al.* 1976). Disseminated disease requires aggressive high dose chemotherapy with agents such as cisplatin, adriamycin, cyclophosphamide, vincristine, carmustine and melphalan, in some cases followed by autologous bone marrow transplantation (Green *et al.* 1976, 1981; Hartmann *et al.* 1987, 1988; Philip *et al.* 1987). Despite the possibility of spontaneous regression of neuroblastoma (Carvalho 1973; Schwartz *et al.* 1974) and recent advances in treatment, the prognosis for affected children remains relatively poor.

Ewing's sarcoma

Ewing's sarcoma is a tumour of primitive mesenchymal cells present in the bone marrow. This malignant tumour usually arises in the long limb bones or bones of the trunk. There is a marked tendency to spread to adjacent soft tissues, other bones and the lungs (Jakobiec & Jones 1983). Usual age of onset is 10–25 years, a period during which neuroblastoma becomes increasingly uncommon.

Albert *et al.* (1967) reported five patients with Ewing's sarcoma metastatic to the orbit. Orbital presentation averaged 14 months after diagnosis of the primary. Presenting signs were rapidly progressive proptosis and orbital haemorrhage.

Treatment of the primary tumour is by surgery or radiotherapy or both, the tumour being highly radiosensitive. Because of the presence of overt or subclinical metastases at the time of diagnosis, these treatments may be supplemented by chemotherapy (Jaffe 1976; Hayes 1987) using agents such as cyclophosphamide and doxorubicin.

Retinoblastoma

Retinoblastoma confined within the eye poses no threat to life and is a curable disease (Jakobiec &

Jones 1983; Abramson 1985). The prognosis is greatly worsened by extension into the orbit or central nervous system or the presence of widespread metastatic disease. This section considers the consequences of transscleral involvement of the orbital tissues (orbital spread) and extension of the tumour into the optic nerve (optic nerve spread).

Orbital spread

Orbital involvement with retinoblastoma was observed in 8% of a series of patients reported by Jakobiec and Jones (1983) but in only 9 out of 268 (3.5%) cases reported by Lennox et al. (1975).

Clinical signs (Fig. 22.8.2) include proptosis a palpable orbital mass, and swelling and ecchymosis. Orbital spread may be discovered as a mass attached to the globe during enucleation or identified by pathological examination of an enucleated eye. Orbital disease may be signalled by a mass arising in the orbit after enucleation. Biopsy is helpful to confirm that this is indeed retinoblastoma rather than a second tumour, such as an osteosarcoma, arising in the field of previous radiotherapy (Abramson et al. 1984). Biopsy may be combined with removal of residual optic nerve but removal of the intracranial nerve back to the chiasm is not advised (Ellsworth 1969).

Optic nerve spread

This is the most common route by which retinoblastoma gains access to the orbit (Henderson 1973). Following invasion of the optic nerve, the tumour may gain access to the cerebrospinal fluid (CSF) and cause widespread central nervous system deposits. Optic nerve spread was identified in 12.7% of the series quoted by Jakobiec and Jones (1983) and 15% of the patients reported by Lennox et al. (1975). Extension into the nerve is most commonly a histological finding; removal of as much optic nerve as possible at the time of enucleation is desirable.

Treatment

Biopsy proven orbital retinoblastoma carries 100% mortality following surgical treatment alone (Ellsworth 1974). Irradiation of the orbital lesions is effective but most patients develop widespread disease within 18 months if radiation is used alone (Abramson 1985). Present treatment of biopsy proven orbital retinoblastoma therefore involves irradiation and systemic chemotherapy with agents such as vincristine,

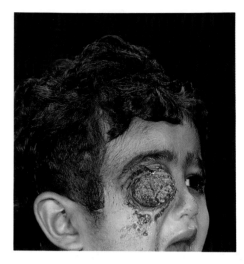

Fig. 22.8.2 Retinoblastoma. This sad picture of a child with extensive orbital involvement with lymphatic spread (note the cervical preauricular gland involvement) is a common presentation in developing countries.

cyclophosphamide, actinomycin D or doxorubicin (White 1983; Abramson 1985). If optic nerve involvement suggests CNS spread, treatment of the central nervous system with radiation or chemotherapy or both is also indicated (White 1983; Keith & Ekert 1987; Zelker 1988).

Lacrimal gland tumours

The most common cause of a lacrimal gland fossa mass in childhood is dermoid cyst, these lesions tending to occur in the upper outer quadrant of the orbit (Nicholson & Green 1981).

Primary epithelial tumours of the lacrimal gland are rare in young children but increase in frequency over the age of 10 years. Benign mixed tumour of the lacrimal gland is unusual and accounted for only one of the 214 childhood orbital tumours reported by Porterfield (1962). Cure is effected by complete removal of the tumour, with a tendency to recurrence if excision is incomplete. These lesions can usually be recognised by their slow progression and the certainty of diagnosis is increased by CT scanning prior to removal (Wright 1979).

Adenoid cystic carcinoma is also uncommon in childhood, although cases have been reported by Porterfield (1962), Wolter and Henderson (1969), Font and Gamel (1978) and Shields et al. (1986). These tumours may not be clinically distinguishable from other lacrimal lesions such as infections, chronic pseudotumour (Kennerdell & Dresner 1984) or leukaemic deposits (Kincaid & Green 1983). Bone erosion on X-rays and presence of calcification in the mass are highly suggestive of malignancy. Biopsy may be required to allow histological confirmation. Adenoid cystic carcinoma is highly invasive and carries a poor prognosis despite surgery, radiotherapy and chemotherapy (Krohel *et al.* 1981).

References

Abramson DH. Treatment of retinoblastoma. In: Blodi FC (Ed.) *Retinoblastoma*. Churchill Livingstone, London 1985; pp. 86–8

Abramson DH, Ellsworth RM, Kitchin FD, Tung G. Second nonocular tumours in retinoblastoma survivors. *Ophthalmology* 1984; **91**: 1351–5

Albert DM, Rubenstein RA, Scheie HG. Tumour metastasis to the eye II. Clinical study in infants and children. *Am J Ophthalmol* 1967; **63**: 727–32

Alfano JE. Ophthalmological aspects of neuroblastomatosis: a study of 53 verified cases. *Trans Am Acad Ophthalmol* 1968; **72**: 830–48

Anonymous. Neuroblastoma (Editorial). *Lancet* 1975; **1**: 379–80

Apple DJ. Wilms' tumour metastatic to the orbit. *Arch Ophthalmol* 1968; **80**: 480–3

Carvalho L. Spontaneous regression of an untreated neuroblastoma. *Br J Ophthalmol* 1973; **57**: 832–5

De Lorimer AA. Neuroblastoma in childhood. *Am J Dis Child* 1969; **118**: 441–50

Ellsworth RM. The practical management of retinoblastoma. *Trans Am Ophthalmol Soc* 1969; **67**: 462–534

Ellsworth RM. Orbital retinoblastoma. *Trans Am Acad Ophthalmol* 1974; **72**: 79–86

Font RL, Gamel JW. Epithelial tumours of the lacrimal gland: an analysis of 256 cases. In: Jakobiec FA (Ed.) *Ocular and Adnexae Tumours*. Aesculapius, Birmingham 1978

Green AA, Hustu HO, Palmer R, Pinkel D. Total-body sequential segmental irradiation and combination chemotherapy for children with disseminated neuroblastoma. *Cancer* 1976; **38**: 2250–7

Green AA, Hayes FA, Husto HO. Sequential cyclophosphamide and doxorubicin for induction of complete remission in children with disseminated neuroblastoma. *Cancer* 1981; **48**: 2310–7

Gross RE, Farber S, Martin LW. Neuroblastoma sympatheticum. A study and report of 217 cases. *Pediatrics* 1959; **23**: 1179–91

Hartmann O, Benhamon E, Beaujean F *et al.* Repeated high-dose chemotherapy followed by purged autologous bone marrow transplantation as consolidation therapy in metastatic neuroblastoma. *J Clin Oncol* 1987; **5**: 1205–11

Hartmann O, Pinkerton CR, Philip T *et al.* Very high-dose cisplatinum and etoposide in children with untreated advanced neuroblastoma. *J Clin Oncol* 1988; **6**: 44–50

Hayes FA, Thompson EI, Parvely L *et al.* Metastatic Ewing's sarcoma: remission, induction and survival. *J Clin Oncol* 1987; **5**: 1199–204

Henderson JW. *Oribital Tumours*. WB Saunders, Philadelphia 1973; pp. 444–94

Jaffe N, Traggis D, Sahan S, Caffady JR. Improved outlook for Ewing's sarcoma with combination chemotherapy (vincristine, actinomycin D and cyclophosphamide) and radiation therapy. *Cancer* 1976; **38**: 1925–30

Jakobiec FA, Jones IS. Metastatic and secondary tumours. In: Duane TD (Ed.) *Clinical Ophthalmology*, Vol. 2. Harper & Row, Hagerstown 1983

Keith CG, Ekert H. The management of retinoblastoma. *Aust NZ J Ophthalmol* 1987; **15**: 359–63

Kennerdell JS, Dresner SC. The non-specific orbital inflammatory syndromes. *Surv Ophthalmol* 1984; **29**: 93–103

Kincaid MC, Green WR. Ocular and orbital involvement in leukaemia. *Surv Ophthalmol* 1983; **15**: 211–32

Krohel GB, Stewart WB, Chavis RM. *Orbital Disease — a Practical Approach*. Grune & Stratton, New York 1981

Lennox EL, Draper GJ, Sanders BM. Retinoblastoma: a study of natural history and prognosis of 268 cases. *Br Med J* 1975; **3**: 731–4

Levy WJ. Neuroblastoma. *Br J Ophthalmol* 1957; **41**: 48–53

Mortada A. Clinical characteristics of early orbital metastatic neuroblastoma. *Am J Ophthalmol* 1967; **63**: 1787–93

Musarella MA, Chan HS, De Boer G, Gallie BL. Ocular involvement in neuroblastoma; prognostic implications. *Ophthalmology* 1984; **91**: 936–40

Nicholson DH, Green WR. *Pediatric Ocular Tumours*. Masson, New York 1981

Philip T, Bernard JL, Zucker JM *et al.* High-dose chemotherapy with bone marrow transplantation as consolidation treatment in neuroblastoma: an unselected group of Stage IV patients over 1 year of age. *J Clin Oncol* 1987; **5**: 266–71

Porterfield J. Orbital tumours in children: a report of 214 cases. *Int Ophthalmol Clin* 1962; **2**: 319–35

Schwartz AD, Dadesu–Zadel M, Lee H, Swaney JJ. Spontaneous regression of disseminated neuroblastoma. *J Pediatr* 1974; **85**: 760–3

Shields JA, Bakewell B, Augsberger JJ *et al.* Space occupying orbital diseases in children. *Ophthalmology* 1986; **93**: 379–84

White L. The role of chemotherapy in the treatment of retinoblastoma. *Retina* 1983; **3**: 194–9

Wolter JR, Henderson JW. Adenoid cystic carcinoma in the orbit of a child. *J Pediatr Ophthalmol Strabismus* 1969; **6**: 47

Wright JE. Symposium on orbital tumours: methods of examination. *Trans Ophthalmol Soc UK* 1979; **99**: 216–9

Zelker M, Gonzalez G, Schwartz L *et al.* Treatment of retinoblastoma. Results obtained from a prospective study of 51 patients. *Cancer* 1988; **61**: 1530–60

22.9 Orbital Trauma and Haemorrhage

JOHN BRAZIER

Blunt trauma to the orbital region may cause fractures of the bony margins or walls of the orbit. In addition, the globe, extraocular muscles, optic nerve, and other orbital structures may be damaged. Orbital haemorrhage, often subperiosteal, may follow orbital injury.

Where orbital damage is severe, there are often other associated facial fractures, head injury and lacerations. In these cases a multidisciplinary approach to treatment is required.

Orbital fractures

Orbital margin fractures ('external' fractures)

The clinical picture and management problems with orbital margin fractures vary with the anatomical location of the fractures (Mustarde 1980; Smith *et al.* 1983; Smith & Lipman 1987).

Fractures of the medial orbital wall often involve the nose (naso-orbital fracture). The lacrimal apparatus and medial canthal tendon may be damaged at the same time. If the ethmoid air cells are involved there may be surgical emphysema of the lids and orbital tissues.

Inferior orbital margin fractures are often comminuted and may involve the infraorbital canal and nerve, giving rise to sensory loss on the cheek and lip.

Fracture dislocation of the zygomatic arch is relatively common and may follow mild trauma. There is depression of the lateral canthus and loss of the bony eminence of the cheek. Surgical reduction of these fractures in the first 24 hours is the most satisfactory treatment.

Fractures of the superior margin may involve the frontal sinus, anterior cranial fossa or trochlea, the latter being associated with superior oblique weakness or a Brown's syndrome.

Treatment of these fractures depends on the anatomical, functional and cosmetic deficits created. The time elapsed since the injury is also crucial: up to 3 weeks after injury bone fragments remain mobile permitting open reduction of the fracture with fixation where needed. Associated injuries to the eye will also need specific attention.

Blowout fractures ('internal' fractures)

Blunt trauma to the orbit may result in marked increase in intraorbital pressure. This force is transmitted to the bony orbital walls. Because they are thin, the medial orbital wall (lamina papyracia) and orbital floor are the surfaces injured. When a fracture occurs in the medial wall or floor of the orbit, connective tissue septae, fat and sometimes extraocular muscles prolapse through the defect and become incarcerated. Such blowout fractures (Smith & Regan 1957) seldom produce functional problems when they involve the medial wall. Restriction of action of the inferior rectus and/or inferior oblique muscles is much more likely to follow an orbital floor blowout. Involvement of the intraorbital groove and canal results in sensory loss in the infraorbital nerve territory.

Orbital floor blowout can usually be diagnosed from the clinical history and signs with plain X-rays of the face. Bony disruption of the orbital floor may be visible and the maxillary sinus is often opaque on the damaged side.

Management (Fells 1982) involves confirmation of diagnosis by X-ray and exclusion of intraocular injury. CT scanning provides detailed information about the position of orbital structures but is not always required. Orthoptic records are made of the field of binocular

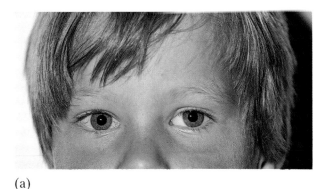

(a)

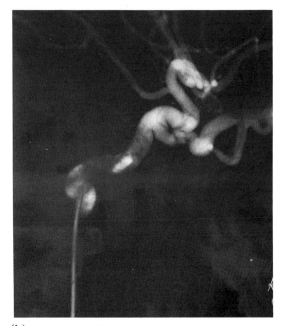

(b)

Fig. 22.9.1 (a) This 5½-year-old boy developed right proptosis and a squeaky bruit a week after a severe road traffic accident. Dilated episcleral veins can be seen. (c, d) Retinal venous congestion and tortuosity with optic disc oedema on the right. (b) Carotid angiogram showing the shunt which was later closed with a balloon catheter. (Same patient a−d.)

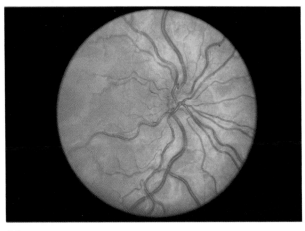

(c)

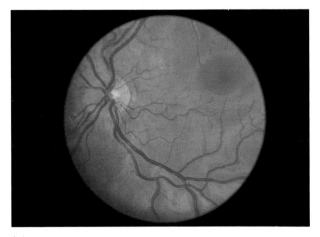

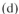(d)

single vision and eye movements with the Lees or Hess screens. The patient is told not to blow the nose and given a course of systemic antibiotics to prevent orbital cellulitis following breach of orbital wall into the sinus. The orthoptic assessment is repeated at 3−4 day intervals. Surgical correction, involving reduction of the prolapsed orbital contents with repair of the orbital floor with bone, cartilage or synthetic implant is undertaken at 10−14 days if (a) there is a large tissue prolapse; (b) enophthalmos is greater than 3 mm; (c) tissue entrapment causes retraction of the globe on attempted upgaze; or (d) diplopia is not improving. At a later stage eye muscle surgery may be undertaken for residual diplopia: some authorities believe that late treatment is preferred except when there is a large tissue prolapse.

Fractures of the optic canal (Hotte 1970)

Unilateral blindness following (sometimes trivial) head or orbital trauma is a well recognized clinical problem. Such indirect optic nerve injuries will be signalled by initial reduction of acuity with an afferent pupillary defect and later optic atrophy. It is generally accepted that the injury in these cases occurs where the optic nerve is fixed in the optic canal.

The role of optic canal fractures following head trauma in pathogenesis of optic nerve damage is unclear. Fractures of the canal may be hard to demonstrate radiologically (Ramsay 1979) and surgical exploration of cases where fracture was suspected has tended to be unrewarding. Sometimes the canal is known to be fractured but the optic nerve is uninjured.

When deterioration of optic nerve function follows head trauma without evidence of canal fracture, systemic steroids are the initial treatment (Anderson *et al.* 1982; Brooks & Cairns 1986). If the response is poor, surgical decompression of the nerve in the canal should be considered (Kennerdell *et al.* 1976; Anderson *et al.* 1982). When marked bony disruption at the orbital apex is associated with optic nerve damage, surgical exploration may be the only hope of salvaging any function.

Carotid—cavernous fistula

This complication of head injury occasionally occurs in children and is usually associated with quite severe injuries, often with a fracture of the skull base. At the time of injury an abnormal communication is formed between the intracavernous internal carotid artery and the cavernous sinus. Over the succeeding days or weeks the patient develops symptoms including subjective bruit, proptosis, a red eye (Fig. 22.9.1), reduced vision, double vision and orbital pain (Sanders & Hoyt 1969). Signs reflect the decreased orbital arterial pressure and increased orbital venous pressure and include proptosis, dilated episcleral vessels, reduced acuity, reduced eye movements, glaucoma, and uveitis.

The severity of the signs depends on the severity of orbital and ocular ischaemia that follows the haemodynamic change.

CT scan of the orbit excludes an orbital mass as a cause of the proptosis and may show non-specific enlargement of the extraocular muscles. Carotid angiography is undertaken both to confirm the site of the fistula and to allow closure of the fistula either by balloon catheter (Debrun *et al.* 1981) or surgical methods. If the fistula can be closed the signs resolve; if closure is not possible, visual reduction persists and may be associated with glaucoma.

Orbital haemorrhage

Orbital haemorrhage may be spontaneous or result from trauma to the orbit or adjacent structures.

Spontaneous haemorrhage is usually due either to a local cause or associated with a systemic disorder such as uraemia, haemophilia, leukaemia, sickle cell disease, or scurvy (Duke-Elder & MacFaul 1974; Jakobiec & Jones 1983). Most common local causes of intraorbital haemorrhages are rhabdomyosarcoma and lymphangioma. The latter may be associated with formation of an orbital blood cyst (Mortada 1969) which may, in turn, cause superior orbital fissure syndrome. Other local causes of haemorrhage, in the orbit include deposits of neuroblastoma (Alfano 1968), Ewing's sarcoma, and leukaemia (Rosenthal 1983).

Traumatic orbital haemorrhage may be localized subperiosteally, giving rise to proptosis and possibly interfering with optic nerve function and ocular motility. Duke-Elder and MacFaul (1974) drew attention to birth trauma as a cause of orbital haemorrhage in otherwise healthy neonates.

References

Alfano JE. Ophthalmological aspects of neuroblastomatosis: a study of 53 verified cases. *Trans Am Acad Ophthalmol* 1968; **72**: 830−48

Anderson RL, Paige WR, Gross CE. Optic nerve blindness following blunt forehead trauma. *Ophthalmology* 1982; **89**: 445−55

Brooks AMV, Cairns JD. Contusion injuries of the optic nerve. *Aust NZ J Ophthalmol* 1986; **14**: 269−73

Debrun G, Lacour P, Vinnela F *et al.* Treatment of 54 traumatic carotid-cavernous fistulae. *J Neurosurg* 1981; **55**: 678−92

Duke-Elder S, MacFaul PA. The ocular adnexa. In: Duke-Elder S (Ed.) *System of Ophthalmology*, Vol. XIII, Part II. Henry Kimpton, London 1974; pp. 819−25

Fells P. Acute enophthalmos. *Trans Ophthalmol Soc UK* 1982; **102**: 88−9

Hotte H. *Orbital Fractures*. Heinemann, London 1970; pp. 196−212

Jakobiec FA, Jones IS. Vascular tumours malformations and degenerations. In: Duane T (Ed.) *Clinical Ophthalmology*, Vol. 2. Harper and Row, Hagerstown 1983

Kennerdell JS, Amsbaugh GA, Myers EN. Transantral-ethmoidal decompression of optic canal fracture. *Arch Ophthalmol* 1976; **94**: 1040−3

Mortada A. Origin of orbital blood cysts. *Br J Ophthalmol* 1969; **53**: 398−402

Mustarde JC. *Repair and Reconstruction in the Orbital Region*. Churchill Livingstone, London 1980

Ramsay JH. Optic nerve injury in fracture of the canal. *Br J Ophthalmol* 1979; **63**: 607−10

Rosenthal AR. Ocular manifestations of leukaemia. *Ophthalmology* 1983; **90**: 899−905

Sanders MD, Hoyt WF. Hypoxic ocular sequelae of carotid-cavernous fistulae. *Br J Ophthalmol* 1969; **53**: 82−97

Smith B, Grove A, Guibor P. Fractures of the orbit. In: Duane T (Ed.) *Clinical Ophthalmology*, Vol. 2. Harper & Row, Hagerstown 1983

Smith B, Lipman RD. Orbital fractures. In: Stark RB (Ed.) *Plastic Surgery of the Head and Neck*, Vol. 1. Churchill Livingstone, London 1987; pp. 366−87

Smith B, Regan WF. Blow-out fracture of the orbit. *Am J Ophthalmol* 1957; **44**: 733−44

23 Uveal Tract

SUSAN DAY

The uveal tract consists of iris, ciliary body, and choroid, each of which has a rich vascular supply and pigment. Its colourful grape-like appearance gives rise to its name 'uvea.' The structure contains two apertures — the pupil and the region of the optic nerve.

The uveal tract's functions are diverse — its pigment acts as a filter; iris musculature forms a 'F-stop' for the eye; the ciliary body secretes aqueous, provides the skeleton for the zonular suspension of the lens as well as the power for focusing, and provides nutrition for the lens. The choroid with its rich vascular supply provides nutrition for 65% of the outer retinal layers (Alm & Bill 1972). Bruch's membrane forms a boundary between retina and choroid; abnormalities in this layer play an important role in various choroidal and retinal disorders (Feeney & Hogan 1961; Hogan 1961).

Embryology

The uveal tract includes contributions from the neural ectoderm, neural crest, and mesoderm. The neural ectoderm gives rise to iris sphincter and dilator muscles, posterior iris epithelium, pigmented and non-pigmented ciliary epithelium. Neural crest cells contribute to iris and choroidal stroma as well as ciliary smooth muscle. Mesodermal tissue forms the endothelium for the many blood vessels (Ozanics & Jakobiec 1982).

The neural ectoderm differentiation occurs within 6–10 weeks of conception whilst definition of the vasculature and pigment migration span the final two trimesters.

Iris formation commences with closure of the fetal cleft at approximately 35 days gestation. The sphincter first is evidenced by neuroectodermal pigment at the optic cup's margin by 10 weeks of gestation (Mund et al. 1972) and differentiation into myofibrils occurs at 11–12 weeks gestation. The dilator forms at approximately 24 weeks gestation.

The neuroectoderm also gives rise to both pigmented and non-pigmented ciliary epithelium. Once the optic cup has invaginated creating the inner and outer layers of neuroectoderm, pigmentation of only the outer layer occurs. At 10–12 weeks, longitudinal ridges form from the outer layer and adhere to inner layers and the ciliary processes form. More posteriorly, the two layers adhere to each other without folding, giving rise to the pars plana.

After the neuroectoderm invaginates, neural crest cells are derived from within the space between neuroectoderm and surface ectoderm. Neural crest cells may be to the head and neck as mesoderm is to somites of the body, since no true somites exist in the head and neck region (O'Rahilly 1965). Tissue derived from these cells is referred to as mesectoderm and its connection to the neuroepithelium remains loose into adulthood, accounting for the iris's porosity to particles of 50 mm to 200 mm by diffusion (Rodrigues et al. 1982). The ciliary smooth muscle is first evident at nearly 4 months gestation just posterior to precursors of the iris stroma. The fibres connect anteriorly to the developing scleral spur during the fifth month, and further increase in size and structure continues after birth.

Finally, neural crest cells also give rise to pigment cell precursors of the uveal tract (in contradistinction to neuroectoderm — derived retinal pigment epithelium). Pigmented cells surrounding the optic cup are visible at 10 weeks gestation. Pigment appears in the peripapillary region after 24 weeks. Migration occurs anteriorly and is nearly complete at birth as mostly mature melanosomes (Rodrigues et al. 1982).

The mesoderm gives rise solely to the endothelium of blood vessels whereas the muscular and support structures of the vessels arise from neural crest cells. These two components combine to form the 'mesenchyme' or connective tissue elements of the head and neck region.

The iris vasculature primordia are present by 6 weeks gestation as loops extending over the anterior surface of the anterior chamber (tunica vasculosa lentis), in association with development of the ciliary body vasculature. By the end of the third month, indentations are created by the radially oriented vessels. The long posterior ciliary arteries are present in the ciliary body, and their terminal branches unite with the peripheral parts of the tunica vasculosa lentis to form the major arterial circle. As the tunica vasculosa lentis regresses, a residual pupillary membrane is created. During the fifth month of gestation the major arterial circle gives rise to radial vessels and branches to the ciliary body.

The choroidal vasculature first differentiates from mesenchymal elements during the second month of gestation, with precursors of the short posterior ciliary arteries which connect posteriorly with the developing choriocapillaris at 3 months, at which time the long posterior ciliary arteries anastomose with the anterior circulation. Further differentiation with intermediate size vessels occurs during the fourth month (Ozanics & Jakobiec 1982). The arterial and venous systems undergo further differentiation into the forerunners of the middle or Sattler's layer during the fifth month (Heimann 1972). The foveal circulation differentiates at approximately the third to fourth month (Heimann 1970).

Postnatal development

At birth, the uveal tract is well differentiated. Two features which are very well scrutinized by the parents are iris colour and pupil size. Of particular concern is: 'What colour will the eyes be?' The ophthalmologist might best observe that (a) the neonate's eyes will never be lighter than they are at birth; (b) pigmentation is usually defined by 6 months of age and always by one year; and (c) it is possible for brown-eyed but heterozygous parents to have a blue-eyed child.

At birth, Caucasions often have blue eyes because there are few melanocytes present with sparse pigment. More darkly pigmented races have irides with already pigmented melanocytes. The pigmentation in all races increases over the first 6 months to 1 year of life.

Pupil size is relatively small at birth, especially in darkly pigmented eyes. As the iris dilator muscle develops postnatally, the pupil correspondingly enlarges. The pupil margin may be accentuated by a prominent ectropion uveae, creating unnecessary concern by the parents or paediatrician.

In the full-term infant, residual pupillary membrane may rarely alter the red reflex, resulting in referral from the primary care physician for further evaluation. In the preterm infant, assessment of the degree of atrophy of the pupillary membrane and its precursor, the tunica vasculosa lentis, has been used to estimate gestational age.

The ciliary muscle is incompletely developed at birth, the increase in accommodation over 3–6 months (Howland 1982) supports further development postnatally.

The clinically significant effects of prematurity on development of retinal circulation are not matched by any effect on choroidal circulation. Choroidal development and pigmentation is relatively complete at birth (Rodrigues et al. 1982); the changing fundus pigmentation is more due to changes in the retinal pigment epithelium.

Developmental abnormalities

Albinism

The term albinism includes any congenital condition in which the apparent pigmentation is reduced involving all of the skin, the skin and eyes, or the eyes alone. The conditions are divided clinically into oculocutaneous albinism and ocular albinism. Histopathologically, however, all forms may be truly oculocutaneous albinism (Green 1985); for patients with oculocutaneous albinism, there is less melanin in each melanosome, whereas the eyes of patients with ocular albinism have fewer melanosomes, and type IV melanosomes in the iris (McCartney *et al.* 1985).

The ocular involvement and clinical significance of albinism varies greatly but nystagmus and reduced vision are usually present. Very rarely patients have normal vision, no nystagmus, and are termed as having albinoidism (Bergsma & Kaiser-Kupfer 1979). These patients have symptoms of photophobia and they have iris transillumination and fundus hypopigmentation.

The reduced acuity associated with albinism is associated with defective fundus pigmentation (Fig. 23.1), and foveal hypoplasia, rods are present within the fovea and cones are distributed away from the fovea (O'Donnell 1984). The chiasm has a decreased proportion of uncrossed fibers, there is abnormal layering of the lateral geniculate nuclei (LGB), and abnormal visual pathways from the LGB to the occipital cortex (Guillery *et al.* 1975). Abnormalities of the visually evoked potentials reflect these anatomical variations (Creel *et al.* 1974; Taylor 1978). Speculation

as to this peculiar association between abnormal pigmentation and chiasmal miswiring includes local interactions between pigmented cells and migrating retinal ganglion cells and an abnormality of a pleotropic gene which controls pigmentation and chiasm formation (Creel 1984).

The diagnosis of the specific type of albinism is largely dependent upon clinical appearance and family history. The severe forms (Fig. 23.2) are inherited as an autosomal recessive trait whereas the milder forms of albinism is inherited in an autosomal dominant fashion. Additionally, an X-linked form of albinism exists in which a characteristic fundus abnormality is present in mothers of affected males (Fig. 23.3) (Forsius & Ericksson 1964). The tyrosinose enzyme test is of limited clinical usefulness (O'Donnell 1984; Green 1985).

Infants with albinism and repeated infections may have the Chediak Higashi syndrome (Bedoya *et al.* 1969) and patients with albinism and easy bruisability may have Hermansky–Pudlak syndrome in which there is an associated platelet defect but are otherwise typical albinos (Summers *et al.* 1988). Although diagnosis is suspected on clinical grounds, consultation with appropriate subspecialists is in order.

Clinical differences exist in the different types of albinism. Ocular albinism most typically is inherited in an X-linked recessive tract and is termed Nettleship–Falls type. Males are photophobic with reduced acuity, nystagmus, iris transillumination defects, foveal hypoplasia, and sparse retinal pigment epithelium (RPE). Carrier females demonstrate partial iris slit defects, and RPE disturbances peripherally (Green 1985). Histologically, macromelanosomes have been demonstrated in the iris, ciliary, and retinal pigment epithelium as well as in skin biopsy of the carrier-stage females (O'Donnell *et al.* 1976). Ocular albinism must be suspected in any child with unexplained congenital nystagmus, especially in darkly pigmented races (Fig. 23.4) (O'Donnell *et al.* 1978).

Patients with oculocutaneous albinism may be 'complete' or 'incomplete', correlating to tyrosine-negative and tyrosine-positive diagnostic testing. Tyrosine-negative individuals include those with Hermansky–Pudlak syndrome. Patients with incomplete albinism, including the Chediak–Higashi syndrome, demonstrate some hair and light skin pigmentation.

Treatment for the ocular involvement with albinism includes symptomatic relief of photophobia with tinted lenses and low vision aids (O'Donnell 1984). Partial occluder contact lenses and prosthetic scleral lenses

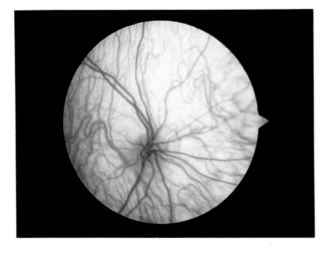

Fig. 23.1 Albinism. Showing the paucity of choroidal and retinal pigment and the foveal hypoplasia.

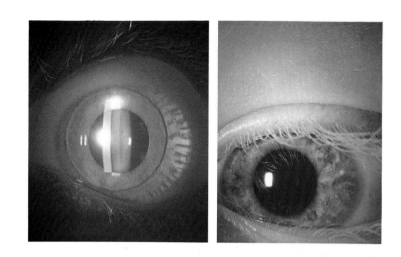

Fig. 23.2 Albinism. Showing iris transillumination in direct light (on the right) and in retro-illumination (on the left). The retro-illumination picture shows details of the lens and ciliary processes seen through the transilluminant iris.

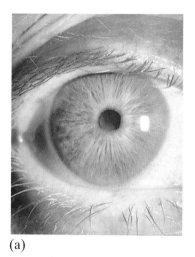

(a)

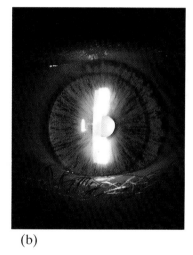

(b)

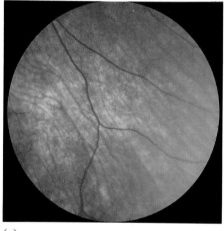

(c)

Fig. 23.3 (a) Female carrier of ocular albinism showing blue iris. (b) The iris is transilluminant on retro-illumination. (c) Female carrier of X-linked ocular albinism, showing the peripheral retina with mottled areas of hypopigmentation.

for infants with albinism and aniridia have been recommended to reduce glare (Stone 1981), but the difficulties in their use often outweigh the benefits.

Coloboma

Congenital coloboma may involve any or all of the iris, ciliary body, choroid, and optic nerve; it occurs when the fetal cleft fails to fuse properly, pointing to an abnormality around the sixth week of gestation (Mann 1964). The defect in isolated iris coloboma may not be due to failure of the fetal cleft since iris development continues after the cleft's closure. Such 'atypical' colobomas and those in atypical sites may be secondary to persistant vascular strands or small ecto-

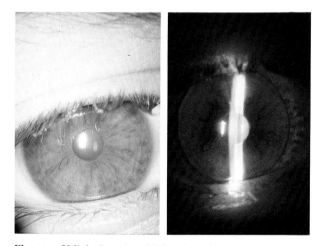

Fig. 23.4 X-linked ocular albinism in a child of Indian origin who presented with nystagmus and poor vision. Showing a brown iris, but marked transillumination.

dermal defects. The abnormality can be associated with more posterior choroidal and optic nerve coloboma as well as with microphthalmos (Cagianut & Theiler 1970; Drews 1973), (see Chapter 17). The colobomas are typically located inferonasally (Fig. 23.5) as is the fetal cleft. Histologically, the stroma is rounded and the pigment epithelium is folded (Green 1985). The defect may involve an entire section of iris or a single layer and ciliary body defects may be associated with lens subluxation (Fig. 23.6).

Iris colobomas represent 2% of congenital eye abnormalities, they are usually bilateral. Mullaney

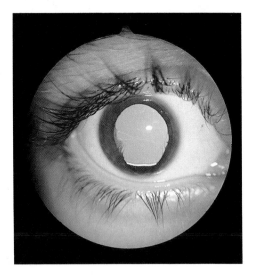

Fig. 23.5 Typical iris coloboma with the margin of the lens visible in the inferior defect. The white fundus reflection is due to an associated choroidal coloboma.

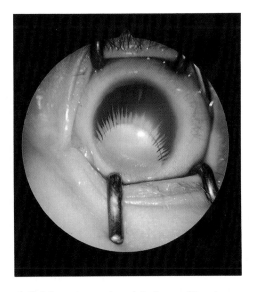

Fig. 23.6 Colobomatous microphthalmos with extreme subluxation of the lens and stretching of the ciliary processes.

(1977) attempted to classify them according to associated pathology including chromosomal defects, systemic abnormalities, phakomatoses, neural tube defects, macular colobomas, and oculorenal abnormalities. Bateman (1984) classifies colobomatous microphthalmos from a more genetic standpoint, separating an isolated ocular malformation related to autosomal dominant and recessive modes of inheritance, from multisystem monogenic syndromes with autosomal dominant and recessive X-linked inheritance, conditions with unknown causes, environmental causes, and chromosomal aberration. (See Chapter 17 and Chapter 28.)

Certain syndromes including uveal colobomas deserve comment. The cat's eye syndrome (Schmid–Fraccaro syndrome) associated iris colobomas with imperforate anus as a consequence of chromosome 22 abnormalities. Variable associations include cardiac defects, mental retardation, urinary tract abnormalities, and preauricular fistulas (Schachenmann et al. 1965; Pfeiffer et al. 1970; Buhler et al. 1972; Freedom & Park 1973; Peterson 1973; Cory & Jamison 1974; Kunze et al. 1975). Patients with a similar clinical appearance without abnormal chromosomes have been observed, including one with a history of parental drug abuse (Spaeth et al. 1982).

The CHARGE syndrome associates colobomas and microphthalmos with heart defects, choanal atresia, retarded growth, genital abnormalities, and ear anomalies (Hall 1979; Pagon et al. 1981). Other syndromes which include coloboma with microphthalmos are the Meckel–Gruber syndrome, microcephaly, occipital encephalocele, congenital heart defects, polydactyly, facial clefts, and polycystic renal, hepatic, and pancreatic disease (Opitz & Howe 1969; MacRae et al. 1972). The Sjögren–Larsson syndrome, colobomatous microphthalmos with mental retardation (Sjögren & Larsson 1949), Lenz microphthalmos syndrome (Goldberg & McKusick 1971), and linear sebaceous naevus syndrome of Jadassohn: linear nevi, severe developmental delay (Marden & Venters 1966); all have associated colobomas.

Congenital iris and ciliary body cysts

These occur when fluid fills an epithelium-lined cyst of the iris. They can either have stratified squamous epithelial or neuroepithelial linings. The former (Fig. 23.7) occur within the stroma and are probably congenital (Grutzmacher et al. 1987), and the latter at or behind the pupillary margin (Fig. 23.8). If the size and location impairs the visual axis, surgical

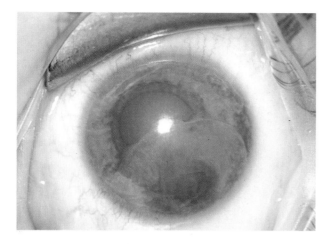

Fig. 23.7 Iris cyst. This stromal cyst recurred after local removal and eventually required a sector iridectomy.

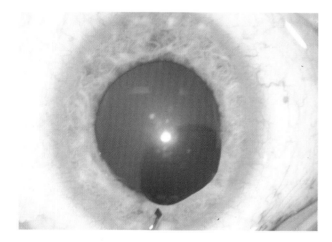

Fig. 23.8 Posterior iris cyst consisting of pigment epithelium. Cysts of this type tend not to recur after simple removal with a vitrectomy machine or puncture with a YAG laser.

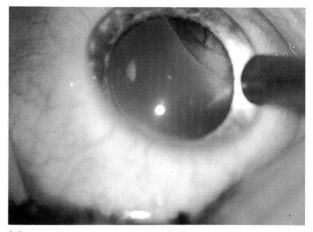

(a)

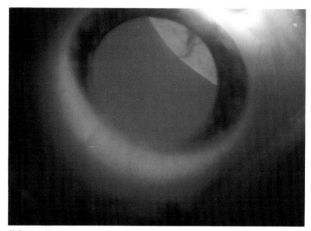

(b)

Fig. 23.9 (a) Ciliary body cyst in direct illumination. It appears brown and solid. (b) Ciliary body cyst in transillumination. Shows that it is semitransparent and fluid filled.

intervention may be necessary. Their size is usually stationary (Shields 1984) but they may recur if incompletely excised. Ciliary body cysts may cause astigmatism and amblyopia (Fig. 23.9).

Brushfield's spots

These are typically found in patients with Down's syndrome, occurring in 85% of persons with trisomy 21 (Brushfield 1924). Donaldson (1961) has found a 24% incidence in normal individuals; the spots were closer to the pupil margin, more numerous, and were distinct in Down's syndrome and he could find no correlation with age or IQ. Histologically, the spots correlate with a normal to hypercellular area of iris tissue with surrounding relative stromal hypoplasia.

Persistent pupillary membranes

Persistent pupillary membranes represent an incomplete involution of the anterior tunica vaculosa lentis. The membranes are attached to the collarette and may be free floating, span the pupil to attach on its opposite side, or attach to the anterior surface of the lens with or without an associated cataract. If extensive, an insult at the fifth month of gestation may be suspected. Autosomal dominant inheritance has been reported (Merin et al. 1971).

They may be substantial but even then may not impair vision (Mader et al. 1988). When more extensive, the red reflex may be altered and rarely they are so extensive as to impair vision (Fig. 23.10) or they may have fibrous remnants (Fig. 23.11); attempts to improve vision with iridectomy have been unsuccessful (Merin et al. 1971, Levy 1957) although with modern intraocular surgery much less of a problem is expected.

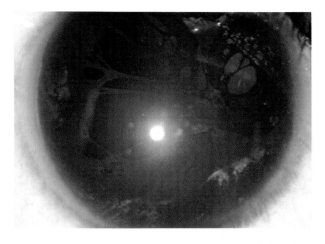

Fig. 23.10 Hyperplastic pupillary membrane in an infant. The acuity in this child was reduced and nystagmus was present.

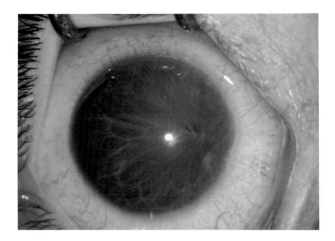

Fig. 23.12 Congenital idiopathic extreme microcoria. The pupil in this case was so small that the eye was potentially amblyopic and a pupil was created surgically.

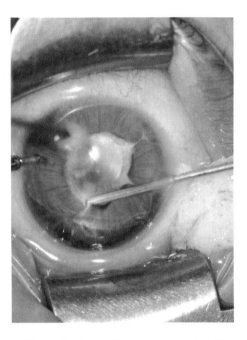

Fig. 23.11 Hyperplastic pupillary membrane stretching across the pupil attached to the collarette. It also involved the anterior capsule of the lens.

Congenital idiopathic microcoria

In this unilateral anomaly the pupil is microscopically small (Fig. 23.12) so that the pupil is nearly or actually obliterated. It is probably related to an abnormality of the development of the fetal pupillary membrane and its main effect is to cause amblyopia and puts the eye at risk from glaucoma. Early surgical treatment and occlusion therapy can result in useful vision (Lambert *et al.* 1988).

Aniridia

Aniridia represents a spectrum of disorders with iris hypoplasia. Its incidence has been estimated between 1 : 64 000 and 1 : 96 000 (Mollenbach 1947; Shaw *et al.* 1960). Both hereditary and sporadic forms exist.

Aniridia may occur due to anomalous development of the neuroectoderm or neural crest cells (Spaeth *et al.* 1982). The neuroectoderm yields a developing optic cup rim at 12–14 weeks gestation (Mann 1964), whilst neural crest cells contribute to iris stroma formation during the second month of gestation. Aniridia has been produced experimentally in mice with maternal vitamin A deficiency (Warkany & Schraffenberger 1946; Kalter & Warkany 1959).

Histologically, the iris is reduced to a small stub, and smooth muscle is usually absent. The angle may be poorly developed, and the retina may be present over portions of the pars plana and pars plicata of the ciliary body. Later changes include development of peripheral anterior synechiae with corneal endothelial growth into the angle (Margo 1983). Other corneal irregularities include epithelial and Bowman's layer abnormalities (Margo 1983) and a thick fibrovascular pannus in patients with glaucoma (Mackman *et al.* 1979).

Aniridia is important as it is associated with poor vision, glaucoma, cataract (Fig. 23.13), and systemic health abnormalities. Decreased vision is usual, with multiple contributory factors including light scatter, corneal and lenticular opacities, severe glaucoma and optic nerve and macular abnormalities. Pedigree studies have found approximately 60% with vision better than 20/30 and 5% with vision worse than 20/

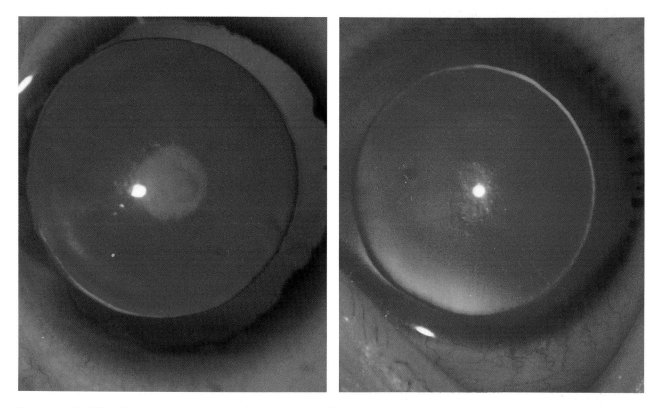

Fig. 23.13 Aniridia. No iris can be seen, revealing the zonules. There is a cataract in both eyes.

200 (Elsas *et al.* 1977; Hittner *et al.* 1980). Others have reported as high an incidence of 86% with vision 20/100 or worse (Grove *et al.* 1961; Jesberg 1962). A lot of the variation in the various studies is accounted for by different inclusion criteria.

Although glaucoma is not typically present at birth, the incidence of childhood glaucoma has been reported between 6 and 75% (Grant & Walton 1974; Shaffer & Cohen 1975; Elsas *et al.* 1977; Walton 1979). The delay in onset of glaucoma is probably due to progressive changes in the angle.

Cataract formation is present in 50–85% of patients by the age of 20 (Layman *et al.* 1974; Elsas *et al.* 1977). The changes are usually progressive. Ectopia lentis (Fig. 23.14) may also occur in conjunction with aniridia (Callahan 1949; Shaw *et al.* 1960), due to an abnormality of the zonular molecular structure (Nelson *et al.* 1984).

The corneal abnormalities are also progressive (Mackman *et al.* 1979); peripheral corneal epithelial irregularities spread to involve the entire cornea. Microcornea has also been reported in association with aniridia (David *et al.* 1978).

Optic nerve hypoplasia was found in nine of 12 patients by Layman *et al.* (1974), contributing to reduced vision.

From one quarter to one third of children with sporadic aniridia will develop Wilms' tumour prior to 3 years of age (Flanagan & DiGeorge 1969; Pilling 1975; François *et al.* 1982). Frequently, mental retardation, genitourinary abnormalities, craniofacial abnormalities, microcephaly, and growth retardation are also present. In the triad of aniridia, genitourinary abnormalities, and mental retardation, in which a short arm deletion of chromosome 11 has been demonstrated (Riccardi & Borges 1978), there is also a high incidence of bilateral Wilms' tumours (Garcia *et al.* 1976; Warburg *et al.* 1980). Aniridia with cerebellar ataxia and mental retardation (Gillespie 1965; Pendergrass 1976), aniridia in association with absent patellae (Mirkinson & Mirkinson 1975) and dominant aniridia with ptosis, obesity and mental retardation (Hamming *et al.* 1986) are other associations.

Gene mapping has supported the 11p13 deletion locus in patients with aniridia and Wilms' tumour. Chromosomes 1 and 2 appear to play an important role in dominant congenital aniridia, suggesting that multiple chromosomes influence iris development (Sloderbeck *et al.* 1975; Ferrel *et al.* 1980).

Elevated intraocular pressure may be better tolerated in aniridic eyes (Callahan 1949; Nelson 1984).

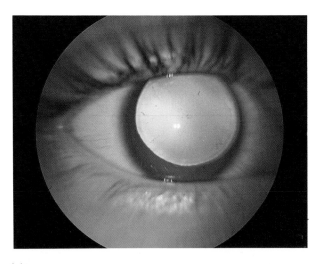

(a)

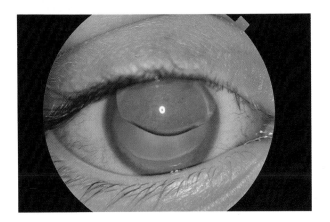

(b)

Fig. 23.14 (a) Aniridia showing the lens in transillumination on 1.11.79. (b) Aniridia showing the lens in retro-illumination (31.10.85). There has been considerable subluxation. A cataract is now present and the eye is glaucomatous. (Same patient.)

Infants with aniridia and glaucoma may not have a normal Schlemm's canal, making goniotiomy an unlikely choice for surgery (Callahan 1949; Barkan 1953). Walton (1979) advocated at least yearly gonioscopy to assess for the presence of increasing iris processes and angle closure with a view to prophylactic goniotomy. Laser trabeculoplasty is not helpful and trabeculectomy may be a better procedure in older patients (Nelson 1984).

Cataract extraction in aniridia patients must also require extra preparation since the lens zonules do not support the lens in a normal fashion. Penetrating keratoplasty may help severe cases of associated corneal involvement but visual expectations must be limited.

Optical correction of significant refractive errors, and a shift to an aphakic refractive error after lens subluxation may be of great help to some affected children. Even though the 'pupil' is large, cycloplegic agents must be used for refraction in young patients since active accommodation is present. The use of occluder contact lenses with a pupillary aperture has been advocated for infants (Stone 1981).

Heterochromia iridis

A difference in iris colour can be congenital or acquired, the abnormal eye being either darker or lighter than the other eye and it may be difficult to decide which is the abnormal eye; skin pigmentation, parental eye colour, assessment of earlier photographs and the history usually resolve this question.

CONGENITAL

Congenital heterochromia with the involved iris darker may point to ocular melanocytosis or oculodermal melanocytosis, or to a sector iris hamartoma syndrome. An iris pigment epithelial hamartoma creates a jet-black superficial lesion which consists of iris pigment epithelium with clumped smooth muscle cells and melanocytes (Jakobiec et al. 1975; Quigley & Stanish 1978).

With congenital heterochromia with the involved iris lighter, Horner's syndrome and Waardenburg's syndrome must be considered. Congenital Horner's syndrome results in ipsilateral hypopigmentation miosis and ptosis (See Chapter 37.)

Waardenburg's syndrome is transmitted as an autosomal dominant trait; it includes lateral displacement of the inner canthi, prominent root of the nose, unusual brows, deafness, and white forelock and heterochromia iridis. Fundus pigmentary heterochromia may also be present. A similar autosomal recessive syndrome includes Hirschsprung's disease which emphasizes the importance of communicating eye findings to primary care physicians; the disorder may involve both eyes with sectoral heterochromia (Fig. 23.15) (Liang et al. 1983).

ACQUIRED

Acquired heterochromia with the involved iris darker results from infiltrative processes (such as naevi and melanomatous tumours) and deposition of material within the iris.

Siderosis results from iron deposition within the

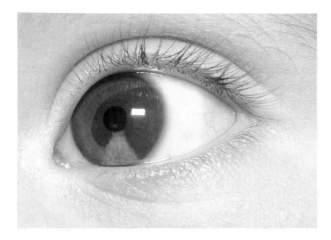

Fig. 23.15 Sector iris hypo-pigmentation.

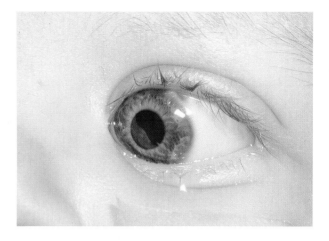

Fig. 23.16 Williams' syndrome. It is said that there is a characteristic 'stellate' iris pattern in these children.

dilator muscles of the iris (Burger & Klintworth 1974). Heterochromia may be the presenting feature of a suspected or unsuspected intraocular foreign body; which may only be found on a CT scan (Barr *et al.* 1984). Haemosiderosis results from deposition of iron derived from blood products as in heterochromia from long standing hyphaema (Sugar *et al.* 1967; Winter 1967).

With an acquired lighter coloured iris, Fuchs' heterochromic iridocyclitis must be strongly considered (See Uveitis section), more rarely infiltrations such as juvenile xanthogranuloma and metastatic malignancies also can be responsible. Acquired Horner's syndrome, when the lesion occurs early in the first year of life, can also lead to heterochromia.

Williams' syndrome

In the Williams' syndrome (prominent lips, hoarse voice, mental and growth retardation, cardiac defect) there is said to be a stellate pattern to the iris (Fig. 23.16) (Jensen *et al.* 1976) often more apparent to dysmorphologists than to ophthalmologists!

Tumours

With the exception of iris naevi, tumours involving the uveal tract are rare in children. Presentation of tumours may be as heterochromia, glaucoma, hyphema, or decreased vision, with or without squint in the case of more posterior masses.

Iris naevi and freckles

Iris naevi consist of localized rests of melanocytes which vary in size and shape, spindle (the most common), epitheloid, and polyhedral. They are common and their association with posterior choroidal melanomas is debatable (Michelson & Shields 1977). Rarely, involvement of angle structures can lead to glaucoma (Nik *et al.* 1981). Iris naevi may also create an irregular pupil, be associated with a sectoral cataract, or 'seed' into the anterior chamber. None of these has any prognostic significance, as iris naevi are benign (Shields 1983).

Iris naevi should be distinguished from iris freckles which are on the anterior surface of the iris without altering the iris structures. Histologically, iris freckles are a cluster of normal iris melanocytes.

Iris and choroidal melanoma

These are uncommon in children (Verdager 1965). Iris melanomas are relatively non-aggressive (Arentson & Green 1975; Jakobiec & Silbert 1981), and all melanomas are rare in blacks (Arentson & Green 1975). Iris melanomas present 10 to 20 years earlier than choroidal melanomas due to their visibility (Friedenwald *et al.* 1952). Whereas less than 10% of all malignant melanomas in the general population arise in the iris, 40–50% of such tumours arise in the iris in patients 20 years old or younger (Apt 1963; Nicholson & Green 1981).

Iris melanomas have a strong bias for presentation inferiorly (Arentson & Green 1975; Cleasby 1958). Due to their vascularity, their presentation may be as a hyphaema (Arentson and Green 1975).

Iris melanoma histologically differs from that of ciliary body and choroidal melanomas, approximately

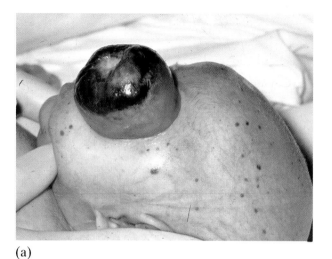

(a)

(b)

Fig. 23.17 (a) Congenital malignant melanoma. This child was born with disseminated melanoma with the eye this size at birth. She was still alive at follow-up 2 years later. (b) Congenital malignant melanoma. Enucleation specimen with forceps on the rectus muscle (Broadway *et al.* 1990).

60% are spindle-cell, 33% mixed cell, and the remainder epitheloid. Only the spindle-cell type behaves in a malignant fashion. A more detailed histologic classification has been made by Jakobiec and Silbert (1981) which includes their view of appropriate treatment.

The differential diagnosis of iris melanomas includes juvenile xanthogranula (Ferry 1965), iris rhabdomyosarcoma (Naumann *et al.* 1972), iris foreign body (Ferry 1965), segmental melanosis oculi (Ferry 1965), iris abscess (Gass 1973), and Fuchs' adenoma in adults (Zaidman *et al.* 1983). Differentiation must also be made from a ciliary body mass since the prognosis differs for this location (Jakobiec & Silbert 1981; Engel *et al.* 1982).

Uveal melanomas are exceedingly rare during childhood, with two thirds of enucleation specimens coming from people 50 years or older (Paul *et al.* 1962). Two case reports of a uveal melanoma in neonates exist (Greer 1966; Broadway *et al.* 1990) both in infants with multiple skin naevi. The slow growth of these tumours may account for their relatively late presentation due to refractive changes and lens distortion, narrowed anterior chamber, prominent episcleral vessels, and slightly reduced intraocular pressure (Foos *et al.* 1969). Later, extension into the anterior chamber, cataracts, and glaucoma may be the presenting features.

Choroidal melanomas are rare in childhood but failure to consider this diagnosis may lead to a delay in treatment (Apt 1963; Leonard *et al.* 1975). The differential diagnosis includes choroidal naevi which are characterized as having a diameter of 7 mm or less, an elevation of 2 mm or less, overlying drusen in older patients, sparse lipofuscin, they are asymptomatic and have no or slow growth. Choroidal naevi may give rise to malignant melanoma (Nicholson & Green 1981). Photographic documentation with careful follow-up is appropriate.

Childhood uveal malignant melanomas do not seem to have a poorer prognosis than adult tumours (Barr *et al.* 1981) the 5-year mortality rate, was 25% in one series of 42 patients. Poorer prognostic indicators include extrocular extension at the time of diagnosis, base diameter greater than 10 mm, and mixed or epitheliod cell type (Barr *et al.* 1981).

Although the enucleation of eyes with suspected malignant melanomas is controversial in adults (Apple & Blodi 1980; Zimmerman & McLean 1980), Nicholson and Green (1981) favour early enucleation in children when unequivocal growth is documented since the expected lifespan is greater, and since they have experienced failure of long-term success with irradiation of a childhood tumour.

Certain congenital disorders are felt to predispose to uveal melanomas. In addition to previously mentioned choroidal melanomas (Yanoff & Zimmerman 1967; Naumann *et al.* 1971), neurofibromatosis may be associated with a greater number of melanocytic naevi and of uveal melanomas (Yanoff & Zimmerman 1967).

Although familial occurrences of malignant melanoma are known (Walker *et al.* 1979), the inverse relationship with skin pigmentation has been much more apparent to clinicians (Scotto *et al.* 1976; Albert *et al.* 1980).

Medulloepithelioma

Medulloepithelioma is a tumour of the ciliary body nonpigmented epithelium; it is a congenital lesion derived from embryonic retina which occasionally includes cartilage, brain, striated muscle, and other elements and are called teratomedulloepitheliomas. Ordinarily they are comprised of membranes, tubules, and rosettes. The arrangement of such networks accounts for their initial designation by Fuchs (1908) as diktyomas. They may undergo malignant transformation (Zimmerman & Broughton 1978). Other structures such as the optic nerve may rarely be involved (Green *et al.* 1974).

They usually present within the first decade as visible iris tumour, leukocoria, glaucoma, hyphaema, or decreased vision with or without strabismus. The average age at enucleation is 5 years (Zimmerman & Broughton 1978), two thirds showed malignancies and metastases occur frequently, and extraocular extension at the time of enucleation was the most important prognostic indicator. Other series have implied a more benign nature (Canning *et al.* 1988).

Enucleation is the recommended treatment unless well localized anteriorly, when local excision or cryotherapy may play a role (Jakobiec *et al.* 1975). The differential diagnosis includes juvenile xanthogranuloma and retinoblastoma, but the cystic nature and rather felt-like appearance and the unilaterality speak heavily for medulloepithelioma. (See Chapter 27.1.)

Choroidal haemangioma

Choroidal haemangiomas may be divided into diffuse and localized lesions. They may include both capillary and cavernous components. Superficial changes, including pigmentation, have resulted in a misdiagnosis with subsequent enucleation for malignant melanoma (Jones & Cleasby 1959; Witschel & Font 1976).

Choroidal haemangiomas carry a risk of associated glaucoma. The diffuse lesions (tomato ketchup fundus) are associated with Sturge–Weber syndrome (Susac *et al.* 1974). Episcleral vascular hamartomas may be the cause of the increased intraocular pressure (Phelps 1978). Retinal detachment may also occur and laser treatment has been advocated for this (Shields 1983) and for small solitary tumours, radiotherapy, using a lens-sparing technique may also be indicated. No treatment is effective for diffuse or large solitary tumours; (see Chapter 25.)

Juvenile xanthogranuloma

See Chapter 22.

Lisch nodules and neurofibromatosis

See Chapter 22.

Spontaneous hyphaema

Trauma is the leading cause of hyphaema and even when there is no history of trauma other signs of trauma, such as recessed angle or contralateral retinal haemorrhages, must be carefully sought. Non-accidental injury may also cause hyphaema.

Truly spontaneous hyphaemas can occur and indicate either underlying pathology of the uveal tract or a bleeding diathesis. Vascular tumours such as juvenile xanthogranuloma, medulloepithelioma, and retinoblastoma are important and retinoschisis, retinopathy of prematurity, persistent hyperplastic primary vitreous, blood dyscrasias such as leukemia, and post-contusion injury or post-surgical intervention have all been implicated (Howard 1962). In older children and adults scurvy, purpura, severe iritis, rubeosis, and migraine may also cause apparently spontaneous hyphaema (Doggart 1950).

Spontaneous hyphaemas deserve immediate concern about elevated intraocular pressure and corneal blood staining, but equal importance must be paid to determination of underlying cause, including studies such as ultrasound and CT scanning. A careful general physical examination may reveal other clues, as might hematologic screening for blood dyscrasias.

Uveal manifestations (non-inflammatory) of systemic disease

Direct leukaemic infiltration of the iris may lead to heterochromia, spontaneous hyphaema, glaucoma, or hypopyon (Perry & Mallen 1979; Ninane *et al.* 1980; Kincaid & Green 1983; Schachat *et al.* 1988), however, a study of 657 children with leukaemia revealed only nine children with anterior segment abnormalities (Ridgeway *et al.* 1976).

Burkitt's lymphoma, with its close association with Epstein–Barr virus, commonly affects children from tropical countries (Burkitt & O'Connor 1961). Although orbital involvement is most common, choroidal findings have been seen on postmortem cases (Green 1985). This tumour may gain further clinical significance since it has been reported in association with acquired immune deficiency syndrome (Fujikawa *et al.* 1983). Although radiotherapy is most frequently used for localized tumour, favourable results may be given with the use of cyclophosphamide (Ziegler 1977).

Uveitis

Inflammation involving the uveal tract is called uveitis with further differentiation based on the primary site of inflammation such as panuveitis, iritis, choroiditis, pars planitis, iridocyclitis or cyclitis.

Uveitis is felt to represent an inflammatory response to a noxious stimulant, be it biological or physical. Polymorphonuclear leukocytes and monocytes respond to the stimulant, and they release chemical factors which can either eliminate the agent, create further inflammatory response, or both (O'Connor 1983).

Uveitis may be classified on the basis of location, clinical characteristics of the inflammatory pathology, or related to the cause or severity and course. Smith and Nozik (1983) have offered a clinical approach which aids the diagnosis in 75–85% cases.

Acute anterior uveitis

This includes symptoms of pain, redness, and photophobia with symptoms lasting days to weeks. Although of no histopathological significance, the terms 'granulomatous' and 'nongranulomatous' may be used on the basis of the slit lamp findings; in the former, symptoms are relatively mild and iris nodules as well as 'mutton fat' keratic precipitates (KPs) are present (Fig. 23.18). In the latter, few KPs are present, and the symptoms are more severe, a fibrinous anterior chamber reaction may be present (Fig. 23.19). When cells are present on slit lamp examination behind the lens, iridocyclitis is present. Slit lamp examination should also assess for corneal changes and iris transillumination defects which may be present with Fuchs' heterochromic cyclitis.

Chronic anterior uveitis

This does not have severe symptoms although milder symptoms may be present months to years. The anterior chamber cellular reaction is usually less, but flare is often prominent. Both granulomatous and non-granulomatous chronic iridocyclitis have KPs. Synechiae, band keratopathy, secondary cataract and glaucoma, are common and cystoid macular edema and vitreous cells may cause decreased vision.

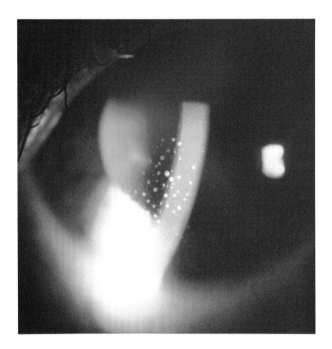

Fig. 23.18 Sarcoidosis. Showing 'mutton fat' KP.

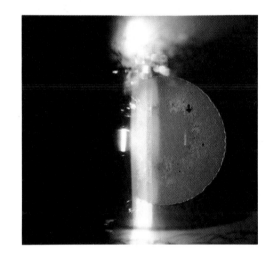

Fig. 23.19 Acute anterior uveitis with fibrinous exudate on the anterior lens surface. There have been repeated attacks of acute iritis in this child and a cataract is present.

Specific causes of anterior uveitis

ACUTE ANTERIOR UVEITIS

Traumatic

Traumatic iridocyclitis is common in childhood. The history usually involves blunt injury to the eye. Symptoms include severe pain, photophobia, and redness. The ophthalmologist must be sure that the pathology is limited to the anterior segment. If the iritis responds to cycloplegia with topical steroids, no further laboratory tests are necessary.

Infectious diseases

Iritis associated with childhood measles, mumps, and chickenpox is typically acute anterior uveitis, sometimes with keratitis. If herpes simplex is possible any steroid used must be covered with antiviral agents (Grayson 1983). Herpes simplex iridocyclitis may be associated with keratitis; corneal involvement is shown by fluorescein or Rose Bengal staining but the iridocyclitis may recur without the corneal lesions (Hogan et al. 1963). Viral particles (Witmer & Iwamoto 1968) and herpes virus antigen (Patterson et al. 1968) have been isolated from the anterior chamber, suggesting a direct infection, but the inflammation could be due to hypersensitivity (Oh 1976).

Infectious mononucleosis has been associated with anterior iritis as well as other forms of uveitis (Stevens et al. 1951; Martenet 1981).

Acute iridocyclitis with keratitis occurs in the lepromatous form of the disease in later stages, contributing significantly to blindness. (Ticho & Ben Sira 1970; ffytche 1981).

Kawasaki's disease (Kawasaki et al. 1974) consists of high fever, stomatitis, palmar erythema, lymphoadenopathy, and erythema multiforme rashes, meningitis, uveitis and myocarditis (Melish 1981). A significant number of these individuals develop secondary coronary or axillary artery aneurysms (Kato et al. 1975) but the uveitis though sometimes severe, usually leaves few sequelae.

Ankylosing spondylitis

Ankylosing spondylitis is characterized by axial skeletal arthritis, but may present at an earlier age. Cystoid macular oedema may limit vision in such patients (Belmont & Michelson 1982). Ocular involvement is often bilateral, and hypopyon or secondary glaucoma may develop. Successful therapy includes intense topical steroids and mydriatics started early in the course of each attack (Smith & Nozik 1983).

Reiter's syndrome

Reiter's syndrome is characterized by recurrent iridocyclitis, mucosal mouth lesions, polyarthritis, conjunctivitis, and urethritis in males after 20 years of age. The iridocyclitis may be very severe with hypo-

pyon and secondary degenerative ocular changes such as cataract and iris atrophy.

Behçet's disease

Behçet's disease is characterized by arthritis, genital ulcerations, aphthous stomatitis, and a usually very severe and refractory recurrent hypopyon iritis, it is rare in children, accounting for only two of 340 children with uveitis in a large series (Kanski & Shun-Shin 1984); it is most frequent in 20–40 year olds (James & Spiteri 1982).

CHRONIC ANTERIOR UVEITIS

Still's disease

Juvenile rheumatoid arthritis (JRA) or Still's disease is a common association of bilateral chronic anterior uveitis in a child 15 years or younger, accounting for 80% of child patients with uveitis in one series (Kanski & Shun-Shin 1984). Children with this condition may have chronic progressive mono- or pauciarticular arthritis, lymphadenopathy, splenomegaly, pericarditis, pleuritis, anaemia, fever, and growth retardation. Since Ohm's (1910) first report of the uveitis, its association has been further defined on the basis of clinical features, serologic test, and HLA antigen typing (Arnett 1982). The acute febrile type and the polyarticular onset type tend not to have associated iritis. With pauciarticular onset, however, eye findings are of importance. These are further subdivided into the following:

1 Pauciarticular, rheumatoid factor-negative; HLA-B27 negative; positive ANA factor. Females are affected more commonly than males (Kanski 1977), and the onset is before 10 years. Chronic iridocyclitis with few symptoms is a significant concern. Some association with HLA-DR5 may be present (Glass et al. 1980).

2 Pauciarticular, ankylosing spondylitis, seronegative rheumatoid factor and ANA; positive HLA-B27; acute iridocyclitis. These patients may evolve into a polyarticular type of rheumatoid arthritis (Arnett et al. 1980).

3 Pauciarticular, seronegative rheumatoid, ANA, HLA-B27 negative; HLA-DW8 and HLA-DRW8 positive.

The pauciarticular forms do not tend to persist into adulthood unlike the polyarticular forms.

The incidence of iridocyclitis approaches 20% in pauciarticular JRA (Bywaters & Ansell 1965; Calabro *et al.* 1970) it occurs especially in females (Kanski 1977). The uveitis is typically bilateral and may precede the onset of the arthritis in which case the visual prognosis is worse than when the arthritis precedes the uveitis (Wolf *et al.* 1987). Band keratopathy, cataract, and secondary glaucoma are common (Fig. 23.20).

Histopathology of the chronic changes includes granulomatous inflammation, plasma cells, and lymphocytic inflammation (Green 1985).

The diagnosis of JRA is made primarily on the basis of clinical history. Positive ANA has been found in 88% of these patients who also have chronic iridocyclitis (Schaller *et al.* 1973). HLA testing is indicated (Stastney & Fink 1979).

Because of the relatively pain-free course of iridocyclitis associated with JRA, follow-up examinations at 3-month intervals are recommended for young patients with pauciarticular JRA.

Treatment includes mydriatics and corticosteroids topically when cells are present in the anterior chamber. Occasionally sub-Tenon's injections of steroids may be required. Band keratopathy may require chelating agents such as EDTA, or removal by corneal scraping. Cataract surgery may be complicated (Smith & Nozik 1983) and a lensectomy/vitrectomy approach is indicated (Flynn *et al.* 1988), together with covering doses of systemic and topical steroids to prevent perioperative flare-up of the uveitis.

Sarcoidosis

Sarcoidosis is an unusual cause of chronic anterior uveitis in children less than 15 years old (Hetherington 1982). Patients younger than 5 years have uveitis, arthropathy and skin rash as the major features (North *et al.* 1970). It is more common in black children (Kendig 1974) and may also involve the orbit simultaneously (Khan *et al.* 1986). Anterior uveitis occurs in 2–48% of child patients in the three largest reported series (Jasper & Denny 1968; Siltzbach & Greenberg 1968; Kendig 1974) it is often granulomatous (Fig. 23.18). In a study of 26 patients of 5 years or less, 20 patients had anterior uveitis (Hoover *et al.* 1986). Diagnosis is made by chest X-ray, biopsy of involved structures (including conjunctiva), Kweim test, the finding of a negative Mantoux test at decreasing dilutions, and the finding of raised levels of serum angiotensin converting enzyme (Baarsma *et al.* 1987).

The treatment of the primary uveitis as well as their sequelae is similar to that of JRA except that more consideration should be given to using systemic steroids (Kendig 1974).

Fuchs' heterochromic iridocyclitis

Fuchs' heterochromic iridocyclitis is characterized by a chronic anterior uveitis with hypopigmentation in the involved eye. It may occur from the second decade onwards but typically starts between 30 and 40 years old as slow painless progressive loss of vision or of heterochromia (Fig. 23.21). Slit lamp findings include small diffuse KPs with a mild anterior chamber re-

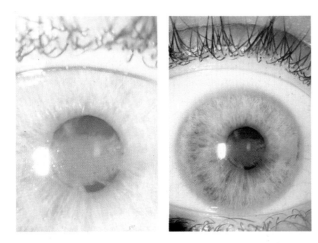

Fig. 23.20 Still's disease. This patient presented because the parents noticed a white spot on the cornea which was due to the band keratopathy associated with chronic uveitis with posterior synechiae. She had the pauciarticular form of Still's disease and later developed cataract which required surgery.

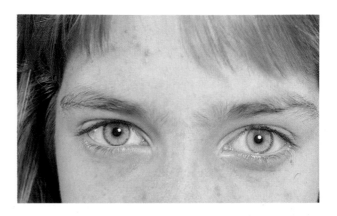

Fig. 23.21 Fuchs' heterochromic iridocyclitis. This girl presented because of mildly blurred vision in the left eye and heterochromia which her parents had noticed. She had a mild chronic anterior uveitis without synechiae and a cataract developed.

action, and iris transillumination defects. Open angle glaucoma develops in 25–50% of the patients. This form of events is considered by some to be the most frequently misdiagnosed form of uveitis (Smith & Nozik 1983; O'Connor 1985).

It has been considered as a degenerative disorder, but evidence now points to an immunologic disorder, perhaps related to depressed suppressor T-cell activity. Occasionally a positive family history is present (O'Connor 1985).

Patients with this condition do not respond favourably to steroids, and glaucoma management is often difficult.

Tuberculosis

Tuberculosis (TB) can cause anterior chronic uveitis in addition to necrotizing retinochoroiditis, choroiditis, and subacute endophthalmitis. Some advocate systemic treatment for TB in patients with positive skin tests and chronic granulomatous uveitis (Schlaegel & O'Connor 1977). Infants with miliary TB may have multiple focal choroidal lesions (Fig. 23.22).

Syphilis

Syphilis typically results in either chorioretinitis or chronic iridocyclitis which may be immunomediated. Iris papules or roseolae may be visible by slit lamp examination (Schwartz & O'Connor 1980).

Anterior uveitis is rarely associated with interstitial keratitis of congenital syphilis (Spicer 1924).

Pars planitis is one of many terms (cyclitis, peripheral uveitis, peripheral cyclitis, and chronic cyclitis) which describes a relatively common entity of non-infectious inflammation of the vitreous secondary to inflammation of the retina, ciliary body and vitreous. Its incidence peaks between 15 and 25 years. The condition is usually bilateral but often asymmetrical and affects both sexes equally. Patients complain of floaters and may note distorted vision if cystoid macular oedema develops. Symptoms of pain, redness, and photophobia are very rare (Smith & Nozik 1983).

The classic finding is 'snowbanking' on the inferior (Aaberg 1987) parts of the pars plana which consists of mononuclear cells (Kenyon 1975); and minimal anterior chamber reaction may be present (Fig. 23.23). Posterior synechiae may be found.

Retinal findings may include vasculitis, peripapillary retinal oedema, and cystoid macular oedema (CME). Complications include cataract, secondary glaucoma, vitreous haemorrhage, retinal detachment band keratopathy, and cyclitic membranes. Overall, visual acuity is 6/12 (20/40) or better in almost 80% of patients with long-term follow-up.

No clearcut cause is known, although viral and immunological causes have been suggested. Laboratory tests including those for TB and syphilis are usually negative.

Treatment with sub-Tenon's steroid should be considered if vision is reduced and CME is present by fluorescein angiography. Topical therapy is not efficacious. If a patient worsens despite treatment, cryo-

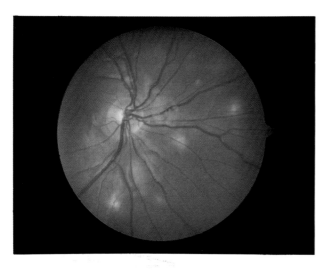

Fig. 23.22 Miliary tuberculosis with focal choroidal lesions.

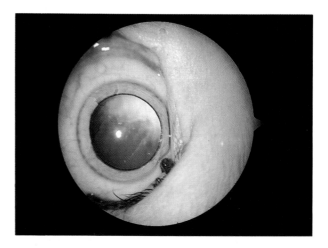

Fig. 23.23 Pars planitis in a 4-year-old girl with no systemic abnormality. The matted white exudate is present mainly in the inferior part of the pars plana.

therapy might be considered and immunosuppressive agents may also have a role.

POSTERIOR UVEITIS

Posterior uveitis refers to inflammation of the choroid; differentiation of choroiditis, chorioretinitis, retinochoroiditis, retinitis and retinal vasculitis is often quite arbitrary.

Posterior uveitis may be either diffuse or focal. Active lesions often trigger an inflammatory response in the overlying vitreous. Inactive lesions may evolve into hypo- or hyperpigmented chorioretinal scars. The manner of presentation is dependent upon which area of the posterior pole is involved and whether the process is unilateral or bilateral.

Toxoplasmosis

See Chapter 11.

Toxocara

Toxocariasis, also traditionally included in discussions of posterior uveitis, is primarily a vitritis. It is common in children and fortunately is usually unilateral, since vision may be greatly impaired in the infected eye. More importantly, its presentation shares many common features with those of unilateral retinoblastoma, making its recognition all the more important. Toxocara seropositivity occurs in a high proportion of asymptomatic kindergarten children (Ellis *et al.* 1986).

Three forms exist: endophthalmitis, macular retinochoroidal granuloma (Fig. 23.24), and peripheral retinochoroidal granuloma.

The condition is caused by the second stage larvae of toxocara canis, and it is the disintegrating organism which evokes eosinophilia and inflammation. Dogs and cats are the natural hosts of the worm, and human infection occurs with ingestion of eggs from contaminated pets, clothes or dirt.

Patients with ocular findings do not usually give a history of systemic disease (visceral larval migrans). Onset is usually between 2 and 3 years, and rare past 12 years. Males are affected more often than females. Presenting features include strabismus and leukocoria or failed screening examination at school.

Toxocara endophthalmitis presenting between 2 and 9 years is most often confused with retinoblastoma, as the red reflex is absent and a complete retinal detachment is present. Macular lesions, presenting slightly later, are solitary and confined to the posterior pole

with few overlying vitreous cells. The lesions are usually single but multiple sites of inflammation have been recorded and may be due to the larva moving in to subretinal space when it is relatively protected from the host's immunological surveillance (Lyness *et al.* 1987). Peripheral chorioretinal granulomas present later since vision is less affected. Rarely, bands of scar tissue may drag the macula and create a pseudoexotropia.

Histopathology will often fail to reveal any organisms but rather be characterized by eosinophilia and granulomatous inflammation.

Laboratory tests include the ELISA for toxocara; when used appropriately, it can help diagnose the condition in over 90% of the cases. Eosinophilia is not usually present. Vitreous aspiration may be helpful in differentiating from retinoblastoma (Smith & Nozik 1983) but only if retinoblastoma is *extremely* unlikely (See Chapter 27.1).

Treatment should only be undertaken once the possibility of retinoblastoma has been eliminated. Toxocara lesions are responsive occasionally to steroids: antihelminthic drugs do not seem to help. Enucleation should only be performed when the diagnosis of retinoblastoma cannot be excluded and/or the eye is blind and painful.

Candidiasis

Candidiasis usually presents as retinitis or vitritis in an immune deficient child (See Chapter 20.2).

Sympathetic ophthalmia

Sympathetic ophthalmia is a disorder in which the uveal tract becomes infiltrated by lymphocytes and epitheloid cells in response to injury to the fellow eye usually involving damage to the uvea.

Most reported high incidences are surrounding war injury, with 14% of eye injuries during the US Civil War associated with sympathetic ophthalmia. It occurs very rarely following intraocular surgery 0.007% according to one series (Liddy & Stuart 1972). It has also been associated with intraocular tumours (Riwchun & DeCoursey 1941).

The interval between trauma and onset of sympathetic ophthalmia has reportedly spanned 5 days (Thies 1947) to 42 years, but usually occurs between 2 weeks and 3 months after insult (Lubin *et al.* 1980).

This condition is characterized by pain, photophobia, decreased vision, and worsening of the traumatized eye. Uveitis may include 'plastic' iritis

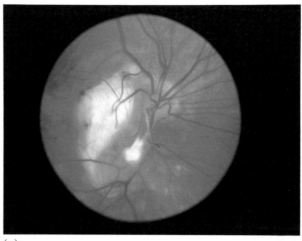

(a)

Fig. 23.24 (a) Toxocara. This 5-year-old child failed his school eye test and was found to have a raised peri-papillary lesion between the disc and the macular in his left eye. At this stage there was minimal active inflammation. (b) Toxocara lesion with minimal leakage at this late stage (same patient).

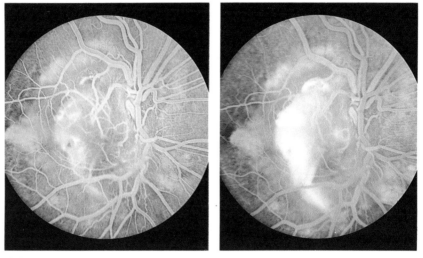

(b)

(i.e. with thick, viscous, exudate) and choroidal infiltration as well as exudative retinal detachment. Vitiligo and poliosis may occur, showing common ground between sympathetic ophthalmia and the Vogt–Koyanagi–Harada syndrome (Schlaegel 1981).

Histopathology reveals similar changes in the 'exciting' and the 'sympathizing' eye (Easom & Zimmerman 1964). Characteristic Dalen–Fuch's nodules represent epitheliod cells just internal to Bruch's membrane (Lubin *et al*. 1980).

The treatment for sympathetic ophthalmia prior to the advent of steroids consisted of enucleation of the injured eye (Lubin *et al*. 1980) but corticosteroids are now the primary mode of treatment (Makley & Leibold 1960).

The extensive literature on sympathetic ophthalmia includes a 30-year follow-up of a child who at 9

months perforated her cornea. After the fellow eye became red, the buphthalmic injured eye was enucleated. Recurrent inflammation with cataract and glaucoma ensued over the following 29 years in the remaining eye. The patient has ambulatory vision after a pars plana lensectomy/vitrectomy (Kinyoun *et al*. 1983).

Sarcoidosis

Sarcoidosis, as mentioned earlier, tends to cause anterior uveitis in children. Posterior involvement can include chorioretinitis, periphlebitis and venous sheathing, chorioretinal nodule, vitreous cells, vitreous haemorrhage and retinal neovascularization (James *et al*. 1964) as well as optic nerve granuloma (Laties & Scheie 1972).

Tuberculosis

Tuberculosis may also present as a posterior segment inflammation (see Fig. 23.22) and pseudoglioma in predisposed children (Saini *et al.* 1986).

References

Aaberg T. The enigma of pars planitis. *Am J Ophthalmol* 1987; **103**: 828–30

Albert DM, Puliafito CA, Fulton AB *et al.* Increased incidence of choroidal malignant melanoma occurring in a single population of chemical workers. *Am J Ophthalmol* 1980; **89**: 323–37

Alm A, Bill A. The oxygen supply to the retina II. Effects of high intraocular pressure and of increased arterial carbon dioxide tension on uveal and retinal blood flow in cats. *Acta Physiol Scand* 1972; **84**: 306–19

Apple DJ, Blodi FC. Pathologic observations and clinical approval to uveal melanoma. In: DH Nicholson (Ed.) *Ocular Pathology Update*, Masson, New York, 1980; p. 213

Apt L. Uveal melanoma in children and adolescents. *Int Ophthalmol Clin* 1963; **2**: 403–10

Arentsen JJ, Green WR. Melanoma of the iris. Report of 72 cases treated surgically. *Ophthalmic Surg* 1975; **6**: 23–37

Arnett FC Jr, Widman LE, Feinstein RS. Clinical conferences at the Johns Hopkins Hospital. Juvenile rheumatoid arthritis. *Johns Hopkins Med J.* 1982; **151**: 313–7

Arnett FC, Bias WB, Stevens MB. Juvenile onset chronic arthritis. Clinical and X-ray features of a unique HLA-B27 subset. *Am J Med* 1980; **69**: 369–76

Baarsma GS, La Hey E, Glasius E, de Vries J, Kijlstra A. The predictive value of serum angiotenisn converting enzyme and lysozyme levels in the diagnosis of ocular sarcoidosis. *Am J Ophthalmol* 1987; **104**: 211–8.

Barkan O. Goniotomy for glaucoma associated with aniridia. *Arch Ophthalmol* 1953; **49**: 1–5

Barr CC, McLean IW, Zimmerman LE. Uveal melanoma in children and adolescents. *Arch Ophthalmol* 1981; **99**: 2133–6

Barr CC, Vine AK, Martonyi CL. Unexplained heterochromia. Intraocular foreign body demonstrated by computed tomography. *Surv Ophthalmol* 1984; **28**: 409–11

Bateman JB. Microphthalmos. *Int Ophthalmol Clin* 1984; **24**: 87–107

Bedoya V, Grimley PH, Dugue O. Chediak–Higashi syndrome. *Arch Pathol* 1969; **88**: 340–9

Belmont JB, Michelson JB, Vitrectomy in uveitis associated with ankylosing spondylitis. *Am J Ophthalmol*; 1982; **94**: 300–4

Bergsma DR, Kaiser-Kupfer M. A new form of albinism. *Am J Ophthalmol* 1979; **77**: 837–44

Broadway D, Lang S, Harper J, Madanot F, Pritchard J, Tarawneh T, Taylor D. Congenital malignant melanoma of the eye. *Cancer* 1990; in press.

Buhler EM, Mehes K, Muller H, Stalder GR. Cat-eye syndrome, a partial trisomy 22. *Humangenetik* 1972; **15**: 150–62

Burger PC, Klintworth GK. Experimental retinal degeneration in the rabbit produced by intraocular iron. *Lab Invest* 1974; **30**: 9–19

Burkitt D, O'Connor GT. Malignant lymphoma in African children. I. A clinical syndrome. *Cancer* 1961; **14**: 258–69

Brushfield T. Mongolism. *Br J Child Dis* 1924; **21**: 241–58

Bywaters EGL, Ansell BM. Monoarticular arthritis in children. *Ann Rheum Dis* 1965; **24**: 116–22

Cagianut B, Theiler K. Bilateral colobomas of iris and choroid. *Arch Ophthalmol* 1970; **83**: 41–4

Calabro JJ, Parrino GR, Atchoo PD, Marchesano JM, Goldberg LS. Chronic iridocyclitis in juvenile rheumatoid arthritis. *Arthritis Rheum* 1970; **13**: 406–13

Callahan A. Aniridia with ectopia lentis and secondary glaucoma, genetic, pathologic, and surgical consideration. *Am J Ophthalmol* 1949; **32**: 28–39

Canning CR, McCartney ACE, Hungerford J. Medulloepithelioma (diktyoma). *Br J Ophthalmol* 1988; **72**: 764–8

Cleasby GW. Malignant melanoma of the iris. *Arch Ophthalmol* 1958; **60**: 403–17

Cory CC, Jamison DL. The cat-eye syndrome. *Arch Ophthalmol* 1974; **92**: 259–62

Creel D. Problems of ocular miswiring in albinism, Duane's syndrome and Marcus Gunn phenomenon. *Int Ophthalmol Clin* 1984; **24**: 165–76

Creel D, Witkop CJ, King RA. Asymmetric visually evoked potentials in human albinos: evidence for visual system anomalies. *Invest Ophthalmol Vis Sci* 1974; **13**: 430–40

David R, MacBeath L, Jenkins T. Aniridia associated with microcornea and subluxated lenses. *Br J Ophthalmol* 1978; **62**: 118–21

Doggart JH. Spontaneous hyphaema XVI *Concil Ophthalmol Acta* 1950; **1**: 450–5

Donaldson DD. The significance of spotting of the iris in Mongoloids Brushfield's spots. *Arch Ophthalmol* 1961; **65**: 26–31

Drews RC. Heterochromia iridum with coloboma of the optic disc. *Arch Ophthalmol* 1973; **90**: 437–42

Easom HA, Zimmerman LE. Sympathetic ophthalmia and bilateral phacoanaphylaxis. A clinicopathologic correlation of the sympathogenic and sympathizing eyes. *Arch Ophthalmol* 1964; **72**: 9–15

Ellis GS, Pakalnis VA, Worley G, Green JA, Frothingham TE, Sturner RA, Walls KW. Toxocara canis infestation: clinical and epidemiological associations with seropositivity in kindergarten children. *Ophthalmology* 1986; **93**: 1032–8

Elsas TJ, Maumenee IH, Kenyon KR, Yodar F. Familial aniridia with preserved ocular function. *Am J Ophthalmol* 1977; **83**: 718–24

Engel HM, de la Cruz ZC, Jimenez-Abalahin LD, Green WR, Michels RG. Cytopreparatory techniques for eye fluid specimens obtained by vitrectomy. *Acta Cytol* 1982; **26**: 551–60

Feeney L, Hogan M. Electron microscopy of the human choroid. *Am J Ophthalmol* 1961; **51**: 1457–83

Ferrell RE, Chakravarti A, Hittner HM, Riccardi VM. Autosomal dominant aniridia: Probable linkage to acid phosphatase – 1 locus on chromosome 2. *Proc Natl Acad Sci USA* 1980; **77**: 1580–2

Ferry AP. Lesions mistaken for malignant melanoma of the iris. *Arch Ophthalmol* 1965; **74**: 9–18

ffytche TJ. Role of iris changes as a cause of blindness in lepromatous leprosy. *Br J Ophthalmol* 1981; **65**: 231–9

Flanagan JC, DiGeorge AM. Sporadic aniridia and Wilms' tumour. *Am J Ophthalmol* 1969; **67**: 558–61

Flynn HW, Davis JL, Culbertson WW. Pars plana lensectomy and vitrectomy for complicated cataracts in juvenile rheumatoid arthritis. *Ophthalmology* 1988; **95**: 1114–9

Foos RY, Hull SN, Straatsma BR. Early diagnosis of ciliary body melanomas. *Arch Ophthalmol* 1969; **81**: 336–44

Forsius H, Eriksson AW. Ein neues augensyndrom mit x-chromosomaler transmission. Eine sippe mit fundusalbinismus, fovea hypoplasie, nustagmus, myopie, astigmatismus und dyschromatopsie. *Klin Monatsbl Augenheilkd* 1964; **144**: 447–57

François J, Verschragen-Spae MR, De Sutter E. The aniridia–Wilms' tumour syndrome and other associations of aniridia. *Ophthalmol Paediatr Genet* 1982; **1**: 125–38

Freedom RM, Park SG. Congenital cardiac disease and the 'cat eye' syndrome. *Am J Dis Child* 1973; **126**: 16

Friedenwald JS, Wilder HC, Maumenee AE *et al. Ophthalmic Pathology: An Atlas and Textbook.* WB Saunders, Philadelphia, 1952

Fuchs E. Wucherungen und geschwulste des ciliarepithels. *Albrecht Von Graefe's Arch Ophthalmol* 1908; **68**: 534–87

Fujikawa LS, Schwartz LK, Rosenbaum EH. Acquired immunodeficiency syndrome associated with Burkitt's lymphoma presenting with ocular findings. *Ophthalmology* 1983; **90**: 50–1

Garcia R, Niero JA, Nistal M. Aniridia associated with gonadoblastoma in the Smith–Lemli–Opitz syndrome. *Ann Esp Pediatr* 1976; **9**: 19–24

Gass JDM. Iris abscess simulating malignant melanoma. *Arch Ophthalmol* 1973; **90**: 300–2

Gillespie FD. Aniridia, cerebellar ataxia, and oligophrenia. *Arch Ophthalmol* 1965; **73**: 338–41

Glass D, Litvin D, Wallace K, Chylack L, Garovoy M, Carpenter CB, Schur PH. Early-onset pauciarticular juvenile rheumatoid arthritis associated with human leukocyte antigen-DRW5, iritis, and antinuclear antibody. *J Clin Invest* 1980; **66**: 426–9

Goldberg MF, McKusick VA. X-linked colobomatous microphthalmos and other congenital anomalies. A disorder resembling Lenz's dysmorphogenetic syndrome. *Am J Ophthalmol* 1971; **71**: 1128–33

Grant WM, Walton DS. Progressive changes in the angle in congenital aniridia, with development of glaucoma. *Am J Ophthalmol* 1974; **18**: 842–7

Grayson M. Viral diseases. In: Grayson M (Ed.) *Diseases of the Cornea.* CV Mosby Co., St Louis 1983; pp. 150–98

Green WR. Ophthalmic pathology. In: Spencer WH (Ed.) WB Saunders, Philadelphia 1985; pp. 607–13

Green WR, Oliff WJ, Trotter RR. Malignant teratoid medulloepithelioma of the optic nerve. *Arch Ophthalmol* 1974; **91**: 451–4

Greer CH. Congenital melanoma of the anterior uvea. *Arch Ophthalmol* 1966; **76**: 77–8

Grove JH, Shaw MW, Bourgue G. A family study of aniridia. *Arch Ophthalmol* 1961; **65**: 81–4

Grutzmacher R, Lindquist T, Chittum M, Bunt-Milam A, Kalina R. Congenital iris cysts. *Br J Ophthalmol* 1987; **71**: 227–35

Guillery RW, Okoro AN, Witkop CJ Jr. Abnormal visual pathways in the brain of a human albino. *Brain Res* 1975; **96**: 373–7

Hall BD. Choanal atresia and associated multiple anomalies. *J Pediatr* 1979; **95**: 395–8

Hamming NA, Miller MT, Rabb M. Unusual variant of familial aniridia. *J Pediatr Ophthalmol Strabismus* 1986; **23**: 195–200

Heimann K. Zur gefassentwicklump der macularen aderhautzone. *Klin Monatsbl Augenheilrd* 1970; **157**: 636–42

Heimann K. The development of the choroid in man: choroidal vascular system. *Ophthalmic Res* 1972; **3**: 257–73

Hetherington S. Sarcoidosis in young children. *Am J Dis Child* 1982; **136**: 13–5

Hittner HM, Riccardi VM, Ferrell RE, Borda RR, Justice J. Variable expressivity in autosomal dominant aniridia by clinical electrophysiologic, and angiographic criteria. *Am J Ophthalmol* 1980; **89**: 531–9

Hogan M. Ultrastructure of the choroid. Its role in the pathogenesis of chorioretinal disease. *Trans Pacific Coast Ophthalmol Soc* 1961; **42**: 61

Hogan MJ, Kimura SJ, Thygeson P. Pathology of herpes simplex kerato-iritis. *Trans Am Ophthalmol Soc* 1963; **61**: 75–99

Hoover DL, Khaim JA, Giangiacomo J. Pediatric ocular sarcoidosis. *Surv Ophthalmol* 1986; **30**: 215–28

Howard GM. Spontaneous hyphema in infancy and childhood. *Arch Ophthalmol* 1962; **68**: 615–20

Howland AC. Infant eyes: optics and accommodation. *Curr Eye Res* 1982; **2**: 217–24

Jakobiec FA, Howard GM, Devoe AG. Sector hamartoma of the iris. *Arch Ophthalmol* 1975; **93**: 614–7

Jakobiec FA, Howard GM, Ellsworth RM, Rosen M. Electron microscopic diagnosis of medulloepithelioma. *Am J Ophthalmol* 1975; **79**: 321–9

Jakobiec FA, Silbert G. Are most iris 'melanomas' really nevi? *Arch Ophthalmol* 1981; **99**: 2117–32

James DG, Anderson R, Langley D, Ainslie D. Ocular sarcoidosis. *Br J Ophthalmol* 1964; **48**: 461–70

James DG, Spiteri M. Systemic ophthalmology, Behçet's disease. *Ophthalmology* 1982; **89**: 1279–85

Jasper L, Denny FW. Sarcoidosis in children with special emphasis on the natural history and treatment. *J Pediatr* 1968; **73**: 499–571

Jensen OA, Marberg M, Dupont A. Ocular pathology in the elfin face syndrome. *Ophthalmologica* 1976; **172**: 434–40

Jesberg DO. Aniridia with retinal lipid deposits. *Arch Ophthalmol* 1962; **68**: 331–6

Jones IS, Cleasby GW. Hemangioma of the choroid, a clinicopathologic analysis. *Am J Ophthalmol* 1959; **48**: 612–20

Kalter H, Warkany J. Experimental production of congenital malformation in mammals by metabolic procedure. *Physiol Res* 1959; **39**: 69–115

Kanski JJ. Anterior uveitis in juvenile rheumatoid arthritis. *Arch Ophthalmol* 1977; **95**: 1794–7

Kanski JJ, Shun-Shin GA. Systemic uveitis syndromes in childhood – an analysis of 340 cases. *Ophthalmology* 1984; 1247–51

Kato H, Koike S, Yamamoto M, Ito Y, Yano E. Coronary aneurysms in infants and young children with acute febrile mucocutaneous lymph node syndrome. *J Pediatr* 1975; **86**: 892–8

Kawasaki T, Kosaki F, Okawa S, Shigematsu I, Yanagawa H. A new infantile acute febrile mucocutaneous lymph node syndrome (MLNS) prevailing in Japan. *Pediatrics* 1974; **54**: 271–6

Kendig EL Jr. The clinical picture of sarcoidosis in childhood. *Pediatrics* 1974; **54**: 289−92

Kenyon KR, Pederson JE, Green WR, Maumenee AE. Fibroglial proliferation in pars planitis. *Trans Ophthalmol Soc UK* 1975; **95**: 391−7

Khan JA, Hoover DL, Giangiacoma J, Singsen BH. Orbital and childhood sarcoidosis. *J Pediatr Ophthalmol Strabismus* 1986; **23**: 190−5

Kincaid MC, Green WR. Ocular and orbital involvement in leukemia. *Surv Ophthalmol* 1983; **27**: 211−32

Kinyoun JL, Bensinger RE, Chuang EL. 30 year history of sympathetic ophthalmia. *Ophthalmology* 1983; **90**: 59−65

Kunze J, Tolksdorf M, Wiedemann HR. Cat eye-syndrome. Klinische und cylogenetische differential diagnose. *Humangenetik* 1975; **26**: 271−89

Lambert SR, Amaya L, Taylor D. Congenital idiopathic microcoria. *Am J Ophthalmol* 1989; **106**: 590−4

Layman PR, Anderson DR, Flynn JT. Frequent occurrence of hypoplastic optic discs in patients with aniridia. *Am J Ophthalmol* 1974; **77**: 573−6

Laties AM, Scheie HG. Evolution of multiple small tumours in sarcoid granuloma of the optic disc. *Am J Ophthalmol* 1972; **74**: 60−6

Leonard BC, Shields JA, McDonald PR. Malignant melanomas of the uveal tract in children and young adults. *Can J Ophthalmol* 1975; **10**: 441−9

Levy WJ. Congenital iris lesion. *Br J Ophthalmol* 1957; **41**: 120−3

Liang JC, Juarez CP, Goldberg MF. Bilateral bicoloured irides with Hirschsprungs disease: a new neural crest syndrome. *Arch Ophthalmol* 1983; **101**: 69−73

Liddy BSL, Stuart J. Sympathetic ophthalmia in Canada. *Can J Ophthalmol* 1972; **7**: 157−9

Lubin JR, Albert DM, Weinstein M. Sixty-five years of sympathetic ophthalmia. A clinicopathologic review of 105 cases (1913−1978). *Ophthalmology* 1980; **87**: 109−21

Lyness R, Earley O, Logan W, Archer D. Ocular larva migrans: a case report. *Br J Ophthalmol* 1987; **71**: 396−401

Mackman G, Brightbell FS, Opitz JM. Corneal changes in aniridia. *Am J Ophthalmol* 1979; **87**: 497−502

MacRae DW, Howard RO, Albert DM, Hsia YE. Ocular manifestations of the Meckel syndrome. *Arch Ophthalmol* 1972; **88**: 106−13

Mader TH, Wergeland FL, Chismire KJ. Enlarged pupillary membranes. *J Pediatr Ophthalmol Strabismus* 1988; **25**: 73−5

Makley TA, Leibold JE. Modern therapy of sympathetic ophthalmia. *Arch Ophthalmol* 1960; **64**: 809−16

Mann I. *The Development of the Human Eye.* British Medical Association, London 1964.

Marden PM, Venters HD. A new neurocutaneous syndrome. *Am J Dis Child* 1966; **112**: 7981

Margo CE. Congenital aniridia: a histopathologic study of the anterior segment in children. *J Pediatr Ophthalmol Strabismus* 1983; **20**: 192−8

Martenet AC. Role of viruses in uveitis. *Trans Ophthalmol Soc UK* 1981; **101**: 308−11

McCartney ACE, Spalton DJ, Bull TB. Type IV melanosomes of the human albino iris. *Br J Ophthalmol* 1985; **69**: 537−42

Melish ME. Kawasaki syndrome: a new infectious disease? *J Infect Dis* 1981; **143**: 317−24

Merin S, Crawford JS, Cardarelli J. Hyperplastic persistent pupillary membrane. *Am J Ophthalmol* 1971; **72**: 717−9

Michelson JB, Shields JA. The relationship of iris nevi to posterior uveal melanomas. *Am J Ophthalmol* 1977; **83**: 694−6

Mirkinson AE, Mirkinson NK. A familial syndrome of aniridia and absence of the patella. *Birth Defects* 1975; **11**: 129−31

Mollenbach CJ. *Congenital Defects in the Internal Membranes of the Eye. Clinical and Genetic Aspects in Opera ex Domo Biologiae Hereditariae Humanae Universitatis Hafniensis,* Vol 15. Ejner Munksgaard, Copenhagen 1947; pp. 1−165

Mullaney J. The Montgomery Lecture 1977. Curious colobomata. *Trans Ophthalmol Soc UK* 1977; **97**: 517−22

Mund ML, Rodrigues MM, Fine BS. Light and electron microscopic observations on the pigmented layers of the developing human eye. *Am J Ophthalmol* 1972; **73**: 167−82

Naumann GOH, Font RC, Zimmerman LE. Electron microscopic verification of primary rhabdomyosarcoma of the iris. *Am J Ophthalmol* 1972; **74**: 110−7

Naumann GOH, Hellnar K, Naumann LR. Pigmented nevi of the choroid. Clinical study of secondary changes in the overlying tissue. *Trans Am Acad Ophthalmol Otolaryngol* 1971; **75**: 110−23

Nelson LB, Spaeth GL, Nowinski TS *et al.* Aniridia, a review. *Surv Ophthalmol* 1984; **28**: 621−42

Nicholson DH, Green WR. *Pediatric Ocular Tumours.* Masson, New York 1981

Nik NA, Hidayat A, Zimmerman LE, Fine BS. Diffuse iris nevus manifested by unilateral open angle glaucoma. *Arch Ophthalmol* 1981; **99**: 125−7

Ninane J, Taylor D, Day S. The eye as a sanctuary in acute lymphoblastic leukaemia. *Lancet* 1980; **1**: 452−3

North AF, Font CW, Gibson WM *et al.* Sarcoid arthritis in children. *Am J Med* 1970; **48**: 449−55

O'Connor GR. Doyne Lecture; heterochromic iridocyclitis. *Trans Ophthalmol Soc UK* 1985; **104**: 219−31

O'Connor GR. Factors related to the initiation and recurrence of uveitis. XL Edward Jackson Memorial Lecture. *Am J Ophthalmol* 1983; **96**: 577−99

O'Donnell FE. Congenital ocular hypopigmentation. In: Kivlin JD (Ed.) *Developmental Abnormalities of the Eye.* International Ophthalmologic Clinic 1984; pp. 133−42

O'Donnell FE, Green WR, Fleischman JA, Hambrick GW. X-linked ocular albinism in blacks. *Arch Ophthalmol* 1978; **96**: 1189−92

O'Donnell FE, Hambrick GW, Green WR *et al.* X-linked ocular albinism. *Clin Genet Arch Ophthalmol* 1976; **94**: 1883−92

Oh JO. Primary and secondary herpes simplex uveitis in rabbits. *Surv Ophthalmol* 1976; **21**: 178−84

Ohm J. Bandformige hornhauttrubung bei einem neunjährigen madchen und ihre Behandlung mit subkonjunktivalen Jodkaliumeinspritzungen. *Klin Monatsbl Augenheikd* 1910; **48**: 243−6

Opitz JM, Howe JJ. The Meckel syndrome (dysencephalia splanchno cystica, the Gruber syndrome). *Birth Defects* 1969; **5**: 167

O'Rahilly R. The optic, vestibulocochlear and terminal vomeronasal neural crest in staged human embryos. In: Rohen JW (Ed.) *Second International Symposium on the Structure of the Eye.* Schattauer verlag, Stuttgart 1965; pp. 557−64

Ozanics V, Jakobiec FA. Prenatal development of the eye and its adnexa. In: FA Jakobiec (Ed.) *Ocular Anatomy, Embryology and Teratology.* Harper & Row, Philadelphia 1982; pp. 11−13

Pagon RA, Graham JM, Zonana J, Yong S-L. Coloboma, congenital heart disease, and choanal atresia with multiple anomalies: CHARGE association. *J Pediatr* 1981; **99**: 223−7

Patterson A, Sommerville RG, Jones BR. Herpetic keratouveitis with herpes virus antigen in the anterior chamber. *Trans Ophthalmol Soc UK* 1968; **88**: 243−9

Paul EV, Parnell BL, Fraker M. Prognosis of malignant melanomas of the choroid and ciliary body. *Int Ophthalmol Clin* 1962; **2**: 487−502

Pendergrass TW. Congenital anomalies in children with Wilm's tumour. A new survey. *Cancer* 1976; **37**: 403−8

Perry HD, Mallen FJ. Iris involvement in granulocytic sarcoma. *Am J Ophthalmol* 1979; **87**: 530−2

Peterson RA. Schmid−Fraccaro syndrome. *Arch Ophthalmol* 1973; **90**: 287−91

Pfeiffer RA, Heimann K, Heiming E. Extra chromosome in 'cat eye' syndrome. *Lancet* 1970; **2**: 97

Phelps CD. The pathogenesis of glaucoma in Sturge−Weber syndrome. *Ophthalmology* 1978; **85**: 276−86

Pilling GP. Wilms' tumour in 7 children with congenital aniridia. *Pediatr Surg* 1975; **10**: 87−96

Quigley HA, Stanish FS. Unilateral congenital iris pigment epithelial hyperplasia associated with late onset glaucoma. *Am J Ophthalmol* 1978; **86**: 182−4

Riccardi VM, Borges W. Aniridia, cataracts, and Wilms' tumour. *Am J Ophthalmol* 1978; **86**: 577−99

Ridgeway EW, Jaffe N, Walton DS. Leukemic ophthalmopathy in children. *Cancer* 1976; **38**: 1744−9

Riwchun MH, De Coursey E. Sympathetic ophthalmia caused by nonperforating intraocular sarcoma. *Arch Ophthalmol* 1941; **25**: 848−58

Rodrigues MM, Hackett J, Donohon P. Iris. In: Jakobiec FA (Ed.) *Ocular Anatomy Embryology and Teratology.* Harper and Row, Philadelphia 1982; pp 285−302

Saini J, Mukherjee A, Nadkarai N. Primary tuberculosis of the retina. *Br J Ophthalmol* 1986; **70**: 533−5

Schachat AP, Jabs DA, Graham ML, Ambinder RF, Green WR, Soral R. Leukemic iris infiltration. *J Pediatr Ophthalmol Strabismus* 1988; **25**: 135−8

Schachenmann G, Schmid W, Fraccaro M, Mannini A, Tiepdo L, Perona GP, Sartori E. Chromosome in coloboma and anal atresia. *Lancet* 1965; **2**: 290

Schaller J, Johnson GJ, Ansell BM, Holborrow EJ. Antinuclear antibodies (ANA) in patients with iridocyclitis and juvenile rheumatoid arthritis (JRA, Still's disease). *Arthritis Rheum* 1973; **16**: 130

Schlaegel TF, O'Connor GR. Tuberculosis and syphilis. *Arch Ophthalmol* 1981; **99**: 2206−97

Schlaegel TF. Uveitis of suspected viral origin. In: Duane TD (Ed.) *Clinical Ophthalmology.* Harper & Row, Hagerstown 1981; p. 9

Schwartz LK, O'Connor GR. Secondary syphilis with iris papules. *Am J Ophthalmol* 1980; **90**: 380−4

Scotto J, Fraumeni JF, Lee JA. Melanoma of the eye and other non cutaneous sites. *J Natl Cancer Inst* 1976; **56**: 489−91

Shaffer RN, Cohen JS. Visual reduction in aniridia. *J Pediatr Ophthalmol Strabismus* 1975; **12**: 220−2

Shaw MW, Falls HF, Neel JV. Congenital aniridia. *Am J Hum Genet* 1960; **12**: 389−415

Shields JA, Kline MUS, Augsburger JJ. Primary iris cysts: a review of the literature and report of 62 cases. *Br J Ophthalmol* 1984; **68**: 152−166

Shields JA. Melanocytic tumours of the iris. In: Shields JA (Ed.) *Diagnosis and Management of Intraocular Tumours,* CV Mosby Co., St Louis 1983; pp. 83−94

Siltzbach LE, Greenberg GM. Childhood sarcoidosis − a study of 18 patients. *N Engl J Med* 1968; **279**: 1239−45

Sjögren T, Larsson T. Microphthalmos and anophthalmos with or without coincident oligophrenia. A clinical and genetic − statistical study. *Acta Psychiat Neurol Scand* (Suppl.) 1949; **56**: 1−103

Sloderbeck JD, Maumenee IH, Elsas FE et al. Linkage assignment of aniridia to chromosome 1. *Am J Genet* 1975; **27**: 83

Smith RE, Nozik RA. Uveitis. In: *A Clinical Approach to Diagnosis and Management* Williams & Wilkins, Baltimore 1983

Spaeth G, Nelson LB, Beaudoin AR. Ocular teratology. In: Jakobiec FA (Ed.) *Ocular Anatomy, Embryology, and Teratology.* Harper & Row, Philadelphia 1982; pp. 1027−56

Spicer WTH. Parenchymatous keratitis: interstitial keratitis: uveitis anterior. *Br J Ophthalmol Monograph* (Suppl.) 1924; **1**: 1−63

Stastny P, Fink CW. Different HLA-D associations in adult and juvenile rheumatoid arthritis. *J Clin Invest* 1979; **63**: 124−130

Stevens JE, Bayrd W, Heck FJ. Infectious mononucleosis: a study of 210 sporadic cases. *Am J Med* 1951; **11**: 202−8

Stone J. Special types of contact lenses and their use. In: Stone J, Phillips AJ (Eds.) *Contact Lenses,* Vol 2. Butterworth, London 1981; p. 667

Sugar HS, Kobernicke SD, Weingarten JE. Hematogenous ocular sclerosis of local cause. *Am J Ophthalmol* 1967; **64**: 749−56

Summers CG, Knobloch WH, Witkop CJ, King RA. Hermansky−Pudlak syndrome: ophthalmic findings. *Ophthalmol* 1988; **95**: 545−55

Susac JO, Smith JL, Scelfo RJ. The 'tomato-catsup' fundus in Sturge−Weber syndrome. *Arch Ophthalmol* 1974; **92**: 69−70

Taylor WOG. Visual disabilities of oculocutaneous albinism and their alleviation. *Trans Ophthalmol Soc UK* 1978; **98**: 423−45

Thies O. Gedanken uber den Ausbruch der sympathischen ophthalmie. *Klin Monatsbl Augenheilkd* 1947; **112**: 185−7

Ticho U, Ben-Sira I. Ocular leprosy in Malawi. Clinical and therapeutic survey of 8325 leprosy patients. *Br J Ophthalmol* 1970; **521**: 107−12

Verdager J. Prepubertal and pubertal melanomas in ophthalmology. *Am J Ophthalmol* 1965; **60**: 1002−11

Walker JP, Weiter JJ, Albert DM et al. Uveal malignant melanoma in 3 generations of the same family. *Am J Ophthalmol* 1979; **88**: 723−6

Walton DS. Aniridia with glaucoma. In: Chandler PA, Grant WM (Eds.) *Glaucoma.* Lea & Feiberger, Philadelphia 1979; pp. 351−4

Warburg M, Mikkelsen M, Andersen SR, Geertinger P, Larsen HW, Vestermark S, Parving A. Aniridia and interstitial deletion of the short arm of chromosome 11. *Metabol Pediatr Ophthalmol* 1980; **4**: 97−102

Warkany J, Schraffenberger E. Congenital malformations induced in rats by maternal vitamin A deficiency. *Arch Ophthalmol* 1946; **35**: 150−69

Winter TC. Ocular hemosiderosis. *Trans Am Acad Ophthalmol Otolaryngol* 1967; **71**: 813−9

Witmer R, Iwamoto T. Electronmicroscopic observation of

herpes like particles in the iris. *Arch Ophthalmol* 1968; **79**: 331−7

Witschel H, Font RL. Hemangioma of the choroid. A clinico-pathologic study of 71 cases and a review of the literature. *Surv Ophthalmol* 1975; **20**: 415−31

Wolf MD, Lichter PR, Ragsdale CG. Discussion by Smith RE. Prognostic factors in the uveitis of juvenile rheumatoid arthritis. *Ophthalmology* 1987; **94**: 1242−7

Yanoff M, Zimmerman LE. The relationship of congenital ocular melanocytosis and neurofibromatosis to uveal melanomas. *Arch Ophthalmol* 1967; **77**: 331−6

Zaidman GW, Johnson BL, Salamon SM, Mondino BJ. Fuchs' adenoma affecting the peripheral iris. *Arch Ophthalmol* 1983; **101**: 771−3

Ziegler JL. Treatment results of 54 American patients with Burkitt's lymphoma are similar to the African experience. *N Engl J Med* 1977; **297**: 75−80

Zimmerman LE, Broughton WL. A clinicopathologic and follow-up study of 56 intraocular medulloepitheliomas. In: Jakobiec FA (Ed.) *Ocular and Adnexal Tumours* Aesculapius, Birmingham Ala, 1978; pp. 181−5

Zimmerman LE, McLean IW. A comparison of progression the management of retinoblastomas and uveal melanomas. In: DH Nicholson (Ed.) *Ocular Pathology Update*. Masson, New York 1980; p. 191

24 Lens

SCOTT LAMBERT AND CREIG HOYT

Anatomy

The crystalline lens is a biconvex optical structure lying posterior to the iris and anterior to the vitreous humor. It is suspended by zonular fibres from the ciliary body. At birth, the lens has an equatorial diameter of 6.5 mm and an anterior−posterior depth of 3.5 mm at its poles. A collagenous capsule surrounds the lens with a monolayer of cuboidal epithelial cells on its anterior inner surface. The cuboidal cells in the equatorial region continue to develop into long spindle-shaped secondary lens fibres throughout life. The addition of secondary lens fibres in the equatorial region accentuates the eliptical shape of the lens in childhood and early adulthood. The lens achieves an equatorial diameter of 9 mm and an anterior−posterior depth of 5 mm by adulthood. The equatorial diameter of the lens stabilizes in early adulthood, with additional growth occurring in the anterior−posterior depth of the lens thereafter. The fetal nucleus is demarcated from the embryonic nucleus by Y-shaped upright sutures anteriorly and inverted Y-shaped sutures posteriorly. Both the embryonic and fetal nuclei are present at birth. Lens fibres developing after birth become the adult nucleus and cortex. The lens nucleus consists of compacted lens fibres which are indistinguishable from one another. The lens fibres in the cortex are less densely packed and individual fibres may be identified by specular microscopy in the superficial layers (Bron & Lambert 1984).

Embryology

The lens develops initially as a thickening of the surface ectoderm overlying the optic vesicle. The thickened surface ectoderm or lens placode then invaginates to form a lens pit which subsequently becomes the lens vesicle. The posterior surface of the lens vesicle is lined by columnar epithelial cells which elongate to become the primary lens fibres. The primary lens fibres gradually fill the lumen of the lens vesicle creating a nearly spherical structure. Only the anterior wall of the lens vesicle retains a monolayer of cuboidal epithelial cells which persists throughout life. Beginning at 7 gestational weeks, cuboidal epithelial cells in the equatorial region begin to develop into secondary lens fibres. The secondary lens fibres elongate in both an anterior and posterior direction inserting over the primary lens fibres. They are thickest equatorially resulting in preferential growth of the equatorial diameter of the foetal lens. Secondary lens fibres insert anteriorly and posteriorly at Y-shaped sutures (Mann 1928).

The lens capsule forms from the deposition of basement membrane material from the lens epithelium. Zonular fibres develop from the nonpigmented epithelium of the ciliary body during the fifth gestational month.

The tunica vasculosa lentis forms from branches of the hyaloid artery posteriorly and the annular vessel laterally. It encircles the developing lens, but begins to regress during the fourth gestational month (Mann 1928) and has disappeared by 28−33 weeks gestation. Remnants of the tunica vasculosa lentis may occasionally be seen in premature infants. Its presence should alert the ophthalmologist to the possibility of retinopathy of prematurity.

Developmental anomalies

Developmental defects of the lens include a wide spectrum of anomalies ranging from primary aphakia to abnormalities in the transparency, position, shape, and size of the lens.

Congenital aphakia occurs when the surface ectoderm in the developing embryo fails to form a lens placode and vesicle. Secondary aphakia occurs when the developing lens is spontaneously absorbed. Both conditions only occur in cases of maldevelopment of the remainder of the eye so that functional vision is rarely possible in these patients (Mann 1957).

Microspherophakia (Fig. 24.1) is a developmental abnormality in which the lens is reduced in diameter and spherical in shape. Although it may occur as an isolated hereditary abnormality, it more frequently occurs as part of the Weill–Marchesani syndrome. Microspherophakia may occur due to an arrest in the development of the secondary lens fibres or the insertion of abnormally thin secondary lens fibres.

Duplication of the lens is an extremely rare anomaly associated with metaplasia of the cornea and colobomas of the iris and chorioretinal tissue (Lyford & Roy 1974). The anomaly is believed to occur secondary to metaplastic changes in the surface ectoderm which prevents the lens placode from invaginating into a single lens vesicle.

Lens colobomas (Fig. 24.2) may be expressed as wedge-shaped defects or indentations in the lens or

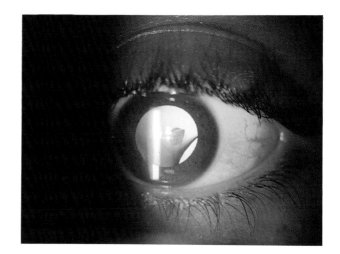

Fig. 24.2 Lens coloboma. Dr S. Day's patient.

only a flattening of a segment of the lens in a region where the zonules have failed to develop. They may occur unilaterally as an isolated anomaly or bilaterally in association with colobomas of the uveal system. A localized lens opacity may often be found in the region of the coloboma. Most colobomas occur in the lower portion of the lens either directly inferiorly or inferotemporally.

Lenticonus and lentiglobus (Fig. 24.3, 24.4, 24.5) are axial deformations of the anterior or posterior lens surfaces. Abnormalities of the posterior surface occur more frequently than those of the anterior surface. The refractive error through the center of the lenses may be highly myopic, while the peripheral lens is emmetropic; the retinoscopy reflex is distorted due to irregular astigmatism. Lentiglobus is more common than lenticonus and is usually unilateral (Crouch & Parks 1978). Anterior lenticonus is frequently associated with Alport syndrome and may be secondary to an abnormally thin anterior capsule centrally (Streeten et al. 1987; Thompson et al. 1987). It is most easily detected by the finding of an abnormal retinoscopy reflex.

Remnants of the tunica vasculosa lentis are residue from the vascular network which surrounds the lens early in foetal life. They usually consist of avascular pigmented pupillary membranes attached to the iris at the collarette. Another vascular remnant, the epicapsular star, appears as a single spot or group of pigmented spots attached to the anterior capsule. A Mittendorf dot is a remnant of the posterior tunica vasculosa lentis and consists of a dense white spot inferonasal to the posterior pole of the lens either adherent to the posterior lens capsule or slightly

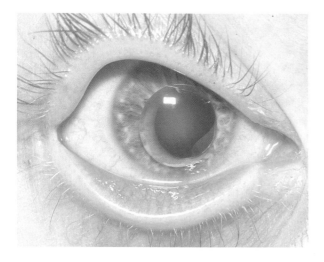

Fig. 24.1 Microspherophakia with anterior dislocation

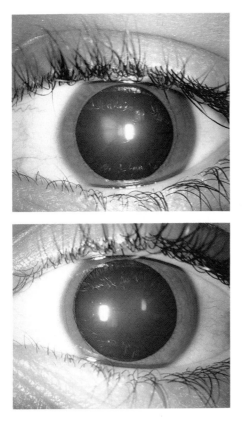

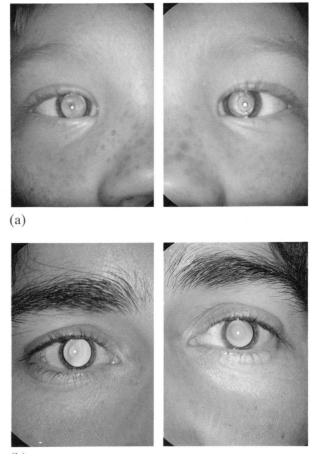

(a)

(b)

Fig. 24.3 Lenticonus with cataract. The characteristic reflex is only visible on retro-illumination.

Fig. 24.4 (a) Lenticonus. Although the reflex is a dynamic phenomenon seen on retinoscopy it can be seen here as a static change in the homogeneity of the red reflex. (b) Mother of patient in Fig. 24.4a. Posterior lenticonus is more frequent in boys and may be X-linked.

posterior to it. The tunica vasculosa lentis may occasionally be seen in significantly premature infants.

Persistent hyperplastic primary vitreous

The term persistent hyperplastic primary vitreous (PHPV) is used to describe a wide spectrum of congenital anomalies. These abnormalities most commonly consist of a retrolental plaque in a microphthalmic eye with prominent blood vessels on the iris, a shallow anterior chamber, elongated ciliary processes, and occasionally intralenticular haemorrhages (Reese 1955; Kazuhiko et al. 1986). They are unilateral in 90% of patients (Karr & Scott 1986). While the lens may be clear initially, with time they usually become cataractous. In some instances, the lens cortex and nucleus may undergo spontaneous absorption through a break in the posterior lens capsule (Fig. 24.6) while in others the lens becomes swollen (Haddad et al. 1978). When the lens becomes swollen the anterior chamber may become shallow and the intraocular pressure elevated. The retrolental fibrovascular plaque may be vascular (Fig. 24.7) and

frequently bleeds if cut surgically in early infancy, but with time becomes avascular. Retinal involvement usually occurs secondary to contraction of the retrolental plaque resulting in traction on the vitreous base and peripheral retina (Fig. 24.8). In most instances the posterior pole of the retina is normal (Haddad et al. 1978).

The differential diagnosis of a retrolental mass must include retinoblastoma, retinopathy of prematurity, retinal dysplasia, posterior uveitis and congenital cataracts as well as PHPV. If the PHPV is bilateral other causes must also be considered in the differential diagnosis. Although it is usually not difficult to distinguish an eye with PHPV from one with other causes of a white pupil, the presence of microphthalmos, a shallow anterior chamber, long ciliary processes, a cataract, and a retrolental opacity with a

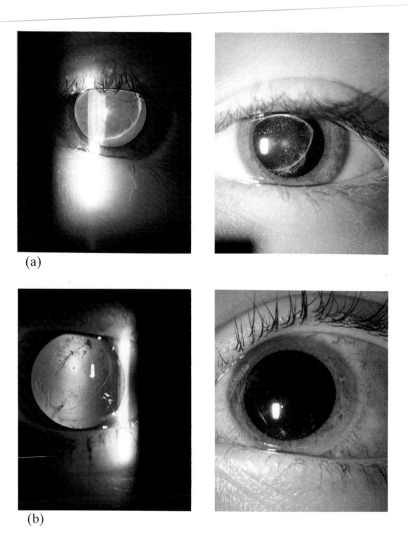

(a)

(b)

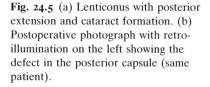

Fig. 24.5 (a) Lenticonus with posterior extension and cataract formation. (b) Postoperative photograph with retro-illumination on the left showing the defect in the posterior capsule (same patient).

persistent hyaloid artery (Fig. 24.9) help to confirm the diagnosis of PHPV.

In certain instances good visual results have been reported in eyes with PHPV after a lensectomy (Fig. 24.10) during the first few months of life. However it remains to be determined if successful visual rehabilitation can be reliably obtained in the majority of these eyes (Karr & Scott 1986). Glaucoma and secluded pupils may develop in eyes with PHPV after lensectomies.

Dislocated lenses

A subluxed lens is partially displaced from its normal position but remains within the pupillary space. In contrast, a luxated or dislocated lens is completely displaced from the pupil implying separation of all or virtually all the zonular attachments. A decrease in the visual acuity is the most common presenting symptom of subluxation or posterior dislocation of the lens. In contradistinction, anterior dislocation of the lens often produces symptoms of pain secondary to pupillary block glaucoma or corneal oedema.

Marfan syndrome is the most common cause of ectopia lentis in childhood. It is an autosomal dominantly inherited disorder characterized by ocular, cardiac, and skeletal abnormalities (Pyeritz & McKusick 1979). It has an incidence of 1 : 15 000 − 25 000 births without a racial or ethnic predilection. Cardiac abnormalities most commonly consist of dilation of the aortic root, mitral valve prolapse, and aortic aneurysms. Skeletal findings include excessive height, arachnodactyly, scoliosis and chest wall deformities. Ectopia lentis, cataracts, high myopia, and retinal detachments are the most common ocular abnormalities. The expressivity of Marfan syndrome is quite variable and the diagnosis may not be suspected until adulthood in some instances. At least two of the four

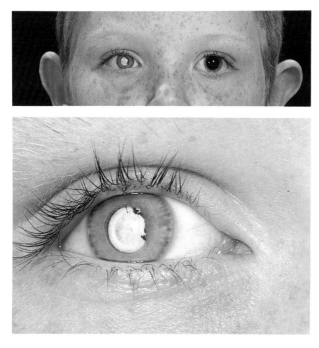

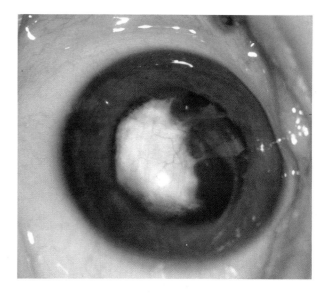

Fig. 24.8 PHPV showing stretched ciliary processes and cataract.

Fig. 24.6 Unilateral PHPV with spontaneous reabsorption of the lens.

criteria (family history, skeletal, cardiovascular, or ocular) of Marfan syndrome should be present to make the diagnosis. Certain 'hard' manifestations such as subluxed lenses, aortic dilation and severe kyphoscoliosis are more reliable than other 'soft' signs such as myopia, mitral valve prolapse, tall stature or joint laxity (Pyeritz & McKusick 1979). Although a defect in collagen or elastin synthesis has been proposed as the basis of the associated abnormalities, the nature of this defect has yet to be characterized.

Subluxation of the lens occurs in 60–80% of affected patients (Cross & Jensen 1973; Maumenee 1981). Lenses most commonly sublux superiorly (Fig. 24.11),

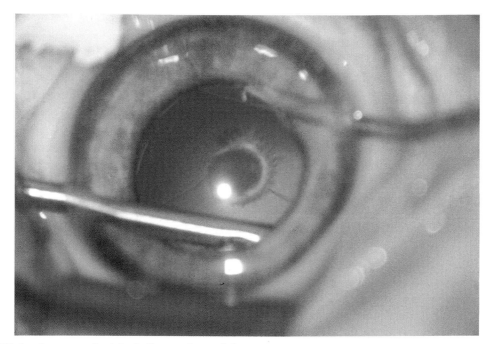

Fig. 24.7 PHPV showing a vascular lake in the membrane fed by a hyaloid artery (seen at 10 o'clock) and drained by a vein to the iris (seen at 2 o'clock).

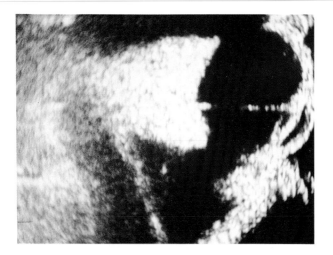

Fig. 24.9 PHPV ultrasound with persistent hyaloid artery.

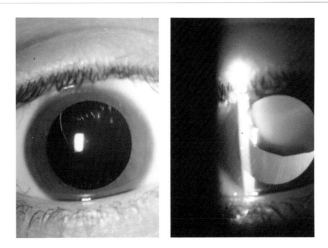

Fig. 24.11 Marfan's syndrome. Upward and nasal lens dislocation with intact zonule.

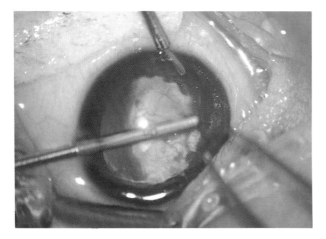

Fig. 24.10 PHPV showing vascularized membrane. Haemorrhages into the lens are not uncommon.

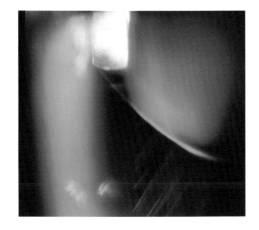

Fig. 24.12 Marfan's syndrome. Dislocated lens with intact zonule.

but may sublux in any direction (Maumenee 1981). The zonules usually remain intact but elongated (Fig. 24.12) and accommodation is occasionally unaffected. Occasionally subluxation may be as subtle as a flattening or notch in one sector of the lens visible only after pupillary dilation. Many patients do not show progression of the lens subluxation. Maumenee observed progression of subluxation in only 7.5% of 193 patients followed longitudinally (Maumenee 1981). Although ectopia lentis is frequently not detected until later in childhood, it is probably congenital in most instances. Many patients with Marfan syndrome also have axial myopia and are at an increased risk of developing retinal detachments. Marfan syndrome has a high intrafamilial concordance rate for the ocular findings (Maumenee 1981).

Homocystinuria is a disease of methionine metab-

olism. Classic homocystinuria (Type 1) is due to a deficiency of the enzyme cystathionine-B-synthetase. Affected individuals develop elevated levels of homocystine and methionine in the blood and other tissues. A urine sodium-nitroprusside test can be used as a rapid screening test for the disorder. A more definite diagnosis can be made by measuring the levels of homocystine in freshly voided urine after ingesting a bolus of methionine, and this technique should be used when the clinical diagnosis is suggestive even in the absence of a positive nitroprusside test (Michalski et al. 1988).

Affected individuals are normal at birth. During infancy they may fail to thrive and are developmentally delayed. The diagnosis is frequently not established until years later when ectopia lentis develops (Mudd et al. 1985). If untreated, 90% of

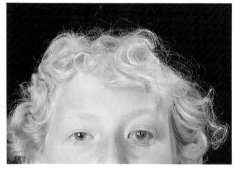

(a)

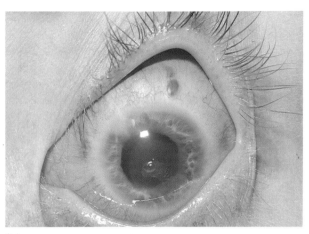

(b)

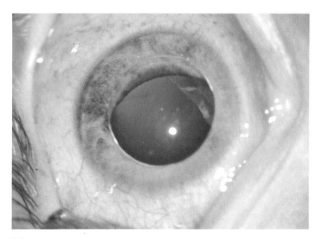

(c)

Fig. 24.13 (a, b) Homocystinuria. Fair-haired boy with chronic glaucoma following unreported anterior dislocation of the lens. Despite his age the left eye had become buphthalmic. (c) Same patient showing anterior dislocation of the lens.

affected patients develop progressive ectopia lentis (Cross & Jensen 1973). Ectopia lentis has been observed in an affected child at 3 years of age but more commonly develops in later childhood or early adulthood. In patients with subluxed lens, the zonules are markedly abnormal with only short broken filaments remaining attached to the lens capsule (Henkind & Ashton 1965). The lens usually subluxes inferiorly (Fig. 24.13) and may dislocate into the anterior chamber. A careful slit lamp examination will usually reveal the irregular distribution of the lens zonules and their matted appearance on the margins of the lens (Ramsey & Dickson 1975).

Patients with homocystinuria are tall with arachnodactyly, a malar flush, and fair hair. Progressive mental retardation frequently occurs if the disorder is not treated, although affected patients with normal intelligence have been reported (Barber & Spaeth 1969). Patients with homocystinuria are also at increased risk of developing thromboembolic episodes, particularly after surgical intervention (Mudd *et al.* 1985). The disorder has been estimated to occur in 1 : 200 000 births, but is more common among some racial groups. In Ireland it has an incidence of 1 : 52 000 births.

Pyridoxine (vitamin B_6) acts as a cofactor with cystathione-B-synthetase and 40–50% of patients with homocystinuria show biochemical improvement after being treated with high doses of pyridoxine (200–1000 mg/24 hours) (Shih & Efron 1970; Mudd *et al.* 1985). Patients unresponsive to pyridoxine may benefit from treatment with betaine (Smolin *et al.* 1981). A low methionine and high cysteine diet is also associated with improved metabolic control in many of these patients (Perry *et al.* 1968) which makes anaesthesia safer (Michalski *et al.* 1988). Alterations in the diet and early treatment with pyridoxine may prevent or delay subluxation of the lens and the development of mental retardation if initiated early in life (Mudd *et al.* 1985; Nelson *et al.* 1986; Burke *et al.* 1989).

The Weill–Marchesani syndrome is a rare disorder characterized by short stature, brachycephaly, stubby fingers and toes, and spherophakia (McGavic 1959). The lens commonly dislocates into the anterior chamber resulting in pupillary block glaucoma (Willi *et al*. 1973). Lenticular myopia also frequently occurs (Jensen *et al*. 1974). It is probably inherited as an autosomal recessive trait, although some pedigrees suggest an autosomal dominant inheritance with variable expressivity (Kloepfer & Rosenthal 1975).

Children with aniridia also commonly develop ectopia lentis. Later in life, they frequently develop cataracts and glaucoma. The removal of subluxed lens in these eyes may compromise the success of subsequent glaucoma filtering operations because of the difficulty in keeping the vitreous away from the filtering site (Callahan 1949). As a consequence, lensectomies should be avoided if at all possible in these eyes but where necessary they should be combined with a vitrectomy.

Ectopia lentis et pupillae is a rare cause of ectopia lentis characterized by the lens and pupil being displaced in opposite directions. The pupil is usually deformed in a slit or oval shape (Townes 1976). They may also have axial myopia, large corneas and transilluminant irides (Goldberg 1988). The inheritance is autosomal recessive. These patients can frequently be treated with their aphakic correction without lensectomies since the lenses are often not in the pupillary space.

In some series trauma is the most common cause of unilateral ectopia lentis (Jarrett 1967). Child abuse should be considered in any child with a traumatic injury.

Sulphite oxidase deficiency is an extremely rare disorder of sulphur metabolism resulting in the accumulation of S-sulfocystine, thiosulphate, and sulphite. Dislocated lenses, progressive muscular rigidity and decerebrate posturing are typical findings. Death usually occurs prior to 5 years of age (Shih *et al*. 1977). Xanthine oxidase deficiency, which is diagnosed by the finding of very low uric acid levels, has also been described as a very rare cause of dislocated lenses.

Ectopia lentis may also occur without any known associated systemic or ocular abnormalities. Some of these children will be found to have Marfan syndrome later in life if followed longitudinally. So-called simple ectopia lentis is usually inherited as an autosomal dominant trait (Falls & Cotterman 1943). The diagnosis is only tenable if all other known causes of ectopia lentis have been excluded. Some of these

patients may have spherophakia and lenticular myopia (Seland 1973).

Treatment of dislocated lenses

Satisfactory visual improvement can frequently be obtained by corrective lenses in patients with ectopia lentis (Alcorn & Maumenee 1987). If the lens is significantly subluxed and the visual acuity fails to improve with the phakic correction, the pupils should be dilated and the child should be given its aphakic correction. If the visual acuity remains inadequate, a lensectomy should then be performed to prevent amblyopia from developing (Reese & Weingeist 1987). Optical correction of a subluxed lens is most difficult when the pupil is bisected by the lens. A posteriorly dislocated lens should only be removed if it results in persistent uveitis, glaucoma, or cystic retinal degeneration. Anterior dislocation of the lens seems to occur most frequently in homocystinuria. It may be treated acutely with pupillary dilatation and manual repositioning of the lens by pressure on the cornea (Elkington *et al*. 1973). A lensectomy is usually advisable after anterior dislocation of the lens because of the risk of irreversible visual loss with each subsequent episode of anterior dislocation of the lens. Patients with homocystinuria are at a higher risk of complications from general anaesthesia due to thromboembolic disease. As a consequence, a more conservative approach is warranted in these patients (Elkington *et al*. 1973), especially whilst waiting for treatment to take effect.

Serious operative and postoperative complications commonly occurred when subluxed lenses were removed before the advent of vitreous cutting instruments (Chandler 1964; Jarrett 1967; Cross & Jensen 1973). However, postoperative complications occur infrequently using vitreous cutting instruments and a closed eye with infusion (Peyman *et al*. 1979; Reese & Weingeist 1987). We prefer to approach these lenses with the vitreous cutting instrument introduced in the area of greatest subluxation using a limbal approach. Precautions should be taken to prevent the lens from falling posteriorly. Subluxed and dislocated lens can also be approached by a pars plana approach combined with a vitrectomy (Peyman *et al*. 1979; Reese & Weingeist 1987). Occasionally minimally subluxed lens may be removed by an extracapsular technique or aspiration, but vitreous loss is a frequent complication (Maumenee & Ryan 1969; Sietner & Crawford 1981). Retinal detachments are the most serious postoperative complication occurring after extraction of subluxed lens. While retinal detachments were a frequent complication with older techniques of lens extraction, they occur infrequently after lensectomies with a vitreous cutting instrument in the short-term (Reese & Weingeist 1987). Longer follow-ups will be necessary to see if this continues to be the case since retinal detachments occur on the average 20–30 years after the removal of congenital cataracts (Toyofuku *et al.* 1980; Jagger *et al.* 1983).

Cataracts

Cataracts are opacities of the crystalline lens. Because they frequently interfere with normal visual development and are time consuming and costly to manage, they represent an important problem in paediatric ophthalmology. Monocular and binocular cataracts during infancy frequently result in significant visual deprivation. Twenty to 30% of children with bilateral cataracts remain legally blind after surgical and optical treatment (Gelbart *et al.* 1982; Parks 1982). Eyes with monocular cataracts seldom regain useful vision in the affected eye. Since early treatment is probably the most important factor in determining the visual outcome, prompt detection of cataracts in neonates is of the utmost importance.

Aetiology

The cause of congenital cataracts can be established in many children by a careful pre-operative assessment (Merin & Crawford 1971; Kohn 1976). Causes include metabolic disorders, genetically transmitted syndromes, intrauterine infections, and ocular conditions with associated anomalies (Table 24.1). In a clinically healthy child, an extensive pre-operative evaluation to establish a cause for the cataract is not routinely necessary. We believe that a paediatrician and an ophthalmologist working together will detect many of the associated ocular and systemic diseases and with a few simple blood tests the others may be diagnosed. An extensive battery of biochemical tests is not routinely necessary.

An intrauterine infection should be suspected in infants with dense unilateral or bilateral central cataracts (Fig. 24.14) and mandates a careful gestational history. A history of a maternal illness accompanied by a rash during the pregnancy would be particularly suggestive of an intrauterine rubella or varicella infection. Rubella IgG and IgM antibody titers should be obtained from the mother and the child. At the time of surgery the lens aspirate can also be sent to the

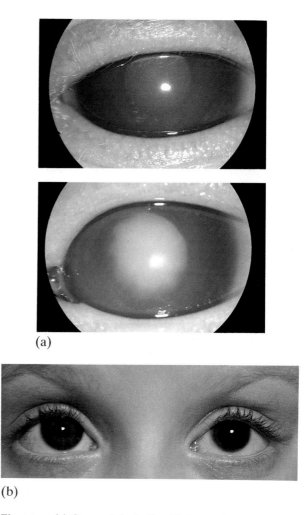

(a)

(b)

Fig. 24.14 (a) Congenital rubella with 'steamy' corneas and a unilateral cataract. Buphthalmos was suspected. (b) Same patient aged 6 showing that the corneas had not enlarged. Buphthalmos does occur in congenital rubella but it is important to be sure that the intraocular pressure is raised because corneal oedema also occurs from a transient keratitis.

laboratory for culture of rubella if the diagnosis is suspected but has not yet been confirmed. The rubella virus has been cultured in the lenses of children with the rubella syndrome up to 4 years of age. Intrauterine varicella infections may also result in congenital cataracts (Lambert *et al.* 1989).

Metabolic disorders do not result in congenital cataracts in otherwise healthy children with the exception of galactokinase deficiency. Galactokinase deficiency is markedly different from classic galactosemia which is characterized by a deficiency of galactose-1-phosphate uridyl-transferase. In classic galactosemia, infants are sick and usually present for medical care early in infancy due to a failure to thrive. Children with galactokinase deficiency are usually entirely well

Idiopathic

Intrauterine infection
  Rubella
  Varicella
  Toxoplasmosis

Uveitis or acquired infection
  Juvenile rheumatoid arthritis
  Pars planitis
  Toxocara canis

Drug induced
  Corticosteroids

Metabolic disorders
  Galactosemia
  Hypocalcemia
  Hypoglycemia
  Lowe's syndrome
  Diabetes mellitus

Trauma

Radiation-induced

Ocular diseases
  Leber's congenital amaurosis
  Aniridia
  Retinitis pigmentosa
  PHPV
  Retinopathy of prematurity

Inherited without systemic
abnormalities
  Autosomal dominant
  Autosomal recessive
  X-linked

Inherited with systemic abnormalities:

Chromosomal
  Trisomy 21
  Turner syndrome
  Trisomy 13
  Trisomy 18
  Cri du chat syndrome

Craniofacial syndromes
  Crouzon's disease
  Apert syndrome
  Engelmann's disease
  Lanzieri syndrome

Skeletal disease
  Conradi syndrome
  Marfan syndrome
  Osteopetrosis
  Weill–Marchesani syndrome
  Stickler syndrome
  Kneist syndrome
  Osteogenesis imperfecta

Syndactyly, polydactyly, or digital anomalies
  Bardet–Biedl syndrome
  Rubenstein–Taybi syndrome
  Ellis-van Creveld syndrome

Central nervous system abnormalities
  Zellweger syndrome
  Meckel–Gruber syndrome
  Sjogren–Larsson syndrome
  Marinesco–Sjogren syndrome
  Norrie's disease

Muscular disease
  Myotonic dystrophy

Dermatological
  Cockayne syndrome
  Goltz syndrome
  Rothmund–Thomson syndrome
  Atopic dermatitis
  Incontinentia pigmenti
  Progeria
  Bonnevie–Ullrich syndrome
  Congenital ichthyosis
  Marshall's ectodermal dysplasia

Table 24.1 Aetiology of cataracts in childhood.

without any evidence of systemic illness. Reducing substances are present in the urine of patients with both types of galactosemia after a galactose containing meal (milk). Enzymatic assays using erythrocytes can then be used to distinguish between the two forms of galactosemia. Both disorders are inherited as autosomal recessive traits. Children with galactosemia develop the 'oil drop' cataract which in reality is not a cataract but a refractive change in the lens nucleus which appears as a yellow drop in the centre of the lens in retro illumination like an oil droplet floating in water (Fig. 24.15a). If galactose is eliminated from the diet 'oil drop' cataracts usually disappear rapidly (Fig. 24.15b). Some patients develop lamellar-like cataracts due to the accumulation of galactitol in the lens (Fig. 24.16) (Kinoshita *et al.* 1962). Eliminating

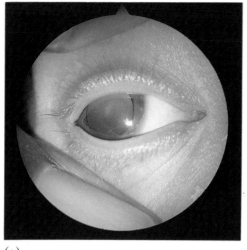

(a)

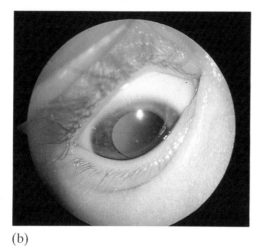

(b)

Fig. 24.15 (a) Galactosaemia — oil drop 'cataract' — it is a change in refractive index of the nucleus. (b) After early dietary control the 'cataract' has disappeared (same patient).

galactose from the diet of these children early in life will frequently prevent the formation or progression of cataracts as well as the other sequelae of classic galactosemia.

In Wilson's disease there may be a subcapsular deposition of copper pigments giving the so-called sunflower cataract (Fig. 24.17).

A decrease in serum calcium can be seen in neonates or infants secondary to surgical trauma or hypoparathyroidism. Cataracts develop as a result of the altered permeability of the lens capsule and are generally lamellar, with fine white punctate opacities (Fig. 24.18). Other signs and symptoms of hypocalcemia are usually present including seizures, failure to thrive, and irritability. Serum calcium and phosphorus levels should be measured in infants with any symptoms of hypocalcemia and cataracts.

Cataracts occur infrequently in children with diabetes mellitus. When they do develop, they usually occur in the teenage years. They frequently begin as cortical opacities but may rapidly progress to maturity.

Hypoglycemia may develop in the perinatal period or in early infancy. Significant hypoglycemia is usually accompanied by seizures and neurologic deficits. Cataracts associated with hypoglycemia may be small, transient, and reversible, or may form several layers of opacification if the hypoglycaemia is recurrent. Occasionally these lens opacities may develop into total cataracts.

Congenital cataracts are frequently inherited as an autosomal dominant trait accompanied by microphthalmos. A slit lamp examination should be performed on the parents and siblings of affected children, since variable expressivity is a characteristic

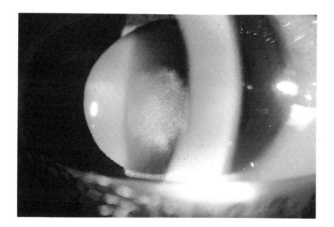

Fig. 24.16 Wilson's disease 'sunflower' cataract. Dr G. Holmstrom's patient.

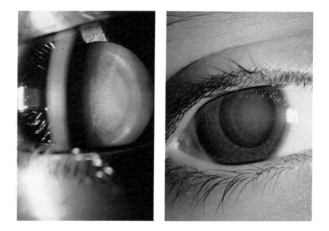

Fig. 24.17 Galactosaemia. In some cases, perhaps related to late treatment a cataract forms which is lamellar but may cause a visual defect.

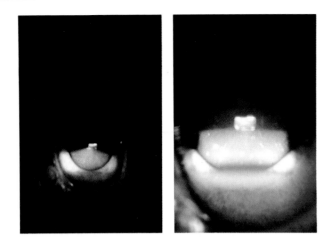

Fig. 24.18 Hypocalcaemic cataract — punctate dots.

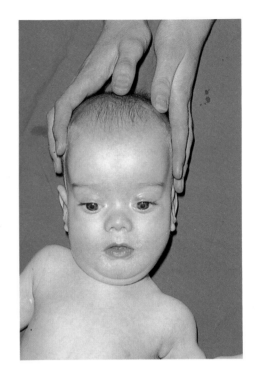

Fig. 24.19 Lowe's syndrome showing 'chubby' cheeks and rounded forehead. He has bilateral cataracts.

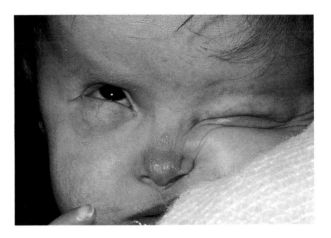

Fig. 24.20 Hallermann—Streiff—François syndrome showing the small nose with prominent veins. Baldness and progenia are common.

of autosomal dominantly inherited cataracts. Thus a parent may have visually insignificant cataracts, while the children may have dense cataracts even in infancy. Autosomal recessive inheritance is less common but should be suspected if there is consanguinity or multiply affected offspring and unaffected parents. Lowe's syndrome is inherited as an X-linked trait. Almost all affected males have cataracts at birth. Carriers usually have multiple fine peripheral cortical punctate lens opacities, which are sparse but increase in number with age (Johnson & Nevin 1976; Delleman *et al.* 1977; Cibis *et al.* 1986). Children with Lowe's syndrome have an abnormal facial appearance with frontal bossing (Fig. 24.19), chubby cheeks, and profound mental retardation. In infancy they are hypotonic. The eyes are abnormal with histological signs suggestive of mesoectodermal dysgenesis; the lens has a reduced anteroposterior diameter (Ginsberg *et al.* 1981; Tripathi *et al.* 1986) with developmental malformations varying from a discoid shape to posterior lentiglobus, and epithelial hyperplasia.

A large number of chromosomal syndromes include cataracts as one of their manifestations (Table 24.1). The most common of these is trisomy 21. Children with trisomy 21 frequently have mature cataracts during infancy (Jaeger 1983). Cataracts have also been reported in a pedigree with reciprocal translocation of chromosomes 3 and 4 (Reese *et al.* 1987). Cataract also occurs with the cri du chat syndrome caused by a partial deletion of short arm of chromosome 5 (Farrell *et al.* 1988). Cataracts may also be the presenting sign of the Hallerman−Streiff−François syndrome (Fig. 24.20) in which there is also thinned hair, a turned up nose with prominent blood vessels and progeria which becomes evident later. Spon-

taneous absorption of the cataract has been described in this syndrome and in a family with aniridia (Yamamoto *et al.* 1988).

Chronic corticosteroid therapy may result in the formation of posterior subcapsular cataracts. Incipient cataracts may be reversible if the corticosteroids are promptly discontinued (Forman *et al.* 1977). However, the associated systemic conditions that prompted the

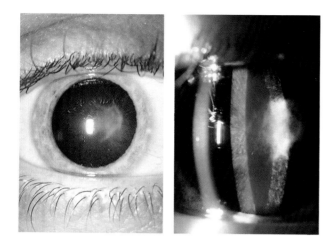

Fig. 24.21 Posterior subcapsular cataracts in a child with treated for leukaemia.

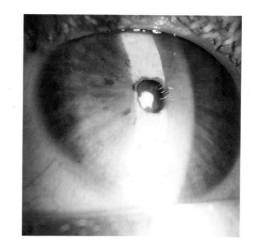

Fig. 24.22 Anterior polar cataract. The acuity is 6/6.

initial steroid therapy are often life threatening, and cessation of steroid therapy may not be possible. Because of the posterior and central location of these cataracts (Fig. 24.21), visual acuity at near is sometimes more severely affected than at distance. Early steroid-induced posterior subcapsular cataracts may be associated with little visual disability and may progress quite slowly (Brocklebank *et al.* 1982).

Posterior subcapsular cataracts also develop in children with uveitis secondary to Still's disease or juvenile rheumatoid arthritis (JRA) and pars planitis. Children with JRA associated cataracts also characteristically develop band keratopathy and posterior synechiae (Key & Kimura 1975). Cystoid macular oedema is a common accompaniment of both conditions.

Transient cataracts have been noted in some premature infants (McCormick 1968). They are usually bilateral and symmetrical opacities beginning as vacuoles along the posterior lens suture. Only rarely do they persist and result in permanent lens opacities.

Morphology

Although it is technically difficult, a slit lamp examination is necessary to define the precise morphology and location of cataracts in infants and young children. Certain morphologic patterns are known to be less likely to progress (e.g. anterior polar cataracts; Fig. 24.22) and in some instances (i.e. in PHPV, trisomy 21, galactosaemia, or rubella) the aetiology of the cataract may be deduced from its morphology alone. The location and density of cataracts deter-

mines their amblyogenic potential. Posteriorly located partial cataracts are particularly amblyogenic and if more than 2–3 mm in diameter are rarely associated with good visual acuity if not treated. Other relatively large partial cataracts may be associated with surprisingly little amblyopia and are compatible with good visual acuity (Fig. 24.23). This is particularly true of bilateral lamellar cataracts and anterior polar catar-

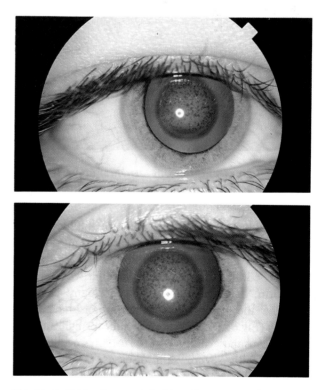

Fig. 24.23 Bilateral symmetrical lamellar cataracts in retro-illumination. The acuity is 6/9 in both eyes.

Management

Although bilateral complete congenital cataracts should be removed as early as possible, partial cataracts should only be extracted after a careful assessment of the morphology of the lens opacity and the visual behaviour of the child. Conservative management is indicated at least until the state of the child's vision becomes obvious. The visual prognosis of bilateral incomplete cataracts correlates better with the density than the size of the opacity. Hence nuclear cataracts, although smaller in size than lamellar cataracts, may have a poorer visual prognosis. If the major blood vessels of the fundus cannot be distinguished through the central portion of the cataract, significant visual deprivation can be expected from even a relatively moderate sized partial cataract; however the ophthalmoscopic clarity of the media is a poor guide to the effect of the opacity on vision.

An attempt should be made to evaluate the integrity of the retina and optic nerve in all children with significant cataracts. Although an objective assessment of visual function is difficult in early infancy, subjective tests such as fixation behaviour are often helpful. It is also important that pupillary reflexes be assessed. An unequivocal afferent pupillary defect indicates that there is a structural anomaly of the optic disc or retina, and is associated with a poor long term visual prognosis. The posterior pole should also be examined by ophthalmoscopy. If the density of the cataracts precludes an adequate view of the fundus, an ultrasound examination should be carried out prior to any surgical intervention. Electroretinography and visual evoked responses may also be helpful in deciding if surgical intervention is indicated. Visual assessment is still carried out by clinical observation, and although this remains the main method for judging whether the cataract is visually significant, the techniques of forced choice preferential looking and pattern visual evoked potentials are playing increasing roles in specialized centres.

Surgery for visually significant bilateral cataracts should be carried out as quickly as possible without jeopardizing the general health of the child. Only a few days should elapse between the removal of the two lenses to prevent monocular amblyopia, and we patch the first operated eye to prevent amblyopia in the second operated eye, until both eyes have been operated upon (Taylor et al. 1979).

The surgical treatment of children's cataracts has evolved considerably since Scheie popularized the aspiration procedure (Scheie 1960). At present, most authorities prefer to perform a lensectomy–vitrectomy utilizing a closed eye vitrectomy system (Lambert et al. 1989). This technique is safe and has greatly reduced the need for secondary surgical procedures on these children (Taylor et al. 1981). Moreover, it provides a clear visual axis which facilitates retinoscopy; preliminary studies of this technique suggest that the incidence of secondary glaucoma and retinal detachment may be markedly reduced by utilizing this technique rather than a standard aspiration procedure (Gelbart et al. 1982; Parks 1982). Phakoemulsification is rarely required in the treatment of paediatric cataracts. Older children, who are less susceptible to amblyopia and in whom posterior capsule opacification is less rapid are often better treated with an aspiration technique, especially in children over 2 years of age or others with lamellar cataract. A Yag laser can be used to create a posterior capsulotomy in co-operative children if the posterior capsule opacifies.

The major obstacle confronting ophthalmologists and the families of infants requiring cataract extraction is the optical treatment of aphakia and the occlusion therapy of amblyopia. Although spectacles may be possible (Fig. 24.26) bilateral aphakia is usually best treated in infancy with contact lenses (Fig. 24.27). Advantages and disadvantages exist for the use of soft, gas-permeable rigid, and silicone aphakic contact lenses (Hoyt 1986). Aphakic soft lenses are relatively inexpensive and easy to fit (Epstein et al. 1988; Levin et al. 1988). They have the disadvantage of being more difficult to insert and do not correct astigmatic refractive errors. Aphakic gas-permeable rigid contact lenses provide a superior optical correction in many instances (Saunders & Ellis 1981) but require greater expertise to fit (Pratt-Johnson & Tillson 1985). Aphakic silicone lenses are easy to fit and easy to insert, but are more expensive than other aphakic contact lenses (Nelson et al. 1985).

The frequent loss of lenses and the need to change the lens power results in numerous lens replacements, particularly during the first 2 years of life (Amaya et al. 1990). Parents are strongly advised to remove the lenses if the child's eye becomes inflamed, irritated, or if excessive discharge develops in order to prevent disabling corneal scarring.

Some investigators have advocated the use of intraocular lenses in aphakic children and isolated reports of good visual acuities have been reported in a few children with monocular congenital cataracts (Ben Ezra & Paez 1983; Hiles 1984; Hiles & Hered 1987). While the correction of paediatric aphakia with intraocular lenses is appealing because of the improved

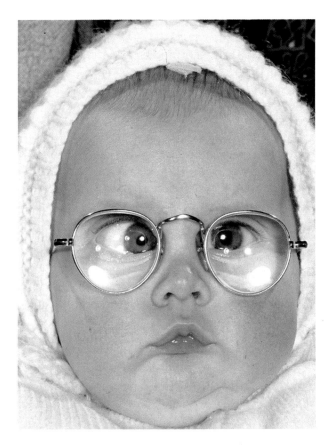

Fig. 24.26 Aphakic spectacles are safe and easily changed but have optical and cosmetic disadvantages.

optics of this form of aphakic correction, their use during infancy also poses several problems. First, the long-term consequences of having an intraocular lens in an eye are not known (Champion *et al.* 1985) (Fig. 24.28). A more immediate concern is the difficulty in coping with the dynamic changes occurring in the refractive power of an infant's eye. Although an intraocular lens with a standard power of 19–20 dioptres could be implanted, an overcorrection would be required for several years until the eye achieves its adult dimensions (Gordon & Donsiz 1985). In addition, many infants with cataracts have microphthalmic eyes and a standard lens would significantly undercorrect these eyes. Removing the lens from a neonatal eye may also affect its growth (Wilson *et al.* 1987).

Aphakic spectacles are better tolerated by some children with bilateral aphakia than contact lenses. This is particularly true of children between 18 months and 4 years of age. Aphakic spectacles also have the cosmetic advantage of improving the appearance of mildly microphthalmic eyes because of the magnification they induce. In addition, a secondary strabismus may be manipulated by the prismatic effect of spectacles.

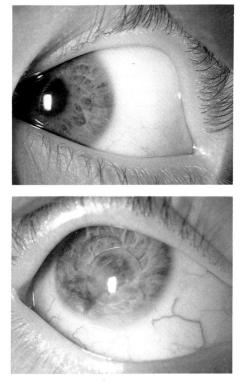

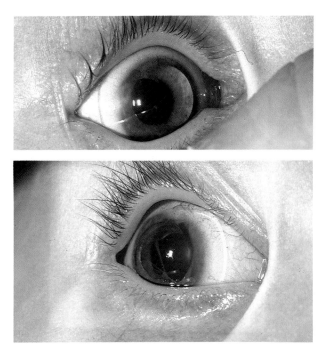

Fig. 24.27 Aphakic contact lenses are the treatment of choice in infant aphakia (see text).

Fig. 24.28 This child had a secondary intraocular lens implant at 18 months. By 2½ years she had a bilateral uveitis with vision in the best eye of perception of hand movements.

Epikeratophakia, the use of a lamellar onlay corneal graft, may be useful in older cases where contact lenses have not been tolerated (Morgan *et al.* 1988; Rostron 1988). Although generally safe they are not without complication (Price & Binder 1987).

No matter what form of aphakic correction is chosen, frequent re-evaluations are necessary. Each examination should include a careful analysis of fixation behaviour to screen for amblyopia. If amblyopia is suspected, occlusion therapy of the preferred eye should be initiated. Frequent retinoscopic measurements of the refractive error and adjustments in the power of the aphakic correction are imperative. The intraocular pressure should also be periodically assessed, particularly if signs or symptoms of glaucoma develop. This may require general anaesthesia in an infant. The importance of encouragement and support for the parents of aphakic children cannot be overemphasized if a continuing successful rehabilitation programme is to be accomplished.

The surgical management of monocular congenital cataracts is more controversial. Although eyes with monocular congenital cataracts may be successfully rehabilitated under certain circumstances, (Beller *et al.* 1981) most eyes with monocular cataracts do not achieve a visual acuity compatible with reading (Kushner 1986; Robb *et al.* 1987; Birch & Stager 1988, Drummond *et al.* 1989). Before a decision is made to perform surgery on a monocular congenital cataract, the difficulties encountered with the use of aphakic contact lenses and occlusion therapy should be described in detail to the parents. If contact lens are not tolerated, epikeratophakia or aphakic spectacles may be of benefit to some children with monocular aphakia (Arffa *et al.* 1986; Kelley *et al.* 1986).

If a decision is made to perform surgery on a monocular congenital cataract, prompt surgical intervention is critical (Rogers *et al.* 1981). Most studies suggest that surgery after the first two months of life is not likely to result in good visual acuity (Vaegan & Taylor 1979; Birch & Stager 1988). Immediate and continued optical correction of the monocular aphakia and occlusion therapy of the phakic eye is crucial in the visual rehabilitation of these eyes.

Visual results

The visual results after the surgical removal of congenital cataracts has improved dramatically over the last two decades (Scheie 1960; Pratt-Johnson & Tillson 1981). Improvements in surgical results may be attributed to better surgical techniques, the avail-

ability of paediatric aphakic contact lens, and the improved screening of children for cataracts by paediatricians and general practitioners at an earlier age. Nevertheless, complete visual rehabilitation is rarely possible, even in the best of circumstances. The visual results of cataract removal in infants and children depend on a number of factors, including the age of onset of the cataracts, the age when the surgery was performed, associated ocular and systemic conditions, and compliance with optical and patching therapy. Older children who develop cataracts after the completion of normal visual development, usually have an excellent visual prognosis after cataract extraction. In contra-distinction, 20–30% of infants remain legally blind after the surgical and optical treatment of bilateral congenital cataracts (Gelbart *et al.* 1982; Parks 1982). Very late operated cases may remain very visually disabled despite optical correction (Synnove *et al.* 1986).

Concomitant ocular abnormalities such as corneal opacities, glaucoma, and retinal abnormalities worsen the visual prognosis of children with congenital cataracts. The presence of manifest nystagmus in children with binocular congenital cataracts or manifest latent nystagmus in children with monocular cataracts is a sign of poor visual potential. Mental retardation is also associated with a poor visual prognosis.

Although mental retardation *per se* is not a contra-indication to cataract surgery, the postoperative care and visual rehabilitation of these children is much more difficult.

References

Alcorn DM, Maumenee IH. Optical correction and visual acuity in patients with the Marfan syndrome and dislocated lenses. *Invest Ophthal Vis Sci* 1987; **28**: 342

Amaya L, Speedwell L, Taylor DSI. Contact lenses for aphakic infants. *Br J Ophthalmol.* 1990. In press.

Arffa RC, Marveille TL, Morgan KS. Long-term follow-up of refractive and keratometric results of paediatric epikeratophakia. *Arch Ophthalmol* 1986; **104**: 668–70

Barber GW, Spaeth GL. The successful treatment of homocystinuria with pyridoxine. *J Pediatr* 1969; **75**: 463–71

Beller R, Hoyt CS, Marg E. Good visual function after neonatal surgery for congenital monocular cataracts. *Am J Ophthalmol* 1981; **91**: 559–65

Ben Ezra D, Paez JH. Congenital cataract in intraocular lenses. *Am J Ophthalmol* 1983; **96**: 311–4

Birch EE, Stager DR. Prevalence of good visual acuity following surgery for congenital unilateral cataract. *Arch Ophthalmol* 1988; **106**: 40–3

Brocklebank JT, Harcourt RB, Meadows SR. Corticosteroid-induced cataracts in idiopathic nephrotic syndrome. *Arch Dis Child* 1982; **57**: 30–5

Bron AJ, Lambert SR. Specular microscopy of the lens. *Ophthalmic Res* 1984; **16**: 209

Burke JP, O'Keefe M, Bowell R, Naughten ER. Ocular complications in homocystinuria — early and late treated. *Br J Ophthalmol* 1989; **73**: 427—31

Callahan A. Aniridia with ectopia lentis and secondary glaucoma. Genetic, pathologic and surgical considerations. *Am J Ophthalmol* 1949; **32**: 28—40

Champion R, McDonnell PJ, Green WR. Intraocular lenses. Histopathologic characteristics of large series of autopsy eyes. *Surv Ophthalmol* 1985; **30**: 1—32

Chandler PA. Choice of treatment in dislocation of the lens. *Arch Ophthalmol* 1964; **71**: 765—86

Cibis GW, Waeltermann JM, Whitcraft CT, Tripathi RC, Harris DJ. Lenticular opacities in carriers of Lowe's syndrome. *Ophthalmology* 1986; **93**: 1041—6

Cross HE, Jensen AD. Ocular manifestations in the Marfan syndrome and homocystinuria. *Am J Ophthalmol* 1973; **75**: 405—20

Crouch ER, Parks MM. Management of posterior lenticonus complicated by unilateral cataracts. *Am J Ophthalmol* 1978; **85**: 503—7

Delleman JW, Bleekers-Wagemakers EM, van Beden AWC. Opacities of the lens indicating carrier status of the oculocerebrorenal syndrome. *J Pediatr Ophthalmol Strabismus* 1977; **14**: 205—7

Drummond GT, Scott WE, Keech RV. Management of monocular congenital cataracts. *Arch Ophthalmol* 1989; **107**: 45—51

Elkington ARL, Freedman SS, Jay B, Wright P. Anterior dislocation of the lens in homocystinuria. *Br J Ophthalmol* 1973; **57**: 325—9

Epstein RJ, Fernandez A, Gammon JA. The correction of aphakia in infants with hydrogel extended-wear contact lenses. *Ophthalmology* 1988; **95**: 1102—6

Falls HF, Cotterman CW. Genetic studies on ectopic lentis. *Arch Ophthalmol* 1943; **30**: 610—20

Farrell JW, Morgan KS, Black S. Lensectomy in an infant with Cri du Chat syndrome and cataracts. *J Pediatr Ophthalmol Strabismus* 1988; **25**: 131—5

Forman AR, Toreto JA, Tina L. Reversibility of corticosteroid-associated cataracts in children with the nephrotic syndrome. *Am J Ophthalmol* 1977; **84**: 75—8

Gelbart SS, Hoyt CS, Jastrbesky G, Marg E. Long term visual results in bilateral congenital cataracts. *Am J Ophthalmol* 1982; **93**: 615—21

Ginsberg J, Bore KE, Fogelson MH. Pathological features of the eye in the oculocerebrorenal (lowe) syndrome. *J Pediatr Ophthalmol Strabismus* 1981; **18(4)**: 16—24

Goldberg MF. Clinical manifestations of ectopia lentis et pupillae in 16 patients. *Ophthalmology* 1988; **95**: 1080—8

Gordon RH, Donsiz PB. Refractive development of the human eye. *Arch Ophthalmol* 1985; **103**: 785—9

Haddad R, Font RL, Reeser F. Persistent hyperplastic primary vitreous. A clinicopathologic study of 62 cases and review of the literature. *Surv Ophthalmol* 1978; **23**: 123—4

Henkind P, Ashton N. Ocular pathology in homocystinuria. *Trans Ophthalmol Soc UK* 1965; **85**: 21—38

Hiles DA. Intraocular lens implantation in children with monocular cataracts. *Ophthalmology* 1984; **91**: 1231—7

Hiles DA, Hered RW. Modern intraocular lens implants in children with new age limitations. *J Cataract Refract Surg* 1987; **13**: 493—7

Hoyt CS. The optical correction of pediatric aphakia. *Arch Ophthalmol* 1986; **104**: 6541—2

Hubel DH, Wiesel TN. The period of susceptibility to the physiological effects of unilateral eye closure in kittens. *J Physiol* 1970; **206**: 419—36

Jaafar MS, Robb RM. Congenital anterior polar cataract. A review of 63 cases. *Ophthalmology* 1984; **91**: 249—52

Jaegar EA. Lens opacities in Down's syndrome. In: *XXIV International Congress of Ophthalmology*. JB Lippincott Co., Philadelphia 1983; pp. 68—71

Jagger JD, Cooling RJ, Fison LG *et al.* Management of retinal detachment following congenital cataract surgery. *Trans Opthalmol Soc UK* 1983; **103**: 103—7

Jarrett WH. Dislocation of the lens: a study of 166 hospitalized cases. *Arch Ophthalmol* 1967; **78**: 289—96

Jensen AD, Cross HE, Paton D. Ocular complications in the Weill—Marchesania syndrome. *Am J Ophthalmol* 1974; **77**: 261—9

Johnson SS, Nevin NC. Ocular manifestations in patients and female relatives of families with the oculocerebrorenal syndrome of Lowe. *Birth Defects* 1976; **12**: 567—72

Karr DJ, Scott WE. Visual acuity results following treatment of persistent hyperplastic primary vitreous. *Arch Ophthalmol* 1986; **104**: 662—7

Kazuhiko U, Kumiko N, Norio O. Haemorrhage in the lens: spontaneous occurrence in congenital cataract *Br J Ophthalmol* 1986; **70**: 593—5

Kelley CG, Keates RH, Lembach RG. Epikeratophakia for pediatric aphakia. *Arch Ophthalmol* 1986; **104**: 680—2

Key SN, Kimura SJ. Iridocyclitis associated with Juvenile rheumatoid arthritis. *Am J Ophthalmol* 1975; **80**: 425—9

Kinoshita JH, Merola LO, Dikmak E. The accumulation of dulcitol and water in rabbit lens incubated with galactose. *Biochem Biophys Acta* 1962; **62**: 176—87

Kloepfer HW, Rosenthal JW. Possible genetic carriers in the spherophakia-brachymorphia syndrome. *Am J Hum Genet* 1975; **7**: 398—420

Kohn BA. A differential diagnosis of cataracts in infants and childhood. *Am J Dis Child* 1976; **130**: 184—91

Kushner BJ. Visual results after surgery for monocular juvenile cataracts of undetermined onset. *Am J Ophthalmol* 1986; **102**: 468—73

Lambert SR, Amaya L, Taylor D. Treatment of infantile cataracts. *Int Ophthalmol Clin* 1989; **29**: 51—6

Lambert SR, Taylor D, Kriss A, Holzel H, Heard S. Ocular features of the congenital varicella syndrome. *Arch Ophthalmol* 1989; **107**: 52—6

Levin AV, Edmonds SA, Nelson LB, Calhoun JH, Harley RD. Extended-wear contact lenses for the treatment of pediatric aphakia. *Ophthalmology* 1988; **95**: 1107—13

Lyford JH, Roy FH. Arrhinencephally Unilateralis, Uveal Coloboma and Lens Reduplication. *Am J Ophthalmol* 1974; **77**: 315—8

Mann I. *The Development of the Human Eye*. Cambridge University Press, Cambridge 1928

Mann I. *Developmental Abnormalities of the Eye*. British Medical Association, London 1957

Maumenee IH. The eye in Marfan syndrome. *Trans Am Ophthalmol Soc* 1981; **79**: 684—733

Maumenee AE, Ryan SJ. Aspiration technique in the management of the dislocated lens. *Am J Ophthalmol* 1969; **68**:

8-08-12

McCormick AQ. Transient cataracts in premature infants: a new clinical entity. *Can J Ophthalmol* 1968; **3**: 302-8

McGavic JS. Marchesani's syndrome. *Am J Ophthalmol* 1959; **47**: 413-20

Merin S, Crawford JS. Etiology of congenital cataracts. *Can J Ophthalmol* 1971; **6**: 178-84

Michalski A, Leonard J, Taylor D. The eye and inherited metabolic disease. *J R Soc Med* 1988; **81**: 286-90

Morgan KS, McDonald MB, Hiles DA *et al*. The nationwide study of epikeratophakia for aphakia in older children. *Ophthalmology* 1988; **95**: 526-31

Mudd SH, Skorby F, Levy HL *et al*. The natural history of homocystinuria due to cystationine-B-synthetase deficiency. *Am J Hum Genet* 1985; **37**: 1-31

Nelson LB, Cutler SI, Calhoun JH. Silsoft extended wear contact lenses in pediatric aphakia. *Ophthalmol* 1985; **92**: 1529-31

Nelson LB, Maumenee IH. Ectopia Lentis. In: Rennie WA (Ed.) *Goldberg's Genetic and Metabolic Eye Diseases*. Little Brown & Co., Boston 1986; pp. 389-410

Parks MM. Visual results in aphakic children. *Am J Ophthalmol* 1982; **94**: 441-9

Perry TL, Hansen S, Love DL, Crawford LE. Treatment of homocystinuria with a low-methionine diet, supplemental cystine and methyl donor. *Lancet* 1968; **2**: 474-8

Peyman GA, Rauchand M, Goldberg MF, Ritacia D. Management of subluxated and dislocated lenses with the vitrophage. *Br J Ophthalmol* 1979; **63**: 771-8

Pratt-Johnson JA, Tillson G. Visual results after removal of congenital cataracts before the age of 1 year. *Can J Ophthalmol* 1981; **16**: 19-21

Pratt-Johnson JA, Tillson G. Hard contact lenses in the management of congenital cataracts. *J Pediatr Ophthalmol Strabismus* 1985; **22**: 94-96

Price FW, Binder PS. Scarring of a recipient cornea following epikeratoplasty. *Arch Ophthalmol* 1987; **105**: 1556-61

Pyeritz RE, McKusick VA. The Marfan syndrome: diagnosis and management. *N Engl J Med* 1979; **300**: 772-7

Ramsey MS, Dickson DH. Lens fringe in homocystinuria. *Br J Ophthalmol* 1975; **59**: 338-42

Rees AB. Persistent hyperplastic primary vitreous. *Am J Ophthalmol* 1955; **40**: 317-28

Reese PD, Tuck-Muller M, Maumenee IH. Autosomal dominant congenital cataract associated with chromosomal translocation. *Arch Ophthalmol* 1987; **105**: 1382-4

Reese PD, Weingeist TA. Pars plana management of ectopia lentis in children. *Arch Ophthalmol* 1987; **105**: 1202-4

Robb R, Luisa MD, Moore B. Results of early treatment of unilateral congenital cataracts *J Pediatr Ophthalmol Strabismus* 1987; **24**: 178-81

Rogers GL, Tishler CL, Tsou BH *et al*. Visual acuities in infants with congenital cataracts operated on prior to 6 months of age. *Arch Ophthalmol* 1981; **99**: 999-1003

Rostron CK. Epikeratophakia: clinical results and experimental development. *Eye* 1988; **2**: 56-63

Salmon JF, Wallis CE, Murray ADN. Variable expressivity of autosomal dominant microcornea with cataract. *Arch Ophthalmol* 1988; **106**: 505-11

Saunders RA, Ellis FD. Empirical fitting of hard contact lenses in infants and young children. *Ophthalmology* 1981; **88**: 127-30

Scheie HG. Aspiration of congenital or soft cataracts: a new tecnique. *Am J Ophthalmol* 1960; **50**: 1048-54

Sietner AA, Crawford JS. Curgical correction of lens dislocation in children. *Am J Ophthalmol* 1981; **91**: 106-10

Seland JH. The lenticular attachment of the zonular apparatus in congenital simple ectopia lentis. *Acta Ophthalmol* 1973; **51**: 520-8

Shih VE, Abrams IF, Johnson IL *et al*. Sulfite oxidase deficiency: biochemical and clinical investigations of a hereditary metabolic disorder in sulfur metabolism. *N Engl J Med* 1977; **297**: 1022-8

Shih VE, Efron ML. Pyridoxine-unresponsive homocystinuria. *N Engl J Med* 1970; **283**: 1206-7

Smolin LA, Benerenga NJ, Berlow S. The use of betaine for the treatment of homocystinuria. *J Pediatr* 1981; **99**: 467-72

Streeten BW, Robinson MR, Wallace R, Jones DB. Lens capsule abnormalities in Alport's syndrome. *Arch Ophthalmol* 1987; **105**: 1693-7

Synnove C, Hyvarinen L, Avitti R. Persistent behavioural blindness after early visual deprivation and active visual rehabilitation: a case report. *Br J Ophthalmol* 1986; **70**: 607-11

Taylor D. Choice of surgical technique in management of congenital cataracts. *Trans Ophthalmol Soc UK* 1981; **101**: 114-8

Taylor D, Vaegan, Morris JA, Rogers JE, Warland J. Amblyopia in bilateral infantile and juvenile cataract. Relationship to timing of treatment. *Trans Ophthalmol Soc UK* 1979; **99**: 170-5

Thompson SM, Deady JP, Willshaw HE, White RH. Ocular signs in Alport's syndrome. *Eye* 1987; **0**: 146-53

Townes PL. Ectopia lentis et pupillae. *Arch Ophthalmol* 1976; **94**: 1126-8

Toyofuku H, Hirose T, Schepens CL. Retinal detachment following congenital cataract surgery. *Arch Ophthalmol* 1980; **98**: 669-75

Tripathi RC, Cibis GW, Tripathi BJ. Pathogenesis of cataracts in patients with Lowe's syndrome. *Ophthalmology* 1986; **93**: 1046-52

Vaegen, Taylor D. Critical period for deprivation amblyopia in children. *Trans Ophthalmol Soc UK* 1979; **99**: 432-9

Wallis & Murray 1988

Willi M, Kut L, Cotlier E. Pupillary-block glaucoma in the Marchesani syndrome. *Arch Ophthalmol* 1973; **90**: 504-8

Wilson JR, Fernandes A, Chandler CV, Tigges M, Boothe R, Gammon JA. Abnormal development of the axial length of aphakic monkey eyes. *Int Ophthalmol Vis Sci* 1987; **28**: 2096-9

Yamamoto Y, Hayasaka S, Setogawa T. Family with aniridia, microcornea, and spontaneously reabsorbed cataract. *Arch Ophthalmol* 1988; **106**: 502-5

25 Childhood Glaucoma

CREIG HOYT AND SCOTT LAMBERT

Childhood glaucoma differs in several important respects from most cases of glaucoma seen in adults.

First, children with glaucoma are often unwell. Secondly, they frequently have coexistent systemic abnormalities. An appreciation of these systemic abnormalities is invaluable in understanding the treatment and prognosis of a child's glaucoma. Finally the mechanism of glaucoma in childhood is often quite different from that seen in older patients. The ophthalmologist needs to work closely with a paediatrician in diagnosing and caring for these patients.

In children with glaucoma, physical signs and symptoms are usually present which suggest the diagnosis. These signs and symptoms vary according to the age of the child and the abruptness and severity of the intraocular pressure elevation (Shaffer 1967). During infancy, but especially in the newborn, corneal changes are often the primary sign of glaucoma. Corneal enlargement and opacification (Fig. 25.1), photophobia and epiphora (Fig. 25.2) commonly accompanies these findings and may be gradual or sudden in onset.

Older children more often present with the loss of vision or symptoms of pain and vomiting related to abrupt intraocular pressure elevation. Though glaucoma may be suspected, by recognizing the appropriate signs and symptoms indicative of childhood glaucoma, the diagnosis remains unproven until an elevation of intraocular pressure is established, or there

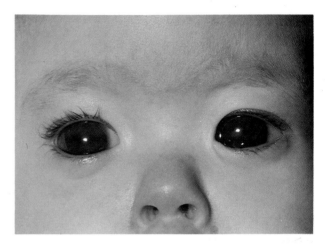

Fig. 25.1 Bilateral buphthalmos. The parents had noticed both eyes watering and photophobia so marked that they did not even take her outdoors on a cloudy day.

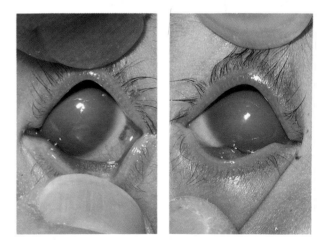

Fig. 25.2 Bilateral severe buphthalmos in a neonate with enlarged 'steamy' corneas.

is clear evidence from a combination of clinical signs that the pressure is raised intermittently; for instance corneal enlargement, worsening of splits in Descemet's membrane (Fig. 25.3, 25.5), increase in corneal asymmetry (Fig. 25.4), increase in the size of optic

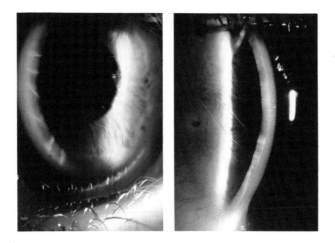

Fig. 25.3 Splits in Descemet's membrane have corneal oedema at their edges for many months giving linear opacities which are present even when the intraocular pressure is controlled.

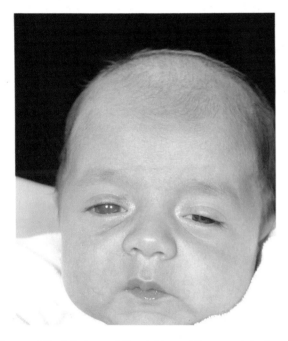

Fig. 25.4 Buphthalmos of the right eye. The parents had thought the left eye was small.

disc cup or in older children, visual field changes. The normal range of intraocular pressure in childhood is approximately that of the normal adult, with pressures rarely in excess of 20 mmHg.

Classification

An attempt to subdivide childhood glaucomas according to the mechanisms responsible for the elevation in intraocular pressure is useful (Hoskins 1984).

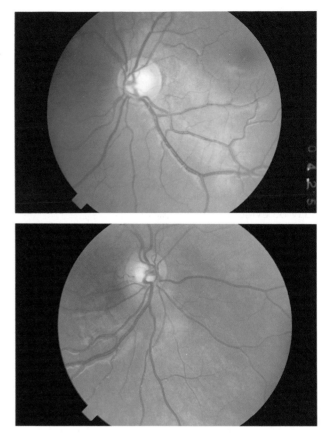

Fig. 25.5 Cupped discs in congenital glaucoma, more marked in the left eye, treated successfully in infancy. Visual function was normal in the right eye but the left eye had slightly reduced acuity, and suppression indicating that the eye is amblyopic.

A primary glaucoma is one considered to be caused by an intrinsic disorder of the aqueous outflow mechanism. A secondary glaucoma is one caused by disease processes in other regions of the eye and body. Both primary and secondary paediatric glaucoma disorders may be associated with important systemic conditions that need to be specifically identified.

Primary congenital glaucoma

This is the most common form of glaucoma in children. It is most often recognized during the first year of life, although cases may occasionally present later in childhood. The underlying disorder is present at birth, but the clinical signs and symptoms may be variable in their presentation (Morin *et al.* 1974); thus, when mild, recognition may be delayed. In most cases, corneal opacification and enlargement will be accompanied by photophobia. Although the term buphthalmos has often been used in association with this condition, enlargement of the globe may occur in other glaucomatous disorders in childhood, as well as in congenital megalocornea without glaucoma. Moreover, corneal opacification may not always be secondary to intraocular pressure elevation in childhood. A number of disorders may present with corneal opacification without any evidence of glaucoma. Posterior polymorphous corneal dystrophy may be especially difficult to distinguish from congenital glaucoma (Cibis *et al.* 1977). This entity is an autosomal dominant condition that is characterized by bilateral defects of the cornea at the level of Descemet's membrane. Rarely a severe expression of this disease may be evident in infancy with corneal opacification secondary to oedema of the stroma and epithelium. In some instances, glaucoma may coexist with polymorphous corneal dystrophy. Other causes of opacification of the infants cornea include rubella embryopathy, congenital hereditary endothelial dystrophy, sclerocornea and anterior segment dysplasia (See Chapter 20.2).

Although primary congenital glaucoma has been previously described as a hereditary condition, usually thought to be due to an autosomal recessive trait, more recent epidemiologic data suggests that the pattern of inheritance is more likely to be polygenic or multifactorial (Merin 1972) at least in its behaviour in North America. In certain countries, most notably in the Middle East the autosomal recessive nature is more clear and it is striking how the nature of the disease appears to differ.

Although the intraocular pressure can usually be adequately controlled in primary congenital glaucoma there is often a residual visual defect. The earlier the onset of glaucoma the poorer the visual prognosis. Less than one third of all eyes with the diagnosis of primary congenital glaucoma will achieve 20/50 or better visual acuity. This decreased visual function occurs secondary to optic nerve damage, corneal opacification and scarring, cataracts and amblyopia. The problem of anisometropic and strabismic amblyopia is especially important in the rehabilitation of monocular congenital glaucoma.

Most eyes having primary congenital open angle glaucoma show abnormalities on gonioscopic examination (Fig. 25.7). Persistence of aberrant mesodermal tissue in and around the chamber angle has been described with various other anomalies of the trabecular meshwork. In the angle the uveal meshwork that sweeps forward from the periphery of the iris towards Schwalbe's line appears to be less well defined and homogenous than in the normal eye. Histologic examination of affected eyes has shown obliteration

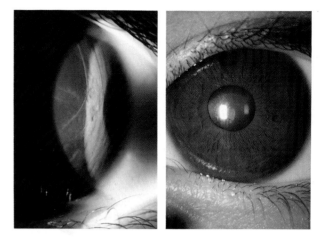

Fig. 25.6 Splits in Descemet's membrane

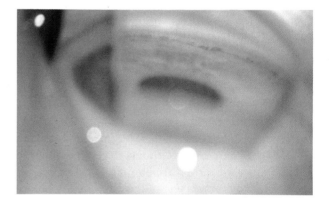

Fig. 25.7 Goniophotograph in primary congenital glaucoma. Schwalbe's line is barely visible anterior to the grey band of the iris insertion posterior to which pigment knuckles project anteriorly from the iris root through bands of fine tissue extending from the anterior iris surface — 'Barkan's membrane'.

or absence of Schlemm's canal. The periphery of the iris in primary congenital glaucoma frequently shows abnormalities. The stroma may be abnormally thin. In approximately 50% of cases, a forward tenting of the portion of the iris to which the uveal meshwork is attached is noted. Usually, neither the iris nor its blood vessels are attached far enough anteriorly to obscure the ciliary band or scleral spur. A number of different aberrations of angle development probably account for the development of primary congenital glaucoma. The severity and pathological mechanisms of this disorder depends in part on how early in embryogenesis the normal angle development is interrupted.

Anterior segment dysgenesis

A number of congenital disorders present with the malformations of the anterior segment of the eye, usually involving the cornea, angle, iris and lens. Glaucoma may occur in some of these disorders as the result of congenital abnormalities of the angle and surrounding structures. These disorders may conveniently be divided into those with peripheral anterior segment anomalies and those with primarily central abnormalities (Waring *et al.* 1975).

The term posterior embryotoxon is used to describe an abnormal thickening of Schwalbe's line at the peripheral termination of Descemet's membrane. In some patients, this is an isolated abnormality without any functional implication, while in others there are associated abnormalities commonly associated with glaucoma (Waring *et al.* 1975). Axenfeld's anomaly is a condition in which the filtration angle is obscured from view by attachments between the iris and a prominent Schwalbe's ring (posterior embryotoxon). The trabeculum may be intermittently visible through these attachments and may be either normal or abnormal in appearance. Glaucoma frequently occurs in such eyes. In Rieger's anomaly similar abnormalities of the chamber angle are noted, but in addition hypoplasia of the anterior iris stroma occurs resulting in pupillary abnormalities (Zauberman 1970).

Systemic abnormalities are most frequently associated with Rieger's anomaly (Fig. 25.8) (Zauberman 1970). Commonly associated systemic abnormalities include maxillary hypoplasia, telecanthus with a broad flat nasal root, dental abnormalities, such as microdontia or anodontia, and umbilical hernia. Less commonly, visceral defects such as congenital heart anomalies, middle ear deafness, mental retardation, and cerebellar vermis hypoplasia may occur. The constellation of anterior segment and systemic abnormalities is dominantly inherited and referred to as Rieger's syndrome. There can be considerable variation in expression of the anterior segment abnormalities in a single family. Glaucoma often does not begin until later in childhood, necessitating careful, periodical examinations, even if the intraocular pressure is initially normal.

Peter's anomaly (Fig. 25.9) represents a variation of the anterior chamber cleavage syndrome which is primarily, although not exclusively, central in location (Waring *et al.* 1975). This anomaly consists of a posterior defect in Descemet's membrane associated with a leukoma that frequently has direct attachment to the iris. These iris adhesions usually occur at the margin

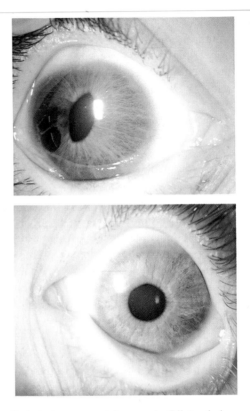

Fig. 25.8 Anterior segment dysgenesis. Bilateral glaucoma in Rieger's anomaly more marked in the left eye.

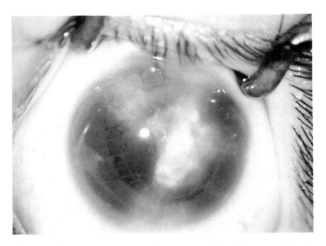

Fig. 25.9 Anterior segment dysgenesis with glaucoma (Peter's anomaly) corneal opacities to the posterior surface of which are attached iris strands. There is a cataract hidden by the corneal opacities.

of the leukoma. A variety of lens abnormalities may occur in Peter's anomaly. These include adhesions of lens cortex to the corneal stroma at the site of the posterior defect, as well as displacement of the lens into the anterior chamber or a central cataract with a normal lens position. Patients with Peter's anomaly and lens abnormalities may also have microphthalmia with vitreoretinal disorganization. Glaucoma may occur in Peter's anomaly as the result of defective development of the angle.

Children with anterior segment dysgenesis syndromes require life-long follow-up, and the prognosis should be guarded (Fig. 25.10).

Glaucoma is a complication in a large proportion of patients with aniridia (See Chapter 23).

A rare but important condition is glaucoma associated with iridotrabecular dysgenesis and ectropion uveae (Fig. 25.11). They have a widespread ocular defect with iris hypoplasia, ectropion uveae and anterior insertion of the iris root on gonioscopy. It is usually unilateral and not associated with systemic disorders. Response to goniotomy is not good (Dowling 1985) but most do well with trabeculectomy.

Paediatric syndromes

Lowe's syndrome, or oculocerebrorenal syndrome is a rare type of congenital glaucoma inherited as an X-linked recessive trait (Lowe 1952). Affected males may develop cataracts, glaucoma, psychomotor retardation, aminoaciduria, and acidosis in infancy. The female carrier state may be recognized by multiple fine punctate lens opacities. Almost all affected males develop congenital cataracts, while the glaucoma is more variable. Investigators attribute the glaucoma to incomplete angle cleavage. Pathologically, the iris

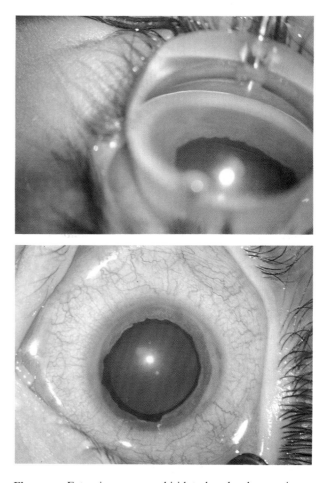

Fig. 25.11 Ectropion uveae and iridotrabecular dysgenesis. The hallmark of these unilateral cases is ectropian uveae (b) with a variable amount of pigment showing at the pupil margin. The anterior chamber angle (a) is abnormal with an anteriorly inserted iris root.

may extend onto the trabecular meshwork and the lens is commonly small (Curtin et al. 1967). Gonioscopy usually reveals an angle which resembles that of primary congenital glaucoma.

The Sturge–Weber syndrome (Fig. 25.12) is a cutaneous haemangiomatous disorder involving the distribution of the Vth cranial nerve and is usually, but not invariably, unilateral. A haemangioma may involve the upper lid as well as other portions of the body, including the leptomeninges. When intracranial involvement occurs, epilepsy, visual field defects, and motor paralysis may occur. Computerized tomography of patients with intracranial involvement frequently shows calcification of the involved areas. Plain X-rays may also show characteristic linear calcification. The glaucoma accompanying this syndrome is unilateral unless the cutaneous haemangiomatous malformation crosses the midline of the face. Increased conjunctival

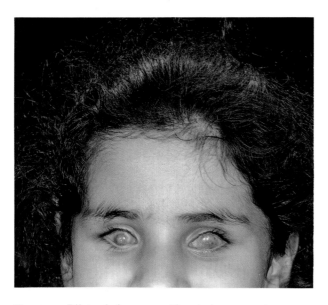

Fig. 25.10 Bilateral glaucoma with anterior segment dysgenesis.

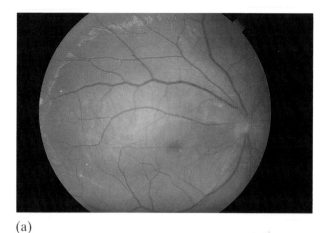

(a)

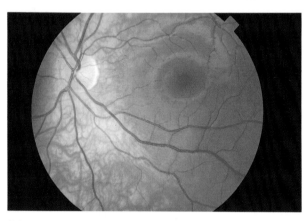

(b)

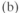

Fig. 25.12 Sturge–Weber syndrome, the right eye (a) shows the choroidal angioma (tomato ketchup fundus) with a homogenous appearance compared with normal left eye (b).

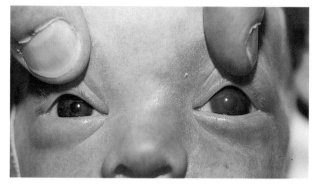

(a)

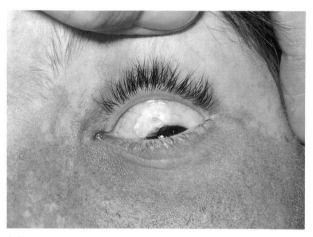

(b)

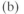

Fig. 25.13 (a) Sturge–Weber syndrome with ipsilateral glaucoma. (b) Same patient aged 13 years. Filtration surgery carried out at 2 years. The conjunctiva, tenons, and sclera are very vascular and the surgical prognosis should be guarded.

vascularity is not a reliable indicator of the coexistence of glaucoma, however, inspection of the conjunctiva may show an increase in the number and tortuosity of blood vessels. The glaucoma may be congenital or acquired in its presentation. Most cases with glaucoma are probably secondary to an attendant angle anomaly (Phelps 1978). Gonioscopy may reveal minor angle abnormalities. Other ocular anomalies that may co-exist include heterochromia, choroidal haemangioma, and abnormal retinal vessels. External fistulizing operations may be complicated by large choroidal effusions and expulsive choroidal haemorrhages (Fig. 25.13).

Neurofibromatosis is a neurocutaneous disorder inherited as an autosomal dominant trait. The main features include café-au-lait spots involving the skin, and tumours of the central nervous system. It may be associated with glaucoma. It is usually unilateral and most often accompanied by an ipsilateral plexiform neuroma involving the upper lid (Fig. 25.14). Facial

hemihypertrophy may also coexist. Enlargement of the involved eye may be grotesque and the marked accelerated growth of these eyes suggest that more than intraocular pressure elevation accounts for this abnormal growth (Hoyt *et al.* 1977). Large areas of deeply pigmented iris surface often extend into the angle and Lisch nodules may be seen on the lids (See Chapter 22.5 and 23). On gonioscopy the iris usually has a high flat insertion, especially in the areas of pigmentation (Grant & Walton 1968). The glaucoma associated with this syndrome may be secondary to abnormal angle development or infiltration of tumour tissue into the trabecular meshwork.

Glaucoma has been identified in some patients with Rubenstein–Taybi syndrome. This syndrome is characterized by mental and motor retardation, broad thumbs and toes (Fig. 25.14b), and an anti-mongoloid slant of the palpebral fissures. Bony anomalies may

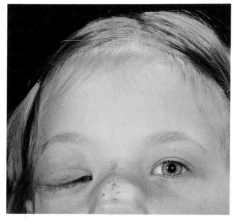

(a)

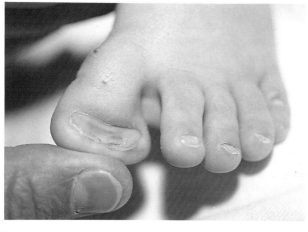

(b)

Fig. 25.14 (a) Neurofibromatosis with plexiform neuroma of the lid and glaucoma. (b) Rubenstein–Taybi syndrome. Broad thumbs and toes are a characteristic feature. See text.

include a high-arched palate and short stature. It's inheritance may be multifactorial. The most common ocular features are the downward slant of the palpebral fissure, strabismus (usually exotropia) and epicanthal folds (Roy *et al.* 1968). Less frequent manifestations include ptosis, cataract, glaucoma, and refractive error.

The Pierre Robin syndrome, which consists of hypoplasia of the mandible, glossoptosis, and usually cleft palate, may occasionally be associated with congenital glaucoma. Common ocular complications include high myopia, cataract, retinal detachment, and microphthalmos (Cosman & Keyser 1974). It would appear that many cases that were described in the past as Pierre Robin syndrome really represented unrecognized Stickler's syndrome (progressive arthroophthalmopathy). It is imperative that these two

syndromes be distinguished from each other since Stickler's syndrome has a serious vitreoretinal disorder associated with it and is inherited as an autosomal dominant with a high degree of penetrance, in contrast to Pierre Robin anomaly that occurs sporadically.

The naevus of Ota is a benign unilateral melanosis of the skin involving the area innervated by the ophthalmic and maxillary divisions of the Vth cranial nerve. It is characterized by irregular pigmentation of the episclera and uveal tract on the involved side, and may extend to the optic disc. It is usually apparent in infancy but occasionally presents later in childhood. Glaucomatous involvement of the affected eye has infrequently been reported.

Trisomy 13 (the Patau syndrome) may have multiple ocular abnormalities; indeed the ocular abnormalities are a cardinal feature of the syndrome (Keith 1966). They include microphthalmia and anophthalmia as well as colobomas, cataracts, corneal opacities, intraocular or epibulbar cartilage, retinal dysplasia, optic atrophy, and defective angle development resulting in glaucoma. Systemic anomalies seen in this syndrome include cardiovascular malformation, polycystic renal cortex, biseptate uterus in females, undescended testes and abnormal insertion of phallus in males, polydactyly of hands and feet, hyperconvex nails, capillary cutaneous defects, and cutaneous scalp defects. The central nervous system is commonly affected. There may be absence of the rhinencephalon, union of ventricles and thalami, and defects of the corpus callosum. Most children with trisomy 13 die before their first birthday. Other associations include trisomy 21 (Traboulsi *et al.* 1988) and cutis marmorata (Sato *et al.* 1988).

Secondary glaucoma

The most important glaucoma in children associated with ocular injury is that caused by an acute or secondary haemorrhage into the anterior chamber (hyphaema). This may occur acutely in association with blunt injury to the eye, and in these patients permanent structural damage to the angle structures may predispose the eye to chronic glaucoma (Spaeth 1967). Children with trauma to the eye should be examined promptly for evidence of serious intraocular injury.

Glaucoma in infants may result from intraocular tumour compromising the angle structures. The most common intraocular tumour causing glaucoma in children is retinoblastoma. The glaucoma is usually secondary to rubeosis iridis and angle closure. These eyes almost invariably show advanced tumour growth within the posterior segment.

Juvenile xanthogranuloma (Fig. 25.15) is an uncommon benign skin disease with its onset in infancy that slowly resolves over a period of years. It is characterized by widespread crops of yellow–orange skin nodules. Ocular involvement includes vascularized lesions in the iris and ciliary body as well as occasional epibulbar masses (Zeuman 1965). A salmon-coloured or yellowish thickening of the iris or angle with vascularization is seen and spontaneous hyphaema may occur. Glaucoma in this syndrome may be secondary to the accumulation of histiocytes within the angle structure, or to spontaneous hyphaema (see Chapter 22.4).

Retrolental fibroplasia may be complicated by glaucoma. Typically these eyes show advanced retinal abnormalities in a cicatricial phase, and possess variable amounts of equatorial, perilenticular, and retrolenticular membrane formation. The corneas are often small and steep. The lenses are usually not cataractous. The onset of glaucoma may be acute with extreme pain in the eye accompanied by nausea and vomiting. Other children may present with less acute symptoms consisting of eye rubbing, photophobia, and tearing. Most authorities attribute glaucoma in this circumstance to the embarrassment of aqueous flow between the lens and iris from the posterior chamber to the anterior chamber. Thus, this represents a form of pupillary block glaucoma that is either precipitated by an increase in lens diameter or movement forward of the lens secondary to the retrolental membrane. The diagnosis may be overlooked in visually impaired infants with retrolental fibroplasia in whom eye rubbing has been attributed to visual impairment alone. Removal of the lens or performance of a peripheral

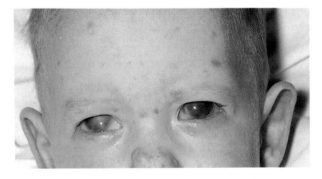

Fig. 25.15 Bilateral juvenile xanthogranuloma. Repeated haemorrhages gave rise to intractable glaucoma. Low dose radiotherapy usually brings about a rapid resolution of the condition.

iridectomy may be effective. Topical steroid therapy has been advocated by some authorities.

Children with ectopia lentis may develop acute glaucoma as the result of pupillary block. This is caused by the anterior movement of the lens into the pupillary aperture obstructing the normal posterior to anterior flow of aqueous humour (Rodman 1963). The glaucoma is usually acute and painful and often associated with vomiting and markedly elevated intraocular pressures. Ectopia lentis occurs most commonly with Marfan's syndrome, an autosomal dominant disorder with variable expressivity. The cardinal features of the syndrome are muscular, cardiovascular, and ocular. Affected patients are usually tall with lax joints and progressive degenerative changes in the walls of the aorta and pulmonary arteries may lead to fatal haemorrhaging. Ocular findings include ectopia lentis, myopia, retinal detachment, and glaucoma. The glaucoma may be secondary to mesodermal abnormalities of the angle or ectopia lentis with secondary angle closure.

Homocystinuria is an inherited metabolic disorder characterized by osteoporosis, arterial venous thrombosis, and mental retardation. Ocular involvement includes spherophakia, retinal detachment, myopia, and ectopia lentis (Presley et al. 1969). Pupil block glaucoma which is more common in this syndrome than in Marfan's syndrome, may occur from the combined effects of the spherophakia and ectopia lentis. Weill–Marchesani syndrome is another disorder in which ectopia lentis may occur. Typically these patients are short and have short hands and fingers. The primary ocular abnormality is spherophakia that may be so marked that the reduced lens diameter may be apparent even through a mid-dilated pupil. High myopia is usually present. Pupillary block and angle closure glaucoma may occur in this syndrome as the result of the spherophakia alone, or in combination with subluxation of the lens.

Treatment of the acute glaucoma secondary to ectopia lentis should be prompt with repositioning of the lens. This may be accomplished with intense mydriasis lying the child on his back and sometimes by indenting the cornea with a squint hook to push the lens back behind the pupil. The subsequent use of miotics and head elevation may be helpful in preventing redisplacement of the lens into the pupil. Iridectomy may be done at a later time to prevent pupillary block, but alone it will not prevent subsequent displacement of the lens into the anterior chamber, and surgical lens removal may be more appropriate.

Acute or chronic glaucoma in children may occur secondary to intraocular inflammation. When acute, the blockage of the aqueous outflow is usually secondary to iris bombé formation and angle closure. Chronic glaucoma secondary to inflammation is more common than the acute form and may be asymptomatic. It is frequently associated with chronic anterior uveitis, especially that accompanying juvenile rheumatoid arthritis (Still's disease) or pars planitis. Peripheral anterior synechia are usually seen on examination of the anterior segment. When evaluating a child with a known uveitis syndrome and glaucoma, the possibility that chronic steroid therapy may have played a role in the precipitation of this glaucoma should be considered. Approximately 4–6% of patients with normal intraocular pressure and no family history of glaucoma can be expected to develop significantly raised intraocular pressure if challenged with 0.1% Dexamethasone drops four times a day for 4–6 weeks (Armaly 1967). The percentage of responders will increase with continued therapy. In some situations it may be appropriate to challenge the uninvolved eye with topical steroids to distinguish between glaucoma secondary to uveitis and that resulting from chronic steroid therapy. Treatment of acute glaucoma associated with iris bombé requires either a laser iridotomy or a surgical iridectomy.

Pigmentary glaucoma may occur in childhood. This form of glaucoma is characterized by elevated intraocular pressure, pigmentary deposit is on the corneal endotheliums in the form of a Krukenberg's spindle, iris atrophy of the pigment epithelium, and signs of pigment dispersion throughout the anterior chamber. This condition generally occurs in young myopic males and is diagnosed on routine ocular examination at the time of evaluation of the refractive error. Levels of intraocular pressure in this syndrome may become quite high and may lead to corneal oedema. Careful evaluation of all children with myopia for signs of pigmentary glaucoma is essential.

Secondary glaucoma may occur in children after successful cataract surgery (Fig. 25.16). This glaucoma may be secondary to the complications of cataract surgery rather than a primary associated defect, but glaucoma may occur after uncomplicated surgery. Children with Lowe's syndrome and the rubella syndrome who frequently require lensectomies, also may have a primary glaucoma. Microphthalmos is a common finding in the congenital rubella syndrome and early corneal enlargement with glaucoma may be unappreciated. The glaucoma that occurs in association with rubella appears to be the result of direct inter-

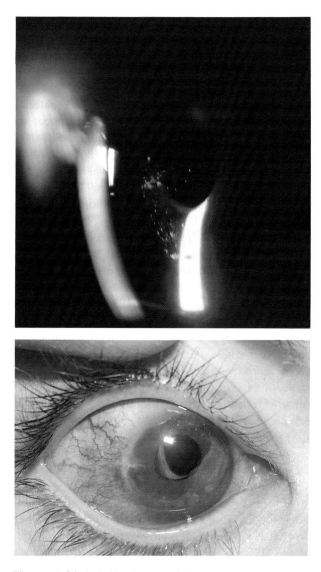

Fig. 25.16 (a) Aphakic glaucoma following lens aspiration in infancy. Vitreous can be seen filling the pupil and covering the anterior surface of the iris (a). Vitrectomy brought about long-term resolution of the condition — the vitreous was adherent to the anterior iris leaf and 'bite' marks can be seen on the iris where the vitrectomy machine cut the anterior leaf.

ference with normal angle development (Weiss *et al.* 1966). To add to the diagnostic difficulty in rubella babies there may be a transient keratopathy with oedema unrelated to glaucoma.

Pupillary block caused by adherence of the iris to residual lens capsule is a frequent cause of glaucoma; this blockage causes closure of the angle and permits peripheral anterior synechiae to form. The possibility of this complication occurring in children undergoing cataract surgery should be considered to be an es-

the patient under 1 year of age or corneal measurements of 13 mm or more at any time in childhood should be strongly suggestive that glaucoma is present (Morin 1980). A difference in diameter of the two corneas is especially noteworthy and usually indicates glaucoma in the larger eye. One should recall that corneal enlargement may have taken place without exceeding the above guidelines.

If the cornea is clear enough to permit it, gonioscopy may provide important additional diagnostic information. We prefer to use a Koeppe glass gonioscopy lens, hand held binocular microscope and a hand held Barkan focal illuminator. We perform gonioscopy with a pair of gonioscopy lenses in order that a direct comparison between the two eyes may be made during this examination. Gonioscopy findings in infants and young children differ significantly from those of adults. The feature of the angle that differs most is the uveal meshwork. In general, the infant's trabecular meshwork appears more translucent than the adult's. Although iris processes may be present, they seldom reach the trabecular meshwork. Most infants have very faintly pigmented iris processes. The angle recess and ciliary body are not a visible in children as they are in adults. A number of abnormal gonioscopic findings occur in different glaucoma syndromes in childhood (Hoskins et al. 1984). These may include (a) iris attachment posterior to the scleral spur appearing indistinctly behind translucent uveal meshwork; (b) iris attachment of the trabecular meshwork anterior to the scleral spur; (c) absence of most iris tissue except for peripheral rim which is attached either posterior or anterior to the scleral spur; (d) the iris and pupil are normal but Schwalbe's line is grossly abnormal and anteriorly displaced; and (e) the iris is congenitally attached to the cornea with progressive atrophic changes in the iris with pupillary distortion occurring.

Evaluation of the appearance of the optic nerve by ophthalmoscopy is an essential feature of the assessment of the glaucoma suspect. This is usually best accomplished using a direct ophthalmoscope. When the cornea is oedematous or has slight residual clouding from previous attacks of oedema, one may be unable to see the details of the fundus by direct ophthalmoscopy but often a great improvement in clarity of view can be obtained by using the indirect ophthalmoscope or by viewing with the direct ophthalmoscope through the Koeppe gonioscope lens after this has been put in place for gonioscopy. This eliminates the optically poor interface between the air and the surface of the cornea, and provides a much clearer view of the fundus details in some cases. The optic nerve may appear slightly more pale in normal infants than it does in adults. In most normal children, there is seldom any apparent central cup in the optic nerve.

Central disc cupping occurs readily and dramatically in infantile glaucoma. However, if the glaucoma is successfully controlled, and the disc is not atrophic, a decrease in cupping may readily occur. Diffuse thinning of the nerve fibre layer and optic nerve atrophy indicate irreparable damage to the optic nerve and permanent visual loss.

SURGICAL OPTIONS

Although some authorities have suggested that goniotomy is the surgical option of choice in the treatment of primary congenital glaucoma, several studies suggest that trabeculotomy is equally effective. The use of goniotomy in the treatment of primary congenital glaucoma dates back to the work of Barkan (1942). In this procedure, an attempt is made to increase filtration at the angle by surgically incising the tissue between the anterior chamber and Schlemm's canal. This is done under direct visualization using an operating microscope and goniolens. The results of goniotomy surgery are best in patients with minimal changes of the angle, a relatively clear cornea, and early treatment (Hoskins et al. 1984). In contrast, newborn patients with glaucoma who have marked enlargement and clouding of the cornea and severe angle anomalies, have a poorer outcome with goniotomy surgery.

Trabeculotomy is utilized by some authorities as the primary procedure in the treatment of primary congenital glaucoma, as well as the procedure of choice when goniotomies have failed to control the intraocular pressure (Quigley 1982). The procedure can be carried out even in the presence of severe corneal opacities since it consists of a slitting open of the trabeculum by external approach. Performance of a trabeculectomy may be indicated in some cases of glaucoma in childhood; although permanent filtration is extremely difficult to achieve in children it may be aided by the use of postoperative 5-fluro-uracil to reduce fistula closure (Ruderman et al. 1987). Full thickness fistulizing procedures also lead to the formation of a staphyloma.

Recently, the use of implanted tube or valve systems have produced promising results in surgical treating infantile glaucoma. The procedure provides direct drainage of the aqueous humor from the eye into the subconjunctival space via the appliance (Hitchings et al. 1987).

Cyclocryotherapy or cyclophotoablation may be helpful in extreme cases of uncontrolled intraocular pressure in childhood where previous uncontrolled intraocular pressure have failed. This procedure involves freezing or lasering the ciliary processes, thereby injuring the ciliary epithelium and decreasing aqueous formation. It has the disadvantage of causing subconjunctival scarring which makes subsequent surgery more difficult.

Surgical removal of the lens is the procedure of choice in some forms of childhood glaucoma. Lens removal is indicated in children with pupillary block associated with persistent hyperplastic primary vitreous and retrolental fibroplasia, as well as some cases when the lens is dislocated. Surgical removal with the newer closed eye vitrectomy techniques offer significant advantages over the techniques involving direct aspiration of the lens.

Glaucoma associated with chronic uveitis is best treated medically, taking care to reduce topical steroid use as much as possible. Surgery by conventional filtration techniques or by trabeculodialysis may be necessary. Trabeculodialysis is performed using a goniotomy knife passed in the usual way across the anterior chamber under direct vision; the anterior synechiae are retracted and an incision made just posterior to Schwalbe's line and the trabeculum is retracted (Kanski & McAllister 1985).

MEDICAL TREATMENT

Though chronic medical therapy is seldom effective in the management of primary congenital glaucoma, there may be circumstances in which various forms of medical therapy are indicated during preparation for surgical treatment, or as an adjunct following surgical procedures. If medical treatment is indicated, miotics, adrenergic agents and carbonic anhydrase agents may be used. The most widely used of these is carbonic anhydrase inhibitor, Acetazolamide, in a dose of 15 mm/kg per day by mouth. Secondary metabolic acidosis may be associated with this form of therapy and may require supplemental sodium bicarbonate. Mitotics such as pilocarpine are often poorly tolerated by children and are generally ineffective in the control of intraocular pressure unless there has been previous surgical correction of an angle defect. Timolol has proven to be frequently efficacious in treating children with glaucoma but has several serious side effects. The most common side effects are bronchospasm and bradycardia. When timolol is used the child's paediatrician should be informed of the possible relationship between this form of therapy and upper respiratory ailments. Several beta-selective adrenergic blocking agents are now available which may have fewer systemic effects.

A major obstacle in the visual rehabilitation of children with glaucoma is amblyopia. Early identification of strabismic and anisometropic amblyopia is imperative to the successful rehabilitation of these patients. Routine retinoscopy should be carried out in order to identify refractive errors that may be important in the visual disability of these children. Spectacle correction should be initiated in these children as soon as they are walking. If the child is predisposed to amblyopia, occlusion therapy should be initiated as soon as possible, sometimes even before successful intraocular pressure control has been achieved. Regrettably a significant proportion of children with glaucoma will be left permanently visually impaired at a level that may require low vision aids. Periodic evaluation of these children by a specialist in this field should be included in the protocol for treatment of these children.

GENETIC ADVICE

Accurate and precise diagnosis of the aetiology of glaucoma in childhood is necessary before specific genetic advice may be given (Demenais *et al.* 1979). In the case of primary congenital glaucoma, this disorder appears to be one inherited in a multifactorial manner. Merin and Morin (1972) have estimated that the risk of a subsequent sibling having primary congenital glaucoma is about 1 in 20 and that a similar risk applies to the likelihood that an affected parent may have an affected child. In cases with consanguineous parents an autosomal recessive inheritance is likely with a 1 in 4 recurrence rate. In contrast, several childhood disorders associated with glaucoma are inherited as autosomal dominant disorders with a 50% recurrence risk. These disorders include aniridia, neurofibromatosis, and Rieger's syndrome. Autosomal recessive inheritance occurs in the Weill–Marchesani syndrome and homocystinuria. Lowe's syndrome is inherited as a sex-linked recessive trait. Appropriate detailed genetic counselling and prediction of risk for subsequent siblings to develop glaucoma may be given in these circumstances.

References

Armaly MS. Inheritance of dexamethasone suppression and glaucoma. *Arch Ophthalmol* 1967; **77**: 747–51

Barkan O. Operation of congenital glaucoma. *Am J Ophthalmol* 1942; **25**: 552−6

Chrousos G, Parks MM, O'Neill JF. Incidence of chronic glaucoma, retinal detachment and secondary membrane surgery in pediatric aphakic patients. *Ophthalmology* 1985; **92**: 856−61

Cibis GW, Kratchmer JH, Phelps CD, Weingeist TE. The clinical spectrum of posterior polymorphous dystrophy. *Arch Ophthalmol* 1977; **95**: 1529−33

Cosmon B, Keyser JJ. Eye abnormalities and skeletal defects in the Pierre Robin syndrome: A balanced evaluation. *Cleft Palate J* 1974; **11**: 404−11

Curtin VT, Joyce EE, Balan N. Ocular pathology in the oculocerebral renal syndrome of Lowe. *Am J Ophthalmol* 1967; **64**: 533−7

Dear G De L, Hammerton M, Hatch DJ, Taylor D. Anaesthesia and intraocular pressure in young children. *Anaesthesia* 1987; **42**: 259−65

Demenais F, Bonatic C, Briard M. Congenital glaucoma: Genetic models. *Human Genetics* 1979; **46**: 205−314

Dowling JL Jr. Primary glaucoma associated with iridotrabecular dysgenesis and ectroplon uveae. *Ophthalmology* 1985; **92**: 912−21

Grant WM, Walton DS. Distinctive gonioscopic findings in glaucoma due to neurofibromatosis. *Arch Ophthalmol* 1968; **79**: 127−34

Hitchings RA, Joseph NH, Sherwood MB, Lattimer J, Miller M. Use of one-piece valved tube and variable surface area explant for glaucoma drainage surgery. *Ophthalmology* 1987; **94**: 1079−84

Hoskins HD, Shaffer RN, Hetherington J. Anatomical classification of development glaucomas. *Arch Ophthalmol* 1984; **102**: 1331−4

Hoskins HD, Shaffer RN, Hetherington J. Goniotomy vs trabeculectomy. *J Pediatr Ophthalmol Strabismus* 1984; **21**: 153−7

Hoyt CS, Billson FA. Buphthalmos in neurofibromatosis: is it an expression of regional giantism? *J Pediatr Ophthalmol Strabismus* 1977; **14**: 228−32

Kanski JJ, McAllister JA. Trabeculodialysis for inflammatory glaucoma in children and young adults. *Ophthalmology* 1985; **92**: 927−30

Keith CG. The ocular manifestations of trisomy 13−15. *Trans Ophthalmol Soc UK* 1966; **86**: 435−9

Lowe CU, Terrey M, MacLachlan EA. Organicaciduria, decreased renal ammonia production, hydrophthalmos, and mental retardation: A clinical entity. *Am J Dis Child* 1952; **83**: 164−7

Merin S, Morin JD. Heredity of congenital glaucoma. *Br J Ophthalmol* 1972; **56**: 414−7

Morin JD, Coughlin WR. Corneal changes in primary congenital glaucoma. *Trans Am Ophthalmol Soc* 1980; **78**: 123−31

Morin JD, Merin S, Sheppard RW. Primary congenital glaucoma; A survey. *Can J Ophthalmol* 1974; **9**: 17−22

Phelps CV. The pathogenesis of glaucoma in Sturge−Weber's syndrome. *Ophthalmology* 1978; **85**: 276−81

Presley GD, Stinson IN, Sidbery JB. Ocular defects associated with homocystinuria. *South Med J* 1969; **62**: 944−7

Quigley HA. Childhood glaucoma: the results with trabeculotomy and the study of irreversible cupping. *Ophthalmology* 1982; **89**: 219−25

Rodman HI. Chronic glaucoma with traumatic dislocation of the lens. *Arch Ophthalmol* 1963; **69**: 445−54

Roy SH, Sunjitt RL, Hiatt RL, Hughes J. Ocular manifestations of the Rubenstein−Taybi syndrome. *Arch Ophthalmol* 1968; **79**: 272−4

Ruderman JM, Welch DB, Smith MF, Shoch DE. A randomized study of 5-fluorouracil and filtration surgery. *Am J Ophthalmology* 1987; **104**: 218−25

Sato SE, Herschler J, Lynch PJ, Hodes BL, Fryczkowski AW, Schlossen HD. Congenital glaucoma associated with cutis marmorata telangiectatica congenita: two case reports. *J Pediatr Ophthalmol Strabismus* 1988; **25**: 13−18

Shaffer RN, Hethington J. New concepts in infantile glaucoma. *Trans Ophthalmol Soc UK* 1967; **87**: 501−90

Spaeth GL. Traumatic hyphaema, angle recession, dexamethasone hypertension and glaucoma. *Arch Ophthalmol* 1967; **78**: 714−21

Traboulsi EI, Levine E, Mets MB, Parelhoff ES, O'Neill JF, Gaasterland DE. Infantile glaucoma in Down's syndrome (trisomy 21). *Am J Ophthalmol* 1988; **105**: 389−95

Waring GO, Rodriguez MM, Laibson PR. Anterior chamber cleavage syndrome: A stepladder classification. *Surv Ophthalmol* 1975; **20**: 3−14

Weiss BI, Cooper LZ, Breen RH. Infantile glaucoma: a manifestation of congenital rubella. *JAMA* 1966; **195**: 727−7

Zauberman H, Sira IB. Glaucoma and Rieger's syndrome. *Acta Ophthalmol* 1970; **48**: 118−26

Zeuman LE. Ocular lesions of juvenile xanthogranuloma. *Trans Am Acad Ophthalmol Otolaryngol* 1965; **69**: 412−22

26 Vitreous

ANTHONY MOORE

The vitreous is a transparent gelatinous structure which fills the posterior four fifths of the globe. It is firmly attached to the pars plana anteriorly and has a loose attachment to the retina and optic nerve posteriorly. In childhood there is also a firm attachment between the vitreous and posterior aspect of the lens.

The development of the vitreous body and zonule can be divided into three stages (Duke-Elder 1963). The primary vitreous is formed during the first month of development and is seen as a vascularized mesodermal tissue separating the developing lens vesicle and the neuroectoderm of the optic cup. This primary vitreous contains the branches of the hyaloid artery which continues to develop in early embryonic life but regresses during the formation of the secondary vitreous.

The secondary vitreous starts to form at 9 weeks (40 mm stage) (Spencer 1985) and continues to develop throughout embryonic life and during the rapid increase in size of the globe in early infancy. The secondary vitreous which ultimately forms the established vitreous body is avascular and transparent and displaces the primary vitreous which becomes condensed into a narrow band (Cloquet's canal) running from the optic disc to the posterior aspect of the lens.

By the third month (70 mm stage) the secondary vitreous fills most of the developing vitreous cavity; the remnants of the primary vitreous are confined to a central area. The vitreous lying between the developing ciliary body and lens become clearly separated from the secondary vitreous and by the 170 mm stage well formed fibrils run from the ciliary processes to the lens; this so called tertiary vitreous later develops into the zonule.

Developmental anomalies of the vitreous

Persistence of the primary vitreous or part of its structure may give rise to a number of abnormalities of the vitreous which may remain in postnatal life.

Persistent hyaloid artery

Persistence of all or more frequently part of the hyaloid artery is one of the commoner congenital abnormalities of the eye. Remnants of the hyaloid artery are seen in about 3% of normal full-term infants but are commonly seen in premature infants (Jones 1963) during examination for retinopathy of prematurity. Most of these will regress: persistence of the whole artery is uncommon. Rarely the whole artery may run from the optic disc to the posterior aspect of the lens. Posterior remnants may give rise to a single vessel running from the centre of the disc or to an elevated bud of glial tissue — the Bergmeister's papilla. Anterior remnants of the hyaloid system may be seen as a small white dot on the posterior lens capsule — the Mittendorf's dot. This does not interfere with vision and does not progress. It is often confused with a posterior cortical lens opacity.

Vitreous cysts

Cysts of the vitreous may be congenital or acquired; acquired cysts may be seen in association with ocular toxoplasmosis or toxocariasis, and rarely with juvenile retinoschisis (Lusky *et al.* 1988). Congenital cysts are usually found in otherwise normal eyes (François 1950; Bullock 1974; Feman & Straatsma 1974). The origin of the cysts is unknown but as blood vessels are sometimes seen within the cyst it has been suggested that they may develop from hyaloid artery remnants (François 1950). No histopathology is available.

Cysts may lie in the anterior vitreous immediately behind the lens (Fig. 26.1) (Hilsdorf 1965) or in the posterior vitreous (François 1950; Bullock 1974; Feman & Straatsma 1974). They may be mobile (Bullock 1974; Elkington & Watson 1974; Feman & Straatsma 1974) or attached to the optic disc (François 1950).

Persistant hyperplastic primary vitreous

Persistant hyperplastic primary vitreous (PHPV), first characterized by Reese in 1949; is a congenital abnormality of the eye caused by failure of the primary vitreous to regress. Most cases are unilateral although there may be minor abnormalities such as a Mittendorf dot in the fellow eye. Bilateral cases have been reported although some of these may be examples of vitreo-retinal dysplasia. Histopathologically a plaque

of fibrous tissue is adherent to the back of the lens and often extends from the ciliary processes in one region to another (Figs. 26.2, 26.3, 26.4). There is a variable degree of vascularization and fat, smooth muscle and cartilagenous material may also be present in the retrolental mass. (Reese 1955; Font *et al.* 1969). Liang *et al.* (1985) have reported an unusual case of a child with unilateral leucocoria who had the affected eye

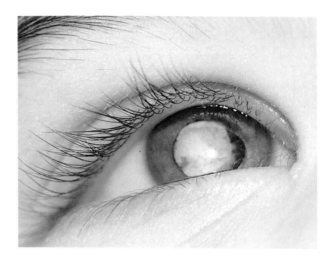

Fig. 26.2 PHPV. A yellowish, partly absorbed cataract is seen in front of a retrolental membrane with the ciliary processes stretched towards it.

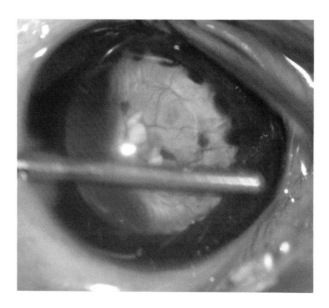

Fig. 26.3 PHPV with vascularised retrolental membrane. There was a large persistent hyaloid artery. If removed sufficiently early, and optically corrected together with occlusion of the fellow eye, useful acuity may sometimes be salvaged.

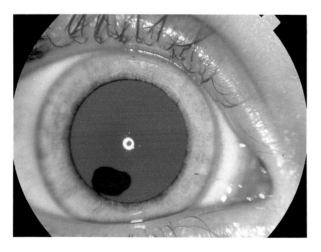

Fig. 26.1 Anterior vitreous cyst seen in retro-illumination. The acuity was 6/5 and the eye otherwise healthy.

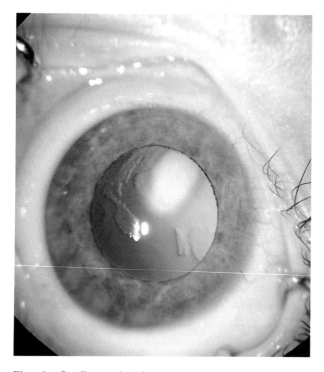

Fig. 26.4 Small posterior plaques in lenses may represent mild forms of PHPV, especially if associated with persistent hyaloid arteries.

enucleated. Pathological examination revealed a diffuse retinoblastoma infiltrating a persistant primary vitreous, this however is an exceptional case and should not lead one to enucleate cases of PHPV.

Pruett and Schepens (1970) have described a posterior form of PHPV (Fig. 26.5). This condition usually presents with strabismus or nystagmus and the ocular abnormality is confined to the posterior segment (Rubinstein 1980). A retinal fold runs from the optic disc to the ora serrata and there is associated condensation of the vitreous and retinal detachment. It is debatable whether this condition described by other authors as congenital retinal fold is really a variant of PHPV or really more closely related to vitreoretinal dysplasia (Fig. 26.6).

CLINICAL FEATURES

The typical presentation of anterior PHPV is with unilateral leucocoria which is recognized by the paediatrician or parent soon after birth. The affected eye is microphthalmic, the anterior chamber is shallow and there may be dilated radial iris vessels. A vascularized retrolental membrane is present and the ciliary processes may be drawn into the fibrous tissue. Although the lens may initially be clear a posterior

cortical cataract often develops. Nystagmus may be present even in unilateral cases and strabismus is common.

The condition often progresses and there may be shallowing of the anterior chamber, cataract formation and pupil block glaucoma. The lens may absorb and haemorrhage into the lens is not infrequent. Other complications include vitreous haemorrhage, retinal detachment and phthisis bulbi.

Posterior PHPV may present with leucocoria, strabismus or nystagmus. The affected eye is often microphthalmic and the lens is usually clear. Further examination usually shows a fold of condensed vitreous and retina running from the disc to the ora serrata and there may be an associated subtotal retinal detachment (Pruett & Schepens 1970; Pollard 1985).

The differential diagnosis of PHPV is that of leucocoria. The presence of microphthalmia and elongated ciliary processes helps to differentiate it from other causes of retrolental mass. Ultrasound and CT scan is useful in differentiating PHPV from retinoblastoma where there is uncertainty about the clinical diagnosis. (Goldberg & Mafee 1983).

MANAGEMENT

The main aim of management in PHPV is to avoid the complications of glaucoma and phthisis bulbi and allow the child to retain the eye. Enucleation should be avoided as not only is the result of a prosthesis less acceptable cosmetically but also enucleation in early infancy is associated with decreased growth of the bony orbit on the affected side and marked facial asymmetry (Kennedy 1965). A limbal or pars plicata approach with vitrectomy instruments may be used to remove the lens and abnormal retrolental tissue (Stark et al. 1983; Pollard 1985). Intraocular scissors may be required to excise dense fibrous tissue and intraocular haemorrhage can be controlled by raising the infusion bottle or the use of intraocular diathermy. In this way it is possible to obtain a clear visual axis, deepen the anterior chamber and prevent angle closure glaucoma. A more controversial aspect of management is whether attempts should be made to obtain a visual result by optical correction of the affected eye and a vigorous patching regime. The good results of surgery in some infants with unilateral congenital cataract (Beller & Hoyt 1981; Lewis et al. 1986) has led to the adoption of a similar approach in the treatment in PHPV and some good visual results have been reported (Stark et al. 1983; Pollard 1985; Karr & Scott 1986). This aggressive approach should be reserved for those in-

frequent finding. The dysplastic retina contains a variety of rosettes which resemble retinoblastoma rosettes but contain Muller cells with an abnormal relationship between the retina and its pigment epithelium (Fulton *et al.* 1978).

Norrie's disease

Norrie's disease is an X-linked recessive disorder in which affected males are blind at birth or early infancy (Norrie 1927; Warburg 1961, 1963; Lieberfarb *et al.* 1985). About 25% of affected males are mentally retarded and about a third develop cochlear-hearing loss which may develop at any time from infancy to adult life (Parving & Warburg 1977). The ocular findings include bilateral retinal folds, retinal detachment, vitreous haemorrhage and bilateral retrolental masses (vitreoretinal dysplasia). Most cases progress to an extensive vitreoretinal mass (Fig. 26.8, 26.9) and bilateral blindness.

Carrier females do not show any ocular abnormality. Recently Warburg *et al.* (1986) have demonstrated close linkage between the gene for Norrie's disease and the DXS7 locus characterized by a restrictive fragment length polymorphism (RFLP) L1.28. It is now possible to use the probe L1.28 in informative families to give improved counselling to possible carrier females. In such families it may also be useful in prenatal diagnosis (See Chapter 9).

Trisomy 13

Trisomy 13 (Patau syndrome) was first characterized by Patau *et al.* (1960); it is the chromosomal abnor-

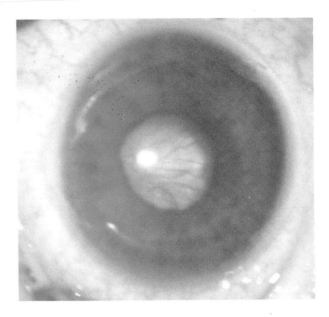

Fig. 26.9 Norrie's disease. Brother of patient in Fig. 26.8a. Showing vascularised white retrolental mass.

mality most consistantly associated with severe ocular defects. The most common systemic abnormalities are microcephaly, cleft palate, congenital cardiac defects, polydactyly, skin haemangiomas, umbilical hernia and malformation of the central nervous system (Patau *et al.* 1960; Smith *et al.* 1963; Taylor 1968). Most affected children die within the first few months of life.

Bilateral ocular abnormalities are seen in almost all cases of trisomy 13 (Smith *et al.* 1963); the common ocular findings are detailed in Table 26.1. Affected infants often show total disorganization of vitreous and retina and histological examination of eyes obtained at postmortem have confirmed the presence of extensive retinal dysplasia (Sergovich *et al.* 1963; Yannoff *et al.* 1963; Cogan & Kuwabara 1964). Intraocular cartilage is frequently found (Cogan & Kuwabara 1964) and may be a characteristic abnormality.

Table 26.1 Ocular abnormalities in trisomy 13.

Microphthalmos
Colobomas of uveal tract
Cataract
Corneal opacities
Retinal dysplasia
PHPV
Dysplastic optic nerves
Cyclopia

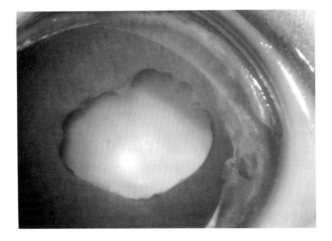

Fig. 26.8 Norrie's disease showing posterior synechiae, shallow anterior chamber and retrolental white mass.

Incontinentia pigmenti

Incontinentia pigmenti (Bloch—Sulzberger syndrome) is an uncommon familial disorder affecting the skin, bones, teeth, central nervous system, and eyes. It is thought to be inherited as an X-linked dominant disorder which is usually lethal in the male leading to a marked female predominance. The skin lesions usually appear soon after birth with a linear eruption of bullae which predominantly affects the extremities. The bullae gradually resolve to leave a linear pattern of pigmentation (Carney & Carney 1970).

Ocular abnormalities occur in about 35% of cases (Carney 1976) and includes strabismus, nystagmus, retinal detachment, and retrolental mass. The most serious complication is retinal dysplasia which, if bilateral, leads to total blindness. Retinovascular abnormalities are common; (Watzkhe et al. 1976; François 1984; Spallone 1987). Arteriovenous anomalies are commonly seen in the temporal periphery often in association with preretinal fibrosis. Fluorescein angiography demonstrates areas of non-perfusion in the temporal periphery (Watzke et al. 1976) and it is possible that these vascular anomalies may represent an early stage in the development of retinal detachment and 'pseudoglioma' (Brown 1988). Affected females should be assessed by an ophthalmologist at regular intervals as it is possible that early cryotherapy or photocoagulation of the retinovascular abnormalities may prevent progression of the ocular disease (Watzke et al. 1976; Brown 1988).

Warburg syndrome

This is an autosomal recessive oculocerebral syndrome characterized by hydrocephalus, agyria of the brain, and retinal dysplasia. Encephalocoele is a variable feature. Death often occurs in the neonatal period and survivors are severely retarded (Warburg 1971; Pagan et al. 1983). The ocular features in this disorder are variable and include micropthalmia, Peter's anomaly, cataract, retinal coloboma and retinal dysplasia.

This rare inherited disorder should be considered in the differential diagnosis of vitreoretinal dysplasia so that appropriate genetic advice may be given.

Autosomal recessive vitreoretinal dysplasia

Vitreoretinal dysplasia may occur as an isolated abnormality in an otherwise healthy child (Lahav et al. 1973; Phillips et al. 1973; Ohba et al. 1981). The usual presentation is with bilateral poor vision in early infancy and nystagmus; examination reveals a shallow anterior chamber and white retrolental mass. Progressive shallowing of the anterior chamber may lead to pupil block glaucoma which if it fails to respond to mydratics may require lensectomy.

Osteoporosis—pseudoglioma—mental retardation syndrome

Neuhauser et al. (1976) delineated a syndrome, thought to be autosomal recessive with osteoporosis, mental retardation and what was probably a form of vitreoretinal dysplasia.

Genetic counselling in the vitreoretinal dysplasias

The vitreoretinal dysplasias are a genetically heterogenous group of disorders which result in a similar ocular abnormality; it is not possible to subdivide the disorders on the basis of the clinical or pathological ocular findings (Lahav et al. 1973) so that the specific diagnosis depends on the presence of associated systemic findings although the family history may suggest the likely mode of inheritance.

For the purposes of genetic counselling families fall into two groups. In the first group the diagnosis (and hence the mode of inheritance) of the affected child is clear. The second more problematic group are those families in which a child is born without family history and with isolated retinal dysplasia and no associated systemic findings.

In the first group counselling is relatively straightforward. When one child has been born with a trisomy the risk of a similar affected child in a future pregnancy is about 1%, but may be higher if one of the parents has a structural chromosome abnormality or mosaicism (Stene et al. 1984). Parents may be offered prenatal diagnosis. In children with the systemic features of Warburg syndrome (Hard± E) or the osteoporosis—pseudoglioma—mental retardation syndrome the inheritance is autosomal recessive and the parents can be counselled accordingly.

In Norrie's disease there are no detectable clinical abnormalities in the carrier female to aid counselling. When there is another affected male relative the mother can be assumed to be a carrier and counselled accordingly. In isolated boys, one third are thought to represent new mutations and in two thirds the mothers are carriers. In the absence of any carrier tests based on DNA analysis there is an overall risk of a further son being affected of one in three.

Counselling a family with an otherwise normal child born with bilateral retinal dysplasia is more difficult. Isolated retinal dysplasia is sufficiently rare that there is insufficient empirical data to aid counselling. If the affected child is female retinal dysplasia may be autosomal recessive or be non-genetic; since autosomal recessive dysplasia is rare so long as there is no parental consanguinity the recurrence risk is likely to be low. In an affected male child the retinal dysplasia may be recessive, X-linked, or non-genetic and the risk of a subsequent affected child is higher. DNA studies should always be performed in affected males as the presence of a deletion of the DXS7 locus on the X chromosome indicates a diagnosis of Norrie's disease (See Chapter 9).

Inherited vitreoretinal dystrophies

Goldmann—Favre disease

This rare autosomal recessive condition was first described by Favre in 1958 (Favre 1958) and since then at least 25 further cases have been reported (Lisch 1983). The usual presentation is with gradual visual loss or night-blindness and the abnormal ocular findings include liquefaction of the vitreous, macular retinoschisis and peripheral retinal pigment epithelial atrophy and pigmentation (Lisch 1983; Carr & Siegel 1970). Peripheral retinoschisis and secondary cataract may also occur. The EOG is subnormal and ERG extinguished, or markedly abnormal. The retinal dystrophy is progressive resulting in extensive visual field loss. Although the macular appearance may be similar, the vitreous changes, peripheral retinopathy, ERG abnormalities and mode of inheritance help differentiate this condition from X-linked juvenile retinoschisis.

Wagner's syndrome

Wagner in 1938 (Wagner 1938) described a dominantly inherited vitreoretinal dystrophy occurring in 13 affected individuals from one Swiss family. The family was subsequently re-examined by Bohringer (1960) and Ricci (1961) and additional affected members were added to the pedigree.

Affected members are myopic and show vitreous and retinal abnormalities. The vitreous appears optically empty apart from scattered translucent membranes; there is usually a posterior vitreous detachment with a thickened posterior hyaloid. Peripheral vascular sheathing is common and is normally as-

sociated with perivascular RPE atrophy and pigment deposition. The electro-retinogram is subnormal.

Cataract commonly develops between the age of 20 and 30 and is the usual cause of visual loss. In Wagner's original family there was no associated retinal detachment or systemic abnormalities.

Inherited vitreoretinal degeneration and systemic disease

Stickler (Stickler et al. 1965) in 1965 described a large autosomal dominant pedigree in which affected members had progressive myopia, retinal detachment and a progressive arthropathy which began in childhood (Fig. 26.10). Patients have a characteristic facial appearance caused by malar hypoplasia and a flattened nasal bridge and also may have sensorineural hearing loss.

Since Stickler's early report it has become clear that vitreoretinal degeneration similar to that seen in Wagner's syndrome may be associated with a variety of bone dysplasias and clefting syndromes. These disorders which probably result from defects in collagen synthesis or metabolism have been reviewed by Deutmann (1977) and Maumenee (1979). Maumenee (1979) has classified them into eight different types on the basis of their ocular and systemic findings. Most of these disorders carry a high risk of retinal detachment which tend to occur at an early age and are associated with giant retinal tears of multiple posterior retinal breaks (Billington et al. 1979). The management of these complex detachments entails the use of closed intraocular microsurgery and silicon oil, and prophylaxis with 360 degree cryotherapy of the fellow eye should be considered.

Juvenile X-linked retinoschisis

This X-linked disorder is seen almost exclusively in males. Foveal retinoschisis is seen in virtually all cases and in 50% is the only funduscopic abnormality

Fig. 26.10 (opposite) (a) Stickler's syndrome. This boy has a flattened nasal bridge, malar hypoplasia, myopia and spondyloepiphyseal dysplasia. (b) Cleft soft palate. (Same patient.) (c) High myopia. He also had vitreoretinal changes in the periphery. (Same patient.) (d,e) Family of the boy in Fig. 26.10(a) showing high incidence of characteristic facies. Spondyloepiphyseal dysplasia in Stickler's syndrome. (f) The vertebral bodies are rounded and flattened, the disc space narrowed.

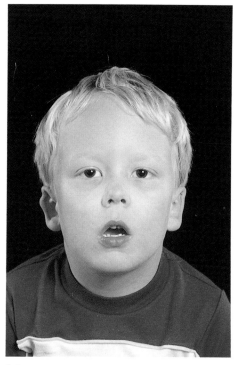

(a)

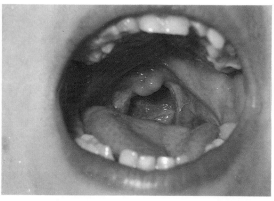

(b)

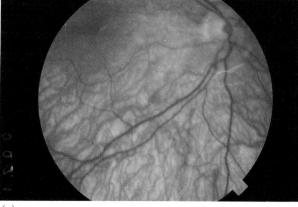

(c)

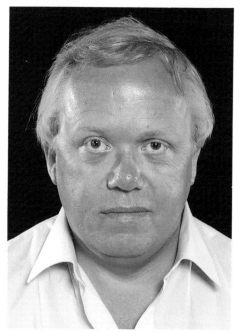

(d)

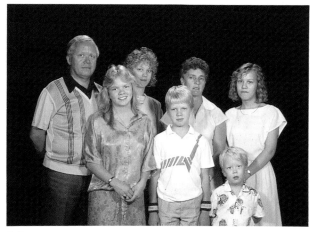

(e)

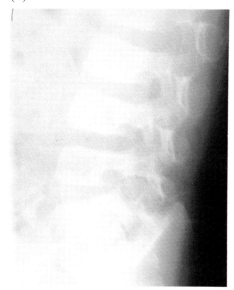

(f)

(Deutman 1971, 1977). The characteristic foveal retinoschisis has been described in early infancy (Pischel 1969), but most children present between the ages of 5–10 years either with reading difficulties or when they fail the school eye test. Asymptomatic individuals may be found on routine examination when a close relative has the disorder. Rarely, sudden vitreous haemorrhage from a ruptured vessel in a vitreous veil may be the presenting sign. The visual acuity is usually in the range 6/12–6/36 at presentation.

The foveal retinoschisis (Fig. 26.11) is easily missed unless a careful examination of the macular region is made with slit lamp biomicroscopy. The schisis is seen as small microcysts associated with radial linear folds running out from the centre of the fovea. These changes are often better appreciated with a red free

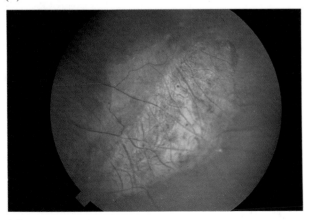

(a)

(b)

(c)

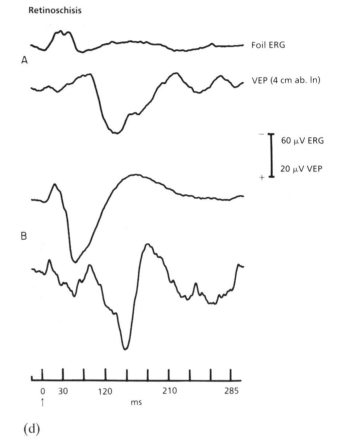

(d)

Fig. 26.11 (a,b) Juvenile X-linked retinoschisis. Bilateral foveal retinoschisis. (c) Same patient showing peripheral pigmentary changes in an area of schisis. (d) The ERG and VEP of the patient (A) compared with his mother (B). The B wave is absent from the ERG whilst the VEP is of only slightly reduced amplitude reflecting good central vision. Studies by Dr A. Kriss

light. Fifty per cent of patients will also show a typical peripheral retinoschisis (Deutman 1977) usually in the lower temporal quadrant (Fig. 26.12); sometimes this is only visible as an unusual sheen to the retinal reflex. Vitreous veils which are often vascularized (Fig. 26.12) are seen in the periphery in about 50% of patients; these vessels may rupture giving rise to vitreous haemorrhage. Other peripheral retinal changes include perivascular sheathing, grey white dendritiform ap-

pearance on the inner surface of the retina (Fig. 26.13) and a glistening reflex from the internal limiting membrane (Deutman 1977).

Fluorescein angiography is usually normal in childhood but progression during adult life may lead to retinal pigment epithelial atrophy and an associated hyperfluorescence. The EOG is normal but the ERG shows a defective or absent B wave (Fig. 26.11d) in the presence of a normal A wave. Female carriers have a normal fundus appearance and normal electro-oculogram (EOG) and electroretinogram (ERG). Arden *et al.* (1988) have recently demonstrated that carrier females show absence of normal rod-cone inter-

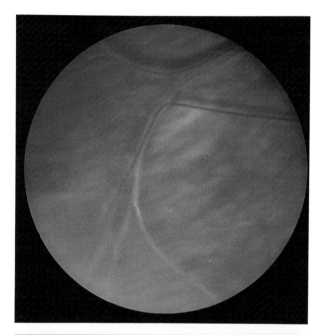

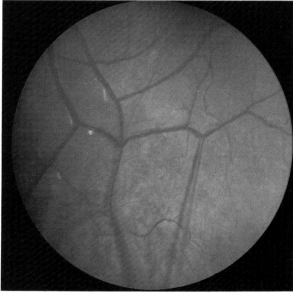

Fig. 26.12 Juvenile X-linked retinoschisis. Peripheral schisis with vessels visible in the schitic strands. Vitreous haemorrhage is not uncommon.

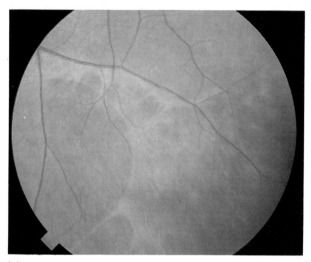

(a)

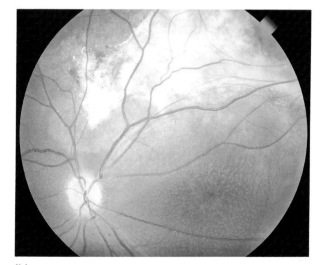

(b)

Fig. 26.13 (a) Juvenile X-linked retinoschisis. Peripheral schisis. (b) Same patient. Arcuate subretinal lesion possibly due to subretinal haemorrhage.

action and this psychophysical investigation may be used to identify the carrier state with a high degree of certainty. DNA probes that flank the retinoschisis locus have been developed (Dahl & Ulf 1988).

Histopathological examination of eyes from patients with X-linked retinoschisis have shown there to be a split occurring in the nerve fibre layer (Yanoff *et al.* 1968; Manschot 1972). Yanoff *et al.* (1968) has suggested that the condition may be caused by a widespread defect in Mueller's cells which would be in keeping both with the histological picture and ERG evidence of an absent B wave.

The visual prognosis in this disorder is relatively good. Central vision deteriorates very slowly and peripheral fields are normal unless there is a peripheral retinoschisis. True retinal detachment is extremely rare.

Dominant exudative vitreoretinopathy (DEVR)

In 1969, Criswick and Schepens (1969) reported six children from two families with a progressive vitreoretinopathy which resembled retrolental fibroplasia. The children were otherwise normal and there was no history of prematurity or oxygen use. Gow and Oliver (1971) were able to demonstrate autosomal dominant inheritance in their family and divided the clinical course into three stages.

Stage I

Mild peripheral retinal changes with abnormal vitreous traction but no evidence of retinal vascular or exudative change.

Stage II

Dilated tortuous vessels between the equator and ora serrata with subretinal exudates and localized retinal detachment. Dragging of disc vessels and macular ectopia is often present.

Stage III

In this advanced stage of the disease a total retinal detachment is usually present with vitreous traction and fibrosis. Other complications include secondary cataract and neovascular glaucoma.

Fluorescein angiography (Canny & Oliver 1976; Ober *et al.* 1980) shows peripheral capillary closure and teliangiectasis in mild cases. In more advanced

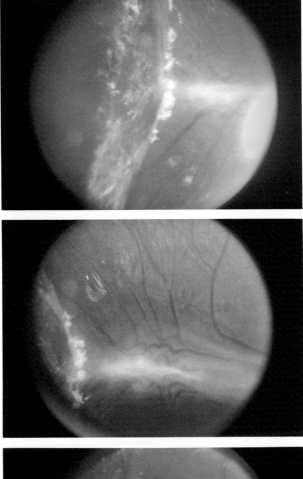

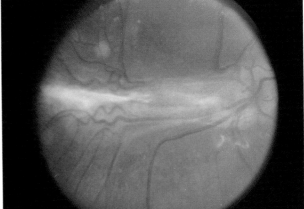

Fig. 26.14 Dominant exudative vitreoretinopathy Stage II. Dr R. McKay's patient.

disease there is an extensive fibrovascular mass in the retinal periphery and angiography demonstrates an abrupt transition at the equator between normal retina and the fibrovascular tissue; vessels at the transition leak fluoroscein.

There is a wide range of expression of the abnormal gene and mild cases may be missed unless fluorescein angiography of the peripheral retina is performed.

Although the retinal changes may progress throughout childhood, progression is rare after the age of 20 years (Ober *et al.* 1980). In children who show progression from Stage I disease cryotherapy of peripheral ischaemic retina may be indicated (Gow & Oliver 1971).

References

Arden GB, Gorin MB, Polkinghorne PJ, Jay M, Bird AC. Detection of carrier state of X-linked retinoschisis. *Am J Ophthalmol* 1988; **105**: 590−95

Beller R, Hoyt CS, Marg E, Odom JV. Good visual function after neonatal surgery for congenital monocular cataracts. *Am J Ophthalmol* 1981; **91**: 559−65

Billington BM, Leaver PK, McLeod D. Management of retinal detachment in the Wagner−Stickler syndrome. *Trans Ophthlamol Soc UK* 1985; **104**: 875−9

Bohringer H, Dieterle P, Landrol E. Zur klinik und pathologie der degeneratio, hyaloideo-retinalis hereditaria (Wagner). *Ophthalmologica (Basel)* 1960; **139**: 330−8

Brown GA. Incontinentia pigmenti: the development of pseudoglioma. *Br J Ophthalmol* 1988; **72**: 452−6

Bullock JD. Developmental vitreous cysts. *Arch Ophthalmol* 1974; **91**: 830−85

Canny CLB, Oliver GL. Fluorescein angiography findings in familial exudative vitreo-retinopathy. *Arch Ophthalmol* 1976; **94**: 1114−20

Carney RG. Incontinentia pigmenti: a world statistical analysis. *Arch Dermatol* 1976; **112**: 535−42

Carney RG, Carnet RG Jr. Incontinentia pigmenti. *Arch Dermatol* 1970; **102**: 157−62

Carr RE, Siegel JM. The vitreo-retinal degenerations. *Arch Ophthalmol* 1970; **84**: 436−45

Cogan DG, Kuwabara T. Ocular pathology of the 13−15 trisomy syndrome. *Arch Ophthalmol* 1964; **72**: 246−53

Criswick VG, Schepens CL. Familial exudative vitreoretinopathy. *Am J Ophthalmol* 1969; **68**: 578−94

Dahl N, Ulf P. Use of linked DNA probes for carrier detection and diagnosis of X-linked juvenile retinoschisis. *Arch Ophthalmol* 1988; **106**: 1414−17.

Deutmann AF. Sex-linked juvenile retinoschisis. In: Deutmann AF. (Ed.) *The Hereditary Dystrophies of the Posterior Pole of the Eye.* Koninklijke Van Gorum Comp NV, Netherlands 1971; pp. 48−99

Deutmann AF. Vitreo-retinal dystrophies. In: Krill AE (Ed.) *Hereditary Retinal and Choridal Diseases*, Vol. II. Harper & Row, London 1977; pp. 1043−108

Duke-Elder S. *System of Ophthalmology.* Duke Elder S. (Ed.) Vol. III. Henry Kimpton, London 1963; pp. 141−52

Elkington AR, Watson DM. Mobile vitreous cysts. *Br J Ophthalmol* 1974; **58**: 103−4

Favre M. A propos de deux cas de degenerescence hyaloideo-retinienne. *Ophthalmologica (Basel)* 1958; **135**: 604−9

Feman SS, Straatsma BR. Cyst of the posterior vitreous. *Arch Ophthalmol* 1974; **91**: 328−9

Font RL, Yanoff M, Zimmerman LE. Intraocular adipose tissue and persistent hyperplastic primary vitreous. *Arch Ophthalmol* 1969; **82**: 43−50

Fulton AB, Croft JL, Howard RO, Albert DM. Human retinal dysplasia. *Am J Ophthalmol* 1978; **85**: 690−8

François J. Prepapillary cysts developed from remnants of the hyaloid artery. *Br J Ophthalmol* 1950; **34**: 365−8

François J. Incontinentia pigmenti (Bloch Sulzberger syndrome) and retinal changes. *Br J Ophthalmol* 1984; **68**: 19−25

Goldberg MF, Mafee M. Computerized tomography for the diagnosis of persistent hyperplastic primary vitreous. *Ophthalmology* 1983; **90**: 442−51

Gow J, Oliver GL. Familial exudative vitreo-retinopathy, an expanded view. *Arch Ophthalmol* 1971; **86**: 150−5

Hilsdorf C. Uber einen fall einer einseitigen glaskorpercyste. *Ophthalmologica (Basel)* 1965; **149**: 12−20

Jones HE. Hyaloid remnants in the eyes of premature babies. *Br J Ophthalmol* 1963; **47**: 39−44

Karr DJ, Scott WE. Visual acuity results following treatment of persistant hyperplastic primary vitreous. *Arch Ophthalmol* 1986; **104**: 662−7

Kennedy RE. The effect of early enucleation on the orbit in animals and humans. *Am J Ophthalmol* 1965; **60**: 277−306

Lahav M, Albert DM, Wyand S. Clinical and histopathologic classification of retinal dysplasia. *Am J Ophthalmol* 1973; **75**: 648−67

Lewis TL, Maurer D, Brent HP. Effects on perceptual development of visual deprivation during infancy. *Br J Ophthalmol* 1986; **70**: 214−20

Liang JC, Augsburger JJ, Shields JA. Diffuse infiltrating retinoblastoma associated with persistent primary vitreous. *J Paediatr Ophthalmol Strabismus* 1985; **22**: 31−3

Lieberfarb RM, Eavey RD, De Long GR *et al.* Norrie's disease: a study of two families. *Ophthalmology* 1985; **92**: 1445−51

Lisch W. Hereditary vitreoretinal degenerations. In: Straub W (Ed.) *Developments in Ophthalmology*, Vol 8. Karger, Basel 1983; pp. 33−8

Lusky M, Weinberger D, Kremer L. Vitreous cyst combined with bilateral juvenile retinoschisis. *J Paediatr Ophthalmol* 1988; **25**: 75−7

Manschot WA. Pathology of hereditary juvenile retinoschisis. *Arch Ophthalmol* 1972; **88**: 131−8

Maumenee IH. Vitreo-retinal degenerations as a sign of generalised connective tissue disease. *Am J Ophthalmol* 1979; **88**: 432−49

Neuhauser G, Kaveggia EG, Opitz JM. Autosomal recessive syndrome of pseudogliomatous blindness, osteoporosis and mild mental retardation. *Clin Genet* 1976; **9**: 324−32

Norrie G. Causes of blindness in children; twenty five years experience of Danish Institutes for the blind. *Acta Ophthalmol* 1927; **5**: 357−86

Ober RR, Bird AC, Hamilton AM, Sehmi K. Autosomal dominant exudative vitreoretinopathy. *Br J Ophthalmol* 1980; **46**: 112−20

Ohba N, Watanabe S, Fujita S. Primary vitreoretinal dysplasia transmitted as an autosomal recessive disorder. *B J Ophthalmol* 1981; **65**: 631−5

Pagon R, Clarren SK, Milam FD, Hendrickson AE. Autosomal recessive eye and brain anomalies: Warburg syndrome. *J Pediatr* 1983; **102**: 542−6

Parving A, Warburg M. Audiological findings in Norrie's disease. *Audiology* 1977; **16**: 124−31

Patau K, Smith DW, Therman E, Inhom SL, Wagner HP. Multiple congenital anomalies caused by an extra autosome. *Lancet* 1960; **1**: 790−3

Phillips CL, Leighton DA, Forrester RM. Congenital hereditary non-attachment of the retina: a sibship of two. *Acta Ophthalmol* 1973; **51**: 425−33

Pischel DK. Three brothers with juvenile retinoschisis. *Mod Probl Ophthalmol* 1969; **8**: 381−9

Pollard Z. Treatment of persistent hyperplastic primary vitreous. *J Pediatr Ophthalmol* 1985; **22**: 180−3

Preslan MW, Beauchamp GR, Zakov ZN. Congenital glaucoma and retinal dysplasia. *J Pediatr Ophthalmol Strabismus* 1985; **22**: 166−70

Pruett RC, Schepens CL. Posterior hyperplastic primary vitreous. *Am J Ophthalmol* 1970; **69**: 535−43

Reese AB. Persistance and hyperplasia of the primary vitreous; retrolental fibroplasia − two entities. *Arch Ophthalmol* 1949; **41**: 527−52

Reese AB. Persistent hyperplastic primary vitreous. *Am J Ophthalmol* 1955; **40**: 317−31

Ricci MA. Clinique et transmission hereditaire des degenerescences vitreoretiennes. *Bull Soc Ophthalmol (Fr)* 1961; **61**: 618−62

Rubinstein K. Posterior hyperplastic primary vitreous. *Br J Ophthalmol* 1980; **64**: 105−11

Sergovich F. The d trisomy syndrome: a case report with description of the ocular pathology. *Can Med Assoc J* 1963; **89**: 151−7

Silverstein AM, Parshall CJ, Osburn BI, Prendergast RA. An experimental virus induced retinal dysplasia in the fetal lamb. *Am J Ophthalmol* 1971; **72**: 22−34

Smith DW, Patau K, Therman E *et al.* The D1 trisomy syndrome. *J Pediatr* 1963; **62**: 326−41

Spallone A. Incontinentia pigmenti (Bloch−Sulzberger syndrome) seven case reports from one family. *Br J Ophthalmol* 1987; **71**: 629−35

Spencer WH. Vitreous. In: *Ophthalmic Pathology. An Atlas and Textbook* 1985; WB Sanders & Co., London pp. 554−6

Stark WJ, Lindsey P, Fagadan WR, Michels RG. Persistent hyperplastic primary vitreous; surgical treatment. *Ophthalmology* 1983; **90**: 452−7

Steve J, Steve E, Mikkelson M. Risk for chromosome abnormality at aminiocentosis following a child with a non-inherited chromosome aberration. *Prenat Diagn* 1984; **4**: 81−95

Stickler GB, Becau PG, Farrel FS *et al.* Hereditary progressive ophthalmo-arthropathy. *Mayo Clin Proc* 1965; **40**: 433−55

Taylor AI. Autosomal trisomy syndromes: a detailed study of 27 cases of Edwards syndrome and 27 cases of Patau syndrome. *J Med Genet* 1968; **5**: 227−52

Wagner H. Ein bisher unbekanntes erbleiden des auges (Degeneratio hyaloideo retinalis hereditaria), beobachtet im Karifon Zurich. *Klin Monatsbl Augenheilkd* 1938; **100**: 840−56

Warburg M. Norrie's disease, a new hereditary bilateral pseudotumour of the retina. *Acta Ophthalmol* 1961; **39**: 757−72

Warburg M. Norrie's disease (atrofia bulborum hereditaria). *Acta Ophthalmol* 1963; **41**: 134−46

Warburg M. The heterogenity of microphthalmia in the mentally retarded. *Birth Defects* 1971; **7**: 136−54

Warburg M, Friedrich U, Bleeker L *et al.* Norrie's disease: delineation of carriers among daughters of obligate carriers by linkage analysis. *Trans Ophthalmol Soc UK* 1986; **105**: 88−93

Watzke RC, Stevens TS, Carney RG. Retinal vascular changes of incontinenti pigmenti. *Arch Ophthalmol* 1976; **94**: 743−6

Yanoff M, Frayer WC, Scheie HG. Ocular findings in a patient with 13−15 trisomy. *Arch Ophthalmol* 1963; **70**: 372−5

Yanoff M, Rahn EK, Zimmerman LE. Histopathology of juvenile retinoschisis. *Arch Ophthalmol* 1968; **79**: 49−53

27 Retina

ANTHONY MOORE

27.1 Retinoblastoma

ANTHONY MOORE

Retinoblastoma is the commonest malignant ocular tumour of childhood; untreated the tumour is almost uniformly fatal but with modern methods of treatment the survival rate is over 90%. The best results are achieved if cases are referred to specialist centres where ophthalmologists, paediatric oncologists and radiotherapists collaborate in management. It occurs in about one in 20 000 live births (François *et al.* 1979; Sanders *et al.* 1988). The tumour arises from primitive retinal cells so the majority of cases occur in children under the age of 4 years. Retinoblastoma is seen in a hereditary and non-hereditary form. In hereditary retinoblastoma there is a germ cell mutation which predisposes the individual to the development of the retinal tumour. In non-hereditary retinoblastoma a somatic mutation in a primative retinal cell gives rise to a solitary, unilateral tumour; as no germinal mutation is involved the disease is not transmitted to any offspring.

Hereditary retinoblastoma

Forty per cent of all cases of retinoblastoma are due to a germinal mutation (Musarella & Gallie 1986) and include those cases with a family history or where the tumour is bilateral or multifocal. However about 15% of sporadic unilateral retinoblastoma are also hereditary. Most new cases of hereditary retinoblastoma are due to a new germinal mutation; familial cases account for less than 10% (François *et al.* 1979) but this proportion may be rising as treatment for retinoblastoma becomes more effective. In familial cases the mode of inheritance is autosomal dominant (Migdal 1976; François *et al.* 1979) with a high degree of penetrance.

Since the initial report of Lele *et al.* (1963) of a deletion of the q14 region of chromosome 13 in a child with retinoblastoma there have been nearly 100 further cases reported; about 1−3% of patients with retinoblastoma have a recognizable deletions of 13q14 (Cowell *et al.* 1986; Musarella & Gallie 1986). The children are usually mentally retarded and may have a variety of other congenital abnormalities (Lele 1963; Howard *et al.* 1974; Knudson *et al.* 1976; Wilson *et al.* 1977).

Survivors of the hereditary form of a retinoblastoma are at a greatly increased risk of developing a second non-ocular malignancy (Abramson *et al.* 1976; Abramson *et al.* 1984). Abramson *et al.* (1984) reviewed 688 patients with hereditary retinoblastoma who survived following treatment with radiotherapy; 89 developed second tumours, 62 within the radiation field and 27 outside. The commonest form of tumour was osteosarcoma. These findings suggest that although radiation may play a part, patients with the hereditary form of retinoblastoma have an increased susceptibility to tumour formation.

Non-hereditary retinoblastoma

This tumour is seen in individuals who have a solitary unilateral tumour and where there is no family history or chromosomal abnormality. Survivors do not pass on the disease to their offspring.

Pathogenesis

Two distinct differences emerge between hereditary and non-hereditary forms of retinoblastoma. Firstly the hereditary form presents earlier and affected children have bilateral or multifocal tumours, rather than the solitary tumour seen in the non-hereditary form. Secondly in hereditary retinoblastoma there is a much increased risk of developing a second non-ocular malignancy. Knudson (1971) and later Gallie and Phillips (1982) plotted the ages of children with bilateral and unilateral retinoblastoma at diagnosis against the logarithm of the proportion in each group not yet diagnosed. The curve for the bilateral cases fitted a simple exponential suggesting that a single event in addition to the germinal mutation was necessary for tumour development. With unilateral cases, the shape of the curve suggested that at least two events are necessary for tumour genesis.

From this data Knudson put forward his 'two hit' hypothesis: in a normal primitive retinal cell two mutational events are needed for tumour formation to occur. In patients with a germinal mutation all retinal cells will carry the abnormal genetic material and only one further mutation is needed for tumour formation. The chances of two or more primitive retinal cells undergoing the second mutation in hereditary

retinoblastomas is sufficiently large for multiple tumours to occur. However the chances of two mutational events occurring in the *same* cell are extremely small so that non-hereditary cases have only a solitary tumour which presents later.

Although this theory helps explain some of the differences between the two forms of retinoblastoma it does not predict which genetic events lead to the development of tumour. The presence of deletions of 13q14 in some patients with retinoblastoma suggests that the first mutation may be a deletion or rearrangement of the normal gene at the retinoblastoma locus at 13q14. The enzyme esterase D which exists in several isomeric forms has also been shown to have its genetic locus at 13q14. Retinoblastoma patients with deletions of chromosome 13 have 50% of the normal levels of esterase D (Sparkes *et al.* 1980; Cowell *et al.* 1986) suggesting that the two loci are closely linked. Furthermore genetic linkage studies in families with hereditary retinoblastoma and a normal karyotype in which two isoenzymes of esterase D are present, the tumour segregates with one isoenzyme suggesting that the locus for the retinoblastoma gene is 13q14 (Sparkes *et al.* 1983). It appears however that as long as the homologous chromosome 13 has a normal gene at the retinoblastoma locus no tumour formation occurs. There is now good evidence (Gallie & Phillips 1984; Murphree & Benedict 1984) that the second mutational event is loss of heterozygosity at the retinoblastoma locus; thus loss, a point mutation, deletion or rearrangement of the normal gene at the retinoblastoma locus on both of a homologous pair of chromosomes 13 leads to tumour formation. This mechanism appears to function in both hereditary and non-hereditary retinoblastoma.

Murphree and Benedict (1984) have suggested that it is the loss of a normal allelic pair of supressor or 'regulating' genes that leads to the development of retinoblastoma and that this mechanism may serve as a model for other forms of malignant tumour formation. It may also explain the increased susceptibility of patients with hereditary retinoblastoma to other malignant tumours.

A DNA sequence thought to represent the normal gene at the retinoblastoma locus has been isolated (Friend *et al.* 1986; Dryja *et al.* 1986) and recently sequenced (Lee *et al.* 1987). The gene, located in the q14 segment of chromosome 13 is transcribed in normal retina, and the messenger RNA transcript is absent or abnormal in most retinoblastomas studied, suggesting that it is in fact the normal gene at the RB locus (Albert & Dryja 1988).

Histopathology

Retinoblastomas are undifferentiated malignant neuro-blastic tumours, composed of cells with large hyperchromatic nuclei and scanty cytoplasm. Mitotic figures are common. In some tumours more differentiated cells form the typical Flexner–Wintersteiner rosettes in which cuboidal cells are uniformly arranged around a lumen into which fine filamentous structures are sometimes seen to project. Electron microscopy shows these projections to be similar to primitive inner segments of photoreceptors (Zimmerman 1985).

Tumour cells often outgrow their blood supply leading to cell necrosis; calcification of necrotic tissue is common. Spontaneous resolution is said to occur more commonly in retinoblastoma than other malignant tumours, but many of such cases may be examples of retinomas, a benign manifestation of the retinoblastoma gene (Gallie *et al.* 1982). True spontaneous resolution is probably due to extensive tumour necrosis and often leads to phthysis bulbi. (Gallie *et al.* 1982).

Two main patterns of growth are seen. Endophtyic tumours (Fig. 27.1.1) tend to grow forward into the vitreous and large tumours may totally fill the vitreous cavity. The tumours are friable and fragments of tumour may float in the vitreous cavity ('seedlings') or may fall onto the retinal surface and attach and grow at their new site. Spread of tumour into the anterior chamber may lead to uveitis, hypopyon, or hyphaema and involvement of the trabecular meshwork may cause secondary glaucoma.

Exophytic tumours (Fig. 27.1.2) grow into the sub-retinal space leading to retinal detachment. Eventually Bruch's membrane is breached and spread into the choroid occurs. Metastatic dissemination via the choroidal vessels or spread along the ciliary vessels and nerves to the orbit may occur in advanced cases.

Retinoblastomas of both types commonly infiltrate the optic nerve head and spread via the nerve to the chiasm or into the subarachnoid space may occur. Involvement of the cut end of the optic nerve is a poor prognostic sign. Diffusely infiltrating retinoblastoma (Fig. 27.1.3) is uncommon and as it rarely give rise to a solid mass or retinal detachment may lead to difficulty with diagnosis. Morgan (1971) reviewed ten such cases and found that they occurred in an older age group, were unilateral and often presented with a hypopyon. Cytology of aqueous was useful in making a diagnosis. In this series the prognosis after enucleation was good.

Metastatic spread may occur in four ways (Zimmerman 1985):

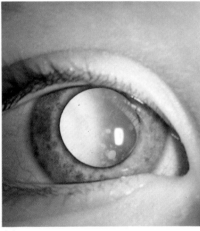

(a)

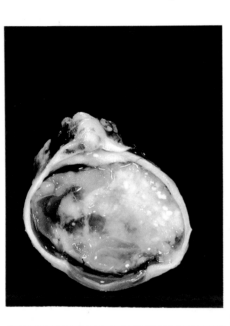

cms 1   2   3

(b)

Fig. 27.1.1 (a) Endophytic retinoblastoma. The tumour has invaded the vitreous and seedlings can be seen behind the lens. (b) Calotte of enucleated eye with tumour filling the eye (same patient).

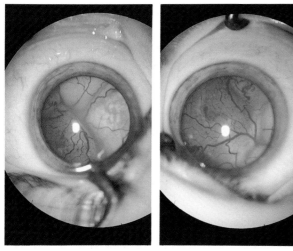

(a)

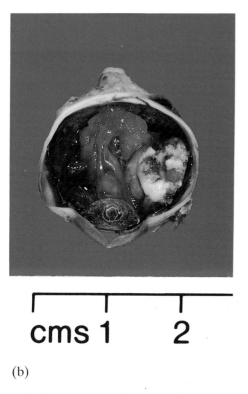

cms 1   2

(b)

Fig. 27.1.2 (a) Exophytic retinoblastoma with retinal detachment and tumour seen in the subretinal space. (b) Calotte of enucleated eye with exophytic retinoblastoma.

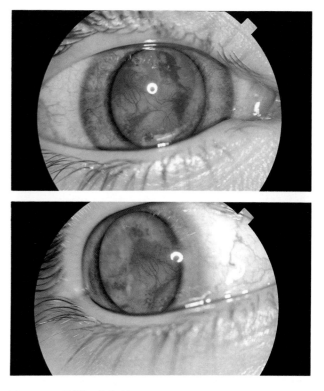

Fig. 27.1.3 Diffusely infiltrating retinoblastoma. The 5-year-old patient had presented with uveitis with hypopyon, retinal detachment and no calcification on the CT scan or ultrasound.

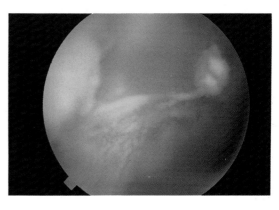

Fig. 27.1.4 Multifocal retinoblastoma with one tumour invading the optic disc.

1 Via the optic nerve (Fig. 27.1.4) to the brain or via the nerve sheath into the CSF of the subarachnoid space and then to the brain and spinal cord.

2 From the optic nerve or via the scleral foraminae into the orbit (Fig. 27.1.5).

3 Haematogenous spread via the choroidal circulation. The bone marrow is commonly involved early and later there may be bone, lymph node, and liver involvement. Lung metastases are rare.

4 Rarely extensive involvement of the anterior segment or adnexae may lead to lymphatic spread (Fig. 27.1.6).

Metastatic spread tends to occur early and is rare later than 3 years following treatment (Sanders *et al*. 1988).

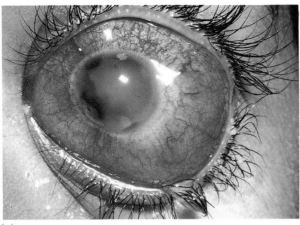

(a)

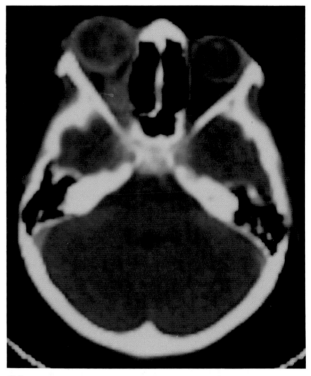

(b)

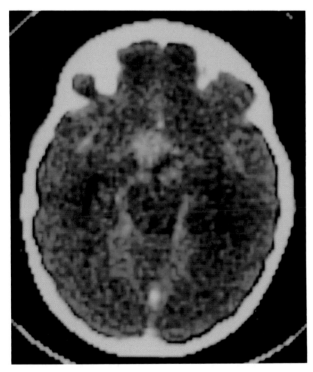

(c)

Fig. 27.1.5 Retinoblastoma. Late diagnosed with orbital optic nerve and intracranial extension.

Other manifestations of the retinoblastoma gene

As well as the retinal tumour other manifestations of the retinoblastoma gene include retinoma, ectopic intracranial retinoblastoma (trilateral retinoblastoma), and second non-ocular malignancies.

Retinoma

A retinoma is a non-malignant manifestation of the retinoblastoma gene. It is seen as an elevated grey retinal mass; calcification is often present and there be surrounding pigment epithelial proliferation and pigmentation (Fig. 27.1.7). Fluorescein angiography usually demonstrates an abnormal retinal circulation over the surface of the mass and in some cases there is associated neovascularisation (Gallie *et al*. 1982).

Retinomas are thought to originate in childhood and do not progress. Gallie *et al*. (1982) have suggested that retinomas develop when the second 'hit' or mutation occurs in a fully developed retinal cell that has lost its potential for malignant change, resulting in a benign disordered growth of the retina.

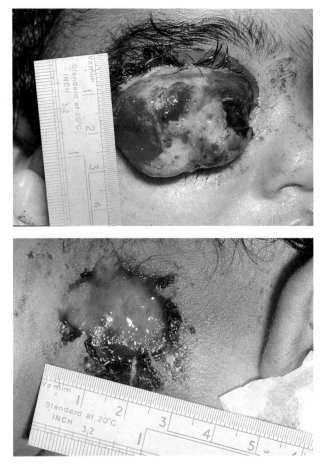

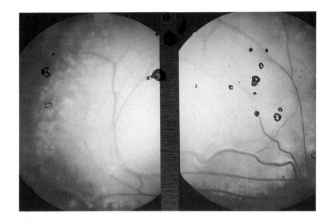

Fig. 27.1.7 Retinoma. Professor A.C. Bird's patient. Slide damaged in reproduction

Fig. 27.1.6 Late diagnosed retinoblastoma with involvement of occipital and other lymph nodes.

The importance of retinoma lies in its significance for genetic counselling; its presence indicates that the individual is carrying the retinoblastoma gene.

Second non-ocular malignancies

Children with the hereditary form of retinoblastoma are at increased risk of developing second non-ocular malignancies (Abramson *et al.* 1976; Abramson *et al.* 1984; Draper *et al.* 1986) which may occur within or outside the radiation field. Osteosarcoma is the commonest tumour seen but a wide variety of other neoplasms have been reported. (Abrahamson 1984; Zimmerman 1985).

Ectopic intracranial retinoblastoma (trilateral retinoblastoma)

The association of a midline tumour and hereditary retinoblastoma was first described by Jakobeic *et al.* in

1977 (1977). Bader *et al.* (1980) later coined the term trilateral retinoblastoma as they believed the intracranial mass to be a new primary tumour rather than metastases. About 2% of cases of retinoblastoma have evidence of ectopic intracranial tumour (Kingston *et al.* 1985) and in most cases the retinoblastoma is familial or bilateral. Affected children usually present with symptoms and signs of raised intracranial pressure and are found to have a pineal or parasellar mass on CT scan (Fig. 27.1.8). Histopathologically they are neuroblastic in origin and often resemble non differentiated retinoblastomas. The prognosis is very poor and ectopic intracranial retinoblastoma is the commonest cause of death in the hereditary form of retinoblastoma in the first 10 years after diagnosis (Kingston *et al.* 1985; Sanders 1988).

Clinical aspects

Presentation

Most children with retinoblastoma present with leucocoria (Fig. 27.1.9) (Ellsworth 1969; Shields 1983). The parents will often notice an odd appearance in their child's eye or see an odd reflex on a colour photograph. The extent of this appearance will depend on the ambient lighting conditions and position of the child's gaze so unless the paediatrician or general practitioner is aware of the importance of this symptom and specifically looks for the 'red reflex' with an ophthalmoscope the diagnosis may be missed.

The next most common presenting sign is strabismus which may be esotropia or exotropia (Ellsworth 1969; Shields 1983); it is constant and unilateral rather than alternating and the vision in the squinting eye is poor. All young children with a constant unilateral squint

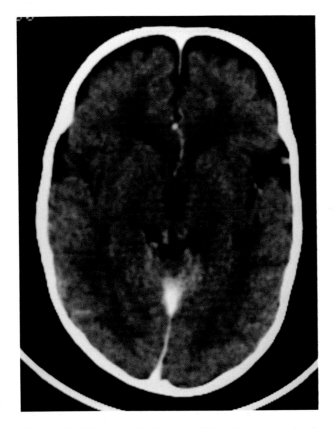

Fig. 27.1.8 Trilateral retinoblastoma. Vascular mass in pineal region.

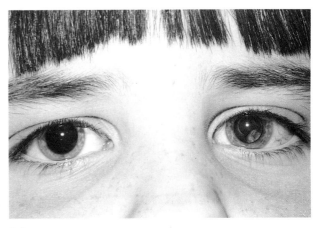

(a)

Fig. 27.1.9 (a) Leukocoria. For 2-years this 5-year-old's mother had noticed a strange white reflex from the pupil in certain combinations of light and positions of gaze. It was only when the tumour became visible in the vitreous through the pupil that the referral was made which led to the diagnosis of retinoblastoma.

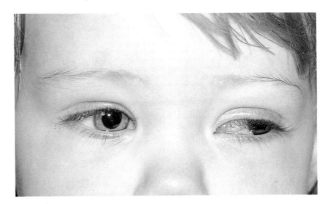

(b)

Fig. 27.1.9 (b) Retinoblastoma presenting with leukocoria and strabismus. The eye is red because of anterior segment involvement and glaucoma.

should have a careful fundus examination to rule out this diagnosis.

Other presenting symptoms and signs (Table 27.1.1) include painful red eye, orbital cellulitis secondary to extensive intraocular tumour necrosis, unilateral mydriasis, heterochromia, hyphaema, hypopyon uveitis, and nystagmus (due to bilateral macular involvement) (Ellsworth 1969). Retinoblastomas may also be found on routine examination of close relatives of children with hereditary retinoblastoma before any symptoms are present. In developing countries many children present late and extensive unilateral proptosis with orbital extension of the tumour is a common presentation (see Fig. 27.1.6).

Diagnosis

When a child is referred with a possible diagnosis of retinoblastoma, a careful history, and thorough ocular and systemic examination should be performed before any specialized investigations are carried out. A

Table 27.1.1 Presenting symptoms and signs of retinoblastoma (Ellsworth 1969).

White reflex	56%
Strabismus	20%
Glaucoma	7%
Poor vision	5%
Routine examination	3%
Orbital cellulitis	3%
Unilateral mydriasis	2%
Heterochromia iridis	1%
Hyphaema	1%
Other	2%

Table 27.1.2 Differential diagnosis of retinoblastoma (modified from Shields & Augsburger 1981).

Hereditary conditions	Inflammatory conditions
Norrie's disease	Toxocariasis
Warburg syndrome	Toxoplasmosis
Autosomal recessive retinal dysplasia	Metastatic endophthalmitis
Dominant exudative vitreoretinopathy	Viral retinitis
Juvenile X-linked retinoschisis	Vitritis
	Orbital cellulitis
Developmental anomolies	
Persistent hyperplastic primary vitreous	Tumours
Cataract	Astrocytic hamartoma
Coloboma	Medullo-epithelioma
Congenital retinal fold	Choroidal haemangioma
Myelinated nerve fibres	Combined hamartoma of retina and pigment epithelium
High myopia	
Morning glory syndrome	Others
	Coats' disease
	Retinopathy of prematurity
	Rhegmatogenous retinal detachment
	Vitreous haemorrhage
	Leukemic infiltration of the iris

number of other ocular conditions may simulate retinoblastoma (Table 27.1.2) and many of these can be excluded by a careful history and examination.

History

A careful history of the pregnancy, labour, delivery, birth weight, and neonatal period should be taken; illnesses in early pregnancy, premature labour and oxygen use in the neonatal period may all be relevant. The onset of the leukocoria should be ascertained as an abnormality present at birth is more likely to be due to a developmental anomaly; leukocoria presents at an average age of 12 months in bilateral retinoblastoma and 24 months in unilateral cases. (Shields & Augsburger 1981). In an older infant with leukocoria the parents should be asked about contact with puppies and other animals. A careful family history of any eye disorder should be obtained and if positive the likely mode of inheritance noted; arrangements should also be made to examine the fundi of both parents, the siblings, and any other affected family members.

Examination

Children presenting with suspected retinoblastoma can be broadly divided into three groups. In the first group there is a clear fundus view and the tumour can readily be visualized. In the second group, an adequate fundus examination is not possible due to vitreous opacity or extensive retinal detachment. The third group includes cases with unusual presentation such

as heterochromia, hypopyon uveitis or orbital cellulitis. It is in the latter two groups that specialized investigations are particularly helpful.

A thorough fundus examination is performed and in infants and young children a full general anaesthetic is necessary. The pupils should be widely dilated and scleral depression used to facilitate visualization of the ora serrata. In atypical cases, transillumination may be helpful in distinguishing solid from serous or rhegmatogenous detachment.

When the tumour is visible the diagnosis is usually straightforward; endophytic growth gives rise to a creamy pink coloured mass (Fig. 27.1.10) projecting into the vitreous with large irregular blood vessels running on the surface and penetrating the tumour. Haemorrhage may be present on the surface of the tumour and clumps of tumour cells may be seen in the adjacent vitreous. Vitreous seeding is virtually pathognomonic of retinoblastoma. Some tumours are surrounded by a halo of proliferating retinal pigment epithelium (Ellsworth 1969). Calcification within the tumour mass is common and is seen clinically as white, 'cottage cheese', appearance (Fig. 27.1.11); the presence of calcification may be confirmed by ultrasound or CT scan (Fig. 27.1.12). Less commonly, retinoblastoma may present as an avascular white mass in the retinal periphery (Ellsworth 1969).

When a clear view of the fundus cannot be obtained other aspects of the examination may give a clue to diagnosis. Retinoblastoma occurs in normal sized eyes; the presence of microphthalmos makes a developmental abnormality much more likely. It is also im-

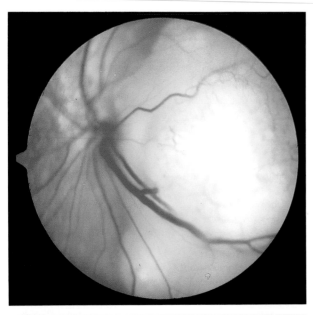

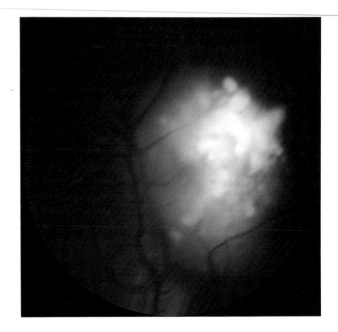

Fig. 27.1.11 Extensive calcification on the surface of an exophytic retinoblastoma seen under the detached retina.

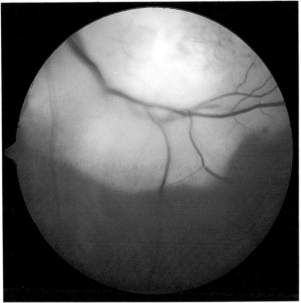

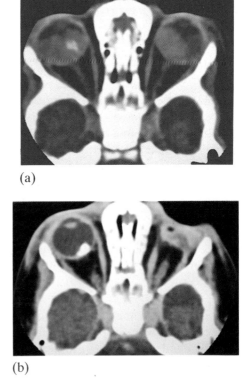

(a)

(b)

Fig. 27.1.10 Retinoblastoma. Creamy raised tumour extending from mid periphery to the optic nerve. The cut end of the nerve was free of tumour at enucleation.

portant to examine the other eye as this may give a clue to diagnosis. The presence of small tumours will confirm the diagnosis of retinoblastoma whereas dragged retinal vessels and peripheral vitreoretinal changes for example may be seen in retinopathy of prematurity and dominant exudative vitreo-retinopathy (DEVR).

Both parents should be examined to exclude a retinoma or other genetic conditions simulating retinoblastoma such as DEVR.

Fig. 27.1.12 (a) Retinoblastoma. CT scan showing calcification within the tumour in both eyes. (b) After enucleation of left eye and radiotherapy to the right eye, showing increase in calcification after treatment (same patient).

Infants with suspected retinoblastoma should be referred to a paediatrician for a careful systemic examination. This is especially important when the diagnosis has been confirmed when a number of specialized investigations will need to be performed to exclude metastatic spread. The systemic evaluation may also suggest alternative diagnoses, for example the findings of typical skin lesions in tuberose sclerosis or incontinentia pigmenti.

Differential diagnosis

The conditions which may simulate retinoblastoma are detailed in Table 27.1.2 Shields and Augsberger have found ocular toxocariasis, PHPV, and Coat's disease to be the three commonest conditions confused with retinoblastoma in referrals to the Oncology Service at the Wills Eye Hospital (Shields & Augsberger 1981). In many cases the true diagnosis may be made after consideration of the history, family history, and findings at examination under anaesthetic. If the retina can be visualized the diagnosis is rarely in doubt although the retinal lesions of tuberose sclerosis may be confused with small tumours especially in young infants. Most difficulties with diagnosis arise in those cases where the retina cannot be easily visualized.

Ocular toxocariasis

Ocular inflammation due to toxocariasis presents either as a chronic endophthalmitis with an opaque vitreous, or as a solitary granuloma in the posterior or peripheral retina in an otherwise healthy child; systemic symptoms or signs are rare (Duguid 1961). In both situations the diagnosis may be confused with retinoblastoma. Several features help to differentiate the two. In toxocariasis where there is marked vitreous inflammation, yellow-grey strands may be seen extending into the vitreous from the chorioretinal lesions; these are rarely seen in retinoblastoma (Ellsworth 1969). CT scan of the eye will often show calcification in retinoblastoma which is not seen in toxocariasis. Solitary granulomas resemble retinoblastoma but in the former there is often a small translucent centre (Ellsworth 1969). If there is doubt about the diagnosis, a period of observation with regular fundus examination of a solitary lesion will usually lead to the correct diagnosis. A positive ELISA test is of limited value as exposure to the organism is common.

Persistent hyperplastic primary vitreous (PHPV) (see Chapter 26)

This condition is usually noted at birth or soon afterwards; it is almost always unilateral. The affected eye is microphthalmic and there is a dense retrolental mass which may be vascularized; the ciliary processes are often prominent and drawn towards the centre of the pupil. Untreated involved eyes may develop pupil block glaucoma, vitreous haemorrhage, retinal detachment or phthysis bulbi; early surgery may prevent many of these complications and some reasonable visual results have been reported. Liang et al. (1985) have reported one infant with unilateral leucocoria who had both PHPV and a diffuse infiltrating retinoblastoma.

Where there is doubt about the diagnosis ultrasound and CT scan of the eyes is helpful.

Coats' disease (see Chapter 27.7)

This condition is almost always unilateral and is much more frequent in boys. An exudative detachment with tortuous dilated telangiectatic vessels is seen and at a later stage there are subretinal lipid and cholesterol crystals. Although telangiectatic vessels may be seen in retinoblastoma, the extensive vascular changes, subretinal lipid and cholesterol and absence of vitreous seeding help to differentiate this from retinoblastoma. Ultrasound and CT scan are helpful in that intraocular calcification is not seen in Coats' disease. Treatment of Coats' disease with cryotherapy or Xenon photocongulation may arrest the disease or result in some improvement (Ridley et al. 1982).

Retinal dysplasia (see Chapter 26)

Retinal dysplasia presents as a bilateral retrolental mass at birth or soon afterwards. There is no history of prematurity or oxygen use. In trisomy 13, it is seen in association with a variety of other serious systemic abnormalities. A similar ocular condition is seen in Norrie's disease, incontinentia pigmenti, Warburg syndrome and it may also occur as an isolated finding in an otherwise normal child. Examination under anaesthetic will reveal a shallow anterior chamber, clear lens and a relatively avascular retrolental mass without any inflammatory signs. There is no calcification on ultrasound or CT scan.

Retinopathy of prematurity (ROP)

Advanced cicatricial ROP may give rise to a dense retrolental mass which may be unilateral or bilateral. It is seen predominantly in very low birth weight infants who have been exposed to oxygen and seldom gives rise to confusion with retinoblastoma.

Metastatic endophthalmitis

Metastatic endophthalmitis results from haematogenous spread of infection from a distant infective locus such as meningitis, endocarditis or abdominal sepsis. *Streptococcus*, *Staphylococcus*, and *Meningococci* are the organisms most commonly involved. The condition may cause marked vitreous opacification but the presence of other inflammatory signs and systemic infection distinguishes this condition from retinoblastoma.

Medullo-epithelioma (diktyoma)

This tumour arises from the ciliary epithelium and is always unilateral. It may present with leucocoria but can be differentiated from retinoblastoma by its later age of onset, anterior origin from the ciliary body and cystic structure (Broughton & Zimmerman 1975).

They are white friable tumours, sometimes with a felt-like structure (Fig. 27.1.13) that are best treated by enucleation since local excision is not usually successful (Canning *et al*. 1988). Life expectancy is good.

OTHER DISORDERS

Extensive myelinated nerve fibres, optic nerve coloboma, high myopia and congenital cataract may all present with leucocoria but a careful examination including a refraction will differentiate them from retinoblastoma.

Occasionally chronic granulomatous uveitis especially if there is a hypopyon may present diagnostic difficulties especially if the posterior segment cannot be visualized. Ultrasound and CT scan is again helpful in ruling out posterior segment tumour. If there is still doubt about the diagnosis, aspiration of aqueous via a corneal paracentesis, for cytology may be performed.

INVESTIGATION

A number of investigations including fluoroscein angiography, ultrasound, CT scan, cytology, and aqueous enzyme studies may be helpful in suspected

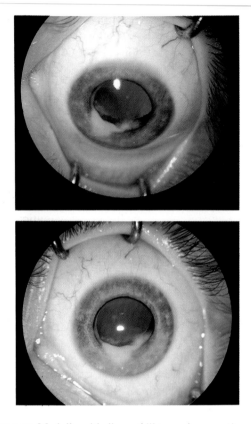

Fig. 27.1.13 Medulloepithelioma (diktyoma) presenting as a felt like structure arising in the ciliary body and involving the iris.

cases of retinoblastoma where the diagnosis is not apparent from clinical examination. Fluoroscein angiography may be helpful in distinguishing retinoblastoma from Coat's disease or DEVR but is not used routinely because of the difficulty in obtaining good quality angiograms in infants. CT scanning is extremely useful in cases where the fundus cannot be visualised (Char *et al*. 1984). Retinoblastoma appears as an intraocular mass with calcification, (see Fig. 27.1.12) an appearance which is almost pathognemonic of retinoblastoma; not all retinoblastomas however show calcification. In addition, CNS involvement or a second tumour such as a pinealoblastoma can be excluded at the same time. Ultrasound is also very useful in differentiating retinoblastoma from other causes of leucocoria (Sterns *et al*. 1974).

The levels of lactate dehydrogenase in the aqueous are elevated in retinoblastoma and in selected cases enzyme studies of the aqueous may be helpful in reaching a diagnosis. However, in about 8% of cases of retinoblastoma, aqueous LDH levels are within the normal range (Abramson *et al*. 1979). In cases of suspected retinoblastoma with anterior segment in-

the offspring of individuals with unilateral retinoblastoma have a 7.5% risk of carrying the abnormal gene, and a 5.7% risk of developing retinoblastoma (Table 27.1.4). The probability of other relatives developing the tumour can be calculated in a similar way to bilateral retinoblastoma (Musarella & Gallie 1987).

The recent advances in the detection of submicroscopic deletions and the recent isolation and sequencing of a candidate gene for retinoblastoma may allow more specific genetic counselling, especially in families with two or more affected individuals. In 95% of such families retinoblastoma gene testing can accurately identify those individuals carrying the retinoblastoma mutation (Wiggs & Dryja 1988). It is hoped that further advances will allow similar techniques to be used in non-familial retinoblastoma.

References

Abramson DH, Ellsworth RM, Kitchin D, Tung G. Second non-ocular tumours in retinoblastoma survivors. Are they radiation induced? *Ophthalmology* 1984; **91**: 1351−5

Abramson DH, Ellsworth RM, Zimmerman LE. Non-ocular cancers in retinoblastoma survivors. *Trans Am Acad Ophthalmol Otolaryngol* 1976; **81**: 454−7

Abramson DH, Piro PA, Ellsworth RM *et al*. Lactate dehydrogenase levels and iso enzyme patterns: measurements in the aqueous humor and serum of retinoblastoma patients. *Arch Ophthalmol* 1979; **97**: 870−1

Albert DM, Dryja TP. Recent studies of the retinoblastoma gene, what it means to the ophthalmologist. *Arch Ophthalmol* 1988; **106**: 181−2

Albert DM, Saulenas AM, Cohen SM. Verhoeffs query: is vitamin D effective against retinoblastoma. *Arch Ophthalmol* 1988; **106**: 536−40

Bader JL, Miller RW, Meadows AT, Zimmerman LE, Champion LAA, Voute PA. Trilateral retinoblastoma. *Lancet* 1980; **ii**: 582−3

Broughton WL, Zimmerman LE. A clinicopathologic study of 56 cases of intraocular medulloepitheliomas. *Am J Ophthalmol* 1978; **85**: 407−18

Canning CR, McCartney ACE, Hungerford J. Medulloepithelioma (diktyoma). *Br J Ophthalmol* 1988; **72**: 764−7

Char DH, Hedges TR, Norman D. Retinoblastoma CT diagnosis. *Ophthalmology* 1984; **91**: 1347−5

Char DH, Miller TR. Fine needle biopsy in retinoblastoma. *Am J Ophthalmol* 1984; **97**: 686−90

Cohen SM, Saulenas AM, Sullivan CR, Albert DM. Further studies on the affect of vitamin D on retinoblastoma. *Arch Ophthalmol* 1988; **106**: 541−3

Cowell JK, Rutland P, Jay M, Hungerford J. Deletions of the esterase D locus from a survey of 200 retinoblastoma patients. *Hum Genet* 1986; **72**: 164−7

Draper GJ, Sanders BM, Kingston JE. Retinoblastoma and second primary tumours. *Br J Cancer* 1986; **53**: 661−71

Dryja TP, Rapaport JM, Joyce JM *et al*. Molecular detection of the deletion involving band q14 on the long arm of chromo-some 13 in retinoblastoma. *Proc Natl Acad Sci USA* 1986; **83**: 7391−4

Duguid IM. Features of ocular infestation by toxocara. *Br J Ophthalmol* 1961; **45**: 789−96

Ellsworth RM. The practical management of retinoblastoma. *Trans Am Ophthalmol Soc* 1969; **67**: 462−534

François J, De Bie S, Multon-Van Leuven MT. Genesis and genetics of retinoblastoma. *J Pediatr Ophthalmol Strabismus* 1979; **16**: 85−100

Friend SH, Bernards R, Regelj S *et al*. A human DNA segment with properties of the gene that predisposes to retinoblastoma and osteosarcoma *Nature* 1986; **323**: 643−6

Gallie BL. Gene carrier detection in retinoblastoma. *Ophthalmology* 1980; **87**: 591−4

Gallie BL, Phillips RA. Retinoblastoma: a model of oncogenesis. *Ophthalmology* 1984; **91**: 666−72

Gallie BL, Phillips RA, Ellsworth RM, Abrahamson DH. Significance of retinoma and phthysis bulbi for retinoblastoma. *Ophthalmology* 1982; **89**: 1393−9

Howard RO, Breg WR, Albert DM, Lesser RL. Retinoblastoma and chromosomal abnormality. *Arch Ophthalmol* 1974; **92**: 490−3

Hungerford JL, Kingston JE, Plowman PN. Orbital recurrence in retinoblastoma. *Ophthalmol Paediatr Genet* 1987; **8**: 63−8

Jacobiec FA, Tso MOM, Zimmerman LE, Danis P. Retinoblastoma and intracranial malignancy. *Cancer* 1977; **39**: 2048−8

Kingston JE, Plowman PN, Hungerford JL. Ectopic intracranial retinoblastoma in childhood. *Br J Ophthalmol* 1985; **69**: 742−8

Knudson AG Jr. Mutation and cancer: a statistical study of retinoblastoma. *Proc Natl Acad Sci USA* 1971; **68**: 820−3

Knudson AG, Meadows AT, Nichols WW, Hill R. Chromosomal deletions and retinoblastoma. *N Engl J Med* 1976; **295**: 1120−3

Lee WH, Bookstein R, Hong F *et al*. Human retinoblastoma susceptibility gene, cloning identification and sequence. *Science* 1987; **235**: 1394−9

Lele KP, Penrose LS, Stallard HB. Chromosome deletion in a case of retinoblastoma. *Ann Hum Genet* 1963; **27**: 171−4

Lennox EL, Draper GJ, Sanders BM. Retinoblastoma: a study of natural history and prognosis of 268 cases. *Br Med J* 1975; **iii**: 731−4

Liang JC, Augsburger JJ, Shields JA. Diffuse infiltrating retinoblastoma associated with persistant primary vitreous. *J Paediatr Ophthalmol Strabismus* 1985; **22**: 31−3

Magramm I, Abramson D, Ellsworth RM. Optic nerve involvement in retinoblastoma. *Ophthalmology* 1989; **96**: 217−23

Migdal C. Retinoblastoma occurring in 4 successive generations. *Br J Ophthalmol* 1976; **60**: 151−2

Morgan G. Diffuse infiltrating retinoblastoma. *Br J Ophthalmol* 1971; **55**: 600−6

Murphree AL, Benedict WF. Retinoblastoma clues to human oncogenesis. *Science* 1985; **223**: 1028−33

Musarella MA, Gallie BL. Retinoblastoma In: Renie WA (Ed.) *Goldberg's Genetic and Metabolic Eye Disease*, 2nd Edn. Little, Brown & Co., Boston 1986; pp. 423−38

Musarella MA, Gallie BL. A simplified scheme for genetic counselling in retinoblastoma. *J Paediatr Ophthalmol Strabismus* 1987; **24**: 124−5

Ridley ME, Shields JA, Brown GC, Tasman W. Coats' disease: evaluation of management. *Ophthalmology* 1982; **89**: 1381−7

Salmonsen PC, Ellsworth RM, Kitchen FD. The occurrence of new retinoblastoma after treatment. *Ophthalmology* 1979; **86**: 840−3

Sanders BM, Draper GJ, Kingston JE. Retinoblastoma in Great Britain 1969−80 incidence, treatment and survival. *Br J Ophthalmol* 1988; **72**: 576−83

Saulenas AM, Cohen SM, Key L *et al.* Vitamin D and retinoblastoma. The presence of receptors and inhibition of growth in vitro. *Arch Ophthalmol* 1988; **106**: 533−5

Shields JA. *Diagnosis and Management of Intraocular Tumours*. CV Mosby Co., St Louis 1983

Shields JA, Augsburger JJ. Current approaches to the diagnosis and management of retinoblastoma. *Survey Ophthalmol* 1981; **25**: 347−71

Sparkes RS, Murphree AL, Lingua RW *et al.* Gene for hereditary retinoblastoma assigned to chromosome 13 by linkeage to esterase D. *Science* 1983; **219**: 971−3

Sparkes RS, Sparkes MC, Wilson MG *et al.* Regional assignment of genes for human esterase D and retinoblastoma to chromosome band 13q14. *Science* 1980; **208**: 1042−4

Sterns GK, Coleman DJ, Ellsworth RM. Ultrasound graphic characteristics of retinoblastoma. *Am J Ophthalmol* 1974; **78**: 608−11

Wiggs JL, Dryja TP. Predicting the risk in hereditary retinoblastoma. *Am J Ophthalmol* 1988; **106**: 346−51

Wilson EG, Ebbin AJ, Towner JW, Spencer WH. Chromosomal anomalies in patients with retinoblastoma. *Clin Genet* 1977; **12**: 1−8

Zimmerman LE. Retinoblastoma and retinocytoma In: Spencer WH (Ed.) *Ophthalmic Pathology*: *An Atlas and Textbook*, 3rd Edn. WB Saunders Co., Philadelphia 1985; pp. 1292−351

27.2 Retinopathy of Prematurity

ANTHONY MOORE

Retinopathy of prematurity (ROP) was first recognized in 1942 when Terry (1942) published a description of the histological findings in advanced cicatricial ROP. As more cases were reported it became evident that the disease was confined to premature infants and retrospective studies showed it to be extremely rare before 1942. Terry (1945) and later Owens and Owens (1948) showed that the retinopathy developed in infants who had a normal fundus examination at birth demonstrating that the disease developed in postnatal life. Retinopathy of prematurity subsequently became the leading cause of blindness in children in the USA and a similar epidemic of ROP was seen in Europe during the 1950s.

Following Campbell's suggestion (Campbell 1951) that the onset of this condition might be related to the introduction of oxygen therapy into the premature nursery, evidence accumulated to support the concept of a toxic effect of oxygen on the immature retinal vaculature. However, subsequent restriction of oxygen use failed to eradicate the disease completely and it is now clear that many factors other than oxygen may play a role in the pathogenesis of ROP (Lucey & Dangman 1984; Ben Sira et al. 1988). The history of the scientific investigation of the pathogenesis of ROP makes fascinating reading and has been comprehensively reviewed by James and Lansman (1976); Silverman (1980); and Lucey and Dangman (1984).

Classification

The international classification of the acute stages of ROP was published in 1984 (Committee for the Classification of ROP 1984) and in 1987 (Committee for the Classification of ROP 1987) a classification of the retinal detachment and other changes of the disease was agreed to replace Reese et al.'s (1953) classification. All stages of ROP are now covered by one internationally agreed classification and the term retrolental fibroplasia is no longer used.

This new classification allows the location, extent and severity of the disease to be specified and has been demonstrated to be useful in clinical practice (Flynn 1985), the findings being recorded on one of various clinical charts (Fig. 27.2.1).

Location

The retina is divided into three zones (Fig. 27.2.1) which are centred on the optic disc, rather than the macula. Zone 1 consists of a circle centred on the disc, the radius of which is twice the distance from the

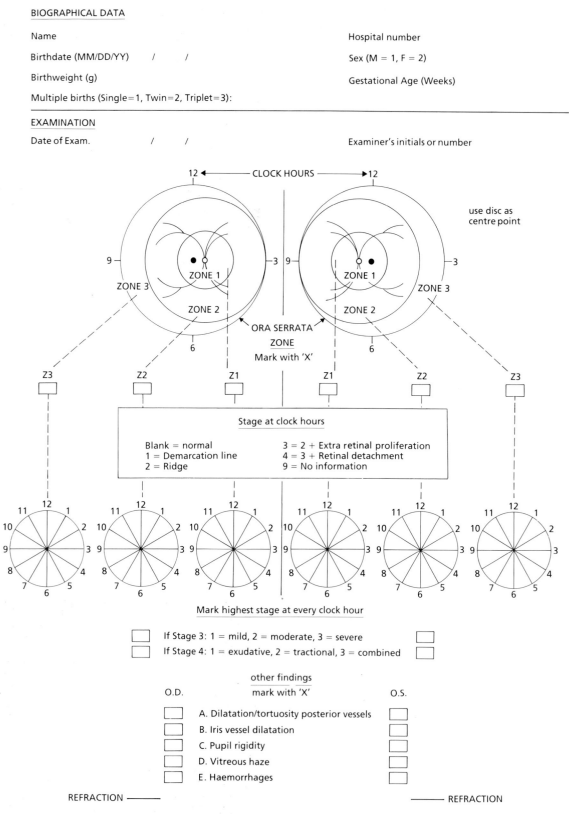

BIOGRAPHICAL DATA

Name   Hospital number

Birthdate (MM/DD/YY)   /   /   Sex (M = 1, F = 2)

Birthweight (g)   Gestational Age (Weeks)

Multiple births (Single=1, Twin=2, Triplet=3):

EXAMINATION

Date of Exam.   /   /   Examiner's initials or number

12 ◄——— CLOCK HOURS ———► 12

use disc as
centre point

9 —   — 3   9 —   — 3
              ZONE 1   ZONE 1
        ZONE 3   ZONE 3
              ZONE 2   ZONE 2
                        6   6

ORA SERRATA
ZONE
Mark with 'X'

Z3   Z2   Z1   Z1   Z2   Z3

Stage at clock hours

Blank = normal   3 = 2 + Extra retinal proliferation
1 = Demarcation line   4 = 3 + Retinal detachment
2 = Ridge   9 = No information

Mark highest stage at every clock hour

If Stage 3: 1 = mild, 2 = moderate, 3 = severe
If Stage 4: 1 = exudative, 2 = tractional, 3 = combined

other findings
mark with 'X'
O.D.   O.S.

A. Dilatation/tortuosity posterior vessels
B. Iris vessel dilatation
C. Pupil rigidity
D. Vitreous haze
E. Haemorrhages

REFRACTION ———   ——— REFRACTION

Fig. 27.2.1 Chart for recording fundus details and staging
ROP. Usually five stages are recorded (see text).

disc to the macula. Zone 2 extends from the edge of Zone 1 to the ora serrata on the nasal side and to the approximate equator on the temporal side. Zone 3 includes all retina temporally, superiorly and inferiorly which is anterior to zone 2.

Extent of disease

The extent of disease is described in clock hours. As the examiner looks at the eyes the 3 o'clock position is on the right, i.e. on the nasal side of the right eye and temporal side of the left eye.

Staging of disease

Retinopathy of prematurity has been divided into five stages (Table 27.2.1). In a normal premature infant the retina is not fully vascularized and the extent of the non-vascularized retina depends on the gestational age. Non-vascularized retina is paler and lacks retinal vessels; usually the vascularized and non-vascularized retina gradually merge into one another, but once a definate demarcation line is seen, stage 1 ROP has developed.

Stage 1

In stage 1 disease there is a definite flat white demarcation line separating vascularized from non-vascularized retina (Fig. 27.2.2, 27.2.3). Retinal vessels may run up to the line but do not cross it.

Stage 2

In stage 2 there is a ridge projecting into the vitreous separating vascularized and non-vascularized retina (Fig. 27.2.4, 27.2.5). The colour of the ridge may be

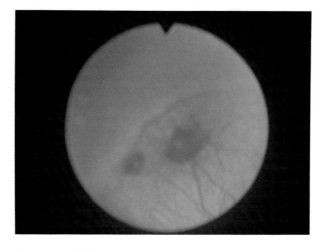

Fig. 27.2.2 ROP Stage 1 demarcation line. The haemorrhages are perinatal and not related to the ROP. Patient of Mr E Schulenburg.

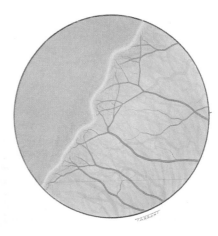

Fig. 27.2.3 ROP Stage 1. Painting showing avascular retina on left with clear non elevated demarcation line between this and the vascularized retina.

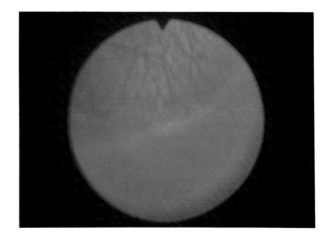

Fig. 27.2.4 ROP Stage II ridge projecting (out of focus) forward into the vitreous. Patient of Mr E. Schulenburg.

Table 27.2.1 Stages of retinopathy of prematurity (from Committee for Classification of ROP 1987).

Stage 1	Demarcation line	
Stage 2	Ridge	
Stage 3	Ridge with extraretinal fibrovascular proliferation	
Stage 4	Subtotal retinal detachment:	
	(a) extrafoveal	
	(b) retinal detachment including fovea	
Stage 5	Total retinal detachment	
Funnel	Anterior	Posterior
	Open	Open
	Narrow	Narrow
	Open	Narrow
	Narrow	Open

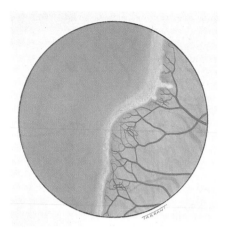

Fig. 27.2.5 ROP Stage II. Painting showing elevated ridge with small dilated vessels in it.

white or pink (Fig. 27.2.6) and small neo-vascular complexes may be seen posterior to the ridge.

Stage 3

At this stage extraretinal neovascularization is seen in addition to the features of stage 3 (Fig. 27.2.7–27.2.9). The new vessels project forwards from the ridge or from the retina posterior to the ridge, into the vitreous.

Stage 4

In this stage a subtotal retinal detachment which may be exudative (Fig. 27.2.10) or tractional is found which may (stage 4b) or may not (stage 4a) involve the fovea.

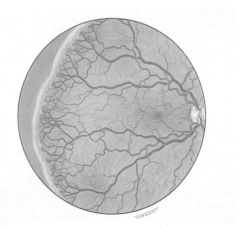

Fig. 27.2.6 ROP Stage II 'plus'. Painting showing vascular ridge with retinal vascular tortuosity.

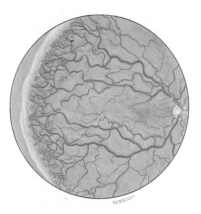

Fig. 27.2.7 ROP Stage III. Painting showing vascularized ridge with some new vessels projecting forwards from posterior to the ridge.

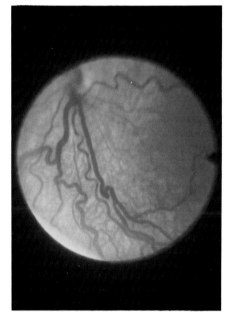

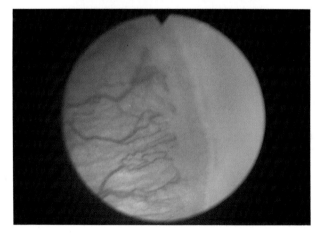

Fig. 27.2.8, 27.2.9 ROP Stage III plus showing ridge with new vessels and marked vascular dilatation and tortuosity. Patient of Mr E Schulenburg.

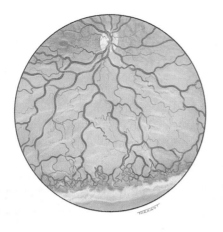

Fig. 27.2.10 ROP Stage IVa. Painting showing ridge and exudative detachment not involving the fovea.

Stage 5

In stage 5 there is a funnel shaped total retinal detachment (Fig. 27.2.11). This stage is further divided according to the characteristics of the funnel, whether it is open or narrowed anteriorly and posteriorly (Table 27.2.1).

PLUS DISEASE

When there is marked dilatation and tortuosity of the retinal veins at the posterior pole, the eye is said to have 'plus disease' (Fig. 27.2.6–27.2.9). Other features often seen in plus disease include vitreous haze, iris vascular engorgement and difficulty in achieving pupillary dilatation.

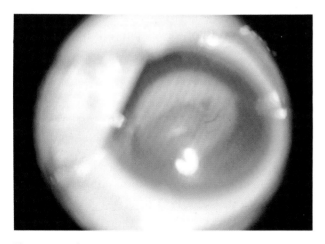

Fig. 27.2.11 Stage 5 funnel shaped retinal detachment. Patient of Mr E Schulenburg.

Other features of involved eyes which are not covered by the classification such as posterior synechiae, corneal oedema and angle closure glaucoma need to be recorded separately.

Pathogenesis

Although the introduction of oxygen therapy for preterm infants played a major role in the epidemic of ROP in the 1950s it is now evident that many different factors may be involved in its pathogenesis. A review of the enormous literature on this subject is outside the scope of this chapter but some of the more important factors related to the development of ROP will be discussed. Several excellent reviews of this subject have been recently published (Lucey & Dangman 1984; Flynn 1987; Ben Sira et al. 1988).

Associated factors

BIRTH WEIGHT AND GESTATIONAL AGE

The incidence and severity of ROP is inversely related to birth weight and gestational age (Kinsey et al. 1977; Flynn 1983; Keith & Kitchen 1983; Reisner et al. 1985, Flynn et al. 1987, Ng et al. 1988). Infants of very low birth weight (<1000 g) are particularly at risk. In the series of Reisner et al. (1985) 72% of infants of birth weight less than 1000 g developed acute ROP which is comparable to Flynn's series (1987) in which 89% of infants weighing less than 900 g at birth developed ROP. Above 1500 g birth weight the incidence falls to less than 10% (Reisner et al. 1985).

OXYGEN

Campbell (1951) was the first to suggest that supplemental oxygen was the cause for the sudden increase in the numbers of infants developing retrolental fibroplasia in the early 1950s. Subsequently Ashton et al. (1953) were able to demonstrate the toxic effect of oxygen on immature vessels in an animal model. Although several controlled trials (Patz et al. 1952; Lanman et al. 1954; Kinsey et al. 1956) comparing high and low supplemental oxygen in premature infants later confirmed the relationship between oxygen therapy and ROP, it has not been possible to define safe level of oxygen usage for clinical practice. When oxygen levels were reduced in the mid and late 1950s, although the incidence of ROP reduced, there was an increase in neonatal mortality (Avery & Oppenheimer 1960) and neurological morbidity (McDonald 1963) in preterm infants.

When arterial blood gas monitoring became available, a multicentre study was set up to try and define the level of arterial oxygen at which ROP would develop. The study (Kinsey *et al.* 1977) which used intermittent sampling from the umbilical artery failed to show any relationship between ROP and arterial blood oxygen tension. More recently Flynn *et al.* (1987) in a randomized controlled trial comparing continuous transcutaneous oxygen monitoring with standard neonatal care failed to show any reduction in ROP in the continuously monitored group, except in the older larger infants in whom ROP is less severe.

It is evident therefore that no direct relationship has been demonstrated between raised levels of arterial oxygen and ROP. In addition, ROP may develop in preterm infants who have never received oxygen and in premature infants with cyanotic heart disease (Lucey & Dangman 1984). Furthermore some studies have established a relationship between neonatal hypoxia and ROP (Lucey & Dangman 1984) and in an animal model retinal ischaemia may lead to the same retinal changes as hyperoxia (Ashton & Henkind 1965). One explanation for these seemingly contradictory findings is that relative hyperoxia may lead to initial vasoconstriction but that it is the subsequent peripheral retinal ischaemia or hypoxia that stimulates vasoproliferation. Generalised systemic hypoxia at this stage may lead to more advanced disease.

VITAMIN E DEFICIENCY

In the developing retina vascularization develops from the optic disc towards the more peripheral retina and is accompanied by the migration of spindle cells which are the precursors of inner retinal endothelial cells (Kretzner & Hittner 1988). It has been suggested that the relative hyperoxic environment (compared to *in utero*) of preterm infants results in free oxygen radical production which inhibits spindle cell migration and stimulates them to produce angiogenic factors responsible for ROP (Kretzner & Hittner 1988). The preterm infant is relatively deficient in vitamin E, a naturally occurring antioxidant, and the immature peripheral retina may lack interstitial retinal binding protein (IRBP) a carrier protein for vitamin E (Johnson *et al.* 1985).

It has been argued that vitamin E supplementation, by increasing the vitamin levels in immature retina will protect spindle cells from free radical damage and hence reduce the incidence of ROP. Anatomical

studies of postmortem eyes from preterm infants have demonstrated changes in spindle cells (Hittner & Kretzner 1983) and in an animal model vitamin E supplementation has been shown to reduce the severity of oxygen induced retinopathy (Phelps & Rosenbaum 1977).

Clinical trials of vitamin E supplementation in preterm infants (Hittner *et al.* 1981; Finer *et al.* 1982; Phelps *et al.* 1987; Johnson *et al.* 1988) have shown that although vitamin E does not appear to affect the frequency of ROP it may reduce its severity. Despite this evidence of a protective effect, concern about possible side effects of treatment, including sepsis (Johnson *et al.* 1985), necrotizing enterocolitis (Johnson *et al.* 1985; Johnson *et al.* 1988) retinal (Rosenbaum *et al.* 1985) and intraventricular haemorrhage (Phelps *et al.* 1987) has meant that high dose vitamin E therapy has yet to be widely accepted. A large multicentre trial may be necessary to answer the question of the efficacy and safety of supplemental vitamin E (Flynn 1987).

EXCHANGE TRANSFUSIONS

Preterm infants given blood transfusions receive adult haemoglobin which binds oxygen less avidly than foetal haemoglobin so more is given up to the tissues. This may result in relative hyperoxia of the retina and increase the risk of developing retinopathy of prematurity. Several studies (Aranda *et al.* 1975; Bard *et al.* 1975; Clark *et al.* 1981; Shohat *et al.* 1983) have demonstrated an association between ROP and blood transfusion but it is unclear whether there is a direct relationship or whether repeated blood transfusion is a marker of high risk infants. Those who need repeated blood transfusions are usually smaller, sicker and require longer duration of oxygen therapy and are therefore at high risk of developing ROP (Lucey & Dangman 1984).

OTHER FACTORS

Other factors which have been found to be associated with ROP include hypercapnia, pregnancy complications, intraventicular haemorrhage, recurrent apnoea, respiratory distress syndrome, and more recently light levels in the preterm nursery (Lucey & Dangman 1984; Flynn 1987; Ben Sira *et al.* 1988).

Clinical aspects

Clinical examination

Although it is agreed that all preterm infants at a significant risk of developing ROP should be examined by an ophthalmologist before discharge, there are no generally accepted guidelines suggesting which infants should be examined and when. It is clear however that the main aim of the examination should be to ensure that all infants with stage 3 ROP, who would benefit from treatment (Cryotherapy for ROP Co-operative Group 1988) and who are at a high risk of developing cicatrization, are recognized.

WHICH INFANTS SHOULD BE EXAMINED AND WHEN?

In the recent study of Ng et al. (1988) no infant of birth weight greater than 1500 g developed acute changes greater than stage 2 and all regressed without cicatrization. Similar findings have been reported by Kingham (1977). Although ideally all premature infants should be screened, if the examination is confined to those weighing less than 1500 g serious disease is unlikely to be missed. A reasonable practicable approach is to routinely examine all infants less than 1500 g or 34 weeks gestation. In addition, older more mature infants who have had particularly complicated medical problems in early life, for example, repeated blood transfusion, sepsis, or prolonged exposure to oxygen, are included.

The timing of the examination is also problematical; the examination should be deferred until the infant is well enough to tolerate it and is no longer requiring ventilation and intensive care, but not so long that the retinopathy is too advanced for treatment. Palmer (1981) has suggested that if a single screening examination is to be performed it is best carried out at age 7–9 weeks when the greatest numbers of cases of acute ROP will be recognized with the least chance of missing serious disease. It is however advisable to carry out more than one examination in high risk infants as with a single examination significant disease may be missed (Ng et al. 1988).

A reasonable approach is to examine infants as soon after 32 weeks post-conceptual age that their general condition permits, and then every 2 weeks while on the special care unit (Flynn 1987). If there is disease within zone 1 or 2 examinations should be performed weekly. In large secondary referral units where infants are often discharged early back to local neonatal units clear arrangements must be made for ophthalmic examinations to be continued locally until the retina is fully vascularized.

Infants with acute ROP should be seen again as outpatients after discharge and may need to be followed-up, long-term because of the increased risk of abnormal refractive errors, strabismus and amblyopia (Kushner 1982; Schaffer et al. 1984).

METHOD OF EXAMINATION

The ophthalmic examination should be performed using the indirect ophthalmoscope, a paediatric lid speculum and dilated pupils. A neonatal scleral indenter may be used if an adequate peripheral view cannot be obtained otherwise. Adequate pupillary dilatation can be achieved by using 1 drop of cyclopentolate 0.5% and phenylephrine 2.5% repeated once if necessary. The infants should be handled gently and it is helpful if a trained nurse is in attendance to help with the examination and to monitor the well being of the infant.

Clinical findings

Acute retinopathy of prematurity

In the mildest form of ROP (stage 1) a white line is seen at the junction between vascularized and non-vascularized retina, and is most commonly observed in the far peripheral retina (zone 3). As the disease advances, the line is replaced by a ridge of tissue projecting into the vitreous and neovascular complexes may be seen posterior to the ridge (stage 2). The vessels supporting the ridge are often dilated and tortuous. Flynn et al (1977) believe the demarcation line or ridge to represent an arteriovenous shunt formed by the anastomosis of primitive retinal vessels in areas of capillary loss and have demonstrated rapid flow and marked vascular leakage on fluorescein angiography (Flynn et al. 1977). Furthermore they have been able to demonstrate the abnormal shunt vessels and capillary circulation histopathologically (Kushner et al. 1978). With more advanced disease new vessels grow forward into the vitreous (stage 3) and retinal detachment, which may be partial (stage 4) or total (stage 5), may be seen. Other findings in advanced disease include marked vitreous haze, iris vascular engorgement, pupillary rigidity and tortuosity of the retinal vessels.

Regression and cicatrization

The acute changes of ROP occur over a limited period of time following which there is regression with or without cicatrization. In most cases there is complete regression without scarring (Ng *et al.* 1988) and in general the more advanced and posterior the disease the greater likelihood of developing significant cicatrisation (Flynn *et al.* 1977).

Early regression can be recognized firstly by a failure of the acute changes to progress and secondly by changes in the appearance of the shunt. The ridge changes colour from white-grey to pink and the neo-vascularization becomes less marked. Fluorescein angiography shows budding of regular capillaries from the shunt vessels which then form capillary complexes growing into the previously avascular retina (Flynn *et al.* 1977). When complete regression occurs the peripheral retina becomes fully vascularized.

Cicatrical changes occur when normal revascularization of the peripheral retina is incomplete. There is persistence of the arteriovenous shunts with related vascular changes and the peripheral retina becomes thin and atrophic. Other fundus abnormalities include retinal pigmentation, dragging of the retinal vessels, macular ectopia, retinal fold (Figs. 27.2.12–27.2.16) and retinal detachment (Table 27.2.2). Cicatrical changes in the vitreous and retina may push the lens forward and cause shallowing of the anterior chamber, glaucoma and corneal decompensation (Fig. 27.2.17). In such cases lensectomy may be indicated to relieve the pupil block glaucoma. In addition infants with cicatrical changes are at greater risk of developing strabismus, amblyopia and high

Table 27.2.2 Cicatrical changes in ROP (from Committee for the Classification of ROP 1987).

Peripheral changes	Posterior changes
Vascular	Vascular
Failure to vascularize peripheral retina	Vascular tortuosity
Abnormal, non-dichotomous branching of retinal vessels	Straightening of blood vessels in temporal arcade
Vascular arcades with circumferential interconnection	Decrease in angle of insertion of major temporal arcade
Telangiectatic vessels.	
Retinal	Retinal
Pigmentary changes	Pigmentary changes
Vitreoretinal interface changes	Distortion of ectopia macula
Thin retina	Stretching and folding of retina in macular region leading to periphery
Peripheral folds	
Vitreous membranes with or without attachment to retina	Vitreoretinal interface changes
Lattice-like degeneration	Vitreous membrane
Retinal breaks	Dragging of retina over disc
Traction/rhegmatogenous retinal detachment	Traction/rhegmetogenous retinal detachment

(usually myopic) refractive errors (Kushner 1982; Schaffer *et al.* 1984).

Treatment

Despite the extensive literature on the management of ROP (Kalina 1980; Ben Sira *et al.* 1988) there are no generally agreed guidelines for treatment. Discussion

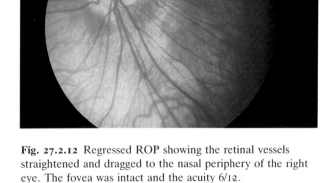

Fig. 27.2.12 Regressed ROP showing the retinal vessels straightened and dragged to the nasal periphery of the right eye. The fovea was intact and the acuity 6/12.

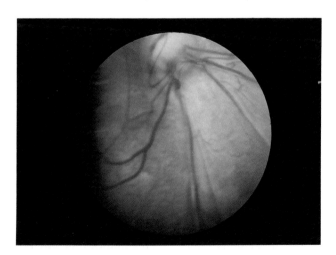

Fig. 27.2.13 Regressed ROP with marked nasal dragging of the vessels.

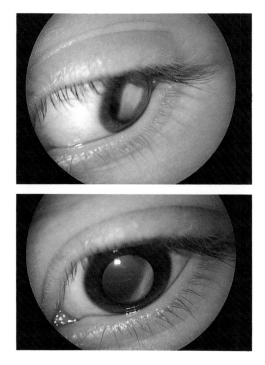

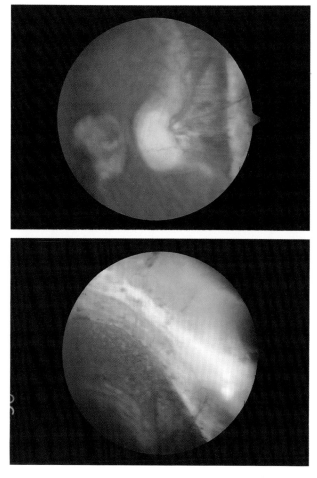

Fig. 27.2.14 Regressed ROP with retrolental membranes with temporal dragging of the retina the acuity in the left eye was 6/60 the right eye saw only hand movements.

Fig. 27.2.15, (top), and 27.2.16 Marked retinal dragging towards an area of chorioretinal atrophy and vitreoretinal fibrosis in the area of what was probably Stage 3 zone 1 disease.

has mainly centered on three areas; vitamin E supplementation, the treatment of acute disease with cryotherapy and the management of retinal detachment.

Vitamin E

Although there is some evidence that vitamin E supplementation may reduce the severity of acute ROP (Hittner *et al.* 1981; Finer *et al.* 1982; Phelps *et al.* 1987; Johnson *et al.* 1988) the failure to show a reduction of the incidence of disease and of cicatrical complications in the treated group and concern about possible side effects (Ben Sira *et al.* 1988; Flynn 1987) of high doses of vitamin E in preterm infants has meant that this form of treatment has not gained widespread acceptance.

Cryotherapy

In stage I and II ROP the most commonest outcome is regression and it is generally agreed that no treatment is necessary until stage III disease is reached. In 1986 a multicentre trial of cryotherapy in stage III disease was started and the preliminary results of the 3 month follow-up of 172 infants have recently been reported (Cryo-ROP Study 1988). An unfavourable outcome

(defined as posterior retinal detachment, retinal fold affecting the macula, or retrolental tissue) was significantly less frequent in eyes treated with cryotherapy compared to untreated eyes. No serious complications were seen and the authors recommend treatment of at least one eye when there is threshold disease (five or more continuous clock hours or eight cumulative clock hours of stage III ROP in zone I or II and 'plus' disease). In such patients 360° cryotherapy of the non-vascularized retina anterior to the ridge should be performed according to the protocol used in the trial (Cryo-ROP Study 1988). A prompt response to treatment is usually seen with resolution of plus disease and gradual resolution of the ridge (Ben Sira 1988). In cases where the disease remains active and there are gaps in the cryo reaction further treatment may be necessary.

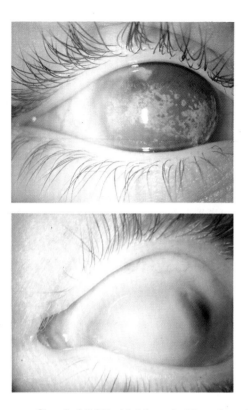

Fig. 27.2.17 Cicatrical ROP with bilateral obliteration of the anterior chamber and angle closure glaucoma with secondary corneal degenerative changes.

Retinal detachment surgery

The management of stage IV and V ROP is controversial. Stage IV ROP has been successfully treated with scleral buckling in older infants (Kalina 1980; McPherson *et al.* 1982) with exudative or tractional detachment but because of the relatively high incidence of spontaneous regression it is difficult to define the precise role of this form of treatment. In more advanced disease with total retinal detachment (stage V) it is clear that spontaneous reattachment will not occur and surgical intervention is more easily justified. Both 'open sky' (Tasman 1987) and closed vitrectomy (Machemer 1983; Chong *et al.* 1986; Trese 1986) approaches have been used. Although anatomical reattachment can be achieved in between 40 and 50% of cases (Chong *et al.* 1986; Trese 1986) the visual results are poor in most infants. This type of complex surgery is clearly at an early stage and it is possible that with more surgical experience, better patient selection and possibly earlier surgery, visual results may improve. In such advanced disease the retention of useful navigating vision could be considered a very successful result.

Prognosis

The prognosis for vision in most preterm infants is excellent; serious ocular disease is now mainly confined to infants of less than 1000 g birth weight (Flynn *et al.* 1987; Ng *et al.* 1988). Between 10 and 15% of these children will develop cicatrical retinal changes (Pape *et al.* 1978; Kitchen *et al.* 1982; Keith & Kitchen 1983) but bilateral blindness due to retinopathy of prematurity is uncommon (Keith & Kitchen 1983). Other ophthalmological findings include high myopic refractive errors, strabismus (commonly infantile esotropia) amblyopia and optic atrophy (Pape *et al.* 1978; Kitchen *et al.* 1982; Kushner 1982; Keith & Kitchen 1983; Nissenkorn *et al.* 1983; Schaffer *et al.* 1984).

Infants who develop acute ROP should be followed up regularly during childhood so that high refractive errors, strabismus and amblyopia can be recognized and treated early.

References

Aranda JV, Clark TE, Maniello R *et al.* Blood transfusions a possible potentiating risk factor in retrolental fibroplasia. *Pediatr Res* 1975; **9**: 362

Ashton N, Henkind P. Experimental occlusion of retinal arterioles. *Br J Ophthalmol* 1965; **49**: 225−234

Ashton N, Ward B, Serpell G. Role of oxygen in the genesis of retrolental fibroplasia. A preliminary report. *Br J Ophthalmol* 1953; **37**: 513−20

Avery ME, Oppenheimer EH. Recent increase in mortality from hyaline membrane disease. *J Pediatr* 1960; **57**: 553−9

Bard H, Cornet A, Orquin J *et al.* Retrolental fibroplasia and exchange transfusions. *Pediatr Res* 1975; **9**: 362

Ben Sira I, Nissenkorn I, Kremer I. Retinopathy of prematurity. *Surv Ophthalmol* 1988; **33**: 1−16

Campbell K. Intensive oxygen therapy as a possible cause for retrolental fibroplasia. A clinical approach. *Med J Austr* 1951; **2**: 48−50

Chong LP, Machemer R, de Juan E. Vitrectomy for advanced stages of retinopathy of prematurity. *Am J Ophthalmol* 1986; **102**: 710−6

Clark C, Gibbs JAH, Maniello R *et al.* Blood transfusions: a possible risk factor in retrolental fibroplasia. *Acta Paediatr Scand* 1981; **70**: 535−9

Committee for the Classification of Retinopathy of Prematurity. The international classification of retinopathy of prematurity. *Br J Ophthalmol* 1984; **68**: 690−7

Committee for the Classification of Retinopathy of Prematurity. II The classification of retinal detachment. *Arch Ophthalmol* 1987; **105**: 906−12

Cryotherapy for Retinopathy of Prematurity Co-operative Group. Multicentre trial of cryotherapy for retinopathy of prematurity (preliminary results). *Arch Ophthalmol* 1988; **106**: 471−9

Finer NN, Grant G, Schindler RF *et al.* Effect of intramuscular vitamin E on frequency and severity of retrolental fibroplasia: a controlled trial. *Lancet* 1982; **i**: 1087–91

Flynn JT. Acute proliferative retrolental fibroplasia: multivariate risk analysis. *Trans Am Ophthalmol Soc* 1983; **81**: 549–81

Flynn JT. An international classification of retinopathy of prematurity. Clinical experience. *Ophthalmology* 1985; **92**: 987–94

Flynn JT. Retinopathy of prematurity. *Pediatr Clin North Am* 1987; **34**: 1487–516

Flynn JT, Bancalari E, Bachynski BN *et al*. Retinopathy of prematurity. Diagnosis, severity and natural history. *Ophthalmology* 1987; **94**: 620–9

Flynn JT, Bancalari E, Bawol R *et al*. Retinopathy of prematurity. A randomised, prospective trial of transcutaneous oxygen monitoring. *Ophthalmology* 1987; **94**: 630–8

Flynn JT, O'Grady GE, Herrera J *et al*. Retrolental fibroplasia I. clinical observations. *Arch Ophthalmol* 1977; **95**: 217–23

Hittner HM, Kretzer FL. Vitamin E and retrolental fibroplasia: ultrastructural mechanism of clinical efficacy. In: *Biology of Vitamin E*, Vol. 10. Ciba Foundation Symposium 1983; pp. 165–85

Hittner HM, Godio LB, Rudolph AJ, *et al*. Retrolental fibroplasia: efficacy of vitamin E in a double blind clinical study of preterm infants. *N Engl J Med* 1981; **305**: 1365–71

James LS, Lansman JT (Eds). History of oxygen and retrolental fibroplasia. *Pediatrics* 1976; **57**: 591–642

Johnson AT, Kretzer JL, Hittner HM *et al*. Development of the subretinal space in the preterm human eye: ultrastructural and immunocytochemical studies. *J Comp Neurol* 1985; **232**: 497–505

Johnson L, Bowen FW, Abbasi S *et al*. Relationship of prolonged pharmocologic serum levels of vitamin E to incidence of sepsis and necrotising enterocolitis in infants with birth weights 1500 gms or less. *Pediatrics* 1985; **75**: 619–38

Johnson L, Quinn GE, Abbasi S *et al*. Vitamin E and retinopathy of prematurity. *Pediatrics* 1988; **81**: 329–31

Kalina RE. Treatment of retrolental fibroplasia. *Surv Ophthalmol* 1980; **24**: 229–36

Keith CG, Kitchen WH. Ocular morbidity in infants of very low birth weight. *Br J Ophthalmol* 1983; **67**: 302–5

Kingham JD. Acute retrolental fibroplasia. *Arch Ophthalmol* 1977; **95**: 39–47

Kinsey VE, Arnold HJ, Kalina *et al*. Pao₂ levels and retrolental fibroplasia: a report of the co-operative study. *Pediatrics* 1977; **60**: 655–68

Kinsey VE, Twomey JT, Hamphill FM. Retrolental fibroplasia. Co-operative study of retrolental fibroplasia and the use of oxygen. *Arch Ophthalmol* 1956; **56**: 481–529

Kitchen WH, Orgill A, Rickards A *et al*. Collaborative study of very low birth weight infants: outcome of 2-year-old survivors. *Lancet* 1982; **i**: 1457–60

Kretzner FL, Hittner HM. Retinopathy of prematurity: clinical implications of retinal development. *Arch Dis Child* 1988; **63**: 1151–67

Kushner BJ. Strabismus and amblyopia associated with regressed retinopathy of prematurity. *Arch Ophthalmol* 1982; **100**: 256–61

Kushner BJ, Essner D, Cohen IJ, Flynn JT. Retrolental fibroplasia II. Pathologic correlation. *Arch Ophthalmol* 1977; **95**: 29–38

Lanman JT, Guy LP, Danus I. Retrolental fibroplasia and oxygen therapy. *JAMA* 1954; **155**: 223–6

Lucey JL, Dangman B. A re-examination of the role of oxygen in retrolental fibroplasia. *Pediatrics* 1984; **73**: 82–96

Machemer R. Closed vitrectomy for severe retrolental fibroplasia in infants. *Ophthalmology* 1983; **90**: 436–41

McDonald AD. Cerebral palsy in children of very low birth weight. *Arch Dis Child* 1963; **38**: 579–88

McPherson AR, Hittner HM, Lemos R. Retinal detachment in young premature infants with acute retrolental fibroplasia. Thirty-two new cases. *Ophthalmology* 1982; **89**: 1160–9

Ng YK, Fielder AR, Shaw DE, Levene DE. Epidemiology of retinopathy of prematurity. *Lancet* 1988; **ii**: 1235–8

Nissenkorn I, Yassur Y, Mashkowski D *et al*. Myopia in premature infants with and without retinopathy of prematurity. *Br J Ophthalmol* 1983; **67**: 170–3

Owens WC, Owens EU. Retrolental fibroplasia in premature infants. *Trans Am Acad Ophthalmol Otolaryngol* 1948; **53**: 18–41

Palmer EA. Optimal timing of examination for acute retrolental fibroplasia. *Ophthalmology* 1981; **88**: 662–8

Pape KE, Buncic RJ, Ashby S, Fitzhardinge PM. The status at two years of low birth weight infants born in 1974 with birth weights of less than 1000 gms. *J Pediatr* 1978; **92**: 253–60

Patz A, Hoeck LE, De La Cruz E. Studies on the effect of high oxygen administration in retrolental fibroplasia: a nursery observation. *Am J Ophthalmol* 1952; **35**: 1248–52

Phelps DL, Rosenbaum A. The role of tocopherol in oxygen induced retinopathy: kitten model. *Pediatrics* 1977; **59**: 998–1005

Phelps DL, Rosenbaum A, Isenberg SJ, Leake RD, Dorey FJ. Tocopherol efficacy and safety for preventing retinopathy of prematurity: a randomised controlled double-masked trial. *Pediatrics* 1987; **79**: 489–500

Reese AB, King MJ, Owens WC. A classification of retrolental fibroplasia. *Am J Ophthalmol* 1953; **36**: 1333–5

Reisner SH, Amir I, Shohat M *et al*. Retinopathy of prematurity: incidence and treatment. *Arch Dis Child* 1985; **60**: 698–701

Rosenbaum AL, Phelps DL, Isenberg SI *et al*. Retinal haemorrhage in retinopathy of prematurity associated with tocopherol treatment. *Ophthalmology* 1985; **92**: 1012–15

Schaffer DB, Quinn GE, Johnson L. Sequelae of arrested mild retinopathy of prematurity. *Arch Ophthalmol* 1984; **102**: 373–6

Shohat M, Reisner SH, Krikler R *et al*. Retinopathy of prematurity. Incidence and risk factors. *Pediatrics* 1983; **72**: 159–163

Silverman WA. *Retrolental Fibroplasia: a Modern Parable*. Grune and Stratton, New York 1980

Tasman W, Borrone RN, Bolling J. Open sky vitrectomy for total retinal detachment in retinopathy of prematurity. *Ophthalmology* 1987; **94**: 449–52

Terry TL. Retrolental fibroplasia in premature infants. Further studies on fibrolastic overgrowth of tunica vasculosa lentis. *Arch Ophthalmol* 1945; **33**: 203–8

Terry TL. Extreme prematurity and fibroblastic overgrowth of persistent vascular sheath behind each crystalline lens. *Am J Ophthalmol* 1942; **25**: 203–4

Trese M. Visual results and prognostic factors for vision following surgery for stage V retinopathy of prematurity. *Ophthalmology* 1986; **93**: 574–9

27.3 Inherited Retinal Dystrophies

ANTHONY MOORE

The inherited retinal dystrophies are a genetically heterogeneous group of disorders many of which become symptomatic in childhood. They may occur as an isolated abnormality in an otherwise normal child or may be associated with other systemic abnormalities. Most are progressive but a few, notably stationary night-blindness, fundus albipunctatus, Oguchi's disease and achromatopsia, are stationary.

Classification of the childhood retinal dystrophies is difficult because of the great heterogeneity even amongst dystrophies which share a common mode of inheritance. It is useful to divide these disorders firstly into those which are stationary or progressive and secondly to consider disorders that present with predominantly rod involvement separately from those with predominantly cone or central receptor disease. The dystrophies that present at birth or in the first few months of life, are considered separately, as they have a different more dramatic presentation and represent a particularly difficult diagnostic problem.

Stationary disorders

This includes (a) night-blindness; and (b) stationary cone disorders.

Stationary night-blindness

Three forms of stationary night-blindness are recognized; in congenital stationary night-blindness (CSNB) the ocular fundus is normal whereas in fundus albipunctatus and Oguchi's disease a distinctive fundus appearance is seen.

Congenital stationary night-blindness

Congenital stationary night-blindness (CSNB) is characterized by night-blindness, variable visual loss and a normal fundus examination. It may be inherited as an autosomal dominant, autosomal recessive, or X-linked disorder (Krill 1977a). The visual acuity is normal in the dominant form whereas in the other two genetic subtypes mild central visual loss is common. Other features that may be seen in X-linked and recessive CSNB include moderate to high myopia, nystagmus, strabismus, and paradoxical pupil responses (Krill 1977; Price et al. 1988). Fundus examination is usually normal but some patients have pale or tilted optic discs (Heckenlively et al. 1983). Although most patients present with symptomatic night-blindness, occasionally in children, nystagmus and visual loss are the predominant symptoms and unless night-blindness is specifically asked for or an ERG performed the diagnosis may be missed (Weleber & Tongue 1987; Price et al. 1988).

As the retinal appearance is normal the diagnosis depends upon demonstrating the characteristic psychophysical and electrophysiological abnormalities seen in this disorder. Most patients show a monophasic dark adaptation curve although in a few there is a recognizable rod component with markedly elevated threshold (Krill 1977). Cone adaptation is also abnormal and other measures of cone function such as flicker fusion and photopic ERG are also abnormal (Krill & Martin 1971).

Patients with CSNB may be divided into two groups on the basis of their ERG findings. The first group which includes most patients with X-linked and autosomal recessive CSNB show a near normal a wave and a substantially reduced b wave on testing under scotopic conditions (negative wave ERG) (Fig. 27.3.1). With increasing intensity of the test stimulus the amplitude of the a wave increases but that of the b wave is unchanged (Schubert & Bornschein 1952). The photopic b wave and oscillatory potentials may also be reduced (Heckenlively et al. 1983; Miyake et al. 1986). This subgroup of CSNB can be further subdivided into two types depending on whether rod function can be demonstrated psychophysically or not (Miyake et al. 1986). Carriers of X-linked CSNB are not night-blind and have a normal fundus examination but may show abnormal oscillatory potentials on ERG (Miyake & Kawase 1984).

A second group of patients with CSNB (predominantly those with the autosomal dominant form) do not show a negative wave ERG, the b wave is larger than the a wave but the amplitude of both is reduced (Auerbach et al. 1969). There is a rod contribution to the dark adaptation curve but it is slowed and the final threshold is elevated (Krill 1977).

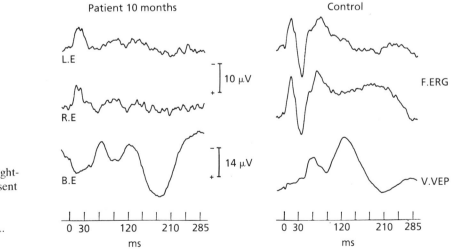

Fig. 27.3.1 Congenital stationary night-blindness. Normal 'a' wave with absent 'b' wave compared to control. (averaged, skin electrodes.) Neurophysiological studies by Dr A. Kriss.

Oguchi's disease

Oguchi's disease is a rare form of stationary night-blindness in which there is a peculiar greyish or green-yellow discolouration of the fundus which reverts to normal on prolonged dark adaptation (Mizuo phenomenon). Although most cases have been reported from Japan it is seen in other races including Europeans (Krill 1977a) and American Negroes (Winn *et al.* 1968). It is inherited as an autosomal recessive trait.

Most patients present with poor night vision. Visual acuity is usually normal or only mildly reduced and photopic visual fields and colour vision are normal. In the light-adapted state the retina has a refractile grey-white appearance which reverts to normal after prolonged dark adaptation. In most patients exposure to light then leads to the gradual reappearance of the abnormal discolouration which may take 10–20 minutes to reach its full effect (Mizuo 1913; Carr & Gouras 1965; Krill 1977a). The abnormal appearance may be confined to the posterior pole or extend beyond the arcades.

Patients with Oguchi's disease have been divided into two types according to the type of abnormality seen on dark adaptation (Krill 1977). In type I rod adaptation is markedly slowed; full recovery of sensitivity takes several hours and the absolute threshold is normal or only minimally elongated. In type II there is no recognizable rod adaptation; the abnormal retinal appearance is less marked and the Mizuo phenomenon may be absent.

Most patients with Oguchi's disease show the 'negative wave' ERG seen in CSNB. Under scotopic conditions the a wave has a normal amplitude but the b wave is markedly reduced or absent. In contrast to fundus albipunctatus the ERG remains abnormal even when full adaptation is complete (Carr & Gouras 1965; Krill 1977a).

Fundus albipunctatus

This autosomal recessive form of stationary night-blindness has a characteristic fundus appearance with multiple white dots scattered throughout the retina. Patients either present with night-blindness or because the abnormal retinal appearance is noted on routine fundoscopy. The visual acuity is normal and the condition non-progressive.

The deposits are discrete dull white lesions which lie at the level of the retinal pigment epithelium. They are most numerous in the mid periphery and are usually absent at the macula (Krill 1977a); the optic discs and retinal vessels are normal. Fluorescein angiography shows multiple areas of hyperfluorescence which may not conform to the deposits seen clinically (Gelber & Shah 1969; Krill 1977a). The differential diagnosis is from other causes of the fleck retina syndrome (see Chapter 27.8).

In fundus albipunctatus both cone and rod dark adaptation is severely delayed. The rod cone break is delayed and full rod adaptation may take several hours (Carr *et al.* 1974; Marmor 1977). The EOG and cone and rod ERG are abnormal in the light adapted eye but after prolonged dark adaptation may reach normal values. In contrast to Oguchi's disease and CSNB rhodopsin regeneration is slow in fundus albipunctatus (Carr *et al.* 1974).

Stationary cone disorders

Monochromatism (achromatopsia)

Rod monochromatism is a stationary retinal dystrophy in which there appears to be an absence of functioning cones in the retina (Sharpe *et al.* 1988). It is characterized by reduced central vision, poor colour vision, photophobia and normal fundus examination; it occurs in typical and atypical forms (Krill 1977a).

Typical rod monochromatism

This condition is inherited as an autosomal recessive trait and results in complete colour blindness. The usual presentation is with reduced vision, nystagmus and marked photophobia in infancy. Parents often comment that vision is very much better in dim illumination. Pupil reactions are sluggish or may show pupillary constriction in the dark; the so-called paradoxical response (Price *et al.* 1985). High hyperopic refractive errors are common and fundus examination is normal. The nystagmus although marked in infancy may improve with age and typically in late childhood there is fine rapid horizontal nystagmus. Photophobia may also improve with age.

In older children the visual acuity is usually about 6/60 and there is complete colour blindness. Peripheral visual field are normal but a small central scotoma can often be detected. Although histopathological studies (Larsen 1921; Harrison *et al.* 1960; Falls *et al.* 1965; Glickstein & Heath 1975) have demonstrated cone-like structures in the retina, psychophysical studies show that the achromat lacks cone vision (Sharpe *et al.* 1988).

The dark adaptation curve is monophasic with no evidence of a cone contribution and spectral sensitivity studies show that rods mediate threshold under both photopic and scotopic conditions (Sharpe *et al.* 1988); there is no evidence of a Purkinge shift.

Electroretinography demonstrates an absence of cone responses to white light, red light and flicker (Krill 1977). The scotopic ERG is normal. In infants, it may be difficult to distinguish achromatopsia from other retinal dystrophies with a flash ERG using only white light. Red and blue light stimuli and flicker responses will however enable a correct diagnosis to be made.

Incomplete typical rod monochromatism

(partial achromatopsia)

The presentation and clinical findings in infancy are similar to the complete form of rod monochromatism but in later childhood and adult life the symptoms are less severe. Visual acuity is often in the range 6/24 to 6/36 and there may be some residual colour perception. This form is also inherited as an autosomal recessive trait (Krill 1977b).

Blue cone monochromatism

Blue cone monochromatism is an X-linked recessive disorder in which affected males have normal rod and blue cone function but lack red and green cone function (Alper *et al.* 1965; Spivey 1965; Krill 1977b). The clinical features are similar to complete rod monochromatism but are less severe. The ERG findings are identical to those seen in complete rod monochromatism (Spivey 1965) but the two disorders may be differentiated by the mode of inheritance and findings on psychophysical testing.

Female carriers of X-linked blue cone monochromatism have abnormal cone electroretinograms (Berson *et al.* 1986) and mild anomalies of colour vision (Krill 1977).

Other stationary cone disorders

The other stationary cone disorders in which there is normal central vision, a normal eye examination but abnormal colour vision will not be considered here. They have however been reviewed in detail by Krill (1977b).

Progressive retinal dystrophies

This includes (a) infantile retinal dystrophies;

(b) childhood onset retinal dystrophies; and (c) cone dystrophies.

Infantile retinal dystrophies

Leber's amaurosis

Leber's amaurosis is a rod-cone dystrophy which presents at birth or the first few months of life and may be progressive in some cases. It is inherited as an autosomal recessive trait (Alstrom & Olson 1957), although it is likely that there are several different genotypes giving rise to the same clinical picture (Waardenberg *et al.* 1963). It has been reported to be inherited as an autosomal dominant trait (Sorsby & Williams 1960) but this has not been confirmed. It is a common cause of blindness in children, accounting for between 10 and 18% of children in institutions for the blind (Alstrom & Olson 1957; Schappert-Kimmijser *et al.* 1959).

Clinical features

The normal presentation is with suspected blindness or poor vision with nystagmus from birth or the first few months of life. Affected infants have roving eye movements and poor pupillary responses to light. Eye poking (the digito-ocular sign) (Fig. 27.3.2) is common (Franceschetti 1947). Fundus examination and fluorescein angiography are often normal but a variety of abnormal fundus appearances may be seen. The optic disc may be pale, the vessels thinned (Fig. 27.3.3, 27.3.4) and there may be a mild peripheral pigmentary retinopathy (Fig. 27.3.4, 27.3.5). Less commonly there may be optic disc oedema or pseudo-papilloedema (Fig. 27.3.6) (Flynn & Cullen 1975), a flecked retina (Fig. 27.3.7) (Mizuno *et al.* 1977), or macular dysplasia (Fig. 27.3.8, 27.3.9) (Margolis *et al.* 1977; Moore *et al.* 1985). Affected infants may have high hyperopic (Foxman *et al.* 1983; Wagner *et al.* 1985) or less commonly high myopic refractive errors, suggesting that the severe visual impairment may interfere with the normal process of emmetropisation.

Although the majority of patients have normal fundi in infancy, in later childhood most develop signs of a pigmentary retinopathy with optic disc pallor and retinal arteriolar narrowing. Rarely yellow flecks may be seen in the equatorial fundus (Chew *et al.* 1984). Other late signs which may be related to eye poking include enophthalmos, keratoconus and cataract (Alstrom 1957). Eventual vision is in the region of 3/

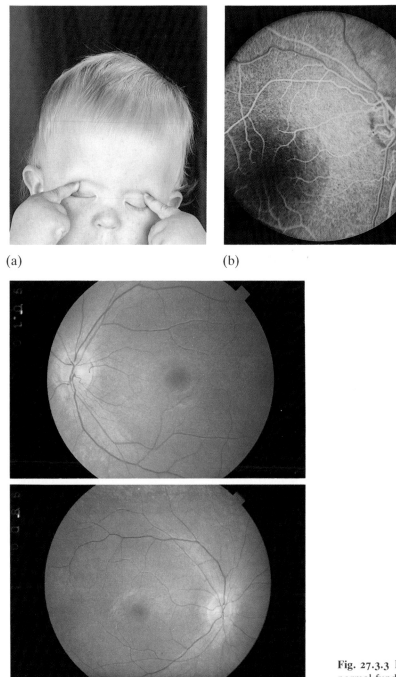

(a)   (b)

Fig. 27.3.2 Leber's amaurosis. (a) Eye poking or the 'digito-ocular sign' of Franceschetti is very common but of unknown cause. It may result in severe atrophy of orbital fat and enophthalmos. (b) Normal fluorescein angiogram. (Same patient.)

Fig. 27.3.3 Leber's amaurosis. Blind 6-year-old with nearly normal fundus — shows retinal arteriolar thinning.

60 to perception of light; only in some cases is deterioration demonstrable (Lambert *et al.* 1989).

Non-ocular features

Most cases of Leber's amaurosis occur in otherwise normal infants. However a variety of associated systemic abnormalities including mental subnormality, neurological disorders, renal and cardiac disease have been reported.

MENTAL SUBNORMALITY AND NEUROLOGICAL DISEASE

Mental retardation and neurological disease are the most frequent of the associations (Schappert-Kimmijser 1959; Vaizey *et al.* 1977; Moore & Taylor 1984; Foxman *et al.* 1985; Lambert *et al.* 1989b) but there is great variation in the incidence of neurological disease in the various series. Several studies (Alstrom & Olson 1957; Nickel & Hoyt 1982) have failed to

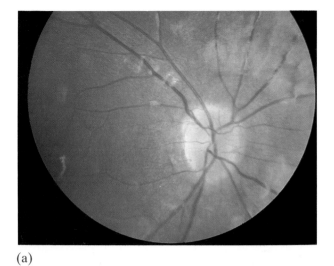

(a)

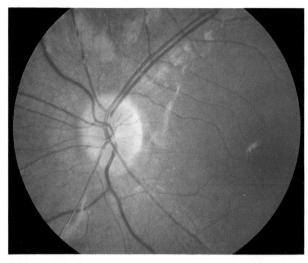

(b)

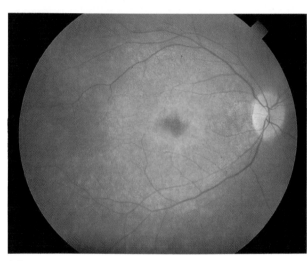

(c)

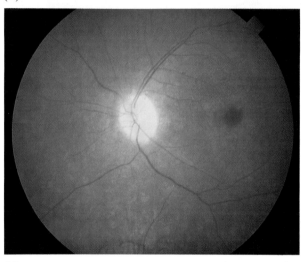

(d)

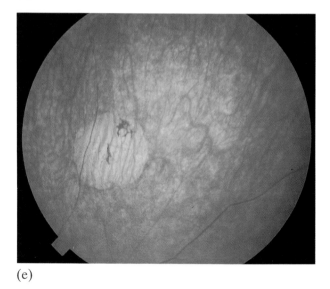

(e)

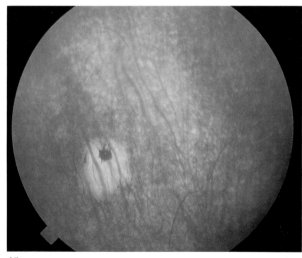

(f)

Fig. 27.3.4 Leber's amaurosis. (a & b) Three-year-old showing mild pigmentary changes and slightly narrow arterioles. (c–e) Same patient 10 years later showing typical retinal pigment epithelial changes, disc pallor and arteriolar thinning with two punched out peripheral pigment epithelial defects.

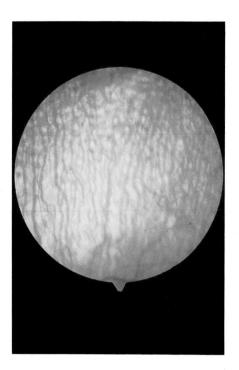

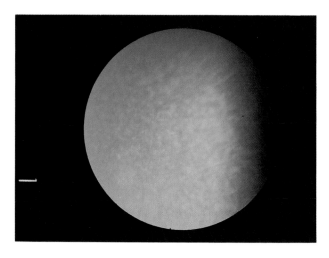

Fig. 27.3.7 Leber's amaurosis — flecked retina appearance.

Fig. 27.3.5 Leber's amaurosis — peripheral pigment mottling.

show a significantly increased incidence of such abnormalities whereas others (Schappert-Kimmijser 1959; Dekaban & Carr 1966; Dekaban 1972; Vaizey 1977; Noble & Carr 1978) have found major neurological or developmental abnormalities in more than 25% of cases. The variation mainly reflects differences in referral patterns to the various centres but the lower incidence in more recent series (Nickel & Hoyt 1982; Lambert et al. 1989b) may reflect the fact that many infants with neurological disease and a retinal dystrophy are now recognized to have specific genetic conditions such as Joubert's syndrome of the peroxisomal

disorders. It is also now evident that normal blind children are often hypotonic and may reach some developmental milestones later than their sighted peers; such delay is not an indication of psychomotor retardation.

Although several different abnormalities of the CNS have been demonstrated on CT scan the only consistent abnormality is hypoplasia of the cerebellar vermis which may be seen in 10% of infants with Leber's amaurosis (Nickel & Hoyt 1982). A retinal dystrophy and cerebellar vermis abnormalities are also seen in Joubert's syndrome and Olivopontocerebellar atrophy.

RENAL DISEASE

Senior et al. (1961) first described the association of a recessively inherited renal disease, juvenile nephronopthysis (medullary cystic disease) and a tape-

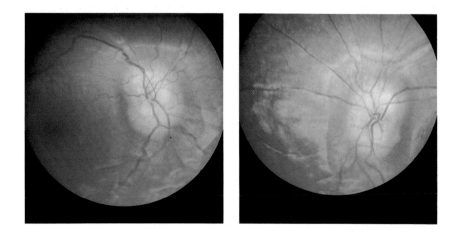

Fig. 27.3.6 Leber's amaurosis — high hypermetropia and pseudopapilloedema.

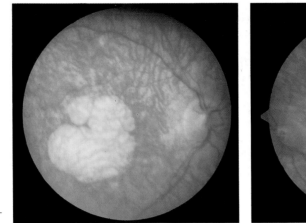

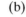

Fig. 27.3.8 Leber's amaurosis —
bilateral macular dysplasia.
(a) Right eye and (b) left eye.   (a)   (b)

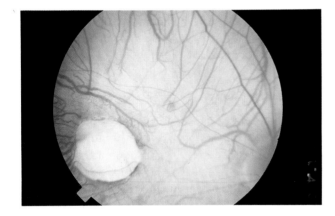

Fig. 27.3.9 Congenital retinal dystrophy, probably Leber's
amaurosis with macular dysplasia.

to-retinal degeneration. Many more cases have since been reported (Loken *et al.* 1961; Fairley *et al.* 1963; Meier & Hess 1965; Herdman *et al.* 1967; Mainzer *et al.* 1970; Abraham *et al.* 1974; Polak *et al.* 1977; Edwards & Grizzard 1981; Ellis *et al.* 1984) and it is evident that the age of onset of the retinal dystrophy is extremely variable. Some children have poor vision and nystagmus from birth and have a retinal dystrophy indistinguishable from Leber's amaurosis (Loken *et al.* 1961; Senior *et al.* 1961; Dekaban 1969) whilst others develop a picture similar to childhood onset retinitis pigmentosa with night-blindness and normal central vision (Mainzer *et al.* 1970; Abraham *et al.* 1974; Polak 1977; Edwards & Grizzard 1981). Loken *et al.* (1961) examined histologically the eye of a child who was blind from infancy and who later died of chronic renal failure. The photoreceptor layer was markedly abnormal with no identifiable rods; the macular region consisted of one layer of large epithelial-like cells and no normal cones could be identified.

Other associations seen in this disorder include cone-shaped epiphyses of the distal interphalangeal joints (Mainzer *et al.* 1970; Ellis *et al.* 1984) cerebellar ataxia (Mainzer *et al.* 1970) and hepatic fibrosis (Stanescu *et al.* 1967), although the latter is more frequently found in peroxisomal disorders.

Other findings

Russell-Eggitt *et al.* (1988) have recently described a group of children with a congenital retinal dystrophy, cardiomyopathy, obesity, and short stature. Photophobia is a prominent symptom and this may represent an early onset cone-rod dystrophy.

Moore and Taylor (1984) described three children with Leber's amaurosis who had a saccadic palsy and head thrusts similar to that seen in ocular motor apraxia. CT scan showed cerebellar vermis hypoplasia. These patients are almost certainly examples of Joubert's syndrome (Joubert *et al.* 1969; King *et al.* 1984).

Sensorineural hearing loss occurs in about 5% of children with Leber's amaurosis (Lambert *et al.* 1989b); this association has not been well characterized but it is important to exclude one of the peroxisomal disorders in infants with hearing loss and a congenital retinal dystrophy.

Electrophysiology

The electroretinogram is extinguished or severely subnormal in infants with Leber's amaurosis. It is important to perform both scotopic and photopic ERGs to distinguish the disorder from CSNB and achromatopsia which may also present in infancy with nystagmus and poor vision. The visual evoked response is usually absent but may be preserved in some infants despite an absent ERG and may indicate a better visual prognosis.

In Senior's syndrome asymptomatic heterozygotes may show an abnormal scotopic ERG and elevated rod thresholds when tested psychophysically (Abraham *et al.* 1974; Polak *et al.* 1977).

Diagnosis

Leber's amaurosis should be suspected in any infant with poor vision, nystagmus, sluggish pupil reactions, and a normal fundus examination. The diagnosis is confirmed by demonstrating an absent or severely subnormal photopic and scotopic ERG. If there are any unusual systemic features other inherited disorders such as the peroxisomal disorders or Joubert's syndrome need to be excluded.

Joubert's syndrome

Joubert's syndrome is an autosomal recessive disorder characterized by cerebellar vermis hypoplasia (Fig. 27.3.10), neonatal breathing difficulties, a retinal dystrophy and ocular motor abnormalities (Joubert 1969; Tomita 1979; King *et al.* 1984; Lambert *et al.* 1989a). In infancy the retinal dystrophy is indistinguishable from Leber's amaurosis but the visual prognosis is better; vision of 6/18 or better has been recorded when the child is old enough to be formally tested (Moore & Taylor 1984; Lambert *et al.* 1988). Although fundus examination is normal in infancy,

disc pallor, arteriolar attenuation and pigmentary retinopathy may develop at a later stage (Lambert *et al.* 1989a). The ERG is absent or markedly attenuated but the VER is usually preserved indicating reasonable macular function.

A wide variety of ocular motor abnormalities have been reported including nystagmus, impaired pursuit and hypometric or absent saccades. In some infants the saccadic palsy is severe and head thrusting similar to that seen in ocular motor apraxia may be used to aid refixation (Moore & Taylor 1984; Lambert *et al.* 1989a). Some infants show frequent hemifacial spasm (King *et al.* 1984). Joubert's syndrome should be suspected in infants with poor vision and nystagmus if there is developmental delay and a history of neonatal breathing difficulties. Electrophysiological testing will show a well preserved visual evoked response (VER) in the presence of a substantially abnormal electroretinogram (ERG) and the finding of cerebellar vermis hypoplasia on CT scan or Nuclear magnetic resonance (NMR) will confirm the diagnosis.

Peroxisomal disorders

Peroxisomes are subcellular organelles that are found in all animal cells and have an important function in the biosynthesis of certain phospholipids and in the catabolism of phytanic acid and pipecolic acid. It is now recognized that dysfunction of peroxisomes may give rise to a variety of inherited metabolic disorders (Schutgens *et al.* 1986; Zellweger 1987; Michalski *et al.* 1988; Naidu *et al.* 1988). The inherited peroxisomal disorders which have eye involvement are listed in Table 27.3.1.

Zellweger's syndrome, infantile Refsum's disease, and neonatal adrenoleucodystrophy may all have an associated retinal dystrophy.

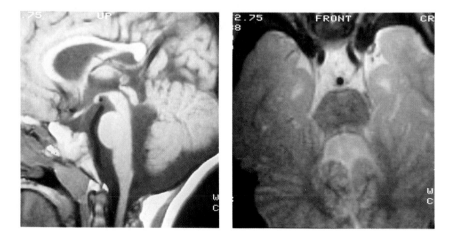

Fig. 27.3.10 Joubert's syndrome. MRI scan shows vermis hypoplasia with large fourth ventricle.

Table 27.3.1 Peroxisomal disorders with eye involvement (modified from Michalski *et al.* 1988)

Disorder	Eye signs
Reduced or absent hepatic peroxisomes	
Zellweger syndrome (ZS)	Corneal clouding
	Cataracts
	Retinal dystrophy
Neonatal adrenoleucodystrophy	Optic atrophy
	Retinal dystrophy
Infantile Refsum's disease	Retinal dystrophy
Reduced activity of peroxisomal enzymes	
Chondrodysplasia punctata	Cataracts
Pseudo-Zellweger	Corneal clouding
	Cataracts
	Retinal dystrophy
X-linked adrenoleucodystrophy	Optic atrophy
Hyperoxaluria type I	Fleck retina syndrome
Adult Refsum's disease	Retinal dystrophy

ZELLWEGER'S SYNDROME

Zellweger's (or the hepato-cerebro-renal) syndrome is characterized by widespread dysmorphic features, neurological abnormalities, renal cysts, and hepatosplenomegaly (Schutgens *et al.* 1986; Zellweger 1987). Affected infants show marked hypotonia, psychomotor retardation, and have frequent seizures. Nystagmus is common and ocular findings include corneal clouding, cataract, and a retinal dystrophy (Stanescu & Draloands 1972; Hittner *et al.* 1981; Garner *et al.* 1982; Cohen *et al.* 1983). The electro-retinogram is absent or severely subnormal (Stanescu & Draloands 1972; Hittner *et al.* 1981; Garner *et al.* 1982). Most patients die in the first year of life. Histopathological studies (Haddad *et al.* 1976; Garner *et al.* 1982; Cohen *et al.* 1983) have demonstrated extensive photoreceptor degeneration and loss of ganglion cells with gliosis of the nerve fibre layer. Biochemical studies of post mortem eyes (Cohen *et al.* 1983) have shown high levels of very long chain fatty acids in the ocular tissues. Inheritance is autosomal recessive and prenatal diagnosis is possible (Hajra *et al.* 1985).

NEONATAL ADRENOLEUKODYSTROPHY

This form of adrenoleukodystrophy affects males and females equally and is thought to be inherited as an autosomal recessive trait. Affected infants are hypotonic, have severe psychomotor retardation, and seizures. Clinically adrenal insufficiency is uncommon but adrenal atrophy is frequently seen at postmortem. Affected children die between 6 months and 7 years.

Most infants show severe visual loss and nystagmus and the ocular findings include cataract, optic atrophy and a pigmentary retinopathy. Histopathology shows marked degeneration of both inner and outer segment of rods and cones and diffuse atrophy of the nerve fibre layer (Cohen *et al* 1983; Glasgow *et al.* 1987).

INFANTILE REFSUM'S DISEASE

Classical Refsum's disease is an autosomal recessive disorder caused by defective oxidation of phytanic acid; the major features are retinitis pigmentosa,

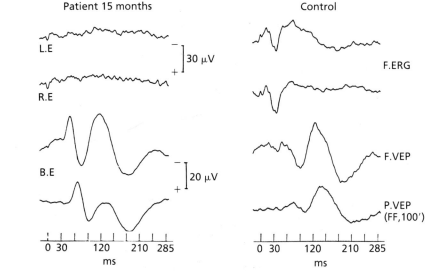

Fig. 27.3.11 Joubert's syndrome. The ERG is attenuated with a well preserved VER (see text). Neurophysiological studies by Dr A. Kriss. (see Lambert *et al.* 1989.)

cerebellar ataxia and peripheral neuropathy. In 1982, Scotto *et al.* described three infants with hepatomegaly, facial dysmorphism, neurosensory deafness, a retinal dystrophy and raised plasma levels of phytanic acid. They suggested that this disorder represented infantile onset Refsum's disease.

Affected infants have poor vision and usually nystagmus from early infancy and on fundus examination have optic atrophy, narrowed vessels and a pigmentary retinopathy (Fig. 27.3.12) (Weleber *et al.* 1984). Fluorescein angiography shows widespread atrophy of the retinal pigment epithelium and choriocapillaries affecting both macula and peripheral retina (Weleber *et al.* 1984).

The ERG shows very small amplitude rod and cone responses and cone B wave implicit times are greatly prolonged to flash and 30 Hz flicker (Weleber *et al.* 1984).

Childhood onset retinal dystrophies

Although there is clearly some overlap between the retinal dystrophies which present in early infancy (described in the last section) and those with a later onset in childhood, the clinical presentation, associated systemic features and visual prognosis are sufficiently different to justify considering these two groups of disorders separately. Most infantile dystrophies have severe rod and cone involvement from the outset but those dystrophies with a later presentation can usefully be divided into those with predominantly rod or cone involvement at presentation. Those children with central receptor dystrophies will be considered separately (see Chapter 27.4).

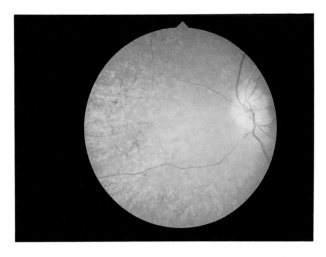

Fig. 27.3.12 Infantile Refsum's disease showing optic atrophy, thinned arterioles, and retinal pigment abnormality.

Progressive rod-cone dystrophies (retinitis pigmentosa)

Retinitis pigmentosa (RP) is a term used for a genetically heterogeneous group of disorders characterized by night-blindness, visual field loss and an abnormal or extinguished ERG. The disease may be confined to the eye or the retinal dystrophy may be part of a more widespread systemic disorder (Table 27.3.2).

GENETICS

Retinitis pigmentosa may be inherited as an autosomal dominant, autosomal recessive or X-linked recessive disorder. There is genetic heterogeneity even within these three classes and it is particularly marked in autosomal recessive RP (Table 27.3.2). The proportion of the different subtypes varies widely in the different series (Amman *et al.* 1965; Jay 1982; Boughman & Fishman 1983; Heckenlively 1988), but in most about half the patients have no family history of RP or evidence of parental consanguinity. It is

Table 27.3.2 Childhood retinal dystrophies with systemic abnormalities

Autosomal dominant
  Olivopontocerebellar atrophy
  Alagille's syndrome
  Myotonic dystrophy
Autosomal recessive
  Abetalipoproteinaemia
  Refsum's disease
  Batten's disease
  Laurence–Moon syndrome
  Biedl–Bardet syndrome
  Usher's syndrome
  Cockayne's syndrome
  Mucopolysaccharidosis (I and II)
  Mucolipidosis IV
  Osteopetrosis
  Alstrom's syndrome
  Peroxisomal disorders
  Joubert's syndrome
  Jeune syndrome
  Hallervorden–Spatz syndrome
  Senior's syndrome
  Idiopathic infantile hypercalcaemia
  Chorio retinopathy and pituitary dysfunction
    (CPD syndrome)
X-linked
  Hunter's syndrome
Mitochondrial inheritance
  Mitochondrial cytopathy

unlikely that all such cases have autosomal recessive disease. Some males may have X-linked disease transmitted via asymptomatic female carriers; other cases may represent new autosomal dominant mutations or autosomal dominant disease in a family with reduced penetrance. It is also possible that some sporadic patients do not have genetic disease.

Jay (1982) using segregation analysis has calculated the proportion of the different genetic subtypes seen in the genetic clinic at Moorfields Eye Hospital, London (Table 27.3.3). Autosomal recessive disease is most frequent with X-linked and autosomal dominant disease occurring in equal proportions. The proportion of X-linked disease is higher than in other series (Heckenlively 1988) and may represent a referral bias as the Moorfields department has a particular interest in X-linked RP (XLRP).

It is evident from clinical experience that X-linked and autosomal recessive RP tend to have an earlier onset and are more severe than dominant disease. The clinical findings may be taken into account when counselling apparently sporadic patients. A severely affected female may be considered more likely to have autosomal recessive disease whereas a severely affected male may have X-linked or autosomal recessive disease. A significant number of patients with sporadic RP however have mild disease and it is likely that a proportion of these will have new autosomal dominant mutations. Before counselling it is clearly important to examine other family members, especially the mothers of severely affected males who may show the fundus abnormalities seen in the X-linked heterozygote.

Since it is not possible to distinguish the different genetic subtypes by clinical examination more accurate genetic counselling will have to await development of biochemical or other markers for the different dis-

orders. The most promising approach appears to be genetic linkage studies using restriction fragment length polymorphisms (RFLPs). Most progress has been made with X-linked RP. Bhattacharia *et al.* (1984) were the first to localize the XLRP gene to the DXS7 region of the short arm of the X-chromosome using a recombinant DNA probe L1.28. In informative families this probe may be used for carrier detection and prenatal counselling (Cooper *et al.* 1987). More recently X-linked RP has also been localized to the Xp21 region using linkage to the OTC gene suggesting there may be two loci for X-linked RP. Until the locus for X-linked RP is definitely established the use of DNA markers, will be confined to large families which show linkage to either L1.28 or the OTC gene (Anandakrishnan & Musarella 1989).

The task of finding markers for the autosomal genes is more daunting because of the greater heterogeneity in dominant and recessive RP. It is evident from the wide variety of associated systemic disorders (Table 27.3.1) that many different autosomal recessive genes may result in a progressive retinal dystrophy. In classical autosomal dominant RP there appears to be at least two distinct subtypes (Massof & Finklestein 1981; Lyness *et al.* 1985; Kemp *et al.* 1988) which can be distinguished using psychophysical and reflectometric techniques. There is also evidence that families showing incomplete penetrance may have a different more severe disease than those showing complete penetrance of the ADRP gene(s) (Berson & Simonoff 1979; Moore *et al.* 1987). In addition sectorial RP when seen in typical form in all family members may represent yet another distinct genetic subtype of ADRP (Moore *et al.* 1988).

Clinical findings

Children with retinitis pigmentosa may present with night-blindness or with symptoms associated with extensive field loss or central retinal involvement. In others there may be no symptomatic night-blindness but the child is referred because of retinal abnormalities seen on routine fundoscopy. When there is a parent or other close relative with RP children may be referred early for examination and investigation to exclude the disease.

In most cases the visual acuity is normal at presentation although later visual loss may occur as a result of posterior cortical cataract, macular oedema or macular involvement in the dystrophic process. Early visual field changes are seen as small scotoma in the mid peripheral retina and are more common in

Table 27.3.3 Frequency of different genetic forms of RP seen at the Moorfields genetic clinic (from Jay 1982.)

	Identified	Calculated
Autosomal dominant	24.4%	24.4%
Autosomal recessive	6.8%	40.8%
X-linked	15.7%	22.3%
Mixed multiplex	6.6%	—
Male multiplex	4.5%	—
Simplex	41.1%	—
Adopted	0.9%	0.9%
Total	100%	88.4%

the upper visual field. These field defects gradually coalesce to give the classical peripheral ring scotoma. In more advanced disease, visual fields become very constricted although there is often a small island of preserved field in the far temporal periphery. In sectorial RP which commonly involves the lower nasal quadrant bilateral upper temporal field loss may lead to unnecessary investigation to exclude a chiasmal lesion.

The appearance of the fundus in the early stages of RP is variable and in young children the changes may be very subtle (Fig. 27.3.13). The earliest change is mild pigment epithelial atrophy in the mid periphery often with small white dots at the level of the retinal pigment epithelium. Later pigment deposition is seen in the equatorial retina and there may be arteriolar narrowing and optic disc pallor (Fig. 27.3.14). In some children pigment may be lacking (RP sine pigmento) and less commonly there may be multiple white deposits scattered throughout the retina (retinitis punctata albescens). It is unlikely that these represent different genetic subtypes as they can each be seen within the same family.

In more advanced disease the classical fundus appearance of optic disc pallor, retinal arteriolar attenuation and peripheral pigment epithelial atrophy and 'bone corpuscle' pigmentation is seen (Fig. 27.3.15, 27.3.16). Other changes include vitreous pigmentation and cells, posterior cortical cataract, optic disc drusen and macular oedema. Occasionally retinovascular changes similar to Coat's disease are seen. Persistant macular oedema may lead to the development of macular holes.

ELECTROPHYSIOLOGY

Electroretinography has been used for many years in the investigation of RP and the introduction of computer averaging techniques combined with the use of variable spectral stimuli and flicker have enabled rod and cone responses to be isolated. These techniques can be used in infants and young children without the need for sedation or general anaesthetic. Rod responses are elicited under conditions of dark adaptation using blue or dim white light and cone responses are seen when high intensity white light or red stimuli are used in the light adapted state (Arden et al. 1983).

The ability to distinguish between scotopic and photopic function allows retinitis pigmentosa to be distinguished from stationary night-blindness and the cone and cone-rod disorders.

Most cases of RP show a reduction in the amplitude

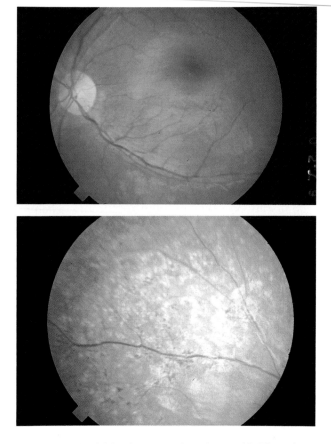

Fig. 27.3.13 Retinitis pigmentosa in a 6-year-old. The only symptom was night-blindness, the acuity was 6/9 in both eyes and the posterior pole is normal. Peripheral pigment clumping is present.

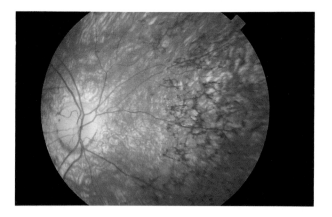

Fig. 27.3.14 Retinitis pigmentosa. 'Bone spicule' formation in the mid-periphery and arteriolar narrowing.

of the rod and cone responses but the responses may vary in different types of RP. For example in ADRP, one (diffuse) subtype shows a complete absence of the rod ERG which is apparent from early childhood

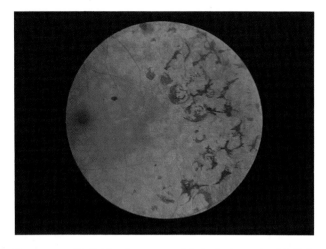

Fig. 27.3.15 Retinitis pigmentosa. Marked pigment epithelial clumping with preservation of a relatively normal macula and good acuity.

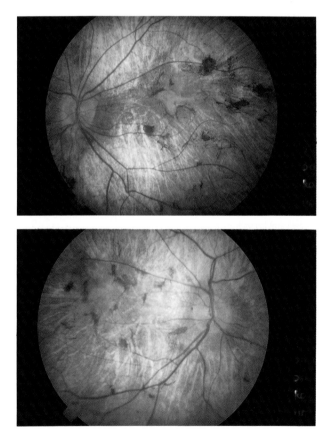

Fig. 27.3.16 Retinitis pigmentosa late stage showing marked pigment abnormalities and chorioretinal atrophy.

whilst in the second (regional subtype) the rod ERG may be recordable even in early adult life (Lyness *et al.* 1985). Similarly individuals from families showing complete penetrance of the RP gene show differences in cone responses from those with incomplete penetrance (Berson *et al.* 1979).

Although the electrooculogram is frequently used in addition to the ERG in the assessment of patients with RP it provides little further information and has the disadvantage that it is difficult to perform in young children. In all types of retinitis pigmentosa there is a reduced or absent light rise.

SECTORIAL RETINITIS PIGMENTOSA

In sectorial RP which is usually inherited as an autosomal dominant trait the abnormalities are confined to one sector of the fundus, usually the lower retina. Children with sectorial RP usually have no symptoms and are referred when the abnormal fundus appearance is noted on routine funduscopy. On Goldmann perimetry field loss is confined to one sector corresponding to the clinically involved retina. However, dark adapted perimetry shows mild rod and cone threshold elevations in the apparently uninvolved retina indicating that there is widespread receptor disease (Massof & Finklestein 1979). Disease progression is slow and confined to the clinically involved sector (Massof & Finklestein 1979). The visual prognosis is excellent.

UNILATERAL RETINITIS PIGMENTOSA

Unilateral retinitis pigmentosa is rare, has yet to be reported in families with RP, and is more likely to be non-hereditary and related to retinal ischaemia, inflammation or infection (Carr & Siegel 1973; Merin & Auerbach 1976).

RECOGNITION OF THE X-LINKED CARRIER STATUS

In X-linked RP the carrier state can be diagnosed with certainty only in females who have affected sons or fathers and are therefore obligate gene carriers. In other female family members carrier detection depends upon recognition of the abnormal fundus appearance seen in the heterozygote or on the results of electrophysiological and psychophysical testing.

Two fundus abnormalities are commonly seen in X-linked heterozygotes. Firstly a prominant tapetal reflex (Fig. 27.3.17) may be seen at the posterior pole or mild pigment epithelial thinning and pigmentation may be present in the equatorial retina (Bird 1975; Krill 1977; Berson *et al.* 1979; Fishman *et al.* 1986). Fluorescein angiography is helpful in confirming the peripheral pigment epithelial atrophy (Bird 1975).

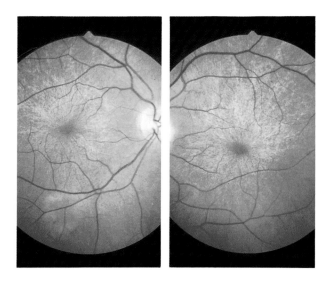

Fig. 27.3.17 X-linked retinitis pigmentosa carrier female showing the 'tapetal reflex'. Professor B. Jay's patient.

Bird (1975) was able to recognize most obligate hetero-zygotes in his series by fundus examination whereas in Berson's series only 60% had an abnormal retinal appearance.

The ERG is often abnormal in heterozygotes with reduced rod and cone amplitudes and delayed cone b wave implicit times. The proportion of obligate heterozygotes with an abnormal ERG varies in different series. Berson *et al.* (1979) were able to identify 22 out of 23 obligate heterozygotes on the basis of an abnormal ERG. Fishman *et al.* (1986) similarly were able to identify 90% of carriers by ERG testing alone and 100% when the results of fundus examination and electrophysiological testing were combined.

Psychophysical testing has demonstrated elevated dark adapted thresholds (Bird 1975) and reduced rod flicker sensitivity (Ernst *et al.* 1981) in X-linked het-erozygotes. In addition, rhodopsin pigment density measured by reflexion densitometry is also reduced (Bird & Hyman 1972). Using a combination of fund-oscopy, electrophysiology and in selected cases psychophysics it is possible to identify X-linked carriers in the majority of cases.

Differential diagnosis

Other disorders may be confused with RP either because there is symptomatic night blindness or be-cause a similar fundus appearance is seen (Table 27.3.4). The other inherited dystrophies can usually be differentiated from RP by the clinical findings and electrophysiological testing. Although a careful history

Table 27.3.4 Differential diagnosis of retinitis pigmentosa

Pigmentary retinopathy	Night-blindness
Blunt trauma (Fig. 27.3.18)	Genetic disorders
Retained intraocular FB	Congenital stationery
Congenital infection	night-blindness
Rubella	Oguchi's disease
Varicella	Fundus albipunctatus
Herpes simplex	Choroideremia
Syphilis	Gyrate atrophy
Acquired infection	Progressive cone–rod
Measles	dystrophy
Onchocerciasis	Acquired
Metabolic	Vitamin A deficiency
Cystinosis	Desferrioxamine toxicity
Oxallosis	
Drugs	
Phenothiazines	
Chloroquine	
Desferroxamine	
Resolved retinal detachment	
(Fig. 27.3.20)	
Ophthalmic artery occlusion	
Other retinal dystrophies	
Cone–rod dystrophy	
Inherited vitreoretinal	
dystrophies	
Unknown aetiology	
Paravenous retinochoroidal	
atrophy (Fig. 27.3.21)	

and examinatic   nay exclude many of the acquired causes of pigmentary retinopathy it is likely that some of the cases of apparently sporadic RP may be due to acquired retinal or pigment epithelial disease.

Management

Although, with the exception of Refsum's disease and abetalipoproteinemia there is no specific treatment for RP, the ophthalmologist has an important role to play in the management of the child and his family.

Once the diagnosis is established it is important that the parents and the child (if old enough) are given a full and sympathetic explanation; most parents will be especially concerned about the visual prognosis and although it is important to give an honest assessment it is better to adopt a cautiously optimistic approach. For example, they can be reassured that most children complete their education at a normal school as central vision is preserved until late in the disease. Parents are often concerned that other children may be at risk of developing the disease; they should be offered genetic counselling and it may be appropriate to

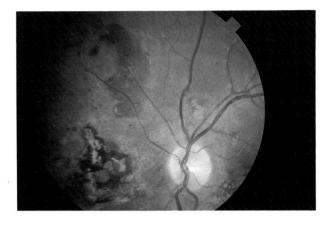

Fig. 27.3.18 Airgun pellet injury with foveal RPE hypertrophy without a definitive history the condition may be diagnosed as a previous infection or, ischaemia or 'unilateral RP' (see text).

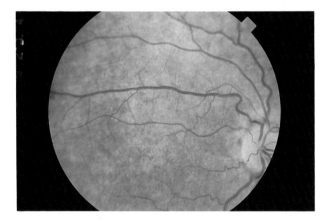

Fig. 27.3.19 Rubella retinopathy showing pigment mottling. Retinal function is usually good and the ERG normal whereas most retinal dystrophies with deafness have severely abnormal ERGs.

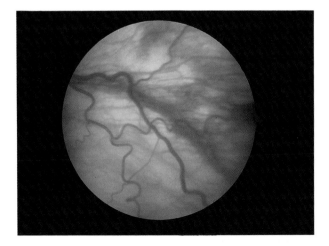

Fig. 27.3.20 Retinal pigment hypertrophy in a child with a resolved retinal detachment. Unless the history is known the diagnosis of sectorial RP or unilateral RP may be made.

examine other family members. It is also helpful to have available the address of patients self-help groups such as the British, American or other RP association.

Practical help can also be given when there are visual difficulties. Many patients with RP have poor vision in bright sunlight and have problems in adapting from bright to dim illumination. It would seem sensible to avoid bright sunlight and tinted lenses may be helpful in summer. If there is macular oedema a trial of diamox (Fishman *et al.* 1989), orbital floor or systemic steroids should be given. In established oedema or macular atrophy low visual aids may be helpful. Visual loss may also develop secondary to posterior cortical cataract and although cataract surgery is often successfully performed in adults with RP it is rarely necessary in childhood.

Prognosis

The prognosis in RP varies according to the type of disease. In X-linked RP affected males are night-blind in early childhood, usually show extensive field loss by their teens and central visual loss in their twenties (Bird 1975). By the fourth decade most have vision reduced to less than an ability to count fingers. Autosomal recessive RP is such a heterogenous condition that it is difficult to give an accurate prognosis. Overall disease is usually of early onset and severe. Most patients have a severely constricted visual field by their teens and may have marked central visual loss by their late twenties.

The prognosis is better in autosomal dominant RP. Although night-blindness and field loss may develop in childhood the prognosis for central vision is much better. Many patients maintain reasonable central visual acuity until the fifth or sixth decade, although they may have extremely constricted visual fields. There is however wide variation within ADRP.

Sector retinitis pigmentosa has the best prognosis of any form of RP. Although there may be a dense scotoma in the field (usually upper) corresponding to the involved retina, involvement of the macula is uncommon. Vision may remain normal throughout life.

Pigmented paravenous atrophy

This is a rare chorioretinal atrophy in which there is paravenous retinal pigment epithelial atrophy and pigment clumping (Fig. 27.3.21). Retinal function may deteriorate quite rapidly (Pearlman *et al.* 1975, 1978) or be more or less static (Skalka 1979; Noble &

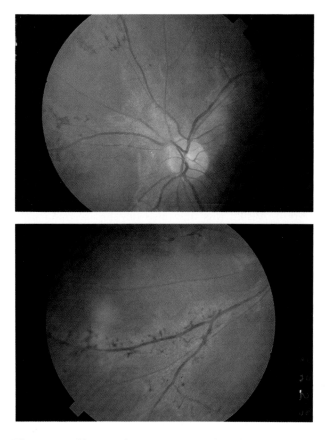

Fig. 27.3.21 Pigmented paravenous atrophy. The veins are surrounded by a band of retinal pigment atrophy and clumping.

Carr 1983; Traboulsi & Maumenee 1986). It is more common in males but the inheritance is as yet uncertain (Traboulsi & Maumenee 1986). It is usually diagnosed in asymptomatic patients who attend for other reasons.

Rod-cone dystrophies with systemic involvement

A progressive retinal dystrophy may be seen in a wide variety of genetic disorders (Table 27.3.1). They have been reviewed by Merin and Auerbach (1978), Francois (1982), and Heckenlively (1988). Lambert *et al.* (1988) have reviewed the systemic associations seen in the congenital retinal dystrophies. In this section it is proposed to give a brief account of the conditions presenting in childhood which have a progressive rod-cone dystrophy as a prominant feature.

ABETALIPOPROTEINAEMIA

Abetalipoproteinaemia is a rare autosomal recessive disorder of lipoprotein metabolism. It is characterized by acanthocytosis of red cells, fat malabsorption, spinocerebellar ataxia, a retinal dystrophy and an absence of beta (low density) lipoproteins from the plasma (Francois 1982; Runge *et al.* 1986b). It has been shown that there is a complete absence of apolipoprotein B a major component of the low density lipoproteins (Gotto *et al.* 1971); this results in defective chylomicron formation and malabsorption of the fat soluble vitamins. The usual presentation is with failure to thrive and steatorrhea in infancy.

Although the retinal dystrophy may occur at any age (Francois 1982; Judisch *et al.* 1984; Runge *et al.* 1986b) it most commonly presents in late childhood. Fundus examination may be normal in the early stages but later there may be a peripheral pigmentary retinopathy or a picture similar to retinitis punctata albescens with scattered white dots at the level of the retinal pigment epithelium (Francois 1982). The ERG may be normal initially but later becomes abnormal with scotopic responses first to be lost (Francois 1982); it is extinguished at a late stage.

Treatment with large doses of vitamin A and E will prevent neurological and retinal complications (Bishara *et al.* 1982; Runge 1986).

REFSUM'S DISEASE

Refsum's disease is a rare autosomal recessive disorder characterized by retinitis pigmentosa, ataxia and polyneuropathy (Refsum 1946). Other abnormalities include anosmia, deafness, icthyosis, and cardiac arrythmias. Plasma phytanic acid levels are markedly elevated.

Although symptoms may be present from late childhood the diagnosis is rarely made until early adult life. As night-blindness is a common early symptom children with sporadic or autosomal recessive RP should be screened to exclude Refsum's disease, especially if there is anosmia or ataxia (Goldman *et al.* 1985; Britton & Gibberd 1988). Dietary treatment to lower the levels of plasma phytanic acid will prevent the development of neuropathy, ataxia, cardiac arrythmias and ichthyosis but the effect on the progression of the retinal dystrophy and deafness is less certain (Britton & Gibberd 1988).

USHER'S SYNDROME

Usher's syndrome is an autosomal recessive disorder characterized by a severe congenital sensorineural hearing loss and retinitis pigmentosa (Usher 1935). It is the most common of the various syndromes associated with RP (Heckenlively 1988). The hearing loss is profound and present from birth and in the typical form normally intelligible speech rarely develops. Night-blindness is first reported in late childhood or early teens, and there is usually visual field loss and an extinguished or severely subnormal ERG at presentation. Visual acuity is good in the early stages but vision may deteriorate to 6/60 or less by the fourth decade (Heckenlively 1988).

It is now evident that there is genetic heterogeneity within Usher's syndrome (Merin *et al.* 1974; Fishman *et al.* 1983). In type 1 Usher's disease there is profound deafness with no intelligible speech; vestibular responses to rotation and calorics are absent or very abnormal. The electroretinogram is usually absent. Ataxia, psychosis, and mental retardation is a variable feature. In type 2 Usher's syndrome the hearing loss is more variable and in some patients it can be quite mild. Speech is often intelligible and vestibular responses are normal. There are rarely any other neurological problems. In type 2 Usher's syndrome the retinal dystrophy is of later onset and is less severe; a small ERG can usually be recorded (Merin *et al.* 1974; Fishman *et al.* 1983). The subtypes of Usher's syndrome seem to 'breed true' in families suggesting that there are two different genes causing this syndrome (Fishman *et al.* 1983).

CNS abnormalities, especially of the posterior fossa, are frequently seen on CT scan (Bloom *et al.* 1983).

Differential diagnosis

In assessing children with deafness and a retinal dystrophy it is important to exclude other genetic disorders before making a diagnosis of Usher's syndrome (Table 27.3.5). Congenital rubella may also cause profound deafness and a pigmentary retinopathy, although the ERG is usually normal.

Table 27.3.5 Deafness and progressive retinal dystrophy in childhood

Usher's syndrome
Cockayne's syndrome
Alstroms syndrome
Refsum's disease
Mitochondrial cytopathy
Peroxisomal disorders
MPS II + III
Leber's amaurosis
Osteopetrosis
Alport's syndrome

MITOCHONDRIAL CYTOPATHY

Mitochondrial cytopathy is an uncommon multisystem disorder in which there are ragged red fibres seen on skeletal muscle biopsy and abnormal mitochondria on electron microscopy. It is likely that there are a number of different disorders each of which result in a disturbance of mitochondrial function and it is hoped that in time structural and biochemical studies will allow these to be specifically identified (Sengers *et al.* 1984). Although most cases are sporadic familial cases are seen and do not seem to follow the pattern of mendelian inheritance (Rosing *et al.* 1985); maternal inheritance is common and may be caused by a mutation of mitochondrial DNA (Rosing *et al.* 1985; Poulton 1988).

Clinical abnormalities begin in childhood and include lactic acidosis, anaemia, myopathy, neurological abnormalities, endocrine disturbance, renal disease, neurosensory hearing loss and a retinal dystrophy (Eggar *et al.* 1981). Cardiac conduction defects are a major cause of premature death. The major ophthalmological abnormalities seen in this disorder are chronic external ophthalmoplegia and a retinal dystrophy similar to retinitis pigmentosa (Kearns & Sayre 1958; Drachman 1968), although early in the course of the disease there is only minimal pigment epithelial atrophy (Fig. 27.3.22).

Histopathology of postmortem eyes have shown marked atrophy and degeneration of the RPE and photoreceptor layer (Runge *et al.* 1986a).

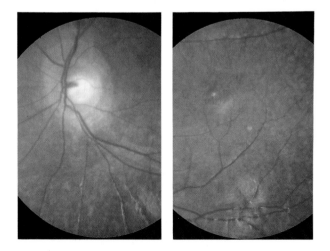

Fig. 27.3.22 Mitochondrial cytopathy in a 15-year-old with a very attenuated ERG and poor vision from 6 years old. There is mild arteriolar thinning and retinal pigment epithelial defects.

COCKAYNE'S SYNDROME

Cockayne's syndrome is a rare autosomal recessive disorder in which there is dwarfism, deafness, presenile appearance, mental retardation, and a progressive retinal dystrophy (Coles 1969; Pearce 1972). In most cases visual and general development is normal in the first year of life following which there is slow physical and intellectual deterioration. There is extensive atrophy of the subcutaneous fat and skeletal muscles and affected patients develop a characteristic bird-like facies. Death usually occurs between the ages of 10 and 30 years. The most consistent ocular feature is a progressive retinal dystrophy with optic atrophy, arteriolar attenuation and peripheral pigmentary retinopathy (Fig. 27.3.23). Other reported findings include enophthalmos, corneal opacities, cataract and nystagmus (Coles 1969; Pearce 1972).

MUCOPOLYSACCHARIDOSIS

A progressive retinal dystrophy may develop in all mucopolysaccharidosis (MPS) except Morquio's, especially in MPS IH (Hurler's disease) MPS IS (Scheie's disease) MPS II (Hunter's syndrome) and MPS III (San Fillipo's disease). The retinal abnormality is a rod-cone dystrophy which is similar in all three types of MPS. Fundus examination may show only mild retinal abnormalities so that the ERG is the best indicator of retinal disease (Caruso et al. 1986). There is a wide range of severity with some patients having a

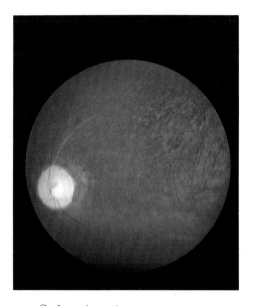

Fig. 27.3.23 Cockayne's syndrome. Severe retinal dystrophy and extreme arteriolar narrowing.

normal ERG whilst in others it is severely abnormal (Caruso 1986). The retinal and other ophthalmic features have been reviewed by François (1982).

BATTEN'S DISEASE (see Chapter 34)

Batten's disease is an autosomal recessive disorder which occurs in an infantile, late infantile and juvenile form. In the infantile and late infantile form neurological deterioration and seizures precede the visual deterioration which is due to a progressive retinal dystrophy. The ERG is extinguished at an early stage and there is marked optic atrophy, arteriolar attenuation and a mild pigmentary retinopathy. A 'Bull's eye' maculopathy is frequently seen (Raitta & Santavouri 1973; Francois 1982).

Juvenile Batten's disease however may present first to the ophthalmologist as the visual deterioration may precede the neurological signs. Visual loss usually starts between 5 and 8 years (Spalton et al. 1980) but this is later followed by intellectual regression, seizures and neurological deterioration. Death usually occurs by the late teens.

The earliest changes are usually seen at the macula where there may be a subtle 'Bull's eye' appearance which is more evident on fluorescein angiography. Later there is optic disc pallor, arteriolar attenuation and macular and peripheral pigmentation and atrophy (Spalton et al. 1980; François 1982). The ERG is substantially abnormal at an early stage. This diagnosis should be excluded in all children who present with visual loss between 5 and 8 years, especially if there is evidence of a mild maculopathy. In contrast to other forms of juvenile macular degeneration the scotopic and photopic ERG is absent or substantially subnormal.

HALLERVORDEN–SPATZ DISEASE

Hallervorden–Spatz disease is an uncommon disorder characterized by extrapyramidal motor signs and dementia which begins in early childhood and is relentlessly progressive leading to death in early adult life (Hallervorden & Spatz 1922). It is thought to be inherited as an autosomal recessive trait. Acanthocytosis and a progressive retinal dystrophy is seen in a proportion of cases (Roth et al. 1971; Newell et al. 1979; Luckenbach 1983). Fundus examination may show a flecked retina and an associated Bull's eye maculopathy (Newell 1979; Luckenbach 1983); the ERG is non-recordable at an early stage (Luckenbach 1983). Postmortem studies of eyes have shown marked loss of rods and cones throughout the retina (Luckenbach 1983).

ALSTROM'S SYNDROME

Alstrom's syndrome is an uncommon autosomal recessive disorder characterised by diabetes mellitus, severe nerve deafness, obesity, and an early onset retinal dystrophy (Alstrom 1959; Goldstein & Fialkow 1973; Sebag *et al.* 1984). Other features may include chronic renal disease, a pigmented skin lesion, acanthosis nigricans, and in males hypogonadism (Goldstein & Fialkow 1973). Visual loss and nystagmus is usually noted in infancy but there is little published information about the ocular examination and electrophysiology at this stage. Most reported cases have been examined in later childhood when there is poor central vision, nystagmus, optic disc pallor, attenuated vessels, and a pigmentary retinopathy. The ERG is absent (Goldstein & Fialkow 1973; Sebag *et al.* 1984). Histopathology in one case revealed an absence of rods and cones (Sebag *et al.* 1984).

Alstrom's syndrome has some similarities with the Biedl−Bardet syndrome but can be distinguished by the absence of mental retardation and polydactyly in the former and the rarity of nerve deafness and diabetes in the latter (Goldstein & Fialkow 1973).

LAURENCE−MOON−BIEDL (BIEDL−BARDET) SYNDROME

The Biedl−Bardet syndrome is an autosomal recessive disorder characterized by obesity, mental retardation, post axial polydactyly (Fig. 27.3.24), hypogonadism and a progressive retinal dystrophy. Renal failure, due to ureteric reflux, and hypertension are common and are the leading cause of death in this condition (Hurley *et al.* 1975). There is a wide variability in expression of the gene so that incomplete forms are seen (Klein & Amman 1969; Schachat & Maumenee 1982). In many cases the mental retardation may be mild and if the extra digits have been excised in infancy the diagnosis may be missed unless a careful history is taken, and the hands and feet examined.

The retinal disease is seen in all cases and is a severe rod-cone dystrophy with onset in childhood (Campo & Aaberg 1982) although rarely it may be present in early infancy (Runge *et al.* 1986a). Early macular involvement is common and a 'Bull's eye' picture may be seen on fundoscopy and fluorescein angiography. Optic disc pallor and arteriolar narrowing is

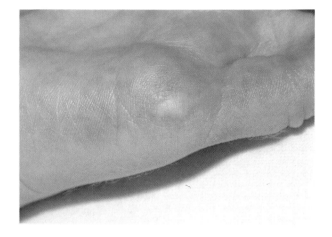

Fig. 27.3.24 Laurence−Moon−Biedl syndrome. Postaxial polydactyly may not be obvious if the extra digit has been removed.

common but peripheral pigmentation is a variable feature (Figs 27.3.25, 27.3.26) (Campo & Aarberg 1982).

The visual prognosis is poor because of early central receptor involvement, most patients have 6/60 vision or less by the third decade (Campo & Aaberg 1982).

In one histological study of the eyes of an infant with the Biedl−Bardet syndrome there was extensive photoreceptor degeneration at the macula with peripheral receptors having shortened outer segments (Runge *et al.* 1986a).

The Laurence−Moon syndrome is a closely related autosomal recessive disorder in which there is no obesity or polydactyly but affected patients have a spinal paraparesis (Campo & Aaberg 1982).

OLIVOPONTOCEREBELLAR ATROPHY

A progressive retinal dystrophy has been described in some families with olivopontocerebellar atrophy (OPCA) a dominantly inherited disorder characterised by progressive cerebellar and brain stem neuronal loss (Weiner *et al.* 1967; Ryan *et al.* 1975; De Jong *et al.* 1980). The onset of cerebellar signs and visual loss is variable but has been reported in early infancy (De Jong *et al.* 1980) and childhood (Weiner *et al.* 1967; Ryan *et al.* 1975). There is optic disc pallor, arteriolar attenuation and a peripheral pigmentary retinopathy. Macular pigment epithelial atrophy and pigmentation is common (Ryan *et al.* 1975; De Jong *et al.* 1980; Traboulsi *et al.* 1988). The ERG is absent or severely abnormal. Histopathological examination of eyes obtained at postmortem have shown marked shortening of the outer segments and receptor loss

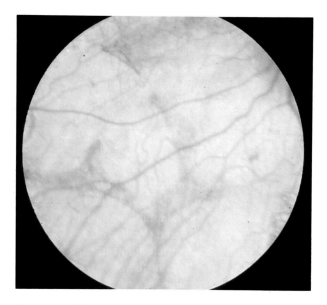

Fig. 27.3.27 Choroideremia. Mid peripheral retinal pigment epithelial atrophy with 'scalloped' appearance.

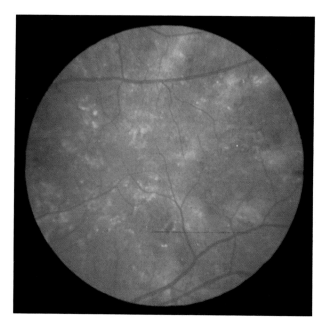

Fig. 27.3.29 Choroideremia carrier: linear depigmented areas in the peripheral retina. Professor B. Jay's patient.

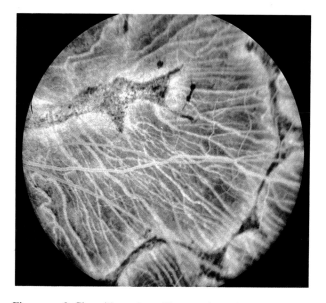

Fig. 27.3.28 Choroideremia — Fluorescein angiogram showing characteristic scalloped appearance given by the surviving RPE and less of choriocapillaris.

appearance of the peripheral retina on fundoscopy (Fig. 27.3.29.)

Male hemizygotes

(a) *Clinical features*: Affected males usually present between the ages of 5 and 10 years with night-blindness. The earliest fundus signs are fine pigment epi-

thelial atrophy and pigmentation in the equatorial retina; at this stage the clinical appearance may be confused with RP. Later focal areas of atrophy of the RPE and choriocapillaries develop, which are particularly well demonstrated on fluorescein angiography (Fig. 27.3.28). These areas coalesce to give a widespread atrophic appearance throughout the equatorial retina (Fig. 27.3.27). This later spreads to involve the peripheral and more posterior retina; the macula is spared until late in the disease.

Visual fields initially show small mid peripheral scotomata corresponding to areas of atrophy but later a typical ring scotoma develops. As the disease progresses marked constriction of the visual field occurs but there is often a small preserved island of field in the far periphery. Visual acuity remains reasonably good until the 5th-6th decade in most patients (Krill 1977; Heckenlively 1988).

(b) *Electrophysiology*: The electroretinogram is abnormal or extinguished at an early stage; in those with a preserved response rod and cone amplitudes are reduced and cone b wave implicit times are prolonged (Heckenlively 1988).

(c) *Histopathology*: Histological examination of the eyes of an 18-year-old male with early disease showed marked degeneration of the outer retina with loss of RPE, Bruch's membrane and choriocapillaris.

Biochemical studies showed reduced levels of inter-receptor retinal binding protein (IRBP) and increased levels of cyclic AMP in the RPE and choroid (Rodrigues *et al.* 1984).

Female heterozygotes

Most female carriers are asymptomatic but the fundus appearance is characteristic (Fig. 27.3.29). There is widespread fine RPE atrophy and granular pigment deposition in the mid peripheral retina. The EOG and ERG are usually normal (Sievring *et al.* 1986). Female carriers with extensive fundus changes may be thought to have RP but the absence of night-blindness and normal ERG help to differentiate this condition from RP.

GYRATE ATROPHY OF THE CHOROID AND RETINA

Gyrate atrophy of the choroid and retina is a rare autosomal recessive disorder characterized by a progressive chorioretinal dystrophy, hyperornithinemia and a deficiency of the enzyme ornithineamino-transferase (OAT) (Simell & Takki 1973; Takki & Simell 1974; Kennaway *et al.* 1977; Weleber & Kennaway 1988). The level of OAT activity in obligate carriers of the gene has been shown to be about 50% of normal (Valle *et al.* 1977). Recently Inana *et al.* (1988) have identified a patient with gyrate atrophy with a partial deletion of the OAT gene on chromosome 10; there was no detectable OAT messenger RNA and by using an antibody directed against the enzyme they were able to demonstrate greatly reduced levels. Gyrate atrophy therefore appears to be caused by a mutation of the OAT gene on chromosome 10 and RFLPs in this area may be useful in prenatal diagnosis and counselling (Inana *et al.* 1988).

Clinical findings

Children may present with night-blindness, progressive myopia or field loss but the diagnosis may be made in early infancy when a raised level of plasma ornithene is found in a child with a family history of gyrate atrophy (Kaiser-Kupfer *et al.* 1985).

The earliest fundus changes are seen as small discrete areas of choroidal and retinal pigment epithelial atrophy in the mid and far peripheral fundus (Fig. 27.3.30) (Takki & Simell 1976; Kaiser-Kupfer *et al.* 1985; Berson *et al.* 1978; Rinaldi *et al.* 1979; Weleber & Kennaway 1988). The adjacent fundus may show evidence of diffuse depigmentation of the RPE and

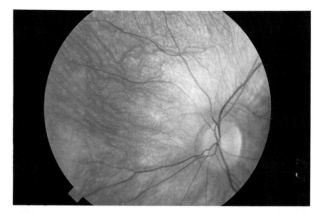

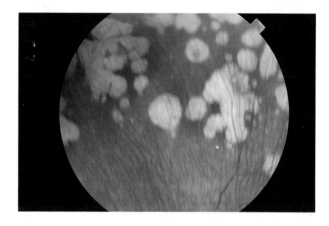

Fig. 27.3.30 Gyrate atrophy with hyperornithinemia. This nine-year-old child presented with night-blindness. The posterior pole (a) shows arteriolar narrowing and some minimal RPE changes. The mid and far periphery (b) show the typical atrophic areas.

atrophic areas are particularly well demonstrated on fluorescein angiography. The atrophic areas subsequently coalesce and enlarge towards the posterior pole with a characteristic scalloped appearance at the leading edge (see Fig. 27.3.31).

Most patients have moderate to high myopia and posterior subcapsular cataracts develop in early adult life. Visual loss may also develop secondary to macular odema or atrophy (Weleber & Kennaway 1988). Most patients maintain a reasonable level of visual acuity until their 40s or 50s, although with a constricted field.

Visual field loss corresponds to the degree of choroidal and RPE atrophy. In the early stages there are small mid peripheral scotomas but progression of disease leads to marked peripheral constriction. Dark adaptation shows markedly elevated rod thresholds in areas of field corresponding to involved retina.

Electrophysiology

The EOG is subnormal in most patients with gyrate atrophy, even in young affected children (Kaiser-Kupfer *et al.* 1985). The ERG responses depend on the severity of disease; early in the disease both rod and cone amplitudes are reduced (Berson *et al.* 1978; Kaiser-Kupfer 1985) but later the ERG may be unrecordable.

Non-ocular features

Although patients with gyrate atrophy show no muscle weakness, muscle biopsy shows atrophy of type 2 fibres with accumulation of tubular aggregates (Sipila *et al.* 1979). Other reported abnormalities include structural abnormalities of hair, EEG abnormalities and mild mental subnormality (Kaiser-Kupfer 1981).

Biochemical findings and treatment

Patients with gyrate atrophy have a deficiency of the pyridoxal phosphate dependent mitochondrial enzyme ornithine-aminotransferase (OAT) which is responsible for the conversion of ornithene to glutamic acid. Ornithene is not present in protein and the major dietary source is arginine which may be converted to ornithene by the arginase reaction of the urea cycle or by the glycine transamidase reaction (Valle *et al.* 1981). Ornithene is an important intermediary in the urea cycle and is necessary for the production of polyamines and in the synthesis of proline and glutamate (Weleber & Kennaway 1988).

It is not clear whether the retinal abnormalities are caused by high levels of ornithene or the reduced levels of proline and glutamate that accompany OAT deficiency. Not all patients with raised ornithene levels develop gyrate atrophy and one patient with gyrate atrophy has been reported who had normal ornithene levels and low plasma proline levels (Tada *et al.* 1983) suggesting that reduced availability of proline may be a contributory factor.

Three different approaches to treatment have been used (Weleber & Kennaway 1988). A minority of patients are responsive to pyridoxine (B6) supplements and show a reduced plasma ornithene levels and improvement in the electroretinogram (Weleber & Kennaway 1988). Vitamin B6 should be used initially in all patients and continued in those who show a positive response. In non-responders plasma ornithene levels may be reduced by adhering to an arginene restricted diet (Valle *et al.* 1981) and proline sup-

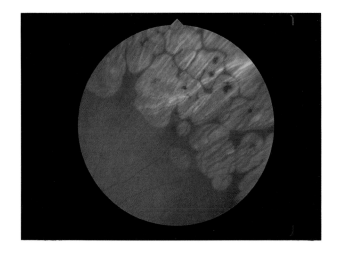

Fig. 27.3.31 Gyrate atrophy with hyperornithinaemia. Mid peripheral coalesced atrophic areas with scalloped edge.

plementation has been reported to prevent retinal degeneration in some patients (Tada *et al.* 1983).

Children with gyrate atrophy are best managed in collaboration with a paediatrician with an interest in clinical biochemistry. Although the present treatment regimes are promising, more long-term studies are needed to assess whether such treatment will prevent retinal deterioration.

Cone dystrophies

The inherited cone dystrophies are a heterogeneous group of disorders characterized by variable photophobia, reduced central vision, abnormal colour vision and an abnormal photopic ERG (Goodman *et al.* 1963). They may be stationary or progressive; the stationary forms (achromatopsia) have already been discussed.

Progressive cone dystrophy

GENETICS

Most cases of progressive cone dystrophy are sporadic but when familial cases are seen the usual mode of inheritance is autosomal dominant (Berson *et al.* 1968; Krill & Deutmann 1972). Most of the sporadic cases probably represent autosomal recessive inheritance. Heckenlively and Weleber (1986) have recently described an X-linked recessive cone dystrophy in which affected males had an abnormal tapetal reflex which disappeared on prolonged dark adaptation (Mizuo phenomenon).

CLINICAL FEATURES

In contrast to achromatopsia which presents in early infancy the progressive cone dystrophies are not usually symptomatic until late childhood or early adult life (Sloan & Brown 1962; Krill 1977). Photophobia is a prominent early symptom and there is progressive loss of central vision and colour vision (Berson *et al.* 1968; Krill & Deutman 1972; Krill 1977c). Fine nystagmus is seen even in older children. A small central scotoma is frequently detected on careful visual field testing but peripheral fields remain full. The rate of visual loss is very variable but visual acuity usually deteriorates to the level of 6/60 or to an ability to count fingers only.

Fundus examination usually shows a typical Bull's eye maculopathy (Figs 27.3.31, 27.3.32) (Berson *et al.* 1968; Krill & Deutman 1972; Krill 1977) although in some cases there may be only minor macular pigment epithelial atrophy and pigmentation. The optic discs show a variable degree of temporal pallor. The retinal periphery is usually normal although rarely white flecks similar to those seen in fundus flavimaculatus may be seen (Krill 1977c). Fluorescein angiography shows typical 'window' defects at the macula in the majority of cases and the so called dark choroid sign is frequently seen (Bonnin 1976; Uliss *et al.* 1988).

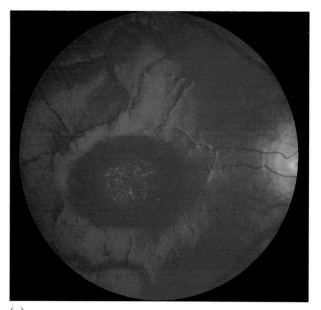

(a)

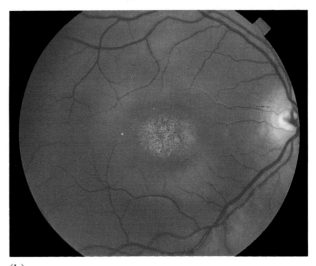

(b)

Fig. 27.3.33 (a) Progressive cone dystrophy in March 1982. (b) July 1985 showing minimal change (same patient).

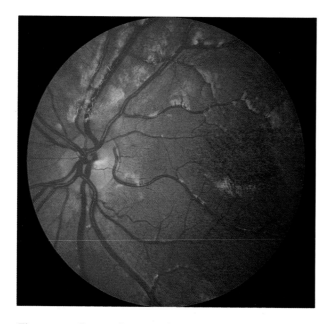

Fig. 27.3.32 Progressive cone dystrophy with 'Bull's eye' maculopathy.

ELECTROPHYSIOLOGY AND PSYCHOPHYSICS

Dark adaptation studies show either a monophasic curve with no recognizable cone component, or a biphasic curve with elevated cone thresholds; rod mediated thresholds are normal (Sloan & Brown 1962; Berson *et al.* 1968; Krill 1977). Spectral sensitivity studies show a typical rod curve under both scotopic and photopic conditions (Krill 1977c).

Electroretinography shows normal rod responses but an absent cone response.

DIFFERENTIAL DIAGNOSIS

Progressive cone dystrophy must be differentiated from the other cone dystrophies notably achromatopsia and progressive cone-rod dystrophies and from other disorders giving rise to Bull's eye maculopathy in childhood (Table 27.3.6). The profoundly abnormal cone ERG allows progressive cone dystrophy to be differentiated from other inherited central receptor dystrophies and the age of onset and lack of rod involvement distinguish this disorder from other cone dystrophies.

Table 27.3.6 Bull's eye maculopathy in childhood

Stargardt's disease
Progressive cone dystrophy
Cone-rod dystrophy
Batten's disease
Hallervorden—Spatz disease
Biedl—Bardet syndrome
Mucolipidosis IV
Drug toxicity (e.g. chloroquine)

Progressive cone-rod dystrophy

In this uncommon disorder affected patients develop the typical findings of a cone dystrophy in early life but later there is evidence of rod involvement with night-blindness and peripheral field loss. Both rod and cone thresholds are elevated and the ERG shows reduced rod and cone amplitudes (Goodman *et al.* 1963). Both autosomal dominant and autosomal recessive inheritance is seen.

Associated findings

Bjork *et al.* (1956) have reported one pedigree of progressive cone-rod dystrophy in which affected members had an associated ataxia of the Pierre—Marie type. Recently Jalili and Smith (1988) have described an autosomal recessive disorder characterized by a cone-rod dystrophy and amelogenesis imperfecta (defective tooth enamel).

References

Abraham FA, Yanko L, Licht A, Visroper RJ. Electrophysiologic study of the visual system in familial juvenile nephronophthisis and tapeto-retinal dystrophy. *Am J Ophthalmol* 1974; **78**: 591−7

Allen AW, Moon JB, Holland KR, Minckley DS. Ocular findings in the thoracic-pelvi-phalangeal dystrophy. *Arch Ophthalmol* 1979; **97**: 489−92

Alpern M, Lee GB, Spivey B. π 1 cone monochromatism. *Arch Ophthalmol* 1965; **74**: 334−7

Alstrom CH, Hallgren B, Nilson LB, Asander H. Retinal degeneration combined with obesity, diabetes mellitus, and neurogenic deafness. *Acta Psychiatr Scand* 1959; **34**: 1−35

Alstrom CH, Olson OA. Heredo-retinopathia congenitalis. Monohybrida recessiva autosomalis. *Hereditas* 1957; **43**: 1−177

Alvarez F, Landrieu P, Laget P *et al.* Nervous and ocular disorders in children with cholestatis and vitamin A and E deficiency. *Hepatology* 1983; **3**: 410−14

Amman F, Klein D, Franceschetti A. Genetic and epidemiological investigations on pigmentary degeneration of the retina and allied disorders in Switzerland. *J Neurol Sci* 1965; **2**: 183−96

Anandakrishnan I, Musarella M. Genetic counselling in X-linked retinitis pigmentosa. Pediatr Ophthalmol Strabismus 1989; **26**: 140−5

Arden GB, Carter RM, Hogg CR *et al.* A modified ERG technique and the results obtained in X-linked retinitis pigmentosa. *Br J Ophthalmol* 1983; **67**: 419−30

Auerbach E, Godel V, Rowe H. An electrophysiological and psychophysical study of two forms of congenital night-blindness. *Invest Ophthalmol* 1969; **8**: 332−45

Bard LA, Bard PA, Owens GW *et al.* Retinal involvement in thoracic-pelvic-phalangeal dystrophy. *Arch Ophthalmol* 1978; **96**: 278−81

Berson EL, Gouras P, Gunkel RD. Progressive cone degeneration dominantly inherited. *Arch Ophthalmol* 1968; **80**: 77−83

Berson EL, Rosen JB, Siminoff EA. Electroretinographic testing as an aid in detection of X chromosome linked retinitis pigmentosa. *Am J Ophthalmol* 1979; **87**: 460−8

Berson EL, Sandberg MA, Maguire A. Electroretinogram in carriers of blue cone monochromatism. *Am J Ophthalmol* 1986; **102**: 254−61

Berson EL, Schmidt SY, Shih VE. Ocular and biochemical abnormalities in gyrate atrophy of the choroid and retina. *Ophthalmology* 1978; **85**: 1018−27

Berson EL, Simonoff EA. Dominant retinitis pigmentosa with reduced penetrance. Further studies of the electroretinogram. *Arch Ophthalmol* 1979; **97**: 1286−91

Bhattacharya JSS, Wright AF, Clayton JF *et al.* Close genetic linkage between X-linked retinitis pigmentosa and a restriction fragment polymorphism identified by recombinant DNA probe. *Nature* 1984; **309**: 253−5

Bird AC. X-linked retinitis pigmentosa. *Br J Ophthalmol* 1975; **59**: 177−99

Bird AC, Hyman V. Detection of heterozygotes in families with X-linked pigmentary retinopathy by measurement of retinal rhodopsin concentration. *Trans Ophthalmol Soc UK* 1972; **92**: 221−8

Bishihara S, Merin S, Cooper M *et al.* Combined vitamin A and E therapy prevents retinal electrophysiological deterioration in abetalipoproteinaemia. Br J Ophthalmol 1982; **66**: 767−70

Bjork A, Lindblau U, Wadensten L. Retinal degeneration in hereditary ataxia. *J Neurol Neurosurg Psychiatr* 1956; **19**: 186−93

Bloom TD, Fishman GA, Matee MF. Ushers syndrome CNS defects determined by computerised tomography. *Retina* 1983; **3**: 108−13

Bonnin J, Passot M, Triolaire M. Le signe du silence choroidien dans les degenerescences tapeto-retiniennes posterieures. *Doc Ophthalmol Proc Ser* 1976; **9**: 461−3

Boughman JA, Fishman GA. A genetic analysis of retinitis pigmentosa. *Br J Ophthalmol* 1983; **67**: 449−54

Britton TC, Gibberd FB. A family with heredopathia atactica polyneuritiformis (Refsum's disease). *J R Soc Med* 1988; **81**: 602−3

Buchanan NM, Atta HR, Crean GJP et al. A case of eye disease due to dietary vitamin A deficiency in Glasgow. *Scott Med J* 1987; **32**: 52−3

Campo RV, Aaberg TM. Ocular and systemic manifestations of the Bardet−Biedl syndrome. *Am J Ophthalmol* 1982; **94**: 750−6

Carr RF, Gouras P. Oguchis disease. *Arch Ophthalmol* 1965; **73**: 646−56

Carr RE, Siegel IM. Unilateral retinitis pigmentosa. *Arch Ophthalmol* 1973; **90**: 21−6

Carr RE, Rupps H, Siegel IM. Visual pigment kinetics and adaptation in fundus albipunctatus. *Doc Ophthalmol Proc Ser* 1974; **4**: 193−204

Caruso RC, Kaiser-Kupfer MI, Muenzerj et al. Electroretinographic findings in the mucopolysaccharidoses. *Ophthalmology* 1986; **93**: 1612−16

Chew E, Deutman A, Pinckers A, DeKirk AA. Yellowish flecks in Leber's congenital amaurosis. *Br J Ophthalmol* 1984; **84**: 727−31

Cohen SMZ, Brown FR, Martyn L et al. Ocular histopathologic and biochemical studies of the cerebrohepatorenal syndrome (Zellweger's syndrome) and its relationship to neonatal adrenoleukodystrophy. *Am J Ophthalmol* 1983; **96**: 488−501

Cohen SMZ, Green WR, De la Cruz ZC et al. Ocular histopathologic studies of neonatal and childhood adrenoleukodystrophy. *Am J Ophthalmol* 1983; **95**: 82−96

Coles WH. Ocular manifestations of Cockayne's syndrome. *Am J Ophthalmol* 1969; **67**: 762−4

Cooper DW, Jay M, Bhattacharya S, Jay B. Molecular genetic approaches to the analysis of human ophthalmic disease *Eye* 1987; **1**: 699−721

Davies S, Marcus RE, Hungerford JL et al. Ocular toxicity of high dose intravenous desferrioxamine. *Lancet* 1983; **ii**: 181−4

de Jong PTVM, de Jong JGY, de Jong−Ten Doeschate JMM, Delleman JW. Olivopontocerebellar atrophy with visual disturbances. An ophthalmological investigation into 4 generations. *Ophthalmology* 1980; 87: 793−804

Dekaban AS. Hereditary syndrome of congenital retinal blindness (Leber), polycystic kidneys and maldevelopment of the brain. *Am J Ophthalmol* 1969; **68**: 1029−36

Dekaban AS. Mental retardation and neurological involvement in patients with congenital retinal blindness. *Dev Med Child Neurol* 1972; **14**: 436−44

Dekaban AS, Carr R. Congenital amaurosis of retinal origin. Frequent association with neurological disorders. *Arch Neurol* 1966; **14**: 294−301

Drachman DA. Ophthalmoplegia plus. The neuro-degenerative disorders associated with progressive external ophthalmoplegia. *Arch Neurol* 1968; **18**: 654−74

Edwards WC, Grizzard WS. Tapeto-retinal degeneration associated with renal disease. *J Pediatr Ophthalmol Strabismus* 1981; **18**: 55−57

Eggar J, Lake BD, Wilson J. Mitochondrial cytopathy. A multysystem disorder with ragged red fibres on muscle biopsy. *Arch Dis Child* 1981; **56**: 741−52

Ellis DS, Heckenlively JR, Martin CL et al. Leber's congenital amaurosis associated with familial juvenile nephronophthisis and cone-shaped epiphyses of the hands (the Saldino−Mainzer syndrome). *Am J Ophthalmol* 1984; **97**: 233−9

Ernst W, Clover G, Faulkner DJ. X-linked retinitis pigmentosa: reduced rod flicker sensitivity in heterozygous females. *Invest Ophthalmol Vis Sci* 1981; **20**: 812−6

Fairley KF, Leighton PW, Kincaid-Smith P. Familial visual defects associated with polycystic kidney and medullary sponge kidney. *Br Med J* 1963; **1**: 1060−3

Falls HF, Wolter JR, Alpern M. Typical total monochromacy. *Arch Ophthalmol* 1965; **74**: 610−6

Fishman GA, Gilbert LD, Fiscella RG et al. Acetazolamide for treatment of chronic macular oedema in retinitis pigmentosa. *Arch Ophthalmol* 1989; **107**: 1445−52

Fishman GA, Kumar A, Joseph ME et al. Usher's syndrome: ophthalmic and neuro-otologic findings suggesting genetic heterogeneity. *Arch Ophthalmol* 1983; **101**: 1367−74

Fishman GA, Weinburg AB, McMahon TT. X-linked recessive retinitis pigmentosa: clinical characteristics of carriers. *Arch Ophthalmol* 1986; **104**: 1329−35

Flynn JT, Cullen RF. Disc oedema in congenital amaurosis of Leber. *Br J Ophthalmol* 1975; **59**: 497−502

Foxman SG, Heckenlively JR, Bateman JB, Wirtschafter JD. Classification of congenital and early onset retinitis pigmentosa. *Arch Ophthalmol* 1985; **103**: 1502−6

Foxman SG, Wirtschafter JD, Letson RD. Leber's congenital amaurosis and high hypermetropia: a discrete entity. In: Henkind P (Ed.) *ACTA XXIV International Congress Ophthalmology*, Vol. 1. JB Lippinicott Co, Philadelphia 1983; pp. 55−8

Franceschetti A. Rubeole pendant la grossese et cataracte congenitale chez l'enfant: accompagne du phenomene digito-oculaire. *Ophthalmologica* 1947; **114**: 332−9

François J. Metabolic tapetoretinal degenerations. *Surv Ophthalmol* 1982; **26**: 293−333

Garner A, Fielder AR, Primavesi R, Steven A. Tapetoretinal degeneration in the cerebro-hepato-renal (Zellweger) syndrome. *Br J Ophthalmol* 1982; **66**: 422−31

Gelber PJ, Shah A. Fluorescein study of albipunctate dystrophy. *Arch Ophthalmol* 1969; **81**: 164−9

Gil-Gilberneau J, Galain A, Callis L, Rodrigo C. Infantile idiopathic hypercalcuria, high congenital myopia and atypical macular coloboma: a new oculorenal syndrome. *J Pediatr Ophthalmol Strabismus* 1982; **19**: 7−11

Glasgow BJ, Brown HH, Hannah JB, Foos RY. Ocular pathologic findings in neonatal adrenoleucodystrophy. *Ophthalmology* 1987; **94**: 1054−60

Glickstein M, Heath GG. Receptors in the monochromat eye. *Vision Res* 1975; **15**: 633−6

Goldman JM, Clemens ME, Gibberd JB, Billimoria JD. Screening of patients with retinitis pigmentosa for heredopathia atactica polyneuritiformis (Refsum's disease). *Br Med J* 1985; **290**: 1109−10

Goldstein JL, Fialkow PJ. The Alstrom syndrome. Report of three cases with further delineation of the clinical, pathophysiological and genetic aspects of the disorder. *Medicine* 1973; **52**: 53−71

Goodman G, Ripps H, Siegel IM. Cone dysfunction syndromes. *Arch Ophthalmol* 1963; **70**: 214−31.

Gotto AM, Levy RI, John K, Fredrickson DS. On the protein

defect in A-betalipoproteinemia. *N Engl J Med* 1971; **284**: 813−5

Haddad R, Font RL, Friendly DS. Cerebro-hepato-renal syndrome of Zellweger. Ocular histopathologic findings. *Arch Ophthalmol* 1976; **94**: 1927−30

Hajra AK, Datta NS, Jackson LG *et al*. Prenatal diagnosis of Zellweger cerebro-hepato-renal syndrome. *N Engl J Med* 1985; **312**: 445−6

Hallervorden J, Spatz H. Eigenartige erkrankung im extrapyramidalen system mit besonderer betelligung des globus pallidus unter der substantia Nigra. *Z Neurol Psychiatr* 1922; **79**: 254−62

Harrison R, Hoefnagel D, Hayward JN. Congenital total colour blindness, a clinicopathological report. *Arch Ophthalmol* 1960; **64**: 685−92

Heckenlively JR. *Retinitis Pigmentosa* JB Lippincott Co, Philadelphia 1988

Heckenlively JR, Martin DA, Rosenbaum AL. Loss of electroretinographic oscillatory potentials, optic atrophy, and dysplasia in congenital stationary night-blindness. *Am J Ophthalmol* 1983; **96**: 526−34

Heckenlively JR, Weleber RG. X-linked recessive cone dystrophy with tapetal-like sheen. *Arch Ophthalmol* 1986; **104**: 1322−28

Herdman RC, Good R, Vernier RL, Anderson LA. Medullary cystic disease in two siblings. *Am J Med* 1967; **43**: 335−44

Hittner HM, Kretzer FL, Mehta RS. Zellwegers syndrome: lenticular opacities indicating carrier status and lens abnormalities characteristic of homozygotes. *Arch Ophthalmol* 1981; **99**: 1977−82

Hurley R, Dery P, Nogrady M, Drummond K. The renal lesion of Laurence-Moon-Biedl syndrome. *J Pediatr* 1975; **87**: 206−9

Inana G, Hotta Y, Zintz C *et al*. Expression defect of Ornithene aminotransferase gene in gyrate atrophy. *Invest Ophthalmol Vis Sci* 1988; **29**: 1001−5

Jalili IK, Smith NJD. A progressive cone-rod dystrophy amelogenesis imperfecta: a new syndrome. *J Med Genet* 1988; **25**: 738−40

Jay M. On the heredity of retinitis pigmentosa. *Br J Ophthalmol* 1982; **66**: 405−16

Jeune M, Beraud C, Canon R. Dystrophie thoracique asphyxiante de caractère familial. *Arch Fr Pediatr* 1955; **12**: 886−91

Joubert M, Eisenring J, Robb JP, Andermann F. Familial agenesis of the cerebellar vermis. *Neurology* 1969; **19**: 813−25

Judisch GF, Lowry B, Hanson JW. Chorioretinopathy and pituitary dysfunction. The CPD syndrome. *Arch Ophthalmol* 1981; **99**: 253−61

Judisch GF, Rhead WJ, Miler DK. Abetalipoproteinemia. *Ophthalmologica* 1984; **189**: 73−9

Kaiser-Kupfer M, Kuwabara T, Askanas *et al*. Systemic manifestations of gyrate atrophy of the choroid and retina. *Ophthalmology* 1981; **88**: 302−6

Kaiser-Kupfer M, Ludwig IH, de Monasterio FM *et al*. Gyrate atrophy of the choroid and retina. Early findings. *Ophthalmology* 1985; **92**: 394−401

Kearns TP, Sayre GP. Retinitis pigmentosa, external ophthalmoplegia and complete heart block. Unusual syndrome with histologic study in one of two cases. *Arch Ophthalmol* 1958; **60**: 280−9

Keith CG. Retinal atrophy in osteopetrosis. *Arch Ophthalmol* 1968; **79**: 234−41

Kemp CM, Jacobson SG, Faulkner DJ. Two types of visual dysfunction in autosomal dominant retinitis pigmentosa. *Invest Ophthalmol Vis Sci* 1988; **29**: 1235−41

Kennaway NG, Weleber RG, Buist NRM. Gyrate atrophy of the choroid and retina: deficient activity of ornithene ketoacid aminotransferase in cultured skin fibroblasts. *N Engl J Med* 1977; **297**: 1180

King MD, Dudgeon J, Stephenson JBP. Joubert's syndrome with retinal dysplasia; neonatal tachypnoea as the clue to a genetic brain−eye malformation. *Arch Dis Child* 1984; **59**: 709−18

Klein D, Amman F. The syndrome of Lawrence-Moon-Biedl Bardet and allied diseases in Switzerland. Clinical genetic and epidemiological studies. *J Neurol Sci* 1969; **9**: 479−89

Krill AE. Congenital stationary night-blindness. In: Krill AE (Ed.) *Hereditary Retinal and Choroidal Disease* Vol. II. Harper & Row, London 1977a pp. 391−417

Krill AE. Congenital colour vision defects. In: Krill AE (Ed.) *Hereditary Retinal and Choroidal Disease* Vol II. Harper & Row, London 1977b pp. 355−90

Krill AE. Cone degenerations. In: Krill AE (Ed.) *Hereditary Retinal and Choroidal Disease* Vol II. Harper & Row, London 1977c pp. 335−90

Krill AE, Deutman AF. Dominant macular degeneration. The cone dystrophies. *Am J Ophthalmol* 1972; **73**: 352−9

Krill AE, Martin D. Photopic abnormalities in congenital stationary night-blindness. *Invest Ophthalmol Vis Sci* 1971; **107**: 625−36

Lakhampal V, Schockett SS, Jiji R. Deferoxamine (Desferol) induced toxic retinal pigmentary degeneration and presumed optic neuropathy. *Ophthalmology* 1984; **91**: 443−51

Lambert SR, Kriss A, Gresty M, Benton S, Taylor D. Joubert syndrome. *Arch Ophthalmol* 1989a; **107**: 109−13

Lambert SR, Kriss A, Taylor D, Coffey R, Pembury M. Leber's congenital amaurosis: a follow-up diagnostic reappraisal of 75 patients. *Am J Ophthalmol* 1989b; **107**: 624−31

Larsen H. Demonstration microskopischer präparate von einem monochromatischen auge. *Ophthalmologica* 1921; **46**: 228−9

Loken AC, Hanssen O, Halvorsen S, Jolster NJ. Hereditary renal dysplasia and blindness. *Acta Paediatr Scand* 1961; **50**: 177−84

Luckenbach MW, Green R, Miller M *et al*. Ocular clinicopathologic correlation of Hallervorden−Spatz syndrome with acanthocytosis and pigmentary retinopathy. *Am J Ophthalmol* 1983; **95**: 369−82

Lyness AL, Ernst W, Quinlan MP *et al*. A clinical, psychophysical and electroretinographic survey of patients with autosomal dominant retinitis pigmentosa. *Br J Ophthalmol* 1985; **69**: 326−39

Mainzer F, Saldino RM, Ozononoff MB, Minagi H. Familial nephropathy associated with retinitis pigmentosa, cerebellar ataxia and skeletal abnormalities. *Am J Med* 1970; **49**: 556−62

Margolis S, Scher BM, Carr RE. Macular colobomas in Leber's congenital amaurosis. *Am J Ophthalmol* 1977; **83**: 27−31

Marmor MF. Defining fundus albipunctatus. *Doc Ophthalmol Proc Ser* 1977; **13**: 227−34

Massoff RW, Finklestein D. Vision threshold profiles in sector retinitis pigmentosa. *Arch Ophthalmol* 1979; **97**: 1899−904

Massof RW, Finkelstein D. Two forms of autosomal dominant

primary retinitis pigmentosa. *Doc ophthalmol* 1981; **51**: 289–346

Mausof FE, Burns CA, Burian HM. Morphological and functional retinal changes in myotonic dystrophy unrelated to Quinine therapy. *Am J Ophthalmol* 1972; **74**: 1141–3

Meier DA, Hess JW. Familial nephropathy with retinitis pigmentosa: a new oculorenal syndrome in adults. *Am J Med* 1965; **39**: 58–69

Meier W, Blumberg A, Imahom W *et al.* Idiopathic hypercalunia with bilateral macular colobomata: a new variant of ocular renal syndrome. *Helv Paediatr Acta* 1979; **34**: 257–69

Merin S, Abraham FA, Auerbach E. Usher's and Hallgren's syndromes. *Acta Genet Med* 1974; **23**: 49–55

Merin S, Auerbach E. Retinitis pigmentosa. *Surv Ophthalmol* 1976; **20**: 303–45

Michalski A, Leonard JV, Taylor DSI. The eye and inherited metabolic disease. *J R Soc Med* 1988; **81**: 286–90

Miyake Y, Kawase Y. Reduced amplitude of oscillatory potentials in female carriers of X-linked recessive congenital stationary night-blindness. *Am J Ophthalmol* 1984; **98**: 208–15

Miyake Y, Yagasaki K, Horiguchi M *et al.* Congenital stationary night-blindness with negative electroretinogram. *Arch Ophthalmol* 1986; **104**: 1013–20

Mizuno K, Takei Y, Sears ML *et al.* Leber's congenital amaurosis. *Am J Ophthalmol* 1977; **83**: 34–42

Mizuo G. On New Discovery in dark adaptation in Ogouchi's disease. *Acta Soc Ophthalmol Jap* 1913; **17**: 1148–50

Modell B. Advances in the use of iron-chelating agents for the treatment of iron overload. *Prog Hematol* 1979; **11**: 267–312

Moore AT, Ernst W, Jay M *et al.* Autosomal dominant retinitis pigmentosa with apparent incomplete penetrance. *Invest Ophthalmol Vis Sci Suppl.* 1987; **28**: 112

Moore AT, Fitzke F, Chen JC, *et al.* Prolonged rod dark adaption in autosonal dominant sector retinitis pigmentosa. *Invest Opthalmol Vis Sci Suppl* 1989; **30**: 45

Moore AT, Taylor DSI. A syndrome of congenital retinal dystrophy and saccade palsy — a subset of Leber's amaurosis. *Br J Ophthalmol* 1984; **68**: 421–31

Moore AT, Taylor DS, Harden A. Bilateral macular dysplasia ('colobomata') and congenital retinal dystrophy. *Br J Ophthalmol* 1985; **69**: 691–9

Naidu S, Moser AE, Moser HW. Phenotypic and genotypic variability of generalized peroxisomal disorders. *Pediatr Neurol* **1988**; **4**: 95–12

Newell FW, Johnson RO, Huttenlocher PR. Pigmentary degeneration of the retina in the Hallervorden–Spatz syndrome. *Am J Ophthalmol* 1979; **88**: 467–71

Nickel B, Hoyt CS. Leber's congenital amaurosis. Is mental retardation a frequent associated defect? *Arch Ophthalmol* 1982; **100**: 1089–92

Noble KG, Carr RE. Leber's congenital amaurosis. A retrospective study of 33 cases and a histopathological study of one case. *Arch Ophthalmol* 1978; **96**: 818–21

Noble KG, Carr RE. Pigmented paravenous chorioretinal atrophy. *Am J Ophthalmol* 1983; **96**: 338–44

Oberklaid F, Danks DM, Mayne V, Campbell P. Asphyxiating thoracic dysplasia. Clinical, radiological, and pathological information on 10 patients. *Arch Dis Child* 1977; **52**: 758–65

O'Donnell MO, Talbot JF. Vitamin A deficiency in treated cystic fibrosis: case report. *Br J Ophthalmol* 1987; **71**: 787–90

Oliver GL, McFarlane DC. Congenital trichomegaly with associated pigmentary degeneration of the retina, dwarfism and mental retardation. *Arch Ophthalmol* 1965; **74**: 169–71

Pearce WG. Ocular and genetic features of Cockayne's syndrome. *Can J Ophthalmol* 1972; **7**: 435–44

Pearlman JT, Heckenlively JR, Bastek JV. Progressive nature of pigmented paravenous retinochoroidal atrophy. *Am J Ophthalmol* 1978; **85**: 215–17

Pearlman JT, Kamin DF, Kopelois SM, Saxton J. Pigmented paravenous retinochoroidal atrophy. *Am J Ophthalmol* 1975; **80**: 630–5

Phillips CI, Stokoe NL, Bartholomew RS. Asphyxiating thoracic dystrophy (Jeune's disease) with retinal aplasia. A sibship of two. *J Pediatr Ophthalmol Strabismus* 1979; **16**: 279–83

Polak BCP, Hogewind BL, Van Lith FHM. Tapetoretinal degeneration associated with recessively inherited medullary cystic disease. *Am J Ophthalmol* 1977; **84**: 645–51

Poulton J. Mitochondrial DNA and genetic disease. *Arch Dis Child* 1988; **63**: 883–5

Price MJ, Judisch GF, Thompson HS. X-linked congenital stationary night blindness with myopia and nystagmus without clinical complaints of nyctalopia. *J Pediatr Ophthalmol Strabismus* 1988; **25**: 33–6

Price MJ, Thompson HS, Judisch FG *et al.* Pupillary constriction to darkness. *Br J Ophthalmol* 1985; **69**: 205–11

Puklin JE, Rielly CA, Simon RM, Cotlier E. Anterior segment and retinal pigmentary abnormalities in arteriohepatic dysplasia. *Ophthalmology* 1981; **88**: 337–47

Rahi AHS, Hungerford JL, Ahmed AI. Ocular toxicity of desferrioxamine: light microscopic, histochemical, and ultrastructural findings. *Br J Ophthalmol* 1986; **70**: 373–81

Raitta C, Santavouri P. Ophthalmological findings in infantile type of so-called neuronal ceroid lipofuscinosis. *Acta Ophthalmol* 1973; **51**: 755–63

Refsum S. Heredopathia atactica polyneuritisformis: a familial syndrome not hitherto described. A contribution to the clinical study of hereditary disorders of the nervous system. *Acta Psychiatr Scand* (Suppl.) 1946; **38**: 1–303

Rinaldi E, Stoppoloni GP, Savastano S *et al.* Gyrate atrophy of choroid associated with hyperornithinemia: report of the first case in Italy. *J Pediatr Ophthalmol Strabismus* 1979; **16**: 133–5

Rodrigues MM, Ballintine EJ, Wiggert B *et al.* Choroideremia: a clinical electron microscopic and biochemical report. *Ophthalmology* 1984; **91**: 873–83

Rosing HS, Hopkins LC, Wallace DC, Epstein CM, Weidenheim K. Maternally inherited mitochondrial myopathy and myoclonic epilepsy. *Ann Neurol* 1985; **17**: 228–37

Roth AM, Hepler RS, Mukoyama M *et al.* Pigmentary retinal dystrophy in Hallervorden–Spatz disease. Clinicopathological report of a case. *Survey Ophthalmol* 1971; **16**: 24–35

Runge P, Calver D, Marshall J, Taylor D. The histopathology of mitochondrial cytopathy and the Laurence–Moon–Biedl syndrome. *Br J Ophthalmol* 1986(a); **70**: 782–96

Runge P, Muller DPR, McAllister J *et al.* Oral vitamin E can prevent the retinopathy of abetalipoproteinaemia. *Br J Ophthalmol* 1986(b); **70**: 166–73

Russell-Eggitt I, Taylor DSI, Clayton PT *et al.* Leber's congenital amaurosis — a new syndrome with cardiomyopathy. *Br J Ophthalmol* 1989; **73**: 250–4.

Ryan SJ, Knox DL, Green WR, Konigsmark BW. Olivopontocerebellar degeneration. Clinicopathologic correlation of the associated retinopathy. *Arch Ophthalmol* 1975; **93**: 169–75

Schachat AP, Maumenee IH. Bardet–Biedl syndrome and related disorders. *Arch Ophthalmol* 1982; **100**: 285–8

Schappert-Kimmijser J, Henkes HE, van den Bosch J. Amaurosis congenita (Leber). *Arch Ophthalmol* 1959; **61**: 211–8

Schubert G, Bornschein H. Beitrag zur analyse des menschlichen elektroretinograms. *Ophthalmologica* 1952; **123**: 396–412

Schutgens RBH, Heymans HSA, Wanders RJA *et al*. Peroxisomal disorders; a newly recognized group of genetic diseases. *Eur J Pediatr* 1986; **144**: 430–40

Scotto JM, Hadehouel M, Odieve M *et al*. Infantile phytanic acid storage disease. A possible variant of Refsum's disease: three cases including ultrastructural studies of the liver. *J Inherited Metab Dis* 1982; **5**: 83–90

Sebag J, Albert DM, Craft JL. The Alstrom syndrome, ophthalmic histopathology and retinal ultrastructure. *Br J Ophthalmol* 1984; **68**: 494–501

Sengers RCS, Stadhouders AM, Trijbels JMF. Mitochondrial myopathies. Clinical, morphological and biochemical aspects. *Eur J Pediatr* 1984; **141**: 192–207

Senior B, Friedmann AI, Braudo JL. Juvenile familial nephropathy with tapetoretinal degeneration. *Am J Ophthalmol* 1961; **52**: 625–33

Sharpe LT, van Norrend D, Nordby K. Pigment regeneration, visual adaptation and spectral sensitivity in the achromat. *Clin Vis Sci* 1988; **3**: 9–17

Sievring PA, Niffenneger JH, Berson EL. Electroretinographic findings in selected pedigrees with choroideremia. *Am J Ophthalmol* 1986; **101**: 361–7

Simell O, Takki K. Raised plasma Ornithene and gyrate atrophy of the choroid and retina. *Lancet* 1973; **1**: 1031–3

Sipila I, Simell O, Rapola J *et al*. Gyrate atrophy of the choroid and retina with hyperomithemia, tubular aggregates and type 2 fibre atrophy in muscle. *Neurology* 1979; **29**: 996–1005

Skalka HW. Hereditary pigmented paravenous retinochoroidal atrophy. *Am J Ophthalmol* 1979; **87**: 286–91

Sloan LL, Brown DJ. Progressive retinal degeneration with selective involvement of the cone mechanism. *Am J Ophthalmol* 1962; **54**: 629–41

Sorsby A, Williams CF. Retinal aplasia as a clinical entity. *Br Med J* 1960; **1**: 293–7

Spalton DJ, Taylor DSI, Sanders MD. Juvenile Batten's disease an ophthalmological assessment of 26 patients. *Br J Ophthalmol* 1980; **64**: 726–32

Spivey BE. The X-linked inheritance of atypical monochromatism. *Arch Ophthalmol* 1965; **74**: 327–33

Stanescu B, Draloands L. Cerebro-hepato-renal (Zellweger's) syndrome: ocular involvement. *Arch Ophthalmol* 1972; **87**: 590–2

Stanescu B, Michaels J, Proesmans W, VanDamme B. Retinal involvement in a case of nephronophthisis associated with liver fibrosis (Senior Boichis syndrome). *Birth Defects* 1967; **12**: 463–9

Tada K, Saito T, Hayasaha S, Mizuno K. Hyperornithemia with gyrate atrophy: pathophysiology and treatment. *J Inherited Metab Dis* 1983; **6**: 105–6

Takki K, Simell O. Genetic aspects of gyrate atrophy of the choroid and retina with hyperomithenemia. *Br J Ophthalmol* 1974; **58**: 907–16

Takki K, Simell O. Gyrate atrophy of the choroid and retina with hyperornithenemia. *Birth Defects* 1976; **12**: 373–84

Tomita H, Ohno K, Tamai A. Joubert syndrome associated with Leber's congenital amaurosis. *Brain Dev* 1979; **11**: 459–65

Traboulsi EI, Maumenee IH. Hereditary pigmented paravenous chorioretinal atrophy. *Arch Ophthalmol* 1986; **104**: 1636–40

Traboulsi EI, Maumenee IH, Green WR *et al*. Olivopontocerebellar atrophy with retinal degeneration. A clinical and ocular histopathologic study. *Arch Ophthalmol* 1988; **106**: 801–6

Uliss A, Moore AT, Bird AC. The dark choroid in posterior retinal dystrophies. *Ophthalmology* 1987; **94**: 1423–8

Usher CH. On a few hereditary eye affections. *Trans Ophthalmol Soc UK* 1935; **55**: 164–245

Vaizey MJ, Sanders MD, Wybar KC, Wilson J. Neurological abnormalities in congenital amaurosis of Leber. Review of 30 cases. *Arch Dis Child* 1977; **52**: 399–402

Valle D, Kaiser–Kupfer MI, Del Valle LA. Gyrate atrophy of the choroid and retina: deficiency of ornithene aminotransferase in transformed lymphocytes. *Proc Natl Acad Sci USA* 1977; **74**: 5159

Valle D, Walser M, Brusilow S *et al*. Gyrate atrophy of the choroid and retina: Biochemical considerations and experience with an arginine restricted diet. *Ophthalmology* 1981; **88**: 325–30

Waardenburg PJ, Schappert-Kimmijser J. On various recessive biotypes of Leber's congenital amaurosis. *Acta Ophthalmologica* 1963; **41**: 317–20

Wagner RS, Caputo AR, Nelson L, Zanoni D. High hyperopia in Leber's congenital amaurosis. *Arch Ophthalmol* 1985; **103**: 1507–9

Walt RP, Kemp CM, Lyness L *et al*. Vitamin A treatment for night-blindness in primary biliary cirrhosis *Br Med J* 1984; **288**: 1030–31

Weiner LP, Konigesmark BW, Stoll J, Magladery JW. Hereditary olivopontocerebellar atrophy with retinal degeneration. Report of a family through six generations. *Arch Neurol* 1967; **16**: 364–76

Weleber RG, Kennaway NG. Clinical trial of vitamin B$_6$ for gyrate atrophy of the choroid and retina. *Ophthalmology* 1981; **88**: 316–24

Weleber RG, Kennaway NG. Gyrate atrophy of the choroid and retina. In: Heckenlively JR (Ed.) *Retinitis Pigmentosa*. JB Lipincott Co, Philadelphia 1988; pp. 198–220

Weleber RG, Tongue AC. Congenital stationary night blindness presenting as Leber's congenital amaurosis. *Arch Ophthalmol* 1987; **105**: 360–4

Weleber RG, Tongue AC, Kennaway NG *et al*. Ophthalmic manifestations of infantile phytanic acid storage disease. *Arch Ophthalmol* 1984; **102**: 1317–21

Wilson DJ, Weleber RLG, Beals RK. Retinal dystrophy of Jeune's syndrome. *Arch Ophthalmol* 1987; **105**: 651–7

Winn S, Tasman JW, Spaeth G *et al*. Ogouchi's disease in negroes. *Arch Ophthalmol* 1968; **81**: 501–7

World Health Organisation (WHO). *Control of Vitamin A Deficiency and Xerophthalmia*. Technical Report Series No. 676 (2). WHO, Geneva 1982

Yamanaka M. Histologic study of Ogouchi's disease: its relationship to pigmentary degeneration of the retina. *Am J Ophthalmol* 1969; **68**: 19–26

Zellweger H. The cerebro-hepato-renal syndrome and other peroxisomal disorders. *Dev Med Child Neurol* 1987; **29**: 821–9

27.4 Inherited Macular Dystrophies

ANTHONY MOORE

Macular abnormalities are seen in several different inherited disorders but these can be broadly divided into four groups (Noble 1986). Firstly, there is a heterogenous group of disorders that primarily affect the macula, and are not associated with any systemic abnormalities. Macular abnormalities are also seen in more generalized receptor dystrophies, particularly in the cone and cone-rod dystrophies. Other ocular disorders, for example albinism and aniridia, have associated hypoplasia of the fovea, which may also be seen as an isolated abnormality. Finally, macular abnormalities are seen in a variety of inherited systemic disorders.

In this chapter only those macular disorders which are seen in childhood will be considered.

Primary hereditary macular dystrophies

This group of disorders is characterized by early onset of bilateral visual loss, usually in the first or second decade of life, and bilateral, generally symmetric, macular abnormalities. Many different disorders have been described (Deutman 1971; Gass 1987).

Many of the disorders are rare and have been incompletely characterized so that classification is unsatisfactory; they may however be subdivided on the basis of the mode of inheritance (Table 27.4.1) or the anatomical site of the primary disease (Noble 1986).

Pigment epithelial disorders

Stargardt's disease (fundus flavimaculatus)

Stargardt's disease and fundus flavimaculatus are now generally considered to be different expressions of the same genetic disorder (Fishman 1976; Noble & Carr 1979; Isashiki & Ohba 1985). It is the commonest of the inherited macular dystrophies. Most cases show autosomal recessive inheritance although dominant forms are occasionally seen (Cibis *et al.* 1980).

CLINICAL FEATURES

The usual presentation is with insidious bilateral visual loss in the first two decades of life; in the early stages

Rod-cone dystrophies

In most of the rod-cone dystrophies macular atrophy is seen at a late stage although macular oedema may be seen at any time. In some patients however, for example those with the Biedl–Bardet syndrome macular involvement may be seen early in the disease. The presence of night-blindness, peripheral field loss and a reduced rod ERG, however, means that these disorders are rarely confused with the primary macular dystrophies.

Macular dysplasia (coloboma)

Bilateral macular dysplasia (coloboma) have been described in association with a variety of inherited retinal dystrophies including Leber's amaurosis (Leighton & Harris 1973; Margolis *et al.* 1977; Moore *et al.* 1985), retinitis pigmentosa (Friedman & Gombos 1971) and idiopathic infantile hypercalcuria, an autosomal recessive disorder with renal abnormalities, high myopia and a rod-cone dystrophy (Meier *et al.* 1979; Gil-Gilberneau *et al.* 1982).

The macular lesions are seen as sharply demarcated areas of retina pigment epithelial and choroidal atrophy; there may be pigmentation at the edge of the lesion and a few large choroidal vessels may cross bare sclera at the base of the coloboma (Fig. 27.4.10, 27.4.11). Scleral ectasia is often present. The ophthalmoscopic appearance may resemble congenital ocular toxoplasmosis but in the latter the toxoplasma serology is positive and the electroretinogram is normal.

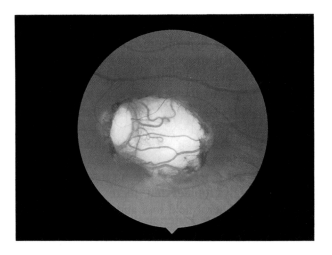

Fig. 27.4.10 Small macular coloboma with large choroidal vessels in its base.

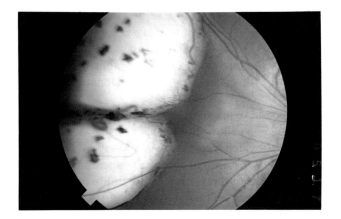

Fig. 27.4.11 Macular coloboma. Large ectatic bilobed macular lesion with pigment clumps in its base and one large central and a few other small choroidal vessels crossing it. Surprisingly the acuity in this eye was 6/36.

Macular abnormalities and inherited systemic disorders

Macular abnormalities may be seen in a variety of other inherited disorders. A cherry red spot due to the accumulation of abnormal material in the ganglion cells is seen in several neurometabolic disorders (see Chapter 34). In addition Bull's eye maculopathy is a frequent finding in certain of the neurodegenerative disorders especially Batten's disease, Hallervorden–Spatz disease and olivopontocerebellar atrophy. These neurometabolic disorders are covered in detail in other chapters.

Macular abnormalities are also seen in several other inherited conditions such as the Sjögren–Larsson syndrome, and oxalosis which will be discussed in the differential diagnosis of the flecked retina syndromes (see Chapter 27.8).

References

Barkman Y. Clinical study of central tapetoretinal degeneration. *Acta Ophthalmol* 1961; **39**: 663–71

Bonnin P, Passet M, Triolaire-Cotten M. Le signe du silence choroidien dans les degenerescences tapeto-retienes posterieures. *Doc Ophthalmol Proc Ser* 1976; **9**: 461–3

Braley AE, Spivey BE. Hereditary vitelline macular degeneration. *Arch Ophthalmol* 1964; 743–62

Chopdar A. Reticular dystrophy of the retina. *Br J Ophthalmol* 1976; **60**: 342–4

Cibis GN, Morey M, Harris DJ. Dominantly inherited macular dystrophy with flecks (Stargardt). *Arch Ophthalmol* 1980; **98**: 1785–89

Curran RE, Robb RM. Isolated foveal hypoplasia. *Arch Ophthalmol* 1976; **94**: 48–50

Curry AF, Moorman LT. Fluorescein photography of vitelliform macular degeneration. *Arch Ophthalmol* 1968; **79**: 705–9.

Daily MJ, Mets BM. Fenestrated sheen macular dystrophy. *Arch Ophthalmol* 1984; **102**: 855–6

Deutman AF. *The Hereditary Dystrophies of the Posterior Pole of the Eye.* Van Gorcum & Co., Netherlands 1971

Deutman AF. Benign concentric annular dystrophy. *Am J Ophthalmol* 1974; **78**: 384–96

Deutman AF, Pinckers AJLG, De Kerk AL. Dominantly inherited cystoid macular oedema. *Am J Ophthalmol* 1976; **82**: 540–8

Deutman AF, Rumke AML. Reticular dystrophy of the retinal pigment epithelium. *Arch Ophthalmol* 1969; **82**: 4–9

Deutman AF, Van Blommenstein, Henkes HE *et al.* Butterfly shaped dystrophy of the fovea. *Arch Ophthalmol* 1970; **83**: 558–69

Fetkenhour CL, Gurney N, Dobbie JG, Choromokos E. Central areolar pigment epithelial dystrophy. *Am J Ophthalmol* 1976; **81**: 745–53

Fish G, Grey R, Sehmi KS, Bird AC. The dark choroid in posterior retinal dystrophies. *Br J Ophthalmol* 1981; **65**: 359–63

Fishman GA. Fundus flavimaculatus. *Arch Ophthalmol* 1976; **94**: 2061–7

Fishman GA, Goldberg MF, Trautmann JC. Dominantly inherited cystoid macular oedema. *Ann Ophthalmol* 1979; **11**: 21–7

Frank RH, Landers MD, Williams RJ, Sidbury JB. A new dominant progressive foveal dystrophy. *Am J Ophthalmol* 1974; **78**: 903–16

Friedman J, Gombos GM. Bilateral macular coloboma keratoconus and retinitis pigmentosa. *Ann Ophthalmol* 1971; **3**: 664–6

Gass JDM. Heredodystrophic disorders affecting the pigment epithelium and retina. In: Gass JDM (Ed.) *Stereoscopic Atlas of Macular Diseases.* 3rd edn. CV Mosby Co., St Louis 1987; pp. 255–331

Gil-Gilberneau J, Galan A, Callis L, Rodrigo C. Infantile idiopathic hypercalcura, high congenital myopia and atypical macular coloboma: A new oculo-renal syndrome. *J Ped Ophthalmol* 1982; **19**: 7–11

Godel V, Chaine G, Regenbogen L, Coscas G. Best's vitelliform macular dystrophy. *Acta Ophthalmol* 1986; **175**: 5–31

Hadden BO, Gass JDM. Fundus flavimaculatus and Stargadt's disease. *Am J Ophthalmol* 1976; **82**: 527–39

Hermsen VM, Judisch GM. Central aerolar pigment epithelial dystrophy. *Ophthalmologica (Basel)* 1984; **189**: 69–72

Isashiki Y, Ohba N. Fundus flavimaculatus. *Br J Ophthalmol* 1985; **69**: 522–4

Kingham JD, Fenzyl RE, Willerson D, Aaberg TM. Reticular dystrophy of the pigment epithelium: a clinical and electrophysiological study of three generations. *Arch Ophthalmol* 1978; **96**: 1177–84

Kraushar MF, Margolis S, Morse P, Nugent ME. Pseudohypopyon in Best's vitelliform macular dystrophy. *Am J Ophthalmol* 1982; **94**: 30–7

Lefler WH, Wadsworth JAC, Sidbury JB, Jr. Hereditary macular degeneration and aminoaciduria. *Am J Ophthalmol* 1971; **71**: 224–30

Leighton D, Harris R. Retinal aplasia in association with macular coloboma keratoconus and cataract. *Clin Genet* 1973; **4**: 270–4

Lewis RA, Lee GB, Martonyi CL *et al.* Familial foveal retinoschisis. *Arch Ophthalmol* 1977; **95**: 1190–6

Margolis S, Sher BM, Carr RE. Macular coloboma in Leber's congenital amaurosis. *Am J Ophthalmol* 1977; **83**: 27–31

Meier W, Blumberg A, Imahorn W *et al.* Idiopathic hypercalcuria with bilateral macular colobomata: a new variant of oculorenal syndrome. *Helv Paediatr Acta* 1979; **34**: 257–69

Mesker RP, Oosterhuis JA, Dellerman JW. A retinal lesion resembling Sjogren's dystrophia reticularis laminae pigmentosae retinae. In: *Perspectives in Ophthalmology.* Exercerpta Medica, Amsterdam 1970 II pp. 40–5

Mohler CW, Fines SL. Long term evaluation of patients with Best's vitelliform dystrophy. *Ophthalmology* 1981; **88**: 688–91

Moore AT, Harden A, Taylor DSI. Bilateral macular dysplasia (Colobomata) and congenital retinal dystrophy. *Br J Ophthalmol* 1985; **69**: 691–9

Noble KG. Hereditary macular dystrophies. In: Renie WA. (Ed.) *Goldberg's Genetic and Metabolic Eye Disease.* Little Brown and Co., Boston/Toronto 1986; pp. 439–64

Noble KG, Carr RE. Stargardt's disease and fundus flavimaculatus. *Arch Ophthalmol* 1979; **97**: 1281–5

Notting JGA, Pinckers AJLG. Dominant cystoid macular oedema. *Am J Ophthalmol* 1977; **83**: 234–41

O'Donnell FE, Jr, Pappas HR. Autosomal dominant foveal hypoplasia and pre-senile cataracts: A new syndrome. *Arch Ophthalmol* 1982; **100**: 279–81

O'Donnell FE, Welch RB. Fenestrated sheen macular dystrophy. *Arch Ophthalmol* 1979; **97**: 1292–6

Oliver MD, Dotan SA, Chemke J, Abraham FA. Isolated foveal hypoplasia. *Br J Ophthalmol* 1987; **71**; 926–30

Pinckers A. Patterned dystrophies of the retinal pigment epithelium. A review. *Ophthalmic Paediatr Genet* 1988; **9**: 77–114

Sjogren H. Dystrophica reticularis laminae pigmentosae retinae. An earlier not described hereditary eye disease. *Acta Ophthalmol (KBH)* 1950; **28**: 279–95

Slagsvold JE. Fenestrated sheen macular dystrophy: A new autosomal dominant maculopathy. *Acta Ophthalmologica* 1981; **59**: 683–8

Slezak H, Hommer K. Fundus pulverulentus. Von Graefe *Arch Klin Exp Ophthalmol* 1969; **178**: 177–182

Uliss A, Moore AT, Bird AC. The dark choroid in posterior retinal dystrophies. *Ophthalmology* 1987; **94**: 1423–8

Van der Biesen PR, Deutmann AF, Pinckers AJL. Evolution of benign concentric annular dystrophy. *Am J Ophthalmol* 1985; **100**: 73–8

Waheed AA, Wyse CT. Progressive bifocal chorioretinal atrophy. *Br J Ophthalmol* 1968; **52**: 742–50

Weingeist TA, Kobrin JL, Watzke RC. Histopathology of Best's macular dystrophy. *Arch Ophthalmol* 1982; **100**: 1108–14

Yassur Y, Nissenkorn I, Ben Sira I *et al.* Autosomal dominant inheritance of retinoschisis. *Am J Ophthalmol* 1982; **94**: 338–43

Yoshizumi MO, Thomas JV, Hirose T. Foveal hypoplasia and bilateral 360 degrees retinal rosettes. *Am J Ophthalmol* 1979; **87**: 186–92

27.5 Congenital and Vascular Abnormalities of the Retina

ANTHONY MOORE

Congenital hamartomatous lesions of the retina and retinal pigment epithelium

Congenital hypertrophy of the retinal pigment epithelium

Congenital hypertrophy of the retinal pigment epithelium (CHRPE) is usually seen as a solitary well circumscribed brown or darkly pigmented, slightly raised lesion about 1−2 disc diameters in size (Fig. 27.5.1). There is often a depigmented halo surrounding the lesion and areas of depigmentation (lacunae) may be present within it (Buettner 1975; Purcell & Shields 1975; Gass 1987). They are most commonly seen as an incidental finding during routine fundus examination and can be found in any area of the retina. Careful perimetry will reveal a relative scotoma in the area of visual field corresponding to the lesion (Buettner 1975). On fluorescein angiography there is masking of the underlying choroidal fluorescein by the hypertrophied RPE but there may be areas of hyperfluorescence within the lesion related to the depigmented lacunae. Cleary *et al.* (1976) have described a number of retinal vascular abnormalities overlying the lesion which are probably secondary to RPE and receptor atrophy.

Histopathologically the lesion is composed of a single layer of hypertrophied retinal pigment epithelial cells containing large pigment granules. In addition there is atrophy of the retinal photoreceptors overlying the lesion (Buettner 1975).

Although most individuals have no systemic abnormality, multiple bilateral pigmented lesions have been reported in association with Gardener's

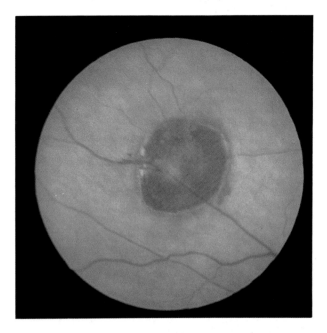

Fig. 27.5.1 Congenital hypertrophy of the retinal pigment epithelium. Slightly raised jet black lesion in the midperiphery with an associated small visual field defect. Professor AC Bird's patient.

syndrome (Blair *et al.* 1980; Romania *et al.* 1989) and with microcephaly (Parke *et al.* 1984).

Grouped pigmentation of the retinal pigment epithelium

Congenital grouped pigmentation of the retinal pigment epithelium (Bear Track pigmentation) is an uncommon disorder in which there are multiple pigmented lesions in the fundus which resemble animal footprints (Fig. 27.5.2). They are usually sporadic unilateral and grouped in one sector of the fundus (Gass 1987); familial cases have only rarely been reported (De Jong & Delleman 1988). Fluorescein angiography shows masking of the underlying choroidal fluorescence (Fig. 27.5.2). Histopathologically they are similar to CHRPE (Shields & Tso 1975) with increased concentration of pigment granules in otherwise normal RPE cells.

Gass (1987) has described a condition of grouped albinotic pigment epithelial spots, closely related to bear track pigmentation in which there are scattered non pigmented lesions in the fundus. Affected patients are asymptomatic and dark adaptation studies, electro-oculography and electroretinography are all normal.

Congenital hyperplasia of the retinal pigment epithelium

Localized hyperplasia of the RPE is usually seen on routine fundus examination as a darkly pigmented small well circumscribed lesion in the peripheral retina. It is usually solitary and extends from the RPE through into the retina. Fluorescein angiography shows early non fluorescence but may show some hyperfluorescence late in the angiogram (Gass 1987). They are not thought to progress and are not associated with any systemic abnormalities.

Combined hamartoma of the retina and retinal pigment epithelium

Gass in 1973 described a series of patients with benign fundus lesions affecting the juxtapapillary, macular or peripheral retina which he believed were hamartomatous disorders of the retina and retinal pigment epithelium. There have been many further reports of similar abnormalities (Laqua & Wessing 1979; Flood *et al.* 1983; Schachat *et al.* 1984; Cosgrove *et al.* 1986). Although they have not been seen in the newborn they have been reported in early infancy (Schachat *et al.* 1984) and it is likely that they are truly congenital in origin. No familial cases have been reported (Gass 1987). Histological examination of enucleated eyes have shown thickened disorganized retina with proliferation of the RPE and glial tissue (Cardell & Starbuck 1961; Vogel *et al.* 1969).

Although rare it is important to recognize these lesions as their appearance may be confused with intraocular tumours such as retinoblastoma or choroidal melanoma and inappropriate treatment given (Gass 1973).

CLINICAL FEATURES

The usual presentation is with unilateral visual loss, or, in young children especially, strabismus (Schachat *et al.* 1984; Gass 1987). Less commonly the retinal abnormality is found on routine fundus examination. Visual acuity is extremely variable and depends on the degree of macular involvement. In one large series (Schachat *et al.* 1984) 45% of patients had vision of 6/12 or better but 40% had 6/60 or worse.

The hamartomas may involve the disc or macula and peripheral retina (Gass 1987). Peripapillary hamartomas are seen as slightly elevated diffuse partly pigmented tumours involving the nerve head and adjacent retina (Fig. 27.5.3a). Wrinkling of the internal limiting membrane and epiretinal membranes are commonly seen (Fig. 27.5.4). Fluorescein angiography shows marked vascular tortuosity and an abnormal capillary circulation which may leak in the late phase (Fig. 27.5.4b).

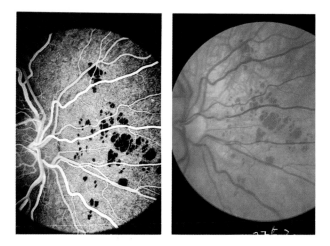

Fig. 27.5.2 Congenital grouped pigmentation ('Bear track'). Unilateral, multiple brown patches in the retinal pigment epithelium of no functional significance. Fluorescein angiography shows masking of the underlying choroidal fluorescense. Professor AC Bird's patient.

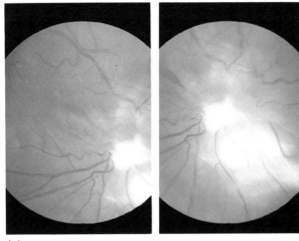

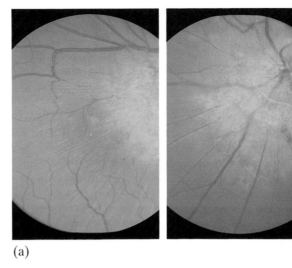

(a)

(a)

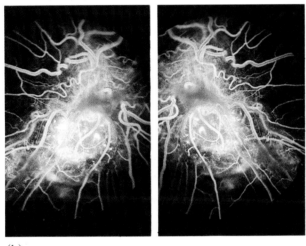

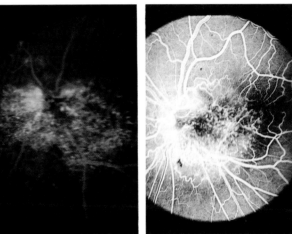

(b)

(b)

Fig. 27.5.3 (a) Combined hamartoma of the retina and retinal pigment epithelium. Elevated peripapillary lesion with retinal traction and exudative detachment. Professor AC Bird's patient. (b) Fluorescein angiogram of the same patient showing the marked vascular tortuousity and distortion.

Fig. 27.5.4 (a) Combined hamartoma of the retina and retinal pigment epithelium. This patient has a marked elevation of the optic disc with radial retinal traction, wrinkled internal limiting membrane and RPE changes around the disc. (b) Fluorescein angiogram showing the capillary beading and late leakage. Professor AC Bird's patient. (Same patient.)

Macula and peripheral retinal hamartomas have a similar appearance; the retina is thickened and hyperpigmented with very tortuous retinal vessels. There is usually associated epiretinal membrane formation and surface traction and less commonly choroidal neovascularization may develop at the edge of the lesion (Gass 1987).

The vision remains stable in most patients but visual loss may develop from exudative detachment or from increasing macular distortion due to surface traction. The hamartomas may rarely show signs of growth (Cardell & Starbuck 1961; Rosenberg & Walsh 1984).

MANAGEMENT

In young children with strabismus a trial of intensive occlusion therapy should be tried, as despite the appearance of the retina, the vision will sometimes improve (Schachat *et al.* 1984). In most cases no surgical treatment is indicated although macula distortion due to epiretinal membrane may be relieved by intraocular microsurgery sometimes with good visual results (Schachat *et al.* 1984).

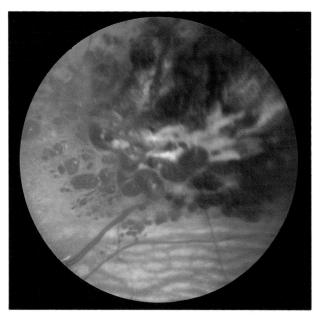

(a)

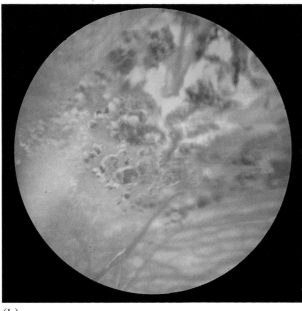

(b)

Fig. 27.5.5 (a) Cavernous haemangioma of the retina. This 11 month old child presented with a squint, but with patching the acuity remained at 6/18. The grape-like cluster of abnormal vessels was adjacent to the macula and regressed over 3 years. (b) Photograph taken few minutes after fluorescein angiogram. The pooling of fluorescein occurs due to the very slow blood flow. No leakage occurred. (Same patient.)

Astrocytic hamartoma

Retinal phakomata or astrocytic hamartoma are a common finding in tuberose sclerosis, occurring in about 40% of cases (Williams & Taylor 1985). Less commonly they are seen in neurofibromatosis (Martyn & Knox 1972), retinitis pigmentosa (Robertson 1972) or as an isolated abnormality (Foos *et al.* 1965; Ramsay *et al.* 1979; Gass 1987). In tuberose sclerosis they are often multiple, may be bilateral and are found at the optic nerve head or peripheral retina (Williams & Taylor 1985). Astrocytic hamartomas are thought to arise from the retinal ganglion cell layer and histopathologically consist of elongated astrocytes with small oval nuclei; the mass is usually vascular and may contain calcium (Green 1985). Although these tumours may grow slowly they do not spread outside the eye. They may rarely be complicated by vitreous haemorrhage (Atkinson *et al.* 1973; Kroll *et al.* 1981). In infants and young children the retinal lesions are seen as translucent grey-white, minimally elevated tumours which may easily be missed unless careful indirect ophthalmoscopy is performed. In older children the more typical raised white 'mulberry' tumours are more common. The early translucent lesions are thought to evolve with time into the more typical 'mulberry' phacomas and intermediate stages may be seen (Williams & Taylor 1985). Calcification may occur at a late stage.

Fluorescein angiography often shows autofluorescence of the phacomata in the control pictures and in the arterial phase there is early filling of the often abnormal capilleries within the lesion. Most show late hyperfluorescence (Williams & Taylor 1985; Gass 1987).

In the majority of patients with astrocytic hamartomas a careful search will reveal other stigmata of tuberous sclerosis (see Chapter 39). The early lucent retinal lesions may be confused with a small retinoblastoma and if there is doubt about the diagnosis it is reasonable to observe the lesion closely for a period; the more rapid growth of retinoblastoma will help differentiate it from an astrocytic hamartoma.

Congenital vascular abnormalities

Persistent hyaloid arteries

See Chapters 26 and 28.

Cilioretinal arteries

See Chapter 28.

Prepapillary vascular loops

See Chapter 28.

Vascular hamartomas

CAPILLARY HAEMANGIOMA

Capillary haemangioma of the optic disc or peripheral retina may be seen as an isolated finding (Von Hippel disease) or in association with angiomatous malformations of the central nervous system or visceral organs (Von Hippel–Lindau disease). It is thought that the ocular and systemic abnormalities result from a single autosomal dominant gene which shows variable expression. The gene for Von Hippel–Lindau disease has recently been mapped to the p 25 region of chromosome 3 (Seizinger *et al.* 1988). The systemic tumours associated with Von Hippel–Lindau disease include cerebellar, medullary and spinal haemangioblastoma, renal cell carcinoma and phaeochromocytoma (Melman & Rosen 1964, Horton *et al.* 1976; Hardwig & Robertson 1984). In addition benign cysts may occur in many organs including pancreas, liver, ovaries and kidney. Retinal angiomatosis occurs in about two thirds of patients and is often the first sign of the condition (Hardwig & Robertson 1984). In genetic counselling it is important to carry out fundus examination and fluorescein angioscopy of all 'at risk' family members as small asymptomatic retinal lesions may be the only sign of disease.

Clinical features

Most patients present with blurred vision but in some the retinal lesions are found during examination of asymptomatic family members.

The retinal haemangioblastomas are most commonly seen in the mid periphery, although papillary or peripapillary lesions are found (Hardwig & Robertson 1984). The tumours are of two main types. Exophytic tumours arise from the outer retinal layers and grow inwards. They are uncommon, are more often seen in the peripapillary area and may present with optic disc swelling or exudative detachment of the macula (Yimoyines *et al.* 1982; Gass 1987). They present problems with diagnosis and the vascular nature of the abnormality may not be recognized unless fluorescein angiography is performed.

Endophytic tumours which arise from the inner retinal layers are more common and give rise to the typical well circumscribed elevated vascular lesion growing forwards into the vitreous cavity. They may be seen at the disc or more commonly in the peripheral retina, where they are often bilateral. Peripheral angiomas often show enlarged feeding and draining vessels and there may be rapid arterio-venous shunting through the lesion. Leakage of fluid from the angioma may give rise to serous retinal detachment and exudate. Continued exudation may lead to total retinal detachment.

Screening of at risk family members may reveal asymptomatic small angiomas (Salazara & Lamiell 1980) which are seen as small pale grey lesions without dilated feeder vessels or exudation. Fluorescein angiography is helpful in confirming the vascular nature of these lesions. (see Chapter 39).

Histopathology

Histopathological examination of eyes with untreated haemangiomas (Nicholson *et al.* 1976; Wing *et al.* 1981) show that the lesions are composed of a fine network of capilleries and small blood vessels which penetrate most of the thickness of the retina. The blood vessels are fenestrated and lack the normal tight junctions so that extensive leakage of fluid occurs, resulting in chronic oedema and atrophy of the surrounding retina.

Management

The treatment of retinal angiomas depend on the type of lesion, its size and location. Small peripheral endophytic lesions can be successfully treated with argon laser and xenon photocoagulation (Sellors & Archer 1969; Apple *et al.* 1974; Goldberg & Koenig 1974). Larger tumours which often have associated detachment are best treated with cryotherapy using a triple freeze–thaw technique but several treatments may be needed (Sellors & Archer 1969; Watzke 1973). Exophytic tumours adjacent to the disc are particularly difficult to treat, argon laser photocoagulation offers the best hope of causing tumour regression without damaging the papillomacular bundle (Yimoyines *et al.* 1982).

Large tumours may not respond to photocoagulation or cryotherapy and Peyman *et al.* (1983) have reported some successful results from transcleral resection of tumour which had failed to respond to conventional treatment. Some eyes, show relentless progression and visual loss despite all forms of treatment (Hardwig & Robertson 1984).

CAVERNOUS HAEMANGIOMA

Cavernous haemangioma is a rare vascular hamartoma which may involve the optic nerve head or peripheral retina (Gass 1971; Lewis *et al.* 1975; Goldberg *et al.* 1979; Messmer *et al.* 1983). Although it has been reported in childhood most cases are seen in young adults; it is commoner in females and is usually unilateral (Lewis *et al.* 1975). In some cases there may be additional cutaneous and intracranial haemangiomas (Gass 1971; Lewis *et al.* 1975; Goldberg *et al.* 1979; Brown & Shields 1985).

The cavernous haemangioma is seen as a grape-like cluster (Fig. 27.5.5a) of aneurysmal dilatations arising from a retinal vein; there is often associated fibrous tissue and small haemorrhages are sometimes seen on the surface of the lesion. There are no prominent feeder vessels as seen in Von Hippel's disease although the draining vein may be dilated (Messmer *et al.* 1983). Visual acuity usually remains good unless the haemangioma is close to the macula (Gass 1971; Lewis *et al.* 1975; Messmer *et al.* 1983). Rarely bleeding from the abnormal vessels may give rise to recurrent vitreous haemorrhage.

Cavernous haemangiomas fill slowly (Fig. 27.5.5b) and often incompletely on fluorescein angiography and there is no evidence of any arteriovenous shunting or extravascular leakage (Brown & Shields 1985). Treatment is only indicated if there is recurrent vitreous haemorrhage when cryotherapy or photocoagulation may be used to cause tumour regression (Brown & Shields 1985; Gass 1987).

Congenital retinal macrovessels (racemose haemangioma)

In this uncommon disorder a large retinal vessel, usually a vein, runs from the disc to the macular region and supplies retina above and below the horizontal raphe (Archer *et al.* 1973; Brown *et al.* 1982). Fluorescein angiography often shows arteriovenous communications and areas of capillary non-perfusion. Archer *et al.* (1973) have divided this disorder into three groups depending on the extent of the arteriovenous anastomosis. In the first group there is a small arteriovenous anastomosis which occurs across a capillary complex; although venous pressure is raised it is well compensated and vision remains good. In the second group there is direct arteriolar–venous communication and high flow between the arterial and venous side of the circulation. This leads to secondary changes such as arteriolar and venous dilatation and capillary non-perfusion in neighbouring vessels.

The third group consist of patients with complex large vessel anastomoses. Many vessels in the fundus may be widely dilated and vision is often poor.

In the Wyburn-Mason's syndrome (Wyburn-Mason 1943) there is large vessel arteriovenous anastomoses of the retinal circulation with similar vascular malformations of the midbrain and cerebrum (Fig. 27.5.6).

Familial retinal arterial tortuosity

This uncommon autosomal dominant disorder is characterized by variable tortuosity of the retinal arterioles and frequently, associated macula or posterior pole retinal haemorrhages (Beyer 1958; Goldberg *et al.* 1972; Boyton & Purnell 1977; Bartlett & Price 1983; Wells & Kalina 1985). The arteriolar tortuosity is apparent in childhood (Wells & Kalina 1985) and may become more marked with age. The macular haemorrhages which lie superficially in the nerve fibre layer, or in the subhyaloid space, may occur spontaneously or follow minor trauma or physical exercise (Goldberg 1985). Although the haemorrhages may be recurrent there is complete resolution with recovery of normal vision. Fluorescein angiography shows no abnormality apart from the arteriolar tortuosity and there are no associated systemic abnormalities (Wells & Kalina 1985).

Inherited retinal venous beading

Meredith (1987) has described one pedigree with probable autosomal dominant inheritance where all affected members had prominent segmental retinal venous beading and other associated retinovascular changes. Two adults from the family developed renal disease in their fourth and fifth decades and it is possible that this may be a variant of Alport's syndrome rather than a distinct inherited retinovascular anomaly.

Coats' disease

Coats' disease is characterized by congenital retinal telangiectasis and exudative retinal detachment (Coats' 1908). It usually presents in late childhood, occurs predominantly in males and is unilateral in over 90% of cases (Morales 1965; Manschot & De Bruijn 1967; Egerer *et al.* 1974). The average age of presentation is about 8 years (Morales 1965; Ridley *et al.* 1982) when the usual presenting features are unilateral visual loss or strabismus. Infants or younger children may present with leucocoria or a painful blind eye (Judisch & Apple 1980; Ridley *et al.* 1982; McGettrick & Loeffler 1987).

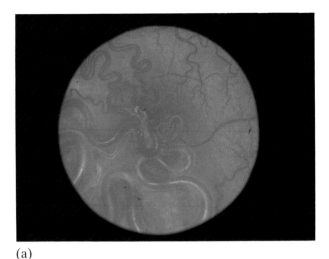

(a)

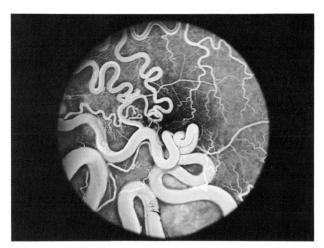

(b)

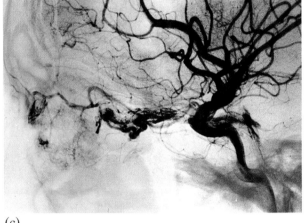

(c)

Fig. 27.5.6 (a) Congenital retinal macro vessels. The acuity was 6/18. (b) The fluorescein angiogram showed no leakage. (Same patient.) (c) Carotid angiogram showing cerebral vascular malformation. (Same patient.)

Fundus examination shows aneurysmal dilation and teliangectasis of the retinal vessels with associated subretinal exudation. (Fig. 27.5.7). There may be extensive retinal detachment with relatively solid yellow exudate and refractile cholesterol crystals in the subretinal space; the subretinal fluid often has a greenish hue. Fluorescein angiography shows aneurysmal dilation of the arterioles, capillaries and veins in the affected area often with associated capillary non-perfusion (Gass 1987). Leakage from the dilated vessels is common.

Histopathological examination of enucleated eyes shows aneurysmal dilation of the retinal vessels with thickening and hyalinization of their walls. The subretinal space contains exudate, cholesterol, and foamy, melanin containing, cells which may be derived from the retinal pigment epithelium (Tripathi & Ashton 1971).

Untreated, most cases show progression of disease (Morales 1965) leading to total retinal detachment,

neovascular glaucoma and pthysis bulbi. Judisch and Apple (1980) reported an unusual case in which an infant with Coats' disease developed an orbital cellulitis secondary to extensive ocular inflammation.

Treatment of the abnormal vessels with photocoagulation or cryotherapy may halt progression of the disease and in early cases result in reabsorption of the exudate and improvement in vision (Ridley *et al.* 1982; McGettrick & Loeffler 1987).

The differential diagnosis of Coats' disease includes other causes of leucocoria and exudative retinal detachment in childhood (see Chapter 27.61). The presence of retinal vascular abnormalities, subretinal exudate and cholestol crystals usually serve to differentiate this disorder from other related conditions. Most cases of Coats' disease are unilateral and sporadic; Tolmie *et al.* (1988) however have recently reported two female siblings with bilateral Coats' disease, intracranial calcification, sparse hair and dysplastic nails and suggest that this may represent a

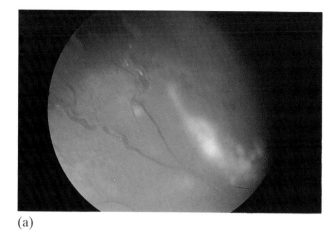

(a)

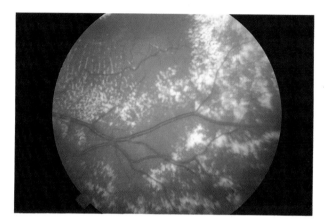

(b)

(c)

Fig. 27.5.7 (a) Coats' disease. Aneurysmal dilation of the retinal arterioles. (b) Coat's disease. Exudative retinal detachment with subretinal solid exudate. (c) Coat's disease. Retinal and subretinal refractile (cholesterol) crystals.

distinct genetic disorder. Retinal telangiectasis similar to Coats' disease has also been reported in patients with retinitis pigmentosa (Khan *et al.* 1988).

Other congenital abnormalities

Other congenital abnormalities of the retina including myelinated nerve fibres, coloboma, and Aicardi's syndrome are covered in the Chapter 28. Albinism is covered in the uvea section.

References

Apple DJ, Goldberg MF, Wyhinny GJ. Argon laser treatment of Von Hippel–Lindau retinal angiomas. II Histopathology of treated lesions. *Arch Ophthalmol* 1974; **92**: 126–30.

Archer DM, Deutman A, Ernst JT, Krill AE. Arteriovenous communication of the retina. *Am J Ophthalmol* 1973; **75**: 224–41

Atkinson A, Sanders MD, Wong V. Vitreous haemorrhage in tuberous sclerosis. *Br J Ophthalmol* 1973; **57**: 773–9

Bartlett WJ, Price J. Familial retinal arteriolar tortuosity with retinal haemorrhage. *Am J Ophthalmol* 1983; **95**: 556–8

Beyer EM. Familiare tortuositas der kleinen wetzhautarterien mit makulablutung. *Klin Monatsbl Augenheilkd* 1958; **132**: 532–9

Blair NP, Trempe CL. Hypertrophy of the retinal pigment epithelium associated with Gardner's syndrome. *Am J Ophthalmol* 1980; **90**: 661–7

Boyton JR, Purnell EW. Congenital tortuosity of the retinal arteries. *Arch Ophthalmol* 1977; **95**: 893

Brown GC, Donoso LA, Magargal LE *et al.* Congenital retinal macrovessels. *Arch Ophthalmol* 1982; **100**: 1430–6

Brown GC, Shields JA. Tumours of the optic nerve head. *Surv Ophthalmol* 1985; **29**: 239–64

Buettner H. Congenital hypertrophy of the retinal pigment epithelium. *Am J Ophthalmol* 1975; **79**: 177–89

Cardell BS, Starbuck MJ. Juxtapapillary hamartoma of the retina. *Br J Ophthalmol* 1961; **45**: 672–7

Cleary PE, Gregor Z, Bird AC. Retinal vascular changes in congenital hypertrophy of the retinal pigment epithelium. *Br*

J Ophthalmol 1976; **60**: 499–503

Coats G. Forms of retinal disease with massive exudation. *R Lond Ophthalmol Rep* 1908; **17**: 440–525

Cosgrove JM, Sharpe DM, Bird AC. Combined hamartoma of the retina and retinal pigment epithelium: the clinical spectrum. *Trans Ophthalmol Soc UK* 1986; **105**: 106–113

De Jong PT, Delleman JW. Familial grouped pigmentation of the retinal pigment epithelium. *Br J Ophthalmol* 1988; **72**: 439–41

Egerer I, Tasman W, Tomer TL. Coat's disease. *Arch Ophthalmol* 1974; **92**: 109–112

Flood TP, Orth DH, Aaberg TM, Marcus DF. Macular hamartomas of the retinal pigment epithelium and retina. *Retina* 1983; **3**: 164–70

Foos RY, Straatsma BR, Allen RA. Astrocytoma of the optic nerve head. *Arch Ophthalmol* 1965; **74**: 319–26

Gass JDM. Cavernous haemangioma of the retina: a neurocutaneous syndrome. *Am J Ophthalmol* 1971; **71**: 799–814

Gass JDM. An unusual hamartoma of the pigment epithelium and retina simulating choroidal melanoma and retinoblastoma. *Trans Am Ophthalmol Soc* 1973; **71**: 175–85

Gass JDM. Retinal and pigment epithelial hamartomas. In: Gass JDM (Ed.) *Stereoscopic Atlas of Macular Diseases*. Mosby Co., St Louis 1987; pp. 605–52

Goldberg MF. Retinal arteriolar tortuosity. Discussion of paper by Wells CG, Kalina FE. *Ophthalmology* 1985; **92**: 1021–4

Goldberg MF, Koenig S. Argon laser treatment of Von Hippel–Lindau retinal angiomas. *Arch Ophthalmol* 1974; **92**: 121–5

Goldberg MF, Pollack IP, Green WR. Familial retinal arteriolar tortuosity with retinal haemorrhage. *Am J Ophthalmol* 1972; **73**: 183–91

Goldberg RE, Pheasant TR, Shields JA. Cavernous haemangioma of the retina. *Arch Ophthalmol* 1979; **97**: 2321–4

Green WR. Congenital variations and abnormalities of the retina. In: Spencer WH (Ed.) *Ophthalmic Pathology: An Atlas and Textbook*. WB Saunders Co., Philadelphia 1985; pp. 607–47

Hardwig P, Robertson DM. Von Hippel–Lindau disease: a familial often fatal phakomatosis. *Ophthalmology* 1984; **91**: 263–70

Horton WA, Wong V, Eldridge R. Von Hippel–Lindau disease: clinical and pathological manifestations in nine families with 50 affected members. *Arch Int Med* 1976; **136**: 769–77

Judisch GF, Appel DJ. Orbital cellulitis in an infant secondary to Coat's disease. *Arch Ophthalmol* 1980; **98**: 2004–6

Khan JA, Ide CA, Strickland MP. Coat's type retinitis pigmentosa. *Surv Ophthalmol* 1988; **32**: 317–32

Kroll AS, Reiken PD, Robb RM, Albert DM. Vitreous haemorrhage complicating retinal astrocytic hamartoma. *Surv Ophthalmol* 1981; **26**: 31–8

Laqua H, Wessing A. Congenital retinal pigment epithelial malformation previously described as hamartoma. *Am J Ophthalmol* 1979; **87**: 34–42

Lewis RA, Cohen MH, Wise GN. Cavernous haemangioma of retina and optic disc. *Br J Ophthalmol* 1975; **59**: 422–4

Manschot WA, De Bruijn WC. Coat's disease: definitions and pathogenesis. *Br J Ophthalmol* 1967; **51**: 145–57

Martyn LJ, Knox DL. Glial hamartoma of the retina in generalized neurofibromatism (Von Recklinghausen's disease). *Br J Ophthalmol* 1972; **56**: 487–91

McGettrick PM, Loeffler KN. Bilateral Coat's disease in an infant (a clinical, light and electron microscopic study). *Eye* 1987; **1**: 136–45

Melmon KL, Rosen SW. Lindau's disease: review of the literature and study of a large kindred. *Am J Med* 1964; **36**: 595–617

Meredith T. Inherited retinal venous beading. *Arch Ophthalmol* 1987; **105**: 949–53

Messmer E, Laqua H, Wessing A *et al*. Nine cases of cavernous haemangioma of the retina. *Am J Ophthalmol* 1983; **45**: 383–90

Morales AG. Coats' disease: natural history and results of treatment. *Am J Ophthalmol* 1965; **60**: 855–65

Nicholson DH, Green WR, Kenyon KR. Light and electron microscopic study of early lesions in angiomatosis retinae. *Am J Ophthalmol* 1976; **82**: 193–204

Parke JT, Riccardi VM, Lewis AR, Ferrel RE. A syndrome of microcephaly and retinal pigmentary abnormalities without mental retardation in a family with coincidental autosomal dominant hyper-reflexia. *Am J Med Genet* 1984; **17**: 585–594

Peyman GA, Rednam KR, Mottow-Lipa L, Flood T. Treatment of large Von Hippel tumours by eye wall resection. *Ophthalmology* 1983; **90**: 840–7

Purcell JJ, Shields JA. Hypertrophy with hyperpigmentation of the retinal pigment epithelium. *Arch Ophthalmol* 1975; **93**: 1122–6

Ramsay RL, Kin Youn JL, Hill CW *et al*. Retinal astrocytoma. *Am J Ophthalmol* 1979; 32–6

Ridley ME, Shields JA, Brown GC, Tasman W. Coat's disease evaluation of management. *Ophthalmology* 1982; **89**: 1381–7

Robertson DM. Hamartomas of the optic disc with retinitis pigmentosa. *Am J Ophthalmol* 1972; **74**: 526–31

Romania A, Zakov N, McGannon E *et al*. Congenital hypertrophy of the retinal pigment epithelium in familial adenomatous polyposis. *Ophthalmology* 1989; **96**: 879–84

Rosenberg PR, Walsh JB. Retinal pigment epithelial hamartoma – unusual manifestation. *Br J Ophthalmol* 1984; **68**: 439–42

Salazar FG, Lamiell JM. Early identification of retinal angiomas in a large kindred with Von Hippel disease. *Am J Ophthalmol* 1980; **89**: 540–5

Schachat AP, Shields JA, Fine SL *et al*. Combined hamartomas of the retina and retinal pigment epithelium. *Ophthalmology* 1984; **91**: 1609–15

Seizinger BR, Rouleau GA, Ozelius LJ *et al*. Von Hippel–Lindau disease maps to the region of chromosome 3 associated with renal cell carcinoma. *Nature* 1983; **332**: 268–9

Sellors PJH, Archer D. The management of retinal angiomatosis. *Trans Ophthalmol Soc UK* 1969; **89**: 529–43

Shields JA, Tso MOM. Congenital grouped pigmentation of the retina: histopathologic description and report of a case. *Arch Ophthalmol* 1975; **93**: 1153–5

Tolmie JL, Browne BH, McGettrick PM, Stephenson JBP. A familial syndrome with Coat's reaction retinal angiomas, hair and nail defects and intracranial calcification. *Eye* 1988; **2**: 297–303

Tripathi R, Ashton N. Electron microscopical study of Coat's disease. *Br J Ophthalmol* 1971; **55**: 289–301

Vogel MH, Zimmerman LE, Gass JDM. Proliferation of the juxtapapillary retinal pigment epithelium simulating malignant melanoma. *Doc Ophthalmol* 1969; **26**: 461–81

Watzke RC. Cryotherapy for retinal angiomatosis: a clinicopathologic report. *Doc Ophthalmol* 1973; **34**: 405−11

Wells CG, Kalina RE. Progressive inherited retinal arteriolar tortuosity with spontaneous retinal haemorrhages. *Ophthalmology* 1985; **92**: 1015−21

Williams R, Taylor D. Tuberous sclerosis. *Surv Ophthalmol* 1985; **30**: 143−54

Wing GL, Weiter JJ, Kelly PJ *et al*. Von Hippel−Lindau disease. Angiomatosis of the retina and central nervous system. *Ophthalmology* 1981; **88**: 1311−4

Wyburn-Mason R. Arterial-venous aneurysm of midbrain and retina, facial naevi and mental changes. *Brain* 1943; **66**: 165−203

Yimoyines DJ, Topilow HW, Abedin S, cMeel JW. Bilateral peripapillary exophytic retinal haemangioblastomas. *Ophthalmology* 1982; **89**: 1388−92

27.6 Retinal Detachment in Childhood

ANTHONY MOORE

Retinal detachment is rare in childhood and often leads to difficulty with diagnosis and management. The presentation is usually late and the disease advanced at the time of diagnosis; furthermore detachments often occur in developmentally abnormal eyes which makes surgical management particularly difficult. Although rare a surprisingly large number of disorders may give rise to detachment in childhood (Table 27.6.1). Detachments may be rhegmatogenous, exudative, tractional or a combination of these. In addition retinoblastoma may give rise to a solid detachment.

Congenital retinal detachment or so called congenital non-attachment of the retina (Foos *et al.* 1968) is now recognized to be part of the spectrum of vitreoretinal dysplasia which may have a variety of causes (see Chapter 26).

Rhegmatogenous retinal detachment

Most cases of rhegmatogenous retinal detachment in children are related to trauma or developmental abnormalities of the eyes (Tasman 1967; Daniel *et al.* 1974a), including high myopia.

Table 27.6.1 Retinal detachment in children.

Rhegmatogenous

Inherited disorders
    X-linked retinoschisis
    Stickler's syndrome (Figs 27.6.1–27.6.3)
    Dominant exudative vitreoretinopathy
    Clefting syndromes
    Incontinentia pigmenti
    Ehlers–Danlos syndrome
    Marfan's syndrome

Developmental anomalies
    Myopia
    Congenital cataract
    Congenital glaucoma
    Ocular coloboma
    Optic nerve anomalies
    Retinopathy of prematurity
    PHPV

Trauma
    Blunt trauma
    Penetrating eye injuries
    Intraocular foreign body
    Nonaccidental injury

Others
    Non-traumatic retinal dialysis

Tractional retinal detachment
    Retinopathy of prematurity
    Incontinentia pigmenti
    Dominant exudative vitreoretinopathy
    Trauma
    Toxocariasis

Exudative retinal detachment
    Retinopathy of prematurity
    Coat's disease
    Retinitis pigmentosa
    Capillery haemangioma of retina
    Posterior scleritis
    Harada's disease
    Choroidal haemangioma

Solid detachment
    Retinoblastoma

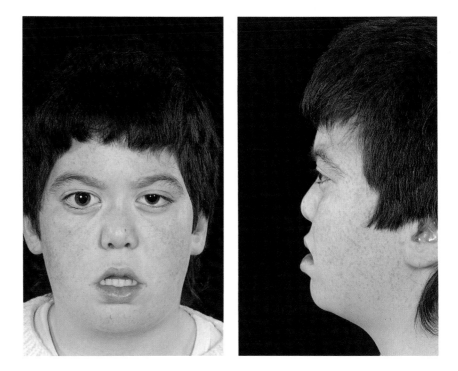

Fig. 27.6.1 Stickler's syndrome. These children have a flat nasal bridge, midfacial hypoplasia and deafness (note hearing aid). Micrognathia, cleft soft palate, and dental abnormalities may also be present.

Traumatic retinal detachment

Traumatic retinal detachment is seen most commonly in older children and is usually caused by blunt trauma (Verdaguer 1982); a rare cause in infancy is non-accidental injury (Mushin & Morgan 1971). Penetrating injuries and retained intraocular foreign bodies are less frequent causes (Percival 1972).

Most traumatic retinal detachments are associated with retinal dialysis (Daniel *et al.* 1974a) which is most commonly seen in the lower temporal quandrant (Chignell 1973; Scott 1977). In some cases the trauma may be trivial or a dialysis may be found in the fellow eye suggesting that there is a predisposing weakness in the ora serrata (Scott 1977). A dialysis may also develop following penetrating trauma with vitreous loss when it tends to occur on the opposite side of the eye to the penetrating wound (Scott 1977).

Detachments associated with dialysis progress slowly and usually present when the macula becomes detached (Chignell 1973). Although the anatomical success rate of surgery is high visual function may remain poor due to the longstanding nature of the detachment.

Penetrating injury is an uncommon cause of detachment in childhood and may rarely follow inadvertent perforation of the globe at strabismus surgery (Basmadjian *et al.* 1975). Intraocular foreign bodies are rarely seen although penetrating injuries from air gun pellets are typically seen in older children and adolescents and have a poor prognosis (Moore *et al.* 1987).

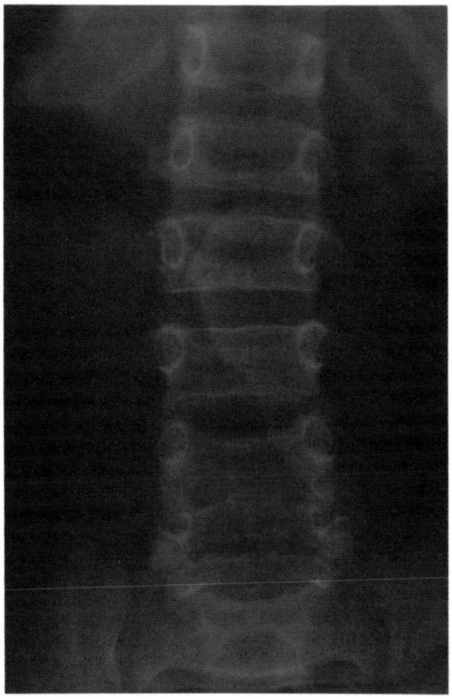

Fig. 27.6.2 Stickler's syndrome. Flat vertebrae as a radiological sign of spondyloepiphyseal dysplasia. These children may be born with an arthropathy and muscular hypotonia.

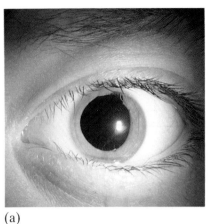

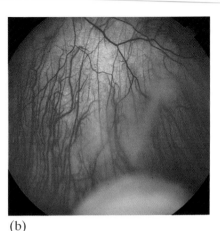

(a)　　　　　　　　　(b)

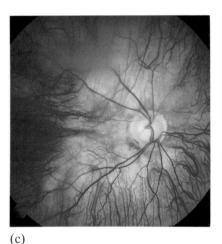

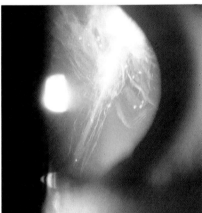

Fig. 27.6.3 Stickler's syndrome.
(a) External eye showing iris defect
following spontaneous lens subluxation
(−25 Dioptre myopia). Same patient as
in Fig. 27.6.1. (b) Fundus showing
dislocated lens inferiorly. (c) Fundus
showing myopic changes and defocussed
areas due to vitreous opacities.
(d) Vitreous opacities and strands. The
vitreo retinal problems in these children
makes them very susceptible to retinal
detachment.

(c)　　　　　　　　　(d)

Familial retinal detachment

Retinal detachment may be seen in a variety of inherited systemic disorders in which there is ocular
involvement (Table 27.6.1). In most cases there is
associated high myopia although in some conditions
for example incontinentia pigmenti and dominant
exudative vitreoretinopathy (DEVR) there is an
underlying retinovascular abnormality. Rarely a true
detachment may complicate juvenile X-linked retinoschisis (Verdaguer 1982; Schulman *et al.* 1985).

High myopia and retinal detachment is seen in
Marfan's syndrome, Ehlers−Danlos syndrome
(Pemberton *et al.* 1966), Stickler's syndrome (Figs
27.6.1−27.6.3) (Billington *et al.* 1985) and in association with mid face clefting syndromes (Delaney *et al.*
1963; Daniel *et al.* 1974b; Feiler-Ofry *et al.* 1980). The
detachments are often complex frequently with associated giant tears (Billington *et al.* 1985).

Detachment in developmental anomalies of the eye

Retinal detachment is more common in eyes which
have other congenital abnormalities, especially high
myopia (Scott 1980). Eyes with ocular colobomata are
at a significantly increased risk of detachment; giant
retinal tears are seen in association with lens colobomata (Hovland *et al.* 1968) and rhegmatogenous
detachment may develop in eyes with choroidal coloboma when small retinal breaks may be found in
thinned retina overlying the coloboma (Jesberg &
Schepens 1960). Retinal detachment may also complicate dysplasia of the optic nerve head, especially the
Morning Glory anomaly. There is usually a total
retinal detachment and often no retinal break can be
found. The cause of the detachment in such cases in
uncertain and rarely spontaneous re-attachment may
occur (Hamada & Ellsworth 1971). Retinal detachment may also occur in eyes with anterior or posterior
hyperplastic primary vitreous (see Chapter 26).

Other ocular abnormalities associated with an increased risk of retinal detachment include congenital cataract (Kanski *et al.* 1974), congenital glaucoma (Cooling *et al.* 1980), and retinopathy of prematurity.

Tractional detachment

Traction on the retina leading to detachment is rare in childhood; it may complicate primary retinovascular disease such as retinopathy of prematurity, DEVR or incontinentia pigmenti or may develop following penetrating trauma, or intraocular inflammation associated with for example ocular toxocariasis. Such traction may lead to retinal detachment directly or cause retinal breaks and subsequent rhegmatogenous detachment. Vitreoretinal traction may also complicate rhegmatogenous detachment and extensive vitreoretinal fibrosis is a common cause of failure of detachment surgery.

Exudative detachment

Exudative detachment although uncommon has a wide variety of causes in childhood, including Coat's disease, retinoblastoma, retinopathy of prematurity, ocular toxocariasis, choroidal haemangioma, capillary haemangioma, posterior scleritis, and Harada's disease. If there is doubt about the diagnosis CT scan or ultrasound and a careful EUA should be performed to rule out retinoblastoma.

Management

In infants and young children with suspected retinal detachment it is important to carry out a thorough examination under general anaesthetic so that the cause of the detachment can be determined and treatment planned. In cases where no retinal breaks are found, scleral transillumination, ultrasound and CT scan are helpful in excluding intraocular tumour or posterior scleral thickening. Fluorescein angiography is helpful in highlighting retinovascular abnormalities in selected cases for example in Coat's disease, DEVR, and choroidal haemangioma. In non-traumatic rhegmatogenous detachment with high myopia a careful ocular and physical examination and on occasion paediatric referral will help exclude systemic disorders such as Stickler's syndrome.

Retinal detachment is rare in childhood and often associated with complex intraocular pathology. Such cases are therefore best referred to specialist centres with experience of dealing with vitreoretinal disorders in children.

References

Basmadjian G, Labelle P, Dumas J. Retinal detachment after strabismus surgery. *Am J Ophthalmol* 1975; **79**: 305–09

Billington BM, Leaver PK, McLeod D. Management of retinal detachment in the Wagner–Stickler syndrome. *Trans Ophthalmol Soc UK* 1985; **104**: 875–9

Chignell AH. Retinal dialysis. *Br J Ophthalmol* 1973; **57**: 572–7

Cooling RJ, Rice NSC, McLeod D. Retinal detachment in congenital glaucoma. *Br J Ophthalmol* 1980; **64**: 417–21

Daniel R, Kanski JJ, Glaspool MG. Retinal detachment in children. *Trans Ophthalmol Soc UK* 1974a; **94**: 325–34

Daniel R, Kanski J, Glaspool MG. Hyalo-retinopathy in the clefting syndrome. *Br J Ophthalmol* 1974b; **58**: 96–102

Delaney WV, Podedworny W, Havener WH. Inherited retinal detachment. *Arch Ophthalmol* 1963; **69**: 44–50

Feiler-Ofry V, Godel V, Nemet P, Lazar M. Retinal detachment in median cleft-face syndrome. *Br J Ophthalmol* 1980; **64**: 121–3

Foos RY, Kiechler RJ, Allen RA. Congenital non-attachment of the retina. *Am J Ophthalmol* 1968; **65**: 202–10

Hamada S, Ellsworth RM. Congenital retinal detachment and the optic disc anomaly. *Am J Ophthalmol* 1971; **71**: 460–3

Hovland KR, Schepens CL, Freeman HM. Developmental giant retinal tears associated with lens coloboma. *Arch Ophthalmol* 1968; **80**: 325–31

Jesberg DO, Schepens CL. Retinal detachment associated with coloboma of the choroid. *Arch Ophthalmol* 1961; **65**: 163–73

Kanski JJ, Elkington AR, Daniel R. Retinal detachment after congenital cataract surgery. *Br J Ophthalmol* 1974; **58**: 92–102

Moore AT, McArtney A, Cooling RJ. Eye injuries associated with the use of air weapons. *Eye* 1987; **1**: 422–9

Mushin A, Morgan G. Ocular injury in the battered baby syndrome. Report of two cases. *Br J Ophthalmol* 1971; **55**: 343–7

Pemberton JW, Freeman HM, Schepens CL. Familial retinal detachment and the Ehlers–Danlos syndrome. *Arch Ophthalmol* 1966; **76**: 817–24

Percival SPB. Late complications from posterior segment intraocular foreign bodies, with particular reference to retinal detachment. *Br J Ophthalmol* 1972; **56**: 462–8

Schulman J, Peyman GA, Jednock N, Larson B. Indications for vitrectomy in congenital retinoschisis. *Br J Ophthalmol* 1985; **69**: 482–6

Scott JD. Retinal dialysis. *Trans Ophthalmol Soc UK* 1977; **97**: 33–5

Scott JD. Congenital myopia and retinal detachment. *Trans Ophthalmol Soc UK* 1980; **100**: 69–71

Tasman W. Retinal detachment in children. *Trans Am Acad Ophthalmol Otolaryngol* 1967; **71**: 455–60

Verdaguer J. Juvenile retinal detachment. *Am J Ophthalmol* 1982; **93**: 145–56

27.7 Flecked Retina Syndromes

ANTHONY MOORE

Table 27.7.1 Flecked retina syndromes

Inherited	Acquired
Stargardt's disease (fundus flavimaculatus)	Vitamin A deficiency
Fundus albipunctatus	Drugs (very rare in children)
Kandori's flecked retina syndrome	tamoxifen
	methoxyfluorane anesthesia
Retinitis punctata albescens	canthaxanthine
Benign familial flecked retina syndrome	
Abetalipoproteinemia	
Dominant drusen	
Bietti's crystalline dystrophy	
Alport's syndrome	
Oxalosis	
Sjögren–Larsson syndrome	

Many different disorders may give rise to multiple white or yellow deposits scattered throughout the retina leading to the appearance of a flecked retina (Table 27.7.1). Most are inherited (and have been considered in detail in other chapters) but vitamin A deficiency and certain drugs may cause a similar appearance. This chapter reviews the differential diagnosis of the flecked retina syndrome in children.

Stargardt's disease (fundus flavimaculatus)

This disorder which is usually inherited as an autosomal recessive trait is characterized by the presence of multiple yellow white 'fish tail' flecks scattered throughout the posterior pole and peripheral retina. There is normally associated macular atrophy. In early disease the flecks may mask the underlying choroidal fluorescence but more commonly there is widespread patchy hyperflourescence due to pigment epithelial atrophy. A 'dark choroid' is a common angiographic finding. The ERG and EOG are usually normal until late in the disease.

Fundus albipunctatus

Fundus albipunctatus is an autosomal recessive form of stationery night-blindness in which there are multiple white dots deposited at the level of the pigment epithelium (Fig. 27.7.1). Fluorescein angiography shows patchy hyperflourescence which doesn't appear to corellate with the distribution of the deposits (Krill 1977). Visual acuity and visual fields are normal. The electroretinogram and electro-oculogram may be abnormal when tested routinely, but revert to normal on prolonged dark adaptation. Dark adaptation is markedly delayed but normal rod thresholds are reached eventually.

The presence of night-blindness with normal visual acuity, visual fields and prolonged dark adaptation help to differentiate this disorder from other flecked retina syndromes.

Kandori's flecked retina syndrome

Kandori (1972) has described a rare stationary dystrophy characterized by onset in childhood, mild slowing of dark adaptation, normal vision and visual

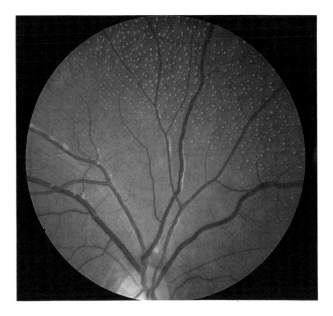

Fig. 27.7.1 Fundus albipunctatus. The child complained of night-blindness, but had normal acuity, colour vision, and visual fields.

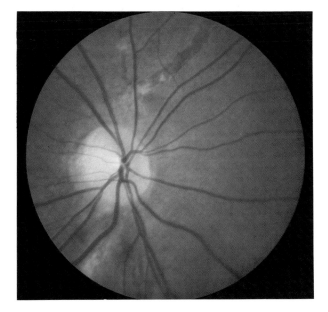

Fig. 27.7.2 Abetalipoproteinaemia. This patient had been treated for 18 years with vitamins A and E and had normal visual function and a normal electroretinogram. Angiods streaks are present; they are also found in some other conditions in which there are deformed red blood cells.

fields and mid peripheral deposition of yellow flecks. These flecks lie at the level of the retinal pigment epithelium and hyperflouresce on fluorescein angiography. The macula is uninvolved. Electro-retinography and electro-oculography are normal and the condition is non progressive.

Retinitis punctata albescens

Some patients with retinitis pigmentosa (RP) have multiple white dots scattered throughout the retina rather than the usual pigment deposition. It is doubtful whether this represents a unique subtype of RP as it may be seen in patients from families where other family members have the classical fundus picture.

This disorder may be distinguished from fundus albipunctatus by its progressive nature, visual field loss and electroretinographic abnormalities.

Abetalipoproteinaemia

Abetalipoproteinaemia is a rare disorder characterized by fat malabsorption, absence of serum beta-lipoprotein, abnormally shaped red cells, ataxic neuropathy, and a retinal dystrophy (Fig. 27.7.2). Untreated patients develop a progressive retinal dystrophy often with white dots deposited at the level of the pigment epithelium. Treatment with vitamin A

and E may prevent the development of the retinal abnormalities (Bishara et al. 1982; Runge et al. 1986).

Dominant drusen

This dominant disorder usually presents in adult life with mild visual loss or metamorphopsia (Krill & Klein 1965). Multiple drusen are seen scattered throughout the fundus but are most numerous at the posterior pole (Krill 1977). The abnormal gene shows a marked variability of expression so that some affected family members have only a few drusen. Although symptoms first appear in adult life the fundus abnormalities have been detected in early childhood (Krill 1977). Fluorescein angiography shows widespread patchy hyperfluorescence which either corresponds to drusen or associated retinal pigment epithelial atrophy.

Since this disorder is asymptomatic in childhood it is rarely diagnosed in children and seldom gives rise to difficulties in diagnosis.

Benign familial flecked retina syndrome

Aish and Dajani (1980) have described a flecked retina syndrome occurring in seven out of ten siblings born to parents who were first cousins. The visual acuity peripheral visual fields and dark adaptation were all normal. The flecks, first seen in infancy, were discrete white yellow lesions at the level of the pigment epithelium and were scattered throughout the fundus. Fluorescein angiography showed multiple areas of hyperflourescence which did not appear to correlate with the flecks. Although there are many similarities with fundus flavimaculatus the lack of macular involvement in all of the seven affected siblings and the good visual prognosis suggest that this disorder may be different.

Alport's syndrome

Alport's syndrome is characterized by chronic renal failure and bilateral sensorineural deafness. X-linked recessive inheritance is usual (Gubler *et al.* 1981). Ocular abnormalities include cataract, lenticonus, corneal arcus and a fleck retinopathy (Govan 1983).

Govan (1983) described 16 patients with Alport's syndrome and 14 had evidence of a flecked retinopathy. The flecks are pale yellow, multiple and lie at the level of the pigment epithelium. Fluorescein angiography showed widespread patchy hyperfluorescence although in some areas the flecks block the underlying choroidal fluorescence (Govan 1983). The electroretinogram and electro-oculogram have been found to be abnormal (Polak & Hogewind 1977; Zylbermann *et al.* 1980) in some patients but interpretation of these results is difficult in the presence of chronic renal failure (Govan 1983).

Primary hereditary oxalosis

Primary hereditary oxalosis is a rare autosomal recessive disorder of glyoxylate metabolism resulting in increased serum and urinary levels of oxalate. As serum levels rise calcium precipitates with oxolate to form insoluble crystals which are deposited in many different tissues. Renal involvement leads to chronic renal failure which is the major cause of death.

Two different types of the disorder have been described each with a specific enzyme deficiency. In type 1 hyperoxaluria there is a deficiency of the enzyme alpha-ketoglutarate : glyoxylate carboligase and its absence leads to increased production of oxalic acid. In type 2 disease a deficiency of D glyceric dehydrogenase results in increased synthesis of oxalic acid. The ocular abnormalities are confined to type 1 disease (Fielder *et al.* 1980; Zak & Buncic 1983; Meredith *et al.* 1984).

Hereditary oxalosis usually presents in early childhood and affected children may show multiple yellow crystals deposited at the level of the pigment epi-

thelium (Fig. 27.7.3). The deposits are more numerous at the posterior pole and with time hyperplasia of the retinal pigment epithelium may develop giving rise to a ring of hyperpigmentation around the macula (Zak & Buncic 1983; Meredith *et al.* 1984). Fluorescein angiography in one case showed hypofluorescence related to the pigmentation and peripheral areas of ring shaped hyperfluorescence surrounding a central area of hypofluorescence — presumably related to the crystal deposition (Meredith *et al.* 1984).

Histopathological examination of involved eyes

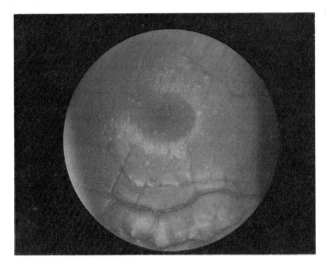

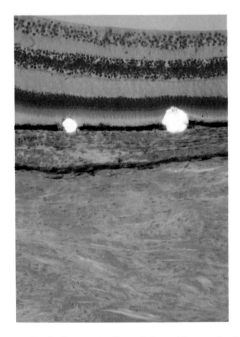

Fig. 27.7.3 Oxalosis type 1. Crystal deposition at the level of the retinal pigment epithelium. Professor A. Fielder's patient.

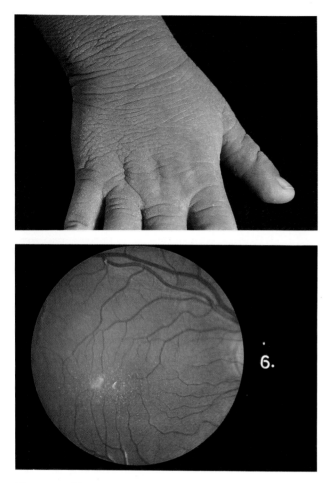

Fig. 27.7.4 Sjögren–Larsson syndrome. Ichthyosis and macular crystal deposition.

have shown deposition of oxalate in the retinal pigment epithelium (Fielder et al. 1980; Meredith et al. 1984).

Oxalosis should be differentiated from other causes of fleck retina and in particular from other causes of crystalline deposition (Grizzard et al. 1978). Oxalate crystal deposition may occur in secondary hyperoxaluria resulting from methoxyflurane anesthesia (Bullock & Albert 1975), when a similar flecked retinopathy is seen. Crystalline deposition has also been reported in cystinosis (Read et al. 1973), Sjögren–Larsson syndrome (Gilbert et al. 1968) Bietti's crystalline dystrophy (Grizzard et al. 1978), tamoxifen retinopathy (McKeown et al. 1981) and canxanthine retinopathy (Daicker et al. 1985).

Sjögren–Larsson syndrome

The Sjögren–Larsson syndrome is a rare autosomal recessive disorder characterized by mental retardation, spastic diplegia, and congenital ichthyosis (Fig. 27.7.4a) (Sjögren & Larsson 1957). Fundus examination shows glistening yellow dots in the macular and paramacular area (Fig. 27.7.4b) (Gilbert et al. 1968; Jagell et al. 1980). Fluorescein angiography shows patchy hyperfluorescence at the macula due to pigment epithelial atrophy (Gilbert et al. 1968). Electroretinography and electrooculography are normal (Gilbert et al. 1968; Jagell 1980).

Histopathological examination of the eyes from one case showed increased lipofuscin levels in the pigment epithelium in the macular area but no evidence of any other retinal or subretinal deposits (Nillson & Jagell 1987)

References

Aish SFS, Dajani B. Benign familial fleck retina. *Br J Ophthalmol* 1980; **64**: 652–9

Bishara S, Merin S, Cooper M *et al.* Combined vitamin A and E therapy prevents retina electrophysiological deterioration in abetalipoproteinemia. *Br J Ophthalmol* 1982; **66**: 767–70

Bullock JD, Albert DM. Flecked retina appearance secondary to oxolate crystals from methoxyfluorane anesthesia. *Arch Ophthalmol* 1975; **93**: 26–31

Daicker B, Schiedt K, Adnet JJ, Bermond P. Canthaxanthine retinopathy. An investigation by light and electron microscopy and physico-chemical analysis. *Graefes Arch Klin Exp Ophthalmol* 1985; **225**: 189–201

Fielder AR, Garner A, Chambers TL. Ophthalmic manifestations of primary oxallosis. *Br J Ophthalmol* 1980; **64**: 782–8

Gibert WR, SR, Smith JL, Nyhan WL. The Sjogren–Larsson syndrome. *Arch Ophthalmol* 1968; **80**: 308–16

Govan JAA. Ocular manifestations of Alport's syndrome. *Br J Ophthalmol* 1983; **67**: 493–503

Grizzard WS, Deutman AF, Nijhuis F *et al.* Crystalline retinopathy. *Am J Ophthalmol* 1978; **86**: 81–8

Gubler M, Levy M, Broyer M *et al.* Alport's syndrome a report of 58 cases and a review of the literature. *Am J Med* 1981; **70**: 493–505

Jagell S, Polland W, Sandgren O. Specific changes in the fundus typical for the Sjögren–Larsson syndrome. *Acta Ophthalmol (KBH)* 1980; **58**: 321–30

Kandori F, Tamai A, Kurimoto S, Fukunaga K. Fleck retina. *Am J Ophthalmol* 1972; **73**: 673–85

Krill AE. Flecked retina diseases. In: Krill AE. (Ed.) *Hereditary Retinal and Choroidal Diseases*, Vol. 2. Harper & Row, Hagerstown 1977: pp. 739–823

Krill AE, Klein BA. Flecked retina syndrome. *Arch Ophthalmol* 1965; **74**: 496–508

McKeown CA, Schwartz M, Blau J *et al.* Tamoxifen retinopathy. *Br J Ophthalmol* 1981; **65**: 177–9

Meredith TA, Wright JD, Gammon JA *et al.* Ocular involvement in primary hyperoxaluria. *Arch Ophthalmol* 1984; **102**: 584–7

Nillson SE, Jagell S. Lipofuscein and melanin content of the retinal pigment epithelium in a case of Sjogren–Larsson syndrome. *Br J Ophthalmol* 1987; **71**: 224−7

Polak BCP, Hogewind BL. Macular lesions in Alport's syndrome. *Am J Ophthalmol* 1977; **84**: 532−5

Read J, Goldberg MF, Fishman G *et al.* Nephropathic cystinosis. *Am J Ophthalmol* 1973; **76**: 791−6

Runge P, Muller DPR, McAllister J *et al.* Oral vitamin E supplements can prevent the retinopathy of abetalipoproteinemia. *Br J Ophthalmol* 1986; **70**: 166−73

Sjögren T, Larsson T. Oligophrenia in combination with congenital ichthyosis and spastic disorders. *Acta Psychiatr Scand* 1957; **32**: 1−113

Zak TA, Buncic R. Primary hereditary oxalosis retinopathy. *Arch Ophthalmol* 1983; **101**: 78−80

Zylberman R, Silverstone BZ, Brandes E *et al.* Retinal lesions in Alport's syndrome. *J Pediatr Ophthalmol* 1980; **17**: 255−60

27.8 Miscellaneous Retinal Disorders

ANTHONY MOORE

Acquired retinovascular disorders

Diabetes mellitus

DIABETIC RETINOPATHY

Diabetic retinopathy in children with Type 1 diabetes is rare early in the disease but the prevalence rises with increasing duration of the disease, and especially after puberty (Burger *et al.* 1986; Weber *et al.* 1986; Lund-Anderson *et al.* 1987). There is some evidence that good glycaemic control may delay the onset of retinopathy (Sterky & Wall 1986; Weber *et al.* 1986). Proliferative retinopathy is rarely seen before late adolescence or early adult life (Malone *et al.* 1984; Burger *et al.* 1986).

Mild background retinopathy may be missed on ophthalmoscopy and early changes are best demonstrated by fluorescein angiography (Frost-Larsen & Starup 1980; Starup *et al.* 1980). In one longtitudinal study only 5% of diabetic children between 10 and 14 years (average duration of diabetes 4–6 years) had evidence of retinopathy at the outset of the study. However at a 5-year follow-up this had increased to 63% and by 8 years over 90% had angiographic evidence of retinopathy (Starup *et al.* 1980). Similar results have been reported by other authors (Burger *et al.* 1986; Sterky & Wall 1986; Weber *et al.* 1986).

Diabetic retinopathy therefore appears to develop gradually with increasing duration of disease and is rare before puberty. From a practical point of view regular screening for treatable disease may be safely confined to the post-pubertal age group but fortunately retinopathy severe enough to require treatment is rare in childhood.

ACUTE DISC SWELLING (see Chapter 28)

Acute optic disc swelling and mild visual loss is a recognized complication of Type 1 diabetes although the mechanism of the optic nerve oedema is unknown. It typically affects adolescents and young adults and may rarely be seen in childhood (Appen *et al.* 1980; Barr *et al.* 1980; Pavan *et al.* 1980). Most patients show mild visual loss and mild unilateral or bilateral disc swelling although less commonly there may be more florid papilloedema with haemorrhages and exudates (Barr *et al.* 1980). The visual prognosis is good with most patients recovering normal acuity within 6 months (Barr *et al.* 1980).

Sickle cell disease

Ocular abnormalities, mainly related to occlusive vascular disease may be seen in homozygous sickle cell (SS) disease, haemoglobin SC disease and sickle cell thalassemia (S-thal). The most frequent complication is peripheral retinal vascular closure which may lead to retinal neovascularization, vitreous haemorrhage, and retinal detachment (Goldberg 1987). Proliferative retinopathy is seen more frequently in SC and S-thal disease (Welch & Goldberg 1966). Other ocular complications include choroidal vascular occlusion (Dizon *et al.* 1979), angioid streaks (Gerde 1974; Hamilton *et al.* 1981), and intractable glaucoma (Goldberg 1979) which may lead to central retinal artery occlusion.

The earliest changes in sickle cell retinopathy are seen in the peripheral retina where there may be multiple small arteriolar occlusions which are clearly demonstrated on fluorescein angiography (Welch & Goldberg 1966; Goldberg 1971, 1987). Occluded arterioles are often seen as white or 'silver wire' vessels within the ischaemic retina. With advancing disease arteriolar-venular anastomoses develop at the junction of normal and ischemic retina and subsequently neovascularizations may develop with the typical 'sea-fan' appearance of the new vessels (Goldberg 1971) which leak profusely on angiography.

Retinal or subretinal haemorrhages (salmon patches) are often seen at the junction of perfused and non-perfused retina and these may resolve to leave a pigmented scar ('sunburst spot') which resembles a focal area of chorioretinitis (Goldberg 1987). Refractile deposits which may represent haemosiderin deposited during the resorptions of retinal haemorrhage are commonly seen in the peripheral retina (Condon & Sergeant 1972). Other findings include retinal venous tortuosity and discoloured retinal patches which may represent areas of ischemia (Talbot et al. 1988).

Peripheral vascular closure begins at an early age and in one study (Talbot et al. 1988) was present in 50% of children with SS and SC disease at age 6 years old, and 90% by age 12. Although vessel closure may be extensive in the older children, proliferative retinopathy is rare in childhood (Talbot et al. 1988). Most children with sickle cell disease retain good visual acuity although rarely macular branch arteriolar occlusion (Knapp 1972; Acacio & Goldberg 1973) or central artery occlusion complicating intractable glaucoma (Michaelson & Pfaffenbach 1972; Goldberg 1979) may cause profound visual loss.

Children with sickle cell disease should be reviewed regularly to document the degree of retinal vascular occlusion but proliferative retinopathy is rare until adolescence or adulthood when treatment may be necessary. Traumatic hyphaema however is a particularly serious problem in children with sickle cell disease as sickled red blood cells in the anterior chamber may cause outflow obstruction and severely elevated intraocular pressure which may be unresponsive to conventional treatment. The pressure should be lowered promptly if necessary by paracentesis to prevent retinal arterial occlusion (Goldberg 1971).

Radiation retinopathy

Radiation retinopathy is most commonly seen in adults who have received radiotherapy for ocular, adnexal, nasopharyngeal, or sinus tumours, but may occur in children treated for retinoblastoma (McFaul & Bedford 1970; Egbert et al. 1978, 1980; Brown et al. 1982a). It may complicate both focal cobalt plaque and external beam therapy. Most patients have received at least 3500 cGy but rarely retinopathy develops following a lower dose (Brown et al. 1982a). The larger the dose and the greater the fractional dose the greater the risk of retinopathy.

The predominant effect is on the retinal vasculature and the clinical abnormalities are usually seen between 6 months and 36 months after therapy (Brown et al. 1982a). The main findings are arteriolar narrowing and sheathing, microaneurysms, telangiectasia, retinal exudates, and cotton wool spots. Cystoid macular oedema is a common cause of visual loss. Other findings include retinal neovascularization, vitreous haemorrhage, and rarely retinal detachment (Brown et al. 1982a; McFaul & Bedford 1970). Involvement of the optic nerve may result in ischaemic optic neuropathy often presenting several years after treatment (Brown et al. 1982b) and loss of the choriocapillaris may lead to retinal pigment atrophy and pigment migration (McFaul & Bedford 1970). Fluorescein angiography usually demonstrates widespread capillary closure, microaneurysms, telangiectasia, and vascular leakage (Brown et al. 1982a). Histological studies have confirmed the extensive damage to retinal and posterior ciliary vessels (Egbert et al. 1980).

Cystoid macular oedema

Cystoid macular oedema (CME) caused by leakage from the perifoveolar capillaries is uncommon in childhood. It may be seen in retinovascular diseases such as diabetes, radiation retinopathy or Coat's disease, in the inherited rod-cone dystrophies and in inflammatory disorders such as juvenile pars planitis or anterior and posterior uveitis. Rarely it may be familial (Deutman et al. 1976).

CME may also complicate intraocular surgery in children (Hoyt & Nickel 1982). Although postoperative aphakic CME was seen in over 30% of infants who had lensectomy and anterior vitrectomy in the study of Hoyt and Nickel (1982) this high incidence has not been confirmed in other studies (Poer et al. 1981; Gilbard et al. 1983; Pinchoff et al. 1988). There appears to be no greater risk of developing CME following one type of surgical procedure than another and the incidence of postoperative CME in cataract surgery in infancy is clearly less than seen in adults (Pinchoff et al. 1988).

Angioid streaks

Angioid streaks are seen as irregular linear streaks of variable pigmentation which radiate out from the peripapillary retina into the more peripheral fundus (Fig. 27.8.1, 27.8.2); the streaks taper towards the disc and may form a circumferential ring around the optic nerve head (Clarkson & Altman 1982). Histopathological examination of involved eyes have shown the streaks to correspond to breaks in Bruch's

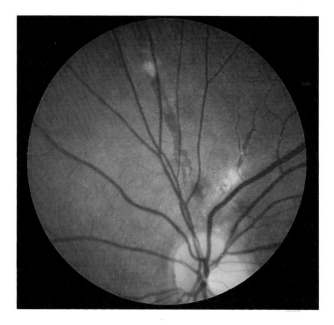

Fig. 27.8.1 Angioid streaks in a 10-year-old girl. The streaks, which represent breaks in Bruch's membrane radiate and taper from the optic disc in this instance above the disc at 11.30 and 1 o'clock.

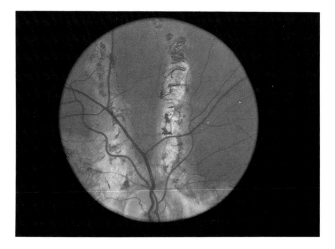

Fig. 27.8.2 Angioid streaks in an adult with pseudoxanthoma elasticum. Choroidal neovascularization and haemorrhages occur at the margins of the streaks.

membrane which may show fibrosis and calcification (Clarkson & Altmann 1982). Choroidal neovascularization may arise from edge of the streaks and may lead to serous detachment of the retina or subretinal haemorrhage.

Angioid streaks have been reported in association with a variety of systemic disorders (Table 27.8.1) but are most commonly found in Paget's disease (Gass & Clarkson 1973), pseudoxanthoma elasticum (Clarkson & Altman 1982), and sickle cell haemoglobinopathy (Nagpal et al. 1976). Even rarer are abetalipoproteinaemia (Runge et al. 1986), beta-thalassaemia (Gibson et al. 1983; Kinsella 1988), and hereditary spherocytosis (McLane et al. 1984; Singerman 1984). They are commonly found in older adults and are rare in childhood. In one series of 50 patients with angioid streaks none were under the age of 30 years old (Clarkson & Altman 1982).

The aetiology, clinical features and management of angioid streaks has recently been reviewed by Newsome (1987).

Disciform macular degeneration

Choroidal neovascularization is uncommon in childhood and is usually seen following traumatic choroidal rupture (Smith et al. 1974) intraocular infections such as congenital rubella (Fig. 27.8.3) (Deutman & Grizzard 1978; Orth et al. 1980), congenital toxoplasmosis (Fine et al. 1981; Cotlier & Friedmann 1982), and toxocariasis or in association with one of the inherited retinal dystrophies most commonly Best's disease (see Chapter 27.4). Other rare causes of childhood disciform degeneration are detailed in Table 27.8.2.

The aetiology, clinical features, and management of choroidal neovascularization in childhood has recently been reviewed by Wilson and Mazur (1988).

Table 27.8.1 Angioid streaks: associated systemic disorders.

Paget's disease
Sickle cell haemoglobinopathy
Thalassemia
Hereditary spherocytosis
Abetalipoproteinaemia
Pseudoxanthoma elasticum
Ehlers–Danlos syndrome
Acromegaly
Hyperparathyroidism
Hyperphosphataemia
Lead poisoning

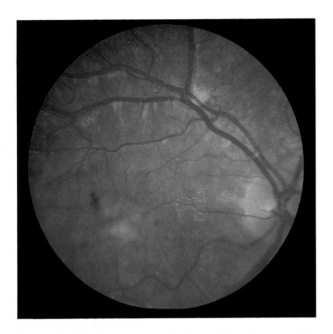

Fig. 27.8.3 Disciform degeneration in rubella retinopathy. This seven-year-old boy had a cataract in the left eye was deaf and noticed a reduction of vision in his right eye. The background pigment mottling usually associated with rubella can be seen surrounding the macular which shows a serous detachment, haemorrhage and a disciform lesion. The acuity fell to 6/60 but recovered to 6/12 over 4 months.

Table 27.8.2 Aetiology of choroidal neovascularization in childhood (modified from Wilson & Mazur 1988).

Trauma
Choroidal rupture

Inflammatory lesions
Congenital rubella
Toxoplasmosis
Toxocariasis
Presumed ocular histoplamosis syndrome
Chronic uveitis

Inherited retinal dystrophies
Vitelliform dystrophy
Choroideremia
Fundus flavimaculatus

Other
Angioid streaks
Optic nerve drusen
Choroidal osteoma
Optic nerve head pits
Combined RPE—retinal hamartoma

References

Acacio I, Goldberg MF. Peripapillary and macular vessel occlusions in sickle cell anaemia. *Am J Ophthalmol* 1973; **75**: 861—6

Appen RE, Chandra SR, Klein R, Myers FL. Diabetic papillopathy. *Am J Ophthalmol* 1980; **90**: 203—9

Barr CC, Glaser JS, Blahkenship G. Acute disc swelling in juvenile diabetes. Clinical profile and natural history of 12 cases. *Arch Ophthalmol* 1980; **98**: 2185—92

Brown GC, Shields JA, Sanborn G *et al*. Radiation retinopathy. *Ophthalmology* 1982a; **89**: 1494—501

Brown GC, Shields JA, Sanborn G *et al*. Radiation optic neuropathy. *Ophthalmology* 1982b; **89**: 1489—93

Burger W, Hovener G, Ousterhus D *et al*. Prevalence and development of retinopathy in children and adolescents with Type I (insulin dependent) diabetes mellitus. A longtitudinal study. *Diabetologica* 1986; **29**: 17—22

Clarkson JG, Altman RD. Angioid streaks. *Survey Ophthalmol* 1982; **26**: 235—46

Condon PI, Sergeant GR. Ocular findings in homozygous sickle cell disease in Jamaica. *Am J Ophthalmol* 1972; **73**: 533—43

Cotlier AM, Friedman AH. Subretinal neovascularization in ocular toxoplasmosis. *Br J Ophthalmol* 1982; **66**: 524—9

Deutman AF, Grizzard WS. Rubella retinopathy and subretinal neovascularization. *Am J Ophthalmol* 1978; **85**: 82—7

Deutman AF, Pinckers AJLG, De Kerk AL. Dominantly inherited cystoid macular oedema. *Am J Ophthalmol* 1976; **82**: 540—8

Dizon RV, Jampol LM, Goldberg MF, Juarez C. Choroidal occlusive disease in sickle cell haemoglobinopathies. *Surv Ophthalmol* 1979; **23**: 297—306

Egbert PR, Donaldson SS, Moazed K. Visual results and ocular complications following radiotherapy for retinoblastoma. *Arch Ophthalmol* 1978; **96**: 1826—30

Egbert PR, Fajardo LF, Donaldson S, Moazed K. Posterior ocular abnormalities after irradiation for retinoblastoma. A histopathological study. *Br J Ophthalmol* 1980; **64**: 660—5

Fine SL, Owens SL, Haller JA *et al*. Choroidal neovascularization as a late complication of ocular toxoplasmosis. *Am J Ophthalmol* 1981; **91**: 318—22

Frost-Larsen K, Starup K. Fluorescein angiography in diabetic children, a follow-up. *Acta Ophthalmol* 1980; **58**: 355—60

Gass JDM, Clarkson JG. Angioid streaks and disciform macular detachment in Paget's disease (osteitis deformans). *Am J Ophthalmol* 1973; **75**: 576—86

Gibson DM, Chaudhuri PR, Rosenthal AR. Angioid streaks in a case of beta thalassaemia major. *Br J Ophthalmol* 1983; **67**: 29—31

Gilbard SM, Peyman G, Goldberg M. Evaluation of cystoid maculopathy after pars plicata lensectomy vitrectomy for congenital cataracts. *Ophthalmology* 1983; **90**: 1201—6

Gerde LS. Angioid streaks in sickle cell trait haemoglobinopathy. *Am J Ophthalmol* 1974; **77**: 462—4

Goldberg MF. Classification and pathogenesis of proliferative sickle cell retinopathy. *Am J Ophthalmol* 1971; **71**: 649—65

Goldberg MF. Sickle cell retinopathy. In: Duane T (Ed.) *Clinical Ophthalmology*. Harper & Row, London 1987; pp. 1—45

Goldberg MF. The diagnosis and treatment of secondary glau-

MISCELLANEOUS RETINAL DISORDERS 439

coma after hyphema in sickle cell patients. *Am J Ophthalmol* 1979; **87**: 43−9

Hamilton AM, Pope FM, Condon PI *et al.* Angioid streaks in Jamaican patients with homozygous sickle cell disease. *Br J Ophthalmol* 1981; **65**: 341−7

Hoyt CS, Nickel D. Aphakic cystoid macular oedema. Occurence in infants and children after transpupillary lensectomy and anterior vitrectomy. *Arch Ophthalmol* 1982; **100**: 746−9

Kinsella FP, Mooney DJ. Angioid streaks in beta thalassaemia minor. *Br J Ophthalmol* 1988; **72**: 303−5

Knapp JW. Isolated macular infarction in sickle cell (SS) disease. *Am J Ophthalmol* 1972; **73**: 857−8

Lund-Anderson C, Larsen KM, Starup K. Natural history of diabetic retinopathy in insulin dependent juvenile diabetics. A longitudinal study. *Acta Ophthalmol* 1987; **65**: 481−6

MacFaul PA, Bedford MA. Ocular complications after therapeutic irradiation. *Br J Ophthalmol* 1970; **54**: 237−47

Malone JI, Grizzard S, Espinoza LR. Risk factors for diabetic retinopathy in youth. *Pediatrics* 1984; **73**: 756−61

McLane KG, Grizzard WS, Kousseff GB, Hartmann RC, Sever RJ. Angioid streaks associated with hereditary spherocytosis. *Am J Ophthalmol* 1984; **97**: 444−9

Michaelson PE, Pfaffenbach D. Retinal artery occlusion following trauma in youths with sickle − trait haemoglobinopathy. *Am J Ophthalmol* 1972; **74**: 494−7

Nagpal KC, Asdourian G, Goldbaum M *et al.* Angioid streaks and sickle cell haemoglobinopathies. *Br J Ophthalmol* 1976; **63**: 31−4

Newsome DA. Angioid streaks and Bruch's membrane degenerations. In: Newsome DA. (Ed.) *Retinal Dystrophies and Degenerations.* Raven Press, New York 1987; pp. 271−83

Orth DH, Fishman GA, Segall M *et al.* Rubella maculopathy. *Br J Ophthalmol* 1980; **64**: 201−5

Pavan PK, Aiello LM, Wafai Z *et al.* Optic disc oedema in juvenile onset diabetes. *Arch Ophthalmol* 1980; **98**: 2193−5

Pinchoff BS, Ellis FD, Helveston EM, Sato SE. Cystoid macular oedema in paediatric aphakia. *J Pediatr Ophthalmol Strabismus* 1988; **25**: 240−7

Poer DV, Helveston EM, Ellis FD. Aphakic cystoid macular oedema in children. *Arch Ophthalmol* 1981; **99**: 249−52

Runge P, Muller DRP, McAllister J, Calver D, Mayo JK, Taylor D. Oral vitamin E supplements can prevent the retinopathy of a-betalipoproteinaemia. *Br J Ophthalmol* 1986; **70**: 166−73

Singerman LJ. Angioid streaks associated with hereditary spherocytosis. *Am J Ophthalmol* 1984; **98**: 647−8

Smith RE, Kelley JS, Harbin TS. Late macular complications of choroidal rupture. *Am J Ophthalmol* 1974; **77**: 650−8

Starup K, Larsen HW, Enk B, Vestermark S. Fluorescein angiography in diabetic children. *Acta Ophthalmol* 1980; **58**: 347−53

Sterky G, Wall S. Determinants of microangiopathy in growth onset diabetes. With special reference to retinopathy and glycemic control. *Acta Paediatr Scand* (Suppl.) 1986; **327**: 1−45

Talbot JF, Bird AC, Maude GH. Sickle cell retinopathy in Jamaican children: further observations from a chart study. *Br J Ophthalmol* 1988; **72**: 727−32

Weber B, Burger W, Hartmann R *et al.* Risk factors for the development of retinopathy in children and adolescents with Type I (insulin dependent) diabetes mellitus. *Diabetologica* 1986; **29**: 23−9

Wilson ME, Mazur DO. Choroidal neovascularization in children. Report of 5 cases and a literature review. *J Pediatr Ophthalmol* 1988; **25**: 23−9

Welch RB, Goldberg MF. Sickle cell haemoglobin and its relation to fundus abnormality. *Arch Ophthalmol* 1966; **75**: 353−62

28 Optic Nerve

DAVID TAYLOR

Normal optic disc in infancy

There are no absolute criteria for normality of the optic disc in infancy but there are important differences between an adult's and an infant's optic disc. It is best to examine the optic disc with the pupil dilated and using both the indirect and the direct ophthalmoscope taking as much time as possible.

The infant disc appears to be about the same size on ophthalmoscopy as that of an adult; the main differences are its colour, the vascular pattern and the size of the physiological cup. The disc, especially in early infancy, is comparatively pale; the fluorescein angiographic appearance is the same as in older children, making vascular changes unlikely as the cause of the pattern. The disc is myelinated at birth, but there may be some difference in the size or optical qualities of the axonal myelin and supporting tissue. The relative whiteness of the infant optic disc makes it easy to misdiagnose optic atrophy and extra information can be gained from examination of the nerve fibre layer of the retina about a half a disc diameter away from the edge of the disc. Normally, the retinal vessels stand out just above the level of the internal limiting membrane which is seen as the surface sheen on the retina. In optic atrophy, the retinal nerve fibres decrease in number leaving the vessels standing up well above the internal limiting membrane. This is best seen by the use of parallax in which the ophthalmoscope is moved from side to side to observe the change in the light reflex over the retinal vessels.

In infancy the physiological cup in the optic disc is smaller than in older children, it is also difficult to see due to lack of sharp definition of it's edge. The retinal vessels may be more tortuous especially in neonates. In the newborn, retinal haemorrhages may occur near or on the disc although they are not necessarily of serious pathological significance, (von Barsewitch 1979).

Grey disc ('myelogenous dysgenesis')

Beauvieux (1926) described a grey appearance of the optic disc in neonates, usually in those born prematurely. He suggested that this may be due to 'myelogenous dysgenesis'. Initially vision appeared defective but improved within a few weeks or months. Several subsequent case reports confirmed the occurrence of this phenomenon and it is now enshrined in the ophthalmological literature, although it does not seem to have been recognized in recent years. It may be that the cases described are analogous to infants with some 'delayed visual development' in whom the occurrence of unexplained poor vision with normal eyes has been associated with a poorly developed visual evoked cortical response (Mellor & Fielder 1980; Harel *et al.* 1983). Both vision and the electrophysiological tests improve with time, but the latter observation is often difficult to evaluate since the electrophysiological tests tend to mature with time in all children, especially in the first few months.

In practice it is reasonable to take a confident line with the parents, especially if there are no other central nervous system signs and if the electrophysiological tests are shown to improve. The literature on the grey disc and experience with delayed visual development both suggest a good outcome.

Pigmentation in and around the optic disc

Disc pigmentation

Congenital pigmentation of the optic disc is rare, although variations of the pigment border of the optic disc are seen quite frequently. Mann (1957) described three types:
1 Dense plaques of pigment overlying a sector of the disc and sometimes extending over the retina. These may be of ectodermal origin, but are more likely to be mesodermal in origin if they surround the optic disc.
2 Linear pigment markings concentric with the disc margin (Fig. 28.1).
3 Lace-like veils of pigment associated with the central retinal vessels and probably of mesodermal origin, like the choroidal pigment.

Shields (1980) has drawn attention to the occurrence of a slate-grey crescent, usually temporal or inferotemporal, in the optic disc which occurs particularly in pigmented races which may be confused with a cupped disc. This is either a congenital anomaly or acquired during the early growth of the eye.

Melanocytomas occasionally occur in children, giving jet black pigmentation to the disc and surrounding tissue together with disc oedema (Haas *et al.* 1986).

In Aicardi's syndrome (Aicardi *et al.* 1965; Hoyt *et al.* 1978) infantile spasms occur with severe retardation, ectopic cerebral grey matter, absence of the corpus callosum (Fig. 28.2a), and characteristic lacunar defects in the retina (Fig. 28.2b, 28.2c). It only occurs in girls. The optic disc may be anomalous with grey pigmentation adjacent to and involving the optic disc, usually associated with a somewhat elevated glial anomaly of the disc.

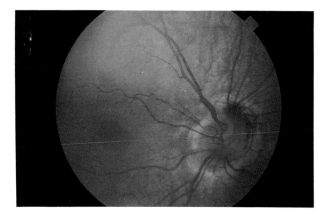

Fig. 28.1 Optic disc pigmentation. Linear pigmentation concentric with the optic disc margin.

Congenital vascular anomalies of, or around, the optic disc

Cilioretinal arteries

These are usually single, occasionally multiple, retinal vessels that arise from the ciliary circulation and appear to bend around the very margin of the optic disc (Fig. 28.6). Usually small, they are occasionally large, supplying a large proportion of the retina. Occasionally they arise in an optic disc pit. They are usually of no significance but they may become selectively occluded causing infarction of the area of retina they supply or they may supply an area of retina that is spared in a central retinal artery occlusion. They may be detected by fluorescein angiography in up to 50% of the population (Justice & Lehman 1976). They occur frequently in patients with optic disc drusen (Erkkila 1976).

Opticociliary veins

These are veins which connect the intraocular retinal venous system via the choroidal veins to the vortex veins.

They are occasionally found in high myopia or in otherwise anomalous optic disc and are usually of no significance. They occur after chronic obstruction of the central retinal vein due to shunting of blood from the retinal to the choroidal veins via the peripapillary capillary plexus (Fig. 28.6). The capillaries enlarge and become venous channels.

Situs inversus

These are tilted optic discs occurring in high myopes with posterior staphylomas in which the vessels are distorted by being dragged towards the staphyloma (Fig. 28.7).

Haemangiomas of the optic disc

These are rare tumours, occurring either alone or in association with the Von Hippel–Lindau syndrome.

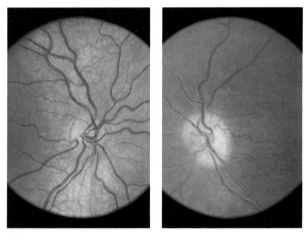

(a)

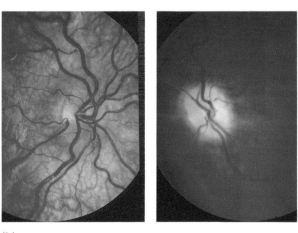

(b)

Fig. 28.6. (a) Cilioretinal arteries and opticociliary veins. In the right eye there is a cilioretinal artery in the infrotemporal quadrant. This patient had a chiasmal and left optic nerve glioma and the left eye shows optico-ciliary shunt vessels. (b) The right eye now shows papilloedema in the upper and lower pole of the optic disc which conforms with the temporal defect in this eye (known as twin peaks papilloedema). The left eye has a totally atrophic optic nerve and the shunt vessels have disappeared. (Same patient 2 years later.)

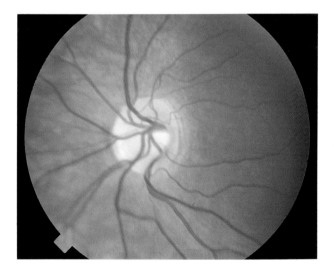

Fig. 28.7 Situs inversus (see text).

They may be sharply defined, reddish, spherical knobs of tumour or diffuse orange coloured tumours that involve the juxta-papillary retina (Fig. 28.8) (Gass 1980). Visual loss with symptoms of blurring and distortion can occur from the formation of exudates and intraretinal or subretinal fluid.

From the literature, untreated tumours seem to show growth and to be associated with a high incidence of visual complications; treatment however is fraught with problems. Schindler and his colleagues (1975) believed (in pre-CT scan days) that an isolated disc haemangioma, diagnosed by fluorescein angiography was not an indication for further neuroradiological studies since without associated retinal lesions they are not usually part of a systemic syndrome. The advent of non-invasive scanning means that it is safer to investigate these patients.

Bergmeister's papilla and pre-papillary vascular loops

These not uncommon abnormalities are remnants of the hyaloid vessels and their glial supporting structures, which regress between the seventh and ninth month of gestation (Apple *et al.* 1982). They may, therefore, be seen in premature babies as a normal feature.

Bergmeister's papilla most frequently appears as a small blue-white or grey conical elevation in front of

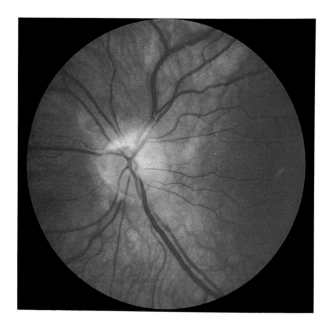

Fig. 28.9 Bergmeister's papilla. In a patient suspected of having raised intracranial pressure with headaches. There was no other abnormality found.

the optic disc. It has no functional or pathological significance. Sometimes the glial element can be quite large, but the retinal vessels are not involved (Fig. 28.9, 28.10). They may be part of a more widespread hyaloid vascular abnormality (Fig. 28.11).

Rarely, vascular loops, sometimes corkscrew in shape (Fig. 28.12), project forwards from the optic disc, occasionally quite far into the vitreous cavity where they sometimes pulsate with each heartbeat

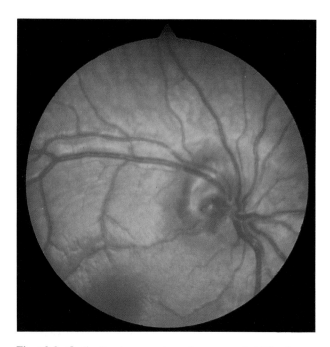

Fig. 28.8. Optic disc haemangioma in a normal child, who presented with a squint.

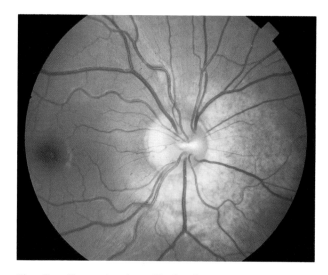

Fig. 28.10 Bergmeister's papilla showing as a more or less solid glial elevation anterior to the optic disc.

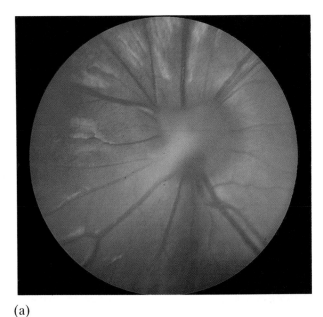

(a)

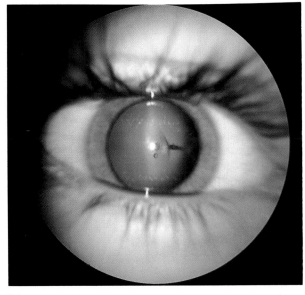

(b)

Fig. 28.11 (a) A glial vascular anomaly associated with a persistent hyaloid artery and retinal abnormalities. (b) The hyaloid artery can be seen extending to the posterior surface of the lens (same patient).

(Degenhart *et al.* 1981). Generally of no local pathological or systemic significance, they have been documented to obstruct in adults with disastrous consequences for the (usually inferior) retinal arteriole which they may supply (Brown 1979). Purely venous loops also occur (Degenhart *et al.* 1981).

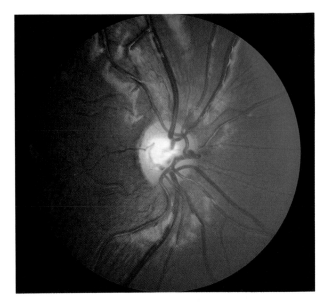

Fig. 28.12 Corkscrew prepapillary vascular loop.

Other vascular anomalies

Patients with Down's syndrome have an unusual number of vessels crossing the optic disc, sometimes in a spoke-like arrangement (Williams *et al.* 1973). The disc vessels are also abnormal in the Wyburn−Mason syndrome (see Chapter 27.5) and in the Klippel−Trenaunay−Weber syndrome (asymmetrical limb hypertrophy with mixed haemangiomas of skin and deep tissue, sometimes with A-V fistulae) where affected patients may have telangiectatic vessels around the disc (O'Connor & Smith 1978). A variety of other unusual A-V malformations and tortuous vessels have also been described (Kottow 1978).

Myelinated nerve fibres

Myelination of the optic nerve begins during fetal life at the lateral geniculate body and reaches the optic disc around the time of birth. Normally the myelin does not extend anterior to the cribriform plate, but in about 1% of the population (Straatsma 1981) the myelination may reach the retina. The commonest appearance, slightly more frequent in males, is of a unilateral, feathery white opacity usually adjacent to but occasionally away from the optic disc (Fig. 28.13). There may be a field defect related to the size and site of the myelinated fibres, but generally central vision is normal. Although most often they occur in normal eyes, they have been found with a variety of ocular malformations. There is an association between

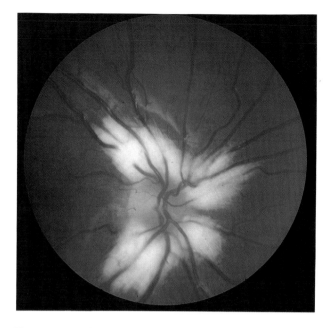

Fig. 28.13 Myelinated nerve fibres adjacent to the optic disc.

widespread demyelinated fibres, high myopia and amblyopia (Levy 1974; Straatsma 1981) (Fig. 28.14). Myelinated fibres may atrophy after an optic neuropathy, with resolution of at least part of the myelinated area (Schachat 1981) and (extraordinarily) have been recorded to develop in adult life (Baarsma 1980). Patients with myelinated fibres are usually otherwise normal, though an association has been reported with craniofacial dysostoses (Franceschetti A 1938) and in the Gorlin–Goltz autosomal dominant multiple basal cell carcinoma syndrome (DeJong et al. 1985). Their

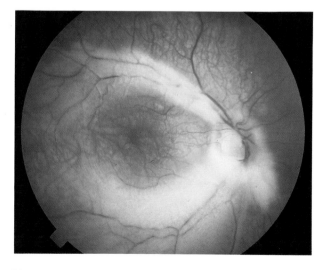

Fig. 28.14 Extensive myelinated nerve fibres associated with amblyopia and high myopia (see text).

cause and origin (Bellhom 1979; Straatsma 1981) is uncertain.

Drusen

Drusen (hyaline bodies) of the optic discs is probably the result of a congenital anomaly of the optic discs, either a vascular anomaly (Sachs et al. 1977) or due to the smallness of the optic nerve head (Rosenberg et al. 1979; Mullie & Sanders 1985) giving rise to a disturbance of axoplasmic transport with axonal degeneration (Spencer 1978). Rare in childhood, they may become quite common in the elderly and were found in between 3.4 (Lorentzen 1966) and 20 (Friedman 1975) per 1000. Drusen may be composed of axoplasmic products (Avendano et al. 1980; Woodford 1980) giving rise to the appearance of a swollen optic disc, often mistaken for papilloedema. Drusen are bilateral in 75% of cases (Lorentzen 1966).

Children with drusen usually present with nonspecific complaints not directly related to the optic disc itself (Erkkila 1974). Occasionally the presentation is related to haemorrhagic or other complications.

Drusen may be inherited as an autosomal dominant trait (Lorentzen 1966) and both parents should be examined when the anomaly is suspected.

In childhood the drusen are not usually visible at first (Fig. 28.15), but the disc has a 'lumpy' appearance There is frequently an anomalous vascular pattern (Erkkila 1974), including the presence of trifurcations of vessels (Rosenberg et al. 1979). The optic disc capillaries are not dilated and do not leak fluorescein as they do in true papilloedema. The drusen may exhibit autofluorescence and glow when illuminated with a blue light before the injection of fluorescein. The peripapillary nerve fibres are normal in drusen, but enlarged in true papilloedema. Haemorrhages are not uncommon and are most often crescentic, appearing at the edge of the disc, in the subretinal layer (Wise et al. 1974), but most types of disc haemorrhage can occur (Harris 1981), including small linear superficial disc haemorrhages (Sanders et al. 1971).

Visual field defects may be detected in older children and these may be progressive (Savino et al. 1979), but loss of acuity should only with caution be attributed to the drusen. The field defects include enlarged blind spots (Hoover et al. 1988) and, when the drusen are visible, nerve fibre bundle defects (Savino et al. 1979) and inferior nasal defects. The buried drusen of childhood become exposed in the late teens (Hoover et al. 1988).

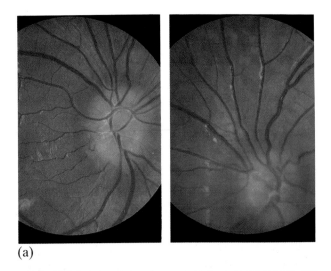

(a)

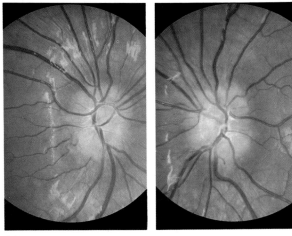

(b)

Fig. 28.15 (a) Optic nerve drusen giving pseudo-papilloedema in a 10-year-old child with headaches — note the anomalous blood vessels in both eyes. (b) Note the increase in clarity with which the drusen bodies can be seen (same patient three years later).

In many cases there seems to be a slowly progressive optic neuropathy with a good prognosis in the absence of serious haemorrhagic complications. Drusen occur in patients with retinitis pigmentosa (Robertson 1972) and other degenerative eye diseases but are not associated with tuberous sclerosis (in which the 'giant drusen' are a form of hamartoma) or with other phakomatoses also. They have been described in hypotelorism (Awan 1977), mandibulofacial dysostoses (Collier 1958) and many ocular diseases (Francois & Veriest 1958).

The calcium in drusen can be detected by CT scanning (Frisen *et al.* 1978) and is characteristically punctate, well-defined, and confined to the disc (Bec 1984).

Pseudopapilloedema (conditions mimicking papilloedema)

Only rarely are patients with myelinated nerve fibres referred to an ophthalmologist in the mistaken belief that they have papilloedema (Fig. 28.16), because the condition is now so widely recognized. But drusen is often testing, even for experienced ophthalmologists most of whom have personal reasons for humility in this area! Substantially hypermetropic eyes may have small crowded optic discs and in myopes with a tilted optic disc or situs inversus the nasal edge may be indistinct due to an overlaying of the retina across the disc margin. Glial anomalies (Fig. 28.17) and Bergmeister's papilla may also give rise to the false appearance of swelling. All of these conditions have a normal peripapillary plexus, normal nerve fibre layer

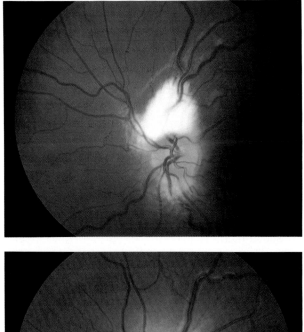

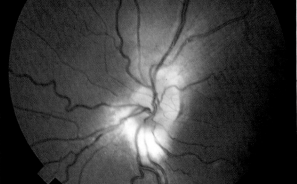

Fig. 28.16 Bilateral peri-papillary myelinated nerve fibres in a patient with hydrocephalus which was mistaken for papilloedema.

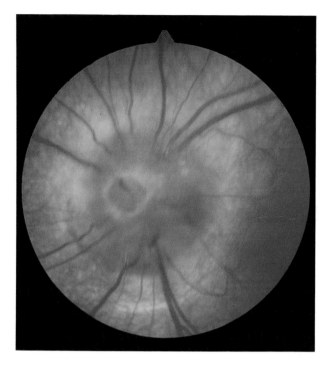

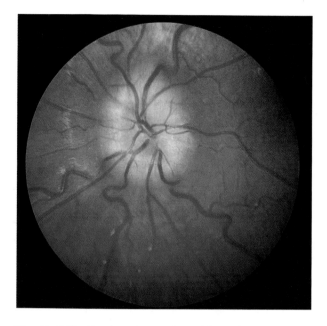

Fig. 28.18 Papilloedema in a patient with craniosynostosis — note the elevated optic disc and tortuous dilated veins.

Fig. 28.17 Anomalous optic disc (unilateral) in a patient presenting with headaches suspected of having unilateral papilloedema by the referring doctor.

and they may have venous pulsation at the disc which, even if it is unilateral, means that raised intracranial pressure is unlikely.

Papilloedema in children

Papilloedema is optic disc swelling associated with raised intracranial pressure (ICP). The vision is usually normal, even when the discs are markedly swollen although in later or very severe cases there may be a progressive loss of visual function.

The swelling is comprised of congested neurones and dilated blood vessels and these spread into the surrounding tissues causing retinal disturbance and choroidal folds. A hypermetropic refractive error is induced, by the raised retina and enlargement of the blind spot is noted on visual field testing (Corbett *et al.* 1988). An enlarged blind spot also occurs in optic nerve infiltration, development anomalies, trauma, as part of a centrocaecal scotoma or as an event of presumed retinal origin in an otherwise normal optic disc (Fletcher *et al.* 1988). If visual loss is progressive nerve fibre bundle field defects and peripheral constriction occur.

The earliest signs of papilloedema include a blurring of the disc margins, an elevated disc (Fig. 28.18), a dilated peripapillary capillary plexus, dilated retinal veins (Fig. 28.19), with absent pulsation at the optic disc and swollen nerve fibre bundles.

Splinter haemorrhages, a more markedly elevated disc (Fig. 28.20), nerve fibre infarcts ('cotton wool

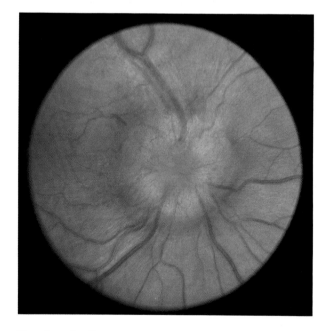

Fig. 28.19 Papilloedema secondary to raised intracranial pressure — note the elevated disc, swollen nerve fibre layer, dilated veins and small haemorrhages radiating around the disc.

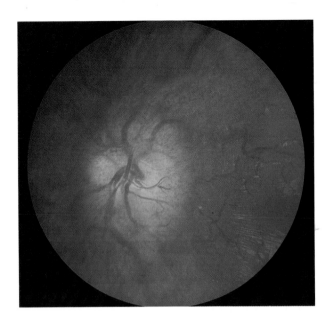

Fig. 28.20 Papilloedema in a patient with neurofibromatosis and a chiasmal glioma. The swelling of the optic disc with dilated veins, haemorrhages, a few exudates and dilated capillaries, is most marked in the upper and lower poles. This eye has a temporal hemianopia and the fibres that are swollen are those subserving the intact nasal field. The horizontal band of relative lack of swelling is in the area of the disc that is atrophic from loss of nerve fibres. The superior poles, although also atrophic, are covered by the fibres from the intact nasal field.

spots') exudates and macular star formation follow (Fig. 28.21). The retinal and disc capillaries become more engorged and tortuous and haemorrhages more widespread (Fig. 28.22a).

Children with a chronic but mildly raised intra-cranial pressure (ICP) (as in craniosynostosis) may have papilloedema for many years. However, if the ICP is very high there is a progressive loss of neurones, accompanied by increasingly frequent visual symptoms. Optic atrophy ensues as the neurones die, the disc becoming flat again after a period of being swollen and pale (Fig. 28.22b).

The symptoms are those of headache and episodic visual loss in the form of obscurations which are posture-related, seconds-long, blackouts or grey outs.

For management of papilloedema see benign intra-cranial hypertension (see Chapter P16).

Swollen optic disc in childhood

Bilateral

1 Papilloedema:
  raised ICP;
  hydrocephalus;
  BIH.
2 Hypertension.

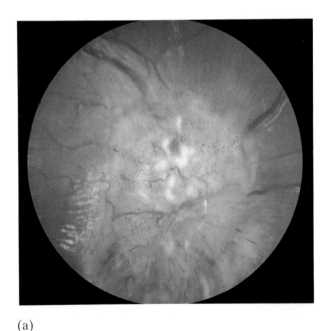

(a)

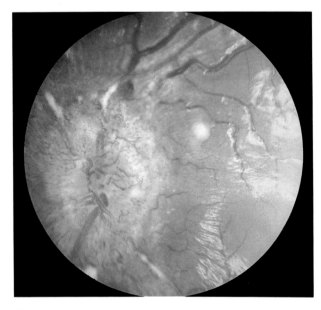

(b)

Fig. 28.21 (a) Severe papilloedema with gross elevation, haemorrhages, exudates, macular star, dilated veins and cotton wool spots on the optic disc. (b) The left eye is less affected. Asymmetry is frequent in papilloedema and may be due to anomalous optic nerve sheaths. (Same patient.)

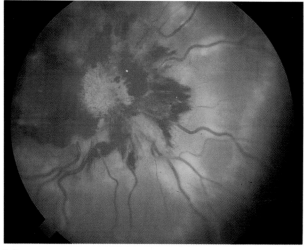

(a)

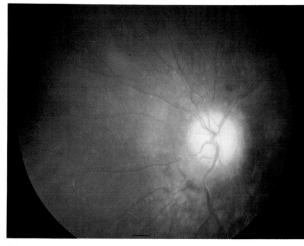

(b)

Fig. 28.22 (a) Severe papilloedema with widespread haemorrhages. (b) The optic nerve has decompensated and there is marked consecutive optic atrophy. The eye is blind. The 7-year-old child had severe papilloedema due to a posterior fossa tumour. (Same eye.)

3 Papillitis (optic neuritis).
4 Bilateral cases of unilateral cases of unilateral disc oedema or pseudopapilloedema.

Unilateral

1 Pseudopapilloedema:
  drusen;
  myelinated nerve fibres;
  hypermetropia;
  myopia;
  glial anomalies.

2 Tumours
  haemangioma;
  mulberry tumour of tuberous sclerosis (Fig. 28.23);
  retinal hamartoma (Fig. 28.3);
  retinoblastoma;
  optic nerve glioma with or without disc invasion (Fig. 28.24);
  leukaemia;
3 Uveitis:
  toxocara involving the disc (Fig. 28.25);
  swollen disc secondary to intraocular inflammation and hypotony (Fig. 28.26);
4 Ischaemic optic neuropathy.
5 Papillitis.
6 Papilloedema.
Papilloedema may be highly asymmetrical due to unilateral acquired or congenital lesions preventing papilloedema in one optic disc.

Optic nerve aplasia

Optic nerve aplasia is a very rare condition in which the optic nerve and, most importantly, its vessels are absent (Yanoff 1978). Many of the reported cases have been found on pathological examination for associated ocular anomalies (Hotchkiss & Greene 1970; Weiter *et al.* 1977) including microphthalmos,

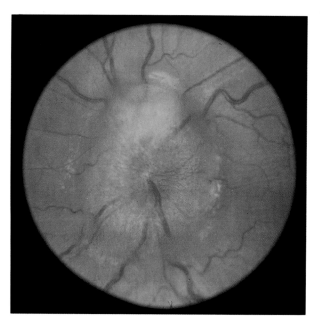

Fig. 28.23 Papilloedema in a child with tuberous sclerosis and hydrocephalus. Note that at the superior pole there is a phakoma which gave rise to a form of pseudopapilloedema in addition to the papilloedematous swelling of the optic disc.

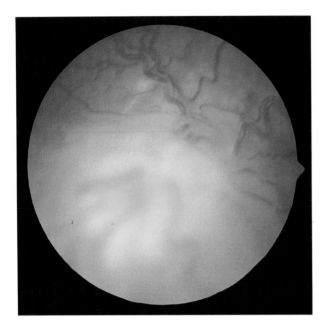

Fig. 28.24 Optic nerve involvement with glioma.

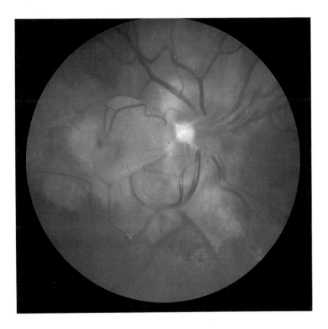

Fig. 28.25 Toxocara involving the optic disc. At presentation there was a marked uveitis and swelling of the optic disc obscuring all details.

retinal dysplasia, coloboma, sclerocornea, and cataract. Clinical descriptions of true optic nerve aplasia are few (Duke-Elder 1964; Francois 1970; Renelt 1972) and clinicopathological correlation (Yanoff *et al.* 1978) even rarer, but they show that the condition is usually unilateral, and is often associated with other central

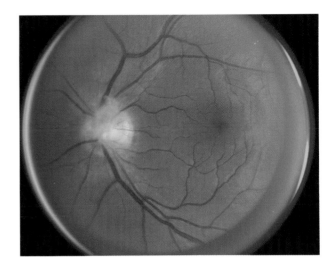

Fig. 28.26 Uveitis with optic disc swelling.

nervous system defects. The eyes are blind and have no direct pupil reaction to light. The fundus, apart from the absence of disc, vessels and retina, may appear normal or there may be other defects including Lacunar retinal defects (Fig. 28.27) (Renelt 1972; Little 1976).

Optic nerve hypoplasia

The paucity of early reports (Cords 1923; Ridley 1938; Boyce 1941; Scheie 1941; Jerome & Forster 1948; Somerville 1962; Edwards & Laydon 1970) suggested that optic nerve hypoplasia (ONH) was a very rare congenital anomaly, but paediatric ophthalmologists in hospital practice see several new cases each year

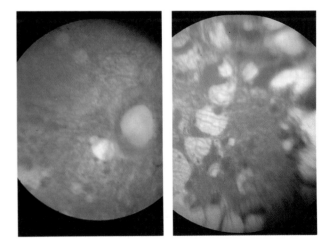

Fig. 28.27 Optic nerve aplasia with chorioretinal defects. In the right eye (left of picture) there was an optic nerve aperture visible, but none was found in the left eye.

and it is a significant cause of blindness in childhood, possibly with an increasing incidence (Jan *et al.* 1977).

PRESENTATION

Bilateral severe ONH presents as blindness in early infancy with roving eye movements and sluggish pupil reactions. Lesser degress of bilateral hypoplasia may cause minor visual defects or squint at any time in childhood and may even be found without symptoms at a routine test. Unilateral ONH usually presents as a squint with a relative afferent pupil defect and unsteady fixation in the affected eye. The eye movement defect may resemble 'see-saw' nystagmus (Davis & Schoch 1975). Amblyopia may contribute to the poor visual acuity and especially if the discs are not markedly hypoplastic the vision may improve with patching.

Affected patients may present because of failure to thrive in infancy or as a result of a variety of endocrine disorders (Skarf 1984; Stanhope *et al.* 1984), such as hypothyroidism, growth hormone deficiency, or neonatal hypoglycaemia.

Hypoplastic discs occur more frequently in males than females, and probably without racial predilection (Zion 1976). The parents of children with optic disc hypoplasia tend to be young primiparae (Elster & McArnarney 1979; Purdy & Friend 1979). Less frequently, children present because of the abnormalities from the associated brain defects.

OPHTHALMOSCOPIC APPEARANCE

The recognition of optic disc hypoplasia should alert the doctor to the associated problems which may arise during development. The diagnosis in the extreme case (Fig. 28.28) is not usually difficult; the true disc substance is minute and often only identifiable as a slightly pink-yellow area from which the retinal vessels emerge. This area is surrounded by an area of exposed sclera which is roughly circular and appears to represent the area of the gap in the retinal pigment epithelium that is present when the disc is of normal size. Sometimes there is proliferation of the retinal pigment epithelium on this normally white ring, but more usually there is a small rim of pigment around part of the margin of the white area. The temporal retinal vessels are often rather straighter than is usual in childhood (Fig. 28.28, 28.29), although Walton and Robb (1970) noticed that some of their cases had tortuous vessels. The retinal nerve fibre layer is variably thinned (Fig. 28.29, 28.30), (Whinery & Blodi

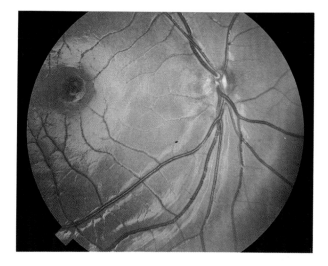

Fig. 28.28 Severe optic nerve phypoplasia with profound retinal nerve fibre layer atrophy.

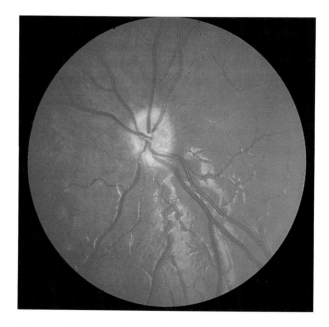

Fig. 28.29 Severe optic nerve hypoplasia with a wide surround of white sclera given by a larger defect in the retinal pigment epithelium than the hypoplastic optic nerve itself. This child had previously been diagnosed as having optic atrophy, but direct ophthalmoscopy revealed the true nature of the disorder.

1963; Manor & Korkzyn 1976), and if the hypoplasia is segmental this thinning is also segmental. It is the white ring of sclera that is so often confused for a normal sized, but atrophic disc and this mistake is more easily made by those who use only indirect ophthalmoscopy.

The chief difficulty in diagnosis arises when optic

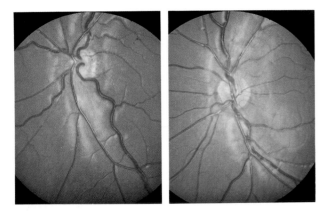

Fig. 28.30 Unilateral optic nerve hypoplasia. Although unilateral, even if there is no CT scan abnormality these children must be followed throughout their childhood for growth defects (see text).

disc hypoplasia is anything less than extreme (Fig. 28.31). Frisen (1978) pointed out that there was a very wide variation in the appearance of hypoplastic optic discs and that their effect on vision is also widely variable; hypoplasia is a non-specific manifestation of damage to the visual system that was sustained at any time before its full development. Notches occur in the disc and nerve fibre layer defects are associated with a relative smallness and irregularity in the outline of the disc in the fellow eye (Fig. 28.32, 28.33). A peripapillary white ring may also be an indication of prenatal damage. Changes may often be very subtle in the less affected optic disc, but may be useful additional clues. The ophthalmoscopic diagnosis is subjective but some objectivity can be introduced by comparing ratios of vessel size and optic disc size or the disc-macula to disc diameter ratio (Alvarez *et al.* 1988).

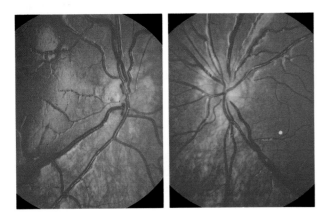

Fig. 28.31 Bilateral asymmetrical optic nerve hypoplasia. The right eye is blind, but the left eye despite significant optic nerve hypoplasia has 6/9 acuity and a useful visual field.

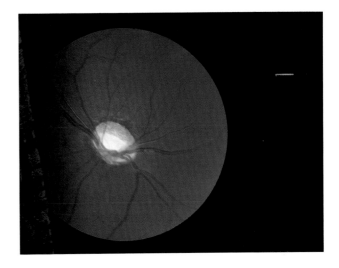

Fig. 28.32 A small irregular optic nerve that is hypoplastic.

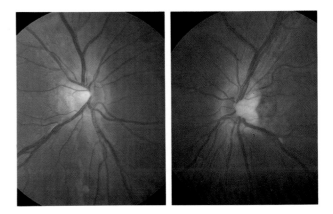

Fig. 28.33 Bilateral segmental optic nerve hypoplasia associated with a bitemporal hemianopia.

Tilted disc (segmental hypoplasia)

Dorrell (1978) pointed out that the familiar tilted disc, in which the optic disc is D-shaped, is accompanied by a defect in the retinal nerve fibre layer adjacent to the flat arm of the 'D', usually inferiorly. He found that nearly half of the patients he tested had non-refractive visual abnormalities associated with the defect, and he pointed out the prenatal origin of the condition suggesting that it represents a form of segmental hypoplasia. These true visual field defects (Rucker 1946; Graham & Wakefield 1973; Young 1976; Dorrell 1978) are frequently bitemporal and this must be remembered in the evaluation of the visual fields when there is no neurological cause found for the defect. The occurrence of suprasellar tumours in patients with tilted optic discs has been considered fortuitous (Rucker 1946; Riise 1975; Young 1976; Keane 1977), but the association may be more than fortuitous as indicated by the developmental nature of the tumours and the frequency of the association (Taylor 1982) (Fig. 28.34). The concurrence of X-linked night-blindness, myopia and tilted optic discs (Fig. 28.35) (Pinckers *et al.* 1978) has been reported.

Situs inversus

Situs inversus is a more widespread defect in which the vessels emerging from the optic disc are so distorted that, together with the appearance resulting from the tilt *per se*, the disc appears to be rotated through approximately 180° (Fig. 28.7). Fuchs (1882) considered this anomaly to be related to coloboma. In patients with these bilateral dysplastic optic discs, upper bitemporal relative visual field defects may occur, which often cross the midline. There may be an associated posterior staphyloma below the disc. In most cases the apparent field defect disappears with appropriate optical correction of the myopia caused by the staphyloma.

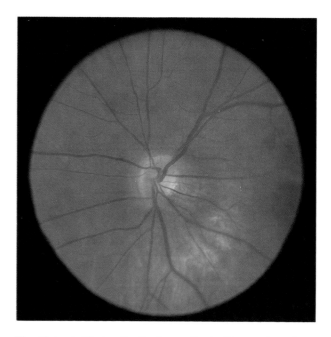

Fig. 28.35 A tilted optic disc in a patient with myopia and congenital stationary night-blindness.

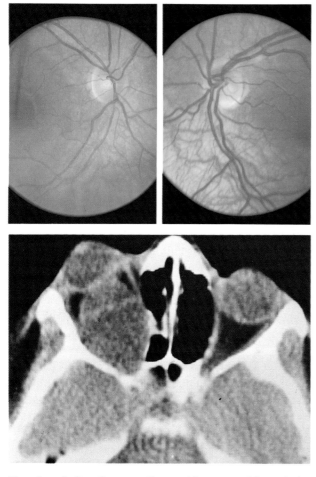

Fig. 28.34 Left optic nerve glioma with segmental hypoplasia of the optic nerve.

OPTIC NERVE HYPOPLASIA IN CNS DEFECTS

Hoyt and Rios-Montenegros (1972) described a case in which trans-synaptic degeneration from a cerebral lesion gave rise to a characteristic pattern of optic disc hypoplasia which reflected the field defect that the lesion caused; they called this appearance homonymous hemioptic hypoplasia. The occurrence of specific patterns of hypoplasia results from local defects throughout the CNS. Novakovic *et al.* (1986) suggest the site of the 'insult' in optic nerve hypoplasia is reflected in the pattern of disc hypoplasia. For instance the appearance of segmental optic disc hypoplasia related to a macular coloboma means the site of the injury is in the eye, whilst optic disc hypoplasia of a 'figure of 8' shape in patients with suprasellar tumour suggests a choroidal site. The optic disc hypoplasia therefore results from an early injury at any site in the developing nervous system (Fig. 28.36).

VISION AND ASSOCIATED FEATURES

Severe hypoplasia causes blindness, but in lesser degrees, a variety of abnormalities have been described with some patients having clinically normal vision, (Gardner 1972; Peterson 1977; Bjork *et al.* 1978) although field defects in these cases with good acuity are common (Peterson 1977).

Frisen *et al.* (1978) pointed out that the diagnostic

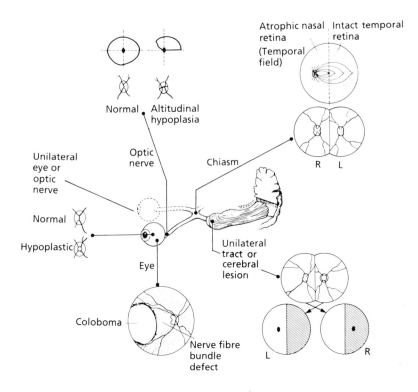

Fig. 28.36 Lesions at any site in the developing nervous system will cause optic nerve hypoplasia if their onset is early enough. Retinal defects may cause a macular coloboma with a segmental optic nerve hypoplasia. Unilateral eye or optic nerve defects cause purely unilateral hypoplasia. Unilateral retinal or anterior optic nerve defects may cause an altitudinal hypoplasia. Chiasmal defects may cause a 'figure of 8' optic disc that is hypoplastic and tract or cerebral lesions will cause homonymous hemioptic hypoplasia (Novakovic *et al.* 1988).

hallmarks of visual field defects due to hypoplasia are that they are static and that there are ophthalmoscopic correlates of the field defects. Patients with a diffuse deficit of nerve fibres have more or less concentric visual field contraction and often a lowered acuity, but when the lack of nerve fibres is focal, the field defects are also focal.

Temporal visual field defects (Seeley & Smith 1971; Davis & Schoch 1975; Buchanan & Hoyt 1981) have been described, and this may indicate a chiasmal location of the primary anomaly (Frisen 1978).

Retrochiasmal lesions associated with hypoplastic discs may also have appropriate homonymous field defects. If unilateral these are clear cut, but if the defect is bilateral the homonymous character is usually lost. Central visual field defects (Ewald 1967; Seeley & Smith 1971) and binasal defects (Missiroli 1947) also occur.

The flash electroretinogram is usually normal in optic disc hypoplasia. Colour vision is usually decreased roughly in proportion to the acuity defect.

OTHER FEATURES

Roving eye movements and unsteady fixation associated with poor vision, and see-saw nystagmus have been described (Davis & Schoch 1975) again suggesting a chiasmal abnormality. Abnormal optokinetic

nystagmus (Hoyt & Rios-Montenegros 1972). A variety of different types of strabismus have been described, usually in patients with poor vision. The optic canal is not necessarily small (Walton & Robb 1970) but small optic nerves are found (Sanders 1980) on CT scanning.

PATHOLOGY

A few pathological studies have been carried out (Manschot 1971, 1972; Anderson 1972; Boniuk 1979). Whinery and Blodi (1963) showed an absence or reduction of ganglion cells and their axons, small optic discs and nerves with abnormal glial tissue. Other parts of the neuroretina were normal and apart from incidental anomalies the eyes were otherwise normal.

PATHOGENESIS

The wide variety of associated central neurodevelopmental anomalies might lead one to conclude that the loss of ganglion cells was secondary to a retrograde degeneration along the visual pathway and the cases of homonymous hemioptic hypoplasia are a dramatic example of this. However, the occurrence of unilateral optic disc hypoplasia and of partial or segmental optic disc hypoplasia must mean that the site in those cases is anterior in the visual system (Novakovic *et al.*

1986). Optic disc hypoplasia is therefore probably a non-specific abnormality resulting from a prenatal insult to any part of the visual system.

The timing of this 'insult' has been of some interest, most authors agreeing that the abnormality has occurred by the 10th week of gestation (Boniuk *et al.* 1979). The retina does not clearly appear until 30 days and therefore the 'insult' must occur after this time. It is, however, difficult to extrapolate from these various pieces of evidence and it is only possible to conclude that the defect occurs early in prenatal development.

There may be a relationship between optic disc hypoplasia and colobomas (Brown 1982)

FAMILY HISTORY AND GENETICS

Familial cases have been described (Missiroli 1947; Kytila & Miettinen 1961; Hackenbruch 1975) but they are rare and not all necessarily genetic. Optic disc hypoplasia, and its systemic associations should therefore be regarded as sporadic in their occurrence. An exception to this rule is in aniridia which has a familial occurrence and has been found to be associated with optic disc hypoplasia (Layman 1974), although usually the optic disc is small rather than truly hypoplastic. Optic nerve hypoplasia may occur in the fetal alcohol syndrome which may affect several children of alcoholic mothers.

ASSOCIATED ANOMALIES AND AETIOLOGICAL FACTORS

Although optic disc hypoplasia may appear to be the result of an isolated event, it occurs in association with certain other developmental anomalies (Fig. 28.37). An association with hydranencephaly (Manschot 1971, 1972; Herman *et al.* 1988), anencephaly (Anderson *et al.* 1972; Manschot 1972; Boniuk 1979), aniridia (Hoyt *et al.* 1972; Layman 1974), congenital hemiplegia with hemianopia (Hoyt *et al.* 1972), porencephaly (Greenfield *et al.* 1980), cerebral atrophy (Rogers 1981), colpocephaly (Garg 1982) have been described. Quinine taken by the mother as an abortifacient early in pregnancy has been associated with optic nerve hypoplasia in the infant (McKinna 1966) as has maternal anticonvulsant ingestion (Hoyt & Billson 1978) and LSD ingestion (Chan *et al.* 1978). Viral infection has been implicated in cattle (Bistner 1973). Diabetic mothers have babies with a higher incidence of neurological anomalies, including optic disc hypoplasia (Patel 1975; Peterson & Walton 1977; Donat 1981; Kim *et al.* 1989). Optic nerve hypoplasia occurs in

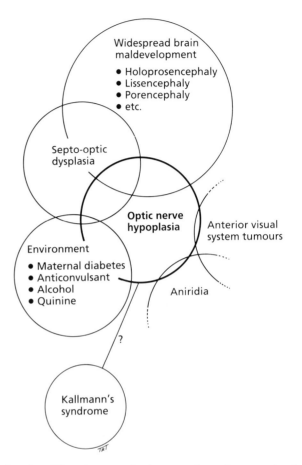

Fig. 28.37 There is an overlap between the various associated defects in optic nerve hypoplasia with only a few environmental causes and a variety of associated brain and anterior visual system disorders (see text).

children with the fetal alcohol syndrome in man (Strömland 1987) and mouse (Cook *et al.* 1987).

SEPTO-OPTIC DYSPLASIA

In 1941 Reeves (1941) described a patient with what was probably ONH and absence of the septum pellucidum but the first clear description of the syndrome of absence of the septum pellucidum and optic disc hypoplasia was by De Morsier (1956). Hoyt *et al.* (1970) were the first to clearly demonstrate hypopituitarism in patients with septo-optic dysplasia and since then a variety of hormonal defects have been described ranging from isolated growth hormone, adrenocorticotrophic or antidiuretic hormone deficiency to panhypopituitarism (Ellenburger 1970; Kaplan 1970; Billson & Hopkins 1972; Brook 1972; Harris 1972; Benoit *et al.* 1978; Krause-Brucker 1980). Hypothyroidism is probably the most common abnormality (Skarf & Hoyt 1984; Stanhope *et al.* 1984).

Pathology in a case (Patel *et al.* 1975) showed an absent posterior lobe of the pituitary gland, with an abnormal ypothalamus. The pituitary defects may occur in optic disc hypoplasia even without evidence of absence of the septum pellucidum (Krause-Brucker 1980).

Whilst many patients have ONH with only an abnormal septum pellucidum or pituitary stalk (Kaufman *et al.* 1989) and hypopituitarism, the associated spectrum of deformities may vary widely in severity up to holoprosencephaly (Fig. 28.38). In holoprosencephaly a variable midline facial defect is associated with a single cerebral ventricle, and absence of the corpus callosum and septum pellucidum; there is also a wide variety of similar brain defects (Ellenberger 1970; Jelliger 1973; Hale & Rice 1974; Donat 1981).

Pathological studies in holoprosencephaly have shown absence of the olfactory apparatus which forms a link with Kallmann's syndrome (1943) in which hypopituitarism and anosmia are associated with forebrain abnormalities (Lightman 1988).

PRACTICAL MANAGEMENT

1 Since optic disc hypoplasia may be bilateral and highly asymmetrical, apparently unilateral optic disc hypoplasia should be considered to be bilateral in terms of the investigation of the patient.
2 Patients found to have optic disc hypoplasia in the first 4 years of life should have neuroradiological studies to confirm or exclude associated cerebral malformations and other defects; those in whom they are present need to be under the care of a paediatrician, or endocrinologist. Whether or not cerebral abnormalities are found, weight and height must be monitored carefully (Skarf & Hoyt 1984). After 4 years of age if the child's general development is proceding normally it is not necessary to perform advanced neuroradiology but it is still necessary to measure height and weight regularly (Lambert *et al.* 1987).
3 Developmental delay may occur in patients with optic disc hypoplasia without structural brain defects (Skarf & Hoyt 1984).
4 In looking for optic disc hypoplasia, a direct ophthalmoscopic examination is preferable, and an examination under anaesthetic should rarely be necessary.
5 A child with optic disc hypoplasia may also be amblyopic in that eye; the vision may be improved by timely and vigorous occlusion (Kushner 1984).
6 The condition is not inherited.

Optic disc anomalies associated with midline defects

Optic disc hypoplasia has been described in association with midline brain defects, facial clefts and other related defects, but there are other optic disc anomalies that occur in these disorders (Fig. 28.39). Such cases are uncommon (Van Noyhuys & Bruyn 1964; Corbett *et al.* 1980; Bullard *et al.* 1981; Goldhammer & Smith 1975; Walsh & Hoyt 1969; Caprioli 1983) but have substantial diagnostic implications.

The patients may present with squint in childhood or with poor vision, or the visual aspects may be overshadowed by the effects of an associated pituitary or hypothalamic defect causing failure to grow. Often there are facial clefts or a midline harelip, a bifid nose, or hypertelorism, though these manifestations may be subtle. Recurrent cerebrospinal fluid rhinorrhoea was the presentation in one case (Bullard *et al.* 1981) and a pulsatile nasal tumour that elicited unwarranted (and rather hazardous!) surgery in another (Goldhammer & Smith 1975). All of the optic disc anomalies described were of a dysplastic type, either frankly colobomatous or having other anomalies including optic disc pits, a Morning Glory anomaly, megalopapilla or hypoplasia. Cryptophthalmos (Goldhammer & Smith 1975) and microphthalmos (Walsh & Hoyt 1969) have also been described; perhaps all of these conditions may be the result of a failure in the proper development and closure of the foetal fissure (see Colobomas, below) and they may all therefore be related to colobomas even if they are rarely typical.

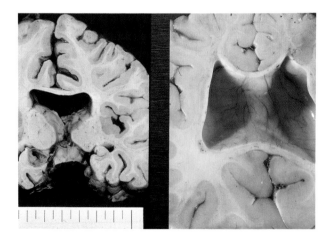

Fig. 28.38 Midline brain defects ranging from holoprosencephaly (common forebrain), absent septum pellucidum or agenesis of the corpus callosum occur in association with optic nerve hypoplasia. They are readily detected by CT or MRI scanning.

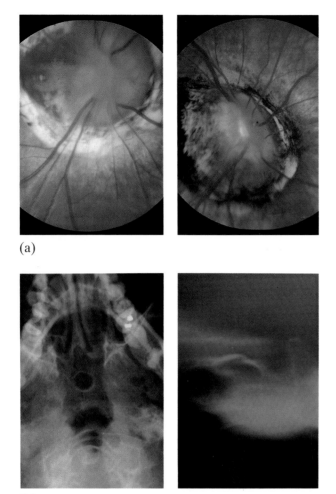

(a)

(b)

Fig.28.39 (a) The optic discs of this child, who presented with a squint and growth defect are dysplastic. (b) The radiological studies show that there is a defect in the floor of the pituitary fossa associated with a midline meningocoele.

Optic disc anomalies with isolated maldevelopment of the anterior visual pathways

Optic disc anomalies with bitemporal hemianopia may be found in a syndrome of apparently isolated maldevelopment of the anterior visual pathways (Taylor 1982) with no abnormalities found on neuroradiological investigation.

Optic disc coloboma and related anomalies

Colobomas result from an abnormality of the closure of the foetal fissure of the embryonic optic cup, and they may comprise a defect of any size from the margin of the pupil to the optic disc. Iris colobomas,

retinochoroidal colobomas and optic disc colobomas probably represent a spectrum of clinical manifestations of a common disease process and microphthalmos and anophthalmos may be extreme manifestations of the same disorder, not least because they occur in syndromes with colobomas in other members of the family (Savell & Cook 1976) and may occur unilaterally with a coloboma in the other eye.

Although the term coloboma is also classically applied to a whole variety of notches, holes or other defects in the iris or choroid it should perhaps be reserved for those anomalies associated with foetal fissure closure defects — 'typical' colobomas. Those colobomas that do not originate in a defect of foetal fissure closure lie in areas other than the infero-nasal quadrant and are designated atypical, as opposed to the typical coloboma of foetal fissure origin. Some atypical disc colobomas may have a similar origin to the typical form and other optic disc anomalies. Colobomas are rare in a general ophthalmology setting, occurring in about 0.25% of 12 000 patients examined ophthalmoscopically (Vossius 1885).

Genetics

Most cases are sporadic or dominantly inherited with variable expressivity (Duke-Elder 1964) so that unless the subtle manifestations (Savell & Cook 1976) are taken into account several generations may appear to be missed. Autosomal recessive (McMillan 1921; François 1968) and X-linked recessive (Goldberg & McKusick 1971) inheritance may occur, but much less frequently. X-linked recessive inheritance also occurs in the Lenz microphthalmia syndrome (p. 00). Microphthalmos, which may be found in families with colobomas occurs less frequently in first born than in subsequent children (Nakajima *et al.* 1979).

Presentation

Children with colobomas present either as a result of the appearance of the iris or the presence of a small eye, or because of apparently poor vision, or especially if unilateral, with a squint. Sometimes the systemic associations of colobomas are the presenting features. The coloboma may only be discovered on routine examination only.

Ophthalmoscopic appearance

The typical optic disc coloboma, associated with an inferonasal chorioretinal defect is familiar to all ophthalmologists (Figs 28.40, 28.41, 28.42). They range from a hugely excavated disc with a cavity so large that it may appear as a retrobulbar swelling on a CT scan through a variety of less obvious malformations to a subtle change in the retinal pigment epithelium (Fig. 28.43, 28.44).

Colobomas of the disc are not invariably associated with choroidal or iris defects but it is important to look for subtle manifestations of these, such as an

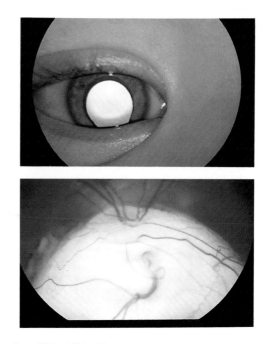

Fig. 28.42 This child with a gross right optic nerve and chorioretinal coloboma presented because of the microphthalmos and the white reflex that the mother could see when she was feeding the child.

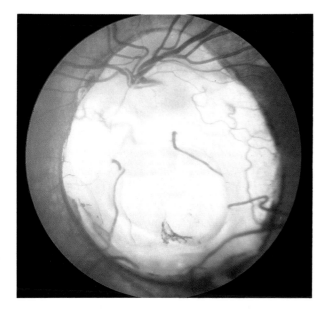

Fig. 28.40 Typical widespread optic nerve coloboma with associated retinal coloboma which gave rise to poor central vision.

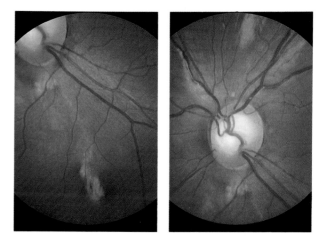

Fig. 28.43 This slightly anomalous optic nerve in a child with the CHARGE association is associated with a mild chorioretinal defect indicating the basically colobomatous nature of the defect.

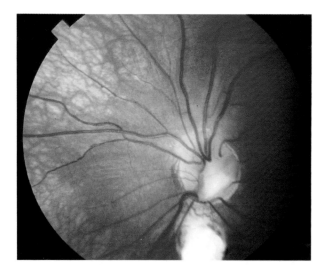

Fig. 28.41 An anomalous optic disc associated with a chorioretinal coloboma in a child with the CHARGE association with preserved central visual functions.

inferonasal area of transillumination of the iris, a notch in the pupil margins, heterochromia of the iris (Drews 1973) or melanosis oculi (Matzkin *et al.* 1970). A notch in the lens, inferonasal lens opacities, or pigment specks on the lens surface may be additional clues (Mann 1957).

Retinal vessels pass over the colobomatous area

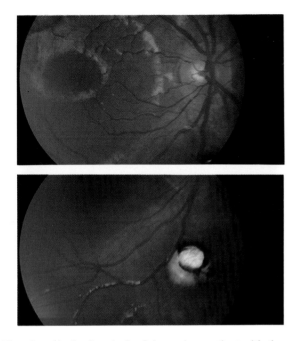

Fig. 28.44 A chorioretinal coloboma in a patient with the CHARGE association.

and there are sometimes large choroidal vessels in the base of the coloboma which may have a smooth surface but usually bulges posteriorly and may be thinned by crater-like areas.

Some developmentally abnormal optic discs, known as axial colobomata, have vessels that radiate from the edge of the disc which itself is surrounded by a rim of choroidal atrophy or thinning, and they have a central area of glial tissue. The occurrence of these in one eye with colobomatous microphthalmos in the other is a strong indication that the basic abnormality is a foetal fissure defect.

Brown (1982) has described a case with an optic disc coloboma in one eye and a small optic disc in the other eye; he suggested that optic disc hypoplasia and coloboma may represent a spectrum of defects with similar cause.

It is important to look for subtle phenotypic expressions since their diagnostic and genetic implications are the same as the most gross manifestations and the liability of a patient to have systemic disease is not dependent on the severity of the expression.

Optic disc pits

Optic disc pits (Weiter 1977) may be of a similar aetiology to colobomas and may occur in one eye with optic disc coloboma either in the same eye or in the other eye (Sugar 1967; Brown 1980; Corbett 1980). They are usually round holes of very variable size that occur usually, but not invariably, temporally near the margin of the disc. They may be associated with visual symptoms from a central serous retinopathy, (Kranenberg 1960; Theodossiadis 1977; Rubinstein & Ali 1978). The origin of subretinal fluid in humans with central serous retinopathy associated with pit is still uncertain (Brown & Tasman 1983). Although often following a benign course, subretinal neovascularisation and other complications may occur (Borodick *et al.* 1984), and some authors advocate aggressive treatment in selected cases (Schatz & McDonald 1988).

Intraocular abnormalities with colobomas

Various intraocular abnormalities may occur in association with colobomas. A preserved hyaloid vascular system has been described (Fig. 28.45) (Bell 1971) and lens notches are not infrequent. Vitreous striae and cataract occurred in one patient (Dascoffe 1975). Glial tissue with abnormal dysplastic retina near the optic disc were described histopathologically (Fig. 28.45) (Takahashi 1979). Mullaney (Mullaney 1978) classified intraocular colobomatous malformations, unassociated with systemic disease, into five groups on histopathological grounds. She drew widely from the literature and her paper serves as a useful review.

Group 1

This group includes lesions with heterotopic intraocular tissue including:
1 Lacrimal tissue.
2 Cartilage with ossification.
3 Adipose and smooth muscle tissue (Pedler 1961; Willis 1972). These cases had a variety of intraocular tissue, usually adipose or glial; in one subgroup (Willis 1972) seven eyes were removed for suspected tumour.

Smooth muscle may be present which may be the basis for the accounts of periodic contraction of colobomas in man and animals, (Wise *et al.* 1966; Sugar & Beckman 1969; Kral & Svarc 1971; Tanaka 1977).

Episodic visual loss has been described (Longfellow *et al.* 1962; Graether 1963; Seybold 1977). The mechanism may be a sphincter-like constriction of the optic nerve entrance by the smooth muscle (Mullaney 1973). One case (Tanaka 1977) showed a three-times-a-minute transient elevation of the optic disc which was thought to be due to rhythmic contraction of smooth muscle around a circular colobomatous cyst.

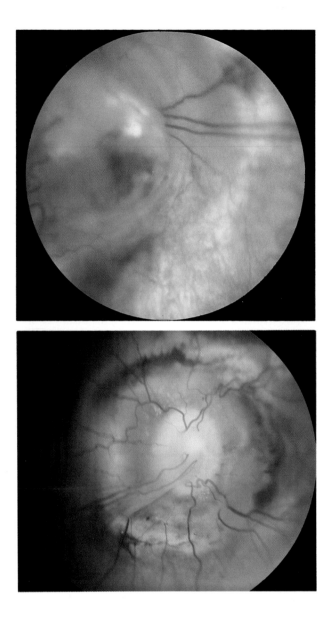

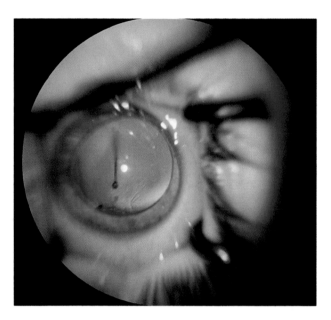

Fig. 28.45 Gross colobomatous defect with preserved hyaloid arteries in a patient with the CHARGE association. There is a wide variety of these defects which often defy exact definition and overlap with Pedler's colobomas.

Group 2

This group includes colobomas associated with cysts. Intraocular cysts associated with colobomatous malformations are rare (Mullaney & Fitzpatrick 1973).

Patients with orbital cysts with colobomas (Fig. 28.46) and colobomatous microphthalmos (Von Arlt 1858; Waring *et al.* 1976) usually present first because of the ocular abnormality and the cyst presents because of its later enlargement. They appear as a swelling in the lower lid which enlarges on crying, or as a thin walled cyst adjacent to the globe; occasionally it may cause a gradual proptosis. The cyst may communicate with the microphthalmic eye. This must be remembered during surgical removal of the cyst since decompression of the cyst may cause an alarming decompression of the eye and, if functionless, the microphthalmic eye may need to be removed.

Group 3

This group includes neoplasms occurring along the line of closure of the foetal fissure including glioneuroma and medulloepithelioma.

Group 4

Group 4 includes colobomatous malformations associated with prenatal infections, particularly cytomegalovirus (CMV). It is difficult to clearly associate these relatively common disorders.

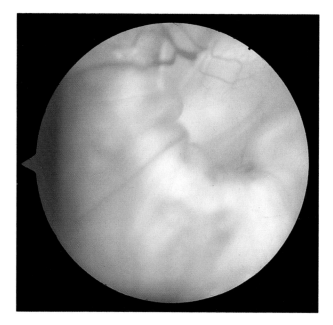

Fig. 28.46 Coloboma of the optic disc with overlay of the peripapillary retina (Pedler's coloboma — see text).

Group 5

This group includes intraocular malformations not directly associated with the coloboma (Foos 1968; Bell 1971; Lyford & Roy 1974; Dascoffe 1975; Rice 1976; Weiter 1977; Takahashi 1979). These include buphthalmos, accessory pupils, lens anomalies and reduplication, optic nerve aplasia, hyaloid vascular anomalies, dysplastic retina and vitreous striae.

Ocular complications and associations of colobomas

The presence of an optic disc coloboma should not blind the ophthalmologist to the presence of other eye malformations, in particular to glaucoma resulting from an anterior chamber anomaly which also causes excavation of the optic disc. Retinal detachment (Savell & Cook 1976) and disciform degeneration may both occur as complications of colobomas of the choroid.

Double optic discs

The earlier literature suggested that a true duplication of the optic disc occurs (Duke-Elder 1964). The second optic disc lies below the main disc and has its own set of retinal vessels, but it may be joined to the main disc by an arteriolar or a venular connection.

The optic nerve itself may be duplicated (Collier 1958), or split by an abnormal artery (Slade & Weekley

1957). Most double discs appear to be a part of the colobomatous malformation (Duke-Elder 1964; Brink 1977; Junge 1978) but the accessory disc is not always below as would be expected in this case (Elbrechtz 1975). Doubling of the optic canal may occur (Lamba 1969). Two brothers with thoracic dystrophy and a renal dystrophy were described by Gallet *et al.* (1973), one of whom had a double optic disc. Brink & Larsen (1977) suggested that the presence of doubling can only be characterized as true doubling (implying two separate nerves each with its own set of nerve fibres, perhaps subserving nasal and temporal vision separately) if it fulfils the following criteria: the nerve fibres should be demonstrated by ophthalmoscopy in the absence of a field defect, the discs should have a largely separate vascular supply, and double nerves must be demonstrated by CT scanning.

Pedler's coloboma (coloboma of the optic disc with overlay of the peripapillary retina)

This description was coined by Cogan (1978) who described the appearance of a uniocular peripapillary lobulated mass in a child of 9 months old. Histopathological studies showed a scleral canal that was about twice the normal size (Fig. 28.46). The central portion of the nerve head was occupied by loosely arranged vascular connective tissue and the peripapillary retina was bunched up to three times the normal thickness, and folded on itself. There was hyperplastic pigment epithelium and glial tissue between the optic nerve and sclera. This case seems to be similar to those described by other authors including Pedler (Seefelder 1909; Pedler 1961; Hogan & Zimmerman 1962; Rack & Wright 1966; Hamada & Ellsworth 1971; Willis *et al.* 1971; Tanaka 1977). Congenitally detached retinas may be found but these should not normally require surgery since they tend to re-attach spontaneously (Hamada & Ellsworth 1971). The presence of muscle in the anomaly is suggested by periodic contractions occasionally observed (Tanaka 1977, Cennamo *et al.* 1983).

Peripapillary staphyloma

In this condition the area of the sclera around the optic disc is ectatic and relatively myopic due to localized increased length of the eyeball. There is often a certain amount of glial tissue in the disc, and the vessels radiate out from the edge of the disc. Hayreh and Cullen (1972) described a case with a long history of undiagnosed visual loss due to a serous detachment of the retina around an atypical coloboma. The colobomatous nature of the problem is attested to by a frequent inferior thinning of the choroid, the usually inferior site of the staphyloma, and by the occurrence of this anomaly in syndromes usually associated with typical coloboma.

Morning Glory anomaly

This is usually a unilateral optic disc anomaly whose appearance is somewhat similar to Pedler's coloboma except there is a raised mass of tissue in the disc. The appearance is variable (Traboulsi & O'Neill 1988) but there is glial tissue in the abnormally large disc and a persistent hyaloid system is present (Fig. 28.47), with the retinal vessels radiating from around the disc. The peripapillary retina may be elevated and detached with radial folds. The vision in the affected eye is usually poor (Krause 1972; Jensen & Kalina 1976). It was probably first described by Handemann (1929) and the term Morning Glory syndrome (after the flower) was coined by Kindler (1970) 40 years later. It is, non-genetic and systemic associations are rare; microtia (Yamaguchi 1975; Grune & Fechner 1978), Duane's retraction syndrome (Kawano & Fujita 1981) and a variety of ocular defects (Kindler 1970; Odagiri 1975; Jensen & Kalina 1976; Steinkuller 1980; Brown 1983) have been described. Sometimes there is a widespread retinal detachment earlier in life which may settle spontaneously (Hamada & Ellsworth 1971) or with treatment where this is deemed necessary (Chang *et al.* 1984; Haik *et al.* 1984). The electro-retinogram (ERG) amplitude is low in proportion to the defect (Giuffre 1986)

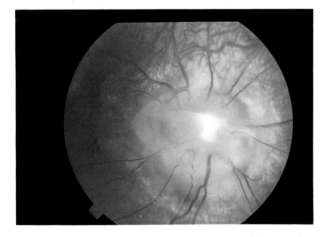

Fig. 28.47 Morning Glory anomaly. There is a glial anomaly with a persistent hyaloid system and the retinal vessels radiate from around the optic disc. At birth the peripapillary retina was detached. It settled spontaneously.

Systemic associations of colobomatous defects

In the earlier literature the association of colobomatous defects with the general health and development of the patient was barely mentioned, perhaps because ophthalmologists were not aware that they are required to look beyond the palpebral fissures! Several surveys have emphasized the systemic aspects (François 1968; James *et al.* 1974; Pagon 1981).

Whilst colobomas are probably most frequently seen by the ophthalmologist as an isolated defect they may occur either as part of a chromosomal syndrome or as a part of a more widespread disorder. In general there is no difference between the ocular aspects of the colobomatous manifestations seen in the various systemic syndromes.

Chromosomal syndromes

Trisomy D (Patau's syndrome)

This is recognized by the combination of a severe colobomatous defect and retinal dysplasia, with a cleft lip and palate, severe cardiac anomalies which cause nearly 80% of affected children to die within a year, and a variety of other defects.

The chromosomal defect is a trisomy (an extra chromosome) in the group D 13–15.

The colobomas usually involve iris, choroid and disc and they may be very large. The child may be clinically anophthalmic microphthalmic or have normal sized eyes. Anterior segment cleavage syndromes also occur and the lens may have posterior lenticonus and cataract. There may be dysplastic retina with cartilage, persistent hyperplastic primary vitreous, congenital retinal folds and detachment (Warburg 1970; Hoepner 1972; Saraux 1972).

Trisomy 18

Although the incidence of trisomy 18 is higher than trisomy D, coloboma is much less frequent. Affected infants are very feeble with characteristic facies, severe mental retardation, and cardiac defects. Coloboma, short palpebral fissure, epicanthus, ptosis cataract and microphthalmos occur (Mullaney 1973).

Cat-eye syndrome (Schmid–Fraccaro syndrome)

As the name implies, colobomas are very frequent in this syndrome (Schachenmann *et al.* 1965). The affected children are mildly mentally deficient; they have anal atresia and they may have microphthalmos, telecanthus, down-slanting palpebral fissures, epicanthic folds, and squint. This is an abnormal small extra chromosome which may be a deleted part of chromosome 22 (Cory 1974; Bofinger 1977; Weleber 1977).

Triploidy

Most affected foetuses abort spontaneously but a few cases have been described in premature babies and even fewer in full-term gestation babies who do not survive.

4p− syndrome

These profoundly mentally defective children have a characteristic face with a 'fish-like' mouth, coloboma, epicanthic folds, hypertelorism, and strabismus.

Coloboma also occurs in monosomy 9 (Sakuma & Sakuma 1976) 11q−, 13q− (more familiar to ophthalmologists on account of its association with retinoblastoma) 18 deletion syndrome (Yanoff 1970), 13 q− and trisomy 22 (Jay 1977; Smith 1976; Pagon 1981). The occurrence of colobomas with a systemic defect may call for chromosome studies.

Coloboma as a part of a multisystem disorder

1 CHARGE association
2 Meckel−Gruber syndrome
3 Golz's focal dermal hypoplasia
4 Lenz microphthalmia syndrome
5 Coloboma with brain defects
6 Others

CHARGE association (Pagon's syndrome)

Although the association between coloboma, choanal atresia, and other systemic defects occurred in both ophthalmological (James *et al.* 1974) and otolaryngological (Evans & McLachlan 1971) literature it was overlooked for many years.

CHARGE (Pagon *et al.* 1980) is an mnemonic for *C*oloboma, *H*eart defect, *A*tresia choanae, *R*etarded growth and development, *G*enital anomalies, and *E*ar anomalies and deafness.

Pagon *et al.* (1981) noted the association of colobomas with a wide variety of anomalies that has no known cause and occurs as an apparently sporadic disorder.

The other anomalies that occur with the CHARGE

association include facial palsy, micrognathia, cleft palate, and pharyngeal incompetence (Hall 1979). Hall (1979) pointed out that two of his 17 patients had a tracheo-oesophogeal fistula (TOF), Pagon (1981) noted this in one of her 21 patients and Lillquist *et al.* (1980) published pathological examinations of a case. It seems likely that TOF is also a part of the spectrum (Fig. 28.48). Chromosome studies have been normal. A wide variety of colobomatous defects occur (Fig. 28.49) from microphthalmos (Hittner *et al.* 1979) to minor disc anomalies. Although very unusual, familial cases have been described (Hittner *et al.* 1979) and the recurrence rate in further children of the same parents is low.

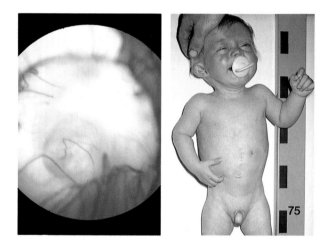

Fig. 28.48 Optic nerve coloboma in a child with tracheo-oesophageal fistula.

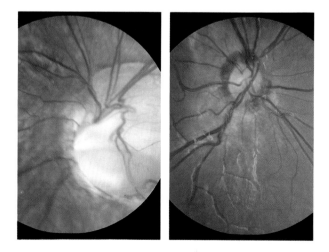

Fig. 28.49 CHARGE association. It is frequent that the optic discs in this syndrome are colobomatous, but often atypical. In this case the right optic disc is hypoplastic with a pigmented surround.

Meckel–Gruber syndrome

This is a severe disorder of presumed autosomal recessive inheritance; affected infants usually have a very short lifespan.

Encephalocoele (Fig. 28.50), (usually occipital), cleft palate and micrognathia, polydactyly, abnormal kidneys, cryptorchidism and microphthalmia or coloboma are the most frequent findings (Meckel 1822; Opitz & Howe 1969).

Goltz focal dermal hypoplasia

The most striking abnormalities in this rare syndrome are atrophic areas of the skin that are pinkish, or pigmented which represent areas of subcutaneous fat prolapsing through the dermis (Fig. 28.51), polysyndactyly (Fig. 28.52), abnormal nails and teeth, and mental retardation. It occurs only in females and is probably lethal in the male. Coloboma and microphthalmos occur (Warburg 1971).

Lenz microphthalmia syndrome

Patients with this X-linked recessive syndrome are born with microphthalmos with or without coloboma. (Hoefnagel *et al. 1963*; Goldberg & McKusick 1971; Baraitser *et al.* 1982). They also have protruding ears, crowded teeth and a variety of skeletal defects.

Coloboma with brain defects

A variety of brain defects have been described together with coloboma: Dandy–Walker cyst (Orcutt & Bunt

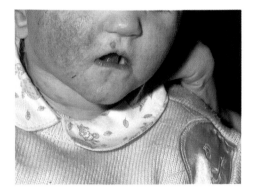

Fig. 28.51 Goltz syndrome showing the atrophic skin lesions. This child had bilateral optic nerve colobomas and marked left microphthalmos.

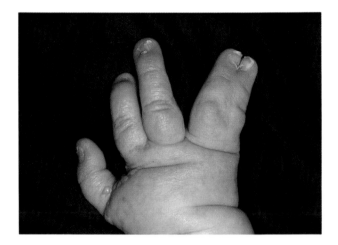

Fig. 28.52 Goltz syndrome showing polysyndactyly.

1982), arrhinencephaly (Lyford & Roy 1974), and others (Warburg 1971; James *et al.* 1974; Chemke *et al.* 1975). The HARD ± (E) syndrome is a more or less clear cut syndrome in which *H*ydrocephalus, *A*gyria, *R*etinal *D*ysplasia, with or without an *E*ncephalocoele occur, probably as an autosomal recessive condition (Pagon *et al.* 1978; Warburg 1978).

Others

Pagon (1981) has carried out a useful survey of other disorders which have occurred with, but are probably not causally related to, colobomas. They include the Laurence–Moon–Biedl syndrome, Stickler syndrome, incontinentia pigmenti, Ellis–Van Creveld syndrome, Hallerman–Strieff syndrome, Pierre Robin anomaly, Crouzon's syndrome, Kartagener's syndrome, Klinefelter's syndrome and tuberous sclerosis. Pagon (1981) also comprehensively listed other cases in which colobomas have occurred.

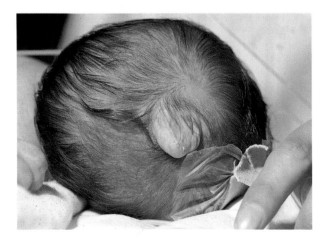

Fig. 28.50 Meckel–Gruber syndrome with occipital encephalocoele.

Coloboma with unilateral mandibulofacial dysostosis or Treacher-Collins—Francescetti syndrome has also been described and is sometimes known as the Weyers—Thier syndrome (Saraux 1966; Cordier *et al.* 1968).

Fuerstein—Mimms syndrome

This is also known as the naevus of Jadassohn, the epidermal naevus syndrome, or Soloman's syndrome. These patients have a non-dermatomal linear pigmented naevus, a variety of other skin defects, skeletal anomalies and usually severe retardation secondary to various brain defects (Jadassohn 1895; Marden 1966; Bianchine 1970; Soloman 1975; Burch 1980). Eye abnormalities (Barth 1977) include ptosis, conjunctival dermoids (Wilkes *et al.* 1981), lid colobomas (Insler & Daulin 1987), and other anterior segment anomalies and several fundus abnormalities have been described including colobomas (of the lids, iris, and optic disc), anomalous discs (Fig. 28.53), peripapillary staphyloma, and Coat's disease (Burch *et al.* 1980), and an osseous choristoma of the choroid (Lambert *et al.* 1987) and optic nerve hypoplasia (Katz *et al.* 1987).

Genetic implications of optic disc anomalies

WITH NO GENETIC IMPLICATIONS

- Optic disc hypoplasia/aplasia.
- Aicardi's syndrome (non-inherited, affects persons with two X chromosomes).
- Morning Glory syndrome.
- Myelinated nerve fibres.

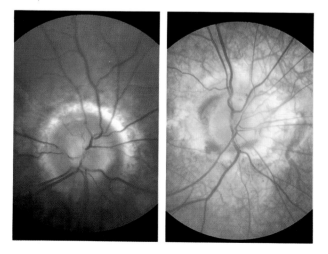

Fig. 28.53 Fuerstein—Mimms syndrome showing the anomalous optic disc.

- Vascular anomalies (except Von Hippel-Lindau).
- Glial anomalies.

WITH GENETIC IMPLICATIONS

- Drusen (sometimes dominant).
- Von Hippel (dominant).
- Phakoma in tuberous sclerosis (dominant);
- Coloboma (a) dominant; (b) recessive; (c) X-linked recessive — Lenz microphthalmic syndrome; and (d) X-dominant — Goltz.

AS A SIGN OF CHROMOSOMAL DISEASE

- Down's syndrome — excess vessels.
- Coloboma — (a) trisomy 13—15, 18, 22; (b) 22 deletion (Schmid Fraccaro); (c) triploidy; (d) 4p—; (e) Monosomy 9; (f) 11q—; (g) 13q—; and (h) 13r—.

References

Aicardi J, Lefebvre J, Lerique-Loechlin A A. A new syndrome: spasm in flexion, collosal agenesis ocular abnormalities. *Electroencephologr Clin Neurophysiol* 1965; **19**: 609—10

Alvarez E, Wakakura M, Khan Z, Dulton GN. The disc-macula distance to disc diameter ratio: a new test for confirming optic nerve hypoplasia in young children. *J Pediatr Ophthalmol Strabismus* 1988; **25**: 151—6

Anderson SR, Bro-Rasmussen F, Tygstrup I. Anencephaly related to ocular development and malformation. *Am J Ophthalmol* 1972; **74**: 967—75

Apple DJ, Rabb MF, Walsh PM. Congenital anomalies of the optic disc. *Surv of Ophthalmol.* 1982; **27**: 3—41

Avendano J, Rodrigues MM, Hackett JJ, Gaskins R. Corpora amylacea of the optic nerve and retina; a form of neuronal degeneration. *Invest Ophthalmol Vis Sci* 1980; **19**: 550—4

Awan KJ. Hypoteleorism and optic disc anomalies: an ignored ocular syndrome. *Ann Ophthalmol* 1977; **9**: 771—7

Baarsma GS. Acquired medullated nerve fibres. *Br J Ophthalmol* 1980; **64**: 651—2

Baraitser M, Winter RM, Taylor DSI. The Lenz microphthalmos syndrome. *Clin Genet* 1982; **22**: 99—101

Barth PG. Organoid nevus syndrome (linear nevus sebaceous of Jadassohn): clinical and radiological study of a case. *Neuropediatrics* 1977; **8**: 418—28

Beauvieux J. La pseudo-atrophie optique des nouveau nes dysgenesie myelinique des voies optique. *Ann Oculist (Paris)* 1926; **163**: 82—92

Bec P, Adam P, Mathis A, Alberge Y, Roulleau J, Arne JHL. Optic nerve head drusen: high resolution CT approach. *Arch Ophthalmol* 1984; **102**: 680—2

Bell RW. Case of total preservation of hyaloid artery with pupillary membrane, cataract, retinal and uveal coloboma and microphthalmos. *Ann Ophthalmol* 1971; **3**: 589—91

Bellhom RW, Hirano A, Henkind P, Johnson PT. Schwann cell proliferations mimicking medullated retinal nerve fibres *Am J Ophthalmol* 1979; **87**: 469—73

Benoit–Gonin JJ, David M, Feit JP, Bourgeois J, Chopart A, Kopp N, Jeune M. La dysplasie septo-optique avec déficit en hormone antidiurétique et insuffisance surrénale centrale. *La Nouvelle Presse Medicale* 1978; **37**: 3327–31

Bianchine JW. The naevus sebaceous of Jadassohn. *Am J Dis Child* 1970; **120**: 223–8

Billson F, Hopkins IJ. Optic nerve hypoplasia and hypopituitarism. *Lancet* 1972; **i**: 905

Bistner S, Rubin L, Aguine G. Development of the bovine eye. *Am J Vet Res* 1973; **34**: 7–12

Björk A, Laurell C-G, Laurell U. Bilateral optic nerve hypoplasia with normal visual acuity. *Am J Ophthalmol* 1978; **86**: 524–9

Bofinger MK, Soukup SW. Cat eye syndrome. *Am J Dis Child* 1977; **131**: 893–7

Boniuk V, Ho PK. Ocular findings in anencephaly. *Am J Ophthalmol* 1979; **88**: 613–17

Borodick GE, Gragoudas ES, Edward WO, Brockhurst RJ. Peripapillary subretinal neovascularisation and serous macular detachment. Association with congenital optic nerve pits. *Arch Ophthalmol* 1984; **102**: 229–32

Boyce DC. Hypoplasia of the optic nerve. *Am J Ophthalmol* 1941; **34**: 888–9

Brink JK, Larsen FE. Pseudodoubling of the optic disc. *Acta Ophthalmol* 1977; **55**: 862–70

Brook GD, Sanders MD, Hoare RD. Septo-optic dysplasia. *Br Med J* 1972; **3**: 811–13

Brown GC. Optic nerve hypoplasia and colobomatous defects. *J Paediatr Ophthalmol Strabismus* 1982; **19**: 90–3

Brown GC, Magargal LE, Augsburger JJ. Pre-retinal arterial loops and retinal arterial occlusion. *Am J Ophthalmol* 1979; **87**: 646–51

Brown GC, Shields JA, Goldberg RE. Congenital pits of the optic nerve head: II clinical studies in humans. *Am Acad Ophthalmol* 1980; **87**: 51–65

Brown GC, Tasman WS. *Congenital Anomalies of the Optic Disc*. Grune & Stratton, New York 1983

Buchanan TAS, Hoyt WF. Temporal visual field defects associated with nasal hypoplasia of the optic disc. *Br J Ophthalmol* 1981; **65**: 636–40

Bullard DE, Crockard HA, McDonald WI. Spontaneous cerebrospinal fluid rhinorrhoea associated with dysplastic optic discs and a basal encephalocade. *J Neurosurg* 1981; **54**: 807–10

Burch JV, Leveille AS, Morse PH. Ichthyosis hystrix (epidermal nevus syndrome) and Coats' disease. *Am J Ophthalmol* 1980; **89**: 25–30

Caprioli J, Lesser RL. Basal encephalocoele and Morning Glory syndrome. *Br J Ophthalmol* 1983; **67**: 349–51

Cennamo G, Sammartino A, Fioretti F. Morning Glory syndrome with contractile peripapillary staphyloma. *Br J Ophthalmol* 1983; **67**: 346–7

Chan CC, Fishman M, Egbert PR. Multiple ocular anomalies associated maternal LSD ingestion. *Arch Ophthalmol* 1978; **96**: 282–4

Chang S, Barrett GH, Ellsworth RM, St Louis L, Berrocal JA. Treatment of total retinal detachment in Morning Glory syndrome. *Am J Ophthalmol* 1984; **97**: 596–606

Chemke J, Czernobilsky B, Mundel G, Barishak YR. A familial syndrome of central nervous system and ocular malformations *Clin Genet* 1975; **7**: 1–7

Cogan DG. Coloboma of optic nerve with overlay of peripapillary retina *Br J Ophthalmol* 1978; **62**: 347–50

Collier M. Les doubles papilles optiques. *Bull Soc Ophthalmol* 1958; **70**: 328–52

Cook CS, Nowotny AZ, Sulik KK. Fetal alcohol syndrome. *Arch Ophthalmol* 1987; **105**: 1576–82

Corbett JJ, Jacobson DM, Maver RC, Thompson HS. Enlargement of the blind spot caused by papilloedema. *Amer J Ophthalmol* 1988; **105**: 261–6

Corbett JJ, Savino PJ, Schatz NJ. Cavitary developmental defects of the optic disc: visual loss associated with pits and colobomas. *Arch Neurol* 1980; **37**: 210–13

Cordier J, Triclon P, Thiriet M, Babut M, Raspiller A. Weyer's oculo-vertebral syndrome. *rev OtoNeurol Ophthalmol* 1968; **40**: 204–11

Cords R. Einseitige kleinheit der papille. *Klin Monatsbl Augenheilkd* 1923; **71**: 414–18

Cory C, Jamison DL. The cat eye syndrome. *Arch Ophthalmol* 1974; **92**: 259–62

Dascoffe JC, Woillez M, Dhoine G. Association of hereditary vitreous striae, iris, coloboma and cataract. *Bull Soc Ophthalmol Fr* 1975; **75**: 335–7

Davis GU, Schoch JP. Septo-optic dysplasia associated with see-saw nystagmus *Arch Ophthalmol* 1975; **93**: 137–9

Degenhart W, Brown GC, Augsburger JJ. Prepapillary vascular loops. *Ophthalmology* 1981; **88**: 1126–31

DeJong P, Bistervels B, Cosgrove J, DeGrip G, Leys A, Goffin M. Medullated nerve fibres. A sign of multiple basal cell nevi (Gorlin's) syndrome. *Arch Ophthalmol* 1985; **103**: 1833–7

De Morsier G. Études sur les dysraphies crânio-encepahliques III. Agénésie du septum lucidum avec malformation du tractus optique. La dysplasie septo-optique. *Schweitz Arch Neurol Psychiatr* 1956; **77**: 267–92

Donat JFG. Septo-optic dysplasia in an infant of a diabetic mother *Arch Neurol* 1981; **38**: 580–91

Dorrell D. The tilted disc. *Br J Ophthalmol* 1978; **62**: 16–20

Drews RC. Heterochromia iridum with coloboma of the optic disc. *Arch Ophthalmol* 1973; **90**: 437–43

Duke-Elder S. System of ophthalmology: normal and abnormal development. *Congenital Deformities*. Vol. III, Part 2. H Kimpton, London 1964

Edwards WC, Layden WE. Optic nerve hypoplasia. *Am J Ophthalmol* 1970; **70**: 950–9

Elbrechtz HC. Über eine doppelle papille im auge. *Klin Monatsbl Augenheilkd* 1975; **166**: 389–91

Ellenberger C, Runyan TE. Holoprosencephaly with hypoplasia of the optic nerves, dwarfism and agenesis of the septum pellucidum. *Am J Ophthalmol* 1970; **70**: 960–7

Elster AB, McAnarney ER. Maternal age re: septo-optic dysplasia. *J Pediatr* 1979; **94**: 162

Erkkila H. Optic disc drusen in children. *Graefes Arch Klin Exp Ophthalmol* 1974; **189**: 1–7

Erkkila H. Optic deisc — congenital anomaly. *Graefes Arch Klin Exp Ophthalmol* 1976; **199**: 1–10

Evans JNG, MacLachlan RF. Choanal atresia. *J Laryngol Otol (Suppl.)* 1971; **85**: 903–29

Ewald RA. Unilateral hypoplasia of the optic nerve: radiologic and electroclinographic findings. *Am J Ophthalmol* 1967; **63**: 763–7

Fletcher WA, Imes RK, Goodman D, Hoyt WF. Acute idiopathic blind spot enlargement. A big blind spot syndrome without optic disc edema. *Arch Ophthalmol* 1988; **106**: 44–9

Foos FY, Kiechler RJ, Allen RA. Congenital non-attachment

of the retina. *Am J Ophthalmol* 1968; **65**: 202−11

François J. *Heredity in Ophthalmology.* CV Mosby, St Louis 1961

François J. Colobomatous malformations of the ocular globe. *Int Ophthalmol Clin* 1968; **8**: 797−816

François J, Hruby K. Uber seltene beobachtungen von hypoplasie der netzhaut. *Klin Monatsbl Augenheilkd* 1970; **157**: 605−10

François J, Verriest G. Les druses de la papille. *Acta Neurol Belg* 1958; **51**: 327−55

Franceschetti A. Fibres à myeline de la rétine et dyscranie *Bull Soc Ophthalmol Fr* 1938; **51**: 573−77

Friedman AH, Gartner S, Modi SS. Drusen of the optic disc: a retrospective study of cadaver eyes. *Br J Ophthalmol* 1975; **59**: 413−21

Frisen L. Visual field defects due to hypoplasia of the optic nerve. *Docum Ophthalmol* 1979; **19**: 81−86

Frisen L, Holmegaard L. Spectrum of optic nerve hypoplasia. *Br J Ophthalmol* 1978; **62**: 7−15

Frisen L, Scholdstrom G, Svendsen P. Drusen in the optic nerve head: verification in the optic nerve head. *Arch Ophthalmol* 1978; **9**: 1611−14

Fuchs E. Beitrag zu den angenborenen Anomalien des schnerven. *Graefes Arch Ophthalmol* 1882; **28**: 139−69

Gallet J-P, Olivier C, Sarrut S. Dystrophie thoracique, malformation oculaire et nèphropathie tubulo-interstitielle chez deux frères. *Ann Pediatr* 1973; **20**: 813−22

Gardner HB, Irvine AE. Optic nerve hypoplasia with good visual acuity. *Arch Ophthalmol* 1972; **88**: 255−8

Garg, B.P. Colpocephaly. *Arch Neurol* 1982; **39**: 243−6

Gass JDM, Braunstein B. Sessile and exophytic capillary angiomas of the juxtapapillary retina and optic nerve head. *Arch Ophthalmol* 1980; **98**: 1790−7

Guiseppe G. Morning Glory syndrome: clinical and electrofunctional study of three cases. *Br J Ophthalmol* 1986; **70**: 229−36

Goldberg MF, McKusick VA. X-linked colobomatous microphthalmos and other congenital anomalies. *Amer J Ophthalmol* 1971; **71**: 1128−33

Goldhammer Y, Smith JL. Optic nerve anomalies in basal encephalocoeles. *Arch Ophthalmol,* 1975; **93**: 115−18

Graether JM. Transient amaurosis in one eye with simultaneous dilatation of retinal veins: in association with a congenital anomaly of the optic nerve head. *Arch Ophthalmol* 1963; **70**: 342−5

Graham MV, Wakefield GJ. Bitemporal visual field defects associated with anomalies of the optic discs. *Br J Ophthalmol* 1973; **57**: 307−14

Greenfield PS, Wilcox LM, Weiter JJ. *et al.* Hypoplasia of the optic nerve in association with porencephaly. *J Pediatr Ophthalmol Strabismus* 1980; **17**: 75−8

Grey RHB, Rice NSC. Congenital duplication of the lens. *Br J Ophthalmol* 1976; **60**: 673−6

Grune HJ, Fechner PU. Über das Morning Glory syndrom. *Klin Monatsbl Augenheilkd* 1978; **172**: 114−15

Haas BD, Jakobiec FA, Iwamoto T, Cox M, Bernacki EG, Pokorny JL. Diffuse choroidal melanocytoma in a child. *Ophthalmology* 1986; **93**: 1632−8

Hackenbruch Y, Meerhoff E, Besio R, Cardoso H. Familial bilateral optic nerve hypoplasia. *Amer J Ophthalmol* 1975; **79**: 314−20

Haik BG, Greenstein SH, Smith ME, Abramson DH,

Elsworth, RM. Retinal detachment in the Morning Glory syndrome. *Ophthalmology* 1984; **91**: 1638−47

Hale BR, Rice P. Septo-optic dysplasia: clinical and embryological aspects. *Dev Med Child Neurol* 1974; **16**: 812−20

Hall BD. Choanal atresia and association multiple anomalies. *J Pediatrics* 1979; **95**: 395−8

Hamada S, Ellsworth RM. Congenital retinal detachment and the optic disc anomaly. *Amer J Ophthalmol* 1971; **71**: 460−4

Handemann M. Erbliche, vermutlich angenborene zentrale gliose Entartung des Sehnerven mit besonderer. Beteilgung der Zentralgefasse. *Klin Monatsbl Augenheilkd* 1929; **83**: 145−54

Harris MJ, Fine SL, Owens SL. Hemorrhagic complications of optic nerve drusen. *Am J Ophthalmol* 1981; **92**: 70−6

Harris RJ, Haas L. Septo-optic dysplasia with growth hormone deficiency (de Morsier syndrome). *Arch Dis Child* 1972; **47**: 973−6

Hayreh SS, Cullen JF. Atypical minimal peri-papillary choroidal colobomata. *Br J Ophthalmol* 1972; **56**: 86−96

Herman DC, Bartley GB, Bullock JD. Ophthalmic findings of hydranencephaly. *J Pediatr Ophthalmology Strabismus* 1988; **25**: 106−12

Hittner HM, Hirsch NJ, Kreh GM, Rudolph AJ. Colobomatous microphthalmia, heart disease, hearing loss and mental retardation: a syndrome. *J Pediatr Ophthalmol Strabismus* 1979; **16**: 122−8

Hoefnagel D, Keenan ME, Cullen FH. Heredofamilial bilateral anophthalmia. *Arch Ophthalmol* 1963; **69**: 760−6

Hoepner J, Yanoff M. Ocular anomalies in trisomy 13−15. *Am J Ophthalmol* 1972; **74**: 729−37

Hogan MJ, Zimmerman LE. *Ophthalmic Pathology*, 2nd edn. Saunders, Philadelphia 1962

Hoover D, Robb R, Petersen R. Optic disc drusen in children. *J Pediatr Ophthalmology Strabismus* 1988; **25**: 191−6

Hotchkiss ML, Green WR. Optic nerve aplasia and hypoplasia. *J Pediatr Ophthalmol*, 1970; **16**: 225−40

Hoyosaki S, Yamaguchi K, Mizuno K, Miyabayashi S, Narisawa K, Taka K. Ocular findings in childhood lactic acidosis. *Arch Ophthalmol* 1986; **104**: 1656−8

Hoyt CS, Billson FA. Maternal anticonvulsants and optic nerve hypoplasia *Br J Ophthalmol* 1978; **62**: 3−6

Hoyt CS, Billson F, Ouvrier R. Ocular features of Aicardi's syndrome. *Arch Ophthalmol* 1978; **96**: 291−5

Hoyt WF, Kaplan SL, Grumbach MM, Glaser J. Septo-optic dysplasia and pituitary dwarfism *Lancet* 1970; **i**: 93

Hoyt WF, Rios−Montenegros EN, Berens MM, Eckelhoff RJ. Homonymous hemioptic hypoplasia. Fundoscopic features in standard and red-free illumination in three patients with congenital hemiplegia. *Br J Ophthalmol* 1972; **56**: 537−45

Insler M, Daulin L. Ocular findings in linear sebaceous naevus syndrome. *Br J Ophthalmol* 1987; **71**: 268−72

Jadassohn J. Bemerkungen zur Histologie der systematisiten naevi under über 'Talgdrusen'-Naevi. *Arch Dermatol Syph* 1895; **33**: 355−7

James PML, Karseras AG, Wybar KC. Systemic associations of uveal coloboma. *Br J Ophthalmol* 1974; **58**: 917−21

Jan JE, Robinson GC, Kinnis C, MacLeod PJM. Blindness due to optic atrophy and hypoplasia in children: an epidemiological study (1944−74). *Dev Med Child Neurol* 1977; **19**: 353−63

Jay M. *The Eye in Chromosome Duplications and Deficiencies.* Marcel Dekker, New York 1977

Jelliger K, Gross H. Congenital telencephalic defects. *Neuropaediatr* 1973; **4**: 446−52

Jensen PE, Kalina RE. Congenital anomalies of the optic disc. *Am J Ophthalmol* 1976; **82**: 27−31

Jerome B, Forster JW. Congenital hypoplasia (partial aplasia) of the optic nerve. *Arch Ophthalmol* 1948; **89**: 669−72

Junge J. Über eine doppelte papille im Augenkolobom. *Klin Mon Augenheilkd* 1978; **172**: 748−50

Justice J, Lehman RP. Cilioretinal artenes. *Arch Ophthalmol* 1976; **94**: 1355−8

Kallmann FJ, Schoenfeld WA, Barrera SE. Genetic aspects or primary eunuchoidism. *Am J Ment Defic* 1943; **48**: 203−28

Kaplan SL, Grumbach MM, Hoyt WF. A syndrome of hypopituitary dwarfism, hypoplasia of the optic nerves and malformation of the prosencephalon. *Pediatr Res* 1970; **4**: 480−6

Katz B, Wiley CA, Lee VW. Optic nerve hypoplasia and the syndrome of nevus sebaceous of Jadassohn. *Ophthalmology* 1987; **94**: 1570−6

Kaufman LM, Miller MT, Mafee MF. Magnetic resonance imaging of pituitary stalk hypoplasia. *Arch Ophthalmol* 1989; **107**: 1485−90

Kawano K, Fujita S. Duanes retraction syndrome associated with Morning Glory syndrome. *J Pediatr Ophthalmol Strabismus* 1981; **18**: 51−4

Keane JR. Suprasellar tumours and incidental optic disc anomalies. *Arch Ophthalmol* 1977; **95**: 2180−3

Kim RY, Hoyt WF, Lessell S, Narahara MH. Superior segmental optic hypoplasia: a sign of maternal diabetes. *Arch Ophthalmol* 1989; **107**: 1312−16

Kindler P. Morning Glory syndrome: unusual congenital optic disc anomaly. *Am J Ophthalmol* 1970; **69**: 376−84

Kottow MH. Congenital malformations of the retinal vessels with primary optic nerve involvement. *Ophthalmologica (Basel)* 1978; **176**: 86−90

Kral K, Svarc D. Contractile peripapillary staphyloma. *Am J Ophthalmol* 1971; **71**: 1090−2

Kranenberg EW Craterlike holes in the optic disc and central serous retinopathy. *Arch Ophthalmol* 1960; **64**: 912−24

Krause U. Three cases of the Morning Glory syndrome *Acta Ophthalmol*, 1972; **50**: 188−98

Krause-Brucker W, Gardner DW. Optic nerve hypoplasia associated with absent septum pellucidum and hypopituitarism. *Am J Ophthalmol* 1980; **89**: 113−20

Kushner BJ. Functional amblyopia associated with abnormalities of the optic nerve. *Arch Ophthalmol* 1984; **102**: 683−5

Kytilä J, Miettinen P. On bilateral aplasia of the optic nerve. *Acta Ophthalmologica* 1961; **39**: 416−9

Lamba PA. Doubling of the papilla. *Acta Ophthalmol (Kbh)* 1969; **47**: 4−9

Lambert HM, Sipperley JO, Shore JW, Dieckert JP, Evans R, Lowd DR. Linear nevus sebaceous syndrome. *Ophthalmol* 1987; **94**: 278−83

Lambert SR, Hoyt CS, Narahara MH. Optic nerve hypoplasia. *Surv Ophthalmol* 1987; **32**: 1−9

Layman PR, Anderson DR, Flynn JT. Frequent occurrence of hypoplastic optic discs in patients with aniridia *Am J Ophthalmol* 1974; **77**: 513−16

Levy NS, Ernest JT. Retinal medullated nerve fibres. *Arch Ophthalmol* 1974; **91**: 330−1

Lightman S. Kallmann's syndrome. *J R Soc Med* 1988; **81**: 315−7

Lillquist K, Warburg M, Anderson SR, Hagerstrand I. Colobomata of the iris, ciliary body and choroid in an infant with oesophagotracheal fistula and congenital heart defects. An unknown malformation complex. *Acta Paediatr Scand* 1980; **69**: 427−30

Little LE, Whitmore PV, Wells TW. Aplasia of the optic nerve. *J Pediatr Ophthalmol* 1976; **13**: 84−88

Longfellow DW, Davis FS, Walsh FB. Unilateral intermittent blindness with dilatation of retinal veins. *Arch Ophthalmol* 1962; **67**: 554−5

Lorentzen SE. Drusen of the optic disc. *Acta Ophthalmologica (Suppl.)* 1966; **90**: 1−66

Lyford JH, Roy FH. Arrhinencephaly unilateralis uveal coloboma and lens reduplication. *Am J Ophthalmol* 1974; **77**: 315−18

McKinna AJ. Quinine induced hypoplasia of the optic nerve *Can J Ophthalmol* 1966; **1**: 261−5

McKusich V. *Mendelian inheritance in man*. Johns Hopkins Univ Press, Baltimore 1978; p 14.

McMillan L. Anophthalmos and maldevelopment of the eyes; 4 cases in the same family. *Br J Ophthalmol* 1921; **5**: 121−2

Mann I. *Developmental Abnormalities of the Eye*. British Medical Association Press, London 1957

Manor RS, Korczyn AD. Retinal red-free light photographs in two congenital conditions. *Ophthalmologica* 1976; **173**: 119−27

Manschot WA. Eye findings in hydranencephaly. *Ophthalmologica* 1971; **162**: 151−9

Manschot WA. *The optic nerve in hydranencephaly and anencephaly. In: Stanley Can J (Ed.) The Optic Nerve.* H. Kimpton, London 1972

Marden PM, Venters HD. A new neurocutaneous syndrome. *Am J Dis Child* 1966; **112**: 79−81

Matzkin GM. Coloboma at the optic nerve entrance and melanosis oculi. *J Pediatr Ophthalmol* 1970; **4**: 222−4

Meckel JR. Beschreibung zweier durch sehr ähnliche bildungsabweichung entsteller Gerchwister. *Dtsch Arch Physiol* 1822; **7**: 99−172

Mellor D, Fielder A. Dissociated visual development: Electrodiagnostic studies in infants who are 'slow to see'. *Dev Med Child Neurol* 1980; **22**: 327−35

Missiroli G. Una nuova sindrome congenita a carattere faningliare, ipoplasia del nervo ottico e emianopsia binasale. *Boll Occul* 1947; **26**: 683−91

Mullaney J. Ocular malformation in trisomy 18 (Edwards' syndrome). *Am J Ophthalmol* 1973; **76**: 246−54

Mullaney J. Complex sporadic colobomata. *Br J Ophthalmol* 1978; **62**: 384−8.

Mullaney J, Fitzpatrick C. Idiopathic cyst of the iris stroma. *Am J Ophthalmol* 1973; **76**: 64−8

Mullie MA, Sanders MD. Sclerol canal size and optic nerve head drusen. *Am J Ophthalmol* 1985; **99**: 356−60

Nakajima A, Fujiki K, Tanabe U. Birth order and parental age in microphthalmos and other ocular conditions. *Am J Ophthalmol* 1979; **88**: 461−8

Novakovic P, Taylor DSI, Hoyt WF. Localising patterns of optic nerve hypoplasia − retina to occipital lobe. *Br J Ophthalmol* 1988; **72**: 176−83

O'Connor PS, Smith JL. Optic nerve variant in the Klippel−Trenaunay−Weber syndrome. *Ann Ophthalmol* 1978; **10**: 131−4

Odagiri Y, Ito T. The Morning Glory syndrome. *J Clin Ophthalmol* 1975; **69**: 483−6

Opitz JM, Howe JJ. The Meckel syndrome. *Birth Defects* 1969; **5**: 167−79

Orcutt JC, Bunt AH. Anomalous optic discs in the patient with a Dandy−Walker cyst. *J Clin Neuro Ophthalmol* 1982; **2**: 42−3

Pagon R. Ocular coloboma. *Surv Ophthalmol* 1981; **25**: 223−36

Pagon RA, Chandler JDV, Collier WR. Hydrocephalus, agyria, retinal dysplasia, encephalocele (Hard± E) syndrome: an autosomal recessive condition. *Birth Defects* 1978; **15**: 233−41

Pagon RA, Graham JM, Sybert VP. The Charge association. *Clin Res* 1980; **28**: 118A

Pagon RA, Graham JM, Zonana J, Yong S-L. Coloboma, congenital heart disease and choanal atresia with multiple anomalies: an association. *J Pediatrics* 1981; **99**: 223−27

Patel H, Tze WJ, Crichton JU, McCormick AQ, Robinson GC, Dolman CL. Optic nerve hypoplasia with hypopituitarism. *Am J Dis Child* 1975; **129**: 175−80

Pedler C. Unusual coloboma of the optic nerve entrance. *Br J Ophthal* 1961; **45**: 803−8

Peterson RA, Walton DS. Optic nerve hypoplasia with good acuity and visual field defects: a study of infants of diabetic mothers. *Arch Ophthalmol* 1977; **95**: 254−8

Pinckers A, Lion F, Notting JGA. X-chromosomal recessive night-blindness and titled disc anomaly. *Ophthalmologica* 1978; **176**: 160−3

Purdy F, Friend JCM. Maternal factors in SOD (letter). *J Pediatrics* 1979; **95**: 661

Rack JH, Wright GF. Coloboma of the optic nerve entrance. *Br J Ophthalmol* 1966; **50**: 705−9

Reese AB. Congenital melanomas. *Am J Ophthalmol* 1974; **77**: 798−808

Reeves DL. Congenital absence of the septum pellucidum. *Johns Hopkins Hospital Bulletin* 1941; **69**: 61−7

Renelt P. Beitrag zur echten Papillenaplasine. *Graefes Arch Klin Exp Ophthalmol* 1972; **184**: 94−8

Ridley H. Aplasia of the optic nerves. *Br J Ophthalmol* 1938; **22**: 669−71

Riise D. The nasal fundus ectasia. *Acta Ophthalmol (Kbh)* (Suppl.) 1975; **26**: 1−108

Robertson DM. Hamartomas of the optic disc with retinitis pigmentosa. *Am J Ophthalmol* 1972; **74**: 526−31

Rogers GL, Brown D, Gray I, Bremer D. Bilateral optic nerve hypoplasia associated with cerebral atrophy. *J Pediatr Ophthalmol Strabismus* 1981; **18**: 18−22

Rosenberg MA, Savino PJ, Glaser JS. A clinical analysis of pseudopapilloedema: population, laterality, acuity, refractive error, ophthalmoscopic characteristics. *Arch Ophthalmol* 1979; **97**: 65−70

Rubinstein K, Ali M. Complications of optic disc pits. *Trans Ophthalmol Soc UK* 1978; **98**: 195−200

Rucker CW. Bitemporal defects in the visual fields resulting from developmental anomalies of the optic discs. *Arch Ophthalmol* 1946; **35**: 546−54

Sachs JG, O'Grady RB, Choromokos E, Leestma J. The pathogenesis of optic nerve drusen: a hypothesis. *Arch Ophthalmol* 1977; **95**: 425−8

Sakuma Y, Sakuma F. A case of monosomy 9 mosaicism with multiple congenital anomalies. *Folia Ophthalmologica Jap* 1976; **27**: 987−91

Sanders MD. CT scanning in diagnosis of orbital disease. *J R Soc Med* 1980; **73**: 284−7

Sanders TE, Gay AJ, Newman M. Hemorrhagic complications of drusen of the optic disc. *Am J Ophthalmol* 1971; **71**: 204−17

Saraux H. Types et contratypes en pathologie chromosomique. *Bull et Mem Soc Fr Ophthalmol* 1972; **85**: 8−16

Saraux H, Lefebure M. Weyers et Thiers oculovertebral syndrome. *Bull Soc Fr Ophthalmol* 1966; **66**: 485−7

Savell J, Cook JR. Optic nerve colobomas of autosomal dominant heredity. *Arch Ophthalmol* 1976; **94**: 395−400

Savino PJ, Glaser JS, Rosenberg MA. A clinical analysis of pseudopapilloedema: visual field defects. *Arch Ophthalmol* 1979; **97**: 71−5

Schachat AP, Miller NR. Atrophy of myelinated retinal nerve fibres after acute optic neuropathy. *Am J Ophthalmol* 1981; **92**: 854−6

Schachenmann G, Schmid W, Fraccaro M *et al.* Chromosomes in coloboma and anal atresia. *Lancet* 1965; **ii**: 290

Schatz H, McDonald HR. Treatment of sensory retinal detachment associated with optic nerve pit or coloboma. *Ophthalmology* 1988; **95**: 178−87

Scheie HG, Adler FH. Aplasia of the optic nerve. *Arch Ophthalmol* 1941; **26**: 61−70

Schindler RF, Sarin LK, MacDonald PR. Hemangiomas of the optic disc. *Can J Ophthalmol* 1975; **10**: 305−18

Seefelder R. Über anomalien im Bereiche der sehnerven und der Netzhaut normaler fötaler augen, ein Beitrag zur Gliomfrage. *Graefes Arch Ophthalmol* 1909; **69**: 463−78

Seeley RL, Smith JL. Visual field defects in optic nerve hypoplasia. *Am J Ophthalmol* 1971; **73**: 882−9

Seybold ME, Rosen PN. Peripapillary staphyloma and amaurosis fugax. *Ann Ophthalmol* 1977; **9**: 1137−41

Shields MB. Gray crescent in the optic nerve head. *Am J Ophthalmol* 1980; **89**: 238−44

Skarf B, Hoyt CS. Optic nerve hypoplasia in children. *Arch Ophthalmol* 1984; **102**: 62−8

Slade HW, Weekley RD. Diastasis of the optic nerve. *J Neurosurg* 1957; **14**: 571−4

Smith DW. *Recognizable Patterns of Human Malformation.* WB Saunders, Philadelphia 1976

Soloman LM. Epidermal nevus syndrome. *Mod Prob Pediatr* 1975; **17**: 27−30

Somerville F. Uniocular aplasia of the optic nerve. *Br J Ophthalmol* 1962; **46**: 51−5

Spencer WH. Drusen of the optic disc and aberrant axoplasmic transport. *Ophthalmology* 1978; **85**: 21−38

Stanhope R, Preece MA, Brook CGD. Hypoplastic optic nerves and pituitary dysfunction. *Arch Dis Child* 1984; **59**: 111−14

Steinkuller PG. The Morning Glory disc anomaly: case report and a review of the literature. *J Pediatr Ophthalmol* 1980; **17**: 81−7

Straatsma BR, Foos RY, Heckenlively JR, Taylor GN. Myelinated retinal nerve fibres. *Am J Ophthalmol* 1981; **91**: 25−38

Stromland K. Ocular involvement in the fetal alcohol syndrome. *Surv Ophthalmol* 1987; **31**: 277−84

Sugar HS. Congenital pits of the optic disc. *Am J Ophthalmol* 1967; **63**: 298−307

Sugar HS, Beckman H. Peripapillary staphyloma with respiratory pulsation. *Am J Ophthalmol* 1969; **68**: 895−7

Takahashi T, Murase T, Hiramatsu K, Asakura S, Okada S. The clinicopathological findings on two cases of coloboma of the optic disc. *Folia Ophthalmol Jap* 1979; **30**: 957−62

Tanaka Y. Contractile coloboma of the optic nerve entrance. *Jpn J Clin Ophthalmol* 1977; **31**: 625−30

Taylor D. Congenital tumours of the anterior visual system with dysplasia of the optic discs. *Br J Ophthalmol* 1982; **66**: 455−63

Theodossiadis G. Evolution of congenital pit of the optic disc with macular detachment in photocoagulated and non-photocoagulated eyes. *Am J Ophthalmol* 1977; **84**: 620−31

Traboulsi EI, O'Neill JF. The spectrum in the morphology of the so-called 'Morning Glory disc anomaly'. *J Pediatr Ophthalmol Strabismus* 1988; **25**: 93−9

Van Noyhuys JM, Bruyn GW. Nasopharyngeal trans-sphenoidal encephalocoele, crater-like hole in the optic disc and agenesis of the corpus callosum. *Psychiatr Neurol Neurochir* 1964; **67**: 243−58

Von Arlt CF. Aux der k.k. *Ges Aertze zu Wien* 1858; 445

Von Barsewisch B. *Perinatal Retinal Haemorrhages*. Springer-Verlag, Berlin 1979

Vossius A. Beitrag zur Lehre von den angenborenen Conis. *Klin Monatsbl Augenheilkd* 1885; **23**: 137−57

Walsh FB, Hoyt WF. In: *Clinical Neuro-ophthalmology*, 3rd edn. Williams & Wilkins, Baltimore 1969, p 716

Walton DS, Robb RM. Optic nerve hypoplasia — a report of 20 cases. *Arch Ophthalmol* 1970; **84**: 572−8

Warburg M, Mikkelsen M. A case of 13−15 trisomy or Bartholin−Patau's syndrome. *Acta Ophthalmol (Kbh)* 1963; **41**: 321−3

Warburg M. Focal dermal hypoplasia: ocular and general manifestations with a survey of the literature. *Acta Ophthalmol (Kbh)* 1970; **48**: 525−36

Warburg M. The heterogenity of microphthalmia in the mentally retarded. *Birth Defects* 1971; **7**: 130−54

Warburg M. Hydrocephaly, congenital retinal non attachment and congenital falciform fold. *Am J Ophthalmol* 1978; **85**: 88−94

Waring GO, Roth AM, Rodrigues M. Microphthalmos with cyst. *Am J Ophthalmol* 1976; **82**: 714−22

Weiter JJ, McLean IW, Zimmerman LE. Aplasia of the optic nerve and disc. *Am J Ophthalmol* 1977; **83**: 569−76

Weleber RG, Walknowska J, Peakman D. Cytogenetic investigation of the cat-eye syndrome. *Am J Ophthalmol* 1977; **84**: 477−86

Whinery RD, Blodi FC. Hypoplasia of the optic nerve: a clinical and histopathologic correlation. *Trans Am Acad Ophthalmol Otol* 1963; **67**: 733−8

Wiethe T. Ein Fall von angeborener Difformitat der Sehnerven papille. *Arch Augenheilkunde*, 1882; **11**: 14−20

Wilkes SB, Campbell BJ, Waller RR. Ocular malformation in association with ipsilateral facial nevus of Jadassohn. *Am J Ophthalmol* 1981; **92**: 344−52

Williams EJ, McCormick AQ, Tischler B. Retinal vessels in Down's syndrome. *Arch Ophthalmol* 1973; **89**: 269−71

Willis R, Zimmerman LE, O'Grady R, Smith RS, Crawford B. Heterotopic adipose tissue and smooth muscle in the optic disc. *Arch Ophthalmol* 1971; **88**: 139−46

Willis R, Zimmerman LE, O'Grady R, Smith RS, Crawford B. Heterotopic adipose tissue and smooth muscle in the optic disc. *Arch Ophthalmol* 1972; **88**: 139−46

Wise JB, MacLean AL, Gass JDM. Contractile peripapillary staphyloma. *Arch Ophthalmol* 1966; **75**: 626−30

Wisek GN, Henkind P, Alterman M. Optic disc drusen and subretinal hemorrhage. *Trans Am Acad Ophthalmol Otolaryngol* 1974; **78**: 211−19

Woodford B, Tso MOM. An ultrastructural study of the corpora amylacea of the optic nerve head and retina. *Am J Ophthalmol* 1980; **90**: 492−502

Yamaguchi Y. Congenital anomalies of the optic nerve head — report of two cases. *Folia Ophthalmol Jpn* 1975; **26**: 1070−4

Yanoff M, Rorke LB, Allman MI. Bilateral Optic system aplasia with relatively normal eyes. *Arch Opthalmol* 1978; **96**: 97−101

Young SE, Walsh FB, Knox DL. The tilted disc syndrome. *Am J Ophthalmol* 1976; **82**: 16−23

Zion V. Optic nerve hypoplasia. *Ophthalmic Seminars* 1976; **1**: 171−96

29 Optic Neuropathies

DAVID TAYLOR

Childhood optic neuritis

Optic neuritis is rare in childhood but of significance because of its quite stunning presentation and the importance of the differential diagnosis. It probably occurs throughout childhood but is rarely recognized in toddlers because any visual defect has to be very profound, and in both eyes, before the child is obviously abnormal to the parents. The most frequent age of onset is 7 years, it occurs more frequently in girls than boys and is usually bilateral (Taylor & Cuendet 1986).

The onset may appear to be sudden but it may, in retrospect, have been developing over a few days with increasing visual difficulty. Smaller children often do not present until they are profoundly affected, with some children complaining that they want lights put on in bright daylight, or that they have been woken by their parents while it is still night time. Other children are referred with the diagnosis of ataxia which is in fact due to blindness. The loss of acuity is usually profound, there is a central scotoma (Fig. 29.1) or diffuse visual field loss and the colour vision is profoundly affected. There is an afferent pupil defect which may be apparent to the parents, if the optic neuritis is bilateral, as dilated pupils even in bright light. The optic discs are swollen in 87% of cases (Fig. 29.2), markedly so in 53% (Taylor & Cuendet 1986). Haemorrhages around the disc are rare (Fig. 29.3, 29.4) and exudates unusual (Fig. 29.5). Fluorescein angiography of the discs in the acute phase shows dilated capillaries and late leakage. When the optic disc is not swollen the condition is known as retrobulbar neuritis, and if it is it may be called papillitis.

The visual prognosis is generally excellent (Hierons & Lyle 1959; Kennedy & Carroll 1960; Meadows 1969; Taylor & Cuendet 1986) although many patients have residual retinal nerve fibre atrophy. Treatment

473

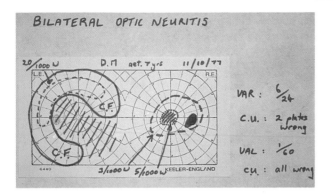

Fig. 29.1 Optic neuritis in a 7-year-old boy. Sudden onset of visual loss to 6/24 acuity right eye 1/60 left eye, central scotomas and colour vision loss.

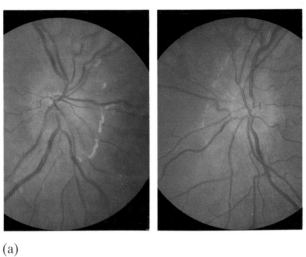

(a)

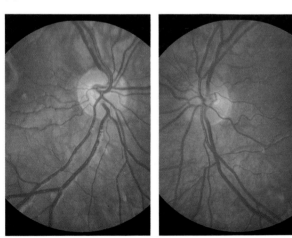

(b)

Fig. 29.2 (a) Bilaterally swollen optic discs. (b) Normal optic discs 2 months later. Complete visual recovery. (Same patient as Fig. 29.1.)

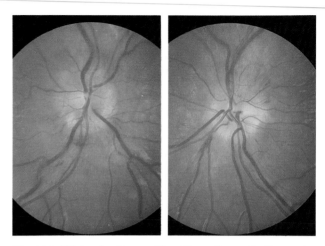

Fig. 29.3 Bilateral optic neuritis with swollen optic discs and a few peripapillary nerve fibre haemorrhages.

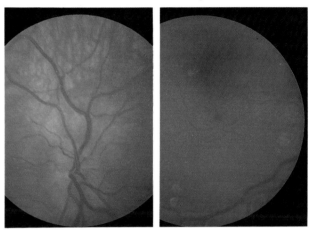

Fig. 29.4 Unilateral optic neuritis with paramacular preretinal haemorrhage.

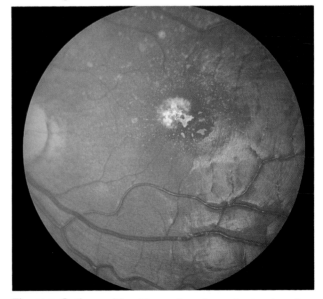

Fig. 29.5 Optic neuritis with remains of macular 'star' — the acuity is 6/9. There are similarities between childhood optic neuritis and neuroretinitis.

with high doses of systemic steroids sometimes brings about a dramatic and rapid improvement in the vision, but there is not yet conclusive evidence that the long term visual prognosis is improved by this treatment. Patients usually improve within several days without any treatment, and the main effect of the steroids seems to be to speed the improvement which is particularly beneficial when the child is profoundly affected.

In contrast to optic neuritis in adults, the systemic prognosis is also good. Eighty per cent of children in one series (Taylor & Cuendet 1986) had no subsequent neurological signs and no recurrence of their optic neuritis. Other series have reported a somewhat higher incidence of neurological problems, including multiple sclerosis (Kennedy & Carter 1961; Parkin et al. 1984). The incidence of neurological problems varies with the method of selection of patients and has been as high as 50% (Haller & Patzold 1979).

Patients with suspected optic neuritis should have a neurologist's opinion, and further investigations including CT scan, CSF studies, sinus X-ray and routine haematology. Visually evoked responses are useful in the acute stage because they are always abnormal (Taylor & Cuendet 1986) but a surprising difference from adults is that even pattern responses are often normal on follow-up.

The aetiology of childhood optic neuritis may be different from adult cases, possibly due to an infectious or parainfectious syndrome.

Neuroretinitis

The symptoms of this condition are virtually the same as in patients with optic neuritis; the difference is in the finding of a macular star which is a collection of intraretinal lipids in a spoke-like arrangement around the fovea (Fig. 29.5), determined by the macular anatomy. It seems likely that the star is merely the sign that there is a very brisk serous exudate from the optic disc and it may well be that it is a similar condition to childhood optic neuritis but that a different part of the neurone is affected (Taylor & Cuendet 1986). The prognosis is good (Dreyer 1984; Maitland 1984).

Optic neuritis in infectious diseases

Exanthemas

Optic neuritis in childhood is often preceeded by a non-specific illness but occasionally it is clearly related to one of the common childhood infectious illnesses,

chickenpox being the most commonly reported. Visual symptoms usually follow the rash by a few days, and although the visual loss may be profound, visual recovery is usually very good, despite the presence of residual optic atrophy (Sellost et al. 1983).

Optic neuritis may follow rubella, measles, mumps, or other vaccination (Kazarian et al. 1979; Kline et al. 1982).

Paranasal sinus disease

Symptoms of optic neuritis may occur in patients with acute or chronic ethmoiditis. The optic canal is extremely close to, or even runs in a bony strut through the ethmoid air cells and the optic nerve may be affected by compression, ischemia or 'toxic' local effects. Sinus X-rays are indicated in all cases of optic neuritis in childhood even in the absence of clinical sinusitis. Treatment is with high doses of antibiotics together with systemic steroids.

Optic neuropathy of malnutrition

It has long been known that patients on near starvation diets are liable to an optic neuropathy, and it is common for hunger-strikers to go through an initially reversible, blinding optic neuropathy before death.

Hoyt and Billson (1979) described two children who had a thiamine-reversable optic neuropathy whilst on a ketogenic diet. One must remember chronic malnutrition as a possible cause of optic neuropathy in any child on an unusual diet, with many gut diseases, from a developing country or from the less priviledged sectors of developed countries.

Optic neuropathy in leukaemia and systemic neoplasms

Optic nerve involvement in leukaemia has long been recognized as a serious complication, especially in acute lymphatic leukaemia, associated with bone marrow involvement in preterminal patients (Rosenthal et al. 1975). Chemotherapy and radiotherapy may have made this prognosis less than totally hopeless (Rosenthal 1983).

Optic nerve compression, not infrequently bilateral, also occurs in histiocytosis X, neuroblastoma (Manschot 1969) and the leukaemias and non-Hodgkin's lymphomas. Rarely patients presenting with clinical optic neuritis may have tumour compression as the cause but the tumour may be corticosteroid responsive producing a temporarily satisfying response to treatment (Hirst *et al.* 1980). Children with neuroblastoma may present with acute visual loss from meningeal infiltration and rapid action must be taken (chemotherapy, irradiation, and systemic steroids) to prevent the blindness which so frequently follows, whether it be from compression or ischaemia (Manschot 1969).

Optic neuritis may rarely occur as a remote effect of tumours (Fig. 29.6).

Radiation optic neuropathy and encephalopathy occur often some weeks or months after the treatment (Shukosky *et al.* 1972; Oliff *et al.* 1978; Brown *et al.* 1982).

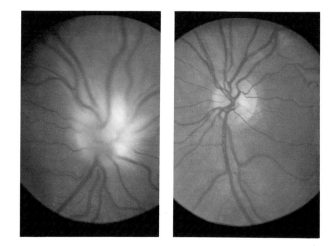

Fig. 29.7 Optic neuropathy from optic nerve glioma with optic disc involvement.

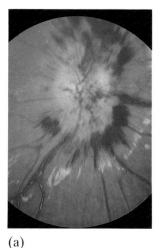

(a)

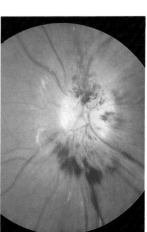

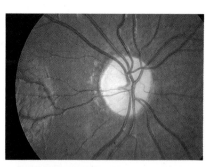

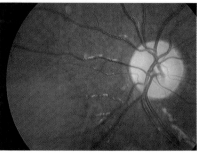

(b)

Fig. 29.6 (a) Acute optic neuropathy in a child with treated neuroblastoma on no therapy for 6 months. There was a bilateral central scotoma, acuities of 1/60 right eye, 4/60 left eye and colour vision loss. The CSF and neuroradiological studies were normal. (b) Same patient 3 months later. The optic neuropathy settled on corticosteroid treatment only and the acuity (despite the obvious optic atrophy) has remained normal for 6 years.

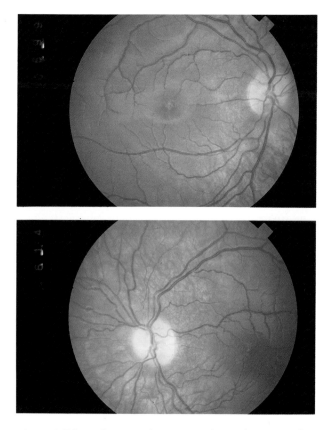

Fig. 29.8 Bilateral progressive compressive optic neuropathy in a child with bone dysplasia. In the left eye the acuity loss was arrested at 6/60 by optic canal decompression.

Compressive optic neuropathy

Optic atrophy from compression occurs from trauma, neoplasm (Fig. 29.7), bone disease (Fig. 29.8), orbital tumours and infections. Optic disc compression/decompression by eye poking may result in chronic disc oedema which resolves when the trauma ceases (Fig. 29.9).

Traumatic optic neuropathy

Soft tissue trauma

Blunt orbital trauma may cause a functional optic nerve transection if the optic nerve is compressed at the orbital apex or if there is a marked orbital haematoma. Optic disc pallor takes several weeks to appear (Fig. 29.10). Eye trauma may cause secondary optic atrophy.

Skull fracture

Fractures of the sphenoid bone resulting from frontal trauma may cause a sudden blindness in one or rarely both eyes. The optic nerve defect is often discovered too late for treatment either because it is unilateral and because the child is restless the relative afferent pupil defect is difficult to detect, or in bilateral cases because the other effects of trauma, including lid swelling are the overwhelming signs. If detected early high dose systemic steroids and transethmoid optic canal decompression may help (Anderson *et al.* 1982), although this active treatment is not universally accepted as being effective. Recovery may be prolonged, Feist *et al.* (1987) described a 16-year-old who had a shotgun injury who had no perception of light for 2 weeks, but who eventually recovered to 20/100 by 4 months.

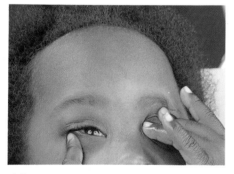

(a)

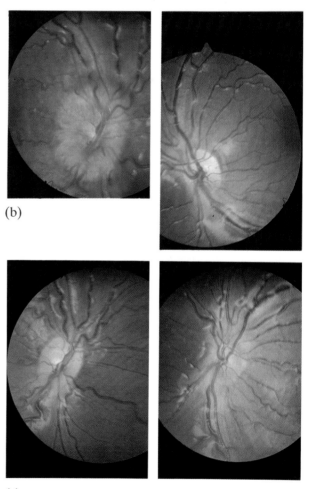

(b)

(c)

Fig. 29.9 (a) Child with severe Down's syndrome who relentlessly poked the right eye. (b) Right optic disc oedema. (c) After 2 weeks of using elbow restraints to stop the eye poking the optic disc oedema had resolved.

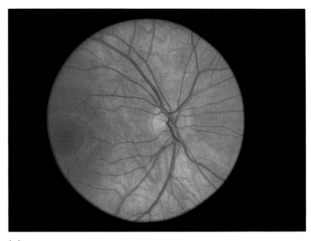

(a)

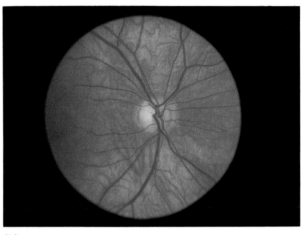

(b)

Fig. **29.10** (a) Right optic disc four hours after the eye was blinded by a billiards cue being accidentally thrust into the orbit of a 10-year-old boy. (b) Same patient 6 weeks later at the first appearance of optic atrophy.

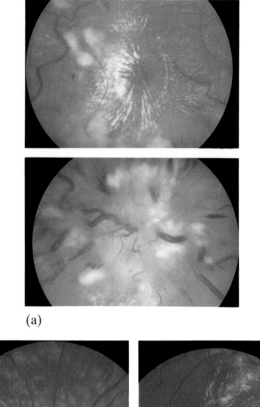

(a)

(b)

Fig. **29.11** (a) Optic neuropathy in malignant hypertension in an 11-year-old boy with reflux nephropathy. The vision had suddenly dropped associated with a gut haemorrhage. This was the presenting symptom. (b) Same patient showing the profound optic atrophy that subsequently occurred.

Ischaemic optic neuropathy

Ischaemic optic neuropathy occurs as a result of hypertension (Fig. 29.11) (Taylor *et al.* 1981), vasculitis, or in anomalous optic discs in profoundly anaemic patients (Fig. 28.12).

Toxic optic neuropathy

In any child presenting with an unexplained optic neuropathy, that is with acuity and colour vision loss and a central scotoma, a careful history of drug and heavy metal ingestion must be taken.

Antituberculous drugs

Ethambutal (Fig. 29.13), streptomycin, and isoniazid have been recorded as having a direct effect on optic nerve neurones. Their use in tuberculosus meningitis affecting the chiasm and optic nerves calls for fine judgement as to the cause of further visual loss.

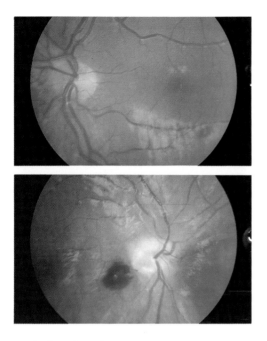

Fig. 29.12 Ischaemic optic neuropathy in the anomalous optic disc of the right eye of a patient with profound anaemia.

Desferrioxamine

High-dose desferrioxamine given for certain refractory anaemias may cause an optic neuropathy (Lakhanpal *et al.* 1984) or retinal pigmentation (Davies *et al.* 1983).

Cardiac drugs

Amiodarone causes largely asymptomatic cornea verticillata (Orlando 1984) and retinal changes which are unusual but usually symptomatic (Ingram *et al.* 1982). A papillopathy with preserved acuity has been described (Gittinger & Asdourian 1987). Propranolol may give an optic neuropathy (Parrish & Todorov 1981) and digitalis is also suspected.

Hydroxyquinolines

Iodochlorhydroxyquin (dioquinol) when used as an antidiarrhoeal and diiodohydroxyquin (iodoquinol) may both give optic atrophy; the former in the form of subacute myelo-optic neuropathy (SMON) (Oakley 1973) and the latter as chronic optic atrophy (Behrens 1974).

Antibiotics

Chloramphenicol and sulphonamides (and their hypo-glycaemic derivatives, tolbutamide and chlorpropomide) may give rise to an optic neuropathy which is reversable if treated early.

Antineoplastic agents

Carmustine (BCNU) and vincristine both give an optic neuropathy (Fraunfelder & Meyer 1983).

Others

Heavy metals, lead in particular, methanol, hexachlorophene (Slamovits *et al.* 1980) and solvents should also be suspected in undiagnosed optic neuropathy.

Hereditary optic neuropathies

Dominant optic atrophy

This is the commonest hereditary optic atrophy. It is inherited as an autosomal dominant trait (Kjer 1959; Brodrick 1974), but penetrance may be low.

The onset is very insidious with children often presenting in their first decade as a result of school eye tests. The acuity is symmetrically and often not severely affected (Smith 1972), 6/9 to 6/24 being most common and 6/36 or worse acuity being unusual. Careful examination of relatives is necessary because they may be very little disabled by their condition (Fig. 29.14), sometimes unaware of it. Flash electro-retinography is usually normal but may show a reduction in the scotopic response (Johnston *et al.* 1975). Blue cone ERG's differentiate dominant optic atrophy from congenital tritanopia, in the latter the blue cone ERG is absent (Miyake *et al.* 1985). The acuity may deteriorate in time, but if it does it is very gradual and not to a marked degree.

Careful visual field testing may show a subtle centro-caecal scotoma when the acuity is poor, the peripheral fields are full. When the acuity is good there is often a blue-yellow colour vision defect, when the acuity is poor there is a more profound and widespread colour defect. Nystagmus probably does not occur with typical dominant optic atrophy even on the rare occasions when it is detected in infancy.

The histopathological finding of ganglion cell loss with loss of myelin and nerve fibres within the optic nerve may suggest the disease is primarily a ganglion

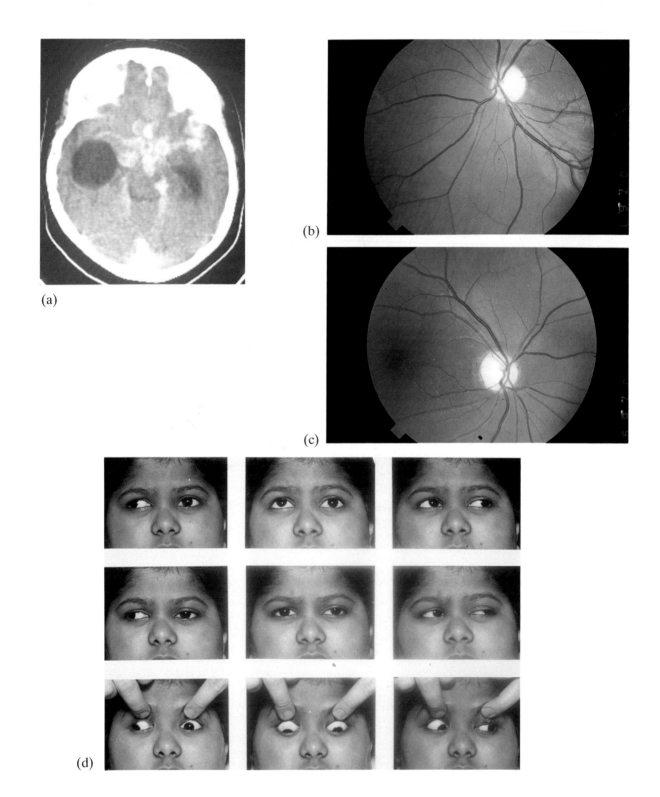

Fig. 29.13 (a) TB meningitis with cystic changes centred on the suprasellar region. (b,c) Same patient bilateral optic atrophy. The organism was only sensitive to Ethambutol which may itself cause a toxic optic neuropathy. (d) Same patient partial left IIIrd nerve palsy.

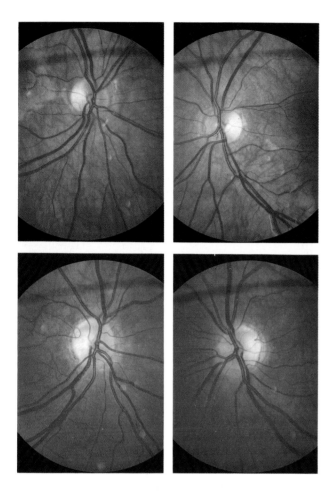

Fig. 29.14 (a) Dominant optic atrophy in a 6-year-old. He had failed the school test because his acuity was 6/12, he had normal red-green discrimination but defective blue-yellow. (b) The optic discs of the asymptomatic mother of the boy in (a). She had 6/9 acuity.

cell degeneration (Johnston *et al.* 1975). The loss of ganglion cells is most marked in the macular region and nerve fibre loss is most marked in the papillo-macular bundle (Johnston *et al.* 1975) which accords with the frequent clinical finding of temporal segment disc pallor with a well defined margin to the nerve fibre layer loss (Fig. 29.14).

The affected patients are usually entirely normal apart from their eyes, but mental retardation has very occasionally been described (Kjer 1959; Johnston *et al.* 1975).

Leber's optic neuropathy

Leber's optic neuropathy rarely occurs in childhood. It is characterized by the onset during late teens to thirties, of a bilateral asynchronous (separated by a few months), loss of central vision occurring over a few days or weeks. This is very profound and is accompanied by a large central scotoma and colour blindness. The visual defect is usually but not necessarily permanent and despite residual optic atrophy and visual defects the improvement in acuity over 2 years may be very useful (Lessell *et al.* 1983). In the presymptomatic phase (Fig. 29.15) a telangiectatic microangiopathy (dilated telangiectatic vessels) of the peripapillary capillaries may be seen which do not leak fluorescein (Nikoskelainen *et al.* 1984). If the acute phase occurs, the optic disc becomes swollen and the peripapillary nerve fibre bundles are easily seen (Smith *et al.* 1973), haemorrhages are unusual and not marked. Inheritance is similar to but different from X-linked recessive disease and is via a mitochondrial inheritance mechanism (see Chapter 9), through a mitochondrial DNA mutation (Wallace *et al.* 1988; Holt *et al.* 1989). Males are mainly but not exclusively affected but they do not transmit the disease (as opposed to X-linked recessive disease where they transmit it through their daughters). Carrier females can transmit the disease to their sons and the carrier trait to their daughters, both having the telangiectatic microangiopathy (Nikoskelainen 1987).

Evidence may point to an as yet unclear association with a disorder in cyanide metabolism (Hulme Adams 1966; Wilson *et al.* 1971; Cagianut *et al.* 1981; Freeman 1988; Berninger *et al.* 1989). Associated cardiac (Nikoskelainen 1987) and myopathic (Uemura *et al.* 1987) lesions have been described.

Optic atrophy in juvenile diabetes

Optic atrophy rarely occurs in diabetic children from the effects of the retinopathy but it may occur as part of a specific syndrome, the Wolfram−Tyrer syndrome (Wolfram 1938, Tyrer 1943) or DIDMOAD (**D**iabetes **I**nsipidus, **D**iabetes **M**ellitus, **O**ptic **A**trophy, and **D**eafness) syndrome.

It is characterized by four main symptoms (François 1975).

1 Optic atrophy of onset between 2 and 24 years, usually before 15 years (Figs 29.16, 29.17). The vision becomes very bad but blindness is rare. The visual fields are constricted and the patient is colour blind. Diabetic retinopathy is rare, perhaps reflecting the loss of nerve fibres. There is no acute stage, the atrophy is relentlessly progressive and the discs do not swell.

2 Juvenile diabetes mellitus which is usually diagnosed before the optic atrophy.

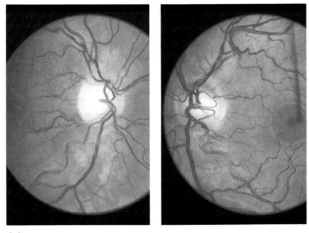

(a)

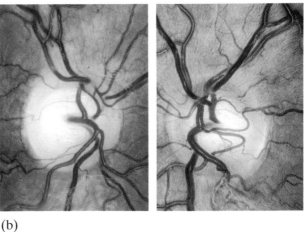

(b)

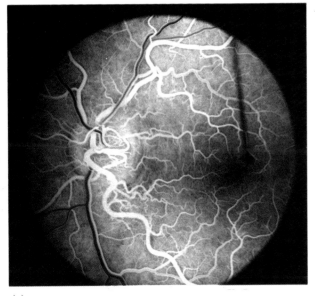

(c)

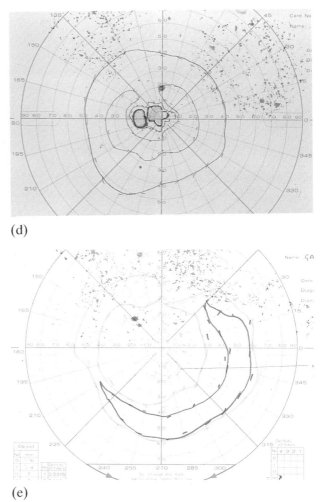

(d)

(e)

Fig. 29.15 (a–d) This 14-year-old boy had optic atrophy (a) with a large central scotoma (e) in the right eye for 2 months when he noticed a field defect in the left eye (d). The left optic disc showed thickened neurones (b, red-free photograph) and a peripapillary telangiectatic microangiopathy in the infero temporal arcades which did not at the onset leak fluorescein (c fluorescein angiogram). His brother and uncle were also affected by Leber's optic neuropathy.

3 Diabetes insipudus is usually undiagnosed until the children have persistent polyuria despite adequate control of the diabetes mellitus (Pilley & Thompson 1976). It usually responds to treatment with vaso-pressin (Bretz *et al.* 1970).

4 There is a bilateral symmetrical, initially partial and affecting high tones, progressive deafness that may need audiometry for presymptomatic detection.

Pigmentary changes at the posterior pole have been described occasionally (Rose *et al.* 1966; Rorsman & Soderstrom 1967) and electroretinography may indicate a more widespread abnormality of the retina than just due to ganglion cell degeneration (Niemeyer & Marquardt 1972).

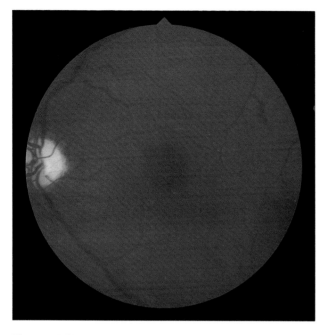

Fig. 29.16 DIDMOAD. There is atrophy and a diabetic retinal haemorrhage.

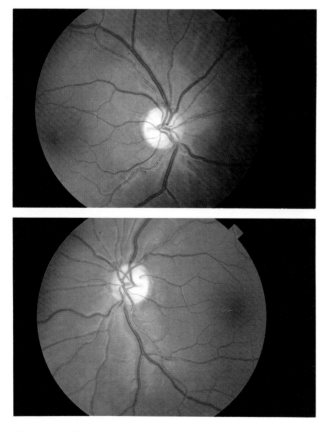

Fig. 29.17 DIDMOAD. Bilateral optic atrophy with profound visual loss.

Anosmia, tonic pupils and optic disc cupping are less frequent findings (Lessell & Rosman 1977) and it is inherited as an autosomal recessive trait.

There are other associations between optic atrophy and diabetes mellitus (Rose *et al.* 1966): (a) Friedrich's ataxia; (b) Refsum's disease; and (c) Laurence–Moon–Biedl syndrome.

SWOLLEN OPTIC DISCS IN DIABETIC CHILDREN

Papilloedema occurs in diabetes as a result of any of the usual causes not directly related to diabetes, but diabetics more frequently have papilloedema for three specific reasons.

1 Transient papilloedema with visual loss, and ensuing optic atrophy but with a good visual prognosis may occur as a result of optic disc ischaemia (Lubow *et al.* 1971).

2 Severe hypertension in diabetic nephropathy.

3 Raised intracranial pressure may occur due to sinus thrombosis or infections.

Recessive optic atrophy

Recessive optic atrophy is extremely rare. It is important to exclude retinal disease as the primary cause since it is likely that a large number of cases in the literature represent undiagnosed autosomal recessive cone dystrophy.

The onset is early, or at birth. The baby may have nystagmus. The optic disc is very pale but otherwise normal. The visual defect is often severe with the child likely to need non-sighted education. The diagnosis is only made by careful clinical, neurophysiological and radiological exclusion of other causes. Often a family history is lacking but consanguinity in the parents and subsequent affected siblings suggest the diagnosis and heredity (Fig. 29.18).

Optic atrophy in heredodegenerative neurological disease

That optic atrophy occurred in some neurological disease was known in the last century; Habershon (1887) referred to optic atrophy in patients with diseases of the spinal cord, locomotor ataxia, and epilepsy, as well as insanity and sexual abuse or excesses. Although not frequently encountered by most ophthalmologists, hereditary neurological diseases are a significant cause of optic atrophy amongst young people (Harding 1984), adding enormously to an existing handicap and requiring a great depth of understanding and empathy by the doctor.

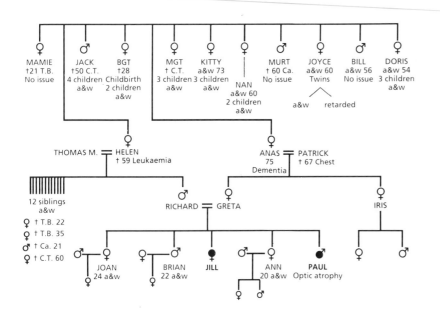

Fig. 29.18 Recessive optic atrophy. Profound optic atrophy occurred in two siblings of a consanguineous marriage. The ERG was normal to flash stimuli.

Behr's disease

Behr (1909) described in children with optic atrophy, poor vision, squint and nystagmus with ataxia, mental retardation, spasticity, urinary incontinence, and pes cavus. It affects both sexes and is inherited as an autosomal recessive trait (Landrigan *et al.* 1973; François 1976), but it may be a common clinical manifestation of a heterogenous group of disorders (Horoupian *et al.* 1979). Pathologically there is loss of central optic nerve axons and widespread neural loss especially in thalamic nuclei (Horoupian *et al.* 1979). The visual and systemic prognosis should be guardedly cautious (Fig. 29.19).

Friedreich's ataxia

Friedreich's ataxia, and the closely related ataxia of Charlevoix–Saguenay are characterized (Barbeau 1978) by:

1 *Genetics*: Autosomal recessive.

2 *Clinical*: Onset is before end of puberty. Ataxia, first of lower limbs, then all four limbs, is relentlessly progressive, usually with muscle wasting.

● Dysarthria.

● Abnormal vibration and position sense in lower limbs.

● Absent deep tendon reflexes in lower limbs.

● Progressive kyphoscoliosis and pes cavus within 2 years of onset.

3 *Paraclinical*: Hypertrophic progressive cardiomyopathy.

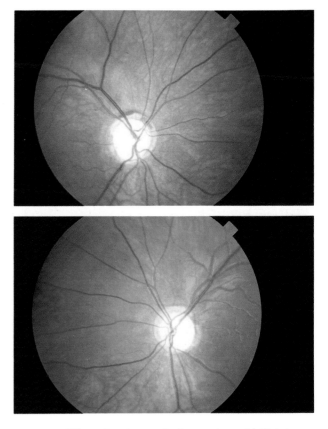

Fig. 29.19 Bilateral optic atrophy in a patient with Behr's disease.

- Abnormal sensory nerve conduction in lower more than upper limbs.
- Essentially normal motor nerve conduction and electromyography.

4 *Neuro-ophthalmic abnormalities*: Optic atrophy occurs frequently in Friedreich's ataxia (Livingstone *et al.* 1981), and a presymptomatic phase may be observed clinically or revealed by visually evoked cortical responses (Carroll *et al.* 1980). Symptomatic, progressive optic neuropathy (Fig. 29.20) that may be disabling occurs in a significant proportion of patients.

Eye movement defects, related to the cerebellar defect are common and occur in patients without a significant visual defect (Kirkham *et al.* 1979). They include downbeat nystagmus, gaze paretic and rebound nystagmus, asymmetrical saccades, reduced vestibulo-ocular reflex (VOR) suppression or unsteady fixation (Zee *et al.* 1976). The finding of decreased VOR responses may be helpful in the differential diagnosis from patients with parenchymal cerebellar disease who usually have increased VORs (Furman *et al.* 1983).

Olivopontocerebellar atrophy

Both autosomal recessive and autosomal dominant heredity has been proposed in various studies of this syndrome in which there is a variably early onset of progressive ataxia, tremor, dysarthria, and visual difficulties which are largely due to a retinal degeneration (Weiner *et al.* 1967) but which may in some cases be due to an optic neuropathy as evidenced by presymptomatic changes in visually evoked potential (Hammond & Wilder 1983).

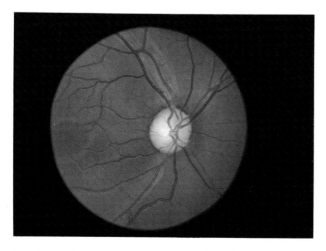

Fig. 29.20 Optic atrophy in a 10-year-old with Friedreich's ataxia. Marked grooves can be seen in the arcuate bundles.

Charcot–Marie Tooth disease (peroneal muscular atrophy)

This is a motor neuropathy predominantly affecting the legs, it is usually inherited as an autosomal dominant trait with an onset in late childhood. Affected children have distal wasting of the legs, pes cavus and foot drop. The hands are only mildly affected and progression is very slow. Optic atrophy, starting in the teenages, with loss of acuity, and central scotomas is an unusual but recognized complication (Hoyt 1960). Similar cases together with deafness have been described (Rosenberg & Chutorian 1967).

Leucodystrophies

METACHROMATIC LEUCODYSTROPHY

This occurs in late infantile, intermediate, and juvenile forms which present with gait disorders, a peripheral neuropathy, behavioural problems and intellectual deterioration. The diagnosis is suspected after finding metachromatic material in the urine and confirmed by the finding of decreased levels of aryl sulphatase A in white blood cells. Optic atrophy is frequent (Libert 1979; Taylor 1983) and may result in severely impaired vision (François 1979).

ADRENOLEUCODYSTROPHY

This X-linked recessive disease occurs in 5–9-year-old boys who have subtle behavioural changes, intellectual deterioration, symptoms of adrenal insufficiency, and a usually severe visual problem which is due to a relatively selective visual cortical defect but optic atrophy also occurs (Wray *et al.* 1976).

KRABBE'S LEUCODYSTROPHY (globoid cell leukodystrophy)

The onset is usually early infancy with rapidly progressive apathy, irritability, neurological regression with clinical evidence of a peripheral neuropathy. Optic atrophy occurs early but is usually overshadowed by the neurological deterioration (François 1975).

Menke's disease

Boys with this X-linked syndrome have psychomotor retardation, progressive spasticity and seizures, and abnormal ('kinky' or 'steely') hair. Plasma copper and caeruloplasmin levels are low. Retinal abnormalities are frequent, with a macular dystrophy, mottled retinal pigment epithelium and tortuous vessels (Taylor 1983) and optic atrophy which probably occurs as an additional feature to, rather than the result of, a retinal degeneration (Seelenfreund *et al.* 1968; Wray 1976).

Neuronal storage diseases and the mucopolysaccharidoses

Batten's disease, clinical Tay Sach's disease and other gangliosidoses, Neimann Pick disease type A, infantile Gaucher's disease, and some of the mucopolysaccharidoses and mucolipidoses such as sialidosis deficiency (cherry red spot−myoclonus syndrome) may all have diffuse affection of their ganglion cells resulting in a cherry red spot. Ganglion cell death eventually results in optic atrophy. In the mucopolysaccharidoses optic atrophy occurs from glaucoma, retinal degeneration, optic nerve involvement directly, compression by thickened bone at the optic canal or hydrocephalus.

Optic atrophy in familial dysautomia

As these children are now living longer, it has become evident that optic atrophy may account for a proportion of their visual loss, as further evidence of central nervous system involvement (Rizzo *et al.* 1986). Nineteen eyes of 12 patients had abnormal pattern VERs, the latency increased with age (Diamond *et al.* 1987).

References

Anderson RL, Danje WR, Gross CE. Optic nerve blindness following blunt forehead trauma. *Am Acad Ophthalmol* 1982; **89**: 445−55

Barbeau A. Quebec Cooperative Study of Friedreich's ataxia. Cooperative Study, Phase Two: Statement of the Problems. *Can J Neurol Sci* 1978; **5**: 57−9

Behr C. Die komplizierte, hereditar-familiare Optikusatrophie des Kindesathers. *Klin Monatsbl Augenheilkd* 1909; **47**: 138−60

Behrens MM. Optic atrophy in children after di-iodohydrxyquin therapy. *J Am Med Assoc* 1974; **228**: 693−4

Berninger TA, Meyer L, Seiss E, Schon O, Goebel F-D, Leber's hereditary optic atrophy: further evidence for a defect in cyanide metabolism. *Br J Ophthalmol* 1989; **73**: 314−6

Bretz GW, Baghadassarian SA, Graber JD, Zacherle B, Norum RA, Blizzard RM. Coexistence of diabetes mellitus and insipidus and optic atrophy in two male siblings. *Am J Med* 1970; **48**: 398−403

Brodrick JD. Hereditary optic atrophy with onset in early childhood. *Br J Ophthalmol* 1974; **58**: 817−24

Brown GC, Shields JA, Sanborn G, Augsburger JJ, Savino PJ,

Schatz N. Radiation optic neuropathy. *J Am Acad Ophthalmol* 1982; **89**: 1489−93

Cagianul B, Rhyner K, Furrer W, Schnebli HP. Thiosulphate-sulphur transferase (rhodanese) deficiency in Leber's hereditary optic atrophy. *Lancet* 1981; **ii**: 981−2

Carrol WM, Kriss A, Baraitser M, Barrett G, Halliday AM. The incidence and nature of visual pathway involvement in Friedreich's ataxia, a clinical and visual evoked potential study of 22 patients. *Brain* 1980; **103**: 413−34

Davies D, Marcys RE, Hungerford JL, Miller MH, Arden GB, Huchns ER. Ocular toxicity of high-dose intravenous desferrioxamine. *Lancet* 1983; **ii**: 181−4

Diamond GA, D'Amico RA, Axelrod FB. Optic nerve dysfunction in familial dysautomonia. *Am J Ophthalmol* 1987; **104**: 645−9

Dreyer RF, Hopen G, Gass JDM, Smith JL. Lebers idiopathic stellate neuroretinitis. *Arch Ophthalmol* 1984; **102**: 1140−5

Feist RM, Kline LB, Morris RE, Witherspoon CD, Michelson MA. Recovery of vision after presumed direct optic nerve injury. *J Am Acad Ophthalmol* 1987; **94**: 1567−70

François J. Ocular manifestations in inborn error of carbohydrate and lipid metabolism. Part II Section G: *Krabbe's Disease*, Part II. S. Karger, Basel 1975; pp. 98−100

François J. Les atrophies optiques héréditaires. *J Genet Hum* 1976; **24**: 183−200

François J. Optico-oto-diabetic syndrome. *Ophthalmologica (Basel)* 1976; **173**: 345−51

François J. Ocular manifestations in demyelinating diseases. *Adv Ophthalmol* 1979; **39**: 391−36

Fraunfelder FT, Meyer SM. Ocular toxicity of antineoplastic agents. *Ophthalmology* 1983; **90**: 1−3

Freeman AG. Optic neuropathy and chronic cyanode intoxication: a review. *J R Soc Med* 1988; **81**: 103−6

Furman JM, Perlman S. Baloh RW. Eye movements in Friedreich's ataxia. *Arch Neurol* 1983; **40**: 343−46

Gittinger JW, Asdourian GK. Papillopathy caused by amiodarone. *Arch Ophthalmol* 1987; **105**: 349−51

Habershon SH. Hereditary optic atrophy. *Trans Ophthalmol Soc UK* 1887; **VIII**: 1−47

Haller P, Patzold U. Die Optikusneuritis im Kindersalter. *Fortschr Neurol Psychiatr* 1979; **47**: 209−16

Hammond EJ, Wilder BJ. Evoked potentials in olivopontocerebellar atrophy. *Arch Neurol* 1983; **40**: 366−9

Harding AE. *The Hereditary Ataxias and Related Disorders*. Churchill Livingstone, London 1984

Heirons R, Lyle TK. Bilateral retrobulbar neuritis. *Brain* 1959; **82**: 56−67

Hirst LW, Miller NR, Kumar AJ, Udvarhelyi GB. Medulloblastoma causing a corticosteroid-responsive optic neuropathy. *Am J Ophthalmol* 1980; **89**: 437−42

Holt IJ, Miller DH, Harding AE. Genetic heterogeneity and mitochondrial DNA heteroplasmy in Leber's hereditary optic neuropathy. *J Med Genet* 1989; **26**: 739−43

Horoupian DS, Zuker DK, Solomon M, Peterson HDC. Behr syndrome; a clinicopathological report. *Neurology* 1979; **29**: 323−7

Hoyt CS, Billson FA. Optic neuropathy in ketogenic diet. *Br J Ophthalmol* 1979; **63**: 191−4

Hoyt WF. Charcot−Marie−Tooth disease with optic atrophy. *Arch Ophthalmol* 1960; **64**: 145−8

Hulme-Adams J, Blackwood W, Wilson J. Further clinical and pathological observations on Lebers optic atrophy. *Brain*

1966; **89**: 15−22

Ingram DV, Jaggarao NSV, Chamberlain DA. Ocular changes resulting from therapy with amiodarone. *Br J Ophthalmology* 1982; **66**: 676−80

Johnston PB, Gaster RN, Smith VC, Tripathi RC. A clinicopathologic study of autosomal dominant optic atrophy. *Am J Ophthalmol* 1975; **88**: 868−75

Kazarian EL, Gager WE. Optic neuritis complicating measles, mumps and rubella vaccination. *Am J Ophthalmol* 1979; **86**: 544−7

Kennedy C, Carroll FD. Optic neuritis in children. *Arch Ophthalmol* 1960; **63**: 747−55

Kennedy C, Carter W. Relation of optic neuritis to multiple sclerosis in children. *Pediatrics* 1961; **28**: 377−87

Kirkham TH, Guitton D, Katsarkis A, Kline LB, Andermann E. oculomotor abnormalities in Friedreich's ataxia. *Can J Neurol Sci* 1979; **6**: 167−72

Kjer P. Infantile optic atrophy with dominant mode of inheritance. *Acta Ophthalmol (Kbh))* (Suppl.) 1959; **54**

Kline LB, Margulies SL, Oh SJ. Optic neuritis and myelitis following rubella vaccination. *Arch Neurol* 1984; **39**: 443−5

Lakhanpal V, Schocket SS, Rouben J. Deferoxamine-induced toxic retinal pigmentary degeneration and presumed optic neuropathy. *Ophthalmology* 1984; **91**: 443−51

Landrigan PJ, Berenberg W, Bresnan M. Behr's syndrome. *Dev Med Child Neurol* 1973; **15**: 41−7

Lessell S, Gise RL, Krohel GB. Bilateral optic neuropathy with remission in young men. *Arch Neurol* 1983; **40**: 2−6

Lessell S, Rosman NP. Juvenile diabetes mellitus and optic atrophy. *Arch Neurol* 1977; **34**: 759−65

Libert J, VanHoof F, Toussant D, Roozitalab H, Kenyon K, Green R. Ocular findings in metachromatic leucodystrophy. *Arch Ophthalmol* 1979; **97**: 1495−1504

Livingstone IR, Mastaglia FL, Edis R, Howe JW. Visual involvement in Friedreich's ataxia and hereditary spastic ataxia. A clinical and visual evoked response study. *Arch Neurol* 1981; **38**: 75−9

Lubow M, Makley TA. Pseudopapilloedema of juvenile diabetes mellitus. *Arch Ophthalmol* 1971; **85**: 417−22

Maitland CG, Miller NR. Neuroretinitis. *Arch Ophthalmol* 1984; **102**: 1146−50

Manschot WA. Transverse ischaemic optic nerve necrosis in neuroblastoma. *Arch Ophthalmol* 1969; **89**: 707−9

Meadows SP. Retrobulbar and optic neuritis in childhood and adolescence. *Trans Ophthalmol Soc UK* 1969; **89**: 603−38

Miyake Y, Yagasaki K, Ichikawa H. Differential diagnosis of congenital tritanopia and dominantly inherited optic atrophy. *Arch Ophthalmol* 1985; **103**: 1496−501

Niemeyer C, Marquardt JL. Wolfram−Tyrer syndrome. *Invest Ophthalmol* 1972; **11**: 617−24

Nikoskelainen E, Hoyt WF, Nummelin K, Schatz H. Fundus findings in Leber's hereditary optic neuroretinopathy. *Arch Ophthalmol* 1984; **102**: 981−9

Nikoskelainen E, Savontaus M-L, Wanni O, Katila MJ, Nummelin KU. Leber's hereditary optic neuroretinopathy, a maternally inherited disease. *Arch Ophthalmol* 1987; **105**: 665−72

Oakley GP. The neurotoxicity of the halogenated hydroxcyquinolines. *J Am Med Assn* 1973; **225**: 395−98

Oliff A, Bleyer WA, Poplack DG. Acute-encephalopathy after initiation of cranial irradiation for meningeal leukaemia. *Lancet* 1978; **ii**: 13

Orlando RG, Dangel ME, School SF. Clinical experience and grading of amiodarone keratopathy. *Ophthalmology* 1984; **91**: 1184−8

Parkin PJ, Heirons R, McDonald WI. Bilateral optic neuritis. A long term follow up. *Brain* 1984; **107**: 951−64

Parrish DO, Todorov AB. Transient bilateral visual reduction and mydriasis after propranolol treatment. *Ann Neurol* 1981; **10**: 583

Pilley SJF, Thompson HS. Familial syndrome of diabetes insipidus, diabetes mellitus, optic atrophy and deafness (didmoad) in childhood. *Br J Ophthalmol* 1976; **60**: 294

Rizzo JF, Lessell S, Liebman S. Optic atrophy in familial dysautomonia. *Am J Ophthalmol* 1986; **102**: 463−7

Rorsman AR, Soderstrom N. Optic atrophy and juvenile diabetes mellitus with familial occurrence. *Ata Med Scand* 1967; **182**: 419−425

Rose FC, Fraser GR, Friedman AI. The association of juvenile diabetes mellitus and optic atrophy: clinical and genetic aspects. *Q J Med* 1966; **35**: 385−405

Rosenberg RN, Chutorian A. Familial opticoacoustic nerve degeneration and polyneuropathy. *Neurology* 1967; **17**: 827−32

Rosenthal AR. Ocular manifestations of leukemia: a review. *Ophthalmol* 1983; **90**: 899−905

Rosenthal AR, Egbert PR, Wilbur JR, Probert JC. Leukemic involvement of the optic nerve. *J Pediatr Ophthalmol Strabismus* 1975; **12**: 84−93

Seelenfreund MH, Gartner S, Vinger F. The ocular pathology of Menke's disease. *Arch Ophthalmol* 1968; **80**: 718−23

Sellost RG, Selhorst JB, Harbison EC. Parainfectious optic neuritis. *Arch Neurol* 1983; **40**: 347−50

Shukovsky LJ, Fletcher GH. Retinal and optic nerve complications in a high dose irradiation technique of ethmoid sinus and nasal cavity. *Radiology* 1972; **104**: 629−34

Slamovits TL, Burde RM, Klingele TG. Bilateral optic atrophy caused by chronic oral ingestion and topical application of hexachlorophene. *Am J Ophthalmol* 1980; **89**: 676−9

Smith DP. Diagnostic criteria in dominantly inherited optic juvenile optic atrophy. *Am J Ophthalmol* 1972; **49**: 183−94

Smith JL, Hoyt WF, Susac JO. Ocular fundus in acute Leber's optic neuropathy. *Arch Ophthalmol* 1973; **90**: 349

Taylor D. Ophthalmological features of some human hereditary disorders with demyelination. *Bull Soc Belge Ophthalmol* 1983; **208**: 405−13

Taylor D, Cuendet F. Optic neuritis in childhood. In: Hess RF, Plant GT (Eds) *Optic neuritis*. Cambridge University Press, Cambridge 1986, pp. 73−85

Taylor D, Ramsay J, Day S, Dillon M. Infarction of the optic nerve head in children with accelerated hypertension. *Br J Ophthalmol* 1981; **65**: 152−60

Tyrer J. A case of infantilism with goitre, diabetes mellitus, mental defect, and primary optic atrophy. *M J Aust* 1943; **II**: 398−401

Uemura A, Osame M, Nakagawa M, Nakahara K, Sameshima M, Obba N. Leber's hereditary optic neuropathy: mitochondrial and biochemical studies on muscle biopsies. *Br J Ophthalmol* 1987; **71**: 531−6

Wallace DC, Singh OG, Lott MT *et al.* Mitochondrial DNA mutation associated with Leber's hereditary optic atrophy (abstract). *Am J Hum Genet* 1988; **43**: abs. no. 0392

Weiner LP, Konigsmark BW, Stoll J, Magladery JW. Hereditary Olivopontocerebellar Atrophy with retinal degeneration. *Arch Neurol* 1967; **16**: 364−376

Wilson J, Linnell JC, Matthews DM. Plasma cobalamins in neuro-ophthalmological diseases. *Lancet* 1971; **i**: 259−61

Wray SH, Cogan DG, Kuwabara T, Schaumberg HH, Powers JM. Adrenoleukodystrophy with disease of the eye and optic nerve atrophy. *Am J Ophthalmol* 1976; **82**: 480−5

Wray SH, Kuwabara T, Sanderson P. Menke's kinky hair disease: a light and electron microscopic study of the eye. *Invest Ophthalmol Vis Sci* 1976; **15**: 128−38

Wolfram DJ. Diabetes mellitus and simple optic atrophy among siblings. Report of 4 cases. *Mayo Clin Proc* 1938; **13**: 715−8

Zee DS, Yee RD, Cogan DG, Robinson DA, Engel WK. Oculomotor abnormalities in hereditary cerebellar atazia. *Brain* 1976; **99**: 207−34

30 Chiasmal Defects

DAVID TAYLOR

Anatomy

The optic nerves and chiasm and the optic tracts extend posteriorly and upwards from the optic canals at an angle of about 45°. The anatomical relationships are not significantly different from those in the adult (Hoyt 1970). The chiasm lies in the suprasellar cystern, above the diaphragma sellae from which it is separated by several millimetres, especially posteriorly, by its oblique course. The anterior cerebral arteries and the anterior communicating arteries lie anteriorly and above the chiasm and optic nerves. The carotid arteries lie laterally with the posterior communicating artery passing underneath the optic tracts. The chiasm lies in the floor of the anterior end of the third ventricle which is above it (expansion of the third ventricle in hydrocephalus is a potent cause of visual damage from chiasmal compression). Posteriorly lies the hypothalamus and the pituitary stalk, the tuber cinerum and the mamillary bodies. The optic nerves emerge from the optic canals where they are fixed; the length of the intracranial portion of the optic nerve varies so that the position of the chiasm in relation to the tuberculum sellae and other structures is different; when the optic nerves are short the chiasm is said to be prefixed, when long it is said to be postfixed.

Development

In a human, the chiasm appears within the first month of life (Barber *et al.* 1954). The precursor of the chiasm appears as a thickening of the floor of the forebrain lying between the optic stalks at the junction of the telencephalon and the diencephalon. Retinal ganglion cells grow down the optic stalks and enter the floor of the third ventricle where they decusate to form the optic chiasm. At first there is a substantial overproduction of neurones which later die back. The lumen of the optic stalk is initially open and in communication with the forebrain cavity. It closes by the end of the second month of gestation, when it elongates and the foetal fissure is formed. Closure of the optic stalk begins distally and proceeds towards the brain. After closure, the nerve fibres fill the whole nerve. The chiasm reaches its definitive form by the fourth month of gestation.

Signs and symptoms

In all children, but in small infants especially, chiasmal disease often presents late because, especially if the process is chronic, the child compensates well and is not suspected of having poor vision until there is a substantial and bilateral visual defect. It is often only when the last remaining vision of the second eye to be affected finally snuffs out that the small child will be noticed to have poor vision by his parents.

The hallmark of chiasmal disease is the bitemporal

hemianopia. In young children, formal visual field testing is not possible but it is still vital to carry out visual field testing even by such apparently crude techniques as the ability to count fingers on either side, or the observation of a child and his response to fingers wiggling, or toys being shown to him in both sides of the visual field of one eye, since these may detect the characteristic bitemporal hemianopia. Lesions from below, usually from the pituitary gland, the surrounding bone or sometimes from the pituitary stalk, for instance craniopharyngiomas, have to grow large before signs of chiasmal compression appear. Inferior lesions compress the lower nasal fibres first and give an upper bitemporal field defect. Similarly lesions from above tend to cause initially an inferior defect. By the time a compressive lesion has caused defects there is usually gross thinning of the chiasm and the pattern of appearance of the field defects is not usually clear-cut.

In a child in whom acuity can be measured, there is often an acuity defect. Purely chiasm splitting lesions, such as trauma, do not affect acuity greatly because the nasal field and the nasal half of the fovea is not affected, but most frequently there is also involvement of the optic nerve or widespread involvement of both crossing and non-crossing fibres in the chiasm, and it is this that gives rise to the acuity defect. Most frequently one eye has a very severe acuity defect and the other is relatively spared, except for a field defect. In very chronic lesions, there is often a most impressive preservation of a high level of acuity in the face of fundoscopic evidence of a profound loss of neurones.

With widespread abnormalities or optic nerve involvement there is a significant colour vision defect. This is best tested for by pseudo-isochromatic plates though in the small child it is often difficult and only gross colour vision defects are detectable.

Stereopsis tends to remain intact in children with pure defects of the decussating fibres (Fisher 1986)

Children with chiasmal disease may present with nystagmus, especially if the onset is early in their life. The classic form of nystagmus is known as see-saw nystagmus. Most patients, however, have a less clear cut abnormality with a compound nystagmus with vertical, horizontal and rotary components. The presence of this sort of nystagmus in a child demands appropriate investigations.

Optic atrophy frequently occurs when there is substantial loss of neurones in the chiasm. Although often there is a generalized loss of neurones. Sometimes there may be a characteristic pattern due to the loss of the fibres subserving the defunct temporal

fields and the relative preservation of those fibres which subserve the intact nasal field (Fig. 30.1). These, because of the temporal retinal location of their ganglion cells, have to arch over the macula and are inserted into the upper and lower quadrants of the

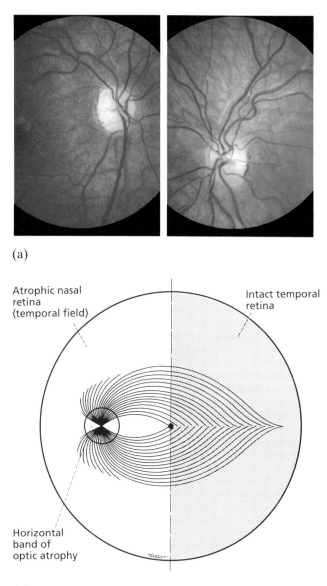

Fig. 30.1 (a) Craniopharyngioma. The right eye has bare perception of hand movements but the left has an absolute temporal hemianopia, normal colour vision and 6/5 acuity. The left optic disc shows band atrophy — there is all-round loss of the nerve fibres that subserve the defunct temporal visual field but preservation of those that subserve the intact nasal field which are inserted into the upper and lower segments of the disc. (b) shows that the origin of the band of atrophy is due to the fact that the horizontal band or bow tie area is the visible area of atrophy where temporal field fibres alone are inserted into the disc.

optic disc. In cases of developmental chiasmal defects and tumours there are often optic disc defects, for instance hypoplasia (Fig. 30.2, 30.3) or coloboma, and the presence of one of these defects should alert the practitioner to the possibility of a chiasmal defect (Taylor 1982).

Because of the proximity of the hypothalamus and pituitary gland, endocrine and growth defects may occur (Fig. 30.4). It is important, therefore, that the paediatric ophthalmologist should have available facilities for measuring and weighing a child and entering his weight and height on an appropriate chart (Fig. 30.5).

In older children there may be odd complaints of visual sensory defects that often sound rather non-organic. These may be due to the bitemporal hemianopia especially if it is absolute with intact acuity. The child may complain of things disappearing because there is a segment of blindness caused by the overlapping temporal fields further away than the point of regard in which objects are not seen. Similarly, the intact nasal fields abut one another and because there are no corresponding retinal points there is little to keep the two together so they may complain of things sliding in their vision (Nachtigaller & Hoyt 1970).

Developmental defects

Unilateral anophthalmos produces an asymmetrical chiasm and bilateral anophthalmos is usually associated with absence of optic nerves, chiasm and lateral geniculate bodies (Recordon 1936; Haberland 1969;

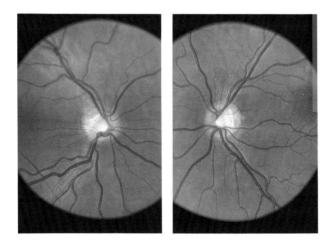

Fig. 30.2 Craniopharyngioma. Bilateral segmental hypoplasia or 'tilted' optic disc. Bitemporal hemianopia with 6/5 acuity right eye (−4.0) 6/4 left (−4.50).

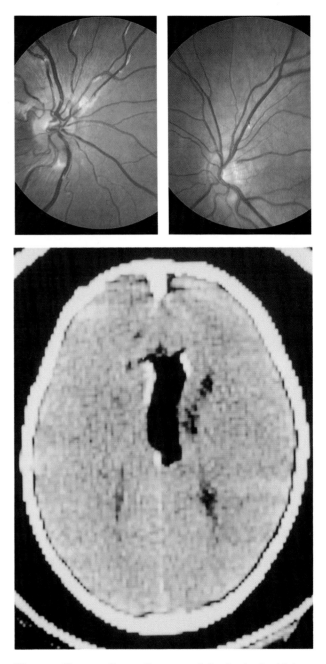

Fig. 30.3 Corpus callosum lipoma, and dysplastic tilted left optic disc in a patient with midline facial defect.

Penner 1976). Sometimes there are remnants of the optic nerve and chiasm (Cagianut 1976). Bilateral optic nerve aplasia is also associated with an absent chiasm.

A chiasmal spur is an anomaly found incidentally at postmortem (Ellis *et al.* 1900). The significance of this anomaly, which consists of a spur projecting anteriorly between the two optic nerves, is not known but the above authors speculated that it may represent the

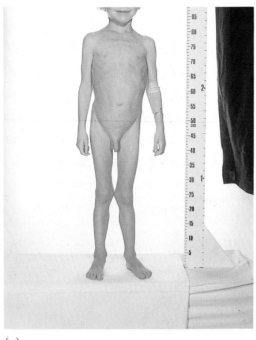

(a)

Fig. 30.4 (a) Chiasmal glioma. This boy presented with poor vision and recent weight loss. Photograph on 12.2.1973.

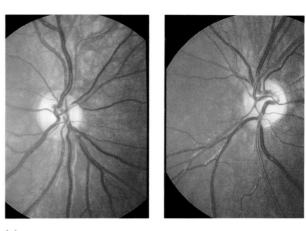

(c)

Fig. 30.4 (b) Photograph on 31.1.1974 showing rapid growth in weight and height. Weight and growth rate fluctuation are common in chiasmal glioma. (c) Bilateral band atrophy. (Same patient a–c.)

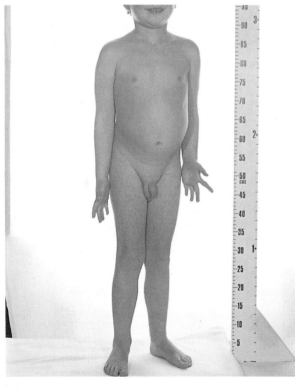

(b)

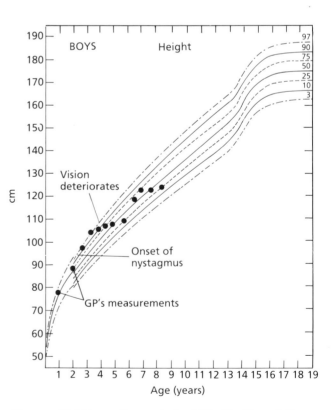

Fig. 30.5 Height growth record of a child with chiasmal glioma showing height growth rate fluctuation. Paediatric ophthalmology clinics need to have these charts available.

fibres that would have made up the anterior knee of von Willebrand.

Chiasmal anomalies as evidenced by clinical findings or by abnormalities on CT scanning have been described in patients with midline defects (Fig. 30.6), for instance septo-optic dysplasia, or mid-facial defects, or basal encephalocoeles. The chiasm may be abnormal in the various midline facial and skull clefting syndromes that are associated with hypertelorism which may also have midline brain anomalies.

A condition of isolated maldevelopment of the anterior visual pathways occurs as the association of an anomalous optic disc with evidence of a chiasmal defect, for instance a bitemporal hemianopia, in otherwise normal people (Taylor 1983).

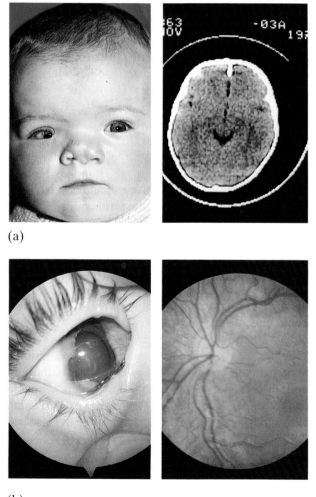

(a)

(b)

Fig. 30.6 (a) Minor midline facial defect with small intracranial lipoma. (b) Left eye has marginally small optic disc. The right eye has iris coloboma, cataract and optic nerve hypoplasia. (Same patient.)

Trauma

Occasionally, following closed head trauma, the child develops a bitemporal hemianopia often associated with other vision defects, together with defects resulting from damage to surrounding structures which may lead to diabetes insipidus, anosmia, CSF rhinorrhoea, growth defects, and mood changes.

Tumours

Chiasmal glioma

Chiasmal glioma, optic nerve glioma, and hypothalamic glioma are closely related tumours, often one indistinguishable from the other and showing common histopathological features and clinical behaviour. All occur with increased frequency in neurofibromatosis and up to a half of patients with chiasmal or optic glioma have this disease (Imes & Hoyt 1986).

Children with chiasmal glioma present in a variety of ways. Small children often present with a compound nystagmus and typically this is see-saw in nature (see Chapter 41). But any child with a compound nystagmus with rotary, vertical and horizontal elements should be suspected of having a chiasmal lesion (Schulman *et al.* 1979). Visual loss is often profound before its presence is noticed by parents of young children but in older children the visual defect may be noticed by the child himself or detected by preschool or school visual testing. Some optic gliomas may be large without gross visual defect (Goodman *et al.* 1975). Chiasmal glioma may reveal itself by its effects on growth and development. An unusual presentation is that of head bobble — the bobble headed doll syndrome (see Chapter 43) — this is usually an indication that the child also has hydrocephalus.

The diagnosis can be made easier by visual field testing or by visual field analysis on visual evoked cortical potential testing. Plain X-rays are seldom used now but the classical finding is an expanded and pear-shaped sella turcica, with chronic bone changes and without calcification. Often one or both optic foramina are enlarged, especially if there is an optic nerve component to the tumour. CT scanning (Figs 30.7, 30.8) (Fletcher *et al.* 1986) shows three diagnostic patterns.

1 A tube-like thickening of optic nerve and chiasm.
2 A suprasellar tumour with contiguous optic nerve expansion.
3 A suprasellar tumour with optic tract involvement.

Cystic or 'globular' suprasellar tumours are not

be profound (Figs 30.10, 30.11). The diagnosis is made by CT or MRI scanning (Fig. 30.10). Calcification occurs in virtually every case in childhood and the tumours are often cystic. Pre- and postoperative endocrine assessment and management is essential. The tumours are usually treated by surgery with or without radiotherapy, total removal is occasionally possible.

Dysgerminoma

The clinical clue to the presence of a dysgerminoma is when diabetes insipidus is the main symptom at presentation together with other chiasmal defects, including acuity and visual field loss and hypothalamic or pituitary disturbances. The tumours are often not large (Takeuchi *et al.* 1978) and occur in older children or young adults (Carmins & Mount 1977).

Other chiasmal tumours

These include arachnoid cysts, ependymomas, epidermoid tumours, leukaemic deposits, ectopic pinaelomas and pituitary gland tumours. These are all rare and do not usually have specific presenting features (Till 1975), but their radiological and associated clinical features together may be suggestive of the underlying pathology.

Granulomas and chronic inflammatory disorders

The chiasm and surrounding structures may be involved in abnormalities of the skull base as in histiocytosis X (see Chapter 22.4), in particular the Hand−Schuller−Christian variant of this condition, which tends to present with diabetes insipidus and visual defects. Sarcoidosis, juvenile xanthogranulomata and pseudotumours similar to those found in adults with the Tolosa−Hunt syndrome may also affect the chiasmal area.

Infections

Tuberculous meningitis, hydatid disease, and cysticercosis together with fungal disorders (especially in debilitated, immunodeficient children, or those affected by AIDS) may all affect the suprasellar cystern with damage to the chiasm and surrounding structures.

Third ventricle distention

In hydrocephalic patients, distention of the third ventricle may cause chiasmal damage and bitemporal or more widespread visual field defects (Sinclair 1931) with sometimes profound vision loss due to stretching or compression of the optic nerves and chiasm to which may be added cortical blindness from posterior cerebral artery stretching and distortion. The exact mechanisms of these defects are not certain but their occurrence due to a distended ventricle is not significantly in doubt. A unilateral visual defect has been described due to compression of one optic nerve against the internal carotid artery (Calogero & Alexander 1971).

Vascular anomalies

Aneurysm is an extremely rare cause of chiasmal defects in children and does not produce specific symptoms or signs. Angiomas of the optic chiasm are also rare and produce symptoms by recurrent haemorrhages (Fermaglich *et al.* 1978). Spontaneous haematomata of the optic chiasm have also been described (Riishede & Seedorff 1974). Perhaps the so-called spontaneous haematoma is related to a pre-existing angiomatous defect.

Empty sella syndrome

When the diaphragma sellae is defective and cerebrospinal fluid is found in the pituitary fossa on a CT scan, this is known as the empty sella syndrome. This may occur for no apparent reason or be associated with surgery, radiotherapy or the presence of an arachnoid cyst. Chiasmal visual field defects occasionally occur and rarely the visual defect may be substantial. Many cases follow hydrocephalus or benign intracranial hypertension.

References

Anderson DR, Spencer. Ultrastructural and histochemical observations of optic nerve gliomas. *Arch Ophthalmol* 1970; **83** 324−38

Barber AN, Ronstrom GN, Muelling RH. Development of the visual pathway; optic chiasm AMA. *Arch Ophthalmol* 1954; **52**: 447−56

Borit A, Richardson EP. The biological and clinical behaviour of pilocytic astrocytomas of the optic pathways. *Brain* 1982; **105**: 161−88

Brand WN, Hoover SV. Optic glioma in children review of 16 cases given megavoltage radiation therapy. *Child's Brain*

1979; **5**: 459–66

Cagianut B, Theiler K. Zur aplaise der sehnerven. *Graefes Arch Klin Exp Ophthalmol* 1076; **200**: 93–8

Calogero JA, Alexander E. Unilateral amaurosis in a hydrocephalic child with an obstructed shunt. *J Neurosurg* 1971; **34**: 236–8

Carmins AB, Mount LA. Primary suprasellar atypical teratoma. *Brain* 1974; **97**: 447–62

Ellis HA, Parish DJ, Hughes B. The chiasmal spur: an anomaly of the human optic chiasm. *J Path Bact* 1900; **81**: 529–32

Fermaglich J, Kattah J, Manz H. Venous angioma of the optic chiasm. *Ann Neurol* 1978; **4**: 470–1

Fisher N. The optic chiasm and the corpus collosum: their relationship to binocular vision. *J Pediatr Ophthalmol Strabismus* 1986; **23**: 126–31

Fletcher WA, Imes RK, Hoyt WF. Chiasmal gliomas: appearance and long-term changes demonstrated by computerized tomography. *J Neurosurg* 1986; **65**: 154–9

Glaser JS, Hoyt WF, Corbett J. Visual morbidity with chiasmal glioma. *Arch Ophthalmol* 1971; **85**: 3–12

Goodman SJ, Rosenbaum AL, Hasso A, Itabashi H. Large optic nerve glioma with normal vision. *Arch Ophthalmol* 1975; **93**: 991–5

Haberland O, Perou M. Primary bilateral anophthalmia. *J Neuropath Exp Neurol* 1969; **28**: 337–51

Holman RE, Grimson BS, Drayer BP, Buckley EG, Brennan MW. Magnetic resonance imaging of optic gliomas. *Am J Ophthalmol* 1985; **100**: 596–601

Hoyt WF. Correlative functional anatomy of the optic chiasm. *Clin Neurosurg* 1970; **17**: 189–202

Hoyt WF, Baghdassarian SB Optic glioma of childhood. *Br J Ophthalmol* 1969; **53**: 793–8

Imes RK, Hoyt WF. Childhood chiasmal gliomas: update on the fate of patients in the 1969 San Francisco study. *Br J Ophthalmol* 1986; **70**: 179–82

MacCarty CS, Boyd AS, Childs DS. Tumours of the optic nerve and optic chiasm. *J Neurosurg* 1970; **33**: 439–44

Nachtigaller H, Hoyt WF. Storungen des Seheindruckes bei bitemporaler Hemianopsie und verscheibung der Schachsen. *Klin Monatsbl Augenheilkd* 1970; **156**: 821–32

Penner H, Schlach HG. Anophthalmie und begleitende fehibildungen. *Klin Paditr* 1976; **188**: 320–30

Recordon E, Griffiths GM. A case of primary bilateral anophthalmia. *Br J Ophthalmol* 1936; **22**: 353–60

Riishede J, Seedorff HH. Spontaneous haematoma of the optic chiasma. *Acta Ophthalmol* 1974; **52**: 317–22

Roberson C, Till K. Hypothalamic gliomas in children. *J Neurol, Neurosurg Psychiatr* 1974; **30**: 1047–52

Rush JA, Younge BR, Campbell RJ, MacCarty CS. Optic glioma: long term follow up of 85 histopathologically verified cases. *Ophthalmology* 1982; **89**: 1213–9

Schulman JA, Shults WT, McAndrew Jones J. Monocular vertical nystagmus as an initial sign of chiasmal glioma. *Am J Ophthalmol* 1979; **87**: 87–9

Sinclair AHH, Doff NM. Hydrocephalus simulating tumour in the production of chiasmal and other parahypophyseal lesions. *Trans Ophthalmol Soc UK* 1931; **51**: 232–40

Takeuchi J, Handa H, Nagata I. Suprasellar germinoma. *J Neurosurg* 1978; **49**: 41–8

Taylor D. Congenital tumours of the anterior visual system with dysplasia of the optic discs. *Br J Ophthalmol* 1982; **66**: 455–63

Taylor D. Chiasmal disease in young children. In: Wybar KC, Taylor D (Eds.) *Paediatric Ophthalmology — Current Aspects*. Dekker, New York 1983 pp. 255–65

Till K. *Paediatric Neurosurgery for Paediatricians and Neurosurgeons*. Blackwell Scientific Publications, Oxford 1975

31 Hydrocephalus

ANTHONY MOORE

Hydrocephalus is a condition in which there is enlargement of the cerebral ventricles secondary to an imbalance between production and reabsorption of cerebrospinal fluid (CSF). CSF is produced mainly by the choroid plexus of the cerebral ventricles and then passes through the ventricular system to reach the subarachnoid space. Reabsorption into the vascular circulation occurs via the arachnoid villi. Hypersecretion is rare and most cases of communicating hydrocephalus are due to impaired reabsorption. In non-communicating hydrocephalus the obstruction to the CSF circulation occurs within the ventricular system and the ventricles proximal to the level of the block are dilated. In communicating hydrocephalus reabsorption of CSF from the subarachnoid space is impaired. Arrested hydrocephalus is a term used to describe a condition in which the hydrocephalic process has stopped spontaneously and although there may be some residual clinical signs, such as enlarged head size, the condition is non-progressive. Normal pressure hydrocephalus, in which there are signs of progressive hydrocephalus with normal CSF pressure, is usually unilateral in childhood, but may be a challenging problem (Stein *et al.* 1971) requiring intracranial pressure monitoring.

Aetiology

Hydrocephalus may be congenital or acquired. It is one of the most frequent congenital abnormalities of the central nervous system and is usually associated with a structural CNS abnormality (Table 31.1). Congenital hydrocephalus is a common complication of spina bifida. Acquired hydrocephalus may follow meningitis, intracranial haemorrhage or tumour and intra-uterine infections such as toxoplasmosis (Fig. 31.1) and cytomegalovirus. Recently there has been a great increase in the incidence of hydrocephalus associated with prematurity with intracranial complications especially intraventricular haemorrhage. In some neurosurgical centres this is now the most common cause for referral of hydrocephalic patients to the centre.

Clinical features

The clinical presentation of hydrocephalus depends on the age of the child and whether the raised intracranial pressure has an acute or more gradual onset.

Table 31.1 Aetiology of hydrocephalus.

Congenital
Aqueduct stenosis
Arnold–Chiari malformation
Dandy–Walker syndrome
Porencephalic cysts
Arachnoid cysts
Acquired
Meningitis
Intracranial haemorrhage
Tumours
Intra-uterine infection

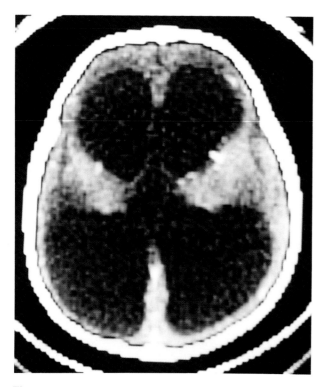

Fig. 31.1 Toxoplasmosis with hydrocephalus. Note the periventricular calcification.

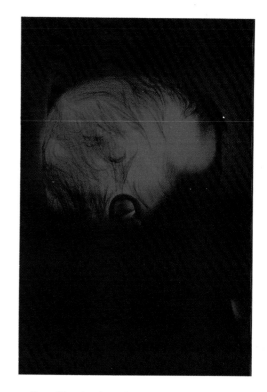

Fig. 31.2 Transillumination of the skull in severe hydrocephalus.

In infants in whom the cranial sutures have not closed, there is a progressive increase in skull growth with separation of the sutures. The fontanelle is tense and scalp veins are dilated due to compression of the cortical veins and sinuses. If the ventricles are greatly enlarged and the cerebral mantle sufficiently thin, the skull may transilluminate (Fig. 31.2). In addition the infant will be irritable and may show signs of failure to thrive or developmental delay. Papilloedema is said to be uncommon in infantile hydrocephalus but the 'setting sun sign' (Fig. 31.3), where the lids are retracted and both eyes deviate downwards in the presence of an up-gaze paresis, is only seen in infants.

In later childhood the usual presentation is with symptoms and signs of raised intracranial pressure, either with an acute or chronic onset. Bilateral papilloedema is usually present and there may be unilateral or bilateral VIth nerve paresis.

Management

There have been two major advances in the management of childhood hydrocephalus in recent years. Firstly the advent of the CT scan (Fig. 31.4) has greatly simplified the investigation of these children and allowed the site and cause of the obstruction to

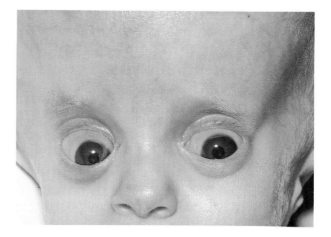

Fig. 31.3 Setting sun sign. This consists of downward deviation of the eyes, an upgaze palsy, and lid retraction.

be easily identified. Furthermore, repeat scans after surgery allow the size of the cerebral ventricles to be monitored radiologically without the need for more invasive techniques. The second advance has been the introduction of valves such as the Spitz–Holter and Pudenz which are designed to give unidirectional flow of CSF from the ventricles into the vascular system (usually the right atrium) or peritoneal cavity

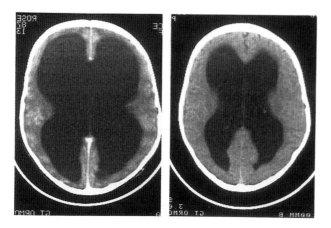

Fig. 31.4 Hydrocephalus. On the left the ventricles are huge with a thin cortical mantle. On the right is the same child after shunting.

(Figs. 31.5, 31.6). Such CSF shunt procedures have greatly improved the prognosis in hydrocephalus but are still subject to complications such as infection or shunt malfunction, necessitating further surgical revision.

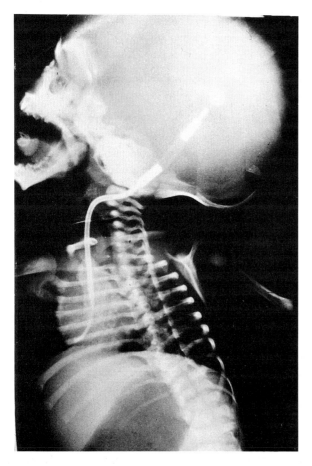

Fig. 31.5 X-ray of a ventriculo-atrial shunt system *in situ*.

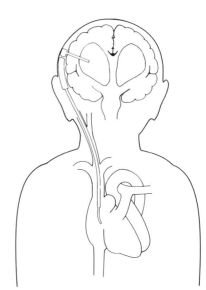

Fig. 31.6 Diagram of shunt system. The valve which can be pumped lies against the skull.

Ocular complications of hydrocephalus

Raised intracranial pressure in hydrocephalus may result in damage to the visual pathway and visual loss may follow optic atrophy or cortical damage (Arroyo *et al*. 1985). Disturbances of ocular motility such as gaze palsies, nystagmus and strabismus are common (Rabinowitz 1974; Rabinowitz & Walker 1975).

Optic nerve

PAPILLOEDEMA

Papilloedema is said to be uncommon in infantile hydrocephalus as the skull is still able to expand but there have been few studies of optic nerve change in this young age group. Ghose (1983) reviewed the optic nerve changes in 200 consecutive cases of congenital hydrocephalus examined before shunt surgery. The optic disc was normal in 56%, optic atrophy was present in 29% and 5.5% had papilloedema. A further 7% had incipient or suspected papilloedema. This study suggests that optic disc oedema is commoner than previously thought in infantile hydrocephalus.

In older children with acquired hydrocephalus or shunt malfunction marked papilloedema is common.

OPTIC ATROPHY

Optic atrophy is common in all forms of hydrocephalus and is a major cause of visual morbidity. Ghose (1983) found that 17% of infants with hydrocephalus had optic atrophy and a further 11% had temporal pallor of the optic disc before shunt surgery. Rabinowitz (1974) reported that 30% of children in his study had optic atrophy. Such children are especially vulnerable to further episodes of raised intracranial pressure which may result in visual loss from damage to an already compromised optic disc. They present further problems in assessment as raised intracranial pressure may not result in optic disc swelling in the presence of atrophy and the diagnosis of shunt malfunction may be more difficult.

Optic atrophy complicating hydrocephalus may result from several mechanisms (Table 31.2). Raised intracranial pressure may result in arterial compression (Lindenberg 1955) and ischaemia of the optic nerve. Shift of the brain stem following shunt surgery may cause traction on the optic nerves and chiasm (Emery & Levick 1966) and optic atrophy may also follow optic nerve (Calgero & Alexander 1977) or chiasmal compression by an enlarged IIIrd ventricle (Tamler 1964; Osher *et al.* 1978; Humphrey *et al.* 1982). Optic atrophy may also develop secondary to longstanding papilloedema. It is also possible in young infants that optic atrophy may follow retrograde transsynaptic neuronal degeneration in the visual pathway secondary to damage to the visual cortex.

Chiasmal disorders

The close anatomical relationship between the third ventricle and the optic chiasm means that the optic chiasm may be distorted by a pathologically enlarged third ventricle. Most cases with evidence of chiasmal dysfunction in hydrocephalus have aqueduct stenosis. Chiasmal compression may result in optic atrophy (Osher *et al.* 1978; Humphrey *et al.* 1982) and field defects including bilateral central scotoma or bitemporal hemianopia (Humphrey 1982). There may be some improvement in visual acuity and fields after a shunt procedure.

Visual cortical abnormalities

Bilateral visual loss or homonymous hemianopic field defects may result from ischaemic damage to the visual cortex in hydrocephalus (Smith *et al.* 1966; Lorber 1967; Arroyo 1985). The mechanism of the visual loss is uncertain but may be related to compression of the posterior cerebral arteries at the edge of the tentorium cerebelli (Lindenberg 1955; Arroyo *et al.* 1985). Visual loss may be associated with shunt

Table 31.2 Causes of optic atrophy in hydrocephalus.

Optic nerve ischaemia
Optic nerve or chiasmal traction
Chiasmal compression
Consecutive optic atrophy
Trans-synaptic neuronal degeneration

malfunction or shunt infections and cortical blindness is usually seen in children who have had multiple shunt revisions (Lawton Smith 1966) often bilaterally. The visual loss may be reversible in some cases if prompt treatment is given (Lorber 1967). Such children may have associated optic atrophy, but the presence of normal pupil reactions and visual loss out of proportion to the degree of optic atrophy allow a diagnosis of cortical blindness to be made. Visual evoked potential measurements and CT scan are helpful in confirming the diagnosis.

Ocular motor abnormalities

The common disorders of ocular motility seen in hydrocephalus are strabismus, supranuclear gaze palsies, and nystagmus.

STRABISMUS

Strabismus is the commonest ocular complication of hydrocephalus occurring in 60–75% of patients (Clements & Kaushal 1970; Rothstein *et al.* 1974; Rabinowitz & Walker 1975). Most have horizontal deviations with esotropia being four times commoner than exotropia (Rabinowitz 1974).

Esotropia

The esotropia may be incomitant or concomitant. Incomitant deviations may follow unilateral or bilateral VIth nerve palsy. The VIth nerve is especially vulnerable to episodes of raised intracranial pressure. Usually a full recovery of function occurs after shunt surgery and corrective squint surgery is rarely necessary.

Most patients with hydrocephalus have concomitant esotropia (Clements & Kaushal 1970; Rabinowitz 1974; France 1975). There is a high incidence of 'A' pattern deviations (France 1975; Rabinowitz & Walker 1975) which in half the cases is associated with bilateral superior oblique overaction (Fig. 31.7). The strabismus is usually alternating and amblyopia is uncommon. The mechanism of the development of

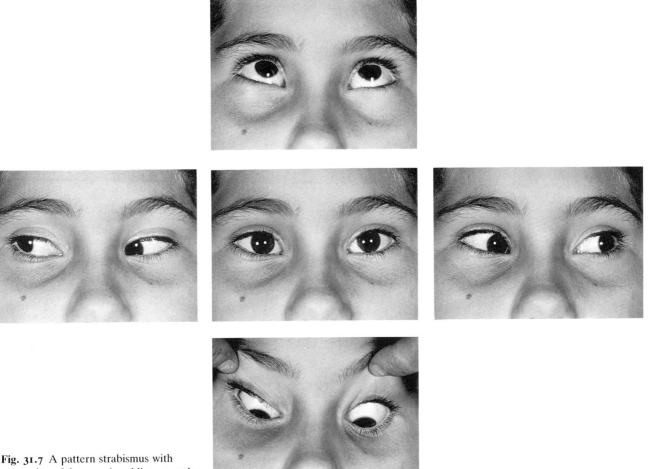

Fig. 31.7 A pattern strabismus with overaction of the superior oblique muscles in a patient with hydrocephalus.

comitant squint in hydrocephalus is uncertain. Wybar (1976) has suggested that the high incidence of strabismus is related to unilateral or bilateral VIth nerve palsies in early childhood and that with time the squint becomes more comitant. However only a minority of infants with hydrocephalus have recognizable lateral rectus palsies (France 1975; Rabinowitz & Walker 1975) and the relative frequency of associated superior oblique overaction suggests that additional factors may be important.

Most children with concomitant esotropia will ultimately require surgical correction. A careful search should be made for an associated 'A' phenomenon before planning surgery. In the absence of an 'A' pattern conventional horizontal surgery is performed but if present the type of surgery depends on whether or not there is associated superior oblique overaction. When this is present horizontal surgery is combined with bilateral superior oblique posterior tenotomies. In the absence of superior oblique over-

action the horizontal surgery is combined with vertical displacement of the horizontal recti, the medial rectus being moved upwards one insertion width and the lateral rectus moved down by a similar amount.

Exotropia

Exotropia in hydrocephalus is usually associated with severe bilateral visual loss and optic atrophy or follows surgical overcorrection of an esotropia (Rabinowitz & Walker 1975). Rarely it may be associated with a IIIrd nerve palsy (Rabinowitz & Walker 1975; France 1975).

Vertical deviations

Vertical deviations are rarely seen in hydrocephalus and when present are associated with a IIIrd nerve palsy or skew deviation (Rabinowitz & Walker 1975).

Gaze palsies

In uncontrolled hydrocephalus two distinct types of vertical gaze palsies may be seen (Swash 1976). In young infants the so-called 'setting sun' sign with bilateral upper lid retraction and downward deviation of the eyes and a vertical gaze palsy affecting both saccadic and pursuit systems is seen (see Fig. 31.3). It is a poor prognostic sign and is often accompanied by visual loss and severe optic atrophy (Rabinowitz 1974). It usually completely resolves following shunt surgery.

In older children with later onset of hydrocephalus or shunt malfunction, a different clinical picture is seen. Episodes of raised intracranial pressure may result in the Sylvian aqueduct (Parinaud's) syndrome with impaired upgaze, light-near dissociation of the pupils, and convergence retraction nystagmus (Shallat *et al.* 1973; Swash 1976; Osher *et al.* 1978). The ocular motor abnormalities usually resolve after shunt surgery but may reappear during shunt malfunction (Shallat *et al.* 1973).

Disorders of vertical gaze in hydrocephalus occur more frequently in aqueduct stenosis than in other forms of non-communicating hydrocephalus (Swash 1976) and are rarely seen in communicating hydrocephalus. There is a close anatomical relationship between the vertical gaze centres of the midbrain and the Sylvian aqueduct and third ventricle. Acquired Sylvian aqueduct syndrome is thought to result from distortion of the periaqueductal structures by an enlarged rostral aqueduct and dilated suprapineal recess of the third ventricle (Swash 1976). The 'setting sun' sign on the other hand is thought to be caused by pressure on the decussating fibres in the posterior commissure by an enlarged third ventricle. In each case decompression of the third ventricle will usually result in recovery of normal vertical gaze.

Horizontal gaze palsies are rarely seen in hydrocephalus, but patients with the Arnold—Chiari malformation may develop internuclear ophthalmoplegia (Woody & Reynolds 1985).

Another rare abnormality seen in hydrocephalus is the bobble headed doll syndrome (Kirkham 1977). In this condition there are flexion—extension movements of the head and neck on the trunk at a rate of about 2—3/second. The condition is almost always associated with a hugely enlarged IIIrd ventricle caused by tumour and usually resolves after shunt surgery (Table 31.3).

Table 31.3 Complications of an enlarged IIIrd ventricle.

Optic nerve compression (Calgero 1971)
Chiasmal syndrome (Tamler 1964; Humphreys *et al.* 1982)
Parinaud's syndrome (Shallat *et al.* 1973; Swash 1976; Osher *et al.* 1978)
Setting sun sign (Swash 1976)
Bobble-headed-doll syndrome (Kirkham 1977)

Nystagmus

Nystagmus in hydrocephalus may have a variety of causes. Pendular nystagmus may follow bilateral visual loss from optic atrophy and gaze evoked nystagmus may be associated with a recovering VIth nerve palsy. Children with hydrocephalus and associated posterior fossa abnormalities may develop nystagmus secondary to cerebellar dysfunction. Downbeat nystagmus is seen in the Arnold—Chiari malformation but has also been reported in hydrocephalus complicating intracranial haemorrhage (Phadke *et al.* 1981).

Advice for parents

The ophthalmologist should warn the parents of a newly diagnosed child with hydrocephalus that, although most children with the disease have only few problems, all are at risk of losing vision and developing squints. Any squint that appears gradually — say over a period of weeks, should be seen promptly by an ophthalmologist and any squint appearing over a period of days or less should be seen immediately by an ophthalmologist or neurosurgeon because it may herald a blocked shunt, especially if accompanied by headache, nausea, vomiting and, in the smaller child, misery. Visual symptoms should prompt immediate referral to an ophthalmologist.

Summary

Children with hydrocephalus who have had shunt surgery should, where possible, be followed-up by both neurosurgeon and ophthalmologist. In the older child a regular assessment of visual acuity, visual fields, colour vision, and optic discs should be performed so that an episode of raised intracranial pressure associated with shunt malfunction is detected early. This is especially important in children with optic atrophy who may not develop papilloedema and in whom the discs are vulnerable to further episodes of raised intracranial pressure. Infants with blocked shunts may also fail to develop papilloedema but may show signs of reduced vision, poor pupillary reactions, or vertical gaze palsy.

Children with hydrocephalus may lose vision from optic atrophy, chiasmal compression or damage to the visual cortex. Although blindness is not common in this condition, the relative frequency of childhood hydrocephalus means that it is a significant cause of visual handicap.

References

Arroyo H, Jan J, McCormick A, Farrel K. Permanent visual loss after shunt malfunction. *Neurology* 1985; **35**: 25–9

Calgero JA, Alexander E. Unilateral amaurosis in a hydrocephalic child with an obstructed shunt. *J Neurosurg* 1971; **34**: 236–40

Clements DB, Kaushal K. A study of the ocular complications of hydrocephalus and myelomeningocele. *Trans Ophthalmol Soc UK* 1970; **90**: 383–90

Emery JL, Levick RK. The movement of the brain stem and vessels around the brain stem in children with hydrocephalus and the Arnold–Chiari deformity. *Ann Radiol (Paris)* 1966; **314**: 141–7

France TJ. The association of 'A' pattern strabismus with hydrocephalus. In: Moore S, Mein J, Stockbridge L (Eds.) Transactions of the Third International Orthoptic Congress 1975; Symposia Specialists, Miami pp. 287–292.

Ghose S. Optic nerve changes in hydrocephalus. *Trans Ophthalmol Soc UK* 1983; **103**: 217–20

Humphrey PRD, Moseley IF, Ross Russell RW. Visual field defects in obstructive hydrocephalus. *J Neurol Neurosurg Psychiatr* 1982; **45**: 251–5

Kirkham TA. Optic atrophy in the Bobble headed doll syndrome. *J Paediatr Ophthalmol* 1977; **14**: 199–301

Lindenberg R. Compresion of brain arteries as a pathogenetic factor for tissue necrosis and their areas of predilation.

J Neuropathol Exp Neurol 1955; **14**: 223–43

Lorber J. Recovery of vision following prolonged blindness in children with hydrocephalus or following pyogenic meningitis. *Clin Pediatr* 1967; **6**: 699–703

Osher RH, Corbett JJ, Schatz NJ. Neuro-ophthalmological complications of enlargement of the IIIrd ventricle. *Br J Ophthalmol* 1978; **62**: 536–42

Phadke JG, Hern JEC, Blaiklock CT. Downbeat nystagmus as a false localising sign due to communicating hydrocephalus (letter). *J Neurol Neurosurg Psychiatr* 1981; **41**: 45a

Rabinowitz IM. Visual function in children with hydrocephalus. *Trans Ophthalmol Soc UK* 1974; **94**: 353–65

Rabinowitz IM, Walker JW. Disorders of ocular motility in children with hydrocephalus. In: Moore, S, Mein J, Stockbridge L (Eds.) Transactions of the Third International Orthoptic Congress 1975; Symposia Specialists, Miami pp. 279–286

Rothstein TB, Romano PE, Shoch D. Myelomeningocele. *Am J Ophthalmol* 1974; **77**: 690–3

Shallat RF, Paul RP, Jerva MJ. Significance of upward gaze palsy (Parinaud's syndrome) in hydrocephalus due to shunt malfunction. *J Neurosurg* 1973; **38**: 717–21

Smith JL, Walsh HTJ, Shipley T. Cortical blindness in congenital hydrocephalus. *Am J Ophthalmol* 1966; **62**: 251–5

Stein BM, Fraser RA, Tenner MS. Normal pressure hydrocephalus – complication of posterior fossa surgery in children. *Pediatrics* 1971; **49**: 50–7

Swash M. Disorders of ocular movement in hydrocephalus. *Proc R Soc Med* 1976; **69**: 480–4

Tamler E. Primary optic atrophy from acquired dilatation of the third ventricle. *Am J Ophthalmol* 1964; **57**: 827–8

Woody RC, Reynolds JD. Association of bilateral internuclear ophthalmoplegia and myelomeningocoele with Arnold–Chiari malformation type II. *J Clin Neuro ophthalmol* 1985; **5**: 124–6

Wybar K. Disorders of ocular motility in hydrocephalus in early childhood. In: Fells P (Ed.) Second Congress of International Strabismological Association 1976; pp. 366–70

32 Brain Problems

SCOTT LAMBERT AND CREIG HOYT

Disorders affecting the posterior visual pathway

Developmental and structural defects

The congenital abnormalities which affect the posterior visual pathway are best understood in the context of the developmental stages in which they occur. During the first month of embryogenesis, a neural plate is formed which invaginates into the neural groove and then fuses into a neural tube. A disturbance of the rostral closure of the neural groove often results in occipital encephaloceles. 75–80% of encephaloceles occur in the occipital region. They are usually filled with portions of the occipital lobe.

During the second month of gestation, the forebrain or prosencephalon is cleaved transversely into the telencephalon and diencephalon and sagitally into the cerebral hemispheres and lateral ventricles. Derangements in these cleavage processes may result in holoprosencephaly which is characterized by a single cerebral structure with a common ventricle. Since the face and optic vessicles are formed during the same developmental period, holoprosencephaly is often associated with facial and ocular anomalies. Optic nerve anomalies, in particular, are frequently associated with holoprosencephaly.

Between the second and fourth gestational months,

the neurones in the ventricular and subventricular zones proliferate and then migrate to the cortical plates. While neurons early in embryogenesis migrate relatively short distances, neurons later in development often migrate long distances across the intermediate zones. Their migration may be facilitated by radial glial cells which appear to serve as guidelines (Rakic 1972). The neurons arriving first in the cortical mantle assume the deepest locations, while neurons arriving later assume a more superficial location.

Aberrations in neuronal migration may result in a variety of neural abnormalities. Lissencephaly (smooth brain) occurs when neurons end their migration in the intermediate zone, resulting in an absence of cortical gyri. Pachygyria is related to lissencephaly, but develops when neuronal migration is disturbed at a later stage; it is characterized by reduced numbers of gyri, abnormally thick cortex and fewer cortical neurons than normal. Polymicrogyria may occur secondary to an even later neuronal migratory disturbance. The gyri are unusually small with a reduced number of cortical layers and a primitive orientation to the neurons. Neuronal heterotopias (ectopic grey matter) are collections of neurons in subcortical white matter; they are a common accompaniment of severe neuronal migratory disorders and also may be found as an incidental finding during autopsies. Their significance is unclear in most cases. Infants with lissencephaly and pachygyria frequently die during infancy and have severe neurological abnormalities including seizures and hypotonia. While children with generalized polymicrogyria are frequently neurologically handicapped, those with focal polymicrogyria will often have only seizures or isolated functional abnormalities. Polymicrogyria localized to the striate cortex may result in homonymous hemianopias, often with incongruous margins not honouring the vertical midline (Hoyt 1985). Polymicrogyria, as well as neuronal ectopias and dysplasias, are also frequently found in the inferior frontal and superior temporal regions of the left hemisphere in dyslexic subjects (Galaburda et al. 1985; Geschwind & Galaburda 1985). Historically,

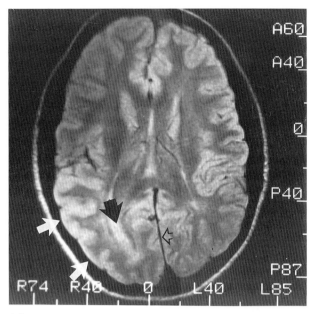

(a)

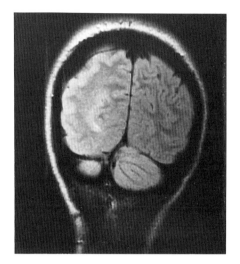

(b)

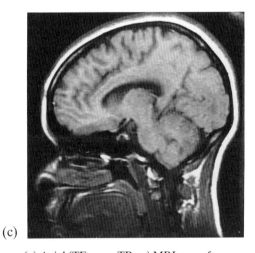

(c)

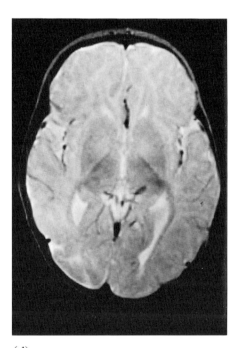

(d)

Fig. 32.1 (a) Axial (TE 2000, TR 35) MRI scan of a 23-year-old woman with a seizure disorder and right occipital polymicrogyri. The visual acuity and fields were normal. The polymicrogyri involve the right occipital lobe laterally (white arrows) but spare the visual cortex medially (open arrow). The white matter in the right occipital lobe is also dysplastic (black arrow). (b) Coronal (TR 2000, TE 35) MRI scan of the same patient. There are polymicrogyri in the right occipital lobe laterally and an absence of normal cortical gyri. The visual cortex medially is normal. (c) Sagittal T1 weighted (TR 400, TE 20) MRI scan of the same patient. The polymicrogyri of the right occipital lobe may be clearly distinguished from the normal cortical gyrations and sulci of the frontal lobe. (d) A 9-month-old child noted to have visual inattention to the left at 6 weeks of age by mother . At 9 months of age the hemianopia was more difficult to detect clinically, but visual evoked potentials recorded from the two hemispheres were grossly asymmetrical. MRI scan shows hypoplasia of the right occipital lobe. The child was the product of a full-term uncomplicated pregnancy and delivery. She is developmentally normal otherwise.

focal cortical gyral anomalies were only identified intraoperatively or at postmortem. In some instances they may now be imaged by high resolution magnetic resonance scanning (Tychsen & Hoyt 1985) (Fig. 32.1.)

The fetal brain responds quite differently to injuries compared with the neonatal or adult brain. Injuries to the brain during foetal development cause total dissolution of the affected parenchyma, often with well circumscribed borders. Insults early in foetal development may result in loss of portions of the brain or schizencephaly, whereas insults later in foetal development result in porencephalic cysts. In contradistinction, full-term infants and children develop encephalomalacia and gliosis after injuries. Schizencephaly and porencephaly may affect large portions of the brain, or only limited regions such as the occipital lobes. The distribution of porencephalic cysts often correspond to a territory perfused by one of the major cerebral vessels suggesting a vascular aetiology (Fig. 32.2).

Occasionally only the occipital horns of the lateral ventricles are dilated with an attendant thinning of the occipital cortex known as colpocephaly. The pathogenesis of colpocephaly is unclear (Garg 1982), but may stem from an *in utero* insult or failure of development of the optic radiations (Fig. 32.3). Colpocephaly is commonly associated with optic disc anomalies.

Congenital vascular anomalies may also occur in

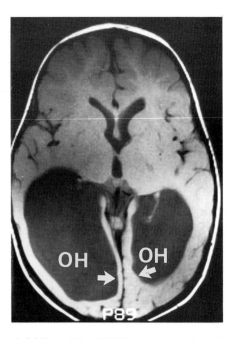

Fig. 32.3 Axial T1 weighted MRI scan of a patient with colpocephaly with dilated occipital horns (OH), but otherwise normal lateral ventricles. There is thinning of the occipital cortex (arrows), but the visual acuity was normal and there were no visual field defects. Prof W.F. Hoyt's patient.

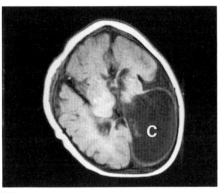

(a)

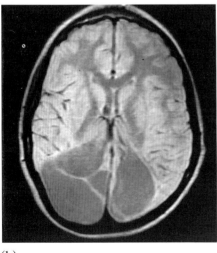

(b)

Fig. 32.2 (a) Axial T1 weighted (TR 600, TE 20) MRI scan of a 6-month-old child with a porencephalic cyst in the left occipital lobe (C). The location of the cyst is suggestive of in utero occlusion or maldevelopment of the left posterior cerebral artery. (b) Bilateral porencephalic cysts.

the occipital lobes resulting in hemianopias or other more subtle field defects. These anomalies may be part of a more widespread vascular disorder such as the Sturge−Weber or Wyburn−Mason syndrome or may occur as isolated arteriovenous malformations (Fig. 32.4). They are often calcified.

Congenital tumours may also occur in the occipital lobes, but are quite uncommon (Fig. 32.5).

Congenital lesions of the geniculostriate pathway may result in trans-synaptic degeneration of the ipsilateral temporal hemiretina which causes thinning of the arcuate nerve fibre bundles inferiorly and superiorly. Trans-synaptic degeneration of the nasal hemiretina contralateral to the lesion produces a horizontal band of atrophy across the optic disc associated with a temporal hemianopia (Hoyt 1985). While ablation of the visual cortex results in striking trans-synaptic degeneration of the retinogeniculate pathway even in adolescent nonhuman primates (Van Buren 1963), the human retinal ganglion cell layer is only known to degenerate after *in utero* insults to the posterior visual pathway (Miller & Newman 1981). Thus an isolated defect of the geniculostriate pathway, associated with either optic nerve atrophy or hypoplasia implies a prenatal injury.

Congenital homonymous hemianopias often remain

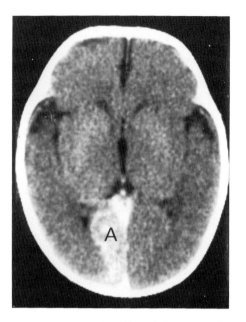

Fig. 32.4 Axial CT scan of a child with Sturge–Weber syndrome and a congenital left homonymous hemianopia. There is an arteriovenous malformation in the right occipital lobe (A). Prof W.F. Hoyt's patient.

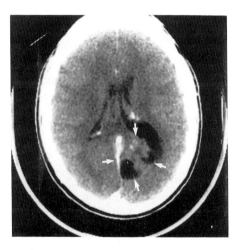

Fig. 32.5 Axial CT scan of a 24-year-old man with a ganglioglioma (arrows) of the left occipital lobe. The patient has a congenital right homonymous hemianopia. Prof W.F. Hoyt's patient.

undetected until early adulthood (Tychsen & Hoyt 1985). Homonymous hemianopias should be suspected in children with lateralized visual evoked potentials (Lambert *et al.* 1990).

Acquired defects

Acquired disorders of the visual cortex may occur secondary to hypoxic, traumatic, infectious, and metabolic insults. Hypoxic-ischaemic encephalopathy

may occur after perinatal asphyxia or later in childhood after cardiorespiratory arrests, intraoperative asphyxia or near-drowning episodes. Although it is often difficult to distinguish the effects of ischaemia (i.e. hypoperfusion) from hypoxaemia (i.e. diminished blood oxygenation), each is associated with specific findings. Generalized ischaemia often results in watershed infarctions of the vulnerable border zones between the areas supplied by the major cerebral arteries. In premature infants, the watershed zone is in the periventricular region between the regions supplied by ventriculopetal and ventriculofugal arteries (De Reuck *et al.* 1972). An ischaemic insult to premature infants most commonly damages the periventricular area resulting first in periventricular cysts and then periventricular leukomalacia several months later (Flodmark *et al.* 1987) (Fig. 32.6). Generalized ischaemic insults to full-term infants and adults commonly result in watershed infarctions in the parasagittal and parieto-occipital regions. The trigone area of the lateral ventricles, comprised largely of the optic radiations, is particularly vulnerable to ischaemia since it is a watershed zone for all three major cerebral arteries. Positron emission tomography has demonstrated that the posterior parasagittal region is the most vulnerable region of the brain to hypoxia-ischaemic insults in full-term infants (Volpe 1985).

Hypoxic-ischaemic insults may also produce diffuse cerebral atrophy and ulegyria (Courville 1971).

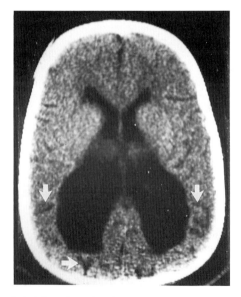

Fig. 32.6 Axial section of a child with severe periventricular leukomalacia who was asphyxiated at birth. The occipital horns of the lateral ventricles are dilated and the cortical sulci impinge directly on the ventricles (arrows).

Ulegyria is the loss of neurons and the formation of gliosis in areas of injured cerebral cortex. Bioccipital lobe infarctions may occur after hypoxic insults presumably secondary to compression of the posterior cerebral arteries against the tentorium by oedematous cerebral tissue.

Moya-Moya disease, an abnormal vascular network in the basilar region caused by bilateral carotid occlusion, may present to ophthalmologists because of homonymous hemianopia, visual agnosia, and a variety of ocular complaints.

Trauma may damage the visual cortex via a coup or contracoup mechanism (Griffith & Dodge 1968; Kaye & Heiskowitz 1986). Traumatic injuries to the posterior visual pathway often occur in children secondary to child abuse (Fig. 32.7a). The injuries may stem from direct trauma as in the battered-child syndrome (Kempe *et al.* 1962) or indirect trauma secondary to vigorous shaking (Frank *et al.* 1985; Lambert *et al.* 1986). Radiographic studies at the time of injury often reveal oedema or haemorrhages in the area of the visual cortex (Fig. 7b).

Meningitis may affect the visual cortex. Haemophilus influenza meningitis has a predilection for damaging the occipital cortex, often resulting in marked areas of radiolucency in the occipital lobes (Acers & Cooper 1965; Desousa *et al.* 1978; Ackroyd 1984). Granulomas and parasitic cysts (Fig. 32.8) also may cause damage to the visual cortex.

Hydrocephalus frequently damages the anterior and the posterior visual pathways (Smith *et al.* 1966; Arroyo *et al.* 1985) (Fig. 32.9). Injuries to the geniculostriate pathway presumably occurs by compression of the posterior cerebral arteries against the tentorium (Lindenberg & Walsh 1964).

Metabolic disease

Leigh's disease (Fig. 32.10), X-linked adrenoleukodystrophy (Fig. 32.11) and others (see Chapter 34) may cause cerebral visual defects.

Cortical blindness

Cortical blindness refers to the loss of vision stemming from injuries to the geniculostriate pathway. Since injuries to both the optic radiations and the visual cortex affect vision, cerebral blindness is perhaps a more accurate term. Clinically, cortical blindness may be identified by the loss of vision and optokinetic nystagmus in a patient with an otherwise normal ocular examination and intact pupillary light re-

sponses. The visual loss may be either transient or permanent (Hoyt & Walsh 1958).

Transient cortical blindness may stem from a number of causes. Hypoxic insults to the posterior visual pathway may result in episodes of no light perception with a subsequent, partial or complete restoration of vision. These episodes may occur as sequelae of generalized hypotension, cardiac surgery, birth

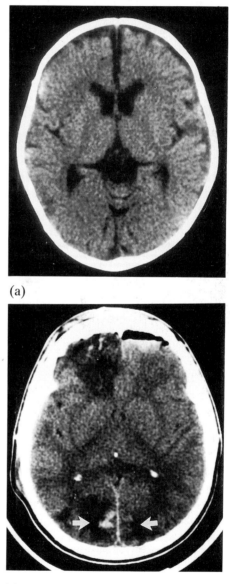

(a)

(b)

Fig. 32.7 (a) CT scan of non-accidental injury shows extensive cortical atrophy in a 6-month-old infant with retinal hemorrhages. (b) Axial CT scan of a youth who fell off a cliff and landed on his face. There are contracoup contusion injuries to both occipital lobes with oedema and haemorrhage involving the visual cortex (arrows). The patient had no light perception for 1 week, but by 2 weeks his vision had returned to normal.

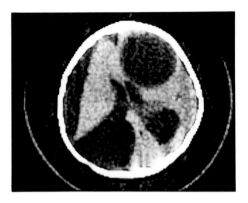

Fig. 32.8 Intracerebral hydatid cysts in an 8-year-old Mexican girl.

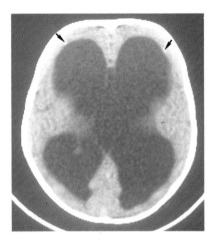

Fig. 32.9 A 10-month-old child with toxoplasmosis chorioretinitis and hydrocephalus. His toxoplasmosis dye test was positive at a 1:512 dilution. Note the calcification in the frontal lobes bilaterally (arrows).

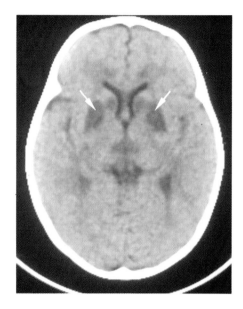

Fig. 32.10 Leigh's disease. The most frequent defect on CT scanning is lucency of the basal ganglia (arrows) seen here. Visual cortical defects also occur.

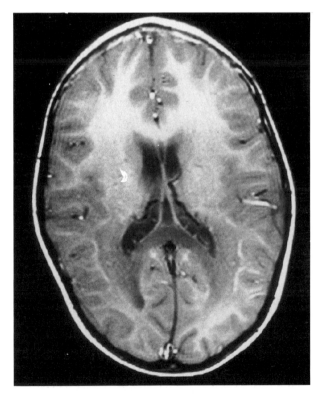

Fig. 32.11 Adrenoleukodystrophy. This 5-year-old boy presented with blindness with normal eyes. The T, weighted MRI scan shows posterior periventricular lucency and enhancement (see Chapter 34).

asphyxia, or metabolic derangements. Hypertensive crises and hydrocephalus may also result in transient episodes of cortical blindness possibly due to occlusion of the posterior cerebral arteries (Tychsen & Hoyt 1984). The cortical blindness associated with trauma is also reversible in certain instances.

A complete restoration of vision is unusual after an episode of cortical blindness (Barnet *et al.* 1970); more commonly some residual vision loss remains which Whiting and co-workers (1985) have termed cortical visual impairment. In two large series of children with cortical blindness, more than half of the children showed a significant improvement in vision over time (Whiting *et al.* 1985; Lambert *et al.* 1987).

The visual recovery was slow, in many instances lasting months to years. Usually the children had no apparent initial light perception, and then with time regained colour vision, form perception and finally improved visual acuity. All the children manifested residual perceptual difficulties, even when there was a recovery of good visual acuity. These difficulties included an apparent preference for touching rather than looking at objects, a reliance on peripheral vision, and a 'crowding' phenomenon with acuity levels better with single letters than when looking at groups of letters. While some had obvious homonymous hemianopias or constricted fields, most did not have easily characterized visual defects, perhaps due to the difficulty of assessing the visual fields of children or to the more diffuse nature of their injuries.

Many tests have been used to try to predict the visual outcome of children with cortical blindness. Visual evoked potentials were initially thought to be quite promising in evaluating cortically blind children (Duchowny *et al.* 1974) but subsequently have been shown to be similar to the visual evoked potentials in neurologically damaged children without visual difficulties (Frank & Torres 1984), or to be normal (Bodis−Wollmer 1977). Electroencephalography is of limited value in evaluating cortically blind children (Robertson *et al.* 1986). Visual evoked potential mapping may be a more accurate way of assessing the visual prognosis of cortically blind children but is still a largely unproven technique (Whiting *et al.* 1985).

Computerized tomography (CT) and magnetic resonance imaging (MRI) are more reliable means of evaluating cortically blind children. In one large series of cortically blind children, normal cranial scans were associated with a good prognosis, but these were quite unusual. Surprisingly, radiographic changes in the visual cortex were not correlated with the visual outcome, while changes in the optic radiations were highly statistically significant (Lambert *et al.* 1987). Presumably the optic radiations lack the plasticity of the visual cortex and are less likely to recover from significant injury. While diffuse atrophy is the most common radiographic abnormality seen in cortically blind children, bioccipital lobe infarctions, periventricular leukomalacia, and parieto-occipital 'watershed' infarctions are also frequently found (Lambert *et al.* 1987). Positron emission tomography may be an even better way of assessing the visual prognosis of children with cortical blindness since it is capable of imaging functional, rather than only structural, changes in the brain (Volpe 1985). Unfortunately, the isotopes currently used for positron emission tomography submit children to significant radiation which limits its use.

Cortically blind children often have other associated neurological deficits including mental retardation, cerebral palsy, seizure disorders, microcephaly or hydrocephalus.

Periventricular and intraventricular haemorrhage

Periventricular and intraventricular haemorrhages occur in many premature infants. The haemorrhages arise from poorly supported small vessels in the subependymal germinal matrix, and frequently occur after hypoxic insults or hypertensive episodes. The haemorrhages usually extend into the ventricular system and severe haemorrhages dilate the ventricles and may dissect into the brain substance. The haemorrhages occur a median of 38 hours after birth and may result in either a catastrophic deterioration or in a more clinically silent, 'saltatory' course. Survival is related to the severity and site of the haemorrhage; hydrocephalus, motor and intellectual deficits commonly occur in survivors.

Periventricular−intraventricular haemorrhages may result in severe damage to the posterior visual pathway by destroying portions of the optic radiations or visual cortex. Porencephalic cysts commonly develop in areas of the brain into which intracerebral haemorrhages have dissected.

Tamura and Hoyt (1987) reported tonic downward and esotropic deviations in 11 infants after severe intraventricular haemorrhages. The downward deviations improved in all cases after 9−21 months, but remained to a limited degree in three patients. The esotropias were permanent. The deviations may have a similar pathogenesis to the downward and convergent deviations adults experience after thalamic haemorrhages.

Extrageniculostriate visual system

In humans and other primates there is evidence suggesting that there is a second visual pathway bypassing the geniculate body and the visual cortex (Weiskrantz 1963). The pathway extends from the superior colliculus, through the pulvinar nucleus to the parastriate cortex (Brodman's areas 18 and 19). The extrageniculate visual pathway seems to mediate the detection of light and movement on a subconscious level (Weiskrantz *et al.* 1974) which has been referred to as 'blindsight'. In neonates some visual responses may be mediated through the extra-geniculate system (Dubowitz *et al.* 1986). After the ablation of the striate cortex, non-human primates gradually regain visual function, possibly by using their extrageniculate visual pathways (Humphrey *et al.* 1967; Denny-Brown & Chambers 1976). It has been proposed that humans utilize the extrageniculate pathway after injuries to their geniculostriate pathway (Barbur *et al.* 1980; Zihl & Von Cramman 1980; Bridgeman & Staggs 1982). Most of the evidence in support of these claims has been derived from testing adults with dense homonymous hemianopias perimetrically. Since fixation and light scattering have been inadequately controlled in some of these tests, the significance of their results are unclear (Campion *et al.* 1983), but children with cortical visual impairment may have a striking dissociation of their visual acuity and function, and Jan *et al.* (1986) suggested that the extra-geniculate pathway may have been responsible for the good navigational skills of a child with severely impaired vision and computerized tomographic injuries largely confined to the visual cortex.

References

Acers TE, Cooper WC. Cortical blindness secondary to bacterial meningitis. *Am J Ophthalmol* 1965; **59**: 226–9

Ackroyd RS. Cortical blindness following bacterial meningitis: a case report with reassessment of prognosis and aetiology. *Dev Med Child Neurol* 1984; **26**: 227–30

Arroyo HA, Jan JE, McCormick AQ *et al.* Permanent visual loss after shunt malfunction. *Neurology* 1985; **35**: 25–9

Barbur JL, Ruddock KH, Waterfield VA. Human visual responses in the absence of the geniculocalcarine projection. *Brain* 1980; **103**: 905–28

Barnet AB, Manson JI, Wilner E. Acute cerebral blindness in childhood. *Neurology* 1970; **20**: 1147–55

Bodis-Wollner I, Atkin A, Raab E *et al.* Visual association cortex and vision in man, pattern evoked potentials in a blind boy. *Science* 1977; **198**: 629–31

Bridgemen B, Staggs D. Plasticity in human blindsight. *Vision Res* 1982; **22**: 1199–203

Campion J, Latlo R, Smith YM. Is blindsight an effect of scattered light, spared cortex and near-threshold vision? *Behav Brain Sci* 1983; **6**: 423–86

Courville CB. *Birth and Brain Damage.* Margaret Courville, Pasadena 1971

Denny-Brown D, Chambers RA. Physiological aspects of visual perception. *Arch Neurol* 1976; **33**: 219–27

De Reuck J, Chatta AS, Richardson EP. Pathogenesis and evolution of periventricular leukomalacia in infancy. *Arch Neurol* 1972; **27**: 229–36

Desousa AL, L Kleiman MB, Mealey J. Quadriplegia and cortical blindness in haemophilis influenzae mengitis. *J Paediatr* 1978; **93**: 253–4

Dubowitz LMS, De Vries L, Mushin J, Arden GB. Visual function in the newborn infant: is it cortically mediated? *Lancet* 1986; **ii**: 1139–41

Duchowny MS, Weiss IP, Majlessi H *et al.* Visual evoked responses in childhood cortical blindness after head trauma and meningitis. *Neurology* 1974; **24**: 933–40

Flodmark O, Raland EH, Hill A *et al.* Periventricular leukomalacia: radiologic diagnosis. *Radiology* 1987; **162**: 231–5

Frank Y, Torres IF. Visual evoked potentials in the evaluation of Cortical Blindness in Children. *Ann Neurol* 1984; **2**: 126–9

Frank Y, Zimmerman R, Leeds NMD. Neurological manifestations in abused children who have been shaken. *Dev Med Child Neurol* 1985; **27**: 312–6

Galaburda AM, Sherman GF, Rosen GD *et al.* Developmental dyslexia: four consecutive patients with cortical anomalies. *Ann Neurol* 1985; **18**: 222–33

Garg BP. Colpocephaly. An error of morphogenesis? *Arch Neurol* 1982; **39**: 243–6

Geschwind N, Galaburda AM. Cerebral lateralisation: biological mechanisms, associations and pathology: a hypothesis and a program for research. *Arch Neurol* 1985; **42**: 428–59

Griffith JF, Dodge PR. Transient blindness following head injury in children. *N Engl J Med* 1968; **278**: 648–51

Hoyt WF. Congenital occipital hemianopia. *Neuro-ophthalmol J* 1985; **2**: 252–9

Hoyt WF, Walsh FB. Cortical blindness with partial recovery following acute cerebral anoxia from cardiac arrest. *Arch Opthalmol* 1958; **60**: 1060–9

Humphrey NK, Weiskrantz L. Vision in monkeys after removal of the striate cortex. *Nature* 1967; **215**: 595–7

Jan JE, Wong PKH, Groenveld M *et al.* Travel vision: 'collicular visual system?' *Pediatr Neurol* 1986; **2**: 359–62

Kaye EM, Heiskowitz J. Transient post-traumatic cortical blindness: brief v prolonged syndromes in childhood. *J Child Neurol* 1986; **1**: 206–10

Kempe GH, Silverman FN, Steele BF *et al.* The battered child syndrome. *JAMA* 1962; **181**: 17–24

Lambert SR, Hoyt CS, Jan JE, Barkovich J, Flodmark O. Visual recovery from hypoxic cortical blindness during childhood: CT and MRI predictors. *Arch Ophthalmol* 1987; **105**: 1371–7

Lambert SR, Johnson TE, Hoyt CS. Optic nerve sheath and retinal hemorrhages associated with the shaken baby syndrome. *Arch Ophthalmol* 1986; **104**: 1509–12

Lambert SR, Kriss A, Taylor D. Detection of isolated occipital lobe anomalies during early childhood. *Dev Med Child Neurol* 1990; **32**: 451–456

Lindeberg R, Walsh FB. Vascular compressions involving intracranial visual pathways. *Tr Am Acad Ophthalmol Otolaryngol* 1964; **68**: 677–94

Miller NR, Newman SA. Transsynaptic degeneration. *Arch Ophthalmol* 1981; **99**: 165–4

Noda S, Mayasalla S, Setogawa T, Matsumoto S, Ocular Symptoms of Moya Moya disease. *Am J Ophthalmol* 1987; **103**: 812–17

Rakic P. Mode of cell migration to the superificial layers of fetal monkey neocortex. *J Comp Neurol* 1972; **145**: 61–83

Robertson R, Jan JE, Wong PKH. Electroencephalograms of children with permanent cortical visual impairment. *Can J Neurol Sci* 1986; **13**: 256–61

Sachiko N, Seiji H, Tomoichi S, Stugeo M. Ocular symptoms of Moya-Moya disease. *Am J Ophthalmol* 1987; **103**: 812–7

Smith JL, Walsh TJ, Shipley T. Cortical blindness in congenital hydrocephalus. *Am J Ophthalmol* 1966; **62**: 251–60

Tamura EE, Hoyt CS. Oculomotor consequences of intraventricular haemorrhages in premature infants. *Arch Ophthalmol* 1987; **105**: 533–5

Tychsen L, Hoyt WF. Hydrocephalus and transient cortical

blindness. *Am J Ophthalmol* 1984; **98**: 819−21

Tychsen L, Hoyt WF. Occipital lobe dysplasia. Magnetic resonance findings in two cases of isolated congenital hemianopia. *Arch Ophthalmol* 1985; **103**: 680−2

Van Buren JM. Trans-synaptic retrograde degeneration in the visual system of primates. *J Neurol Neurosurg Psychiatry* 1963; **26**: 402−9

Volpe JJ. Neonatal intraventricular haemorrhage. *N Engl J Med* 1985; **304**: 886−91

Weiskrantz L. Contour discrimination in a young monkey with striate cortex ablation. *Neuropsychologia.* 1963; **1**: 134−64

Weiskrantz L, Warrington E, Sanders MD, Marshall J. Visual capacity in the hemianopic field following a restricted cortical ablation. *Brain* 1974; **97**: 709−28

Whiting S, Jan JE, Wong PKH *et al.* Permanent cortical visual impairment in children. *Dev Med Child Neurol* 1985; **27**: 730−9

Zihl J, Von Cramon D. The contribution of the 'second' visual system to directed visual attention in man. *Brain* 1980; **102**: 835−56

Section 5
Selected Topics in Paediatric Ophthalmology

33 Non-Organic Ocular Disorders

DAVID TAYLOR

What is it that causes otherwise well children to have symptoms, the reality of which cannot be doubted, without evidence of organic disease and why is the visual system so often chosen as the site for these manifestations?

Association with organic disease

Non-organic symptoms are common amongst children referred to a paediatric ophthalmology service (Schlaegel & Quilala 1955), and their prompt and correct diagnosis, with appropriate management, saves the doctor, and child and his parents much heartache and time and saves the discomfort and risk of unnecessary investigations.

'The fear of missing organic disease means that doctors have become more cautious about diagnosing hysteria. Several conditions previously regarded as hysterical are now thought to have an organic basis including spasmodic torticollis, blepharospasm, and writers cramp, there may be some more to come. Nevertheless, there is

a nucleus of patients for whom no diagnosis, other than hysteria, seems right (Lloyd 1986)'.

The concept of hysteria in the eyes of the public has achieved such a distorted and variable meaning that its use has been criticized and the American Paediatric Association's classification now does not use the term. But the clinical subdivisions that were included in the catch-all term hysteria are used instead, the most relevant of which to childhood ocular disorders is 'conversion disorder'. Marsden (1986) defines conversion disorder as a loss or distortion of neurological function not fully explained by organic disease. In psychiatry, it is well recognized that the presence of organic disease may be associated with non-organic disease with the classic situation being the occurrence of pseudoseizures in epileptics (Fenton 1986). The same may well be true of ocular hysterics, but in childhood the symptoms usually occur free of organic disease, or psychiatric disease (Jones & Levy 1983; Catalano *et al.* 1986). In adults, organic disease may be found in a substantial proportion of hysterics (Kathol *et al.* 1983) and a significant proportion may be deliberate deceivers. Thompson (1985) described this type as 'The Deliberate Malingerer — this patient is a villain who, with malicious intent, deliberately feigns visual loss'. Patients with self-inflicted injuries, known as the ocular Munchausen's syndrome (Rosenberg *et al.* 1986) and malingerers are rare in childhood. The child who has nonorganic ocular symptoms seems to be very different from the adult. He is a normal child, usually not from a very disturbed background (although serious underlying social problems may co-exist), and he does not have any eye or psychiatric disease.

Freud, nurtured by Charcot, developed the forerunner of the conversion theory. He believed that the patient had an internal conflict (usually sexual) of which he was unaware, which became converted into a symptom as a means of expression after a process of dissociation, which is a mental mechanism whereby underlying feelings and the symptoms are separated.

Clinical presentation and symptoms

Mersky (1986) made a useful clinical definition of conversion symptoms:

1 They correspond to an idea in the mind of the patient concerning physical or sensory changes or psychological dysfunction.

2 They are definable, if somatic, in terms of positive evidence and, if psychological, by techniques of clinical examination.

3 They are related to emotional conflict.

Three terms are commonly applied to this situation, one is hysterical visual loss and the others are functional and nonorganic visual loss. The latter two are used rather loosely to describe the same phenomenon, implying that the impairment is a result of a disorder of function rather than structure and is, therefore, restorable (Thompson 1985). Hysterical visual loss is a more specific description of one form of functional visual loss.

The child with a non-organic ocular defect is aged between 6 and 16 years, most frequently 10 years old (Jones & Levy 1983), girls are more frequently affected than boys (Yasuna 1951). The symptoms seem to come on gradually in most cases, often the first problem being a marginal failure at a school eye test. Subsequent examinations by optometrists or ophthalmologists reveal varying degrees of acuity and visual field loss, often worsening as time goes on, but rarely to the extent that the child becomes bilaterally blind. The remarkable thing is how little most children are inconvenienced by an apparently marked visual loss. Repeated objective examinations and further examinations, including neurophysiology and radiology, are all normal. The condition is usually bilateral (Yasuna 1951), the commonest complaints are of 'just not seeing', blurred vision, distorted or small images, occasionally visual field defects are described as 'tunnel vision' which is the commonest, but hemianopias are occasionally encountered (Keane 1979). Central scotomas are rare and should make one think of associated organic disease. Non-ocular defects occasionally occur, including spasm of the near reflex, headaches, voluntary nystagmus (Catalano et al. 1986), horizontal gaze paresis has occurred in an adult (Troost & Troost 1979) and accommodation paralysis has also been described.

Psychological background

Enquiry into the background, looking for the underlying stress that produces the symptoms should centre on two main areas, the home and family, and the school. Conflict between children, sibling rivalry, the child who needs more attention, an unhappy marriage, overcrowding, sexual abuse or harrassment by relatives or others, or conflict with neighbours and their children may all be predisposing factors. In the school it is the slow child who is being overstretched, or the bright child who is being understretched who may produce visual symptoms, but unsympathetic or agressive teachers, teasing or bullying, sexual or non-sexual harrassment are all factors to look for as predisposing to hysterical visual loss. It is of utmost importance to enlist the help of the parents, and to tell them explicitly of the possible underlying problems so that they can best help their own child, because it is by relieving underlying factors that the symptoms are best treated.

Detection of hysterical ocular disorders in children

It is of crucial importance that the diagnosis is made positively, with the clear demonstration of signs that are widely outside the bounds of physiological possibility. Marginal anomalies should be treated with the greatest of caution.

There are certain situations that are particularly suggestive of hysteria.

1 A severe functional defect in the presence of a normal physical examination and especially when there is a severe unilateral defect with normal pupil reactions and no refractive error.

2 The sudden onset of a disorder related to an emotionally significant event or situation.

3 Step-like deterioration, with the patient's acuity becoming one or two lines worse on each examination but with no objective abnormalities.

4 The ability of a patient to achieve a better acuity or better visual fields with coaxing or cajoling.

5 A monotonous and excessively slow reading of all the letters on a letter chart, regardless of whether they are large or small.

6 A single symptom is most frequent in hysterics whereas psycho-neurotic patients will tend to have numerous symptoms. Children rarely have substantial ocular complaints.

7 A previous history of hysterical manifestations, ocular or non-ocular, is a recognized predisposing factor to further hysterical disorders.

8 The occurrence of visual problems in other members of the family, especially if serious.

Bilateral total blindness

Although unusual, this severe disturbance is usually easy to detect as being non-organic.

1 Direct threat or throwing a ball on a string at the patient while the eyes are open invariably produces a blink (Fig. 33.1). By asking the patient to close his eyes, the string can be concealed before the ball is thrown, making the test more effective.

2 When facing a mirror a patient will involuntarily move his eyes when the mirror is rotated about a vertical axis running through the centre of the mirror. The velocity of the eye movement is proportional to the velocity of rotation of the mirror and the only way in which the patient can inhibit the eye movement is by 'looking through' the mirror, usually easily detected by a change in convergence of the eyes and an associated pupil reaction. (Fig. 33.2).

3 An optokinetic drum or tape, subtending a large angle at the eye can be held in front of the patient and the drum rotated to elicit visually evoked movement

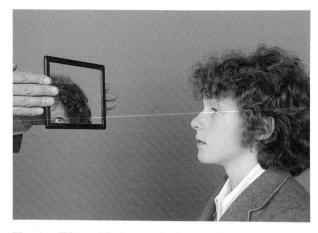

Fig. 33.2 When a blind person looks at a mirror no movement takes place when the mirror is rotated. The sighted person's eyes will move as the mirror rotates although he feels he is looking straight ahead.

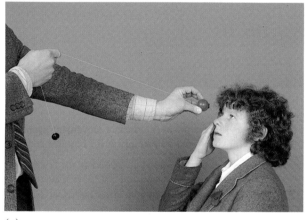

(a)

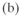

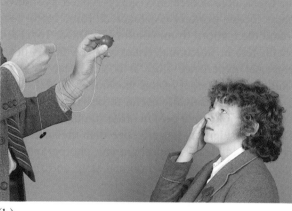

(b)

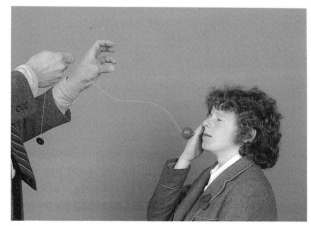

(c)

Fig. 33.1 Bilateral non-organic blindness. The ball on a string is measured for distance (a), withdrawn (b) and then thrown at the child, eliciting a blink if she is indeed sighted (c).

Unilateral partial acuity loss

In this group the same tests that are used for unilateral complete visual loss are applicable. The results, however, are often less easy to interpret. Pupil reactions are rarely helpful and since there are no clear norms for the correlation between acuity and stereo-acuity, the stereo-acuity tests are difficult to interpret. The pseudoscope and the confusion-refraction test are most useful in this situation.

Bilateral partial acuity loss

This group is the most difficult to diagnose as being non-organic but they nearly always have associated functional field defects that can establish the diagnosis.
1 The finding of an acuity that greatly varies in terms of the angle subtended, at different distances is an indicator of the hysterical defect. The patient may sometimes, by the use of a second chart with different sized figures or a mirror placed so as to decimate the increased distance between the patient and the chart, be induced to read letters of a size that he was not previously able to read. Similarly, near vision testers, using Snellen near equivalent letters, may show a disparity.
2 A severe bilateral loss of acuity due to organic disease is not compatible with a high level of stereo-acuity.
3 Similarly it is unusual for a patient to make fusional movement when a 5 dioptre prism is placed base out in front of the other eye, if that eye has organically reduced acuity.

Visual field defects

When having their visual fields tested, even normals may apparently perform in a non-organic manner if the examination is not carefully conducted. Abnormal fields are often associated with an apparently reduced acuity in functional visual loss, or sometimes with other symptoms including reading disability (Leary & Van Selm 1987).

Tunnel vision is the commonest of hysterical field defects (Eames 1947; Yasuna 1951). In tunnel vision the size of the field is the same at all distances; usually the field is also small. Purely constricted fields, for instance in retinitis pigmentosa, are conical becoming larger as the patient moves away from the testing screen. The defect is always gross; there is an apparently dense defect involving the whole visual field only a few degrees away from the fixation point and this is

the same size whether tested at 1, 2 or more metres away from the screen.

The defect, characterized by the piling of isoptres, is usually 'sharp edged' so that both large and small targets are perceived at the same point which is often remarkably constant. This 'piling up' of the isoptres may occur even in the face of gross changes in the contrast between the brightness of the background and the target; a distinctly unphysiological effect!

The absolute nature of the defect may make it easier to detect as being hysterical.
1 In a confrontation technique, if the patient alternates fixation between the examiner's eye and a fixation point on a stick held by the examiner, and at a time when he is fixing the examiner's eye, the fixation point is moved. If the patient has organic disease with constricted fields, he will have difficulty in relocating the spot, whereas a hysteric will find it accurately (Fig. 33.8).
2 On parting the examiner fixes the patient in the eye and, without speaking, raises his hand from the elbow as though to shake hands. Given the variations of social backgrounds, most patients with organically constricted fields do not see the examiner's hand, while the hysteric will.

Using large targets, one may obtain a square visual field. The target when moved inwards from one direction being detected in areas previously blind.

On successive testing the field may become smaller. If the target is moved inwards as though around a clockface the target becomes detectable at an ever decreasing distance from fixation giving rise to 'spiraling'.

A binasal field defect is rare and may be a hysterical phenomenon (Pilley & Thompson 1975). Pilley and Thompson pointed out that with a binasal hemianopia, if the patient fixes the examiner, there is a blind area between the two which is wedge-shaped, with a base between the patient's eyes and the apex at the examiner's nose. In organic disease targets that were not visible in this wedge are visible and hysteric, therefore, may see them. Hysterical binasal defects are usually clear-cut, organic ones are not.

In the very rare bitemporal hysterical visual field defect there is a wedge of blindness extending away from the fixation point. Therefore, if the patient fixes the examiner's nose and then fixes a point between the examiner's nose and himself, if the bitemporal hemianopia is complete there will be a loss or blurring of the central features of the examiners face. Obviously this does not occur in hysterical amblyopia.

De Schweinitz (1906) stressed the importance of

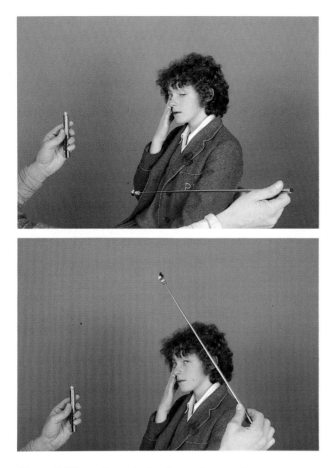

Fig. 33.8 The patient who has been shown to have very constricted visual fields looks accurately between the light and the mobile target which moves in the apparently blind part of the visual field.

inverted colour fields in hysteria. In this, the red targets are detected more peripherally than the blue targets of identical size and brightness, whereas the reverse is normal. This is not a test frequently done today but may be a useful adjunct.

Lastly it must be emphasized that an examiner skilled in testing for hysteria should not let his enthusiasm for testing to allow him either to overlook co-existing organic disease, or to encourage the patient to give apparently hysterical results when none are normally present, and do not forget that Eames (1947) demonstrated tunnel vision in 9% of 193 normal school children! The visual field testing is best done with a tangent screen but defects can be detected even using automated perimetry (Smith & Baker 1987).

Confirmatory studies

Once the clinician has made a positive diagnosis of non-organic visual loss and has not found evidence of any disease, there remains little to do from the point of view of diagnosis and one can easily argue that the more one investigates the child the more stress one creates and the more one reinforces his underlying problem. If there is any doubt in the mind of the doctor, parent or the older child, about the possibility of organic disease detailed neurophysiological studies, including an electroretinogram and pattern visually evoked responses may be very reassuring and may inspire sufficient confidence to base the treatment only on reassurance. Hysterical symptoms may also occur in brain disorders such as Batten's disease or adrenoleukodystrophy, many of which are accompanied by neurophysiological changes. So these are useful confirmatory studies in many cases and are risk free. Further investigations such as a CT or MRI scan are not completely risk free and are, therefore, only indicated if the neurophysiological tests are abnormal or if there is real doubt in the doctor's mind.

Management

The most important thing is to try to find the underlying cause and this is possible in most cases; appropriate and sensitive modification of these underlying predisposing factors will abolish the symptom. It is useful to demonstrate the non-organic nature of the defect to the parents and to reassure them strongly that it is such a common problem that it could almost be regarded as a 'normal stress reaction'. There is a very strong need to discuss the condition in full with both child and parents, in language appropriate to both; it is this that makes most paediatric ophthalmologists hearts fall when they make the diagnosis in the middle of a busy clinic!

Prognosis

The prognosis is good (Jones & Levy 1983; Catalano et al. 1986) and strong reassurance with minimal follow-up is indicated. Psychiatric help may be useful in certain cases. If there is any indication of an underlying psychiatric disorder, or of a more widespread psycho-neurosis, or if the patient has not responded to treatment, or if there have been other hysterical symptoms, the psychiatrist's expert help is mandatory.

References

Aichner H, Rubi E. Objective Seh Scharf Bentimmung bei Kleinstkmdern. *Klin Mbl Augenheilkd* 1976; **169**: 255–9
Catalano RA, Simon JW, Krohel GB, Rosenburg PN. Func-

tional visual loss in children. *J Am Acad Ophthalmol* 1986; **93**: 385−91

Catford GV, Oliver A. A method of visual acuity detection. Proc 2nd Intl Orthoptic Cong Amsterdam. *Exerpta Medica* 1971; 183−00

De Schweinitz GW. Neuroses and Psychoses. In: Posey WC, Spiller WG, (eds). *The Eye and the Nervous System.* Lippincott, 1906; pp. 614−96

Eames TH. A study of tubular and spiral central fields. *Am J Ophthalmol* 1947; **30**: 610−1

Fenton GW. Epilepsy and hysteria. *Br J Psychiatry* 1986; **149**: 28−37

Hinchcliff H. Clinical evaluation of stereopsis. *Br Orthopt J* 1978; **35**: 46−50

Jones RB, Levy IS. Hysterical blindness in pediatric ophthalmology. In: Wybar KC, Taylor DSI (eds) *Pediatric Ophthalmology* Marcel Dekker, New York 1983; pp. 399−405

Kathol RG, Cox TA, Corbett JJ, Thompson HS. Functional visual loss. *Arch Ophthalmol* 1983; **101**: 729−35

Keane JR. Hysterical hemianopia. *Arch Ophthamol* 1979; **97**: 865−6

Leary PM, Van Selm JL. Tunnel vision presenting as reading disability. *J Roy Soc Med* 1987; **80**: 585−7

Lloyd GG. Hysteria: a case for conservation. *Br Med J* 1986; **293**: 1255−6

Marsden CD. Hysteria: a neurologist's view. *Psychol Med* 1986; **149**: 28−37

Mersky H. Disorders of conscious awareness hysterical phenomena. *Br J Hosp Med* 1986; **19**: 305−9

Pilley SJH, Thompson HS. Binasal field loss and prefixation blindness. In: Glaser J, Smith JL (eds) *Neuro-ophthalmology*, Vol. 8 CV Mosby, St Louis 1975; pp. 277−84

Rosenberg PN, Krohel GB, Webb RM, Hepler RS. Ocular Munchausen's syndrome. *Ophthalmology* 1986; **93**: 1120−4

Schlaegel TD Jr, Quilala FU. Hysterical amblyopia; statistical analysis of 42 cases found in a survey of 800 unselected eye patients at a state medical centre. *Arch Ophthalmol* 1955; **54**: 875−44

Smith TJ, Baker RS. Perimetric findings in functional disorders using automated techniques. *J Am Acad Ophthalmol* 1987; **94**: 1562−7

Thompson SH. Functional visual loss. *Am J Ophthalmol* 1985: **100**: 209−13

Troost TB, Troost GE. Functional paralysis of horizontal gaze. *Neurol* 1979; **29**: 82−5

Yasuna ER. Hysterical amblyopia in children and young adults. *Arch Ophthalmol* 1951; **45**: 70−6

34 Neurometabolic Disease

DAVID TAYLOR

Gangliosidoses

Amaurotic family idiocy is a term which used to be applied to a variety of neurometabolic diseases. It has outlived its usefulness because it is inappropriately non-specific and often hurtful to parents.

GM2 gangliosidoses

TAY–SACHS DISEASE (GM2 type I)

Warren Tay, a London ophthalmologist first described this disease but the frequency of the gene in people of Ashkenazi Jewish stock led to the finding of the disease in New York where it was described as 'amaurotic family idiocy' by Bernard Sachs in 1887. It is an autosomal recessive disorder in which a deficiency of hexosaminidase A leads to an accumulation of GM2 ganglioside in neurones of brain and elsewhere. Children with the disease present early in their first year of life with a loss of skills already acquired, blindness, seizures, spasticity, and an exaggerated startle response to sound and light flash stimuli which may be the first abnormality noted by the parents. The head enlarges and the child usually dies by 4 years of age.

Ophthalmoscopy at an early stage reveals the characteristic cherry red spot which is due to ganglioside accumulation in the retinal ganglion cells (Cogan & Kuwabara 1959). The absence of ganglion cells at the fovea gives rise to the red spot surrounded by white diseased cells.

As the ganglion cells die the cherry red spot fades and optic atrophy become apparent. The electroretinogram is normal or large (Godel et al. 1978) but the VER extinguished (Honda & Sudo 1976) and the injection of placental hexasaminidase A enzyme did "ot improve these neurophysiological parameters in three patients (Godel et al. 1978).

SANDHOFF'S DISEASE (GM2 type II)

These children have a clinical disease similar to that of Tay–Sachs patients, but have a defect of both hexaminidase A and B. The gene frequency in the Jewish population is 1/1000, but in this case, the disease is more frequent in non-Jews, in whom the frequency is probably 1/600 (Canter & Kabach 1985).

JUVENILE (GM2 type III)

This is a very rare variant with an onset of ataxia between 2 and 6 years with late onset of blindness which may lead to it being misdiagnosed as Batten's disease. The electroretinogram is normal in gangliosidoses and should therefore avoid this mistake. There is a partial defect of hexaminidose A. A faint cherry red spot sometimes occurs (Brett et al. 1973). Patients may have eye movement defects including pursuit and vestibulo-ocular reflex suppression defects and saccadic dysmetria; the ERG and VER are normal (Musarella ET AL. 1982).

GM1 gangliosidoses

INFANTILE (GM1 type I)

This is a rare autosomal recessive trait with deficient beta-galactosidose leading to the accumulation of GM1 gangliosides. There is no racial predilection.

Children are affected at birth or very early in infancy with:

1 Severe cerebral degeneration and regression with death by 2 years.
2 Seizures in some patients.
3 Visceral involvement of liver, spleen, and bone marrow, and kidney.
4 Coarse features with a Hurler's syndrome-like appearance.
5 A cherry red spot, retinal haemorrhages, and occasionally corneal clouding (Emery et al. 1971).

The diagnosis may be suspected by finding large foamy histiocytes in bone marrow aspirate but clinicians usually seek confirmation by enzyme analysis as a first procedure.

LATE INFANTILE (GM1 type II and type III)

This autosomal recessive disease presents in older children with mental and motor regression and seizures, followed by spasticity and decerebrate rigidity. Their facial features appear normal, but they may have kyphoscoliosis. They have abnormal marrow histiocytes and deficient beta galactosidase. Neuro-ophthalmological problems are not dominant in the clinical picture.

Prenatal diagnosis in the gangliosidoses

Prenatal diagnosis is available by measuring the enzymes from cultured amniotic cells or chorionic villus biopsy and is applicable to parents with one or more affected children but the gene frequency is not sufficiently high for screening in most populations.

Batten's disease (neuronal ceroid lipofuscinosis)

In childhood, four forms of Batten's disease occur. All are characterized by visual deterioration with retinal degeneration and a severely abnormal ERG, seizures and mental regression. Because the infantile and late infantile types have a rapid downhill course and are already diagnosed by the neurologist, the paediatric ophthalmologist rarely has a role to play.

Infantile

- Santavuori disease.
- Infantile neuronal ceroid lipofuscinosis.

These babies present between 8 and 18 months of age with myoclonus, mental and motor regression, and visual failure (Santavouri *et al.* 1973). There is severe neuronal destruction with phagocytosis by often binucleated cells, and fibrillary astrocytes are found in the cerebral cortex (Haltia *et al.* 1973) which leads to microcephaly. Blindness occurs early in the course of the disease with an absent ERG or a low amplitude ERG which later becomes isoelectric (Pampiglione & Harden 1977). The flash VER is diminished in amplitude. Death occurs by 4 years. First described in Finland, cases have been recognized around the world in several racial groups. The retinas show narrow blood vessels, some pigment epithelial changes around the macular and later optic atrophy and clumped retinal pigmentation (Raitta & Santavouri 1973; Bateman & Phillipart 1986). Cherry red spots are not seen. Neurones contain granular osmophilic deposits known by the acronym 'GROD' or as 'Finish snow-balls' and the diagnosis can be made on ultrastructural studies of rectal neurones or of peripheral leukocytes (Baumann & Markesbery 1982). It is inherited as an autosomal recessive trait and there is no racial predilection.

Late infantile

- Janski–Bielschowski disease.
- Late infantile neuronal ceroid lipofuscinosis.

These children present from 2 to 4 years with mental deterioration, ataxia, myoclonic jerks, and epilepsy with death by 7 years. They become blind early from retinal degeneration most marked at the macula but later the whole retina is affected and appears thinned with clumped pigment, narrow arterioles, and optic atrophy. The ERG is extinguished early but there is an extraordinarily enlarged VER amplitude; many times the normal. The EEG shows large spikes at low rates of photic stimulation (Pampiglione & Harden 1977).

Diagnosis is established by the finding of characteristic electron microscopic curvilinear bodies in rectal neurones, lymphocytes (Markesbury *et al.* 1976) or in sural nerve (Bolmers *et al.* 1973). It is inherited as an autosomal recessive trait and there is no racial predilection.

Juvenile

- Batten–Mayou disease.
- Vogt–Spielmeyer disease.
- Spielmeyer–Sjögren disease.
- Juvenile neuronal ceroid lipofuscinosis.

Frederick Batten (1903) a pathologist of the National Hospitals, Queen Square, and later a physician at the Hospital for Sick Children, Great Ormond Street, London, described two siblings with a maculopathy and progressive mental retardation and he later (Batten 1914) cited another family described by Vogt in 1905. Other cases were described at this time (Mayou 1904; Spielmeyer 1905). Mayou gave a good description of the retinae when he noted granular pigmentation with a reddish–black spot at the macula. In the discussion following the presentation of Mayou's paper, Mr Sidney Stephenson said 'a number of such cases have been recorded in the last few years and it must be a gratification to the Society (the Ophthalmological Society of the United Kingdom) that the first case of this kind was shown at the Society by Mr Rayner Batten in 1897'. RE Batten was FE Batten's older brother, but it may be that he described patients with only a retinal and not a combined retinal and cerebral degeneration. Not just for chauvinistic reasons has the name Batten stuck!

Juvenile Batten's disease is the commonest neuro-degenerative disease seen at the Hospital for Sick Children today, and it represents a small but important cause of child blindness in the UK. Perhaps 25–30% of the ten children each year registered are blind with acquired retinal or macular disease (Spalton *et al.* 1980).

Children with juvenile Batten's disease present with visual failure between 4 and 10 years, with a peak incidence at 6 years (Spalton *et al.* 1980). The earliest change is a bull's eye maculopathy (Fig. 34.1) but the whole retina is affected early as shown by the ERG changes which are present early in the disease (Pampiglione & Harden 1977). Attenuation of the B wave of the ERG, with initial preservation of the EOG, and later involvement of all elements of the

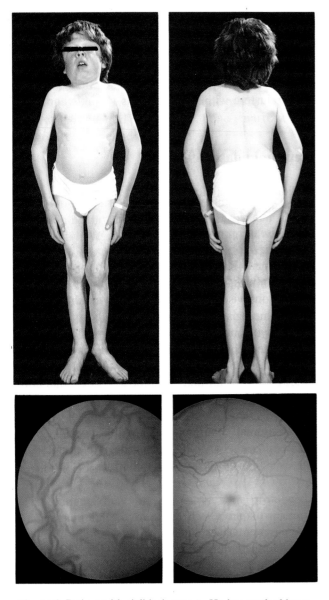

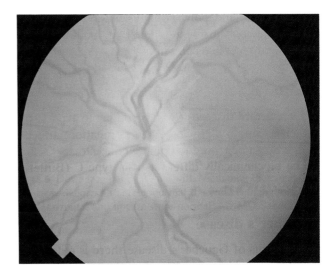

Fig. 34.9 Cherry red spot and optic desk swelling in a patient with sialidosis type 2. The picture is hazy due to corneal clouding.

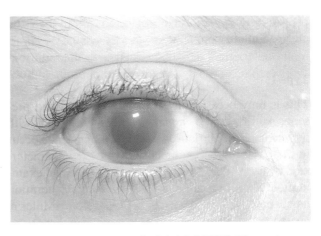

Fig. 34.10 Opaque cornea in Scheie's MPSIS. The acuity was 6/12 at this stage.

Fig. 34.8 Patient with sialidosis type 2. He has marked bony changes and a cherry red spot.

glycosamioglycan excretion and enzyme analysis. The old term gargoylism is too offensive to the patients and their parents to be retained.

A quick clinical guide to diagnosis for the ophthalmologist can be based on the facial features, bony, and eye changes.

1 Hurler's-like with cloudy cornea, retinal degeneration and optic atrophy. It can be subdivided into:

(a) MPSIH — Hurler's syndrome.

(b) MPS VII — Maroteaux–Lamy syndrome (mentally normal) (Fig. 34.9).

(c) MPSVII — Beta-glucuranidase deficiency (eye findings not reported).

2 Mild facial changes and cloudy cornea. It can be subdivided into:

(a) MPSIS — Scheie's disease: hand deformity, aortic incompetence, retinal degeneration, normal intelligence (Fig. 34.10).

(b) MPSIV — Morquio's disease: severe skeletal changes and dwarfing. Normal intelligence and no retinal degeneration (Fig. 34.11).

3 Mental retardation, facial changes without cloudy cornea.

(a) MPSII Hunter's: occasional mild corneal changes, severe skeletal changes, retinal degeneration, mental retardation.

(b) MPSIII Sanfillipo: severe mental retardation, mild facial changes, moderate skeletal changes, and retinal degeneration present.

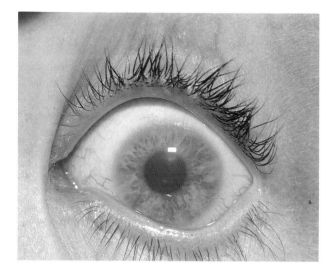

Fig. 34.11 Very mild corneal cloudiness in Morquio's disease MPSIV. Normal vision.

The above classification is incomplete, but serves as an *aide mémoire*. MPSV is not present; it is now MPSIS (Scheie's syndrome).

The paediatric ophthalmologist is rarely involved with Hunter's, Hurler's, Sanfillipo or MPSVII because their mental retardation and short lives often preclude treatment for their corneas, but not infrequently is asked to see patients with Maroteaux–Lamy, Morquio's and Scheie's disease whose pathological and ocular clinical features have many similarities, although they are not identical.

Ocular findings and management

CORNEAL CLOUDING

When the corneas are affected they take on a 'ground glass' appearance that in some instances is better seen with transillumination from the side, than on slit lamp examination. All layers of the corneas are symmetrically infiltrated, both within cells and in the extracellular space with acid mucopolysaccharide. Although not clinically affected, the conjunctiva (which is readily biopsied) also shows intracellular inclusions which are mucopolysaccharide containing lysosomes (Kenyon 1976). The only treatment for the cloudy cornea is by corneal transplantation unfortunately the coexistence of retinal degeneration, optic atrophy, severe mental retardation or a markedly shortened lifespan often contraindicate treatment. Careful assessment of the patient's needs together with neurophysiological studies and MRI scanning to

establish the viability of the retina and postretinal pathways are mandatory before embarking on surgery. The visual improvement is rarely long lived but sometimes give an extended period of vision to children who would otherwise be blind. Reports vary but we have found corneal grafts may remain clear for months, rejection is unusual, the graft re-opacifies by involvement with the original process. Provided the cases are carefully selected the procedure can benefit the child even if the ophthalmologist finds it tiresome that his perfect graft become opacified more quickly than he is used to! They can always be regrafted provided that retinal degeneration or optic atrophy has not supervened.

RETINAL DEGENERATION

This is seen in forms but has not yet been recorded in Morquios disease. It has a very insidious onset and is usually overshadowed by the corneal opacities. The more intelligent child with MPSIS, or MPSVI may note onset of night-blindness or dimness in addition to the blurring of the corneal disease. Histopathologically most tissues of the eye, are affected especially the retinal pigment epithelium (RPE) (Delmonte *et al.* 1983; Lavery *et al.* 1983, McDonnell *et al.* 1983). Kenyan (1976) found the RPE cells were filled with mucopolysaccharide but were generally intact. The outer retina is also affected.

No treatment is available and detection of the retinal degeneration is mandatory before corneal grafting is undertaken.

OPTIC ATROPHY

Histopathological studies show that both the ganglion cells and the nerve fibre layer of the retina, and optic nerve itself are severely affected. Kenyon (1976) thought that the optic nerve axons might be compressed or nutritionally compromised by the infiltration of glial cells but there has been no substantiation of this. Optic atrophy can also be caused by glaucoma. Neurophysiological studies help to delineate optic nerve and cortical visual defect.

GLAUCOMA

Glaucoma probably occurs in all of the mucopolysaccharidoses and some other metabolic diseases with cloudy corneas. It was clearly described by Spellacy *et al.* (1980), with histopathological studies of a trabeculectomy specimen showing MPS laden cells in the disease. A not infrequent symptom, usually only elicited by direct questioning is that the patient's summer suntan failed to fade. The visual symptoms are easily dismissed as being hysterical because initially the eye examination is normal and there are quite marked behavioural changes. Boys with hysterical blindness should always be suspected of having adrenoleukodystrophy; neurophysiological studies are very helpful (Battaglia *et al.* 1981); the ERG is normal, the VER reduced and the EEG showed irregular slow activity over the posterior parts of the brain. The auditary evoked response can be used to detect carriers (Moloney & Masterson 1982). Somatosensory evoked responses may be more sensitive for carrier detection (Garg *et al.* 1983).

Computed tomography is extremely helpful in making the diagnosis in the early stages (Quisling and Andriola 1979) as it shows low density zones in the periventricular white matter, especially posteriorly (Fig. 34.15). The grey matter is spared and the lesions are remarkably symmetrical and confluent, contiguous over the midline via the splenium.

Optic atrophy occurs later. Ocular histopathology showed inclusions in optic nerve macrophages, retinal

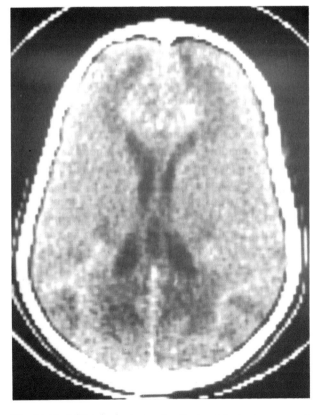

Fig. 34.15 Adrenoleukodystrophy. Periventricular lucency and enhancement on CT.

neurones and macrophages, and, retinal photoreceptor and pigment epithelial degeneration (Cohen *et al.* 1983; Glasgow *et al.* 1987). One of Cohen *et al*'s (1983) cases had a cataract and cystoid macular oedema. The inclusions in optic nerve macrophages are not invariable (Wray *et al.* 1976).

Progressive neurological deterioration occurs with death within a few years.

The diagnosis is made by a combination of the clinical, CT, neurophysiological endocrine studies, and measurement of long chain fatty acids.

Canavan's disease and Alexander's leukodystrophy

These are two rare diseases with progressive neurological deterioration which occurs in childhood, with a rapid downhill course. Ophthalmological symptoms are overshadowed by the overwhelming neurological deterioration. Canavan's disease is autosomal recessive, occurring particularly in Ashkenazi Jewish families and the only good thing that can be said for Alexander's leukodystrophy is that it is non genetic.

They are probably the only two conditions in which brain biopsy may be still indicated (Brett 1983). Cogan (1976) described two cases of Canavan's disease who had flutter-like oscillations of the eyes and these together with another case without nystagmus. The two cases with nystagmus were blind with optic atrophy.

Other metabolic diseases

Organic acidaemias

This is a group of disorders including maple syrup urine disease, propionic acidaemia, glutaric aciduria, methyl malonic aciduria, and multiple acyl CoA dehydrogenase deficiency that are autosomal recessive enzyme disorders of amino acid catabolism. They present in infancy with a severe metabolic acidosis with rapid deterioration and ketosis or as failure to thrive or a variety of neurological problems including seizures, dystonia or as an ataxia in older children. Most of the ophthalmological problems have been recorded in infants with maple syrup urine disease.

A variety of gaze pareses occur, both vertical (Zee *et al.* 1974; McDonald & Sher 1977) and horizontal and vertical mixed gaze pareses (Mainardi 1966; Schwartz & Kolendrianos 1969; Chhabria *et al.* 1979). Ptosis is frequent (Lonsdale *et al.* 1963; Zee *et al.* 1974; Chhabria 1979).

Before diagnosis the infant is hypotonic with a

divergent squint, poor eye movements, and ptosis. As treatment is started, before recovery takes place, there are bursts of wild eye movements and eyelid movements (Dickinson et al. 1969). Older children may present with nystagmus (Morris et al. 1961).

Rapid diagnosis is essential to reduce the permanent neurological defects, since the outcome becomes worse after the first 24 hours with progressively severe permanent neurological sequelae (Naughten et al. 1982).

Diabetes

See Chapter 27.

Urea cycle disorders

This is a group of diseases which may present at any age but occurs particularly severely in the neonatal period when they present with the gradual onset of lethargy, seizures, and liver failure. They have abnormal liver enzymes, raised ammonia, and excess urinary orotic acid.

Later onset disorders present in a much more chronic fashion; papilloedema has been described in late onset citrullinaemia (Hayasaka et al. 1974). Ornithine carbamyl transferase deficiency is inherited as an X-linked dominant condition in which the male infants usually die but the females survive and thrive poorly. One male has been recorded as having survived with marked myopia vitiligo and, hyperammonaemia and transient visual disturbances (Snebold et al. 1987).

Menke's disease

- Kinky hair syndrome
- Steely hair syndrome
- Tricholipodystrophy

This is an X-lined recessive disease of copper metabolism. Serum copper and caeruloplasmin levels are extremely low.

The babies are often premature but slow to mature with failure to grow. When the second hair grows it is stubbly, stiff, fractures easily, and feels like wire wool. They progressively deteriorate with increasing spasticity and seizures.

The eyebrows are sparse, twisted and white with the eyelashes better preserved and pigmented than the brain (Horn & Warburg 1978). There is a retinal dystrophy affecting the outer nuclear layer and photoreceptors in the macular area (Toussaint & Davis 1978) or more widespread (Horn & Warburg 1976; Wray et al. 1976; Billings & Degnam 1971; Seelenfreund et al. 1968). Tortuous retinal vessels are frequent (Billings & Degnan 1971; Levy et al. 1974;); the ERG becomes extinguished (Billings and Degnan 1971; Levy et al. 1974; Horn & Warburg 1976). The ERG is unaffected by raising the copper levels (Levy et al. 1974). Optic atrophy is probably secondary to retinal degeneration.

Demyelination is found in the optic nerve histopathologically (Wray et al. 1976).

Amino acid and protein disorders

For cross-references, see list of sub-headings at beginning of chapter.

PHENYLKETONURIA

Phenylketonuria is a rare autosomal recessive disorder of phenylalanine metabolism to tyrosine, because of the lack of the enzyme phenylalanine hydroxylase.

Despite the gene frequency of about one in 50 of the population, untreated cases are rare because of neonatal screening which is universal in the western world. Sadly a few cases each year have false negative results or are missed for one reason or another and they present with a gradual mental deterioration, sometimes with seizures and they are often fair haired blue eyed and with a pale rough skin. Treatment is by a diet low in phenylalanine which should be continued for the first decade of life. Phenylketanuric mothers have a high incidence of congenital anomalies and microcephaly in their children. In late-diagnosed cases the eyes have blue irides even in those of dark skinned stock but the hypopigmentation does not seem to have the same associations, i.e. strabismus as in albinos (Zwaan 1983). High refractive errors are common (Cotticelli et al. 1985). Cataracts are quite frequent: they may occur in older children or in adult life and may be related to trauma and treatment (Zwaan 1983); they may be congenital (Cotticelli et al. 1985; Parks & Schwilk 1963).

Lipid metabolism disorders

Hyperlipoproteinaemias

The hyperlipoprotcinaemias may occasionally cause corneal arcus (type IIa, IIb), xanthomas (type I, IIa, IIb), and lipaemia retinatis may very rarely be found in occasional children with type IV.

Lecithin cholesterol acyltransferase deficiency
(LCAT deficiency)

Homozygotes with this disease which is autosomal recessive have central corneal clouding and arcus-like changes. The central corneal changes are grey dots occupying the full thickness of the stroma mainly centrally, with peripheral condensation to form the arcus-like changes (Vrabec *et al.* 1988). Patients have a haemolytic anaemia which may lead to renal failure.

Tangier disease (an alpha-lipoproteinaemia)

This rare autosomal recessive disease may present in childhood with a neuropathy including facial diplegia and orange coloured tonsils and sometimes a yellowish tinge to the conjunctiva, and stromal corneal clouding (Hoffman & Fredrickson 1965)

Fish eye disease

This very rare disease was described in a man and his three daughters by Carlson and Philipson (1979). They had eyes like those of a boiled fish; normal serum cholesterol, raised triglycerides and very low-density lipoprotein (VLDL), and very high density lipoprotein (VHDL).

Urbach–Wiethe syndrome (lipoid proteinosis)

This autosomal recessive disease is characterized by nodules and plaques in skin and mucus membranes. Laryngeal nodules and thickening give rise to hoarseness and the skin changes consist of:
1 Multiple pigmented varioliform scarring on the face, elbows, and knees resulting from vesicular eruptions (Feiler-Ofry *et al.* 1979).
2 Nodules at the margins of the lids (Blodi *et al.* 1960) and mucus membranes of the mouth and pharynx.

The lid nodules rarely give rise to problems but corneal changes (Muirhead & Jackson 1963; Newton *et al.* 1971; Charlin & Fernandez 1978), glaucoma and cataract (Francois *et al.* 1968; Charlin & Fernandez 1978), and retinal changes including a pigmentary retinopathy (Schilovitz *et al.* 1973) and drusen (Charlin & Fernandez 1978) occur.

Metabolic diseases with ophthalmological presentation

CORNEAL ABNORMALITIES

Those presenting with this include:

- Mucopolysaccharidoses (all except MPS II and MPS III)
- Mucolipidoses
- Fucosidosis
- Mannosidosis
- Farbers disease (one case)
- Sialidosis II
- LCAT disease
- Tangier disease
- Fish eye disease
- Cystinosis
- Tyrosinaemia
- Wilson's disease

CORNEAL DISEASE AND ANGIOKERATOMA CORPORIS DIFFUSUM

Those presenting with this include:
- Fabry's disease
- Mucolipidosis 1
- Fucosidosis type II

VISUAL FAILURE

Those associated with this include:
- Juvenile Batten's disease
- Leukodystrophies
- Gangliosidoses
- A beta-lipoproteinaemia

EYE MOVEMENT DISORDERS

Those associated with this include:
- *Niemann–Pick type C* (vertical gaze palsy)
- *Sialidosis type I* (periodic alternating nystagmus, myoclonus)
- *Gaucher's disease type III* (congenital oculomotor apraxia)
- *Pelizaeus–Merzbacher disease* (see Chapters 42, 43)
- Organic acidaemias
- Urea cycle disorders (bursts of chaotic eye movements)
- Sialidosis type II (nystagmus)
- GM2 type III (Pursuit + VOR defects)
- Canavan's disease (flutter-like oscillations)

CHERRY RED SPOT

This occurs in
- GM2 type I, II, III
- GM1 type I
- Niemann–Pick type A

- Sialidosis type I, II
  A faint or irregular cherry red spot occurs in:
- Niemann–Pick type C, type B
- Metachromatic leukodystrophy
- Farber's disease
- Mucolipidosis III.

References

Allen RJ, McCusker JJ, Tourtelotte WW. Metachromatic leukodystrophy. Clinical, histochemical and cerebrospinal fluid abnormalities. *Pediatrics* 1962; **30**: 629–38

Arbisser AI, Murphree AL, Garcia CA, Howell RR. Ocular findings in mannosidosis. *Am J Ophthalmol* 1976; **82**: 465–71

Barrone R, Gatti R, Trias X, Durnad P. Fucosidosis. *J Pediatr* 1974; **84**: 727–35

Bateman J, Philippart M. Ocular features of the Hagberg–Santavuori syndrome. *Am J Ophthalmology* 1986; **102**: 262–72

Bateman J, Philippart M, Isenberg SJ. Ocular features of multiple sulfatase deficiency and a new variant of metachromatic leukodystrophy. *J Pediatr Ophthalmol* 1984; **21**: 133–40

Battaglia A, Harden A, Pampiglione G, Walsh PJ. Adrenoleucodystrophy: neurophysiological aspects. *J Neurol Neurosurg Psychiat* 1981; **44**: 781–5.

Batten FE. Cerebral degeneration with symmetrical changes in the maculae in two members of a family. *Trans Ophthalmol Soc UK* 1903; **23**: 386–90.

Batten FE. Family cerebral degeneration with macular change (so-called juvenile form of family amaurotic idiocy). *Quart J Med* 1914; **7**: 444–54

Baumann RJ, Markesbery WR. Juvenile amaurotic idiocy (neuronal ceroid lipofuscinosis) and lymphocyte fingerprint profiles. *Ann Neurol* 1978; **4**: 531–6

Baumann RJ, Makersbery WR. Santavuori disease: diagnosis by leukocyte ultrastructure. *Neurology* 1982; **32**: 1277–81

Beck M. Papilloedema in association with Hunter's syndrome. *Br J Ophthalmol* 1983; **67**: 174–7

Beck M, Cole G. Disc oedema in association with Hunter's syndrome: ocular histopathological findings. *Br J Ophthalmol* 1984; **68**: 590–5

Billings DM, Degnam M. Kinky hair syndrome: a new case and review. *Am J Dis Child* 1971; **121**: 447–52

Blodi FC, Whinery RD, Hendricles CA. Lipoid proteinosis (Urbach–Wiette) involving the lids. *Trans Am Ophthalmol Soc* 1960; **58**: 155–6

Bolmers DJM, Gabreels FJM, Joosten EMG, Gabreeles–Festen A. Ceroid lipofuscinosis (Batten's disease), first ophthalmological report of cytoplasmic inclusions in Schwann's cell of the sural nerve in two patients with an amaurotic familial idiosy. *Acta Ophthalmol* 1973; **51**: 47–57.

Bolthauser E, Schirmert G, Gitzelmann R, Henn V. *Ocular apraxia in Gaucher's disease type III.* Presented at V International Neuro-ophthalmological Society, Elsevier Antwerp, Belgium 1984.

Bosch EP, Hart MN. Late adult-onset metachromatic leukodystrophy. *Arch Neurol* 1978; **35**: 475–81

Brett EM. *Paediatric Neurology.* Churchill Livingstone, London 1983

Brett EM, Ellis RB, Haas L, Ikonne JN, Lake BD, Patrick AD, Stevens R. Late onset GM2 gangliosidosis. Clinical pathological and biochemical studies in eight patients. *Arch Dis Child* 1973; **48**: 775–85

Brod RD, Packer AJ, Van Dyk JL. Diagnosis of neuronal ceroid lipofuscinosis by ultrastructural examination of peripheral blood lymphocytes. *Arch Ophthalmol* 1987; **105**: 1388–93

Brownstein S, Meagher–Villemure K, Polomeno RC, Little JM. Optic nerve in globoid leukodystrophy (Krabbe's disease). *Arch Ophthalmol* 1978; **96**: 864–70

Butler J De B, Camly M, Kruth H, Vanier M *et al.* Niemann–Pick variant disorders: comparison of errors of cellular cholesterol hemeostasis in Group D and Group C fibroblasts. *Proc Natl Acad Sci USA* 1987; **84**: 556–60

Calmettes L, Deodati F, Dupre A, Bec P. Manifestations oculaires du syndrome de Fabry. *Bull Soc Ophthalmol* 1967; **59**: 513–17.

Canter RM, Kabach MM. Sandhoff disease, heterozygate frequency in North American Jewish and non-Jewish populations: implications for carrier screening. *Am J Hum Genet* 1985; **37**: A48

Carlson LA, Philipson B. Fish-eye disease. *Lancet* 1979; **ii**: 921–3

Chhabria S, Tomasi LG, Wong PWK. Ophthalmoplegia and bulbar palsy in variant form of maple syrup urine disease. *Ann Neurol* 1979; **6**: 71–81

Charlin C, Fernandez FL. The Urbach–Wiethe syndrome. *Arch Ophthalmol Paris* 1978; **35**: 521–26

Cibis GW, Harris DJ, Chapman AL, Tripathi RC. Neurolipidosis I. *Arch Ophthalmol* 1983; **101**: 933–9

Cogan DG. Ocular manifestations of spongy degeneration. *Birth Defects: Original Article Series* Year Book Medical Publishers, Chicago 1976; **12**: 527–34

Cogan DG, Kuwabara T. Histochemistry of the retina in Tay–Sachs disease. *Arch Ophthalmol* 1959; **61**: 414–23

Cogan DG, Kuwabara T. The sphingolipidoses and the eye. *Arch Ophthalmol* 1968; **79**: 437–52

Cogan DG, Kuwabara T, Moser H. Metachromatic leucodystrophy. *Ophthalmologica* 1970; **180**: 2–17

Cogan DG, Kuwabara T, Moser H, Hazard GW. Retinopathy in a case of Farber's lipogranulomatosis. *Arch Ophthalmol* 1966; **75**: 752–58

Cohen SMZ, Green WR, Cruz C de la, *et al.* Ocular histopathologic studies of neonatal and childhood adrenoleukodystrophy. *Am J of Ophthalmol* 1983; **95**: 82–96.

Collier MM. Dégénéréscence maculaire d'un type special dans un cas de maladie de Gaucher. *Bull Soc Ophthalmol Franc* 1961; **7**: 497–500

Cotticelli L, Costagliola C, Rinaldi E, DiMeo A *et al.* Ophthalmological findings in phenylketonuria: a survey of 14 cases. *J Pediatr Ophthalmol & Strabismus* 1985; **22**: 78–9

Dangel ME, Bremer DL, Rogers GL. Treatment of corneal opacification in mucolipidosis IV with conjunctival transplantation. *Am J Ophthalmol* 1985; **99**: 137–42

De Venecia G, Shapiro M. Neuronal ceroid lipofuscinosis — a retinal trypsin digest study. *Ophthalmology* 1984; **91**: 1406–11

Del Monte MA, Maumenee IH, Green WR, Kenyon KR. Histopathology of Sanfilippo's syndrome. *Arch Ophthalmol* 1983; **101**: 1255–62

Den Tandt WR, Van Martin JJ. Peroxidase in ceroid lipofuscinosis. *J Neurol Sci* 1978; **38**: 191−3

Dickinson JP, Holton JB, Lewis OM *et al*. Maple syrup urine disease: four years experience with dietary treatment of a case. *Acta Pediatr Scand* 1969; **58**: 341−3

Dreborg S, Erikson A, Hagberg B. Gaucher's disease − Norrbothnian type: 1. General clinical description. *Eur J Pediatr* 1980; **133**: 107−18

Dunn HC, Sweeney VP. Progressive supranuclear palsy, an unusual juvenile variant of Niemann. Pick disease. *Neurology* 1971; **21**: 442−43

Elleder M, Jirasek A. International symposium on Niemann Pick disease. *Eur J Pediatr* 1983; **140**: 90−1

Emery JM, Green WR, Huff DS. Krabbe's disease. *Am J Ophthalmol* 1972; **74**: 400−6

Emery JM, Green WR, Wyllie RG, Howell RR. GM(1) gangliosidosis, ocular and pathological manifestations. *Arch Ophthalmol* 1971; **85**: 177−87

Eyb C. Augenhintergrundveranderungen bei der Rindlichen gaucherschen Erkrankurg. *Wen Klin Wochtenschr* 1952; **64**: 38

Feiler-Ofry V, Lewy A, Regenbogen L *et al*. Lipid proteinosis (Urbach−Wiethe syndrome). *Br J Ophthalmol* 1979; **63**: 694−8.

Fettes I, Killinger D, Volpe R. Adrenoleukodystrophy − report of a familial case. *Clin Endocrinol* 1979; **11**: 151−60

Franceschetti A Th. Fabry disease: ocular manifestations. *Birth Defects: Original Article Series*, Year Book Medical Publishers, Chicago 1976; **12**: 195−208

Francois J. Ocular manifestations in inborn errors of carbohydrate and lipid metabolism. *Krabbe's disease*, Part II, Section G. S. Karger, Basel 1975; pp. 98−100

Francois J. Ocular manifestations in demyelinating disease. *Adv Ophthalmol* 1979; **39**: 1−36

Francois J, Backulin J, Follmann P. Ocular manifestations of Urbach Wiethe syndrome. *Ophthalmologica (Basel)* 1968; **155**: 433−48

Garg BP, Markand ON, Dellyer WE, Warren C Jr. Evoked response studies in patients with adrenoleukodystrophy and heterozygous relatives. *Arch Neurol* 1983; **40**: 356−59

Glasgow BJ, Brown HH, Hannah JB, Foos RY. Ocular pathologic findings in neonatal adrenoleukodystrophy. *J Am Acad Ophthalmol* 1987; **94**: 1054−61

Goebel HH, Shimokawa K, Argyrakis A, Pilz H. The ultrastructure of the retina in adult metachromatic leukodystrophy. *Am J Ophthalmol* 1978; **85**: 841−9

Godel V, Blumenthal M, Goldman B *et al*. Visual functions in Tay Sachs diseased patients following enzyme replacement therapy. *Metab Ophthalmol* 1978; **2**: 27−32

Goldberg MF, Cotlier E, Fichenscher LG *et al*. Macular cherry red spot, corneal clouding and beta galactosidase deficiency. *Arch Int Med* 1971; **138**: 387−9.

Goldstein E, Wexler D. Niemann Pick disease with cherry-red spots in the macula. *Arch Ophthalmol* 1931; **5**: 704−06

Goutieres F, Arsenio-Nunes M-L, Aicardi J. Mucolipidosis IV. *Neuropediatrics* 1979; **10**: 321−31

Hall NA, Patrick AD. Accumulation of phosphorylated dolichol in several tissues in ceroid − lipofuscinosis (Batten's disease). *Clin Chim Acta* 1987; **170**: 323−36

Haltia M, Rapola J, Santavuori P, Keranen A. Infantile type of socalled neuronal ceroid lipofuscinosis − Part 2. Morphological and biochemical studies. *J Neurol Sci* 1973; **18**: 269−85

Hammami H, Daicker B, Streiff E *et al*. Leucodystrophie metachromatique associes au syndrome de Lowe. *Bull Mem Soc Fr Ophthalmol* 1973: **86**: 106−7

Hara S, Hayasaka S, Mizuno K. Distribution and some properties of lysosomal arylsulfatases in the bovine eye. *Exp Eye Res* 1979; **28**: 641−50

Harcourt B, Ashton N. Ultrastructure of the optic nerve in Krabbes leucodystrophy. *Br J Ophthalmol* 1973; **57**: 885−91

Harcourt B, Hopkins D. Tapeto-retinal degeneration in childhood presenting as a disturbance of behaviour. *Br Med J* 1962; **1**: 202−5

Harzer K, Ruprecht KW, Seuffer-Schulze D, Jans U. Morbus Niemann−Pick Type B − enzymatisch giesichert-mit unerwarteter retinaler Beteiligung. *Grafes Arch Clin Exp Ophthalmol* 1978; **296**: 79−88

Hayasaka S, Kiyosawa M, Nomura H, Takase S. Papilledema in late-onset citrullinemia. *Am J Ophthalmol* 1974; **97**: 242−3

Hobbs JR, Hugh-Jones K, Barrett AJ *et al*. Reversal of clinical features of Hurler's disease and biochemical improvement after treatment by bone-marrow transplantation. *Lancet* 1981: **ii**: 709−11

Hoffmann H, Fredrickson DS. Tangier disease. *Am J Ophthalmol* 1965; **39**: 582−5

Honda Y, Sudo M. Electroretinogram and visually evoked cortical potential in Tay−Sachs disease; a report of two cases. *J Pediatr Ophthal* 1976; **13**: 226−9

Hormia M. Diffuse cerebral sclerosis, melanoderma and adrenal insufficiency (Adreno-leukodystrophy). *Acta Neurol Scand* 1978; **58**: 128−33

Horn M, Warburg M. Menke's disease. *Birth Defects: Original Article Series* 1976; **12**: 557−62

Jaben SL, Flynn JT, Parker JC. Neuronal ceroid lipofuscinosis: diagnosis from peripheral blood smear. *Ophthalmology* 1983; **90**: 1373−7

Kenyon KR. Ocular manifestations and pathology of systemic mucopolysaccharidoses. *Birth Defects: Original Article Series* 1976; **12**: 133−53

Kenyon KR, Maumenee IH, Green WR, Libert J, Hiatt RL. Mucolipidosis IV. *Arch Ophthalmol* 1979; **97**: 1106−12

Kocen RS, Thomas PK. Peripheral nerve involvement in Fabry's disease. *Arch Neurol* 1970; **22**: 81−8

Lake BD. The differential diagnosis of the various forms of Batten's disease by rectal biopsy. *Birth Defects: Original Article Series* 1976; **12**: 455−64

Lake BD. Lysosomal enzyme deficiencies. In: Adams JH, Corsellis JAN, Duchen LW (Eds.) *Greenfields Neuropathology*, 4th edn. Edward Arnold, London 1984; pp. 491−572

Lake BD, Cavanagh NPC. Early Juvenile Batten's disease. *J Neurol Sci* 1978; **36**: 265−71

Lake BD, Milla PJ, Taylor DSI, Young EP. A mild variant of ML4. *Birth Defects: Original Article Series* Year Book Medical Publishers, Chicago 1982; **18**: 391−404

Lavery MA, Green WR, Jabs EW, Luckenbach MW, Cox JL. Ocular histopathology and ultrastructure of Sanfilippo's syndrome, Type III-B. *Arch Ophthalmol* 1983; **101**: 1263−74

Letson RD, Desnick RJ. Punctate lenticular opacities in Type II mannosidosis. *Am J Ophthalmol* 1978; **85**: 218−24

Levy NS, Dawson WW, Rhodes BJ, Garnica A. Ocular abnormalities in Menke's kinky hair syndrome. *Am J Ophthalmol* 1974; **77**: 319−25

Libert J, Kenyon KR, Maumenee IH. Mucolopidosis III

(pseudo-Hurler polydystrophy) ultrastructure of conjunctival biopsies. *Metab Ophthalmol* 1977b; **1**: 145−48

Libert J, Tandeur M, Van Hoof F. The use of conjunctival biopsy and enzyme analysis in tears for the diagnosis of homozygotes and heterozygotes with Fabry's disease. *Birth Defects: Original Article Series* 1976a; **12**: 221−39

Libert J, Toussaint D. Tortuosities of retinal and conjunctival vessels in lysosomal storage disorders. *Birth Defects: Original Article Series* 1982; **18**: 347−58

Libert J, Van Hoof F, Farriaux J-P, Toussaint D. Ocular findings in I-cell disease (mucolipidosis type II). *Am J Ophthalmol* 1977a; **83**: 617−28

Libert J, Van Hoof F, Tandeur M. Fucocidosis: ultrastructural Study of conjunctiva and skin and enzyme analysis of tears. *Invest Ophthalmol Vis Sci* 1976b; **15**: 626−39

Libert J, Van Hoof F, Toussaint D *et al.* Ocular findings in Metachromatic leucodystrophy. *Arch Ophthalmol* 1979; **97**: 1495−504

Lonsdale D, Mercer RD, Faulkner WR. Maple syrup urine disease. *Am J Dis Child* 1963; **106**: 258−66

Lowden JA, O'Brien JS. Sialidosis: a review of human neuraminidase deficiency. *Am J Hum Genet* 1979; **31**: 18−24

MacFaul R, Cavanagh N, Lake BD, Stephens R, Whitfield AE. Metachromatic leucodystrophy: review of 38 cases. *Arch Dis Child* 1982; **57**: 168−75

Mainardi P. Un caso di malattia dello sciroppo d'acero. *Pediatr Minerva* 1966; **18**: 1969−72

Markesbery WR, Shield LK, Egel RT, Jameson MD. Late infantile neuronal ceroid-lipofuscinosis: an ultrastructural study of lymphocyte inclusions. *Arch Neurol* 1976; **33**: 630−5

Matthews JD, Weiter JJ, Kolodry EH. Macular halos associated with Niemann−Pick type B disease. *Ophthalmology* 1986; **93**: 933−938

Mayou MS. Cerebral degeneration with symmetrical changes in the maculae in three members of a family. *Trans Ophthalmol Soc UK* 1904; **24**: 142−5

McDonald JT, Sher PK. Ophthalmoplegia as a sign of metabolic disease in the newborn. *Neurology (Minn)* 1977; **27**: 971−73

McDonell J, Green W, Maumenee I. Ocular histopathology of systemic mucopolysaccharidosis, Type II-A Hunter syndrome, severe. *Ophthalmology* 1983; **92**: 1772−80

McKeran RO, Bradbury P, Taylor D, Stern G. Neurological involvement in Type I (adult) Gaucher's disease. *J Neurol Neurosurg Psychiatr* 1985; **48**: 172−5

McKusic VA. *Mendelian Inheritance in Man.* John Hopkins University Press, Baltimore 1986

Merin S, Livini N, Berman ER, Yatziv S. Mucolipidosis IV; ocular, systemic, and ultrastructural findings. *Invest Ophthalmol* 1975; **14**: 437−48

Miller JD, McCliver R, Kanfer J. Gaucher's disease: neurologic disorder in adult siblings. *Ann Int Med* 1973; **78**: 883−7

Moloney J, Masterson JG. Detection of adrenoleucodystrophy carriers by means of evoked potentials. *Lancet* 1982; **i**: 852−00

Montgomery TR, Thomas GH, Valle DL. Mannosidosis in an adult. *Johns Hopkins Med J* 1982; **151**: 113−7

Morgan SH, Crawford M d'A. Anderson−Fabry disease. *Br Med J* 1988; **297**: 872−3

Morris MD, Lewis BD, Doolan PD, Harper HA. Clinical and biochemical observations of an apparently non fatal variant of branched-chain ketoaciduria. *Pediatrics* 1961; **28**: 918−23

Muirhead JF, Jackson P. Urbach Wiethe disease. *Arch Ophthalmol* 1963; **69**: 174−79

Murphree AL, Beaudet AL, Palmer EA, Nichols BL. Cataract in mannosidosis. *Birth Defects: Original Article Series* 1976; **12**: 319−25

Musarella MA, Raab EI, Rudolph S, Grabowski GA, Desnick RJ. Oculomotor abnormalities in chronic GM2 gangliosidosis. *J Pediatr Ophthalmol Strabismus* 1982; **19**: 80−9

Naughten ER, Jenkins J, Francis DEM, Leonard JV. Outcome of maple syrup urine disease. *Arch Dis Child* 1982; **57**: 918−21

Neville BGR, Lake BD, Stevens R, Sanders MD. A neurovisceral storage disease with vertical supranuclear ophthalmoplegia and its relationship to Niemann−Pick disease − a report of nine patients. *Brain* 1973; **96**: 97−120

Newell FW, Matalon R, Meyer S. A new mucolipidosis with psychomotor retardation, corneal clouding, and retinal degeneration. *Am J Ophthalmol* 1975; **80**: 440−49

Newton FH, Rosenberg RN, Laupert PW, O'Brien JS. neurologic involvement in Urbach−Wiette's disease (lipid proteinosis). *Neurology* 1971; **21**: 1205−13

Norman RM, Forrester RM, Tingey AH. The juvenile form of Niemann−Pick disease. *Arch Dis Child* 1967; **42**: 91−96

Ozaki H, Mizutani M, Hayashi H. Farber's disease. *Acta Med Okayama* 1978; **32**: 69−79

Pampiglione G, Harden A. So-called neuronal ceroid lipofuscinosis. Neurophysiological studies in 60 children. *J Neurol Neurosurg Psychiatr* 1977; **40**: 323−30

Parks MM, Schwilk Bilateral lamellar-type cataracts in a case of phenylketonuria. *Am J Ophthalmol* 1963; **56**: 140−2

Petrochelos M, Tricoules D, Kotziras T, Vauzoukos A. Ocular manifestations of Gaucher's disease. *Am J Ophthalmol* 1975; **80**: 1006−1011

Pinckers A, Bolmers D. Neuronal ceroidlipofuscinosis (ERG et EOG). *Ann Oculist (Paris)* 1974; **207**: 523−9

Pullarkat RK, Patel UK, Brokerhoff H. Leukocyte docosahexanoic acid in juvenile form of ceroid lipofuscinosis. *Neuropediatrics* 1978; **9**: 127−30

Quigley MA, Green WR. Clinical and ultrastructural ocular histopathologic studies of adult-onset metachromatic leukodystrophy. *Am J Ophthalmol* 1972; **82**: 472−9

Quisling RG, Andriola MR. Computed tomographic evaluation of the early phase of Adrenoleukodystrophy. *Neuroradiology* 1979; **17**: 285−8

Raitta C, Santavuori P. Ophthalmological findings in infantile type of so-called neuronal ceroidlipofuscinosis. *Acta Ophthalmol* 1973; **51**: 755−63

Rapin I, Katzmann R, Engel J Jr. Cherry red spots and myoclonus without dementia: a distinct syndrome with neuronal storage. *Arch Neurol* 1975; **32**: 349−54

Reich C, Scife M, Kessler B. Gaucher's disease: a review and discussion of 20 cases. *Medicine* 1951; **30**: 1−20

Renard G, Bargeton E, Dhermy P, Aran J-J. Etude histologique des deterations de la retine et du nerf optique au cours de la leucodystrophie metachromatique. *Bull Mem Soc Fr Ophthalmol* 1963; **76**: 40−58

Riedel KG, Zwaan J, Kenyon KR *et al.* Ocular abnormalities in mucolipidosis IV. *Am J Ophthalmol* 1985; **99**: 125−37

Santavuori P, Haltia M, Rapola J, Raitta C. Infantile type of so-called neuronal ceroid lipofuscinosis I. A Clinical study of 15 cases. *J Neurol Sci* 1973; **18**: 257−67

Santavuori P, Moren R. Experience of antioxidant treatment in neuronal ceroid-lipofuscinosis of Spielmeyer–Sjogren type I. *Neuropediatric* 1977; **8**: 333–4

Schaumberg HH, Powers JM, Raine CS, Suzuki K, Richardson JCP. Adrenoleukodystrophy: a clinical and pathological study of 17 cases. *Arch Neurol* 1975; **32**: 577–91

Schilovitz G, Grupper Ch, Payran P. Urbach–Wiethe's disease. Association with retinitis pigmentosa. *Ann Oculist (Paris)* 1973; **206**: 105–14

Schwartz JF, Kolendrianos ET. Maple syrup urine disease. A review with a report of an additional case. *Dev Med Child Neurol* 1969; **11**: 460–70

Seelenfreund MH, Gartner S, Vinger F. The ocular pathology of Menke's disease. *Arch Ophthalmol* 1968; **80**: 718–23

Sher NA, Letson RD, Desnick RJ. The ocular manifestations in Fabry's disease. *Arch Ophthalmol* 1979; **97**: 671–6

Sher NA, Reiff W, Letson RD, Desnick RJ. Central retinal artery occlusion complicating Fabry's disease. *Arch Ophthalmol* 1978; **96**: 815–7

Snebold NG, Rizzo JF, Lessell S, Pruett RC. Transient visual loss in ornithine trans carbamoylase deficiency. *Am J Ophthalmol* 1987; **104**: 407–12

Snodgrass M. Ocular findings in fucosidosis. *Br J Ophthalmol* 1976; **60**: 508–513

Snyder RO, Carlow TJ, Ledman J, Wenger DA. Ocular findings in fucosidosis. *Birth Defects* 1976; **12**: 241–6

Spaeth GK, Frost P. Fabry's disease, its ocular manifestations. *Arch Ophthalmol* 1965; **74**: 760–9

Spalton DJ, Taylor DSI, Sanders MD. Juvenile Batten's disease; an ophthalmological assessment of 26 patients. *Br J Ophthalmol* 1980; **64**: 726–32

Spellacy E, Kennerly-Bankes JL, Crow J, Dourmashkin R, Shah D, Watts RWE. Glaucoma in a case of Hurler disease. *Br J Ophthalmol* 1980; **94**: 773–9

Spielmeyer W. Weitere Mittheilung uber eine besondere form von familiarer amaurotischer idiotie. *Neurol Centralbl* 1905; **24**: 1131–2

Spranger JW, Wiedemann HR. The genetic mucolipidoses: diagnosis and differential diagnosis. *Hum Genet* 1970; **9**: 113–9

Swallow DM, Evans L, Stewart G, Thomas PK, Abrahams JD. Sialidosis type I. *Ann Hum Genet* 1979; **43**: 27–35

Taylor D, Lake BD, Marshall J, Garner A. Retinal abnormalities in ophthalmoplegic lipidosis. *Br J Ophthalmol* 1981; **65**: 484–9

Thomas PK, Abrams JD, Swallow D, Stewart G. Sialidosis type I: cherry-red spot myoclonus syndrome with sialidase deficiency and altered electrophoretic mobilities of some enzymes known to be glycoproteins. *J Neurol Neurosurg Psychiatr* 1979; **42**: 873–80

Toussaint D, Davis P. Dystrophie maculaire dans une maladie de Menkes. Etude histologique oculaire. *J Fr Ophthalmol* 1978; **1**: 457–60

Traboulsi EI, Maumenee IH. Ophthalmologic findings in mucolipidosis III (psuedo-Hurler polydystrophy). *Am J Ophthalmol* 1986; **102**: 592–7

Tripp JH, Lake BD, Young E. Ngu J, Brett EM. Juvenile Gaucher's disease with horizontal gaze palsy in three siblings. *J Neurol Neurosurg Psychiatr* 1977; **40**: 470–68

Valavanis A, Friede RL, Schubiger O, Hayek J. Computed tomography in neuronal ceroid lipofuscinosis. *Neuroradiology* 1980; **19**: 35–8

Vellodi A, Hobbs JR, O'Donnell NM, Coulter BS, Hugh-Jones K. Treatment of Niemann–Pick disease type B by allogenic bone marrow transplantation. *Br Med J* 1987; **295**: 1375–6

Vrabec MP, Shapiro MB, Koller E, Wiebe DA, Henricks J, Albers JJ. Ophthalmic observations in lecithin cholesterol acyltransferase deficiency. *Arch Ophthalmol* 1988; **106**: 225–30

Walton DS, Robb RM, Crocker AC. Ocular manifestations of group A Niemann–Pick disease. *Am J Ophthalmol* 1978; **85**: 174–80

Weicksel J. Angiomatosis bzw: Angiokeratosis universalis. *Dtsch Med Wochenschr* 1925; **51**: 890–900

Weingeist TA, Blodi FC. Fabry's disease — ocular findings in a female carrier. A light-and electron-microscopic study. *Arch Ophthalmol* 1971; **85**: 169–76

Weiter JJ, Feingold M, Kolodny EH, Raghaven SA. Retinal pigment epithelial degeneration associated with leukocytic arylsulfatase A deficiency. *Am J Ophthalmol* 1980; **90**: 768–72

Westmoreland BF, Groover RV, Sharbrough FW. Electrographic findings in three types of cerebromacular degeneration. *Mayo Clin Proc* 1979; **54**: 12–21

Winkelman MD, Banber BQ, Victor M, Moser HW. Noninfantile neuronopathic Gaucher's disease: a clinicopathologic study. *Neurology* 1983; **33**: 394–8

Wolfe LS, Ng Ying Kin NMK, Baker RR, Carpenter S, Anderman F. Identification of retinoyl complexes as the autofluorescent component of the neuronal storage material in Batten disease. *Science* 1977; **195**: 1360–64

Wray SH, Cogan DG, Kuwabara T, Schaumberg HH, Powers JM. Adrenoleukodystrophy with disease of the eye and optic nerve. *Am J Ophthalmol* 1976; **82**: 480–5

Wray SH, Kuwabara T, Sanderson P. Menke's kinky hair disease: a light and electron microscopic study of the eye. *Invest Ophthalmol Vis Sci* 1976; **15**: 128–38

Yunis EJ, Led RE. Further observations on the fine structure of globoid leucodystrophy. *Hum Pathol* 1972; **3**: 371–88

Zarbin MA, Green WR, Moser HW, Morton SJ. Farber's disease. *Arch Ophthalmol* 1985; **103**: 73–80

Zee DS, Freeman JM, Holtzman NA. Ophthalmoplegia in maple syrup urine disease. *J Pediatrics* 1974; **84**: 113–15

Zetterstrom R. Disseminated lipogranulomatosis (Farber's disease). *Acta Paediatr* 1958; **47**: 501–10

Zlotgora J, Schaap T, Bach G. Retinal pigment epithelial degeneration and arylsulfotase A deficiency. *Am J Ophthalmol* 1981; **92**: 136–8

Zwann J. Eye findings in patients with phenylketonuria. *Arch Ophthalmol* 1983; **101**: 1236–7

35 Non-Accidental Injury

NICHOLAS CAVANAGH

Non-accidental injury (NAI) is a serious problem with a significant mortality and substantial long-term physical and emotional sequelae (Rosenbloom & Hensey 1985). NAI in children was first identified by Caffey (1946) from the radiological findings of unexplained multiple fractures. Kempe *et al.* (1962) coined the phrase of the 'battered child syndrome', but with time it has become clear that other forms of injury, apart from battering, may take place. These include nutritional deficiency, poisoning, neglect of medical care, neglect of safety (e.g. drowning), chronic eye injury (Taylor & Bentovim 1979) (Fig. 35.1), Munchausen by proxy (Meadow 1982), emotional and sexual. Munchausen by proxy is a term coined by Meadow (1982) in which the mother is involved in elaborate rituals of deception (Lancet Editorial 1983) including repeated caustic applications to skin, adding salt to urine or blood samples, giving sedatives or tranquillizers to the children. Reece and Grodin (1985) expressed caution concerning the use of emotive lables such as 'battered', 'abused', etc. The borderline between accidental and non-accidental, injurious and non-injurious, normal and abnormal sexuality between adults and children, and children and children, of individual versus society guilt, is often very fine indeed, and we need less moral criticism, but more to think in terms of prevention (DHSS 1988).

All forms of non-accidental injury are likely to be underdiagnosed (Strauss *et al.* 1980), but Schmitt and Krugman (1987) give the following statistics for the USA. One percent of children are reported to be injured: 33% of these are under 1 year; 33% 1—6 years and the remaining one third are over 6 years. The mortality is about 3%. A related caretaker of the child is involved in 90% of cases. There are a number of features that may characterize the affected child such as premature birth, misery, overactivity, features that differentiate him from his siblings, and from the normal, e.g. soiling or congenital abnormalities.

Diagnosis

History

Often the injury is unexplained. If an explanation is offered, it may be implausible or inconsistent, or conflict with that of either the child's or another involved person. The demeanour of the history-giver may be inappropriate to the story given. There may be a delay between the time of injury and the presentation of the injured child to hospital.

Examination

CUTANEOUS INJURIES

These are the commonest manifestation of non-accidental injury and may be recognized as such by their location, pattern and number.

Accidental injuries typically involve the forehead, anterior tibia and other bony prominences, such as chin or hips. Other affected areas of the face and

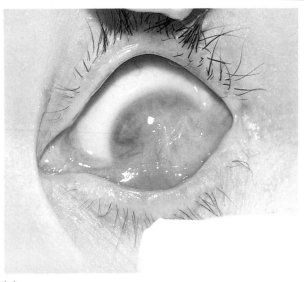

(a)

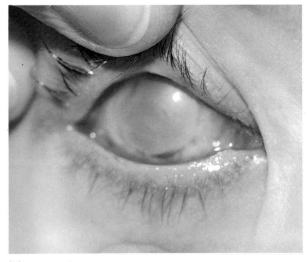

(b)

Fig. 35.1 This child had had recurrent attacks of keratoconjunctivitis in the left eye which had in the early stages resolved on admission to hospital but later resulted in an axial pseudopterygium. (b) The right eye became suddenly inflamed 2 years after the left eye had started to have keratitis. This picture shows the eye 4 days after the onset of the abnormality which was when it was reported. Both injuries were later found to be caused by the mother.

involvement of the trunk, thorax, buttocks and genitalia, suggest non-accidental injury (Pascoe *et al.* 1979). The appearance of certain injuries may be diagnostic, e.g. the slap on the face with the hand, leaving a bruise with two or three parallel lines through it, human bite marks leave paired, opposing, semi-circular bruises, buckle marks from a belt, elliptical welts from flex, thick welts from a strap, finger and

thumb-prints on the thorax of a shaken child or on the upper arm of a grabbed child, burns on the neck from a rope, etc. Non-accidental burns may be distinguished from accidental ones, both by location (the latter usually occur on the front of the body) and appearance (the accidental ones are often single, asymmetrical and partial thickness). Multiple bruises of different colours should arouse suspicion of repetitive injuries. Red-purple colour suggests injury inflicted 24−48 hours ago, brown colour 2−3 days, green colour 4−10 days, yellow colour 10 days plus (Reece & Grodin 1985), but the observations that the presence of up to five bruises at any one time on an individual child may be within normal limits must always be borne in mind.

HEAD INJURY

Intracranial damage in NAI leads to the greatest number of abuse-related deaths. There are many indicators of head injury which include fractures of various kinds, intracranial bleeding of various kinds, non-specific signs of intracranial pressure, scalp wounds and bruising, CSF leak, bleeding from the ears, etc.

EYE INJURIES

These may be evident in up to 40% of non-accidentally injured children. Kiffney (1964) may have been the first to describe the eye of the non-accidentally injured child. The commonest ocular abnormality is retinal haemorrhage (Jensen *et al.* 1971; Harley & Spaeth 1982), often in association with intracranial bleeding, but also resulting from thoracic compression (Fig. 34.2, 34.3, 34.4). Other posterior segment haemorrhage, such as pre-retinal and vitreous bleeding, does occur and, in contrast to the retinal haemorrhages which usually resolve without sequelae, may be associated with macular scarring, raised intraocular pressure or subsequent retinal traction. The origin of the haemorrhages is uncertain, the more peripheral retinal haemorrhages, isolated from the optic disc may be due solely to raised retinal venous pressure together with the trauma of shaking. The finding of optic nerve sheath haemorrhages (Lambert *et al.* 1986) suggests that the haemorrhages found surrounding the optic disc may have an origin from the subarachnoid space. Peripheral white lesions may represent previous retinal haemorrhages.

The next most common ocular manifestation of NAI is peri-orbital oedema and subconjunctival haemorrhage (Fig. 34.5), and if accompanied by bleeding, is usually associated with forehead and scalp

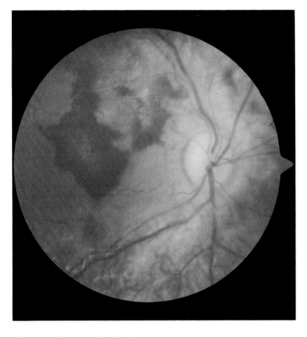

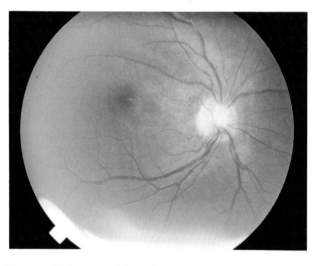

Fig. 35.4 This 4-year-old child had been seen with bilateral exudative retinal detachments, now resolved leaving poor acuity, nystagmus and peripheral subretinal white masses (not visible on the photographs).

Fig. 35.2 Intraretinal and subhyaloid haemorrhages in NAI.

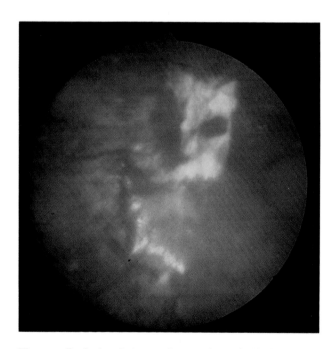

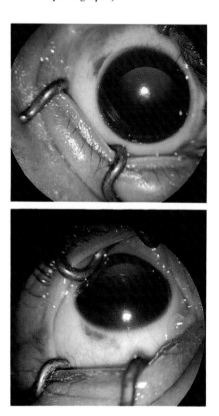

Fig. 35.3 Retinal and vitreous haemorrhages in NAI. The white areas represent partially organised haemorrhage.

Fig. 35.5 Conjunctival haemorrhages associated with shaking.

contusions. Other manifestations include retinal detachment (Weidenthal & Levin 1976), choroidol-retinal atrophy, retinoschisis (Greenwald *et al.* 1986), and from direct trauma, cataracts, subluxated lenses, traumatic mydriasis and corneal enlargement with scarring (Harley 1980). Long-term follow-up of non-

accidentally injured infants has shown considerable visual handicap due to optic nerve, optic radiation and cortical injuries (Harcourt & Hopkins 1971). Whilst occult NAI may be associated with retinal haemorrhages and more widespread CNS disorders

(Giangiacomo & Barkett 1985) it is most important that retinal haemorrhages should not be taken as being pathognomonic of NAI: they occur in a wide variety of other causes of raised central venous pressure including epileptic fits, asphyxia, and subarachnoid haemorrhage and are present in a large proportion of normal neonates. The presence of haemorrhages at different stages of resolution is more suspicious of NAI but may still occur from natural causes.

OTHER INJURIES

These may include tears in the floor of the mouth from trauma due to forced-feeding, and rupture of intra-abdominal organs, e.g. spleen and liver.

Investigations

Plain X-rays

A full skeletal survey is indicated in all infants under 1 year of age suspected of being injured by any means. Between the ages of 1 and 3 years, a skeletal survey is probably only indicated if there is suspicion of physical abuse and in the older child a skeletal survey must be performed selectively (Merton et al. 1983). Fractures are most commonly present in the under-3 age group (particularly under the age of 1), in boys, and involving extremities, skull and ribs. Bony injuries which are characteristically produced by abuse include epiphyseal-diaphyseal fractures both spiral and transverse, metaphyseal injuries resulting from shaking or jerking, posterior rib fractures from blunt injuries, occult (often in infants) or occult multiple or multiple fractures at various stages of repair (Merton et al. 1983). Ninety per cent of skull fractures in NAI occur in children under the age of 2 and intent to injure is suggested by one or more of the following features: (a) multiple or complex fractures; (b) depressed fracture; (c) a fracture with a maximum width of greater than 3 mm; (d) a growing fracture; (e) involvement of more than one cranial bone; (f) non-parietal fracture; or all fractures associated with intracranial injury (Hobbs 1984). Linear fractures of the calvarium are best seen on plain X-ray of skull, fractures of the skull-base or depressed fractures are best visualized by CT scan (Hershey & Zimmermann 1985).

CT or MRI scanning

In addition to showing skull-base or depressed fractures, these may reveal evidence of cerebral swelling and/or intracranial haemorrhage. Cerebral swelling occurs acutely due both to increased cerebral blood flow and oedema, and shows with evidence of absence or compression of the ventricles and increased density in brain substance. Vasogenic oedema may be focal or multifocal and is seen in haemorrhagic contusion and intracerebral haematoma and extends along axon pathways into white matter. It may be evident for as long as 2 months after the injury.

Brain contusion may result directly from the injury or from contrecoup, and shows as a non-homogeneous area of high density (haemorrhage) and low density (necrosis) areas.

Intracranial bleeding may be of several kinds. Intracerebral haemorrhage occurs at the site of contusion or from blood vessels torn by shearing forces. Often this kind of bleeding occurs at juncture points between cortex and white matter and shows as little areas of focal haemorrhage.

Non-intracerebral haemorrhage may be epidural when it can be associated with skull fracture, e.g. in the temporoparietal regions when the bleeding does not then cross suture lines. Alternatively, the bleeding may be subdural, which is often associated with underlying brain damage. Bilateral subdurals strongly suggest a whiplash injury leading to shearing of bridging veins at fixed sites of attachment to the walls of the sagittal sutures. Shaking may lead to parieto-occipital interhemispheric subdural haematoma. Infants under the age of 6 months with subdurals often present with coma, but in the older age-group the signs are less specific, such as lethargy, vomiting, crying, etc. Concomitant subdural hygroma and atrophy may be indicative of earlier traumatic episodes.

Subarachnoid haemorrhage often occurs in association with the other kinds of bleeding mentioned above and shows as an increased density in the region of the falx. Communicating hydrocephalus may be a sequel to this.

Bleeding and clotting studies

The types of bruising and the manner in which they are said to occur may be very similar in NAI and in bleeding disorders (Schwer et al. 1982). The tests which must be done to exclude a bleeding disorder are (O'Hare & Eden 1984) (a) full blood count and film; (b) platelet count size and shape; (c) partial thromboplastin time; (d) prothrombin time; (e) thrombin time; and (f) fibrinogen and bleeding time. It is, of course, possible that a bleeding diathesis and non accidental injury may co-exist.

Drug history

It is important to enquire about salicylate and other drug ingestion both around the time that bruises are thought to have occurred and when bleeding and clotting studies are being performed, since they may affect test results. It is also important to be aware of circulating antibodies after minor viral infections in children (O'Hare & Eden 1984).

Radio nucleotide bone scanning

This may be a useful addition to plain radiography and increase the detection rate of hair line fractures. It should, perhaps, be reserved for occasions where plain X-rays are negative and there is a strong suspicion of NAI. It should be noted that bone scans and plain X-rays may give false-negative results.

Differential diagnosis

Osteogenesis imperfecta

This condition has to be actively considered in any child suspected of NAI, since very mild forms may present with fractures in the toddler age group up to adolescence. The clinical features include blue sclera, large fontanelle, excess joint laxity, small stature, and poor dentition. The distinguishing radiological features of osteogenesis imperfecta that help to distinguish fractures caused in the condition from non-accidental injuries include the following: the fractures are mainly in the diaphyses of long bones and are rare in the metaphyses. Wormian bones are usually present, and generally there are radiological signs of osteoporosis (Carty 1988).

Copper deficiency

This most commonly has to be considered in the under 2 age group. The clinical features include a predisposing cause (low birth weight, dietary deficiency, malnutrition) and anaemia, neutropaenia, pallor, hypotonia, hyperpigmentation, prominent scalp veins, and finally plasma copper concentrations, usually below 40 mg/dl and caeruloplasmin less than 13 mg/dl. The radiological features include osteoporosis, fraying and cupping of the metaphyscs, spur formation, periosteal reactions and fractures. These findings are in contrast to the non-accidentally injured child where the bone texture is normal and there is no cupping or fraying of the metaphysis where a fracture has occurred (Shaw 1988).

Scurvy

In this condition, too, spur formation and corner fractures may occur, but there is no fraying of the metaphyses to distinguish this from copper deficiency and the epiphyses have distinctive etched appearances to distinguish them from both copper deficiency and the bones of the non-accidentally injured child (Carty 1988).

Management

Although details of management of suspected non-accidental injury will vary in different parts of the world according to specific legal requirements, there are a number of guiding principles of universal application. These include (a) that all professionals involved must actively guard themselves against feelings of vindictiveness, moral superiority, sexism, and any personal crusade; (b) that the aims are to correctly recognize non-accidental injury, help the child and the family in the immediate and long-term, and prevent recurrence; and (c) that any system designed to achieve these aims will have to strike a balance between extremes. On the one hand it must not result in the false accusation of innocent people and the disruption of innocent families, and on the other that it does not miss actual cases.

In practice, a case of suspected NAI might be managed as follows:

1 Admit the child to hospital under the care of a paediatrician. It may be necessary at that stage to express to the parents what your concerns are. Only resort to legal placement of the child in hospital if the patients refuse their consent.

2 Take a full history including details of the pregnancy, delivery, new born period, developmental milestones, previous illnesses, family history, social history, educational history, drug ingestion, as well as details of the circumstances of the particular injury/injuries in question.

3 Examine the child fully, paying particular attention to the physical injuries, nutritional state, intellectual and developmental progress, and growth. Record all findings, make drawings where possible and photograph injuries.

4 Obtain a social services report.

5 The paediatrician should keep in frequent informing contact with parents.

6 The paediatrician should decide on the basis of all the information received whether NAI has occurred. It would be the policy of some doctors to hold a case conference of all the parties involved with the child including, perhaps, the police. This author would not because he shares the concerns expressed by James and Ward (1988) about case conferences, and particularly deplores the tendency for these to be held without the parents of the child being present. He would, though, keep in close contact with all the involved professionals.

7 If the decision is made that NAI has occurred then the police must be informed. Some doctors might then place the child on Child Protection Registers, but this author would not, again sharing the concerns expressed by James & Ward (1988).

8 It would be hoped that good liaison with the police would allow for as little punitive intervention on their part as possible.

9 Full liaison should be maintained with the Social Services department which have a statutory duty to promote the welfare of that child, and to appoint a 'key worker' (DHSS 1988).

10 The aim, whenever possible would be to maintain the family together, and support them in such a way as to prevent re-occurrence. This might involve (a) various agencies, e.g. the family doctor, The National Society for the Prevention of Cruelty to Children, the Local Education Authority, the health visitor, or the Housing department etc.; (b) regular outpatient review; and (c) the offer of respite care from time to time, etc.

11 On-going liaison at all levels between all the parties involved.

12 Particular attention has to be paid to enable the family to provide the environment that prevents the emotional disturbances which so often persist long after the accidental injury has stopped (Oates 1984).

References

Caffey J. Multiple fractures in long bones of children suffering from chronic subdural haematomata. *Am J Radio* 1964; **56**: 163–73

Carty H. Brittle or battered? *Arch Dis Child* 1988; **63**: 50–352

DHSS (Department of Health & Social Security) and Welsh Office. *Working Together: A Guide to Arrangements for Inter-agency Co-operation for the Protection of Children from Abuse.* Her Majesty's Stationery Office, London 1988

Editorial. Lancet 1983; **i**: 456

Giangiacomo J, Barkett KJ. Ophthalmoscopic findings in occult child abuse. *J Pediatr Ophthalmol Strabismus* **1985**; 22: 234–8

Greenwald MJ, Weiss A, Osterle CS, Friendly DS. Traumatic retinoschisis in battered babies. *Ophthalmology* 1986; **93**: 618–25

Harcourt RB, Hopkins D. Ophthalmic manifestations of the battered baby syndrome. *Br Med J* 1971; **3**: 398–403

Harley RD. Ocular manifestations of child abuse. *J Pediatr Ophthalmol Strabismus* 1980; **17**: 5–13

Harley RG, Spaeth GL. Ocular manifestations of child abuse. In: François J, Maione M (eds) *Pediatric Ophthalmology.* John Wiley, Chichester 1982; pp 141–5

Hershey BL, Zimmermann RA. Paediatric brain computed tomography. *Pediatr Clin N Am* 1985; **32**: 1477–508.

Hobbs CJ. Skull fracture and the diagnosis of abuse. *Arch Dis Child* 1984; **59**: 246–52

James D, Ward K. Child abuse registers (letter). *Lancet* 1988; **i**: 1398

Jensen AD, Smith RE, Olson MI, Ocular clues to child abuse. *J Pediatr Ophthalmol Strabismus* 1971; **8**: 270–2

Kempe CH, Silverman FN, Steele BF, Droegemuller W, Silver HH. The battered child syndrome. *J Am Med Assn* 1962; **181**: 17–24

Kiffney GT. The eye of the battered child. *Arch Ophthalmol* 1964; **72**: 231–4

Lambert SR, Johnson TE, Hoyt CS. Optic nerve sheath and retinal haemorrhage associated with the shaken baby syndrome. *Arch Ophthalmol* 1986; **104**: 1509–12

Meadow SR. Munchausen syndrome by proxy. *Arch Dis Child* 1982; **57**: 92–8

Merton DF, Radkowski MA, Leonidas JC. The abused child, a radiological re-appraisal. *Radiology* 1983; **146**: 377–82

Oates RK. Personality development and physical abuse. *Arch Dis Child* 1984; **59**: 147–50

O'Hare AE, Eden OB. Bleeding disorders and non-accidental injury. *Arch Dis Child* 1984; **59**: 860–4

Pascoe JM, Hildebrandt HM, Tarrier A *et al.* Patterns of skin injury in non-accidental and accidental injury. *Pediatr* 1979; **64**: 245–7

Reece RM, Grodin MA. Recognition of non-accidental injury. *Pediatr Clin N Am* 1985; **32**: 41–60

Rosenbloom L, Hensey OJ. Outcome for children subject to non-accidental injury. *Arch Dis Child* 1985; **60**: 191–3

Schmitt BD, Krugman RD. Abuse and neglect of children. In: Behrman RE, Vaughan VC (Eds.) *Nelson's Textbook of Pediatrics*, WB Saunders, Philadelphia 13th edn. 1987: 79–84

Schwer B, Brueschke EE, Dent T. Haemophilia. *J Fam Pract* 1982; **14**: 661–74

Shaw JCL. Copper deficiency and non-accidental injury. *Arch Dis Child* 1988; **63**: 350–2

Strauss MA, Gelles RJ, Steinmetz SK. *Behind Closed Doors: Violence in the American Family.* Anchor Double Pay, Garden City, New York 1980

Taylor D, Bentovim A. Recurrent non-accidentally inflicted chemical eye injuries to siblings. *J Pediatr Ophthalmol* 1979; **13**: 238–42

Weidenthal DT, Levin DB. Retinal detachment in a battered infant. *Am J Ophthalmol* 1976; **81**: 727–31

36 Specific Learning Disorders (Dyslexia)

NICHOLAS CAVANAGH

Practical aspects

Reasons for academic failure in childhood include mental retardation, a sensory disability such as blindness or deafness, a primary emotional disturbance, or inadequate education. In addition there is a small but significant proportion (perhaps 5%) of children who, in the absence of any of the above explanations, show profound difficulties in one or more of listening, thinking, talking, reading, writing, spelling or mathematics. In this book these children will be referred to as having specific learning difficulties, but there is considerable confusion and disagreement about terminology and in another context they might be described as having dyslexia, specific developmental dyslexia, minimal brain dysfunction, the attention deficit syndrome, hyperactive child syndrome, perceptual handi-caps, the chronic brain syndrome, developmental dyspraxia, etc (Wheeler & Watkins 1978). Even the term specific learning disability has its critics (Crystal 1982). What is abundantly clear from this proliferation of terms is that there are many facets to the problem and that the affected children may present in a variety of ways.

Presentation

Usually the difficulties manifest for the first time soon after schooling begins, though sometimes there are overt problems much earlier. Some children are slow to learn to dress, have problems knowing which way round things go, or may be slow to show hand preference (usually this is becoming evident around 18 months to 2 years of age). They have great difficulty using scissors, eat messily, appear clumsy, and unable to cope with buttons and buckles; they seem to trip over 'nothing' and fall frequently, and drop things excessively. These are the children who later on may be shown to have a relatively low performance intelligence (IQ) on the Wechsler Intelligence Scale for Children (Revised) (WISCR) compared with higher verbal abilities. They go on to have problems learning to write smoothly and efficiently. Their writing is slow, untidy and messy. They cannot take down dictation. They fail examinations because they cannot commit their knowledge to paper. They have difficulty in distinguishing left from right. They tend to lose their place on the page.

A relationship between early speech delay and impaired language development, and subsequent learning difficulties has been suspected for a long time (McCready 1910). By 1979 Vellutino claimed that there was moderately suggestive evidence for this, and both the Dunedin (Silva 1980; Silva *et al.* 1983) and Waltham Forest (Graham *et al.* 1980) longitudinal studies of language delay in children, show significant reading and spelling delay compared with controls. However, it is Stevenson's opinion (1984) that it is not possible to establish from the published data why the results represented a specific learning difficulty with reading that is not accounted for by the low intelligence scores of the children. Such children may show a discrepancy between their poor ability to express themselves and their ideas, and their normal or superior understanding of what is said to them. Alternatively, the problems may be the reverse with good expressive language, but inability to receive information and act on it or respond to it appropriately. These children may appear in a dream and forget messages or what they've been asked to do.

Problems of concentration, distractability or overactivity are often present from an early age. Sometimes as babies they have been noticeably wriggly even when breastfeeding, have required very little sleep, have been very light sleepers, and have been constantly on the go.

It is on a background of such problems early in life that the children then go on to have difficulties reading and writing, show bizarre spelling, confusion of b and d, saw and was, and more profound problems of syntax and semantics. Difficulties in memorising may be more for visual input than auditory or vice versa, or some times both, manifesting with difficulty in learning by heart. Sometimes short-term memory deficits are paramount, and sometimes the difficulties are more to do with numbers than letters.

Finally all these problems commonly lead to behavioural disturbance. The children may lose confidence in themselves, and feel they are stupid. These feelings may be reinforced by their peers and ignorant teachers. They may become withdrawn and depressed. Aggression is a common consequence. Alternatively they may cease to try and become deliberately inattentive to the teaching of what they find hard to understand.

Diagnosis

The majority of children with specific learning difficulties are undetected until they start school, and even if their parents or preschool teachers have been concerned, it is unlikely that their problems will be investigated earlier. This delay results from a combination of factors: it may not be appreciated that the presenting symptoms portend learning difficulties and instead they may be attributed to immaturity; there may be a fear of making the problem worse by emphasizing it; there may be a belief that the child will compensate for it; and finally it may be asked what could be done anyway at such a young age? This important question will be addressed later.

The role of the paediatrician

In most educational systems, even if the parent or teacher decides that a child does have learning difficulties, the sequence of events in establishing the diagnosis is still exceedingly haphazard and there is considerable uncertainty both in the lay, educational and medical spheres about the ideal course of action. Some of this uncertainty results from the variability of the presenting symptoms, but partly reflects the ambivalence of some professionals about the validity of the concept of specific learning difficulties. This ambivalence is not shared by the British Paediatric Association or the British Neurological Association (Gordon et al. 1983) or in the editorial column of the Journal of Paediatrics (Deuel 1981). They contended that the paediatrician is ideally suited to be in overall charge of management, seeking to correlate the essential contributions of educationalist and psychologist and referring when necessary to their ophthalmological, audiological, neurological and psychiatric colleagues. They might also seek the help, when appropriate, of a number of therapists; physiotherapists, occupational therapists, specialists in perceptual problems, speech and language therapists, or remedial teachers, etc. In many societies a greater problem seems to be to find anyone with appropriate skills and interests to care for the child with specific learning difficulties.

The role of the psychologist

Although specific learning difficulties may be suspected by parent, teacher or doctor, the diagnosis of such problems can only be made by the psychologist; a detailed review of the tests needed to do this is beyond the scope of this text. Although the age of the child concerned will determine to some extent the tests used, any assessment will need to measure the overall level of intelligence, reading ability (including both accuracy and comprehension), spelling age, mathematical ability, visual, and auditory discrimination, etc. If over 6 years of age, the WISC (R) is the most useful test of general intellectual functioning since it provides information about both verbal and performance abilities. On the verbal scale, the subtests assess vocabulary, abstract verbal concepts, general knowledge, verbal reasoning, auditory sequential memory, and mental arithmetic. On the performance scale, the sub-tests assess spatial organisation and reasoning, visual perception, conceptual sequencing and visual associative learning and memory.

The role of the ophthalmologist

The attitude of the American Academy of Paediatrics, the American Association of Ophthalmology, and American Association of Paediatric Ophthalmology and Strabismus, is unequivocal about this (1983).

'*Children with dyslexia or related learning difficulties have the same instance of ocular abnormalities as children without. There is no peripheral eye defect which produces dyslexia and associated learning disabilities. There is no scientific evidence to support claims for improving the academic abilities of dyslexic or learning disabled children with treatment based on (a) visual training including muscular exercises, ocular pursuit or tracking exercises or glasses (with or without bifocals or prisms); or (b) neurological organisational training (laterality training, balance board, perceptual training.)*'

Two recent studies by ophthalmologists have underlined this view (Helveston *et al.* 1985; Aasved 1987) but point out, however, that although not causative, any eye problems should be treated appropriately so that they do not compound the problem.

These views do not meet with universal acceptance. For example Dunlop (1972). an orthoptist, points to a higher instance of esophoria in reading disabled children compared with normals and advocates orthoptic intervention, and Stein and Fowler (1982) claim that just over 50% of dyslexics 'show unstable ocular motor dominance with possible consequent failure to develop dependable association between retinal and ocular motor signals' and recommend treatment with uniocular occlusion (see Chapters 7 & 44).From the practical point of view the ophthalmologist's role with children with learning difficulties is the simple one of excluding or treating refractive errors and significant eye movement or eye defects whilst those with a greater interest in the problem may feel that occlusion based on the results of the Dunlop test may be beneficial to some of their patients.

Audiological assessment

The same uncertainty that exists about the role of the eyes in specific learning difficulties also attends the ears. By definition 'dyslexia' can only be diagnosed in the absence of significant hearing impairment, but this requirement does not rcfer to the possible role of transient, though significant, auditory difficulties during the early, critical years of life when language is being developed. Glass' findings (1981) indicated that there is a connection between early conductive hearing loss and several measures of auditory learning (auditory perception, auditory vocal associations and auditory sequential memory). Zinkus *et al.* (1978) point out the language and auditory processing deficits experienced by children aged 6–11 years of age who in the first 3 years of life had chronic severe otitis media; they also found evidence that children with history of severe otitis media experience difficulty in performing tasks that require the integration of visual and auditory processing skills.

The question of which ear is dominant for language has been nearly as much a matter of study as eye dominance and vision. There seems to be unequivocal evidence of right ear dominance (left hemisphere) in right handed normal people, fairly good evidence that it is established by the age of 5 years, and recent evidence that in children with dyslexia there is a strong left ear dominance (Chasty 1982).

The role of the paediatric neurologist

One of the problems of managing children with specific learning difficulties is that their problems often transcend the conventional speciality boundaries or remain at the periphery of several. An example of this is clumsiness which is usually a dyspraxia but may be due to a neurological disorder of cerebellar or extra pyramidal pathways or be due to unsuspected hemiplegia. Other examples are children with wide verbal/performance discrepancies and children with the attention deficit syndrome. It would be beneficial for all such children to be referred at least once to a paediatric neurologist for a full neurological history, examination and, if indicated, investigation (e.g. neuroradiology) and treatment, e.g. with methylphenidate or Piracetam. Of course, it does not take a neurologist to recognize 'soft' neurological signs e.g. the fine involuntary movements of the out stretched fingers, right/left confusion, confused laterality, synkinesis, clumsiness with fine manipulative tasks, etc., nor does it need a neurologist to confirm that the significance of such findings is uncertain and not specific to children with specific learning difficulties. But in many instances an authoritative analysis of the signs and symptoms and firm advice on their meaning and relevance, and on the role of treatment or necessity of further investigation makes a neurological consultation helpful to parent, child and those trying to help them.

Differential diagnosis

Some of the differential diagnoses of specific learning disabilities are mentioned in the first paragraph of this chapter. Distinction between mild to moderate mental retardation and specific learning difficulties depends upon the results of psychological testing. If mental retardation is found it may be present by itself or be part of a recognizable syndrome with genetic and possibly therapeutic implications: these children should always be referred to a paediatric neurologist. There are some dysmorphic features that might alert the ophthalmologist to possible mental handicap, e.g. macrocephaly (large head circumference), large stature as found in Soto's syndrome, cutaneous naevi such as achromic naevi or café-au-lait patches as found in tuberous sclerosis and neurofibromatosis respectively, coarse features as may be present in mucopolysaccharidosis, short stature as may be found in hypothyroidism, or hypertelorism signifying underlying agenesis of the corpus callosum, etc. This further emphasises the role of the ophthalmologist in the detection and management of systemic disease and the fact that the paediatric ophthalmologist needs to have appropriate measuring apparatus and developmental scales readily available.

Progressive degenerative disease of the central nervous system may be so insidious as to masquerade as a static disorder or result in deterioration that is matched in tempo by natural adaptation and therefore be unrecognised in the early stages. Slowing down in acquisition of skills rather than frank loss of them may be the main indication of this but a careful developmental history will alert the physician (Cavanagh & Lobascher 1983).

Finally, it is important not to overlook the gifted child who, if unrecognized, may express his boredom with disturbed behaviour, withdrawal, depression and failing to progress at school (Lobascher & Cavanagh 1977).

Management

General management

A significant aspect of the management of a problem is its recognition and delineation. Sometimes this is all that can be done but the beneficial effect in terms of relief by the patient or parents that there is not something more sinister afoot, that the problems are often partly self-limiting, that the child is not 'repeated' or that there are many other children with similar problems, must not be under-rated. Evidence is emerging that there is a stage beyond the diagnosis, and that 'treatment' can be offered, its efficacy monitored and its benefits measured. Such optimism is relatively new. Yule (1976) asked 'does remedial-help, help in relation to the school-aged child' and concluded that there was no good evidence that it did confer any long-term benefits. Six years' later a review of the intervening literature led Hewitson (1982) to the same conclusion, but Hicks (1986) pointed out some promising results with the combined strength-deficit orientated approach, i.e. remedial help which both capitalizes on a child's strengths as well as improves weaknesses (Hicks 1980). She refers to the study by Hicks and Spurgeon (1982) which characterized patterns of error in reading and spelling of the child with 'auditory' problems and the child who has difficulty attaching a verbal label to visual stimuli.

There are now widespread efforts to provide perceptual motor training for 'clumsy children', i.e. those with a relatively low performance compared with verbal IQ and showing a motor dyspraxia. The experience of Lobascher et al. (personal communication) at the Hospital for Sick Children, Great Ormond Street, London, with 80 such children, has shown that where there is good verbal function (VIQ greater than 105), expert therapy will lead to a closing of the V/P gap over a 6 month period with the performance IQ coming up to the verbal IQ, though sometimes the latter may also slightly reduce to meet the elevating performance IQ. This effect, as measured by formal psychological assessment, is mirrored by a marked functional improvement but for this to be maintained the child has to continue to work to a 'recipe' and needs refresher courses in perceptual motor training.

Drug treatment

Hyperactivity, impulsiveness, and distractibility are behavioural disturbances which are difficult to quantitate and, when attributed to a child, often raise the question of whether the observation is simply in the eye of the beholder. Nevertheless, there are a number of children with specific learning difficulties who appear to their teachers to have a very short attention span and to be unduly susceptible to environmental distractions. Treatment of such children with Methylphenidate (Ritalin) may bring about a great improvement in their concentration, which on occasions has meant the difference between the child being accepted at his school as opposed to being expelled for unmanageable behaviour (Ottenbacher & Cooper 1983). There are two important criticisms to the use of this medication: (a) the danger of side effects; and (b) there is no proof of long-term academic benefit to children so treated.

In the author's experience, using this medication in a dose of 0.6 mg/kg body weight per day in two divided doses (the second dose not being given after 3 o'clock in the afternoon), there have been no extra-pyramidal side effects nor depression of appetite, nor misery. In order to prevent the potential (but not proven) side effects of growth inhibition, it is recommended that the medication is prescribed only from Monday to Friday and only during the school term. There is not yet any evidence that children treated with Ritalin perform any better academically in the long-term, though Sebrecht et al. (1986) have shown its effectiveness in producing benefits in performance of a number of basic cognitive tasks.

The author has no personal experience in the use of piracetam, which is claimed (Chase et al. 1984) to improve reading accuracy and comprehension, reading speed and writing accuracy as compared with a placebo controlled group.

Psychological and psychiatric problems

Depression, behavioural disturbances and hyperactivity may be very substantial problems for the child with specific learning disability; given improvement in the child's academic performance there will usually be a spontaneous improvement in these problems but sometimes the help of a child psychiatrist or psychologist may be useful.

Theoretical considerations

Genetic aspects

The belief that there is an inherited basis to specific learning difficulties goes back many years. Hermann's (1959) classic study on twins with dyslexia showed that in 12 monozygotic twins there was 100% concordance and in 33 dizygotic twins, a 33% concordance. An earlier study by Hallgren (1950) had shown a very high familial incidence in 116 cases with parent–sibling or first-degree relative involvement in all but 12 cases and he had concluded that there was an autosomal dominant pattern of inheritance. This is difficult to reconcile with the universal observations that boys are four times more commonly affected than girls.

Other view points have been expressed, e.g. Rutter et al. (1970) who points to the greater importance of biological rather than hereditary factors and by Finucci et al. (1976) who concluded that there is no single mode of inheritance and urged more accurate sub-grouping and categorization. Recently, Smith et al. (1977) have demonstrated a linkage with chromosome 15 in a family with dominantly inherited reading disability.

Neuropathology and neuroradiological findings

Hier et al. (1978) performed a CT brain scan on 24 patients with dyslexia and found that in ten there was a reversal in the normal pattern of cerebral asymmetry in that the right temporo-parietal-occipital region was larger than the left. Even allowing for the fact that six of the 24 patients were left-handed, this figure was statistically significant.

The first postmortem report on the brain of a dyslexic child (Drake 1968), indicated excess subcortical white matter neurones. A number of more recent postmortem studies show disorders of neuronal migration in the left cortex, particularly around the sylvian fissure and left planum temporale, foci of ectopic neurones in the subcortical white matter, and bilateral abnormalities of the thalami (Galaburda & Kempner 1979; Galaburda et al. 1983). Whilst these studies do not indicate the precise aetiology of the neuronal disturbance, they do point to an organic rather than purely behavioural explanation for specific learning difficulties, and to a disturbance affecting early brain development.

Immunology

Geschwind and Behan (1984) reported an association between childhood dyslexia and immune disorders. A further study (Behan et al. 1985) has shown the presence of raised anti-Ro antibody titres in the serum of mothers with dyslexic children in a significantly greater proportion than in controls, raising the possibility that the antibody may play a role in the pathogenesis of dyslexia, perhaps synergistically with the male hormone (Geschwind & Behan 1982).

Electroencephalogram (imaging brain electrical activity)

The electroencephalogram (EEG) recorded conventionally in the form of a continuously fluctuating tracing on a polygraph, does not have any significant role in the investigation or management of children with specific learning difficulties. However, re-displaying the EEG in terms of the amount of energy or power occurring at a given moment in time for each of the frequencies of the EEG across the entire spectrum of frequencies (quantitative topographic mapping) and in colour has demonstrated a difference between dyslexia and normal controls that can be used diagnostically and which points to aberrant neurophysiology in dyslexia (Duffy *et al.* 1979, 1980a, 1980b).

Ocular aspects

The literature relating to ocular movements and reading disability is a confusing one, partly because of the difficulty in defining reading disability and partly because of lack of normal controls. These problems of interpretation are discussed by Pavlides (1981) who in his own studies takes great care to define what he means by dyslexia and to include controls. His studies confirmed the observations that dyslexic children show abnormalities of duration of eye fixation, perceptual span, ocular sweeps and increased regressions of the eyes during reading. By comparing dyslexic children with backward readers with the same chronological and reading age, he was able to discount the effect of patient difficulties with textual comprehension. His development of a test to assess a child's ability to follow sequentially illuminated lights, aimed to overcome environmental, psychological, and intellectual factors by avoiding the use of a text, and he has shown that dyslexic children demonstrate specific difficulties. The question then posed is whether the difficulties derive from impaired oculomotor control of the eyes or from an inability to sequence. Causality is always difficult to prove, which has been one of the reasons why many ophthalmologists and others have felt that the eye movement and some other problems seen in dyslexic children may be the effect of the reading difficulties rather than the cause. Stein *et al.* (1987, 1988) however, feel that a defect in vergence control

is an important cause, but not the only cause of dyslexia. They note that some children make mainly phonological errors and that others do not improve with the occlusion that may help those with vergence defects, and speculate that the underlying cause may exert its effect by a combination of vergence defect and by disturbing phonemic segmentation.

The Dunlop test is a synoptophore test (Fig. 36.1) in which foveal sized fusion slides are placed in the synoptophore tubes with the controls towards the examiner and they are viewed with each eye separately (a and b). The child is asked to move the tubes to join (fuse) the two slides so that he sees one house and two trees (c).

Whilst the child is concentrating on the door of the house the examiner abducts the synoptophore tubes and asks the child to tell him whether the large or the small tree moves. The tree that moves indicates the non-dominant eye. This is carried out at least six times then repeated with the positioning of the slides reversed.

Results

1   If the tree in front of the right eye always moves, this is recorded:

Right ||||||||||||||||||||||||

Left

i.e., left dominant.

2   If one or other moves but more often the right, this is recorded:

Right ||||||||||||||||||

Left ||||||

i.e., partial left dominant.

3   If there is no clearly dominant eye this is known as mixed dominance:

Right ||||||||||||||

Left |||||||||||

Stein *et al.* (1986) have shown that 30% of a group of 753 school children have an unstable reference eye

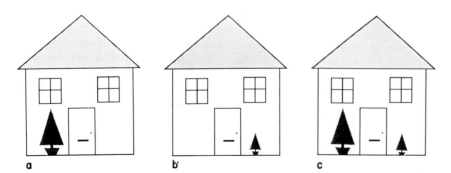

a   b   c   **Fig. 36.1** The Dunlop Test (see text).

on the Dunlop test, the incidence falling with increasing age. Children with unstable responses were much more likely to be backward readers. One very valid point is that in reading-aged children, a treatment by supervised monocular occlusion is very unlikely to do harm.

References

Aasved A. Ophthalmological status of school children with dyslexia. *Eye* 1987; **1**: 61–8

American Academy of Paediatrics/American Academy of Ophthalmology. *Ad hoc* working group of the American Association for Paediatric Ophthalmology and Strabismus. *Learning Disabilities, Dyslexia and Vision.* American Academy of Ophthalmology, San Francisco 1983

Behan M, Behan P, Geschwind N. Anti-Ro antibodies in mothers of dyslexic children. *Dev Med Child Neurol* 1985; **27**: 538–42

Cavanagh, N, Lobascher M. Childhood dementia. *Med Internat* 1983; **31**: 1682–5

Chase CH, Schmitt RL, Russell G, Tablal P. A new chemotherapeutic investigation: piracetam effects on dyslexia. *Ann Dyslexia* 1984; **34**: 29–48

Chasty H. Dichotic listening techniques and brain specialisation. In: *Current Research into Specific Learning Difficulties: Neurological Aspects.* Better Books, 1982 pp. 50–9

Crystal D. Linguistic factors in specific learning difficulty. In: *Current Research into Specific Learning Difficulties: Neurological Aspects.* Better Books, 1982 pp. 1–14

Deuel R. Minimal brain dysfunction, hyperkinesis, learning difficulties and attention deficit disorder. *J Pediatr* 1981; **98**: 912–5

Drake WE. Clinical and pathological findings in a child with developmental learning disability. *J Learn Disab* 1968; **1**: 9–25

Duffy F, Burchfield J, Lombroso C. Brain electrical activity mapping (BEAM): a method for extending the clinical utility of EEG and evoked potential data. *Ann Neurol* 1979; **5**: 309–321

Duffy FH, Denckla MB, Bartels P, Sandini E. Dyslexia: regional differences in brain electrical activity by topographic mapping. *Ann Neurol* 1980a; **7**: 412–20

Duffy FH, Denckla MB, Bartels P, Sandini G, Kiessling LS. Dyslexia: automated diagnosis by computerised classification of brain electrical activity. *Ann Neurol* 1980b; **7**: 421–8

Dunlop P. Dyslexia. The orthoptic approach. *Aust Orthop J* 1972; **12**: 16–20

Finucci JM, Guthrie JT, Childs AL, Abbey H, Childs B. The genetics of specific reading disability. *Ann Hum Genet* 1976; **40**: 1–23

Galaburda AM, Kempner TL. Cytoarchitectonic abnormalities in developmental dyslexia: a case study. *Ann Neurol* 1979; **6**: 94–100

Galaburda AM, Sherman GF, Geschwind N. Developmental dyslexia: third consecutive case with cortical anomalies. *Neurosci Abstr* 1983; **9**: 940

Geschwind N, Behan P. Left handedness: association with immune disease, migraine and developmental learning disorders. *Proc Nat Acad Sci USA* 1982; **79**: 5097–100

Geschwind N, Behan P. Laterality, hormones and immunity. In: Geschwind N, Galaburda A (eds) *Cerebral Dominance: The Biological Foundations.* Harvard University Press Harvard 1984 pp. 211–24

Glass R. The association of middle-ear effusion and auditory learning difficulties in children. *Rehab Lit* 1981; **42**: 81–5

Gordon N, McKinlay I, Rosenbloom R. Medical contribution to: *The Management of Children with Dyslexia* Report of a working party set up by the British Paediatric Neurology Association 1983.

Graham P, Stevenson J, Richman N. Epidemiology of language delay in childhood. In: Rose FC (ed.) *Clinical Neuroepidemiology.* Pitman Medical, Tunbridge 1980

Hallgren B. Specific dyslexia: a clinical and genetic study. *Acta Psychiatr Neurol* (suppl.) 1950; **65**: 1–287

Helveston EM, Weber J, Miller K *et al.* Visual function and academic performance. *Am J Ophthalmol* 1985; **99**: 346–56

Hermann K. *Reading Disability: A Medical Study of Blindness and Related Handicap.* CC Thomas, Springfield, Illinois 1959

Hewitson J. The current status of remedial intervention for children with remedial problems. *Dev Med Child Neurol* 1982; **24**: 183–93

Hicks C. Modality preference and the teaching of reading and spelling to dyslexic children. *Br Educat Res J* 1980; **6(2)**: 175–87

Hicks C. Remediating specific reading disabilities: a review of approaches. *J Res Read* 1986; **9**: 39–55

Hicks C, Spurgeon M. Two-factor analytic studies of dyslexic sub-types. *Br J Ed Psychol* 1982; **52**: 289–300

Hier DB, Le May M, Rosenberger PB, Perlo VP. Developmental dyslexia. *Arch Neurol* 1978; **35**: 90–2

Lobascher M, Cavanagh N. The other handicap: brightness. *Br Med J* 1977; **2**: 1269–71

McCready EB. Biological variations in the higher cerebral centres causing retardation. *Arch Pediatr* 1910; **27**: 506–13

Ottenbacher KJ, Cooper HM. Drug treatment of hyperactivity in children. *Dev Med Child Neurol* 1983; **25**: 358–66

Pavlides G, Miles TR (eds). *Dyslexic Research and its Application to Education.* Wiley, Chichester 1981

Rutter M, Tizard J, Whitmore K. *Education, Health and Behaviour.* Longmans, London 1970. (Reprinted Krieler, Huntington (New York) 1981)

Sebrecht M, Shaynitz S, Shaynitz B, Jatlan P, Anderav G, Cohen D. Components of attention: methylphenidate dosage and blood levels in children with attention deficit syndrome. *Pediatrics* 1986; **77**: 222–8

Silva PA. The prevalence, stability and significance of developmental language delay in pre-school children. *Dev Med Child Neurol* 1980; **22**: 768–77

Silva PA, McGee R, Williams SM. Developmental language delay from three to seven years and its significance for low intelligence and reading difficulties at age seven. *Dev Med Child Neurol* 1983; **25**: 783–93

Smith SD, Kimberling WJ, Lubs HA. Family studies in specific dyslexia. *Am J Hum Genet* 1977; **29**: 101

Stein JF, Fowler S. Diagnosis of dyslexia by means of a new indication of eye dominance. *Br J Ophthalmol* 1982; **66**: 332–6

Stein JF, Riddell PM, Fowler MS. The Dunlop test and reading in primary school children. *Br J Ophthalmol* 1986; **70**: 317–20

Stein, JF, Riddell PM, Fowler MS. Fine binocular control in

dyslexic children. *Eye* 1987; **1**: 433−9

Stein JF, Riddell PM, Fowler MS. Disordered vergence control in dyslexic children. *Br J Ophthalmol* 1988; **72**: 162−7

Stevenson J. Predictive value of speech and language screening. A review article. *Dev Med Child Neurol* 1984; **26**: 528−38

Vellutino FR. Dyslexia. In: *Theory and Research*. MIT Press, Cambridge, Mass 1979, p. 237

Wheeler TJ, Watkins EJ. Dyslexia: the problem of definition. *Dyslexia Rev* 1978; **1**: 1−4

Yule W. Issues and problems in remedial education. *Dev Med Child Neurol* 1976; **18**: 674−82

Zinkus P, Gottlieb M, Schapiro M. Developmental and psycho-educational sequelae of chronic otitis media. *Am J Dis Child* 1978; **132**: 1100−4

Despite the above list of causes, it must be said that most children with congenital Horner's syndrome have no abnormality found despite extensive investigation.

Acquired

Where there is no obvious cause, such as trauma or surgery, a child with acquired Horner's syndrome should be investigated by or in conjunction with a neurologist and the further investigations should include a chest X-ray, CT or MRI scan and 24-hour catecholamine assay. Some authors (Sauer & Levinsohn 1976) have emphasized the seriousness of the causes of acquired Horner's syndrome in childhood.

Pupil changes from high sympathetic 'tone'

Cases have been described in which an intermittent dilated pupil, with or without widening of the palpebral fissure, occur associated with a cervicomedullary syrinx (Lowenstein & Levine 1944), lung tumours, seizures (Gadoth *et al.* 1981) or migraine. In seizures and migraine (Pant *et al.* 1966) there may well be a lowering of parasympathetic tone at the same time, but sympathetic induced spasm is suggested by pallor and sweating (Jammes 1980).

Pupil changes from damage to the parasympathetic system

Internal ophthalmoplegia (paralysis of the sphincter pupillae and accommodation) are occasionally seen without external ophthalmoplegia from nuclear lesions. It is bilateral and often associated with other oculomotor palsies (Daroff 1971).

Damage to the IIIrd nerve in the interpeduncular fossa, where the pupillomotor fibres are confined to the superomedial aspect of the nerve, may occur from aneurysm or tumour when it is usually associated with external ophthalmoplegia, but meningitic lesions can cause an isolated internal ophthalmoplegia.

In uncal herniation the comatose patient develops a dilated pupil on the side of the herniation, together with an asymmetrically sluggish reaction to light. The pupil signs may be the only abnormality other than coma for a period of some hours. Flexion of the neck, by stretching the brainstem, may worsen the dilatation or even cause both pupils to dilate but this is not a recommended procedure! Later ispilateral external ophthalmoplegia and hemiplegia develop, contralateral ophthalmoplegia and then more profound brain-

stem signs. The syndrome is caused by the uncus of the temporal lobe herniating under the tentorial edge to compress the posterior cerebral artery, IIIrd nerve and the midbrain with the opposite tentorial edge cutting into the cerebral peduncle. Midbrain compression occludes the Sylvian acqueduct worsening the already raised supratentorial pressure.

Pharmacological agents

Numerous pharmacological agents affect pupil size and reactivity. Systemic agents usually affect the pupils symmetrically whilst topical agents are often only instilled into one eye and may be asymmetrical.

PUPIL-DILATING AGENTS

Parasympatholytic agents

Atropine 0.5–1%, homatropine 2%, cyclopentolate 0.5–1%, tropicamide 1% are all commonly used agents to dilate the pupil and cause cycloplegia. Homatropine and atropine have a prolonged action and are not often indicated diagnostically or therapeutically unless their long action is desirable. Hyoscine 0.5% has an action similar to atropine but is less long-lived.

Sympathomimetics

Adrenaline 0.1–1% or phenylephrine 2.5–10% maybe used to dilate the pupil in association with a parasympatholytic. They have no action on accommodation but are not sufficient by themselves to produce good dilatation. They must be used with great care, and at lowest dilution, if at all, in premature babies, those with cardiac or vascular disease or with hypertension.

PUPIL-CONSTRICTING AGENTS

Cholinergic drugs

Pilocarpine 1–4%, is commonly used to constrict the pupil and as treatment for glaucoma. It has little effect on infantile glaucoma.

Anticholinesterases

Phospholine iodide (ecothiopate) 0.03–0.125%, eserine 0.5% and isofluorophate 0.025% are occasionally for treatment of glaucoma. Isofluorophate is used in the USA and phospholine iodide was used in Europe to cause peripheral accommodation and 'unlink' the association between accommodative convergence and accommodation in some high AC:A ratio squints (see Chapter 44.45).

Sympatholytic agents

Guanethidine 5% (ismelin) can be used to counter lid retraction in hyperthyroidism. Thymoxamine 1% may also cause pupillo-constriction.

SYSTEMIC AGENTS

Atropine, scopolamine and benztropine can cause pupil dilatation and paralysis of accommodation in sufficient quantities. The seeds of jimson weed, the berries of deadly nightshade and henbane have all been known to cause a serious or fatal poisoning. The symptoms have been described as 'hot as a hare, blind as a bat, dry as a bone, red as a beet, mad as a hen'. When proof of atropine poisoning is needed in the absence of facilities for assay it is said that a few drops of the child's urine put into one eye of a cat may suggest the diagnosis. Mydriasis from topical atropine or atropine-like drugs is not counteracted by pilocarpine 1% but in systemic poisoning it may be.

Antihistamines and some antidepressants produce a mydriasis.

Heroin, morphine and other opiates, marijuana and some other psychotropic drugs cause bilateral pupil constriction.

Abnormalities of the near reflex

Congenital absence

Children may be born with a defect in the near reflex. They have absent accommodation and poor convergence and the pupil fails to constrict to a near stimulus, but it constricts to light (Chrousos *et al.* 1985).

Familial cases of accommodation defect occur (Karseras *et al.* 1974, Hibbert *et al.* 1975). The cause is unknown but it may be peripheral (Hibbert *et al.* 1975), in the ciliary body or lens.

Acquired defects

PSYCHOGENIC

Children in the second decade may present with symptoms of difficulty with reading due to non-organic causes. They can usually be cajaoled into a normal near response or tricked by prisms and minus lenses; the synoptophore is particularly useful here. In older persons, malingering may be suspected especially when compensation for injury is a possibility.

SYLVIAN AQUEDUCT (PARINAUD'S) SYNDROME

Premature presbyopia is one of the signs of tumours encroaching on the dorsal midbrain together with the more classic signs of convergence, i.e. retraction nystagmus, vertical gaze defects, eyelid retraction, convergence defect, and pupil light-near dissocation.

SYSTEMIC DISEASE

Botulism, diphtheria, diabetes, head and neck trauma may all give rise to accommodation defects either isolated or associated with eye movement and vergence defects. Wilson's disease has been shown to be associated with a defect in the near response in some cases. It is not yet clear but the cause may be central rather than in the eye (Curran *et al.* 1982).

PHARMACOLOGICAL AGENTS

Accommodation defect, see p. 567.

EYE DISEASE

Defective accommodation occurs in children with severe iridocyclitis, dislocated lenses, large colobomas, buphthalmos, very high myopia, and direct eye trauma including retinal detachment surgery.

OTHER NEUROLOGICAL CAUSES

Adie's tonic pupil syndrome and IIIrd nerve paralysis may cause defective accommodation. Sinus disease, presumably by affecting the short ciliary nerves, may cause cycloplegia and accommodation defect (Hein 1961).

ACCOMMODATION IN SCHOOL CHILDREN

One expects a school child to have a high amplitude of accommodation irrespective of refractive error (Donders 1864). Low amplitudes of accommodation occur in children who specialize in music as opposed to sport (Mantyjarvi 1988) and it has been suggested that there is a causal relationship between a defective near response and some cases dyslexia (Hammerberg & Norn 1974).

It is important, however, to distinguish clearly between reading difficulties due to a defective near response, which can be improved by exercises, and dyslexia which is a specific defect in the perceptual processes involved with reading and writing and which cannot be remedied by simple exercises. Stein *et al.* (1987) have suggested that because they found that 67% of dyslexics had electro-oculographic evidence of poor or 'unstable' vergence control in response to a small fusion stimulus, associated with low stereoacuity; whilst most good readers had good vergence control that, there may be a causal link. It was difficult for them to show a direct causal link but 51% of the dyslexics with unstable vergence movements improved after monocular occlusion as opposed to 24% who had no occlusion. Occlusion is, if nothing else, a harmless treatment in the older child.

Spasm of the near reflex

Spasm of the near reflex consists of episodes of a combination of:
1 Accommodation-induced myopia.
2 Convergence of the eyes.
3 Miosis.

The symptoms are usually of blurred, double vision, and ocular pain or headache. These cases are rarely due to organic disease and truly causal relationship with organic pathology is often not easy to establish. Safran *et al.* (1982) described three cases with pre-existing eye movement defects and a small number of other associations have been described including neurosyphilis, myasthenia gravis, and multiple sclerosis. Upper brainstem pathology is often suspected but rarely found.

In most cases it is not possible to demonstrate any organic disease and the phenomenon is assumed to be psychogenic. The episodes have a sudden onset and can last many hours and may be very variable. It is usually associated with considerable discomfort, blurred vision and photophobia. The eyes are crossed and may mimic a bilateral VIth nerve paresis but the essential finding is of the pupils constricting increasingly as the deviation increases. It is unusual in childhood but may occur. We have seen a teenager who had recurrent symptoms for 3 years.

The treatment is to reassure the patient and parents and sometimes they are helped by miotics but more usually by a combination of cycloplegia with bifocal glasses. Unless there are any neurological signs no investigations are required and the prognosis is good.

Anisocoria

Anisocoria, (unequal pupils), occurs when there is a local abnormality in the iris, or its musculature, or when there is an asymmetric abnormality in the efferent pathways that drive pupil constriction or dilatation. Afferent (visual) defects never cause anisocoria, even if they are highly asymmetrical, unless they are associated with an efferent defect. Apart from the size abnormality there is usually a change in reactivity which is usually the clue to the diagnosis.

PHYSIOLOGICAL ANISOCORIA

This is also known as simple anisocoria or occasionally as central anisocoria. The difference is rarely more than 1 mm between the two sides and may vary from time to time. The size difference is usually apparent in light and dark and the pupil reactions are normal. Direct clinical measurements are often difficult in children and this may be avoided by making measurements from polaroid photographs.

Anisocoria during reflex responses to unilateral light stimulation, with the direct light reaction exceeding the consensual, can be shown by pupillometry in a significant number of normals (Smith *et al.* 1979) This 'contraction anisocoria' was repeatable and the difference was about 6%.

DIAGNOSIS

The diagnosis of anisocoria can be difficult. It is frequently found that the patient and the doctor mistake which is the abnormal pupil, especially in Horner's syndrome in which there are no associated visual or oculomotor symptoms.

The abnormality is usually sorted out in three simple stages:
1 The reactions to light and accommodation. If these are abnormal, whether unilateral or bilateral the diagnosis is of an efferent, parasympathetic or local cause.
2 Slit lamp examination will show sinuous pupil reactions and iris anomalies, uveitis, etc.
3 The size difference in light and dark will help to diagnose sympathetic and parasympathetic lesions. In Horner's syndrome the anisocoria is greater in the dark because the dilator pupillae fails to function (Fig. 37.7). In a parasympathetic lesion the difference is greatest in the light because of the failure of the sphincter pupillae.

In nearly all situations the pupil abnormality can be

diagnosed by looking at the pupil and by looking for accompanying clinical signs. Drug testing may occasionally help but often it is difficult to decide on clinicial grounds. It is usually difficult even with the aid of drug testing, especially in small wriggling children who never seem to want to be still at the time you want to measure. The flow chart in Chapter P. 20 summarizes the clinical approach and has some notes on drug testing for completeness. It is not meant to be absolutely complete or totally foolproof but acts as a guide to diagnosis and is not helpful when both pupils are abnormal.

References

Barricks ME, Flynn JT, Kushner BJ. Paradoxical pupillary responses in congenital stationary night blindness. *Arch Ophthalmol* 1977; **95**: 1800.

Bell RA, Thompson SA. Ciliary muscle dysfunction in Adie's syndrome. *Arch Ophthalmol* 1978; **96**: 638−42

Borzyskowski M, Harris R, Jones R. The congenital varicella syndrome. *Eur J Pediatr* 1981; 137: 335−338

Bourgon P, Pilley SFJ, Thompson SH. Cholinergic supersensitivity of the iris sphincter in Adie's tonic pupil. *Am J Ophthalmol* 1978; **85**: 373−377, 63

Braddick O, Atkinson J, French J, Howland H. A photorefractive study of infant accommodation. *Vision Res* 1979; **19**: 1319−30.

Burde RM. The pupil. *Int Ophthalmol Clinics* 1967; **7**: 839−55

Campbell WW, Hill TA. A good treatment for Horner's syndrome. *N Engl J Med* 1978; **299**: 835−00

Chrousos GA, O'Neill JF, Cogan DG, Absence of the near reflex in a healthy adolescent. *J Pediatr Ophthalmol Strabisnus* 1985; **22**: 76−77

Curran RE, Hedges TR III, Boger WP III. Loss of accommodation and the near response in Wilson's disease. *J Pediatr Ophthalmol Strabismus* 1982; **19**: 157−60

Czarneki JSC, Thompson HS. The iris sphincter in aberrant regeneration of the third nerve. *Arch Ophthalmol* 1978; **96**: 1606−10

Daroff RB. Ocular motor manifestations of brainstem and cerebellar dysfunction. In: Smith JL (ed.) *Neuroophthalmology*, Vol. 5. CV Mosby & Co. St Louis 1971: 104−18

Donders FC. *Accommodation and Refraction of the Eye.* New Sydenham Society, London 1864

Fisher CM. Oval pupils. *Arch Neurol* 1980; **37**: 502−3

Fison PN, Garlick DJ, Smith SE. Assessment of unilateral afferent pupillary defects by pupillography. *Br J Ophthalmol* 1979; **63**: 195−9

Gadoth N, Margalith D Bechar M. Unilateral pupillary dilatation during focal seizures. *J Neurol* 1981: **225**: 227−30

Giles CL, Henderson DA. Horner's syndrome, an analysis of 216 cases. *Am J Ophthalmol* 1958; **46**: 289−301

Greenwald MJ, Folk ER. Afferent pupillary defects in amblyopia. *J Pediatr Ophthalmol Strabismus* 1983; **20**: 63−7

Hammerberg E, Norn MS. Defective dissociation of accommodation and convergence in dyslexic children. *Br Orthoptic J* 1974; **31**: 96−8

Haynes H, White BL, Held R. Visual accommodation in human infants. *Science* 1965; **148**: 528−30

Hein P.A. Unilateral paralysis of accommodation. *Am J Ophthalmol* 1961; **52**: 711−2

Hibbert FG, Goldstein V, Oborne SM. Defective accommodation in members of one family. *Tr Ophthalmol Soc UK* 1975; **95**: 455−61

Jaffe H, Cassady JR, Filler RM, Petersen R, Traggis D. Heterochromia and Horner's syndrome associated with cervical and mediastinal neuroblastoma. *J Pediatr* 1975; **87**: 75−7

Jammes JL. Fixed dilated pupils in petit mal attacks. *Neuro Ophthalmol* 1980; **1**: 155−9

Karseras A, Unwin B, Wybar KC. Defective accommodation in young people. *Brit Orthoptic J* 1974; **31**: 91−95

Klumpke A. Contribution a l'etude des paralyses du plexus brachial. *Revue du medecin (Paris)* 1885; **5**: 591−616

Korczyn AD, Rubenstein AE, Yahr MD, Axelrod FB. The pupil in familial dysautonomia. *Neurology* 1981; **31**: 628−9

Leone CR, Russell DA. Congenital Horner's syndrome. *J Pediatr Ophthalmol Strabismus* 1970; 7: 152−156

Lhermitte F, Guillaumat L, Lyon-Caen O. Monocular blindness with preserved direct and consensual pupillary reflex in multiple sclerosis. *Arch Neurol* 1984; **41**: 993−4

Loewenfeld IE, Thompson HS. Mechanism of tonic pupil. *Ann Neurol* 1981; **10**: 275−6

Loewenfeld IE, Thompson HS. The tonic pupil: a re-evaluation. *Am J Ophthalmol* 1967; **63**: 46−87

Lowenstein O, Levine AS. Periodic sympathetic spasm and relaxation and role of sympathetic system in pupillary innervation. *Arch Ophthalmol* 1944; **31**: 74−94

Manor RS, Yassur Y, Siegal R, Ben-Sira L. The pupil cycle time test; age variations in normal subjects. *Br J Ophthalmol* 1981; **65**: 750−3

Mantyjarvi MI. Accommodation in school children with music or sports activities. *J Ped Ophthalmol Strabismus* 1988; **25**: 3−7

Marshall LF, Barba D, Toole BM, Bowers SA. The oval pupil. *J Neurosurg* 1983; **58**: 566−8

Miller RG, Nielsen SL, Sumner AJ. Hereditary sensory neuropathy and tonic pupils. *Neurology* 1976; **26**: 931−3

Miller NR. *Walsh and Hoyt's Clinical Neuro-ophthalmology*, 4th edn, Vol. 2. 1985 Williams & Wilkins, Baltimore p. 385−469

Miller SD, Thompson HS. Edge light pupil cycle time. *Br J Ophthalmol* 1978a; **62**: 495−500

Miller SD, Thompson HS. Pupil cycle time. *Am J Ophthalmol* 1978b; **83**: 635−42

Mobius PJ. Zur pathologie des halssympathikus. *Klin Wochenschr* 1884; pp. 15−18

Newman SA, Miller NR. The optic tract syndrome: neuroophthalmologic considerations. *Arch Ophthalmol* 1983; **101**: 1241−50

Nielsen PJ. Upside down ptosis in Horner's syndrome. *Acta Ophthalmologica* 1983a; **61**: 952−8

Nielsen PJ. The corneal thickness and Horner's syndrome. *Acta Ophthalmologica* 1983b; **61**: 467−73

Pant SS, Benton JW, Dodge PR. Unilateral pupillary dilatation during and immediately following seizures. *Neurology* 1966; **16**: 837−40

Portnoy JZ, Thompson HS, Lennarson L, Corbett JJ. Pupillary

defects in amblyopia. *Am J Ophthalmol* 1983; **96**: 609–14

Price MJ, Thompson HS, Judisch F, Corbett JJ. Pupillary constriction to darkness. *Br J Ophthalmol* 1985; **69**: 205–12

Purcell JJ, Krachmer JH, Thompson HS. Corneal sensation in Adie's syndrome. *Am J Ophthalmol* 1977; **84**: 496–500

Robinson GC, Dikrainian DA, Roseborough GF. Congenital Horner's syndrome and heterochromia iridum: their association with congenital foregut and vertebral anomalies. *Pediatrics* 1965; **35**: 103–7

Safran AB, Roth A, Gauthier G. Le syndrome des spasmes de convergence 'plus'. *Klin Monatsbl Augenheilkd* 1982; **180**: 471–3

Sauer C, Levinsohn MN. Horner's syndrome in childhood. *Neurology* 1976; **26**: 216–21

Sayed AK, Miller BA, Lack EE, Sallan SE, Levey RH. Heterochromia iridis and Horner's syndrome due to paravertebral neurolemmoma. *J Surg Oncol* 1983; **22**: 15–16

Selhorst JB, Hoyt WF, Feinsod M, Hosobuchi Y. Midbrain corectopia. *Arch Neurol* 1976; **33**: 193–5

Selhorst JB, Madge G, Ghatak N. The neuropathology of the Holmes–Adie syndrome. *Ann Neurol* 1984; **16**: 138–9

Smith SA, Ellis CJK, Smith SE. Inequality of the direct and consensual light reflexes in normal subjects. *Br J Ophthalmol* 1979; **63**: 523–7

Stein JF, Riddell PM, Fowler MS. Fine binocular control in dyslexic children. *Eye* 1987; **1**: 433–9

Stewman DA. Unilateral straight hair in congenital Horner's syndrome due to stellate ganglion tumour. *Ann Neurol* 1983; **13**: 345–6

Taylor D. Congenital tumours of the anterior visual system with dysplasia of the optic discs. *Br J Ophthalmol* 1982; **66**: 455–63

Thompson HS. Adie's syndrome: some new observations. *Trans Am Ophthalmol Soc* 1977a; **75**: 587–626

Thompson HS. Diagnosing Horner's syndrome. *Trans Am Acad Ophthalmol Otolar* 1977b; **83**: 840–842

Thompson HS. Segmental palsy of the iris sphincter in Adie's syndrome. *Arch Ophthalmol* 1978; **96**: 1615–20

Thompson HS, Bell RA, Bourgon P. The natural history of Adie's syndrome. In: Thompson HS, Daroff R, Frisen L, Glaser JS, Sanders MD (eds) *Topics in Neuro-ophthalmology*. Williams & Wilkins, Baltimore 1979 pp. 96–9

Thompson HS, Corbett JJ, Cox TA. How to measure the relative afferent pupillary defect. *Surv Ophthalmol* 1981; **26**: 39–42

Thompson BM, Corbett JJ, Kline LB, Thompson HS. Pseudo-Horner's syndrome. *Arch Neurol* 1982; **39**: 108–11

Thompson HS, Zackon J, Czarnecki SC. Tadpole-shaped pupils caused by segmental spasm of the iris dilator muscle. *Am J Ophthalmol* 1983; **96**: 467–76

Weinstein J, Zweifel TJ, Thompson HS. Congenital Horner's syndrome. *Arch Ophthalmol* 1980; **98**: 1074–8

Woodruff G, Buncic JR, Morin JD. Horner's syndrome in children. *J Ped Ophthalmol Strabismus* 1988; **25**: 40–4

Yinon U, Urinowsky E, Barishak Y-TR. Paradoxical pupillary constriction in dark reared chicks. *Vision Res* 1981; **21**: 1319–22

38 Leukaemia

DAVID TAYLOR

Incidence

Although the ophthalmic manifestations of leukaemia in childhood may be memorably dramatic, a prospective study Hoover *et al.* (1988) showed that serious eye involvement is rather unusual. Only one of their 82 patients had reduced vision due to the leukaemia from bilateral retinal detachments and vitritis and although half of their surviving patients had cataracts these were of little visual significance.

Nonetheless, ocular involvement when it occurs is important and demands prompt diagnosis and treatment. Now that survival rates of 50–70% are usual (Niemeyer *et al.* 1985) the eye complications of the disease and its treatment become more significant. Children dying of leukaemia have a high incidence of eye involvement (Allen & Straatsma 1961).

Eye involvement in leukaemia is particularly interesting because it is the only site where the leukaemic involvement of nerves and blood vessels can be directly observed, because the eye may act as a 'sanctuary' for leukaemic cells against chemotherapy, and because in the occasional patient the eye complications may be the major residual disability (Taylor & Day 1982).

Acute lymphoblastic leukaemia is the most common leukaemia in childhood.

Orbit

Oakhill *et al.* 1981) found that of 27 children presenting with unilateral proptosis over an 8.5-year-period, three had leukaemia. The incidence in other series, i.e. Porterfield (1962), has varied probably mainly because of varying referral patterns, but leukaemia is probably a small, but significant cause of proptosis in children. In Kincaid and Green's (1983) postmortem study of patients of all ages orbital involvement was found in 14% of eyes with chronic leukaemia and 7.3% in acute leukaemia. It was more common in lymphatic leukaemia (12%) than in myeloid leukaemia (8%).

Orbital involvement may be due to soft tissue infiltration or tumour formation, or due to haemorrhage. Orbital presentation may occur without ocular involvement and it may be the only manifestation, especially in myeloid leukaemia (Zimmerman & Font 1975).

In orbital involvement with some forms of myeloid leukaemia in childhood the tumour takes on a greenish tinge which has given rise to the name chloroma; the colour is said to be due to the enzyme myeloperoxidase, but probably also results from the presence of altered blood products. Children with orbital involvement present with proptosis, chemosis, rarely with muscle involvement and these may occur early in the course of the disease. Because it may be difficult to differentiate between primary leukaemia infiltration and complications such as haemorrhage or opportunistic infection a biopsy may be necessary (Rubinfield *et al.* 1988).

Lids

The lids are usually only involved as a part of orbital infiltration, but Kincaid and Green (1983) saw a 4-year-old girl who relapsed with lid swelling due to leukaemic infiltration.

Conjunctiva

The conjunctival vessels may be involved by haemorrhage, infiltration (Allen & Straatsma 1961) or by hyperviscosity when the vessels are tortuous or comma-shaped (Swartz & Jampol 1975). Conjunctival mass formation is rare, but can be the presenting sign in acute leukaemia (Kincaid & Green 1983).

Cornea and sclera

Being avascular, the cornea is not often involved in the leukaemias, but it may be involved by herpes simplex or zoster in the immune-compromized child or by other inflammatory disease.

Corneal ring ulcers may be the presenting sign in acute leukaemia (Bhadresa 1971; Wood and Nicholson 1973) or in chronic leukaemia in adults (Eiferman *et al.* 1988). They may respond to topical antibiotics and

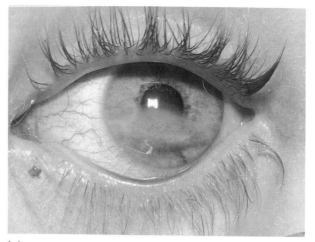

(a)

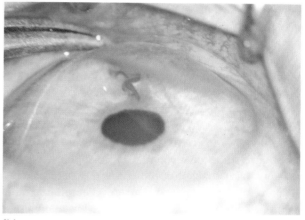

(b)

Fig. 38.2 (a) Corneal inflammatory infiltrate in patient with ALL who had a bone marrow transplant. The infiltrate started with symptoms and signs similar to a recurrent erosion. (b) After 2 years the same patient had an infiltrated cornea fed by an iris vessel.

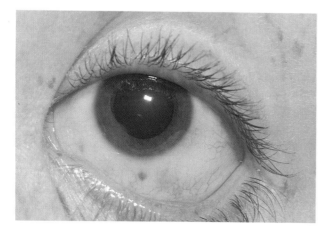

Fig. 38.1 Conjunctival haemorrhages and infiltration in ALL.

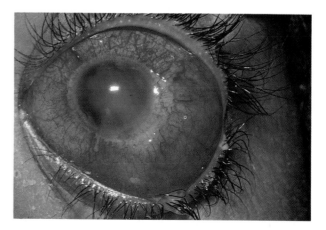

Fig. 38.3 ALL in relapse with iris, subconjunctival and scleral invasion and glaucoma.

steroids. Perilimbal infiltrates have been described in a young adult with acute monocytic leukaemia (Font *et al.* 1985). Scleral involvement has mainly been an autopsy finding (Kincaid & Green 1983).

Anterior chamber, iris, and intraocular pressure

The anterior segment is an uncommon site of extramedullary relapse accounting for between 0.5% and 2.6% of all relapses (Allen & Straatsma 1961; Kincaid & Green 1983; Bunin *et al.* 1987), it is seen most frequently in lymphoblastic leukaemia, but occasionally occurs in other forms of leukaemia (Perry & Mallen 1979; Tabbara & Beckstead 1980; Novakovic *et al.* 1989). Most reported cases have been in acute lymphoblastic leukaemic in relapse, but rarely children may present with a leukaemic hyphaema or hypopyon (Tabbara & Beckstead 1980).

The pathogenesis of anterior segment disease is unknown, but the relative infrequency of concurrent central nervous system (CNS) relapse suggests that seeding from the CNS is not an important mechanism (Novakovic *et al.* 1989). The infiltration is most likely to be bloodborne and the relatively frequent occurence of isolated anterior segment relapse supports Ninane *et al.*'s (1980) concept of the eye as a 'sanctuary' site. Because of the blood−eye barrier, chemotherapeutic agents do not penetrate the eye as well as many other sites and this, together with the avoidance of the eye in cranial irradiation, allows the survival of leukaemia cells which most frequently cause symptoms after chemotherapy has been stopped.

Symptoms include redness, watering, photophobia and the parents may notice changes in the shape or reactions of the pupil or in the colour and appearance of the iris. Pain and visual loss may occasionally occur.

Clinical findings are variable with iritis and hypopyon being the most common. Ciliary injection, keratic precipitates (KP), anterior chamber cells and flare (Zakka *et al.* 1980). Posterior synechiae are unusual, but a greyish hypopyon which may be streaked with blood (Hinzpeter *et al.* 1978) is common.

Other causes of hyphaema include juvenile xanthogranuloma, retinoblastoma, retrolental fibroplasia, persistent hyperplastic primary vitreous, iridoschisis, unsuspected trauma, iris vascular malformations, rubeosis iridis and other blood dyscrasias.

Secondary glaucoma is common and is associated with corneal oedema, pain and redness (Tabbara & Beckstead 1980).

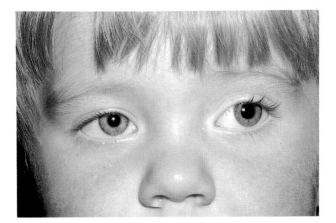

Fig. 38.4 Heterochromia iridis due to iris relapse in the left eye.

The iris may be thickened either diffusely or in the form of one or more nodules or a mass of variable size; the iris may also be thinned with loss of pigment. This iris colour may be changed, usually by a brownish discolouration and the thickening of the iris obliterates the iris crypts and may give a rather featureless iris. Rubeosis may occur. It is often the failure of standard uveitis treatment that draws the ophthalmologist's attention to the underlying leukaemia. It should not, however, be assumed because a child has leukaemia any uveitis is leukaemic, this is not necessarily the case and histological confirmation must be obtained. The diagnosis is best established by a combination of an anterior chamber paracentesis and an iridectomy. Novakovic *et al.* (1989) pointed out that a paracentesis alone may not be sufficient to give an accurate diagnosis. Pathological studies show leukaemic infiltration of the iris and trabecular meshwork (Kincaid & Green 1983; Jankovic *et al.* 1986) and the hypopion consists of leukaemic cells, necrotic tissue and proteinaceous exudate. Leukaemic cells may be difficult to find. Patients with glaucoma have histological evidence of leukaemic obstruction of the outflow channels and episcleral vessels (Glaser & Smith 1966). The latter case was an adult, reported by J Lawton Smith and Dr B. Glaser (the father of Dr Joel Glaser), who presented with limbal injection and raised intraocular pressure which failed to respond to acetazolamide. The leukaemia was discovered on routine investigation after admission and the glaucoma responded well to low dose radiotherapy.

Choroid

The choroid is the part of the eye most frequently involved in all types of leukaemia (Allen & Straatsma

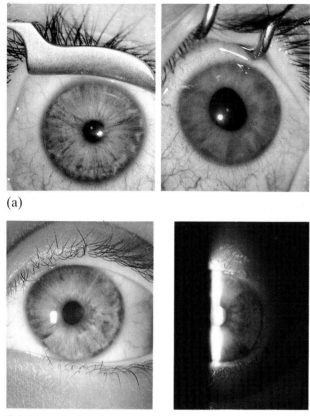

(a)

(b)

Fig. 38.5 (a) Iris relapse with heterochromia, infiltrated iris and sluggish pupil reactions. The other eye on the right for comparison. (b)After treatment with 2500 cGy there is iris transilluminance

1961; Kincaid & Green, 1983), but it only rarely becomes clinically apparent. The clinical manifestations are the result of a serous retinal detachment (Burns *et al.* 1965) caused by infarction in ophthalmic artery occlusion or retinal pigment epithelial defects and clumping (Clayman *et al.* 1972). Fluorescein angiography demonstrates myriads of diffuse leakage points at the level of the retinal pigment epithelium (Kincaid *et al.* 1979). Similar fluorescein patterns are seen in serous detachments with melanoma, metastatic tumour, Vogt–Koyanagi–Harada disease and posterior scleritis. Leukaemic choroidopathy can be detected by ultrasound even when there is no abnormality on clinical examination (Abramson *et al.* 1983).

Retina and vitreous

The retina, because of its ready visibility is the part of the eye most frequently found to be involved clinically, and fundoscopy is part of the routine follow-up examination of leukaemic patients.

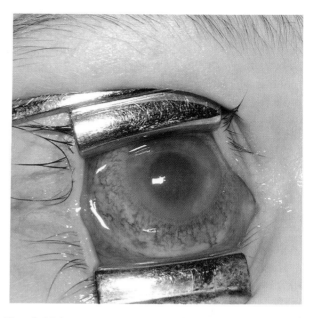

Fig. 38.6 Iris relapse with glaucoma in ALL.

Hyperviscosity changes

Hyperviscosity of the blood occurs at some stage in most cases of leukaemia, but reaches its most pronounced manifestations in the chronic leukaemias which are more common in adults.

Vascular tortuosity and dilatation with irregularity or even 'beading' of the veins, sheathing and haemorrhages are probably the earliest manifestations.

Fluorescein angiography (Jampol *et al.* 1975) and trypsin digests (Duke *et al.* 1960; Kincaid & Green 1983) show capillary saccular and fusiform micro-

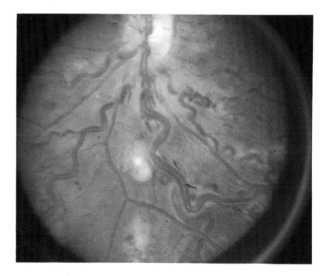

Fig. 38.7 Hyperviscosity changes in chronic myeloid leukaemia in a 20-year-old. Dr S. Day's patient.

aneurysms, and neovascularization has also been observed in some cases of chronic myeloid leukaemia in adults; it seems to be more closely related to the longevity of the disease and the increased amounts of blood cells giving rise to a prolonged hyperviscosity, reduced flow with capillary closure, microaneurysm formation and neovascularisation (Rosenthal 1983). Microaneurysms do not occur in acute leukaemia (Duke *et al.* 1968).

Retinal haemorrhages

Haemorrhages occur as a result of a combination of hyperviscosity, coagulation, infiltration and defective damage to retinal vessel walls and vessel occlusion.

Haemorrhages occur throughout the retina and may involve the vitreous. They may be massive and involve the whole eye.

Nerve fibre layer haemorrhages are seen as bright red haemorrhages with at least one margin being 'flame-shaped'. Deeper haemorrhages are not quite so red and usually more rounded. Subhyaloid haemorrhages have sharply defined margins and can form a fluid level in which there may be a layer of white cells.

Some haemorrhages are white centred, this should not be confused with the pinpoint white light reflex from the apex of a haemorrhage, or with haemorrhage around a leukaemic deposit. The white area consists of platelet and fibrin deposits which occlude the vessel or septic emboli (Duane *et al.* 1980). The haemorrhage occurs because of infarction and weakening of the vessel wall, which can also be damaged by leukaemic deposits.

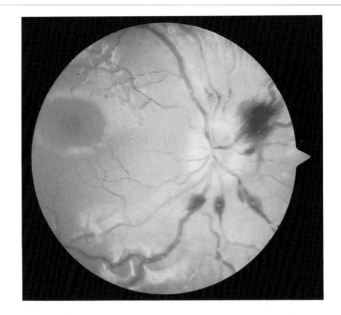

Fig. 38.9 Retinal nerve fibre layer haemorrhages in ALL. The tiny white centres to the haemorrhages are light reflexes.

White patches

White areas in the retinas of leukaemic children may be caused by:
1 Vessel sheathing.
2 Retinal infiltrates — these are nodular deposits which before the era of modern chemotherapy were commonly seen. They are unusual in acute leukaemia today. The are often associated with haemorrhage.

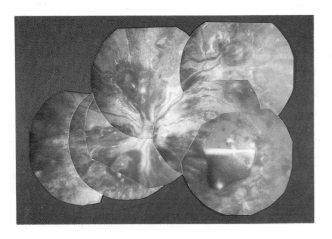

Fig. 38.8 Widespread retinal infiltrates and haemorrhages in all layers of the retina in ALL.

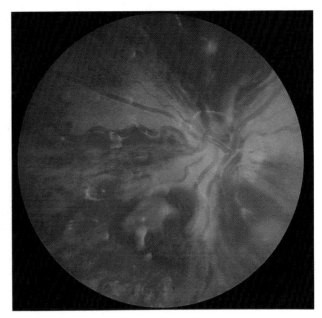

Fig. 38.10 White centred and nerve fibre retinal haemorrhages in ALL.

3 Cotton wool spots — these are retinal nerve fibre layer infarcts and occur frequently in acute leukaemia (Kincaid & Green 1983). They presumably occur because of retinal vascular occlusion.

4 Hard exudates. These small yellowish lesions are seen in relation to vessels that are chronically leaking non-cellular blood elements and are most frequently seen in chronic leukaemias with hyperviscosity.

5 Opportunistic infections with cytomegolovirus or fungus may occur in the immunosuppressed patient.

6 Retinal infarction, in the acute stage gives rise to large areas of cloudy swelling of the retinal nerve fibres and ganglion cell layer.

Retinal infarction

Occlusion of larger retinal arterioles or of the ophthalmic artery occasionally occurs as a preterminal event (Taylor & Day 1982) (Fig. 38.15).

Vitreous cells

Vitreous involvement with leukaemic or blood cells is usually secondary to retinal infiltration or haemorrhage (Kincaid & Green 1983), but may occur without obvious involvement of the retina (Reese & Guy 1933). Occasionally vitreous aspiration may be needed to confirm the diagnosis (Swartz & Schumann 1980) especially if the patient is apparently in remission and

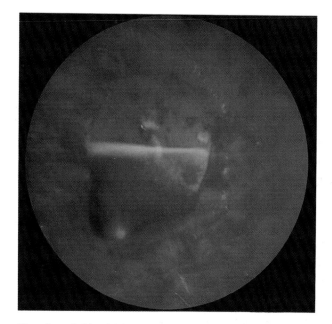

Fig. 38.12 Subhyaloid haemorrhage with gross leukaemic cell content.

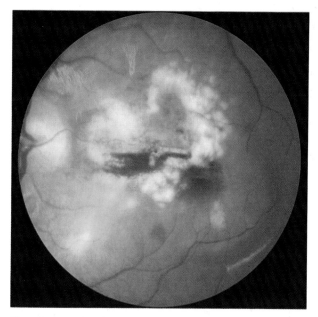

Fig. 38.13 Retinal infiltrates in ALL.

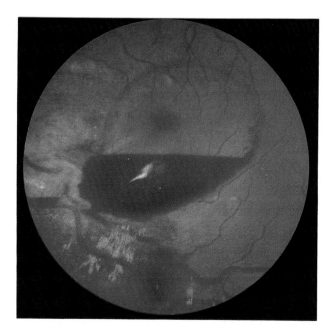

Fig. 38.11 Subhyaloid haemorrhage with ALL, profound anaemia and thrombocytopenia.

there is a possibility of an opportunistic infection. Vitreous organisation is an unusual but serious sequel to widespread retinal or optic nerve infiltration.

Other retinal manifestations

Serous retinopathy (Burns *et al.* 1965; Kincaid *et al.* 1979) and retinal pigment clumping (Clayman *et al.* 1972) occur as manifestations of choroidal involvement.

Optic nerve

Optic nerve involvement in postmortem cases occurs in nearly one-fifth of acute or chronic leukaemia (Kincaid & Green 1983), although in clinical series it is more frequently seen in acute lymphatic leukaemia (Ellis & Little, 1973; Rosenthal *et al.* 1975; Brown *et al.* 1981) Optic nerve involvement, which used to presage death is now less frequently seen presumably due to aggressive chemotherapy (Rosenthal 1983).

Leukaemic optic neuropathy may have only minimal visual symptoms despite even massive involvement, but often marked loss of central vision is observed, especially with infiltration behind the lamina cribrosa (Rosenthal 1983). With prelaminar infiltration there is ophthalmoscopically visible fluffy white infiltration with haemorrhage, but on occasion, especially if the infiltration is bilateral the differentiation from papilloedema may be difficult and a lumbar puncture may be necessary.

The response to irradiation with 2000 cGy of radiotherapy may be dramatic (Rosenthal *et al.* 1975); whatever the treatment optic atrophy is a frequent sequel (Nikaido *et al.* 1988).

An optic neuropathy may also be caused by vincristine treatment (Sanderson *et al.* 1976) or by radiotherapy.

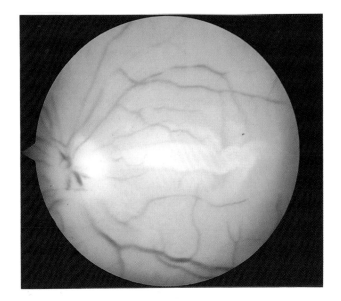

Fig. 38.15 Ophthalmic artery occlusion as a preterminal event.

Other neuro-ophthalmic involvement

Neurological complications of leukaemia and its treatment are common. Campbell *et al.* (1977) found that 61 of 438 children had significant complications including haemorrhage, which occurred in 1% of children with lymphoblastic leukaemia, and 7% of children with myeloblastic leukaemia. Infection by measles, varicella or mumps occurred in 11 patients and left permanent defects in many. Bacterial infections were less frequent. Methotrexate, vincristine and other drugs may cause significant defects.

Communicating hydrocephalus (De Reuck *et al.* 1979), chiasmal infiltration (Zimmerman & Thorenson 1964) and VIth nerve palsies (Abbassidum 1979) have also been described.

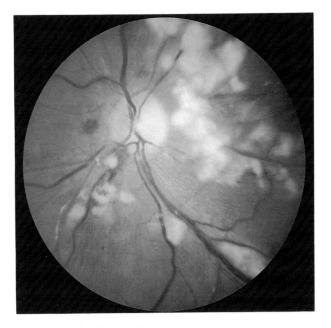

Fig. 38.14 Transient multiple cotton wool spots after bone marrow transplant.

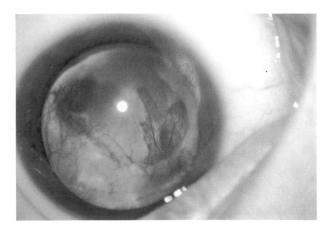

Fig. 38.16 Vitreous organization in ALL following leukaemic retinopathy and choroidopathy.

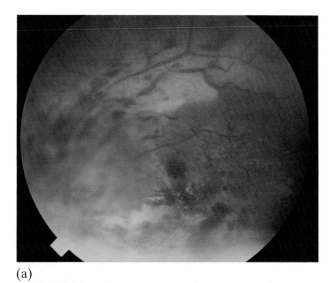

(a)

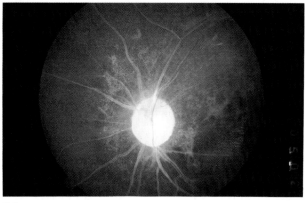

(b)

Fig. 38.17 (a) Gross optic nerve head and retinal involvement in ALL. (b) Profound optic atrophy and vascular attenuation following treatment with radiotherapy (same patient).

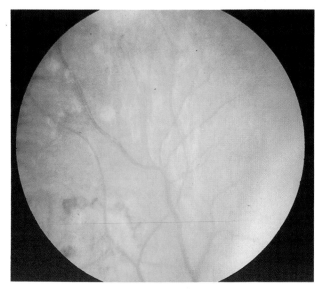

Fig. 38.18 Cytomegalovirus retinitis in ALL in relapse.

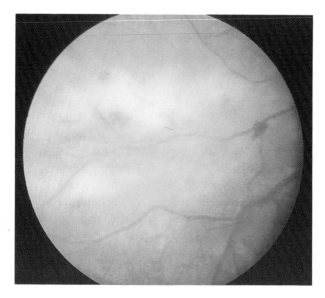

Fig. 38.19 Cytomegalovirus retinitis in ALL in relapse.

Complications of treatment

Drugs

Vincristine may cause corneal hypo-aesthesia, ptosis, IIIrd. VIth and VIIth nerve palsies (Albert *et al.* 1967), optic neuropathy (Sanderson *et al.* 1976) which may be reversible if the treatment is stopped early. The neuropathy is dose related (Sandler *et al.* 1969) and is most frequently seen initially as a peripheral neuropathy with abnormal deep tendon reflexes. Fits also occur (Campbell *et al.* 1977).

Cytarabine may cause blurred vision from corneal epithelial opacities and microcysts (Hopen *et al.* 1981).

Methotrexate is a significant cause of neurological problems including arachnoiditis from intrathecal administration, fits, depression, ataxia and dementia (Campbell *et al.* 1977).

Steroids may cause posterior subcapsular cataracts. Elliott *et al.* (1985) found cataracts in 32% of 37 children who had been treated with steroids and cranial irradiation, but they were not of great visual significance.

Rapid withdrawal of steroid therapy may cause benign intracranial hypertension (pseudotumour cerebri).

Immunosuppression

Antileukaemia chemotherapy, steroids and radiotherapy all contribute to the immunosuppression which allows infection by opportunistic bacteria, viruses, fungi or protozoa some of which do not usually cause significant infection in humans.

Herpes simplex and zoster affect the cornea, conjunctiva and lids. Herpes simplex and cytomegalovirus, which have an affinity for neural tissue may cause a severe necrotising retinochoroiditis which may be difficult to differentiate from leukaemic infiltrates, a distinction which can be helped by chorioretinal biopsy (Taylor *et al.* 1981), but can usually be made by culture of urine or saliva.

Yeast and fungus infections are rare, but important complications of immunosuppression (Michaelson 1971; Greene & Wiernick 1972; Avenda *et al.* 1978) and, if possible, biopsy is necessary to establish the diagnosis and to plan appropriate treatment. Other infections include mucormycosis, toxoplasmosis and aspergillus (Cogan 1977).

Graft-versus-host disease (GVHD)

In some children with leukaemia in relapse, and in some aplastic anaemias, following total body irradiation and chemotherapy to destroy the existing marrow, a bone marrow transplant is performed (Chessells 1988) to give a new population of bone marrow cells. Because of failure to recognize the transplant recipient as 'self', the transplanted lymphocytes may attack the recipient and cause GVHD.

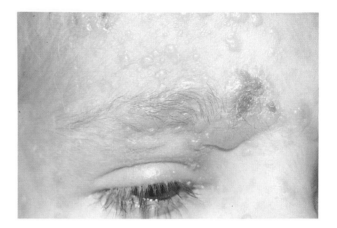

Fig. 38.21 Confluent varicella in a patient with ALL in relapse.

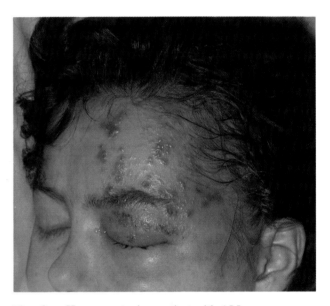

Fig. 38.22 Herpes zoster in a patient with ALL on chemotherapy.

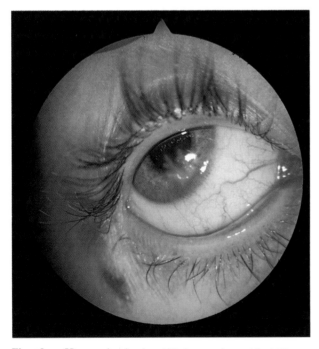

Fig. 38.20 Herpes simplex keratitis in a patient with ALL on chemotherapy.

GVHD is characterized by the occurrence within 4 months of the transplant of weight loss, fever, rash, liver dysfunction, and a dry mouth.

Ocular manifestations are common in GVHD (Franklin *et al.* 1983; Jack *et al.* 1983) and include dry eye, cicatricial lagophthalmos, sterile conjunctivitis and uveitis. The eye problems are frequently severe and test the ophthalmologist's management of the dry eye. In our experience these patients, who have all had previous chemotherapy and radiotherapy, have a high incidence of visually significant cataract.

An interesting occurrence of unknown significance is the transient appearance of multiple white cotton wool spots in bone marrow transplant recipients (Gratwahl *et al.* 1983).

The ophthalmologist's role

Since ocular complications are rare (Hoover *et al.* 1988) there is probably no need for routine ophthalmological surveillance in these children and the ophthalmologist usually only becomes involved by the referring oncologist or paediatrician, from whom most ophthalmologists can learn a lot about communication and patient management!

References

Abbassidum K. Headaches, vomiting and diplopia in a 16 year-old child. *Clin Pediatr* 1979; **18**: 191–2

Abramson DH, Jereb B, Wollner N, Murphy L, Ellsworth RM. Leukemia ophthalmopathy detected by ultrasound. *J Pediatr Ophthalmol Strabismus* 1983; **20**: 92–7

Albert DM, Wong VG, Henderson ES. Ocular complications of vincristine therapy *Arch Ophthalmol* 1967; **78**: 709–13

Allen RA, Straatsma BR. Ocular involvement in leukaemia and allied disorders. *Arch Ophthalmol* 1961; **66**: 490–509

Avenda NJ, Tanishima T, Kuwabara T. Ocular cryptococcosis. *Am J Ophthalmol* 1978; **86**: 110–3

Bhadresa GN. Changes in the anterior segment as a presenting feature in leukaemia. *Br J Ophthalmol* 1971; **55**: 133–5

Brown GC, Shields JA, Augsburger JJ, Serota FT, Koch P. Leukaemic optic neuropathy. *Int Ophthalmol* 1981; **3**: 111–6

Bunin N, Rivera G, Goode F, Hustu HO. Ocular relapse in the anterior chamber in childhood acute lymphoblastic leukaemia. *J Clin Oncol* 1987; **5**: 299–303

Burns CA, Blodi FC, Williamsen BK. Acute lymphocytic leukaemia and central serous retinopathy. *Trans Am Acad Ophthalmol Otol* 1965; **69**: 307–9

Campbell RHA, Marshall WC, Chessels JM. Neurological complications of childhood leukaemia. *Arch Dis Child* 1977; **52**: 850–8

Chessels JMS. Bone marrow transplantation for leukaemia. *Arch Dis Child* 1988; **63**: 879–82

Clayman HM, Flynn JT, Koch K, Israel C. Retinal pigment epithelial abnormalities in leukemic disease. *Am J Ophthalmol* 1972; **74**: 416–9

Cogan DG. Immunosuppression and eye disease. *Am J Ophthalmol* 1977; **83**: 777–88

De Reuck J, De Coster W, Vander Eecken H. Communicating hydrocephalus in treated leukaemic patients. *Eur Neurol* 1979; **18**: 8–14

Duane TD. Osher RH, Green WR. White centered haemorrhages: their significance. *Ophthalmology* 1980; **87**: 66–9

Duke JR, Wilkinson CP, Sigelman S. Retinal microaneurysms in leukaemia. *Br J Ophthalmol* 1968; **52**: 368–74

Eiferman RA, Levartovsky S, Schulz JC. Leukemic corneal infiltrates. *Am J Ophthalmol* 1988; **105**: 318–9

Ellis W, Little HL. Leukaemic infiltration of the optic nerve head. *Am J Ophthalmol* 1973; **75**: 867–71

Elliott AJ, Oakhill A, Goodman S. Cataracts in childhood leukaemia. *Br J Ophthalmol* 1985; **69**: 459–61

Font R, Mackay B, Tang R. Acute monocytic leukaemia recurring as bilateral perilimbal infiltrates: immunohistochemical and ultrastructural confirmation. *Ophthalmology* 1985; **92**: 1681–6

Franklin RM, Kenneth R, Kenyon PS *et al*. Ocular manifestations of graft-vs-host disease. *J Am Acad Ophthalmol* 1983; **90**: 4–13

Glaser B, Smith JL. Leukaemic glaucoma. *Br J Ophthalmol* 1966; **50**: 92–4.

Gloor B, Gratwohl A, Hahn H, Kretschmar S, Robert Y, Speck B, Daicker B. Multiple cotten wool spots following bone marrow transplantation for treatment of acute lymphotic leukaemia. *Br J Ophthalmol* 320–5

Gratwahl A, Gloor D, Hann H, Speck B. Retinal cotton-wool patches in bone-marrow-transplant recipients. *N Engl J Med* 1983; **308**: 110–11

Greene WH, Wiernick PH. Candida endophthalmitis. Successful treatment in a patient with acute leukaemia. *Am J Ophthalmol* 1972; **74**: 1100–4

Hinzpeter EN, Knoeber H, Freund J. Spontaneous haemophthalmos in leukaemia. *Ophthalmologica* 1978; **177**: 224–8

Hoover DL, Smith LEH, Turner SJ, Gelber RD, Sallan SE. Ophthalmic evaluation of survivors of acute lymphoblastic leukaemia. *Ophthalmology* 1988; **95**: 151–5.

Hopen G, Mandino BJ, Johnson BL *et al*. Corneal toxicity with systemic cytarabine. *Amer J Ophthalmol* 1981; **95**: 500–5

Jack MK, Kack GM, Sale GE *et al*: Ocular manifestations of graft-v-host disease. *Arch Ophthalmol* 1983; **101**: 1080–4.

Jampol LM, Goldberg MF, Busse B. Peripheral retinal microaneurysms in chronic leukaemia. *Am J Ophthalmol* 1975; **80**: 242–8

Jankovic M, Masera G, Uderzo C. Recurrences of isolated leukaemic hypopyon in a child with acute lymphoblastic leukaemia. *Cancer* 1986; **57**: 380–4

Kincaid MC, Green WR. Ocular and orbital involvement in leukaemia. *Surv Ophthalmol* 1983; **27**: 211–32

Kincaid MC, Green WR, Kelley JS. Acute ocular leukaemia. *Am J Ophthalmol* 1979; **87**: 698–702

Michelson PE, Stark W, Reeser F *et al*. Endogenous *candida* endophthalmitis. *Int Ophthalmol Clin* 1971; **11**: 125–47

Niemeyer CM, Hitchcock-Bryan S, Sallan SE. Comparative analysis of treatment programs for childhood acute lymphoblastic leukaemia. *Semin Oncol* 1985; **12**: 122–30

Nikaido H, Mishima H, Ono H, Choshi K, Dohy H. Leukemic involvement of the optic nerve. *Am J Ophthalmology* 1988; **105**: 294–9

Ninane J, Taylor D, Day S. The eye as a sanctuary in acute lymphoblastic leukaemia. *Lancet* 1980; **i**: 452–3

Novakovic P, Kellie S, Taylor D. Childhood leukaemia: relapse in the anterior segment of the eye. *Br J Ophthalmol* 1989; **73**: 354–9

Oakhill A, Willshard H, Mann JR. Unilateral proptosis. *Arch Dis Child* 1981; **56**: 549–51

Perry HD, Mallen FJ. Iris involvement in granulocytic sarcoma. *Am J Ophthalmol* 1979; **87**: 530–2

Porterfield JF. Orbital tumours in children: a report of 214 cases. *Int Ophthalmol Clin* 1962; **2**: 319–35

Reese AB, Guy L. Exophthalmos in leukaemia. *Am J Ophthalmol* 1933; **16**: 476–8

Rosenthal AR. Ocular manifestations of leukaemia: a review. *Ophthalmology* 1983; **90**: 899–905

Rosenthal AR, Egbert PR, Wilbur JR, Probert JC. Leukaemic involvement of the optic nerve. *J Pediatr Ophthalmol* 1975; **12**: 84–93

Rubinfeld RS, Gootenberg JE, Charis R M, Zimmerman LE. Early onset acute orbital involvement in childhood acute lymphoblastic leukaemia. *J Am Acad Ophthalmol* 1988; **95**: 116–21

Sanderson PA, Kuwabara T, Cogan DG. Optic neuropathy presumably caused by vincristine therapy. *Am J Ophthalmol* 1976; **81**: 146–50

Sandler SG, Tobin W, Henderson ES. Vincristine-induced neuropathy. *Neurology* 1969; **19**: 367–74

Swartz M, Jampol LM. Comma-shaped venular segments of conjunctiva in chronic granulocytic leukaemia. *Can J Ophthalmol* 1975; **10**: 458–61

Swartz M, Schumann OB. Acute leukaemic infiltration of the vitreous diagnosed by pars plana aspiration. *Am J Ophthalmol* 1980; **90**: 326–30

Tabbara KF, Beckstead JH. Acute promonocytic leukaemia with ocular involvement. *Arch Ophthalmol* 1980; **98**: 1055–9

Taylor DSI, Day SH. Neuroophthalmologic aspects of childhood leukaemia. In: Smith JL (ed.) *Neuroophthalmology Focus*. Massan, New York 1982; pp. 281–90

Taylor D, Day S, Constable I, Marshall W, Tiedemann K. Chorioretinal biopsy in a patient with leukaemia. *Br J Ophthalmol* 1981; **65**: 489–93

Wood WJ, Nicholson DH. Corneal ring ulcer as the presenting manifestation of acute monocytic leukaemia. *Am J Ophthalmol* 1973; **76**: 69–72

Zakka KA, Yee RD, Shorr N *et al*. Leukaemic iris infiltration. *Am J Ophthalmol* 1980; **89**: 204–9

Zimmerman LE, Font RL. Ophthalmologic manifestations of granulocytic sarcoma (myeloid sarcoma or chloroma). *Am J Ophthalmol* 1975; **80**: 975–90

Zimmerman LE, Thoreson HT. Sudden loss of vision in acute leukaemia. *Surv Ophthalmol* 1964; **9**: 467–73

39 Phakomatoses

CREIG HOYT

A hamartoma is a tumour mass arising as an anomaly of tissue formation. It is composed of tissue elements normally present in the involved organ or site. Several important syndromes with clinical manifestations in children, involving the neurologic, ocular, and cutaneous tissues, are characterized by the presence of such hamartomas. These hamartoses are frequently also referred to as phakomatoses (Font & Ferry 1972). The most important of these hamartoses in the practice of paediatric ophthalmology are Neurofibromatosis, Tuberous sclerosis, Sturge—Weber syndrome, and von Hippel—Lindau syndrome, although others sometimes included in this group are Klippel—Trenaunay—Weber and, previously, ataxia telangiectasia.

Neurofibromatosis

See Chapter 22.5.

Tuberous sclerosis

In 1908 Vogt presented the classic trad of epilepsy, mental retardation, and specific skin lesions in tuberous sclerosis (TS). Skin lesions are an early manifestation of the disease and most diagnostic are angiofibromas occurring in a 'butterfly' distribution over the nose and cheeks (Fig. 39.1) (Nichol & Reed 1962). However, these cutaneous manifestations are rarely seen in the first 2 years of life and, for that reason, careful ophthalmic evaluation of suspected patients may be

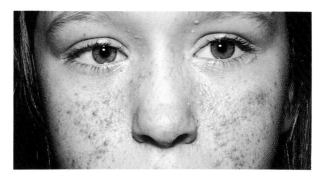

Fig. 39.1 Tuberous sclerosis. Angiofibromas of the face — most characteristically seen, as here, over the malar region.

essential in establishing the diagnosis (Williams & Taylor 1985). Tuberous sclerosis occurs in about one per 30—60 000 live births; the disorder may be inherited as an autosomal dominant; it may also occur as a sporadic condition.

By far the most common manifestation of this disorder is seizures. In infancy, the seizure disorder often takes on the picture of so-called infantile spasms. These may occur up to several hundred times a day and quite typically involve flexion and extension movements of the arms and legs. The major neurologic signs and symptoms in tuberous sclerosis are related to cortical and subependymal astrocytic hamartomas (Fig. 39.2). These occur most commonly in the region of the basal ganglia and protrude into the lateral and third ventricles. These may be seen on CT scan or MRI scanning; visible intracranial calcification can be identified in 50% of patients with tuberous sclerosis. However, calcification is much less frequently seen in infancy. Brain tumours occur occasionally in tuberous sclerosis but with much less frequency than in neurofibromatosis, most commonly, these are subependymal giant cell astrocytomas which are usually benign (Fig. 39.2). Other characteristic cutaneous lesions include Shagreen patches (Fig. 39.3) usually seen on the trunk, periungual fibromas, and white depigmented areas known as ash leaf spots (Fig. 39.4) which are best seen with a Woods lamp.

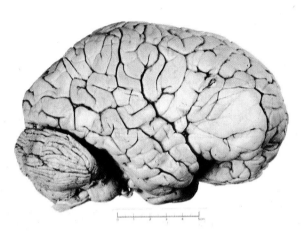

(a)

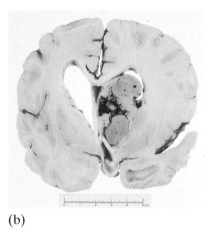

(b)

Fig. 39.2 Tuberous sclerosis. (a) Brain hamartomas show as smooth, firm pale areas on the gyri. These superficial foci of cortical gliomas (cortical tubers) may appear on the ventricular surfaces as linear lumpy strands or 'candle guttering.' (b) Benign astrocytoma with hydrocephalus.

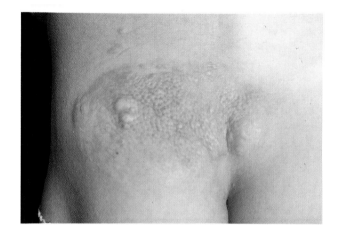

Fig. 39.3 Tuberous sclerosis. Shagreen patch on the skin of the lower back. Shagreen is a name used for a rough form of untanned leather or sharkskin.

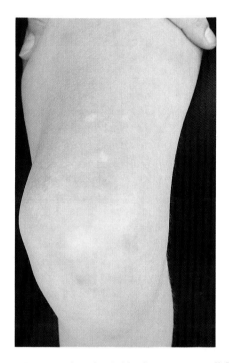

Fig. 39.4 Tuberous sclerosis. Ashleaf spots are small flat depigmented areas on the skin which occur anywhere on the body, are usually lanceolate in shape and are best seen with a Wood's (UV) light.

Ocular involvement occurs in at least 50% of patients, and although this may not be evident in infancy. The primary ocular manifestation of tuberous sclerosis is hamartomas of the retina and optic nerve (Fig. 39.5–39.10). Although these lesions are typically described as being elevated, highly refractile, yellowish, multinodular, or cystic masses resembling mulberries or clumps of tapioca, this description is not usually appropriate for these lesions in the first few years of life. Characteristically these lesions evolve from a stage of a poorly defined, flat, even, translucent lesion. They are not calcified in infancy but become so later in life. There may be single or multiple lesions occurring throughout the fundus, although typically they appear clustered around the optic nerve. These ocular hamartomas rarely interfere with visual func-

tion; their presence is of great diagnostic importance, particularly in the evaluation of a child with seizures and evidence of retardation. Rarely, vitreous hemorrhages have been reported presumably as the result of bleeding from the abnormal blood vessels involved in the tumour (Atkinson *et al.* 1973). Papilloedema and/or optic atrophy may occur in these patients as signs of associated intracranial lesions, es-

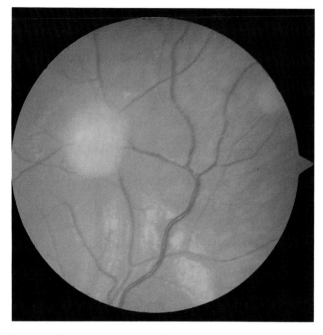

Fig. 39.5 Tuberous sclerosis. Almost flat translucent retinal lesions overlying blood vessels.

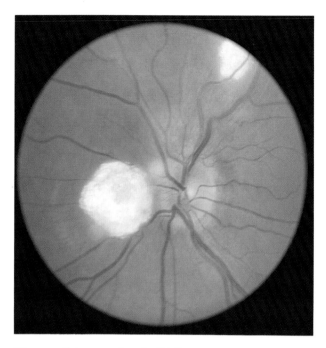

Fig. 39.7 Tuberous sclerosis. 'Mulberry tumours' — these white elevated refractile hamartomas probably evolve from flat translucent lesions.

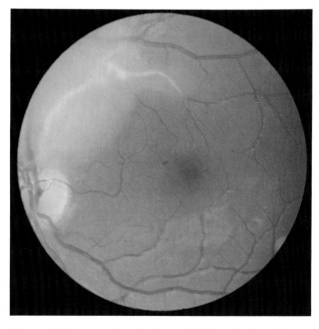

Fig. 39.6 Tuberous sclerosis. Large slightly raised translucent lesions with 'pseudosheathing'. (Williams & Taylor 1985.)

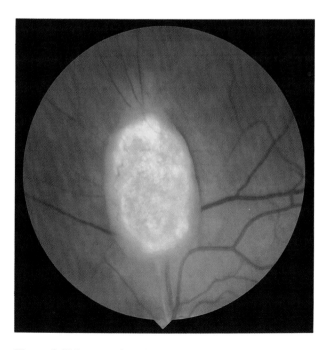

Fig. 39.8 Tuberous sclerosis. Fundus lesion transitional between a flat lesion (Fig. 39.5, 39.6) and a mulberry tumour (Fig. 39.7).

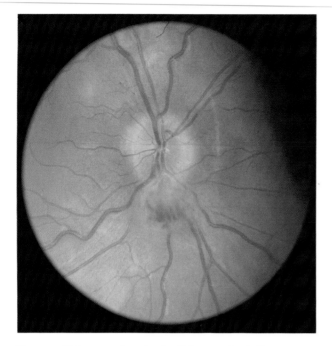

Fig. 39.9 Tuberous sclerosis. Small haemorrhagic flat hamartoma above the disc. Vitreous haemorrhage may occur from these lesions.

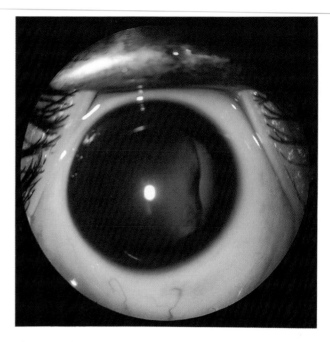

Fig. 39.11 Tuberous sclerosis. Lens pseudocoloboma.

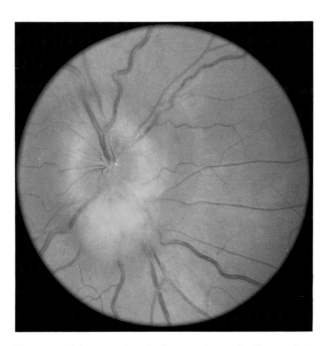

Fig. 39.10 Tuberous sclerosis. Same patient as in Fig. 39.9 but during a period of raised intracranial pressure showing papilloedema and the hamartoma (Williams & Taylor 1985).

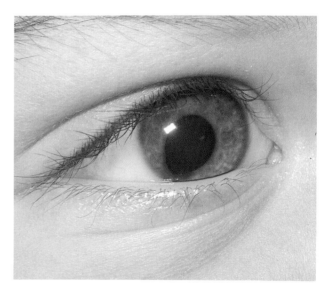

Fig. 39.12 Tuberous sclerosis. Iris pseudocoloboma.

commonly seen as renal cysts or angiomyolipomas of the kidney. Rhabdomyomas of the heart and cystic lesions of the lung and bone may also occur. For a fuller review see Williams and Taylor (1985).

Sturge–Weber syndrome

This syndrome includes ipsilateral glaucoma, facial hemangioma, and contralateral epileptic attacks. Facial involvement may occur, however, without

pecially if hydrocephalus has developed. Other ocular lesions include pseudocolobomas (Fig. 39.11, Fig. 39.12) and depigmented fundus lesions (Fig. 39.13).

Visceral involvement in tuberous sclerosis is most

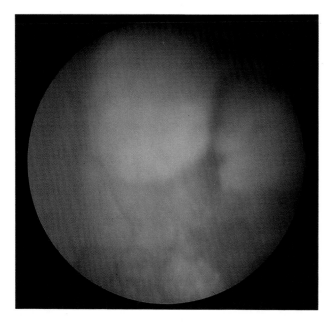

Fig. 39.13 Tuberous sclerosis. Peripheral fundus lesions showing depigmentation. In a girl with seizures the main differential diagnosis is with Aicardi's syndrome.

either eye or brain involvement. The Sturge–Weber syndrome is not familial and generally affects both sexes equally.

Cutaneous involvement is usually noticed at birth. The typical port wine stain or facial hemangioma is usually unilateral and located along the first and second divisions of the trigeminal nerve. It is evident at birth and does not increase in extent but does become darker in colour with age. Hypertrophy of the face may occur on the same side as the hemangioma and the globe on the affected side may be enlarged even without glaucoma. The process may extend to the gingiva and may involve palate and tongue. The cutaneous lesion consists of large dilated capillaries in the dermis and subcutaneous tissues. It does not undergo malignant change or degeneration. Central nervous system involvement is manifest as ipsilateral leptomeningeal hemangiomas present over the occipital and/or temporal lobes. These lesions may calcify and they are seen easily on CT scanning. The cerebral tissue on the side of the meningeal haemangioma is often atrophic. Seizures occur commonly in these patients. In addition, up to 60% of patients show some degree of mental retardation. Visceral involvement is less common than in other phakomatoses but tumours of the lung, gastrointestinal tract, pituitary, ovaries, and pancreas have been reported.

The two primary ocular complications of this syndrome are glaucoma and choroidal hemangiomas. Glaucoma occurs almost exclusively in those patients with ipsilateral eyelid and conjunctival involvement (Phelps 1978). One third of patients with the Sturge–Weber syndrome develop glaucoma at some time. Infrequently this may be contralateral to the cutaneous lesions. Pathophysiology of the glaucoma may be either due to malformation of the anterior chamber angle with anterior insertion of the ciliary muscle and uveal tissue or due to a mechnism very similar to those seen in cases of congenital glaucoma with no neurocutaneous disorders (Phelps 1978). Elevated episcleral venous pressure may also play a role in the genesis of glaucoma in these patients (Phelps 1978). Treatment of the glaucoma in these patients is difficult and expulsive choroidal hemorrhage may occur when the intraocular pressure is surgically lowered.

Approximately 40% of patients with the Sturge–Weber syndrome develop choroidal hemangiomas. This is usually seen as flat choroidal lesions lacking pigmentation and showing poorly defined borders. In those cases in which the haemangioma is diffuse, a deep red colour may appear and has been described as the so-called 'tomato ketchup' fundus (Susac et al. 1974). These haemangiomas grow slowly and may lead to degenerative changes of the overlying retina with serous retinal detachment. Ultimately neovascular glaucoma may ensue. Radiotherapy may using lens-sparing technique have some role in their treatment (Plowman & Harnett 1988).

Other ocular involvement includes heterochromia with the darker iris being ipsilateral to the cutaneous lesions, as well as colobomas and ectopia lentis.

For illustrations see Chapter 25.

Von Hippel–Lindau syndrome

This syndrome consists of haemangiomatous tumours of the cerebellum with retinal angiomatosis (Mellman & Rosen 1964). It may be inherited as an autosomal dominant disorder with irregular penetrance, but most cases are sporadic and show no familial tendency (Mellman & Rosen 1964). No racial or sexual predelictions are known.

Central nervous system involvement in this syndrome is seen primarily as cerebellar haemangioblastomas (Fig. 39.14) (Bech & Jenson 1961). These space occupying posterior fossa tumours present with typical signs of raised increased intracranial pressure. Less frequently, these tumours may involve the medulla or upper spinal cord. Patients may also pre-

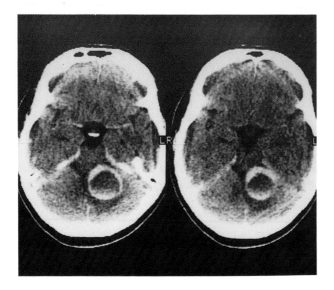

Fig. 39.14 Von Hippel—Lindau disease. CT scan showing posterior fossa lesions of haemangioblastomas.

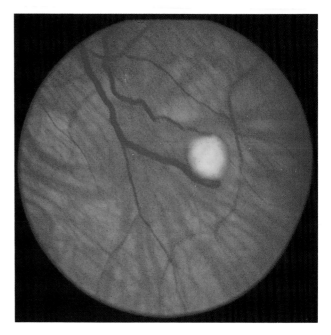

Fig. 39.15 Von Hippel—Lindau disease. Haemangioblastoma with large feeding and draining vessels.

sent with classic signs of cerebellar dysfunction, including ataxia, clumsiness, and nystagmus. These central nervous system tumours are usually amenable to surgical treatment.

Other visceral manifestations occur not infrequently in this syndrome. Some of these are life-threatening and account for the premature death of these patients. These include angiomas of the kidney, pancreas, liver, and spleen, as well as cystic involvement of bone, omentum, ovary, and epididimus. The life-threatening lesions associated with this syndrome include hypernephromas, pheochromocytomas, and cystadenomas of abdominal organs.

The typical ocular lesions of the Von Hippel—Lindau syndrome are haemangioblastomas (Welch 1970). These tumours are composed thin walled capillaries and solid masses of endothelial cells often showing cystic degeneration (Jessberg et al. 1968). These tumours are often multiple with both eyes involved in more than 50% of cases. Patients rarely present with ocular complaints in the first two decades of life. Early involvement is seen as a smooth domed tumour fed by an enlarged tortuous artery and drainage by an arterialized vein (Fig. 39.15) (Jessberg et al. 1968). As these lesions grow, the feeding and drainage vessels become more prominent and massive exudative change may take place surrounding the lesion (Welch 1970). This may closely mimic Coat's disease. Once subretinal exudation takes place the possibility of retinal detachment occurring becomes much more likely and neovascular glaucoma may be the ultimate

threat to the involved eye. Treatment of the early ocular lesions with cryotherapy and/or photocoagulation is frequently successful, especially in small lesions (Annesley et al. 1977). In the late stages of this disease these are largely unsuccessful (Annesley et al. 1977). When a patient is discovered to have a retinal angioma, all the members of his family should be carefully studied for the presence of additional ocular lesions so that early treatment may be initiated if necessary (Welch 1970).

Klippel—Trenaunay—Weber syndrome

The Klippel—Trenaunay—Weber syndrome has been recognized as a separate clinical entity (Troost et al. 1975). It consists of a port-wine lesion on the extremities, varicosities on the affected side, and local hypertrophy of bone and soft tissue on the affected part. It is said by some authorities that glaucoma occurs much less commonly in this syndrome; many of the cases reported have features in common with the Sturge—Weber syndrome.

References

Annesley WH, Leonard BC, Shields JA, Tasman WS. Fifteen year review of treated cases of retinal angiomatosis. *Ophthalmology* 1977; **83**: 446—51

Atkinson A, Sanders MD, Wong V. Vitreous haemorrhage in

tuberous sclerosis. *Br J Ophthalmol* 1973; **57**: 773−9

Bech K, Jenson OA. On the frequency of coexisting racemose hemangiomata of the retina and brain. *Acta Psychiatr Scand* 1961; **36**: 47−50

Font RL, Ferry AP. The phakomatoses. *Int Ophthalmol Clin* 1972; **12**: 44−63

Jesberg DO, Spencer WH, Hoyt WF. Incipient lesions of Von Hippel−Lindau disease. *Arch Ophthalmol* 1968; **80**: 632−36

MacDonald P, Miller NR. Chiasmatic and hypothalmic extension of optic nerve glioma. *Arch Ophthalmol* 1968; **101**: 1412−14

Mellman K, Rosen SW. Lindau's disease: review of the literature and a study of a large kindred. *Am J Med* 1964; **36**: 595−8

Nichol WR, Reed WB. Tuberous sclerosis: special reference to the microscopic alterations in cutaneous hamartomas. *Arch Dermatol* 1962; **85**: 209−13

Phelps CD. The pathogenesis of glaucoma in Sturge−Weber syndrome. *Ophthalmology* 1978; **85**: 276−81

Plowman PN, Harnett AN. Radiotherapy in benign orbital disease. 1. Complicated ocular angiomas. *Br J Ophthalmol* 1988; **72**: 286−8

Susac JO, Smith JL, Scello RJ. The tomato ketchup fundus in Sturge−Weber syndrome. *Arch Ophthalmol* 1974; **92**: 69−70

Troost BT, Savino PJ, Lozito JC. Tuberous sclerosis and the Klippel−Trenaunay−Weber syndrome. *J Neurol Neurosurg Psych* 1975; **38**: 500−03

Welch RB. Von Hippel−Lindau disease. *Trans Am Ophthalmol Soc* 1970; **68**: 367−71

Williams R, Taylor D. Tuberous sclerosis. *Surv Ophthalmol* 1985; **30**: 143−54

40 Polydactyly and the Eye

DAVID TAYLOR

Laurence—Moon—Biedl syndrome (LMB)

The Laurence—Moon and the Bardet—Biedl syndromes are similar but polydactyly and obesity are absent in the Laurence—Moon syndrome. Many authors lump them together as the LMB syndrome.

The most common features are (Bell 1958): retinal dystrophy (93%); obesity (91%); mental retardation, often mild (87%); hypogenitalism (74%) and polydactyly (73%).

It is autosomal recessive. Many cases of incomplete forms have been described and many cases have urological or renal abnormalities, deafness is unusual and diabetes has been described.

The retinal dystrophy may be severe in early life (Schachat & Maumenee 1982; Runge et al. 1986) but more frequently presents later in life usually in the teenages or twenties (Rizzo et al. 1986; Campo & Aaberg 1982). It is described as a typical retinitis pig-mentosa often with early macular involvement which may have a 'Bulls-eye' appearance. In the early stages there is no pigment clumping; the retina has a nearly normal appearance despite a severely abnormal elec-troretinogram (Runge et al. 1986). The prognosis is highly variable and unpredictable, with some cases showing little deterioration over many years (Rizzo et al. 1986), others becoming rapidly worse (Runge et al. 1986).

The retinal defect seems to be primarily in the photoreceptor cells (Runge et al. 1986).

Alström's syndrome

Alström's syndrome (Alström et al. 1959) is not usually associated with polydactyly although Alström de-scribed an unaffected relative with an extra digit. Alström's syndrome comprises diabetes mellitus, acanthosis nigricans, hypogenitalism, obesity, nerve deafness, and a retinal dystrophy that is somewhat different to retinitis pigmentosa (Sebag et al. 1984). It is autosomal recessive.

Carpenter's syndrome

The main features include preaxial (thumb or big toe side) or postaxial (little finger or little toe side) poly-dactyly, brachycephaly with synostosis, shallow supra-orbital ridges, laterally placed inner canthi, obesity, and mental retardation (Carpenter 1901; Temtamy 1966; Robinson et al. 1984). It is autosomal recessive.

Biemond syndrome

Biemond described a syndrome similar to LMB with short stature, iris coloboma, mental retardation, obes-ity, hypogenitalism, and polydactyly. Schachat and Maumenee (1982) found four other cases in the litera-ture. It is probably autosomal recessive.

Schachat and Maumenee's patient

Schachat and Maumenee (1982) described a patient with congenital cataracts, mental retardation, obesity hypogenitalism, skull deformities, and polydactyly.

Meckel–Gruber syndrome

This autosomal recessive syndrome includes an occipital encephalocoele, coloboma, microphthalmos, cleft palate, polycystic kidneys and abnormal genitalia with polydactyly (Hsia *et al.* 1971; Altman *et al.* 1977; Salomen & Norio 1984).

Jeune's syndrome (asphyxiating thoracic dystrophy, ATD)

These children are born with hypoplastic lungs and rib cage abnormalities that often lead to asphyxia and death, if they survive they are of moderate short stature. Renal dystrophy (Donaldson 1985), hepatic changes and a retinal dystrophy (Bard *et al.* 1978; Allen *et al.* 1979; Phillips *et al.* 1979). Polydactyly is an inconstant feature, when present it affects both hands and feet. It is autosomal recessive.

Ellis–Van Creveld syndrome

In this autosomal recessive disease polydactyly of the hands is a constant feature together with hypoplastic nails, small thorax, heart defect, short upper lip. Cases described as having retinal disease probably represent cases of Jeune's syndrome (Calver *et al.* 1981).

Rubenstein–Taybi syndrome

This probably autosomal recessive syndrome is characterized by broad thumbs and great toes which may occasionally be bifid giving polydactyly. The maxillae are hypoplastic and the palpebral fissures downward slanted. Ocular abnormalities include epicanthic folds, strabismus, refractive error, cataract and coloboma (Roy *et al.* 1968; Filippi 1972; Volker & Haase 1975). It is said that Scoline should be avoided in these children (Stirt 1982).

Smith–Lemli–Opitz syndrome

This not uncommon autosomal recessive syndrome features a broad nasal tip with anteverted nostrils, moderate or severe mental retardation, microcephaly,

ptosis, epicanthus, strabismus, cataract (Kretzer *et al.* 1981), post-lenticular membrane (Freedman & Baum 1979), and sclerocornea (Harbin *et al.* 1977).

Chromosomal defects

Trisomy 13

Polydactyly is a constant feature of the trisomy 13 syndrome. It is a syndrome which is usually fatal in the first days or months of life. Other features are coloboma, microphthalmos, glaucoma, and retinal dysplasia (Zimmerman & Font 1966; Hoepner & Yanoff 1972; Ginsberg & Bove 1974; Lichter & Schmickel 1975).

Partial trisomy 10q

Although camptodactyly (bent finger) is the more frequent finding, extra digits are a feature of 10q partial trisomy together with severe mental and growth deficieny, microcephaly. A variety of ocular defects have been described including narrow palpebral fissures, microphthalmos, anti-mongoloid slant, cataract (Jay 1977).

References

Allen AW, Moon JB, Hovland KR, Minckler DS. Ocular findings in thoracic–pelvic–phalangeal dystrophy. *Arch Ophthalmol* 1979; **97**: 489–92

Alström CH, Hallgren B, Nilson LB *et al.* Retinal degeneration combined with obesity, diabetes mellitus and deafness. *Acta Psychiatr Neurol Scand* 1959; **129**: 1–35

Altmann P, Wegenbichler P, Schaller A. A causistic report on the Gruber or Meckel syndrome. *Hum Genet* 1977; **38**: 357–63

Bard LA, Bard PA, Owens GW, Hall BD. Retinal involvement in thoracic–pelvic–phalangeal dystrophy. *Arch Ophthalmol* 1978; **96**: 278–81

Bell J. The Laurence–Moon syndrome. In: Enrose LS (Ed.) *The Treasury of Human Inheritance*. Cambridge University Press, London 1958; pp. 51–69

Calver D, Keast-Butler J, Taylor D. The extra digit. *Trans Ophthalmol Soc UK* 1981; **101**: 35–8

Campo RV, Aaberg TM. Bardet–Biedl syndrome. *Am J Ophthalmol* 1982; **94**: 750–6

Carpenter G. Two sisters sharing malformation of the skull and other congenital abnormalities. *Rep Soc Study Dis Child London* 1901; **1**: 110

Donaldson MDC, Warner AA, Trompeter RS, Haycock CB, Chantler, C. Familial juvenile nephronopthisis, Jeune's syndrome, and associated disorders. *Arch Dis Child* 1985; **60**: 426–434

Filipi G. The Rubenstein–Taybi syndrome. Report of 7 cases. *Clin Genet* 1972; **3**: 303–18

Freedman RA, Baum JL. Postlenticular membrane associated with Smith−Lemli−Optiz syndrome. *Am J Ophthalmol* 1979; **87**: 675−7

Ginsberg J, Bove KE. Ocular pathology of trisomy 13. *Ann Ophthalmol (Chic)* 1974; **6**: 113−22

Harbin RL, Katz JI, Frias JL, Rabinowicz IM, Kaufman HE. Sclerocornea associated with the Smith−Lemli−Optiz syndrome. *Am J Ophthalmol* 1977; **84**: 72−4

Hoepner J, Yanoff M. Ocular M. Ocular anomalies in trisomy 13−15. *Am J Ophthalmol* 1972; **74**: 729−37

Hsia YE, Bratu M, Herbordt A. Genetics of the Meckel syndrome. *Pediatrics* 1971; **48**: 237−47

Jay M. *The Eye in Chromosome Duplications and Deficiencies.* Marcel Dekker, New York 1977

Kretzer FL, Hittner HM, Mehta RS. Ocular manifestations of the Smith−Lemli−Opitz syndrome. *Arch Ophthalmol* 1981; **99**: 2000−6

Lichter PR, Schmickel RD. Posterior vortex vein and glaucoma in a patient with Trisomy 13 syndrome. *Am J Ophthalmol* 1975; **80**: 939−42

Phillips CI, Stokoe NK, Bartholomew RS. Asphyxiating thoracic dystrophy. *J Pediatr Ophthalmol Shabismus* 1979; **16**: 279−83

Rizzo JF, Berson EL, Lessell S. Retinal and neurologic findings in the Laurence−Moon−Bardet−Biedl phenotype.

Ophthalmology 1986; **93**: 1452−6

Robinson LK, James HE, Mubarak S, Allen EJ, Jones KL. Carpenter syndrome: natural history and clinical spectrum. *Am J Med Genet* 1985; **20**: 461−9

Roy FH, Summitt RL, Hiall RL, Hughes JG. Ocular manifestations of the Rubinstein−Taybi syndrome. *Arch Ophthalmol* 1968; **79**: 292−8

Runge P, Calver D, Marshall J, Taylor D. Histopathology of mitochondrial cytopathy and the Laurence−Moon−Biedl syndrome. *Br J Ophthalmol* 1986; **70**: 782−96

Salomen R, Norio R. The Mecker syndrome in Finland. *Am J Med Genet* 1984; **18**: 691−8

Schachat AP, Maumenee IM. Bardet−Biedl syndrome and related disorders. *Arch Ophthalmol* 1982; **100**: 285−8

Sebag J, Albert DM, Croft JL. The Alstrom syndrome: ophthalmic histopathology and retinal ultrastructure. *Br J Ophthalmol* 1984; **68**: 494−501

Stirt JA. Succinylcholine in Rubinstein−Taybi syndrome. *Anaesthesiology* 1982; **57**: 49

Temtamy SA. Carpenter's syndrome. *J Pediatr* 1966; **69**: 111−20

Volker HE, Haase W. Augensymptomatik bein R-T syndrome. *Klin Monatsbl Augenheilkd* 1975; **167**: 478−83

Zimmerman LE, Font RL. Trisomy 13. *J Am Med Assn* 1966; **196**: 694−7

Section 6
Eye Movements and Strabismus

41 Nystagmus

DAVID TAYLOR

Nystagmus is a rhythmic oscillation of the eyes which is usually bilateral affecting the two eyes equally, and is usually involuntary.

Nystagmus is characterized by its various components which can be detected clinically but are best delineated by nystagmography. Since the calibration of nystagmography devices is difficult in infancy and in the uncooperative child, detailed clinical observations and recordings are vital to diagnosis and management.

Characteristics

Amplitude

This is the length of excursion of the eyes from the fixation point; it is measured by nystagmography in degrees of arc but clinically as large, medium or small.

Frequency

This is the number of oscillations the eyes make per second and is clinically noted as high or low.

Velocity

The velocity of an eye movement is impossible to judge clinically except as an overall impression: by nystagmography it is measured in degrees per second.

Rapid eye movements are known as saccades, which have velocities of up to 500 degrees per second or more, the larger velocities being for larger amplitude movements. The relationship between amplitude and velocity is relatively close and if a movement falls within the normal range it is known as a main sequence (normal) saccade. Saccades are used in refixation, in the quick phases of nystagmus, and are the result of bursts of neuronal activity in brainstem nuclei.

Slow (pursuit) movements are initiated by the desire to follow a moving object, by a shift in the environment by movement of the body or by movement of the head which, via the vestibuloocular reflex, brings about an equal and opposite movement of the eyes. Intensity of nystagmus represents the amplitude multiplied by the frequency.

Waveform

When one phase of the oscillation is of higher velocity than the other, the nystagmus is known as jerk; when the two phases are equal it is called pendular or sinusoidal. More complex analysis of waveform is not clinically possible and nystagmography is necessary.

Direction

By convention, the direction noted is the direction of the fast phase in nystagmus. In jerk nystagmus the amplitude is usually greatest when the eye looks towards the direction of the fast component (Alexander's Law). The direction of the nystagmus can be horizontal (to the right or left of the patient), vertical, rotary (with rotation around the anteroposterior axis of the eye) or circumrotary (where the oscillation of the eye is a wide ranging combination of vertical and horizontal movements).

Recording

Nystagmus can be graphically documented by using an arrow to show the direction of the fast phase and the recording made in a box for each of the nine positions of gaze (Fig. 41.1).

The notation is really for descriptive purposes and clinical comparison, and has little use in the localization of underlying neurological, oculomotor or ocular defects.

Clinical examination of eye movement defects

History

1 The onset, progression and characteristics as they appear to the parent.
2 The family history.
3 The effect of any treatment.

GENERAL OCULAR EXAMINATION

1 The child's general development and neurological state.
2 The best corrected acuity, monocular and binocular, near and distance.
3 A general examination of the eyes including fundos-

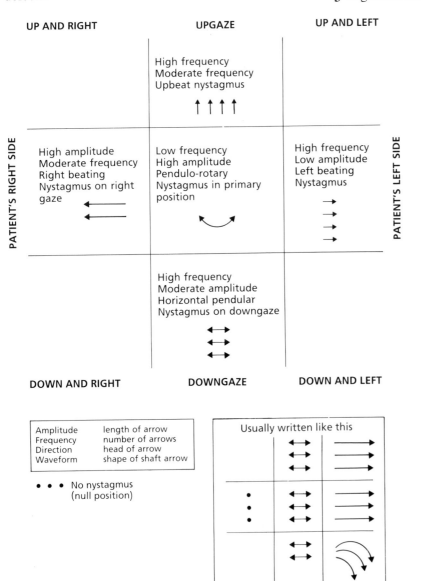

Fig. 41.1 Recording of nystagmus.

copy and slit lamp examination including transillumination of the iris.

SPECIFIC EXAMINATION

Examination of eye movements

1 With and without abnormal head posture or head movements.
2 In nine positions of gaze.
3 Monocular (ductions) and binocular (versions).
4 Near and distance (use an interesting fixation target, e.g., a toy).

Examination for disorders of eye position (squint)

Observe and note velocity of eye movements on command and when freely looking around the room, note the direction of the nystagmus. Note the smoothness of slow pursuit or following movements.

High frequency low amplitude nystagmus can sometimes only be detected by direct ophthalmoscopy.

Test the vestibulo-ocular reflex (VOR) by the doll's head manoeuvre. Encourage the child to fix an object while the parent moves his head from side to side; usually the movements of the head and eye are equal and opposite.

Test the child's ability to inhibit his VOR by spinning him and at the same time getting him to fix the examiner.

Convergence is tested by getting the child to fix an interesting near object and noting the smoothness, velocity and extent of the eye movements and the reaction of the pupils.

Assess optokinetic nystagmus (OKN) by using a large tape or drum. This is often difficult because the sighted child usually finds more interest in the examiner than in the test; a decorated drum or tape may help to regain the interest of an older child, and a numerate child can be asked to count the stripes. Optokinetic nystagmus consists of a slow phase in the direction of the tape's movement and a rapid movement back. If a baby is unable to make slow movements he will not follow the tape; if he cannot make rapid movements (saccade palsy) he will follow the tape across but not back.

Examination of head posture and movements

1 Does the head shake, vertically or horizontally?
2 Does it shake when the child is looking at something or when he is not concentrating?

3 Does it affect his vision?
4 If there is an abnormal head posture, note its characteristics — tilt, turn and chin elevation or depression. Does the eye position change when the head is tilted?

Congenital nystagmus

Congenital nystagmus (CN) is a description used for all forms of nystagmus present at birth or at around the time the child should show visual awareness. This occurs within the first 4 months of life except in very premature babies. Congenital nystagmus therefore may encompass a large variety of serious pathological processes with vision or life threatening potential as well as the benign condition that the term is usually associated with. Usually, however, clinicians use the term congenital nystagmus when meaning idiopathic congenital nystagmus, thus implying that the pathological causes for CN have been excluded by appropriate examinations.

It is of utmost importance that infants with nystagmus are not given the label CN until any pathological cause has been excluded by clinical, neurophysiological and neuroradiological examinations.

Congenital nystagmus occurs in up to one in 1000 of the population (Forssman & Ringner 1971). Although idiopathic CN may have a variety of eye movement characteristics a majority have sufficient in common to be called 'typical CN', the others being grouped as 'atypical CN'. This distinction is important since if an infant has typical CN he can be spared the rigorous investigations which are indicated for atypical CN because of their clinical overlap with the signs associated with secondary CN.

Congenital nystagmus can, therefore, be divided into:
1 Idiopathic CN — typical CN and atypical CN.
2 Secondary CN — where the nystagmus is due to ocular or neurological disease.

Typical congenital nystagmus

ONSET

The onset of the nystagmus, in an otherwise normal baby, is usually within the first 3 months of life: it is unusual but not exceptional for it to be present at birth and the nystagmus amplitude is usually greatest shortly after onset, sometimes the amplitude at onset may be very high.

FUNCTIONAL CHARACTERISTICS

The characteristic that is the hallmark of typical CN and which is rarely present in secondary CN is that its direction is purely horizontal, whether the child is looking in the straight ahead position, up, down, right or left.

It may be pendular or jerk or pendular becoming jerky on lateral gaze. Distinguishing pendular from jerk nystagmus may be very difficult clinically and probably has little relevance: it is the direction and amplitude that are the more important parameters. Typical CN is always conjugate.

In infancy the lack of control over the eye movements may give a falsely bad impression of the baby's vision, and there may also be a delay in apparent visual maturation (Fielder *et al.* 1985). As the infant grows his vision appears to improve and be good despite the continuing presence of the nystagmus, albeit of a smaller amplitude. A 2-year-old child may appear normal to his parents because his navigating ability is normal and it is only when he starts to require detail vision in childhood for reading, that the visual defect becomes apparent. Once acuity measurements are possible it is found that most children have acuities in the range 6/12 to 6/36. However, the measured acuity improves with age and may even reach normal (Forssman 1963). Patients with typical CN rarely have acuities of less than 6/36 and if they do the ophthalmologist must be extra careful to exclude pathological causes. Patients with lower amplitude nystagmus usually have the best vision, especially if they show adaptive mechanisms such as a head shake or abnormal head posture. Patients with CN typically have better near than distance acuity. This may not be due to reducing the intensity of nystagmus by the near reflex but to other mechanisms such as alteration in waveform or the ability of the child to use the fovea better in adduction (Von Noorden & La Roche 1983). Surprisingly there does not seem to be a particularly high incidence of specific learning (especially reading) disorders in this condition.

Apart from a reduction in Snellen acuity, both pattern and movement detection sensitivities are also reduced (Abadi & Sandikcioglou 1975).

The amplitude of the nystagmus is often highest soon after the onset of the nystagmus and it reduces in amplitude over some months or years. There is an improvement in acuity over the first two decades.

Patients with typical CN never experience oscillopsia except occasionally on extremes of gaze of if they acquire an additional eye movement disorder in adult life, even if this lessens the nystagmus amplitude.

One characteristic that seems to be unique to CN is the occurrence of 'inverted OKN', the fast phases of OKN are in the direction of rotation of the drum, instead of the opposite which is normal. The mechanism is not clear (Halmagyi 1980) but it is not found in other conditions.

The intensity of the nystagmus may be altered by getting the patient to view black and white stripes at varying orientation. It is interesting that most patients with CN have hypermetropic astigmatism (Gamble 1934) and it may be that there is a meridional amblyopia related to the astigmatism which has some effect in decreasing the visual feedback necessary for stable fixation along the meridian of the amblyopia. Colour vision is normal in typical CN. Typical CN is suppressed by eyelid closure, probably not specifically by blocking fixation but by the act of lid closure itself Shibasaki *et al.* (1978), and it disappears in sleep.

About one third of patients have a null zone on eccentric gaze (Forssman 1963); as they look to one side the amplitude of nystagmus becomes lower and the acuity may improve. In order to make use of this, the child may turn his head to the opposite side so that his null point is more or less straight ahead with regard to his body. This is a useful adaptive phenomenon which in most cases is of no harm to the child (although it may lead him to being scolded by an unthinking teacher!).

MANAGEMENT

The most important first stage is to carry out a full clinical examination to ensure that the eyes are normal in all respects other than the eye movements. If the nystagmus is horizontal in all directions of gaze and the eyes are normal and the child is normal the diagnosis of typical congenital nystagmus is acceptable and no further investigations need to be carried out. If there is any doubt the child should be investigated neurophysiologically and by CT or MR scanning.

However old the child, the clinical investigations should include slit lamp examination for iris transillumination and fundoscopy with direct and indirect ophthalmoscopy to exclude retinal or optic disc disease.

Cycloplegic refraction is very important at all ages because of the high incidence of astigmatism. Glasses should be prescribed early to fully correct this.

CHARACTERISTICS OF CONGENITAL NYSTAGMUS
EYE MOVEMENTS

Accurate eye movement recording techniques have enabled over 40 different varieties of congenital nystagmus to be identified (Dell'Osso 1982) on the basis of the waveform. By using eye movement recordings and high speed cinematography of the eye movements it has been possible to shown that in CN the eyes oscillate away from and back to the target, so that at one stage of the oscillation the eye is relatively stable in space and it is probably at this time that the best acuity is achieved, together with any damping effect that headshake or abnormal head position achieves (Dell'Osso & Daroff 1975). The flattened peaks, troughs or other part of the waveforms in CN probably represents the period during which the fovea is brought to bear on the target. The multitude of waveforms is unfortunately no clue to the aetiology of the nystagmus (Yee et al. 1976), and it does not even run true in a family with CN (Dell'Osso & Flynn 1979). Waveform analysis may show the nystagmus to be pendular, jerk or a mixture of the two, there is marked variation in space and time and the waveforms and foveation strategies are not related to the diagnosis, (i.e. albino or idiopathic) (Abadi & Dickson 1986).

AETIOLOGY

The aetiology is unknown. The contention (Cogan 1967) that pendular nystagmus has a sensory basis whilst jerk nystagmus has a 'motor defect' basis is no longer tenable on clinical or neurophysiological grounds. CN is a defect in the complex neurological substrate for maintaining steady fixation but there are few clues as to the site or nature of the abnormality. The similarity of CN to some cases who have an obvious sensory defect such as partial congenital cataract, or to central nervous system defects such as in albinism give few direct clues. Whilst the lessening of nystagmus by meridional stimulation (Daroff et al. 1973) and the occurrence of astigmatism and meridional amblyopia (Abadi & King-Smith 1979) are also sensory abnormalities there is probably little to be gained by trying to lay the blame on one or other side of a very complex reflex.

Optokinetic responses serve to maintain the eyes in a steady position relative to a moving environment and CN may be a defect in the optokinetic reflex. There are several abnormalities in the optokinetic nystagmus (OKN). It may be reversed (Halmagyi et al. 1979), it may have abnormal gain (the eye movements may be greater or less than the OKN drum movements), the nystagmus waveforms may be superimposed (Yee et al. 1980), or OKN may be so disturbed as to be barely recognizable as such (Kommerell & Mehdorn 1982), especially with regard to the slow phase. This may imply that a defect in the slow phase of OKN at a very early stage in development might give rise to a longlasting defect, even if the initial defect is transient.

CN is often inherited (Dell'Osso et al. 1974; Forssman 1968) but inheritance is not the only factor as indicated by the large number of non-familial cases, the intrafamilial differences in the type of nystagmus (Dell'Osso et al. 1974) and the occurrence of different forms of nystagmus in identical twins (Abadi et al. 1983).

TREATMENT DIRECTED TOWARDS IMPROVING THE
NULL POINT

Prismatic spectacles may be prescribed so that the eyes are maintained in an eccentric null position without an abnormal head posture, the base of the prism away from the null position, the two eyes having the base on the same side. Bilaterally base-out prisms can be used, sometimes combined with minus lenses to induce a false near response which sometimes damps nystagmus and improves acuity. Unfortunately, the prism lenses usually have to be very thick and are heavy and ugly; Fresnel prisms tend to interfere with vision unacceptably.

If the abnormal head position is marked it is possible to improve it by eye muscle surgery. If for instance the null position is to the left, the head will be turned to the right to bring the eyes in the null position nearer to the midline of the body. The surgery therefore consists of left lateral rectus and right medial rectus recession and left medial rectus and right lateral rectus resection. In principle this treatment was first advocated in 1953 by J.R. Anderson, who recommended a bilateral recession of muscles responsible for the slow phase of the nystagmus. It is instructive to follow the development of this treatment because of each author's method has produced less than perfect results the next authority to publish has replied with his (same) solution to the problem — more and more surgery! Kestenbaum (Kestenbaum 1954) introduced the combined recession and resection and Parks (Parks 1973) increased the amounts of surgery done so that 13 mm of surgery were done on each eye, i.e. a lateral rectus recession of 7 mm combined with a medial rectus resection of 6 mm and a medial rectus resection of 5 mm combined with a lateral rectus recession of 8 mm, this being known as 5, 6, 7, 8 procedure. Over the years the numbers have increased until Nelson *et al.* (1984) carried out Parks' procedure augmented by 60%, i.e. 9, 9.6, 11.2, 12.8 with evident satisfaction in their results, albeit with the acceptance that some patients have a residual gaze palsy! One wonders where we will be in the year 2000! It is interesting how opinion varies; some paediatric ophthalmologists rarely find it necessary to operate for nystagmus whilst others operate frequently. One reason which is frequently given for surgery is to prevent the development of bony abnormalities in the neck; it seems unlikely that these would develop unless the abnormal head posture is constantly present and marked, which is a fairly unusual combination. As well as improving the null point position itself the surgery may also improve visual acuity at angles of gaze away from the null point (Dell'Osso & Flynn 1979).

Other treatment

A sceptic might be tempted to say that any form of treatment which involves training the patient with CN to concentrate on detailed objects will improve his vision but there is evidence that one such treatment, auditory biofeedback, does improve vision (Abadi *et al.* 1980) and the improvement persists (Ciuffreda 1981).

The movements of nystagmus, recorded by infrared or other oculography, are 'converted' into noise and the patient tries to maintain a tone in the noise that is associated with the least intensity of nystagmus.

Drug treatment by phenobarbitone, hydroxytryptamine, phenytoin, and baclofen (Yee *et al.* 1980) have all been used with success but without widespread acceptance.

Visual improvement greater than would be expected solely from the correction of corneal astigmatism is achieved by the use of contact lenses (Allen & Davies 1983; Dell'Osso *et al.* 1988) and there seems every reason for a trial of contact lenses in cases where small but significant improvement is needed for social or occupational reasons, e.g. passing the driving test.

Visual stimulation by acupuncture (Ishikawa *et al.* 1987) pleoptics or other devices (Mallett 1986) probably have little effect beyond that engendered by concentrating the patient's mind on the subject, and are not yet of proven value.

EDUCATIONAL IMPLICATIONS

Most children with congenital nystagmus have few problems in the early years of their education as their acuity is usually reasonable, say 6/12 to 6/36, but as more demanding tasks are required of them their difficulties become more profound and they require more help in the classroom. Parents can usually be reassured that their child will not be severely handicapped, there are people with congenital nystagmus in all walks of life — engineers, doctors and musicians and even an eye-movement scientist amongst them!

Atypical congenital nystagmus

Any patient with congenital nystagmus which is not strictly horizontal in all positions of gaze is designated atypical. The main purpose of this separation is to make it clear that in this clinical group there may be patients with nystagmus secondary to brain or eye disease; they, therefore, require more detailed clinical, neurophysiological and radiological investigation.

Where no abnormalities are found on further investigation other than the eye movement defect the characteristics and behaviour of the nystagmus and the visual abnormalities and prognosis are similar to those in typical CN.

The nystagmus can be vertical or oblique, may vary from one to the other or be compound, and it may vary within a family with atypical CN (Marmor 1973). The more compound the nystagmus is (i.e. if it has more vectors) and especially if there is a 'see saw' element to it (see p. 610), the more one should be diligent to exclude eye or visual pathway disease.

Secondary infantile nystagmus

Almost any condition which causes poor vision in early childhood, (before about 2 years of age), will cause unsteady fixation and nystagmus. If the visual defect is partial, the nystagmus starts before the child has substantial difficulty with navigation which is why so many are thought initially to be atypical CN.

Commoner retinal causes include retinal dystrophies, including cone dystrophy, disc anomalies and albinism. Visual pathways disease giving rise to nystagmus without obvious cause includes chiasmal and optic nerve glioma, craniopharyngioma and optic nerve compression by other tumour or bony anomalies.

Systemic disorders associated with congenital nystagmus include Down's syndrome, hypothyroidism

(Shulman & Crawford 1969; McFaul *et al.* 1978), maple syrup urine disease (in which the nystagmus usually occurs in the recovery phase) (Zee *et al.* 1974), and in Pelizaeus–Merzbacher disease (Begaux 1966). Pelizaeus–Merzbacher disease is an X-linked recessive condition in which nystagmus is acquired in early childhood and is usually a horizontal pendular nystagmus of greater amplitude on attempted fixation and on lateral gaze (Taylor 1983). Retinal degeneration also occurs.

Magnesium depletion gives rise to a vertical nystagmus in adults (Saul & Selhorst 1981). Young children with profound malnutrition may present with an acquired gaze-evoked nystagmus with a Wernicke type of encephalopathy that is responsive to B group vitamins (Zak & D'Ambrosio 1985); in Leigh's disease a similar eye movement defect occurs.

Monocular or asymmetrical congenital nystagmus

One of the main characteristics of congenital nystagmus is that it is conjugate, but occasionally cases are encountered where the nystagmus is highly asymmetrical or even unilateral. They should be considered as highly suspicious of being secondary nystagmus.

Uniocular visual loss may rarely give rise to uniocular nystagmus (Yee *et al.* 1979) but when there is uniocular nystagmus it usually implies that the defect is retro-ocular, such as a chiasmal abnormality or optic nerve defect (Farmer & Hoyt 1984; Donin 1967).

Unfortunately the term 'spasmus nutans' has become enshrined in the literature as a condition which spontaneously resolves, characterized by dissociated (different in the two eyes) nystagmus, head nodding and sometimes an abnormal head posture. It is really only made retrospectively but the unquestioning acceptance of diagnosis has caused many chiasmal tumours in children to be overlooked. (See spasmus nutans, p. 614.)

Monocular nystagmus occurs associated with epileptiform seizures (Jacome & Fitzgerald 1982). Congenital or acquired monocular or asymmetrical nystagmus in childhood warrants full neuroradiological investigation (Farmer & Hoyt 1984; Lavery *et al.* 1984).

Children, such as those with Arnold–Chiari malformation, demyelinating disease, vasculitis or brainstem tumours may have an internuclear ophthalmoplegia with nystagmus of the abducting eye.

Latent nystagmus

Latent nystagmus (LN) occurs when one eye is covered, closed or subjected to reduced illumination. It does not occur in binocular vision except as part of another form of nystagmus when it may be described as nystagmus with latent worsening. In fact, most patients designated as having LN, on careful inspection or on eye movement recordings, have manifest nystagmus (Dell'Osso *et al.* 1979). It is very frequent in patients with congenital strabismus and although it can be seen in the very young infant it is often not detected until they are much older. It very frequently occurs with dissociated vertical deviation (see Chapter 44).

LN is a jerk nystagmus with the fast phase away from the occluded eye. By the use of a pseudoscopy (a system of mirrors through which the patient looks and is unaware of which eye he is having covered), Van Vliet (1973) showed that it was the intention to cover the eye that determined the nystagmus so that if the patient thought he was covering the left eye, but was in fact covering the right eye the nystagmus still beat with fast phase to the right. This apparently mysterious finding must imply that LN occurs as a disorder of central visual processing.

Latent nystagmus may become 'manifest' in patients with LN who fix with an amblyopic eye and it is present in what appears to be binocular viewing. This may also account for the high incidence of nystagmus in patients with monocular congenital nystagmus.

References

Abadi RV, Carden D, Simpson J. A new treatment for congenital nystagmus. *Br J Ophthalmol* 1980; **64**: 2–6

Abadi RV, Dickinson C. Waveform characteristics in congenital nystagmus. *Doc Ophthalmol* 1986; **64**: 153–67

Abadi RV, Dickinson DM, Lomas M, Ackerley R. Congenital idiopathic nystagmus in identical twins. *Br J Ophthalmol* 1983; **67**: 693–5

Abadi RV, King-Smith RP. Congenital nystagmus modified orientational detection. *Vision Res* 1979; **19**: 1409–11

Abadi RV, Sandikcioglu M. Visual resolution in congenital pendular nystagmus. *Am J Optomtr Physiol Optics* 1975; **52**: 573–81

Allen ED, Davies PD. Role of contact lenses in the management of congenital nystagmus. *Br J Ophthalmol* 1983; **67**: 834–6

Anderson JR. Latent nystagmus and alternating hyperphorias. *Br J Ophthalmol* 1953; **38**; 217–31

Begaux C, Decock G, Van Bogart L. Séméiologie Ophthalmologique des leucodystrophies ou maladies apparentes et leurs bases histopathologiques. *J Genet Hum* 1966; **15**: 221–62

Cogan DG. Congenital nystagmus. *Can J Ophthalmol* 1967; **2**: 4−10

Cuiffreda KJ, Goldrich SG, Neary C. Control of nystagmus using eye movement auditory biofeedback. In: Lennardstrand G, Zee DS, Keller EL (eds) *Functional Basis of Ocular Motility Disorders*. Permanon Press, Oxford 1981; pp. 147−50

Darroff RB, Hoyt WF, Bettman JW, Lessell S. Suppression and facilitation of congenital nystagmus by vertical lines. *Neurology* 1973; **23**: 530−4

Dell'Osso LF. Congenital nystagmus: basic aspects. In: Lennerstrand G, Zee D, Keller EL (eds) *Functional Basis of Ocular Motility Disorders*. Pergamon Press, Oxford 1982; pp. 129−38

Dell'Osso LF, Darroff RB. Congenital nystagmus waveforms and foveation strategy. *Doc Ophthalmol* 1975; **19**: 155−9

Dell'Osso LF, Flynn JT. Congenital nystagmus surgery − a quantitative evaluation of the effects. *Arch Ophthalmol* 1979; **97**: 462−9

Dell'Osso LF, Flynn JT, Darroff RB. Hereditary congenital nystagmus. *Arch Ophthalmol* 1974; **92**: 366−74

Dell'Osso LF, Schmidt D, Darroff RB. Latent, manifest latent and congenital nystagmus *Arch Ophthalmol* 1979; **97**: 1877−85

Dell'Osso LF, Traccis S, Abel LA, Erzurum SI, Donin JF. Contact lenses and congenital nystagmus. *Clin Vis Sci* 1988; **3**: 229−32

Donin JF. Acquired monocular nystagmus in children. *Can J Ophthalmol* 1967; **2**: 212−5

Farmer J, Hoyt CS. Monocular nystagmus in infancy and early childhood. *Am J Ophthalmol* 1984; **98**: 504−9

Fielder AR, Russell-Eggitt I, Dodd KL, Mellor DH. Delayed visual maturation. *Trans Ophthalmol Soc UK* 1985; **104**: 653−61

Forssman B. A study of congenital nystagmus. *Acta Otolaryngol* 1963; **57**: 139−47

Forssman B, Ringner B. Prevalence and inheritance of congenital nystagmus in a Swedish population. *Ann Hum Genet* 1971; **35**: 139−47

Gamble RC. The visual prognosis for children with congenital nystagmus. A statistical study. *Trans Am Ophthalmol Soc* 1934; **32**: 485−96

Halmagyi GM, Gresty MA, Leach J. Reversed optokinetic nystagmus (OKN). *Ann Neurol* 1980; **7**: 429−31

Ishikawa S, Ozawa H, Fujiyama Y. Treatment of nygtagmus by acupuncture. In: *Highlights in neuro-ophthalmology*. Aeolus Press, Amsterdam 1987; 227−33

Jacome DE, Fitzgerald R. Monocular ictal nystagmus. *Arch Neurol* 1982; **39**: 653−6

Kestenbaum A. Nouvelle operation de nystagmus. *Bull Soc Ophthalmol Fr* 1954; **2**: 1071−8

Kommerell G, Mehdorn E. Is an optokinetic defect the cause of congenital and latent nystagmus? In: Lennerstrand G, Zee DS, Keller EL (eds) *Functional Basis of Ocular Motility Disorders*. Oxford, Pergamon Press 1982; pp. 159−67

Lavery MA, O'Neill JF, Chu FC, Lab JM. Acquired nystagmus in early childhood: A presenting sign of intracranial tumour. *Ophthalmology* 1984; **91**: 425−35

Mallett RFJ. The treatment of congenital idiopathic nystagmus by intermittent photic stimulation. *J Physiol Optics* 1986; **3**: 341−56

Marmor M. Hereditary vertical nystagmus. *Arch Ophthalmol* 1973; **90**: 107−11

McFaul R, Dorner S, Brett EM, Grant DG. Neurological abnormalities in patients treated for hypothyroidism from early life. *Arch Dis Childhood* 1978; **53**: 611−9

Nelson LD, Ervin-Mulvey LD, Calhoun JH, Harley RD, Keisler MS. Surgical management for abnormal head position in nystagmus. The augmented modified Kestenbaum procedure. *Br J Ophthalmol* 1984; **68**: 796−801

Parks MM. Congenital nystagmus surgery. *Am Orthop J* 1973; **23**: 35−9

Saul RF, Selhorst JB. Downbeat nystagmus with magnesium depletion. *Arch Neurol* 1981; **10**: 650−3

Shibasaki H, Yamashita Y, and Motomura S. Suppression of congenital nystagmus. *J Neurol Neurosurg Psychiatr* 1978; **41**: 1078−83

Shulman JD, Crawford JD. Congenital nystagmus in hyopthyroidism. *New Engl Med J* 1969; **280**: 708−13

Taylor D. Ophthalmological features of some human hereditary disorders with demyelination. *Bull Soc Belge Ophthalmol* 1983; **208**: 405−13

Van Vliet AGM. On the Central mechanism of latent nystagmus. *Acta Ophthalmol* 1973; **51**: 772−5

Von Noorden GK, La Roche R. Visual acuity and motor characteristics in congenital nystagmus. *Am J Ophthalmol* 1983; **95**: 748−51

Yee RD, Baloh RW, Honrubia V. Study of congenital nystagmus: optokinetic nystagmus. *Br J Ophthalmol* 1980; **64**: 926−32

Yee RD, Baloh RW, Honrubia V. Effect of Baclofen on congenital nystagmus. In: Lennarstrand G, Zee DS, Keller EL (eds) *Functional Basis of Ocular Motility Disorders*. Pergamon Press, Oxford 1981; pp. 151−57

Yee RD, Jelks GW, Baloh RW, Honrubia V. Unioncular nystagmus in monocular visual loss. *Ophthalmology* 1979; **86**: 511−5

Yee RD, Wong EK, Baloh RW, Honrubia V. A study of congenital nystagmus waveform. *Neurology* 1976; **26**: 326−33

Zak TA, D'Ambrosio A Jr. Nutritional nystagmus in infants. *J Pediatr Ophthalmol Strabismus* 1985; **22**: 141−2

Zee DS, Freeman JM. Holtzman NA. Ophthalmoplegia in maple syrup urine disease. *J Pediatr* 1974; **84**: 113−15

42 Acquired Eye Movement Disorders

DAVID TAYLOR

Eye movement disorders due to poor vision

Any acquired nystagmus, especially a compound nystagmus, in early life may presage visual failure. If the visual failure is prenatal or perinatal the nystagmus will occur in the first months of life and is discussed in the section on secondary congenital nystagmus p. 600.

In infancy, the nystagmus or unsteady fixation often occurs before visual failure; it is only when the vision in the least affected eye becomes poor that there is evidence of poor vision from the child's behaviour. The nystagmus consists of anything from a few jerks on fixation, through a compound (multidirectional) nystagmus, to roving eye movements. Roving eye movements (REM) are the large amplitude, relatively low frequency multidirectional movements seen in children who are born behind or become blind within the first few years of life. The more peripheral the cause of the blindness the greater the amplitude of the eye movements. REM also occur in early onset cortical blindness, but it is striking how much less marked the nystagmus is in cortically blind infants compared with those blind from an ocular cause.

When the cause of the poor vision is chiasmal compression, as in craniopharyngioma, chiasmal glioma or other tumours, the nystagmus may take on a rotary form reminiscent of see-saw nystagmus.

Cerebellar disease

Chronic

Cerebellar lesions rarely occur in isolation so the clinical picture is frequently complicated by brainstem involvement. Experimental lesions in primates and signs in isolated cerebellar degenerative lesions give a clear picture of some of the clinical eye movement disorders occurring in human cerebellar disease. Most of the abnormal eye movements that occur however are not specific and the clinical diagnosis is made by the occurrence of combinations of abnormal eye movements and non-ocular signs of loss of the cerebellar influence on movements.

SQUARE WAVE JERKS

Probably the commonest abnormality in cerebellar disease is the occurrence of barely visible jerks on steady fixation or of smooth pursuit. They consist of a 1–5 degree saccade away from the fixation point followed, after an interval of about 200 ms during which the position disorder is visually detected, by a refixation movement. The larger movements may be easily detectable clinically.

DYSMETRIA

In cerebellar disease saccades usually, but not always, have normal velocity but do not accurately achieve their target, either overshooting (hypermetria) or undershooting (hypometria); the inaccurate saccade is followed by one or more corrective saccades, often themselves dysmetric.

GAZE EVOKED NYSTAGMUS

The patient with cerebellar disease has difficulty maintaining eccentric gaze; the eyes drift back from the eccentric position and a series of corrective saccades are made to refixate, the nystagmus may be upbeat, downbeat, or horizontal.

SMOOTH PURSUIT DISORDERS

Slow movements, whether pursuit movements, VOR slow movements, or slow phases of nystagmus including optokinetic nystagmus, become jerky and irregular.

REBOUND NYSTAGMUS (Hood *et al.* 1978)

Occasionally in children, frequently in adults it is possible to demonstrate a reversal in the direction of nystagmus brought about by holding eccentric gaze. If, for instance, the patient is made to look to the left he will develop a left beating nystagmus which decreases in amplitude and may even reverse. It reverses in direction on refixating to the straight ahead position. It is probably due to the imperfect working of a system used to correct the drifting of the eyes away from the fixation point.

VESTIBULO-OCULAR REFLEX DISORDERS

Slow phases of vestibular movements may be jerky and the fast phases subject to dysmetria but one of the most pronounced abnormalities is the failure to suppress VOR during head movements with fixation. To test this, the child turns his head while looking at a pin stuck in the end of a tongue–depressor held in his teeth. Normally the eyes fix steadily on the pin but when the child is unable to suppress the VOR his eyes drift away from the pin, only to make saccades back to it in order to attempt fixation, i.e. he develops nystagmus.

In a small baby, as in older children, one can test the ability of the child to inhibit post-rotational nystagmus by spinning the baby and stopping suddenly. Normally there are one or two beats of post rotational nystagmus, but in cerebellar disorders (and also in some other disorders including occipital blindness) the nystagmus induced by rotation continues after the rotation has ceased.

OTHERS

Skew deviation (a vertical incomitant squint secondary to supranuclear or vestibular defect implying brainstem or cerebellar disease) and positional nystagmus (nystagmus in which direction changes with shift in head position) are only occasionally seen in children.

Acute

Acute damage to a cerebellar hemisphere causes ipsilateral gaze paresis, disturbed smooth pursuit, and gaze evoked nystagmus. This acute phase rapidly improves in children and is often not seen by the doctor in hospital who sees the more long-term effects of the damage in the posterior fossa and the compensation for this. In the acute phase all the chronic findings may be present but often are much more marked.

In the normal newborn, a variety of abnormal eye movements including spontaneous downward deviations, skew deviation and opsoclonus may occur transiently (Hoyt *et al.* 1980).

OPSOCLONUS

Opsoclonus is an extraordinary eye movement disorder mainly occurring in children with a sudden onset in the first 5 years of life, it may also be known as the dancing eye syndrome (Kinsbourne 1962). Usually it occurs for no clear reason, but there is often a vague or sometimes a clear relationship to a variety of infectious illnesses including coxackie B, St Louis encephalitis, varicella, or polio (Marmion & Sandilands 1947; Estrin 1977; Evans & Welch 1981; Kuban *et al.* 1983).

There is also a clear association of some cases with neuroblastoma (Moe & Nellhaus 1970) and it is known that the finding of opsoclonus imparts a favourable prognosis (Altman & Baehner 1976), and the removal of the tumour may coincide with clinical improvement.

The term opsoclonus first appeared in the Polish literature about 1920 (Orzechowski 1927) and it is now recognized as a diffuse cerebellar system disorder. The eye movements are wild with vertical, horizontal oblique and circumrotary eye movements occurring in bursts often excited by attempted fixation, and they may still be present during sleep. There is an associated truncal and limb ataxia, and emotional or behavioural instability is frequent in older children. The symptoms may sometimes be improved with ACTH (Kinsbourne 1962).

After a variable period of a few weeks to many months the child begins to improve; residual defects depend on the length and severity of the disease but many children are left with some cerebellar defects (Savino & Glaser 1975) and some with intellectual, emotional and non-ocular motor defects.

OCULAR FLUTTER AND MACROSACCADIC OSCILLATIONS

Ocular flutter consists of bursts of purely horizontal spontaneous eye movements rapidly rising to a crescendo, then decreasing as control is established the whole burst lasting less than 2 seconds, usually less than 1 second. It is often associated with other cerebellar abnormalities (Cogan 1954) especially dysmetria (which is not a spontaneous movement but an abnormality that occurs on attempted refixation) and it occurs as part of the process of improvement in eye movement control from the wild movements of opsoclonus (Savino & Glaser 1975).

In ocular flutter there is no intersaccadic latency, the movements are 'preprogrammed' whereas in the closely related macrosaccadic oscillations there is an intersaccadic latency of about 200 ms suggesting that visual reprocessing is taking place.

Opsoclonus and flutter occur also in hydrocephalus (Shetty & Rosman 1972), trauma, and in normal neonates (Hoyt et al. 1980); they are not a specific or localizing sign but an indication of disordered inhibition of saccade generation.

Vestibular disease

Diseases which affect the peripheral vestibular apparatus present with symptoms of dizziness, vertigo, tilting or leaning of the environment, oscillopsia, and abnormal eye movements. In childhood it is most commonly ascribed to a viral illness either labyrinthitis or neuronitis. Mumps, measles, herpes zoster, and infectious mononucleosis have all been implicated as well as trauma resulting in a perilymph fistula. In older children, the Cogan syndrome (Cogan 1945) of acute keratitis, deafness and vertigo, associated with widespread vasculitic disease (Bicknell & Holland 1978), may occur.

Nystagmus in vestibular disease is usually a mixture of horizontal and vertical jerk nystagmus with a torsional component, worse in the dark or without fixation, often influenced by head posture, it is said that the axis around which the eye rotates is related to the plane of one of the semicircular canals.

Disease affecting the central vestibular nuclei is more likely to cause pure horizontal or vertical nystagmus than peripheral lesions, but rotary or torsional nystagmus also frequently occurs. Associated symptoms occur due to the relation of other brainstem structures. Children may wander to the side of the lesion, and may make larger saccades to the side of the lesion; this is the child equivalent of the Wallenberg syndrome of adult neurology. Skew deviation often occurs.

Children with damage to the inferior olivary nucleus may develop a pendular horizontal, vertical or torsional nystagmus that may be dysconjugate but with synchronous movements of the palate or pharynx occurring at 1−3 cycles per second, and which is usually still present during sleep (Guillain 1938; Gresty et al. 1982), it is known as palatal myoclonus. Patients with posterior fossa malformations including the Arnold−Chiari malformation may develop similar abnormalities but they are also found in tumours, vascular anomalies, demyelinating disease, and as a part of a brainstem encephalitis.

Brainstem disease

Midbrain disorders

In infancy midbrain eye movement defects are most commonly seen in hydrocephalus, probably due to distortion of the upper parts of the midbrain, especially the posterior commissure. This is associated with the classic 'setting sun' sign in hydrocephalus which is due to a combination of lid retraction and an upgaze palsy with a tonic downward deviation of the eyes. The setting sun sign is rapidly reversed by lowering of the intracranial pressure. Brief transient downward deviation of the eyes occurs in healthy neonates (Hoyt et al. 1980) but is longer lasting, and associated with an esotropia in premature babies with intraventricular haemorrhage.

Lid retraction (Collier's sign) occurs isolated in hydrocephalus or in other midbrain abnormalities including tumour.

Lesions around the Aqueduct of Sylvius give rise to a syndrome (also known as Parinauds syndrome when applied to some of the specific manifestations of the dorsal midbrain syndrome) of impaired vertical, especially upward, gaze, and large pupils that react poorly to light but relatively well to accommodation. Attempts at upward gaze give rise to adducting saccades (Ochs *et al.* 1979) which are known as convergence retraction nystagmus. Rapid upward saccades such as those brought about by downwards OKN are the most effective at bringing about convergence retraction nystagmus, which may be quite uncomfortable.

In childhood, hydrocephalus, pinealoma, and vascular anomalies are the most common structural lesions giving rise to the syndrome. A variety of metabolic diseases have a similar presentation but usually confined to the vertical gaze abnormalities. These include neurolipidoses especially Niemann−Pick type C (ophthalmoplegic lipidosis), Tay−Sachs disease, infantile Gaucher's disease, kernicterus, Wilson's disease (in older children), and maple syrup urine disease. Tuberculoma, encephalitis, Whipple's disease, and demyelination can also give rise to variants of the dorsal midbrain syndrome.

Pontine disorders

Nuclear abducens abnormalities are not common in childhood but developmental anomalies, brainstem involvement by cerebellar tumour, and encephalitis are occasional causes. The abducens nuclei contain not only fibres going to the ipsilateral VIth nerve but also gaze neurones and those with fibres going via the medial longitudinal fasciculus (MLF) to the contralateral medial rectus, so lesions of the nucleus give rise to a gaze palsy with sparing of vergence movements of the affected medial rectus. Lesions in this area also very frequently affect the ipsilateral VIIth nerve.

Lesions affecting the medial longitudinal fasciculos (MLF) are rare in early childhood but internuclear ophthalmoplegia (INO) affects older children with demyelinating disease. Younger children do develop INO's as part of a parainfectious vasculitis or from tumours and malformations (including the Arnold−Chiari malformation) but these are rare. Unilateral INOs result from damage to the ipsilateral MLF which connects the contralateral gaze (abducens nucleus) centre to the medial rectus motor pool in the midbrain. The medial rectus action may be spared for convergence if the lesion is caudal in the pathway of the MLF. The abducting eye usually shows nystagmus, and especially in bilateral INOs there is often vertical nystagmus and sometimes a skew deviation.

Disorders of the medulla

A variety of disorders affect the medulla including developmental anomalies, encephalitis, demyelination, and extrinsic or intrinsic tumours. The Arnold−Chiari malformation is a developmental anomaly affecting to a varying degree the contents of the posterior fossa. Cyst formation as part of the malformation, may be treatable by decompressive surgery. Many children with hydrocephalus have the Arnold−Chiari malformation and in addition to the oculomotor signs from the hydrocephalus itself have a variety of brainstem signs from medullary involvement, including internuclear ophthalmoplegia, and downbeat nystagmus.

Downbeat nystagmus can result from many causes, the commonest being drugs and alcohol and cerebellar abnormalities. But downbeat nystagmus from medullary disease has special characteristics: it is worse on downgaze, usually less marked on upgaze but greatest in amplitude on looking down and laterally and sometimes on neck extension. There is often a torsional component to the nystagmus.

Primary position upbeat nystagmus has a much less close association with medullary disease and is less specific. It is sometimes seen with drug and alcohol or other intoxication (Jay *et al.* 1982). Primary position upbeat nystagmus that increases on upgaze and is usually of large amplitude implies midline cerebellar disease but can be due to medullary disease (Gilman *et al.* 1977), whilst upbeat nystagmus that increases in intensity on downgaze implies medullary disease (Darroff & Troost 1973).

Thalamic disorders

Tamura and Hoyt (1987) described 11 premature infants who had intraventricular haemorrhage and who developed a slowly resolving tonic downward deviation of the eyes and an upgaze palsy. Although a secondary hydrocephalus may have been implicated only two babies required a shunt and direct thalamic involvement was suspected. Nearly all the affected

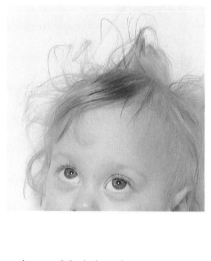
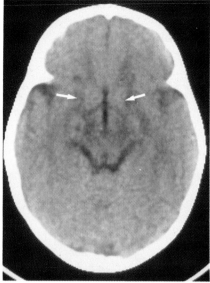

Fig. 42.1 (a) Leigh's disease. The child has forced upward deviation of gaze, nystagmus, and optic atrophy (b) Leigh's disease. CT scan showing lucencies in the basal ganglia.

babies had large angle infantile esotropia which required surgery.

Leigh's disease (subacute necrotizing encephalomyelopathy) is an autosomal recessive disease of unknown cause with an onset in infancy, rarely older. They present with tachypnoea, weight loss, psychomotor retardation, a peripheral neuropathy, and occasionally seizures. Spontaneous improvement may occur. Eye symptoms and signs are common (Montpetit *et al.* 1971) and include nystagmus, ophthalmoplegia (Fig. 42.1), ptosis, and optic atrophy (Howard & Albert 1972). Retinal macular changes have been described (Dunn & Dolman 1969).

Cerebral hemisphere disease

Unilateral hemisphere lesions are most frequently seen in small infants as a result of a haemorrhage due to prematurity, non-accidental injury, developmental abnormalities and hydrocephalus or its treatment by shunting.

Acute lesions give rise to gaze weakness to the side opposite the lesion and if the lesion is severe there may be tonic deviation of gaze to the side of the lesion, with relatively intact movements to spinning or caloric stimulation. On spinning the infant the slow or the quick phases of nystagmus or both to the side opposite the lesion may be defective.

These gaze abnormalities in acute lesions are transient, lasting days or a few weeks, a high proportion of affected babies have a residual strabismus.

Bilateral hemispheric lesions give rise to bilateral but often asymmetrical abnormalities. The abnormality of voluntary movements can give rise to a false impression of poor vision; this happens especially in hydrocephalic babies.

As the acute phase passes there are often residual defects that are more specific for the side of the damage. A gaze palsy becomes a gaze paresis with nystagmus on the gaze to the side opposite the lesion, and smooth pursuit movements away from the side of the lesion may be slow. After loss of a hemisphere (for instance in hemispherectomy in Sturge–Weber syndrome) there are permanent asymmetrical defects in eye movements to both sides (Sharpe *et al.* 1979; Sharpe & Lo 1981).

Occipital damage with an homonymous hemianopia results in inaccurate saccades into the blind hemifield with compensatory searching strategies designed to overcome the defect. Bilateral occipital cortical defects result in varying degrees of blindness which may recover over a period of some years. The preservation of some visual responses, occasionally the selective preservation of OKN, has been taken as evidence of extra-geniculostriate vision. The preservation of any visually evoked cortical responses on neurophysiological testing should allow a very cautiously optimistic prognosis. The infant and young child with cortical blindness is less likely to develop nystagmus or roving eye movements than when the damage is due to anterior visual pathway disease. Causes of occipital lesions include hydrocephalus (in which sudden blindness from posterior cerebral artery occlusion occurs in children with markedly enlarged heads), hypertension,

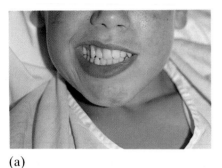
(a)

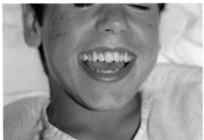
(b)

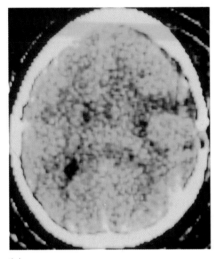
(c)

Fig. 42.2 (a) Supranuclear VIIth nerve palsy. (a) On command he can only move the right side of his face but; (b) when he spontaneously laughed both eyes shut and he moved both halves of the face. He also had a voluntary gaze palsy to the right. (c) CT scan shows the infiltrating tumour in the fronto-parietal area.

vasculitis, trauma including NAI, perinatal anoxia, cardiac surgery, and meningitis.

Frontal lesions are usually associated with a supranuclear disorder of contralateral gaze that resolves almost completely but frontoparietal lesions may give rise to residual defects of voluntary gaze similar to oculomotor apraxia. Supranuclear cranial nerve palsies also occur (Fig 42.2).

Parietal and temporal lobe defects, unless associated with a midline shift in cerebral contents do not usually have specific eye movement defects, but a defect in pursuit and slow OKN movements towards the side of the lesion may be present in parietal lobe damage.

Vergence disorders

Anomalies of the vergence mechanisms play an important role in the genesis of many forms of squint, and manipulation of vergence is important in the treatment. Non-strabismic vergence eye movement disorders however are very rare in childhood.

Convergence insufficiency

Convergence insufficiency is not uncommon in teenagers; it gives rise to symptoms of eye strain after near work especially related to examinations, and on examination by the cover test a poorly controlled exophoria is found for near fixation. Eye movements are full and the reading acuity is normal and there should be no other neurological abnormalities. Treatment consists of reassurance that the symptoms are not an indication of harm being done to the eyes by excessive work, and that they are not due to eye disease. The child's reading habits should be modified so that they read at a bent-arm distance, in a bright light and that they do not read for more than a page or so without breaking concentration. Most cases improve on simple treatment but occasional cases are linked with more deep-rooted psychological problems and where really necessary appropriate aid should be sought from a clinical psychologist.

It should be remembered that dorsal midbrain problems may present with similar symptoms but they will usually be a defect of accommodation and other symptoms and signs of the acqueduct of Sylvius syndrome.

Spasm of the near reflex

Spasm of the near reflex is most frequently seen in young women but may occur in older girls. We have seen one case lasting 4 years in an 8-year-old girl. They complain of attacks of blurring and diplopia together with eye ache, and friends or relatives report the presence of a marked cross-eye. The patients often produce an attack for the examiner, but they seem, and probably are, genuinely unable to control its onset and offset. There are no neuriligical abnormalities but there is a marked convergent squint and so great is the convergence effect that there may be an apparent inability to abduct with either eye associated with a variable gaze directed nystagmus of the eye that is attempting to abduct. The eyes can usually be induced to abduct in monocular viewing or by using optokinetic targets. Together with the convergence there is miosis and accommodation giving rise to blurring. The spasms may last a long time, sometimes many minutes, but they are usually momentary. It is interesting how infrequently an underlying psychological factor is discovered either by an ophthalmologist or by his psychologist colleagues but if such factors are found the prognosis is better. Treatment with cycloplegics, which prevent the worrysome change in refraction and the pain, may help and miotics may act by causing an 'ocular' miosis and spasm of accommodation, reducing the central drive. Providing that the distinction from VIth nerve palsy is made (Griffin et al. 1976) further investigations are not necessary (Sarkies & Sanders 1985), but because occasional underlying abnormalities have been described; pituitary tumours, cerebellar tumours, Arnold–Chiari malformation, a careful neurological and neuroophthalmolgical examination is mandatory (Dagi et al. 1987).

Divergence paralysis

In divergence paralysis, when the patient looks in the distance there is a convergent squint whilst when they look near they do not squint. A criterion is that they have totally normal eye movements on abduction. Many cases suspected of having divergence paresis have in fact a partial bilateral VIth nerve palsy and underlying hydrocephalus, and any convergent squint that is greater for distance than near should be suspect.

Miscellaneous eye and lid movement disorders

Ping-pong gaze

Ping-pong gaze consists of a rhythmic horizontal conjugate movement of the eyes occurring every second or so; it therefore must be named after the movements seen during the slowest game of ping-pong ever! It is usually seen in severely ill patients with a variety of causes (Selenich 1976; Von Cramon & Zihl 1977; Stewart et al. 1979). It probably has no localizing value but may imply a poor prognosis in that many of the described cases were profoundly and often irrecoverably obtunded. Its mechanism is unknown.

Ocular bobbing and dipping

Ocular bobbing is a sign of severe posterior fossa structural disease especially affecting the pons and is most often seen in comatose patients. Typical bobbing (Susac et al. 1970) consists of rapid conjugate downward jerks followed by a slow drift upwards with absent horizontal movements; it is usually due to intrinsic pontine lesions but extra-axial disease and sometimes diffuse CNS disease may also be responsible (Daroff & Waldman 1965; Finelli & McEntee 1977; Sherman & Salmon 1977). Monocular and atypical forms, with convergence movements, or intact horizontal movements also occur (Susac et al. 1970).

In ocular dipping (reversed ocular bobbing) there is a slow downward movement with a rapid return phase (Knobler et al. 1981); it may be that dipping is caused by an anoxic insult to the cerebral hemispheres and possibly basal ganglia (Ropper 1981).

Skew deviation

Skew deviation is a non-specific sign of posterior fossa disease probably reflecting damage to vestibular connections in which a vertical squint becomes evident on lateral gaze without muscle paresis. There is usually asymmetry on right or left gaze, but sometimes the vertical deviation is comitant. Skew deviation has no specific localizing value by itself, localization may be achieved from its neurological accompaniments.

Voluntary nystagmus

Voluntary nystagmus is a trick acquired by a few young people, possibly from their relatives (Zahn 1978). It is usually horizontal, high frequency and appears to be pendular; it may be vertical (Krohel & Griffin 1979) and sometimes circumrotary. Unless there is another oculomotor palsy in addition the movements are conjugate. The movements consist of multiple saccades (Shults *et al.* 1977) that are difficult to sustain for more than a few seconds. It is often associated with fluttering of the lids and sometimes with a facial expression of concentration. Subjects have the normal suppression of vision during saccades but still have oscillopsia (Nagle *et al.* 1980).

Lid nystagmus

Children with vertical nystagmus frequently have associated lid movements. A rare form of nystagmus (Pick's nystagmus) is occasionally seen in posterior fossa disorders. On convergence there is a bilateral conjugate upper lid nystagmus without eye nystagmus (Sanders *et al.* 1968; Safran *et al.* 1982).

Periodic alternating nystagmus

Nystagmus that alters in direction over a period of minutes, or occasionally at shorter intervals is known as periodic alternating nystagmus (PAN). It may be congenital, or occurs in blindness from demyelination or with anti-epileptic drug intoxication. It may result from abnormal vestibular−optokinetic interaction (Leigh *et al* 1981) and in acquired cases may be relieved by baclofen (Halmagyi *et al.* 1980). Periodic alternating gaze deviation is a closely related condition in which instead of the direction of nystagmus altering, there is a periodic alteration in the direction of gaze (Kennard *et al.* 1981).

See-saw nystagmus

Maddox (1914), the father of the founder of orthoptics, described beautifully a case of bitemporal hemianopia with a peculiar nystagmus with the eyes alternately rising and falling, and as the eye rose it intorted and as it fell it extorted. He likened the movement to that of a see-saw.

There is a very clear relationship to chiasmal disorders with bitemporal hemianopias. The movement is often asymmetrical with the eye with the worst vision having the larger excursion, and the amplitude may vary with gaze usually being greater in downgaze.

Although the onset may be quite sudden, the commonest cause in early childhood is a slow growing suprasellar tumour, in particular a glioma. It may be detected in the first year of life but usually presents later unless the child is seen because of other effects of the frequency of the nystagmus. Any rotary or torsional and vertical element in a patient with early onset nystagmus should raise suspicions about the presence of a suprasellar defect. Not all patients with congenital see saw nystagmus have suprasellar tumours however, it has been described in an otherwise normal child (Zelt & Bigan 1985) in septo optic dysplasia (Davis & Schoch 1975) in trauma (Schmidt & Kommerell 1969), neck extension injury (Keane 1978). In childhood the clinician first thinks of suprasellar tumour. It may start suddenly after squint surgery for exodeviations in known craniopharyngioma (Mewis 1982) and there appears to be a high incidence of exodeviation, possibly due to the poor vision that many patients have (Arnott & Miller 1970).

The mechanism is not known but it may imply that the upper midbrain is involved (Daroff 1965); destruction of the interstitial nucleus of Cajal in the upper midbrain abolished nystagmus in one case (Sano *et al.* 1972) and stimulation in this area produces an elevation and intorsion of the contralateral eye (Westheimer & Blair 1975). Alcohol at a dose of 1.2 g/kg reduced the nystagmus and its symptoms (Frisen & Wikkelso 1986).

References

Altman AJ, Baehner RL. Favourable prognosis for survival in children with coincident opso-myoclonus and neuroblastoma. *Cancer* 1976; **37**: 846−8

Arnott EJ, Miller SJH. See saw nystagmus. *Trans Ophthalmol Soc UK* 1970; **90**: 491−6

Bicknell JM, Holland JV. Neurologic manifestations of Cogan syndrome. *Neurology* 1978; **28**: 218−23

Cogan DG. Syndrome of non-syphilitic interstitial keratitis and vestibulo auditory symptoms. *Arch Ophthalmol* 1945; **33**: 144−9

Cogan DG. Ocular dysmetria, flutterlike oscillations of the eyes and opsoclonus. *Arch Ophthalmol* 1954; **51**: 318−23

Dagi LR, Chrousos GA, Cogan DG. Spasm of the near reflex associated with organic disease. *Am J Ophthalmol* 1987; **103**: 582−5

Daroff RG. See saw nystagmus. *Neurology* 1965; **15**: 874−7

Daroff RB, Troost T. Upbeat nystagmus. *JAMA* 1973; **225**: 312−7

Daroff RB, Woldman AL. Ocular bobbing. *J Neurol Neurosurg Psychiatr* 1965; **28**: 375−7

Davis GU, Schoch JP. Septo-optic dysplasia associated with see-saw nystagmus. *Arch Ophthalmol* 1975; **93**: 137−9

Dunn HG, Dolman CL. Necrotising encephalomyelopathy. *Neurology* 1969; **19**: 536−50

Estrin WJ. The serological diagnosis of St Louis encephalitis in a patient with the syndrome of opsoclonia, body tremulousness, and benign encephalitis. *Ann Neurol* 1977; **1**: 596−8

Evans RW, Welch KWA. Opsoclonus in a confirmed case of St

Louis encephalitis. *J Neurol Neurosurg Psychiatr* 1981; **45**: 660—1

Finelli PF, McEntee WJ. Ocular bobbing with extra-axial haematoma of posterior fossa. *J Neurol Neurosurg Psychiatr* 1977; **40**: 386—8

Frisen L, Wikkelso C. Post traumatic see saw nystagmus abolished by ethanol engestion. *Neurology* 1986; **36**: 841—4

Gilman N, Baloh RW, Tomiyasu H. Primary position of upbeat nystagmus, a clinicopathologic study. *Neurol* 1977; **27**: 294—8

Gresty MA, Ell JJ, Findley L. Acquired pendular nystagmus. *J Neurol Neurosurg Psychiatr* 1982; **45**: 431—5

Grifin JF, Wray SH, Anderson D. Misdiagnosis of spasm of the near reflex. *Neurology* 1976; **26**: 1018—20

Guillain G. The syndrome of synchronous rhythmic palato-pharyngo-laryngo-ocular-diapragmatic myoclonus. *Proc R Soc Med* 1938; **31**: 1031—5

Halmagyi GM, Rudge P, Gresty MA, Leigh RJ, Zee DS. Treatment of periodic alternating nystagmus. *Ann Neurol* 1980; **8**: 609—11

Hood JD, Kayan A, Leech J. Rebound nystagmus. *Brain* 1978; **96**: 507—15

Howard RO, Albert DM. Ocular manifestations of subacute necrotising encephalomyelopathy. *Am J Ophthalmol* 1972; **74**: 386—92

Hoyt CS, Mousel DK, Weber AA. Transient supranuclear disorders of gaze in healthy neonates. *Am J Ophthalmol* 1980; **89**: 708—11

Jay WM, Marcus RW, Jay MS. Primary position upbeat nystagmus with organophosphate poisoning. *J Pediatric Ophthalmol Strabismus* 1982; **19**: 318—9

Keane JR. Intermittent see-saw eye movements. Report of a patient in coma after hyperextension head injury. *Arch Neurol* 1978; **35**: 173—4

Kennard C, Barger G, Hoyt WF. The association of periodic alternating nystagmus with periodic alternating gaze. *J Clin Neuroophthalmol* 1981; **1**: 191—4

Kinsbourne M. Myoclonic encephalopathy in infants. *J Neurol Neurosurg Psychiatr* 1962; **25**: 271—5

Knobler RL, Somasundaram M, Schutta HS. Inverse ocular bobbing. *Ann Neurol* 1981; **9**: 194—7

Krohel G, Griffin JF. Voluntary vertical nystagmus. *Neurology* 1979; **29**: 1153—4

Kuban KC, Ephros MA, Freeman RL, Laffell LB, Bressnan MJ. Syndrome of opsoclonus-myoclonus caused by coxsackie B3 infection *Ann Neurol* 1983; **13**: 69—72

Leigh RJ, Robinson DA, Zee DA. A hypothetical explanation for periodic alternating nystagmus: instability in the optokinetic vestibular system. *Ann NY Acad Sci* 1981; **347**: 619—29

Maddox EE. See saw nystagmus with bitemporal hemianopia. *Proc R Soc Med* 1914; **7**: 12—13

Marmion D, Sandilands J. Opsoclonia — a rare sign in polioencephalitis. *Lancet* 1947; **II**: 508—9

Mewis L, Tang RA, Maxow ML. See-saw nystagmus after strabismus surgery. *J Pediatric Ophthalmol Strabismus* 1982; **19**: 302—5

Moe PG, Nellhaus G. Infantile polymyoclonia—opsoclonus syndrome and neural crest tumours. *Neurology* 1970; **20**: 756—62

Montpetit JVA, Andermann S, Carpenter S, Fawcett JS,

Zobrowska—Sluis D, Giberson HR. Subacute necrotising encephalomyelopathy. *Brain* 1971; **94**: 1—30

Nagle M, Bridgeman B, Stark L. Voluntary nystagmus saccadic suppression, and stabilization of the visual world. *Vision Res* 1980; **20**: 717—21

Ochs AL, Stark L, Hoyt WF, D'Amico D. Opposed adducting saccades in convergence retraction nystagmus. *Brain* 1979; **102**: 497—503

Orzechowski K. De l'ataxie dysmetrique des yeux: rémarques sur l'ataxie des yeux dite myoclonique (opsoclonie, opsochorie). *J Psychol Neurol* 1927; **35**: 1—18

Safran AB, Berney J, Safran E. Convergence-evoked eyelid nystagmus. *Am J Ophthalmol* 1982; **93**: 48—51

Sanders MD, Hoyt WF, Daroff RB. Lid nystagmus evoked by ocular convergence: an ocular EMG study. *J Neurol Neurosurg Psychiatr* 1968; **31**: 368—71

Sano K, Yoshimasu N, Ishijima B, Sekino H, Tsukamoto Y. Stimulation and destruction of the region of the interstitial nucleus in cases of torticollis and see-saw nystagmus. *Confin Neurol* 1972; **34**: 331—8

Sarkies NJC, Sanders MD. Convergence spasm. *Trans Ophthalmol Soc UK* 1985; **104**: 782—6

Savino PJ, Glaser JS. Opsoclonus — a pattern of regression in a child with neuroblastoma. *Br J Ophthalmol* 1975; **59**: 696—9

Schmidt D, Kommerell G. See-saw nystagmus and bitemporal hemianopia as sequels of cerebral and cranial trauma. *Graefes Arch Clin Exp Ophthalmol* 1969; **178**: 349—66

Selenich RC. Ping-pong Gaze. *Neurology* 1976; **26**: 532—5

Sharpe JA, Lo AW. Voluntary and visual control of the vestibulo-ocular reflex after cerebral hemi de cortication. *Ann-Neurol* 1981; **102**: 387—96

Sharpe JA, Lo AW, Rabinovitch HE. Control of the saccadic and smooth pursuit movements after cerebral hemidecortication. *Brain* 1979; **102**: 387—98

Sherman DG, Salmon JH. Ocular bobbing with superior cerebellar artery aneurysm — case report. *J Neurosurg* 1977; **47**: 596—8

Shetty T, Rosman NP. Opsoclonus in hydrocephalus. *Arch Ophthalmol* 1972; **88**: 585—90

Shults WT, Stark L, Hoyt WF, Ochs AL. Normal saccadic structure of voluntary nsytagmus. *Arch Ophthalmol* 1977; **95**: 1399—404

Stewart JD, Kirkham TH, Mathieson G. Periodic alternating gaze. *Neurology* 1979; **29**: 222—4

Susac JO, Hoyt WF, Daroff RB, Lawrence W. Clinical spectrum of ocular bobbing. *J Neurol Neurosurg Psychiatr* 1970; **33**: 771—5

Tamura E, Hoyt CS. Oculomotor consequences of intraventricular haemorrhages in premature infants. *Arch Ophthalmol* 1987; **105**: 533—5

Von Cramon D, Zihl J. Das Phänomenon der periodisch altiemiernden Bulbus deviation. *Arch Psychiatr Nervenkr* 1977; **224**: 247—57

Westheimer G, Blair SM. The ocular tilt reaction. *Invest Ophthalmol* 1975; **14**: 833—41

Zahn JR. Incidence and characteristics of voluntary nystagmus. *J Neurol Neurosurg Psychiat* 1978; **41**: 617—23

Zelt RP, Bigan AW. Congenital see saw nystagmus. *J Pediatr Ophthalmol Strabismus* 1985; **22**: 13—17

43 Head and Eye Movement Disorders

DAVID TAYLOR

One of the most important functions of head movement is the directional orientation of the special senses and there is an intimate and complementary relationship between head movement and eye movements (Gresty 1974). When a normal subject's attention is drawn to a new eccentric area, head movements are preceded by eye movements, the two resulting in a combined displacement; small amplitude shifts of gaze are achieved by eye movement alone. Head movements are complicated because of the nature of the articulation and the natural resonance of the cervical spine (Gresty & Halmagyi 1979).

In order to maintain a constant relationship between the eyes and surroundings despite movements of the head or the environment, two main mechanisms exist.

Optokinetic movements

Movement of the environment brings about a slow pursuit eye movement after a latency of about 125 ms with a maximum velocity of up about 150 degrees per second. The stimulus for pursuit eye movements is 'retinal slip' (a disparity between the target image position and its predicted position on the retina), and the movements are conjugate, smooth and continuously modified in velocity. A moving target is usually required to generate pursuit movements, otherwise the eye movements are broken into a series of small saccades. In a pursuit sequence there may be initially a 'catch up' saccade, and large amplitude changes are often accompanied by head movements. Optokinetic nystagmus (OKN) occurs when there is continuous movement of the visual environment; a slow following movement is followed by a saccade in the opposite direction, the reflex being a feedback system to which the input signal is retinal slip. The following phase of optokinetic nystagmus maintains a stable relationship between the eye and the environment, allowing relatively high resolution of objects in the moving field. The movement of the retinal image during the fast phase of optokinetic nsytagmus is perceptually suppressed and is not therefore perceived as movement.

Vestibulo-ocular reflex

Mammals have a sophisticated vestibulo-ocular reflex (VOR) which maintains the relationship between the head and eye during rotation in the horizontal, frontal and sagittal planes, and their vectors. The control signal for the vestibulo-ocular reflex is angular head acceleration around an axis passing through the head and this is transduced by the semi-circular canals into a neural signal proportional to the head velocity (Robinson, 1972). The effect of this is that a head movement in any direction is accompanied by an equal and opposite eye movement, thus stabilizing the eye relative to its target despite head movement, not only in the three primary planes, but also in their vectors.

Vestibulo-ocular, neck and body reflexes combine with optokinetic reflexes to stabilize the retinal image. A very important aspect of these reflexes is the ability of normal persons to inhibit them. These vital reflexes and their inhibition reach a high level of sophistication, as shown by commuters who daily read their newspapers while holding onto the strap of a badly sprung and damped bus or train.

When there is central nervous system disease that affects the oculomotor system, head-eye movement may be disrupted, with head movements sometimes preceding eye movements.

Abnormal head movements in disorders of saccades

Congenital oculomotor apraxia

This abnormality presents in the early months or years of life. Often it is noticed by the parents because the child does not appear to look around the room; this is because he cannot make saccades (rapid eye movements), or makes saccades only intermittently. Once the development of head movement control is achieved, thrusting head movements appear, sometimes associated with a blink at the beginning of the movements. The children are sometimes delayed in other spheres. Boys are more frequently affected and the condition is sometimes familial (Vassella et al. 1972). In later life congenital oculomotor apraxia appears to improve, possibly as the affected person develops adaptive mechanisms to get round the disorder of saccades. Cerebral abnormalities such as agenesis of the corpus calosum and cerebral atrophy (Fielder et al. 1986) or cerebral lipoma (Summers et al. 1987) have been described, but probably do not represent a specific lesion. The abnormal head and eye movements are variable and asymmetrical (Catalano et al. 1989), sometimes normal saccades and head and eye movement sequences are achieved, whereas at other times severe abnormalities are present, which often are said to be worse with the head immobilized. They take several patterns:

1 Cogan (1953), Altrocchi and Menkes (1960), and Vasella et al. (1972) describe what is now taken as the typical pattern of congenital oculomotor apraxia. The patients have a severe disorder of saccades, either voluntarily, by reflex, or both. Instead of using saccades to shift their eyes they move the head in the direction of attention, often at an unusually high velocity (the head thrust), with the effect that the eye is jammed into extreme deviation in the opposite direction by the vestibulo-ocular reflex and it is then mechanically swept round towards the target. This produces the head thrusts so characteristic of the condition. Once fixation had been achieved the head rotates back to bring the eyes into the straight ahead position, the eyes being kept still in space by the vestibulo-ocular reflex.

2 Zee et al. (1977) described two children with congenital oculomotor apraxia who showed a somewhat different pattern of head–eye co-ordination; their patients had delayed initiation and hypometria of voluntary saccades while the fast phases of vestibular and optokinetic nystagmus were less severely affected. Their head movements began either approximately synchronously with or before the saccades, and in the former, the authors postulated that the head movements were an adaptive attempt to trigger an improvement in the saccadic velocity.

Normal people moving their heads from side to side in the dark generate a saccade which begins synchronously with the head movement (Barnes 1979). The amplitude of the saccade is related to the amplitude and velocity of the head movement, suggesting a link between the mechanisms for generating head movement and rapid eye movement, which thus may be used to advantage by patients with at least one form of oculomotor apraxia.

On some occasions in one patient (Zee et al. 1977) in whom the head movement clearly preceded any eye movement the eye initially made an opposite (presumably vestibulo-ocular reflex) movement and then made a series of quick eye movements which the authors felt might be an adaptive use of vestibular nystagmus.

3 It may be that the vestibulo-ocular reflex, the effects of which are so easily suppressed by normal subjects, could be inhibited by patients with abnormal saccades, in doing so the patient might be able to add head movements to improve eye velocity and amplitude. This has never been clearly demonstrated, however, although patients with a more global loss of eye movements may make what may be described as additive head thrusts which more frequently occur in acquired saccade disorders.

Conjugate eye deviation is initiated first, followed by a blink, when the lids reopen the eyes have reached their target. The function of the blink is not certain; it is not seen in normal persons, but may function to break fixation and allow eye deviation behind the closed lids; it also occurs in many cases of congenital oculomotor apraxia. It is possible that a learned suppression of the vestibulo-ocular reflex enables the patient with defective saccades to increase the velocity and amplitude of the eye movement in space by additive head thrusts. Suppression of the vestibulo-ocular reflex is necessary to prevent the physiological contraversion of the eyes negating the effect of the head thrusts.

MANAGEMENT

Despite the finding of (non-progressive) cerebral abnormalities in some cases, neuroradiological investigations are not necessary in most cases unless there is evidence of associated developmental or neurological problems. Neurophysiological studies of vision should be normal.

OTHER SACCADE PALSIES

Abnormal head movements occur frequently in patients with acquired disorders of rapid eye movements. Saccades and following pursuit movements are the only way in which eyes are moved in space and since in predominantly pursuit system disorders multiple saccades are substituted for the lost smooth pursuit, saccadic disorders are the only ones associated with compensatory head movements. Smith and Cogan (1959) have described an oculomotor apraxia-like syndrome in ataxia-telangiectasia, and disordered saccades have also been described in Wilson's disease (Kirkham & Kamin 1974), Huntingdon's chorea (Starr 1967; Avanzini et al. 1979), in spinocerebellar degenerations (Zee 1976) and olivopontocerebellar degeneration (Koeppen & Hans 1976). Patients with olivopontocerebellar palsy may be very handicapped by a combination of retinal dystrophy giving constricted fields (Weiner et al. 1967) and saccade palsy.

Head shaking and nodding in congenital nystagmus

Spasmus nutans

Many patients who have congenital nystagmus also tend to nod or shake their head. The term spasmus nutans has become associated with the triad nystagmus, head nodding and an abnormal head posture. The onset is in infancy, the nystagmus is often asymmetrical, sometimes being monocular, and it is of high frequency and low amplitude. It remits spontaneously within a few years of life. In many ways it is preferable to treat subjects with congenital nystagmus associated with abnormal head movements as a single group and not to identify those who, by virtue of having a combination of nystagmus, head nodding, head turning and good prognosis, as having the separate condition of spasmus nutans. Spasmus nutans is a diagnosis that depends on the symptoms and signs improving and must therefore be made retrospectively. There are no factors which can predict the resolution of the symptoms to allow the diagnosis of Spasmus nutans to be made (Jayalakshmi et al. 1970). The main reason why it is important not to use the term Spasmus nutans, except perhaps in retrospect, is that it encourages the clinician to think no further about the possible underlying causes of asymmetrical nystagmus in childhood; these include especially abnormalities of the anterior visual pathway including glioma and craniopharyngioma.

The pathogenesis of head shaking with congenital nystagmus is obscure, but Raudnitz (1897), who originated the term Spasmus nutans, noted that children who had the syndrome came from a very dark area of Prague, and he suggested that this rearing in the dark damaged the fixation mechanism during the development of ganglion cells in the visual pathways. Raudnitz produced nystagmus and head shaking in dark-reared dogs. Still (1906) felt that malnutrition may play a role. There has been little evidence to support these hypotheses and the non-specific nature of spasmus nutans is underlined by its occurrence as the presenting sign in patients with optic glioma, or other anterior visual pathway tumour.

Three mechanisms underlie the combination of head nodding and congenital nystagmus (Gresty et al. 1978; Gresty & Ell 1982):

Suppressive head nodding

The head shaking and nodding may be not only of a different amplitude and frequency to the nystagmus, but it may be in a different direction. The nystagmus may be asymmetrical, dissociated or even uniocular. The presence of the head movement reduces or abolishes the nystagmus through an unclear mechanism which may be related to stimulation of the powerful vestibulo-ocular reflexes which 'over-ride' the nystagmus. The child learns that his vision is better during head shaking and thus shakes his head when concentrating.

Compensatory head shaking

In this situation the patient uses head movements directly to counter the movements of the eyes, thus steadying the eyes in space and enabling relatively constant fixation. For instance, if the eyes are moving to the right the head moves to the left to counter the eye movement (Metz *et al.* 1972). In a normal person the vestibulo-ocular reflex would cause an equal and opposite eye movement to the head movement cancelling what would have been a compensatory head movement. The patient who makes compensatory head shakes must therefore either have an abnormal vestibulo-ocular reflex or be able to manipulate a normal VOR. The opposite head movements do not perfectly counteract the eye movements, but produce plateaus of stability during which fixation is improved.

Compensatory head shaking and suppressive head nodding are adaptive mechanisms which the child uses in order to improve his vision. They are, therefore, seen when he is concentrating on an object and this is a useful clue because it is these cases which tend to improve with time and would have been called Spasmus nutans in years gone by.

Head shaking and nystagmus of common genesis

The nystagmus and head movements sometimes appear to have a common pathological mechanism. In such patients the amplitude, frequency, and waveform of the nystagmus and the head movements are similar to each other, and the vestibulo-ocular reflexes are normal. In most cases the eye and head movements do not compensate for each other and these tremors can in no way be interpreted as being adaptive or a technique adopted to improve vision. They can only be regarded as primarily pathological. In these cases the head shaking occurs at any time, sometimes continuously, but most frequently when the child is not concentrating on a detailed object.

Myoclonus with eye and head movement disorders

Halliday (1975) described three forms of myoclonus: jerk, rhythmical, and extrapyramidal. The jerk form are shock-like contractions involving one part of the body at a time, sometimes triggered by sensory input, and disappearing in sleep. In some, a loud noise sets off a crescendo-decrescendo oscillation of the head. The 'nystagmus' for which these patients may be referred, is in fact a normal eye movement mediated by a normal vestibulo-ocular reflex in response to the head oscillations. Head tremor and nystagmus may also occur in a 'phase-locked' manner to tremors of the palate; the so-called palatal myoclonus (Jacobs & Bender 1976) and in rhythmical myoclonus. Both of these may be present in some stages of sleep. In cases of suspected congenital nystagmus it is a worthwhile

clue to look for movements of the palate and pharynx which may help to direct appropriate investigations.

Eye and head movements in acute cerebellar syndromes

Flutter-like oscillations, opsoclonus, and other eye movement disorders associated with acute cerebellar syndromes are frequently associated with head movement disorders, in particular head tremors. Both abnormalities probably have a common cause.

The bobble-headed doll syndrome

Children with large third ventricular tumours or cysts and hydrocephalus may develop a fairly rapid antero-posterior temor of the head and trunk which is not present during sleep and which they can sometimes voluntarily inhibit. The children have cycles of head and trunk rotation in the sagittal plane around an axis through the neck giving rise to the appearance of a weak-necked puppet or doll (Benton *et al.* 1966.

Jensen *et al.* (1978) described one case and alluded to 17 others, of whom 15 had a slow-growing supra-sellar space-occupying lesion and two had aqueduct stenosis. In all cases the symptoms started in childhood. The tremor disappeared after surgery in five cases. The eye movements in this syndrome represent normal vestibulo-ocular reflex activity, unless there is a visual defect when nystagmus may be superadded. One patient whom we have seen had poor vision and bilateral compound eye movement disorder resembling see-saw nystagmus, together with the classic bobble movement of the head and upper trunk. Although the movement disorder is usually associated with chronic lesions it has been described as a transient manifestation during one of many episodes of raised intracranial pressure in an infant with hydrocephalus (Dell 1981).

References

Altrocchi PH, Menkes JH. Congenital oculomotor apraxia. *Brain* 1960; **83**: 579–88

Avanzini G, Girotti F, Caraceni T, Spreafico R. Oculomotor disorders in Huntington's Chorea. *J Neurol Neurosurg Psychiatr* 1979; **42**: 581–9

Barnes GR. Vestibulo-ocular function during co-ordinated head and eye movements to acquire usual targets. *J Physiol* 1979; **287**: 127–33

Benton JW, Nellhaus G, Huttenlocher PR, Ojemann RG, Dodge PR. The bobble-headed doll Syndrome. *Neurology* 1966; **16**: 725–9

Catalano RA, Calhoun VH, Reinecke RO. Asymmetry in congenital oculomotor apraxia. *Surv Ophthalmol* 1989; **34**: 149

Cogan DG. A type of congenital ocular motor apraxia presenting jerky head movements. *Trans Am Acad Ophthalmol Otol* 1953; **56**: 853−8

Dell S. Further observations on the 'bobble-headed doll syndrome'. *J Neurol Neurosurg Psychiatr.* 1981; **44**: 1046−52

Fielder AR, Gresty MA, Dodd KL, Mellor DH, Levene MI. Congenital oculomotor apraxia. *Trans Ophthalmol Soc UK* 1986; **105**: 589−98

Gresty MA. Co-ordination of head and eye movements to fixate continuous and intermittent targets. *Vision Res* 1974; **14**: 395−401

Gresty MA, Ell JJ. Normal modes of head and eye co-ordination and their symptomatology. In: Lennerstrand G, Zee DS, Keller EL (Eds.) *Functional Basis of Ocular Motility Disorders*. Pergaman Press, Oxford 1982; pp. 391−406

Gresty MA, Halmagyi GM. Abnormal head movements. *J Neurol Neurosurg Psychiatr* 1979; **41**: 705−14

Gresty MA, Halmagyi GM, Leech J. The relationship between head and eye movements in congenital nsytagmus with head shaking. *Br J Ophthalmol* 1978; **62**: 533−8

Halliday Am. The neurophysiology of myodonic jerking. (Charlton M. Ed.) *Exerpta Medica Int Cong Ser* No 307 1975; p 1−30

Jacobs L, Bender MB. Palato-ocular synchrony during eyelid closure. *Arch Neurol* 1976; **33**: 289−91

Jayalakshmi P, Scott TFM, Tucker JSH, Schaffer DB. Infantile nystagmus: A prospective study of Spasmus nutans, congenital nystagmus and unclassified nystagmus of infancy. *J Pediatrics* 1970; **77**: 177−84

Jensen HP, Pendle G, Goerke W. Head bobbing in a patient with a cyst of the third ventricle. *Child's Brain* 1978; **4**: 235−43

Kirkham TH, Kamin DF. Slow saccadic eye movements in Wilson's disease. *J Neurol Neurosurg Psychiatr* 1974; **37**: 191−4

Koeppen HH, Hans MB. Supranuclear ophthalmoplegia in olivopontocerebellar degeneration. *Neurology* 1976; **26**: 764−8

Metz HS, Jampolsky A, O'Meara DM. Congenital ocular nystagmus and nystagmoid head movements. *Am J Ophthalmol* 1972; **74**: 1131−33

Raudnitz RW. Zur lehre von Spasmus nutans. *Jahrb Kinderheilk* 1897; **45**: 145−7

Robinson DA. On the nature of visual oculomotor connections. *Invest Ophthalmol* 1972; **11**: 497−503

Smith JL, Cogan DG. Ataxia telangiectasia. *Arch Ophthalmol* 1959; **62**: 364−9

Starr A. A disorder of rapid eye movements in Huntington's chorea. *Brain* 1967; **90**: 545−64

Still GF. Head nodding with nystagmus in infancy. *Lancet* 1906; **ii**: 207−09

Summers CG, MacDonald JT, Wirtschafter JS. Ocular motor apraxia associated with intracranial lipoma. *J Pediatr Ophthalmol Strabismus* 1987; **24**: 267−71

Vasella F, Lutschg J, Mumenthaler M. Cogan's congenital ocular motor apraxia in two successive generations. *Dev Med Child Neurol* 1972; **14**: 788−803

Weiner LP, Konigsmark BW, Stoll J Jr, Magladery JW. Hereditary olivopontocerebellar atrophy with retinal degeneration. *Arch Neurol* 1967; **16**: 364−76

Zee DS, Optican LM, Cook JD, Robinson DA, Engel WK. Slow saccades in spinocerebellar degeneration. *Arch Neurol* 1976; **33**: 243−8

Zee DS, Yee RD, Singer HS. Congenital ocular motor apraxia. *Brain* 1977; **100**: 581−600

44 Concomitant Strabismus

JOHN ELSTON

Epidemiology

Strabismus, or misalignment of the visual axes, is a common condition, with prevalence estimates ranging from 3.8% (Friedman *et al.* 1980) to 5% (Simons & Reinecke 1978) of the population. There is a spectrum of abnormality, ranging from large manifest strabismus, convergent or divergent, through stable microtropia with reduced binocular functions, to intermittent deviations. The epidemiology is therefore difficult, and depends on the criteria used as well as the sampling methods, diagnostic techniques and age at examination. Graham (1974) examined 4784 children, 99% of all those born in Cardiff (UK) during 1 year, at the age of 4–5 years. The cover test was in some way abnormal in 7.1%, and these children were referred for more detailed examination, a manifest strabismus being confirmed in 5.3% of the total. The onset was in the first year in 22%, with a second peak of incidence in the third year. There is evidence from other studies for the existence of two main groups of disorder with different clinical features, making up most of the population of childhood strabismus. In considering cases of strabismus under treatment, Crone & Velzeboer (1956) extended the early onset group to 18 months of age; these cases of infantile strabismus represented 42% of the total; 94% had convergent squints, most were emmetropic, and there was a significant association with birth trauma. The clinical features included free alternation of fixation and alternating hypertropia (i.e. a combined horizontal and vertical strabismus.) In contrast, those of later onset were associated with hypermetropia (or in 7%, mostly divergent, myopia), anisometropia and amblyopia, and the strabismus was often triggered by an intercurrent illness, such as measles. The first group, infantile esotropia, can be divided clinically on various grounds, for example some cases have nystagmus compensation or blockage (von Noorden 1976), whilst in the second group, subdivision on the basis of refraction, amblyopia, and the dynamics of the near synkinesis is possible. Untreated, both groups will have either absent or deficient binocular functions. The fundamental aetiology of the condition is therefore closely related to the factors that influence the development of binocularity.

Aetiology

Neurophysiology of binocularity and amblyopia

ANIMAL EXPERIMENTS

The neurophysiology of binocularity has been extensively investigated in experimental animals. Hubel and Wiesel (1961) introduced the concept of 'receptive fields' to designate the group of photoreceptors controlling the firing of a retinal ganglion cell. It is also applied to the region of the retina that controls a particular lateral geniculate body cell, or cell in the visual cortex. There is no binocular interaction in the lateral geniculate body, but the majority (85%) of striate cortical cells are binocular, and here the receptive fields are of two types: simple cortical receptive fields have afferents directly from the lateral geniculate body, and show axis orientation, whilst complex receptive fields have afferents from a number of cortical cells with simple fields, and respond to variously shaped stationary or moving forms (Hubel & Wiesel 1962). The receptive fields of all binocularly driven cortical cells occupy corresponding positions on the two retinas. This complex and orderly projection of receptive fields onto the striate cortex is present in visually inexperienced kittens, and is therefore the substrate for normal binocular vision (Wiesel & Hubel 1963a). In kittens, visual deprivation of one eye from birth by suturing the eyelid produces a reduction in visual function in that eye that is accompanied by profound histological changes in the lateral geniculate body, where the number of cells driven by the deprived eye falls by 40% (Wiesel & Hubel 1963b). In the striate cortex, the vast majority of cells become driven by the undeprived eye (Wiesel & Hubel 1963c).

Normal binocular visual experience for the first 2–3 months of life protects against these anatomical and functional changes, but reverse suturing after the age of 3 months cannot alter the established abnormalities (Wiesel & Hubel 1965a). There is therefore a 'sensitive period' for the establishment of the permanence of the innate potential for binocularity, and it has behavioural, physiological, and morphological correlates in the visual system. The sensitive period has a sudden onset, a period of high susceptibility to disruption, and then a slow decline, with the possibility of limited recovery of structure and function if the disruption is not too severe, or for too long (Dews & Wiesel 1970; Hubel & Wiesel 1970). The system appears to have a degree of innate plasticity (Blakemore & Van Sluyters 1974a); Blakemore and Cummings 1975). Likewise, in man, visual deprivation of one eye from birth by for example, untreated unilateral congenital cataract, invariably produces profound amblyopia with strabismus and absent binocularity.

An artificial divergent squint produced in kittens by medial rectus tenotomy quickly reduces the number of binocularly driven cortical cells, whilst preserving good vision in each eye (Hubel & Wiesel 1965). Alternate day patching of each eye has the same effect, but binocular visual deprivation leads to less

cortical abnormality. Competition between the two eyes is eliminated, and binocularity remains largely intact (Wiesel & Hubel 1965b; Kratz & Spear 1976).

Integrating the concepts of innate potential binocularity, competition for cortical dominance, and the sensitive period, a model of the neural mechanism of binocularity in the normal animal, and in man, can be devised (Barlow et al. 1967). The slight disparity between what is seen by the two eyes leads to a summation effect when binocularly driven cortical cells are stimulated. Some features that are nearly the same are transmitted by each eye separately, and the differences are integrated in the visual cortex to achieve stereopsis.

More recent work in non-human primates has determined that in these animals also, strabismus and amblyopia represent a decline from a pre-existing binocular neuronal substrate (Von Noorden et al. 1970; Baker et al. 1974; Wiesel & Hubel 1974; Hendrikson & Boothe 1976). It is apparent that interference with the developing nervous system, involving either the afferent or efferent visual systems, can compromise the normal development of the innate capacity for binocularity (Blakemore & Van Sluyters 1974b). Permanent electrophysiological and histological changes are rapidly produced, and largely irreversible, since complex cortical receptive field properties degrade by a process of active inhibition (Blakemore & Van Sluyters 1975).

EVIDENCE IN MAN

Although there are inter-species differences, particularly in the influence of age on neuronal plasticity, and the length of the sensitive period, there is good evidence that the development of vision in humans is the same as in other mammals. In bilateral infantile and juvenile cataract, for example, the visual results are worse the longer surgery is delayed, and the first operated eye always develops better vision (Taylor et al. 1979). The sensitivity to visual deprivation is at its height between 3 and 8 months, but a unilateral cataract developing even up to 8 years of age will cause amblyopia and deterioration of binocular function. Human amblyopia, however caused, disrupts binocularity in exactly the same way as in animals (Von Noorden 1974).

Normal neonates show some evidence of their presumed innate binocular potential. The eyes are either intermittently exotropic or straight (Rethy 1969; Nixon et al. 1985: Sondhi et al. 1988) and, notably, never convergent. Esodeviations may be seen in infants who do not go on to develop congenital esotropia, but not after 2 months of age (Sondhi *et al.* 1988). Some behavioural evidence of binocular fixation and conjugate following may be demonstrated in full-term neonates at 2 days old (Dayton *et al.* 1964) and more consistently in 2 and 16-week-old infants (Bower 1966, 1971). Random dot stereopsis, probably the most sensitive indicator of binocular function, is demonstrable in 98% of normal infants over the age of 28 weeks (Bechtoldt & Hutz 1979; Fox *et al.* 1980).

There is good experimental and clinical evidence, therefore, for regarding early onset strabismus not due to anatomical factors (such as unilateral cataract) as an acquired disorder of maturation of the visual system. Features such as amblyopia and the absence of binocular functions are secondary neural anomalies consequent on a primary disruption of the visual axes (Bechtoldt & Hutz 1979). The fundamental stability of neonatal binocularity is illustrated by its persistence in conditions where ocular movements are abnormal and a full field of binocular single vision is therefore not possible. This may be temporary, as in transient neonatal lateral rectus palsy, an isolated abnormality in otherwise neurologically normal babies (Benson 1962; Reisner *et al.* 1971). Full recovery of eye movements occurs by 6 weeks and normal binocularity develops (de Grauw *et al.* 1983). In a congenital IVth nerve lesion, however, full recovery does not take place, but despite a persistent vertical squint, compensated for by a head posture, full binocularity develops, and neuronal plasticity allows the development of a large vertical fusion range (Reynolds *et al.* 1984). In Duane's retraction syndrome, despite evidence of paradoxical innervation of the lateral rectus dependent on the position of gaze, binocularity is frequently maintained, often with a head posture in unilateral cases (Huber 1984), and even in bilateral cases (Hotchkiss *et al.* 1980). Duane's syndrome indicates an anatomical and functional brain stem abnormality (Jay & Hoyt 1980; Ramsey & Taylor 1980; Miller *et al.* 1983). Even an isolated total unilateral gaze palsy of presumed pontine origin did not prevent the development of normal binocular functions in the case reported by Hoyt *et al.* (1977).

Aetiology of strabismus

VISUAL, REFRACTIVE AND EYE MOVEMENT FACTORS

A normal central nervous system, therefore, can allow the maturation of the innate potential for binocularity even in the presence of quite severe abnormalities of eye movement. This is not always the case however, and infantile or childhood strabismus may therefore be the presenting sign of an underlying eye movement disorder, due for example to neurological or neuromuscular disease. It is important in assessing a case to ensure the child's eye movements are full, and look for signs of restriction or fatigue of movement. On the other hand, even subtle abnormalities of the afferent visual system are likely to compromise binocularity. Strabismus is invariable in unilateral or severe bilateral visual deprivation by congenital cataract, and the response to surgical treatment closely follows the pattern predicted from animal experiments. Strabismus may be the presenting sign of unilateral optic nerve hypoplasia or coloboma. Anisometropia of greater than one dioptre, especially if associated with astigmatism is a potent cause of disruption of the binocular reflexes, producing amblyopia and strabismus. In ocular or oculo-cutaneous albinism, because of the abnormal decussation of the visual pathways, the anatomical substrate for binocularity is missing, and strabismus invariable (Fonda 1962; Coleman *et al.* 1979). A similar, visual pathway projection abnormality has been suggested as the cause of infantile strabismus in some non-albinos (Tsutsui & Fukai 1978) but the evidence is unconvincing (Hoyt and Caltrider 1984).

NEUROLOGICAL DYSFUNCTION

Between 20 and 40% of cases of cerebral palsy have early onset esotropia without individual ocular muscle palsy (Breakey 1955; Levy *et al.* 1976; Losseff 1962). Moreover, specific features of the cerebral palsy such as athetosis, suggesting damage to the basal ganglia, are associated with a specific type of dyskinetic strabismus (Buckley & Seaber 1981). Strabismus is also very common in hydrocephalus, occurring in 44% of cases of meningomyelocoele who needed shunting (Rothstein *et al.* 1974). The squint generally appears as the intracranial pressure rises (Rabinowitz 1974) but lateral rectus weakness is often not demonstrable (although classically a convergent deviation greater for distance than near is a sign of bilateral VIth nerve paresis). The eye movements characteristically show an A pattern (increase in convergent deviation on upgaze), with bilateral superior oblique overaction, (Fig. 44.1) which may merge into or be superceded by the setting sun sign of tonic downward deviation of the eyes with lid retraction and upgaze palsy, if the intracranial pressure is uncontrolled (Rabinowitz &

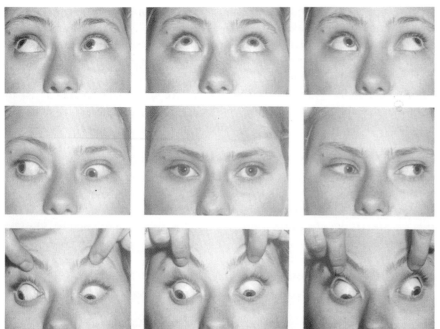

Fig. 44.1 'A' phenomenon with overaction of the superior obliques in a patient with hydrocephalus.

Walker 1975). It is interesting that a similar pattern of ocular movement has been induced in adults treated with unilateral stereotactic thermal lesions in the midbrain pretectum for the relief of intractable pain (Nashold and Seaber 1972). The esotropia and A pattern of hydrocephalus probably has a similar origin, and is virtually pathognomonic of the condition.

VERY LOW BIRTH WEIGHT

Prematurity or very low birth weight is not in itself associated with an increased incidence of strabismus, if the central nervous system, investigated by cranial ultrasound, is normal. If, however, there is evidence of peri- or intraventricular haemorrhage, strabismus occurs in 7% whilst if there is in addition, ventricular dilation, it is seen in 25% (Palmer *et al*. 1982; Fawer *et al*. 1985). Children with evidence of regressed retinopathy of prematurity without detectable developmental delay also have a high incidence of strabismus, amblyopia and high refractive (myopic) error (Kalina 1969; Kushner 1982). Any evidence, therefore, of neurological dysfunction complicating very low birth weight makes strabismus very likely (Keith & Kitchen 1984).

OTHER HANDICAPS

Apart from specific neurological dysfunction, a number of diffuse neurological insults, such as head injury can disrupt central binocular functions (Pratt-Johnson 1973; Stanworth 1974). Strabismus is a common finding in children with multiple handicaps (Harcourt 1974), in congenital heart disease, particularly if it is cyanotic (Gardiner & Joseph 1968), in 30% of Turner's syndrome (Chrousos *et al*. 1984) and 45% of Down's syndrome (Eissler & Longenecker 1962) where the poorer the general neurological development, the more likely is a squint. There may also be an increased incidence of binocular abnormalities, including manifest squint, in otherwise normal boys showing minor learning disabilities (Cassin 1975). More detailed psychometric testing in those with a manifest strabismus (6%) showed that 73% had definite but minimal neurological dysfunction. Such children, although of normal intelligence and at normal schools, may also show behavioural abnormalities such as poor attention, and some evidence of vestibular dysfunction (Steinberg & Rendle-Short 1977).

OTHER FACTORS

A constant, usually convergent, strabismus may be the presenting sign of a visual deficit. Developmental abnormalities such as unilateral cataract, optic nerve hypoplasia or high myopia may be responsible. Amblyopia secondary to the ocular deviation may contribute to the poor vision in these cases, and patching treatment may be indicated. Acquired visual deficit producing strabismus may be due a tumour (retinoblastoma), trauma or infection (e.g. toxocara) or other cause.

Stereotyped patterns of strabismus and eye movement disorder may result from purely anatomical factors. Orbital depth, and orientation, and the number and structure of the extraocular muscles play a role in the aetiology of strabismus in the craniofacial dysostoses (Fig. 44.2) (Urrets-Zavalia *et al.* 1961; Diamond *et al.* 1980). Attempts to implicate extraocular muscle histopathology as a significant factor are unconvincing (Margolis *et al.* 1977).

The evidence presented above is of great interest in determining the aetiology of strabismus. However, the vast majority of children with either infantile esotropia or other forms of childhood strabismus do not have any overt signs of neurological dysfunction.

Diagnosis and assessment

The history is important in the diagnosis of strabismus, since many deviations are intermittent initially. A child's mother is very rarely wrong if she says that she has definitely seen an inward or outward turn of the eyes at times. Occurrence during a period of illness, particularly a neurotropic virus infection such as chicken pox, should also be taken seriously, as it may indicate an underlying susceptibility to strabismus. A family history of strabismus or amblyopia, hypermetropia or anisometropia (patches, glasses or operations in childhood amongst parents or siblings) should also be sought. The adoption of a consistent head posture may also be a clue to an underlying ocular

muscle imbalance and is found from the time head control is gained in congenital IVth nerve palsy and Duane's syndrome if binocularity is present. An A or V phenomenon may also be responsible, as may manifest nystagmus with a null point.

The gross appearance of ocular alignment is an unreliable guide to the presence or absence of manifest strabismus. Variations in facial skin disposition such as the common epicanthic folds of infancy may be mistaken for convergent strabismus, whilst other orbital and ocular factors may either mask or simulate a squint. Testing the visual acuity of each eye separately using either letter charts or clinical assessment of fixation is important to exclude amblyopia, but equal vision does not exclude strabismus.

Since normally developed stereoscopic vision requires normal optical, motor and neural functions of both eyes, a reliable test for absent or reduced stereopsis should detect all strabismus. The randomdot stereogram provides such a test, and is reliable down to the age of about 3 years. Although randomdot stereogram presentations are now available that may be usable in even younger patients, a properly administered cover test is probably more accurate. In older children it may be augmented by repeated alternate cover testing, with fixation controlled at near and distance to demonstrate a latent deviation.

Classification

Many different classifications of strabismus in infancy and childhood are available, none universally accepted. Having eliminated pseudostrabismus, usually

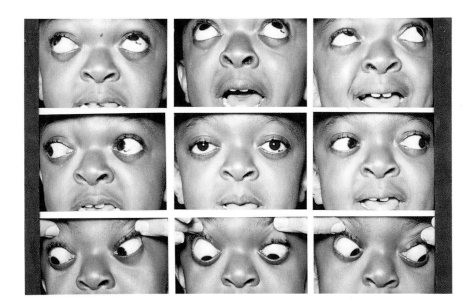

Fig. 44.2 Apert's syndrome with shallow orbits, a 'V' exotropia with overacting inferior obliques.

due to epicanthus or an exaggeration of the baby's broad nasal root, the following practical categorization is suggested.

1 *Concomitant strabismus* may be intermittent (from the history or examination), latent (apparent only on repeated alternate cover testing) or manifest. The term concomitant implies that the angle of deviation between the two eyes is the same for all positions of gaze, provided accommodation is controlled. Many cases of concomitant strabismus have an incomitant element.

(a) Esodeviation may be classified according to the age of onset (see above) as infantile (0–18 months) or childhood (18 months or older). In either category the horizontal deviation may be accompanied by a vertical one, usually in association with oblique muscle dysfunction and an A or V pattern of eye movement (Fig. 44.1, 44.2). Microesotropia is discussed in this section.

(b) Exodeviations in infancy or childhood may be considered as a single category (see full discussion below): again an A or V pattern may also be found.

3 Vertical strabismus is a frequent accompaniment of eso or exodeviations, but may also rarely be a primary disorder.

4 Incomitant strabismus: (See Chapter 45): In this group are considered (a) special categories of strabismus, usually of developmental origin (e.g. Duane's and Möbius' syndrome), sometimes of peripheral or mechanical origin, and (b) oculomotor palsies: infranuclear III, IV and VIth nerve palsies, and combinations.

Concomitant strabismus

Esodeviations

INFANTILE ESOTROPIA

As indicated above, although it seem likely that the fundamental cause of infantile esotropia is an acquired abnormality of central eye movement control systems, children with this condition are usually neurologically and developmentally normal (Fig. 44.3).

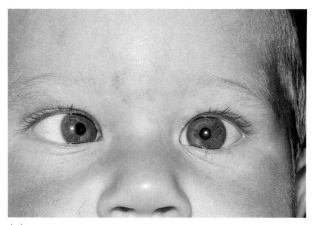

(a)

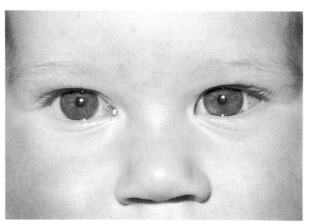

(c)

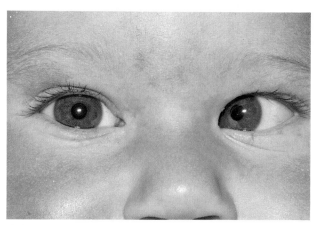

(b)

Fig. 44.3(a,b) Infantile esotropia showing alternating fixation. (c) Same patient immediately following surgery showing small residual esotropia.

Special examination techniques, however, may reveal subtle or temporary abnormalities that have been enough to disrupt binocular functions at the height of the sensitive period. Once disruption has occurred, strabismus is likely. For example, 56 out of 242 healthy neonates examined showed transient supranuclear disturbances of gaze, including 22 with skew deviation, indicative of brain stem dysfunction (Hoyt *et al.* 1980). Five of these 22 subsequently developed a typical infantile esotropia. Again, 24/32 infantile esotropes showed moderate or severe reduction in the vestibulo-ocular response (VOR), possible evidence of brain stem dysfunction (Hoyt 1982). The eight children in this study with a normal VOR showed the clinical features of the nystagmus blockage syndrome (Von Noorden & Avilla 1984), a specific subtype of infantile esotropia with features such as sudden onset and abducting nystagmus with higher amplitude in abduction, perhaps suggesting an acute neurological origin. It represents 12% of all cases of infantile esotropia, and the incidence is high in Down's syndrome, hydrocephalus and cerebral palsy (Hoyt 1977; Von Noorden & Avilla 1984).

Directional asymmetry of optokinetic nystagmus (OKN), with defective monocular responses when the stimulus is from the nasal to the temporal side, but not temporal to nasal, is reported in infantile esotropia. The optokinetic system is an image-stabilization mechanism producing a smooth pursuit eye movement followed by a saccade in the opposite direction. The neuronal circuitry involved includes the visual cortex and the accessory optic system, including the nucleus of the optic tract; the vestibular nuclei appear to generate the slow phases. Directional asymmetry is seen in normal neonates, and it has been suggested that its persistence in infantile esotropia may be of aetiological significance, reflecting an imbalance in brain stem ocular alignment factors. The abnormality is however also seen in congenital and latent nystagmus, and in both esotropia and primary exotropia where binocularity is absent (Van Hof-Van Duin & Mohn 1982). The asymmetry may be secondary to the absence of cortical binocularity, a suggestion supported by its occurrence in non-strabismic subjects who have had bilateral occipital infarcts (Kommerel & Mehdorn 1982).

Because of the rapidity with which anatomical abnormality develops in the nervous system following disruption of the visual axes, a brain stem aetiology for infantile esotropia does not necessarily imply continuing neurological dysfunction. After the initial appearance of the strabismus, however, further physical signs may develop in some cases. Dissociated vertical deviation (DVD), for example, a bilateral, often asymmetrical abnormality consisting of elevation and extorsion of one eye when retinal illumination is made unequal by either an occluder or neutral density filter, probably occurs exclusively in infantile esotropia (Parks 1982). Up to 85% of cases show it, and although it may be seen as early as at 8 months, it is usually only detectable from 18 months onwards (Anderson 1954) that is, a year or more after the original appearance of the squint. It is particularly common in patients with abducting nystagmus, and may represent some form of nystagmus blockage or compensation, or alternatively both abnormalities may have a common underlying central nervous system origin (Harcourt *et al.* 1980). An A-pattern of eye movement, indicating, as suggested above, possible pretectal dysfunction is usual in DVD (Helveston 1969) although a V-pattern may be seen. Abnormal visual pathway projection has been suggested in some cases (Fitzgerald & Billson 1984), but refuted by recent observations (Kriss *et al.* 1988, 1989). The rarity of a detectably abnormal afferent visual system in infantile esotropia (Tsutsui & Fukai 1978) argues against this an an important causative factor. There is no evidence for spontaneous resolution of DVD (Harcourt *et al.* 1980).

Latent nystagmus is another ill-understood clinical phenomenon that is often, but not exclusively associated with dissociated vertical deviation; both cortical and brain stem factors seem to be involved in the aetiology (Van Vliet 1973). In 'manifest' latent nystagmus, a horizontal strabismus is invariable and a vertical one common; half the cases have an abnormal head posture (Dell 'Osso *et al.* 1979). Although there is no overt neurological disease in dissociated vertical deviation, latent or 'manifest' latent nystagmus, these abnormalities appear to be acquired supranuclear eye movement abnormalities and may suggest continuing brain stem dysfunction in some cases of infantile esotropia. (See Chapter 41.)

CHILDHOOD ESOTROPIA AND MICROTROPIA

Whilst infantile esotropia may be a physical sign of brain stem dysfunction, strabismus that develops after the age of 18 months, with a peak at between 3 and 4 years may result from several different aetiologies (Adelstein & Scully 1967). Esotropia remains more common than exotropia, but the proportions change (Fletcher 1971). Amblyopia increases as the age at presentation rises, as do refractive errors, especially anisometropia and high hypermetropia (Crone & Velzeboer 1956; Stevens 1960). Specific subtypes such as the microtropia syndrome can be identified (Parks 1969). Microesotropia is best considered as a small (less than 5°), stable, cosmetically insignificant convergent strabismus that is associated with mild amblyopia and reduced binocularity. It may occur primarily, or secondary to surgical or optical treatment of a larger esotropia. The fundamental abnormality in primary cases is usually anisometropia, producing amblyopia and a central scotoma; sensory adaptations nevertheless result in the development of stereopsis, maintained by binocular motor responses. At the smallest angles of esodeviation the cover test may be negative if the amblyopic eye fixes with a high acuity extrafoveal point (Helveston & Von Noorden 1967). In most cases, a small abducting movement is seen when the eye with better vision is covered (Lang 1969). Primary microesotropia may be genetically determined, and in childhood esotropia as a whole, genetic factors become more important. A consistent sex difference is found in all surveys with girls more commonly affected than boys (Crone & Velzeboer 1956; Waardenburg 1963), and 25% of affected children have either a parent or sibling with strabismus (Graham 1974). Twin and genealogical data suggest however that multiple modifying factors are involved (François 1961; McKussick 1978). Refractive error,

for example, is itself to a large extent genetically determined with evidence for both autosomal dominant and recessive pedigrees in high myopia, hypermetropia and anisometropia, and even the degree and axis of astigmatism may be inherited (Waardenburg 1963). The broad categories of esotropia, exotropia, hypermetropia and myopia certainly seem to be under some genetic control, and strabismus may even appear at the same age in twins (Chimonidou *et al.* 1977). Reduced divergence fusional amplitudes may be found in families of patients with accommodative convergent squint (Nash *et al.* 1975). The overall evidence is that both microtropia and other forms of childhood onset strabismus (Cross 1975), are transmitted in a multifactorial genetic pattern (Cantolino & Von Noorden 1969).

Whereas in infantile esotropia, the accommodative convergence: accommodation ratio (AC:A ratio) is usually normal, in childhood esotropia, up to 59% have an abnormal ratio (Fig. 44.4), in most cases very high (Parks 1958). The ratio is also to some extent under genetic control, and in families with an esotropic propositus, it is on average significantly higher in unaffected family members than in normals (Franeschetti & Burian 1970). The near synkinesis of accommodation, convergence and pupillary constriction originates in the transitional region from temporal to occipital lobes, and is mediated, via the corticotectal

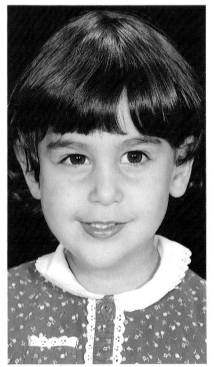

(a)

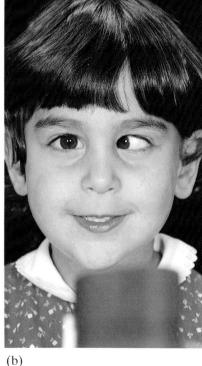

(b)

Fig. 44.4(a) Childhood esotropia when fixing light. No refractive error (b) Childhood esotropia fixing an 'accommodative' target.

tracts, through the IIIrd, and via the medial longitudinal fasciculus, the VIth nerve nuclei (Jampel 1959). It is a complex neurological function, found only in primates, and the range of the normal AC:A ration is wide (Parks 1958). The high reported incidence of an infectious disease precipitating a squint in childhood may result from decompensation of this function under stress, and the development of a manifest from a latent deviation when tired may be the same phenomenon. In some cases, a subclinical encephalitis in neurotropic viral infection (most commonly measles or chickenpox) may permanently disrupt the near response. An acquired disorder of the near synkinesis with insufficiency of convergence associated with reduced near point of accommodation may be due to closed head trauma (Von Noorden et al. 1973).

COMBINED HORIZONTAL AND VERTICAL DEVIATIONS

A high proportion of patients with both infantile and childhood esotropia develop, in addition, a vertical deviation (Knapp 1971). In certain specific situations orbital anatomical factors may be responsible, such as the V-pattern with bilateral superior oblique underaction and inferior oblique overaction seen in the craniofacial dysostoses (Fig. 44.2) (Collin 1983). These cannot be invoked in the majority, and attempts to correlate oblique muscle dysfunction with facial anthropometry have been unsuccessful (Urrets-Zavalia et al. 1961; Ruttum & Von Noorden 1984). Horizontal muscle dysfunction may be responsible, and since the medial recti are more active in downgaze, for near viewing, a V-esotropia may be due to their 'overaction', whilst an A-esotropia could be due to their 'underaction'. The lateral recti, more effective in upgaze, would, by 'overacting', cause a V-exotropia and 'underacting', an A-exotropia (Urist 1958; Wybar & Walker 1980). In most cases, however, oblique muscle dysfunction is demonstrable, either primarily (Fig. 44.4), as an 'overacting' muscle, or secondary to underaction of the ipsilateral antagonist, as seen in an acquired superior oblique palsy (Parks 1974). Theoretically, a muscle may primarily overact because of a developmental abnormality, for example an insertion which favours one muscle against its antagonist (Fink 1955). In the case of the inferior oblique, its elevating fibres may thereby have a mechanical advantage against the depressing fibres of the superior oblique (Gobin 1964).

Arguing from the results of surgical treatment, the concept of sagitallization (leading to overaction) of the offending oblique muscle as the primary abnormality in an A and V pattern has been advanced (Gobin 1968a, 1968b). On the other hand, a primary torsional abnormality has been suggested, with an 'overacting' inferior oblique causing excessive excyclotropia, raising the medial rectus insertion, lowering that of the lateral rectus and enhancing the V pattern (Kushner 1985).

A and V patterns usually develop after the onset of the horizontal strabismus and present a stereotyped appearance difficult to reconcile with a primary insertional abnormality in which a congenital, variable pattern would be expected. The A pattern of hydrocephalus is probably a supranuclear abnormality (France 1975) and reproducible by stereotactic pretectal lesions (Nashold & Seaber 1972). It can also be acquired in exaggerated form in children with progressive restriction of ocular motility, and ptosis of probably supranuclear origin (Fells et al. 1984), and it may be that most A patterns have this fundamental aetiology. The evidence for a supranuclear origin for V patterns is less clear, but it can be seen after traumatic lesions of the upper brain stem in the absence of superior oblique weakness (Stanworth 1974) and rarely with other brain stem pathology (alternating skew deviation). It is such a constant feature of acquired strabismus that a peripheral origin seems unlikely.

PRINCIPLES OF TREATMENT OF ESODEVIATIONS

Infantile esotropia

The therapeutic aim in the management of this condition is bifoveal fixation with full binocular function. Because of the rapid, and irreversible, adaptation of the developing visual system to misalignment of the visual axes, however caused, there is no convincing evidence that this has ever been achieved. As indicated above, multiple aetiological factors, mostly ill-understood, are probably relevant in producing the syndrome, and there are subgroups, for example nystagmus blockage, within it. Although it is generally agreed, therefore, that surgical treatment is necessary, no single treatment plan, in terms of either the age of the patient or surgical technique is likely to be appropriate in all cases. Refraction, full clinical examination and exclusion of any ocular and neurological defects are a mandatory preliminary to the long-term management: the children rarely require glasses, and they are usually healthy.

There are good neurophysiological reasons, backed

up by some clinical evidence, for believing that early surgery is likely to result in better quality binocular function on both sensory and motor testing (Taylor 1974; Ing 1981). It is also true that from the cosmetic point of view and possibly that of the developing parent–child relationship, early surgery is preferable. There are, however, disadvantages in operating too early. Although the anterior segment of the neonatal eye is well developed, the diameter of the globe is only 17 mm compared to 24 mm in the adult; maximum growth occurs in the first 6 months of life, mostly in the posterior segment. A standard 5 mm recession of a medial rectus muscle in the first few months of life, therefore, could result in reduced eye movement in later life. Moreover, the inferior oblique inserts very close to both the macula and optic nerve, and surgery may damage these structures. The size of the ocular deviation may be difficult to measure in infancy and it may be hard to assess the range of eye movement. A or V patterns (see above) may either not be present or difficult to detect when the esotropia first develops. Since both the horizontal and vertical elements of the strabismus must be corrected to achieve binocularity, it may be preferable to postpone surgery until oblique muscle dysfunction can be assessed. Because spectacle correction will be required in some infantile esotropes and refraction may be difficult in small babies, surgery should be delayed until consistent results are obtained. Cross-fixating infantile esotropes very frequently become amblyopic in one eye after surgery (Hoyt *et al.* 1984): this may be difficult to detect after surgery in infancy, although it is probably easier to treat by patching than it is in older children.

A balance between the theoretical requirements of early ocular alignment and its practical difficulties has to be struck. Clinical evidence from various centres suggests that the results in terms of binocularity are better if the eyes are straight by the age of 1 (Deller 1988) or 2 years (Robb & Rodier 1987; Von Noorden

1988). The diagnosis of infantile esotropia will be made in the first few months of life. At this stage, a full explanation to the parents of the condition and its treatment is required. Emphasis should be placed on the inevitability of repeated visits to the clinic, the likelihood of patching treatment for amblyopia at some stage, and the possibility of glasses. The child will definitely need one operation, probably on both eyes, with a 30% chance of a second operation on one or both eyes being required. Patching of alternate eyes for half an hour each day is sensible prior to surgery, since it will ensure that there is no amblyopia before operation, and make subsequent patching treatment easier. The first operation may be around the first birthday, and consist of bimedial recessions to 10.5 mm from the limbus often combined with oblique muscle surgery and sometimes a lateral rectus resection. The number of children requiring a second operation at some stage varies between 15 and 30%. Special categories of infantile esotropia, such as nystagmus blockage syndrome, require specific treatment strategies, including the use of a posterior fixation (faden) suture on the medial rectus. (Von Noorden 1976; Von Noorden & Avilla 1984; Von Noorden *et al.* 1986). Dissociated vertical deviation may be treated with a superior rectus recession, with or without a faden suture or by a combination of superior rectus and inferior, oblique muscle surgery (James 1987). Unilateral cases must be treated with caution and a faden suture without recession may be indicated.

Childhood esotropia

These patients overlap to some extent with those with infantile esotropia, and in some the treatment plan above will be appropriate. Dependant on the age of onset and the underlying aetiology, however, variable degrees of amblyopia will be present, and variable development of binocular functions. In anisometropia

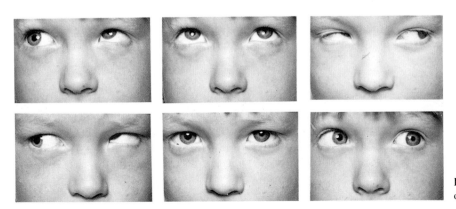

Fig. 44.5 'V' esotropia with inferior oblique overaction.

with amblyopia and constant strabismus, the initial management is with spectacle correction and occlusion of the normal-seeing eye; in children with a dynamic strabismus due to abnormal development of accommodative convergence, spectacles alone (sometimes bifocals) may be required. At the initial consultation, the parents and the child need an explanation of the disorder, and an outline of the treatment proposed. Parents often do not appreciate that spectacles and patching are the mainstay of management, and not something that is tried before surgery. The importance of refraction and appropriate optical correction is emphasized by cases such as the curing of cyclic esotropia by intraocular lens implantation (Cole *et al.* 1988). Many childhood esotropes, however, will require muscle surgery, and the technique adopted will depend on the orthoptic measurements, the AC : A ratio (Ludwig *et al.* 1988), and the underlying aetiology. Oblique muscle dysfunction should be corrected at the same time as the horizontal deviation. (Fig. 44.5).

Exodeviations

The term exodeviation encompasses both the spectrum of divergent strabismus (exotropia) and the latent tendency to divergence of the visual axes (exophoria). Exodeviations in childhood therefore consist of exophoria, intermittent exotropia (in which the strabismus may be manifest either at near or distant fixation, or both) and constant exotropia. Secondary and consecutive exotropia is less common than in adults.

Exodeviations are relatively unusual; in Graham's (1974) study, of the 339 children (7.1% of the total) with an abnormal cover test, 20.3% had an exodeviation nearly half of which were exophorias. On this basis, convergent strabismus is 5 times more common than divergent in childhood. There are other differences: exodeviations do not have the bimodal distribution of age of onset seen in esodeviations, but 50% occur in the first year of life (Hall 1961). All studies show a consistent sex difference, with between 65–70% of exodeviations occurring in girls (Hall 1961; Hiles *et al.* 1968; Gregerson 1969). Exodeviations are characteristically intermittent. They are usually regarded as getting progressively worse, in other words, an intermittent deviation becoming constant, (Jampolsky 1964) but they may also, unlike esodeviations, spontaneously improve with age. (Hiles *et al.* 1968). The disturbance of the normal development of binocular vision associated with exodeviations differs

from that seen in esodeviations and children often do not show any fixation preference. Amblyopia is therefore less prominent. In exophoria and intermittent deviations, sensory aspects of binocularity are usually well developed, whilst motor aspects of binocularity are characterized by reduced or absent divergence fusional amplitudes. Despite having one eye intermittently divergent and good vision in each eye, double vision is not usually a problem, implying that suppression of vision in the deviating eye is complete, and occurs over the whole temporal hemiretina. By contrast, esodeviations tend to be constant, and associated with amblyopia and a central (facultative) scotoma in the deviating eye.

The final distinguishing feature of exodeviations is their association with photophobia or worsening in bright light; children characteristically shut the deviating eye under these conditions, and this may be a useful diagnostic clue. The reason is not understood.

AETIOLOGY

The fundamental abnormality in exodeviations is an imbalance between influences responsible for the active divergence of the visual axes, and those responsible for convergence. Unlike esodeviations, genetic factors do not seem to be important (Gregerson 1969). The range of refraction in a representative group of children with exodeviations was the same as that in controls. Unlike esodeviations, an abnormality of the AC : A ratio is not of aetiological significance; the ratio is frequently high, however, in intermittent deviations, but this is a secondary response to achieve binocularity for near fixation.

Structural factors involving the overall size, depth and relative disposition of the orbits may produce an exotropia. In hypertelorism, the wide lateral displacement of the orbits may be accompanied by an exodeviation. In Crouzon's syndrome, maxillary hypoplasia is associated with shallow, laterally directed orbits and an exotropia, to which abnormalities of the number and insertions of the extraocular muscles may contribute (Collin 1983).

In the vast majority of cases, however, these considerations do not apply, and the underlying pathophysiology is presumed to be an innervational abnormality. There is no doubt that divergence is an active process. Both binocular convergence and divergence eye movements involve active participation of the lateral and medial rectus muscles. (Breinin 1957; Miller 1967; Tamler & Jampolsky 1967). Since all fibre types in the muscles contribute to these movements, it is assumed that the same motoneurones are involved as in versional movements; in other words that the final common pathway for both vergence and versional movements is the same. The supranuclear control systems are independent however, as is demonstrated by, for example, the preservation of convergence in some cases of bilateral internuclear ophthalmoplegia. Different neuronal circuitry responding to either a retinal binocular disparity signal, or blurred vision (accommodative convergence) directly influences the medial and lateral rectus motoneurons without involving the medial longitudinal fasciculus. In experimental animals, groups of mid-brain neurons have been identified with activities related to both convergence and divergence although anatomical localization is relatively sparse. (Malp & Porter 1984) It is reasonable to suggest, however, that the 'innervation-free' position of the eyes is modified, amongst other influences, by active divergence and convergence input, reciprocally and binocularly integrated. The corollary is that divergence abnormalities, that is exodeviations, are centrally generated, and that the alterations in vision and sensory and motor fusion (see above) are secondary functional changes.

The birth and general medical history in children with exodeviations is usually unremarkable, with no over-representation of prematurity with intraventricular haemorrhage, birth trauma or chromosomal abnormalities.

It is likely therefore that the central abnormality producing an exodeviation is more subtle than that required to produce an esodeviation. Truly congenital exotropia however may be associated with neurological defects (Fig. 44.6).

Oblique muscle dysfunction may also occur in exodeviations, producing A and V patterns. Children characteristically find more difficulty controlling an exophoria on upgaze, so that eye movement testing may suggest a V pattern without oblique dysfunction.

CLASSIFICATION

The generally agreed classification of exodeviations provides information that is useful both for the treatment of the individual case and the overall prognosis. (Burian & Franceschetti 1970). Five categories are recognized: basic, divergence excess (real or simulated), convergence insufficiency, secondary, and consecutive exodeviations. The last two are uncommon in early childhood.

1 In basic exodeviation, the size of the strabismus is

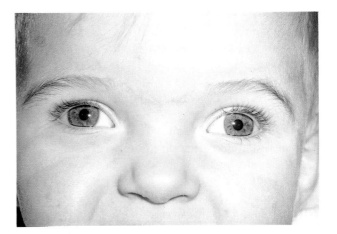

Fig. 44.6 Congenital exotropia. Neurological defects are more frequently found in congenital exotropia then in congenital esotropia.

the same at near and distance fixation. In Burian and Franceschetti's series, 50% of cases were in this category.

2 Divergence excess implies an innervational abnormality: (17% cases). The deviation is greater at distance than near fixation. The difference between these two measurements may be real (8.5%) or simulated (8.5%) by excessive accommodative convergence reducing the near measurement, (i.e. a basic exodeviation mimicking divergence excess). The two can be differentiated by substituting + 3 lenses for the accommodation at near fixation and repeating the measurements.

3 Convergence insufficiency, when the near deviation is greater than that at distance represented 33% of the series quoted, and has the same aetiological implications as divergence excess.

4 Secondary exodeviations occur due to defective vision in one or both eyes.

5 Consecutive exodeviations follow an esodeviation, most commonly after surgery.

DIAGNOSIS

Helpful clues from the history that make a diagnosis of exodeviation likely include an intermittent strabismus, perhaps noticed by the parents only when the child is reading or drawing, and shutting one eye in bright sunlight. In order to ensure correct classification, assessment should include measurement of the exodeviation at a far distance fixation of 100 feet (Burian & Smith 1971), and the use of plus 3 lenses to eliminate accommodation in divergence excess. Prolonged (several hours) patching of the deviating eye to disrupt binocularity that is being maintained by active convergence mechanisms may also help to clarify the diagnosis. In some cases it may be helpful to measure the AC:A ratio for the same reason.

PRINCIPLES OF TREATMENT

The treatment of exodeviations is complicated by the fact that correction of the results of the presumed motor deficit (exotropia) has no effect on the secondary sensory abnormality (temporal hemi-retinal suppression), and the deviation is therefore very likely to recurr. Other variables must also be taken into account: although the prognosis depends on the category, long term follow up of patients for whom surgery was recommended, but, for a variety of reasons, not carried out, indicates that there is a tendency for spontaneous improvement with age (Hiles et al. 1968). Larger deviations tended to decrease more, and divergence excess has a better prognosis than convergence insufficiency. The age at which the diagnosis is made and treatment instituted is important, since neuronal plasticity in the younger age group may allow more manipulation of the developing visual system. It is probably better not to base a programme of treatment on the results of a single examination since variation in the measurements and binocular control may depend on the child's general health and tiredness.

The treatment of a constant exotropia is relatively straightforward. After optical correction and patching for amblyopia, if necessary, surgery should be carried out as soon as is feasible. If there is a constant unilateral divergence, this eye should be operated with simultaneous correction of any oblique dysfunction. If the exotropia is bilateral (alternating), symmetrical bilateral surgery is indicated. In intermittent exodeviation, the treatment programme depends on whether the child is visually mature or not. In a young child, too cautious an operation in terms of millimetres of recession and resection of the rectus muscles will be followed by recurrence of the deviation; too much surgery will produce an esotropia and be followed by the development of amblyopia and the loss of binocular functions. The margin between benefit and permanent damage to the developing visual system is narrow, and because of the absence of divergence fusional amplitudes, even in the best hands, esotropia may occur in over 10% of cases (Pratt-Johnson et al. 1977). A good result appears to follow the production of a small esotropia in the immediate post-operative

period, although there is disagreement about the importance of this.

The first step in intermittent exodeviations of all ages is the correction of refractive error: if the child is myopic, with divergence excess, this may be all that is needed to control the strabismus. Small degrees of symmetrical hypermetropia (less than 3 dioptres) need not be treated, but because of the possibility of developing bilateral amblyopia, higher hypermetropia, especially with astigmatism, must be corrected. Simulated divergence excess will be thereby revealed as a basic exodeviation and need appropriate treatment. Amblyopia should be managed conventionally.

Orthoptic treatment is particularly valuable in divergence excess where the recognition of pathological diplopia (i.e. when the visual axes diverge) may be achieved by alternate patching. Convergence insufficiency may respond to some extent to convergence exercises. Surgical treatment, even in the visually immature, has traditionally been carried out later in exo- than in esodeviations, but Pratt-Johnson (1977) has demonstrated better results in younger patients (median age 2.5 years). Divergence excess should be treated with bilateral lateral rectus recessions, convergence insufficiency with bilateral medial rectus resections, and a basic deviation with recession of the lateral and resection of the medial. Appropriate oblique muscle surgery will also required.

In older, visually mature children of 8 or 9 years orthoptic treatment to teach the recognition of pathological diplopia should be followed by surgery. (Durran 1961).

Another form of treatment that may have a role in individual cases is the use of prisms base-in, in front of each eye to produce an esodeviation with diplopia in the hope of developing active fusional divergence. Minus lenses in the lower segment of bifocal glasses may help in some cases of convergence insufficiency.

References

Adelstein AM, Scully J. Epidemiological aspects of squint. *Br Med J* 1967; **3**: 334−8

Anderson JR. Latent nystagmus and alternating hyperphoria. *Br J Ophthalmol* 1954; **38**: 217−31

Baker FH, Grigg P, Von Noorden GK. Effect of visual deprivation and strabismus on the response of neurones in the visual cortex of the monkey, including studies on the striate and pre-striate cortex in the normal animal. *Brain Res* 1974; **66**: 185−208

Barlow HB, Blakemore C, Pettigrew JP. The neural mechanism of binocular depth discrimination. *J Physiol (London)* 1967; **193**: 327−42

Bechtoldt HP, Hutz CS. Stereopsis in young infants and

stereopsis in an infant with congenital esotropia. *J Pediatr Ophthalmol Strabismus* 1979; **16**: 49−54

Benson PF. Transient unilateral external rectus muscle palsy in newborn infants. *Br Med J* 1962; **1**: 1054−5

Blakemore C, Cummings RM. Eye opening in kittens. *Vision Res* 1975; **15**: 1417−18

Blakemore C, Van Sluyters RC. Reversal of the physiological effects of monocular deprivation in kittens: further evidence for a sensitive period. *J Physiol (London)* 1974a; **237**: 195−216

Blakemore C, Van Sluyters RC. Experimental analysis of amblyopia and strabismus. *Br J Ophthalmol* 1974; **58**: 176−82

Blakemore C, Van Sluyters RC. Innate and environmental factors in the development of the kitten's visual cortex. *J Physiol (London)* 1975; **248**: 663−16

Breakey AS. Ocular findings in cerebral palsy. *Arch Ophthalmol* 1955; **52**: 852−6

Breinin GM. The nature of vergence revealed by electromyography. *Arch Ophthalmol* 1957; **58**: 623−31

Bower TGR. The visual world of infants. *Scientific Am* 1966; **215**(4): 80−92

Bower TGR. The object in the world of the infant. *Scientific Am* 1971; 225 (4): 30−38

Buckley E, Seaber JH. Dyskinetic strabismus as a sign of cerebral palsy. *Am J Ophthalmol* 1981; **91**: 652−7

Burian HM, Franceschetti AT. Evaluation of diagnostic methods for the classification of exodeviations. *Trans Am Ophthalmol Soc* 1970; **68**: 56−71

Burian HM, Smith DR. Comparative measurement of exodeviations at 30 and 100 feet. *Trans Am Ophthalmol Soc* 1971; **69**: 188−199

Cantolino SJ, Von Noorden GK. Heredity in microtropia. *Arch Ophthalmol* 1969; **81**: 753−7

Cassin B. Strabismus and hearing disabilities. *Am Orthopt J* 1975; **25**: 38−45

Chimonidou E, Palimeris G, Koliopoulos J, Velissaropoulos Z. Family distribution of concomitant squint in Greece. *Br J Ophthalmol* 1977; **61**: 27−9

Chrousos GA, Ross JL, Chrousos G *et al.* Ocular findings in Turner syndrome: a prospective study. *Ophthalmol* 1984; **91**: 926−8

Cole MD, Hay A, Eagling EM. Cyclic esotropia in a patient with unilateral traumatic aphakia: case report. *Br J Ophthalmol* 1988; **72**: 305−9

Coleman J, Sydnar CF, Wolbarsht ML, Creel DJ. Abnormal visual pathways in human albinos studied with visually evoked potentials. *Exp Neurol* 1979; **65**: 667−79

Collin JRO. The craniofacial dysostoses. In: Wybar KC, Taylor D *Pediatric Ophthalmology*. Marcel Dekker, New York. 1983; **381**−96

Crone RA, Velzeboer CMJ. Statistics on strabismus in the Amsterdam youth. *Arch Ophthalmol* 1956; **55**: 455−470

Cross HE, The heritablity of strabismus. *Am Orthopt J* 1975; **25**: 11−17

Dayton GO, Jones MH, Steele B, Rose M. Developmental study of co-ordinated eye movements in the human infant. *Arch Ophthalmol* 1964; **71**: 871−5

Deller M. Why should surgery for early-onset strabismus be postponed? *Br J Ophthalmol* 1988; **72**: 110−6

Dell'Osso LF, Schmidt D, Daroff RB. Latent, manifest latent,

and congenital nystagmus. *Arch Ophthalmol* 1979; **97**: 1877−85

Dews PB, Wiesel TN. Consequences of monocular deprivation on visual behaviour in kittens. *J Physiol (London)* 1970; **206**: 437−55

Diamond GR, Katowitz JA, Whitaker LA, Quinn GE, Schaffer DB. Variations in extraocular muscle number and structure in craniofacial dysostosis. *Am J Ophthalmol* 1980; **90**: 416−18

Durran I. Orthoptic treatment of intermittent divergent strabismus of the divergence excess type. *Br Orthopt J* 1961; **18**: 110−13

Eissler R, Longenecker LP. The common eye findings in mongolism. *Am J Ophthalmol* 1962; **54**: 398−406

Fawer C-L, Calarne A, Furrer M-T. Neurodevelopmental outcome at 12 months of age related to cerebral ultrasound appearances of high risk preterm infants. *Early Hum Dev* 1985; **11**: 123−32

Fells P, Waddell E, Alvares M. Progressive, exaggerated A-pattern strabismus with presumed fibrosis of extraocular muscles. In: Reinecke RD (ed) *Strabismus II: Proceedings of the Fourth Meeting of The International Strabismological Association.* Grune & Stratton, Orlando, 1984; p. 335−43

Fink WH. The role of developmental anomalies in vertical muscle defects. *Am J Ophthalmol* 1955; **40**: 529−33

Fitzgerald BA, Billson FA. Dissociated vertical deviation: evidence for abnormal visual pathway projection. *Br J Ophthalmol* 1984; **68**: 801−06

Fletcher ML. Natural History of idiopathic strabismus. In: Burian HM, Dunlap EA, Dyer JA *et al.* (eds) *Symposium on Strabismus: Transactions of the New Orleans Academy of Ophthalmology.* CV Mosby Co., St Louis 1971; pp. 15−333

Fonda G. Characteristics and low-vision corrections in albinism. *Arch Ophthalmol* 1962; **68**: 754−61

Fox F, Albin RN, Shea SL, Dumais ST. Stereopsis in human infants. *Science* 1980; **207**: 323−4

France TD. The association of A pattern strabismus with hydrocephalus. *Trans 3rd Int Orthoptic Congress* 1975; pp. 287−92

Franceschetti AT, Burian HM. Gradient accommodative convergence/accommodation ratio in families with and without esotropia. *Am J Ophthalmol* 1970; **70**: 558−62

Francois J. *Heredity in Ophthalmology.* CV Mosby Co., St Louis 1961; pp. 255−69

Friedman L, Biedner B, David R, Sachs V. Screening for refractive errors, strabismus and other ocular anomalies from ages 6 months to 3 years. *J Pediatr Ophthalmol Strabismus* 1980; **17**: 315−17

Gardiner PA, Joseph M. Eye defects in children with congenital heart lesions: a preliminary study. *Dev Med Child Neurol* 1968; **10**: 42−8

Gobin MH. Anteroposition of the inferior oblique muscle in V-esotropia. *Ophthalmologica* 1964; **148**: 325−41

Gobin MH. Cyclotropia as a possible cause of squint particularly in V- and A- syndromes. In: *Transactions of the 1st International Congress of Orthoptics* Henry Kimpton, London 1968(a); 142−48

Gobin MH. Sagittalization of the oblique muscles as a possible cause for the 'A', 'V', and 'X' phenomena. *Br J Ophthalmol* 1968(b); **52**: 13−18

Graham PA. Epidemiology of strabismus. *Br J Ophthalmol*

1974; **58**: 224–31

de Grauw AJC, Rotteveel JJ, Cruysberg JRM. Transient sixth cranial nerve paralysis in the newborn infant. *Neuropediatr* 1983; **14**: 164–5

Gregerson E. The polymorphous exo patient. *Acta Ophthalmologica* 1969; **47**: 579–90

Gunter K, Von Noorden GK, Wong SY. Surgical results in nystagmus blockage syndrome. *Ophthalmology* 1986; **93**: 1028–32

Hall IB. Primary divergent strabismus. *Br Orthopt J* 1961; **18**: 106–9

Harcourt B. Strabismus affecting children with multiple handicaps. *Br J Ophthalmol* 1974; **58**: 272–9

Harcourt B, Mein J, Johnson F. Natural history and associations of dissociated vertical divergence. *Trans Ophthalmol Soc UK* 1980; **100**: 495–97

Helveston EM. A-exotropia, alternating sursumduction and superior oblique overaction. *Am J Ophthalmol* 1969; **67**: 377–80

Helveston EM, Von Noorden GK. Microtropia: a newly defined entity. *Arch Ophthalmol* 1967; **78**: 272–81

Hendrickson A, Boothe R. Morphology of the retina and dorsal lateral geniculate nucleus in dark-reared monkeys (*Macaca nemestrina*). *Vision Res* 1976; **16**: 517–21

Hiles DA, Davies GT, Costenbader FD. Long-term observations on unoperated intermittent exotropia. *Arch Ophthalmol* 1968; **80**: 436–42

Hotchkiss MD, Miller NR, Clark AW, Green WR. Bilateral Duanes Retraction Syndrome. *Arch Ophthalmol* 1980; **98**: 870–4

Hoyt CS. Nystagmus compensation (blockage) syndrome. *Am J Ophthalmol* 1977; **83**: 423–4

Hoyt CS. Abnormalities of the vestibulo-ocular response in congenital esotropia. *Am J Ophthalmol* 1982; **93**: 704–8

Hoyt CS. Billson FA, Taylor H. Isolated unilateral gaze palsy. *J Pediatr Ophthalmol* 1977; **14**: 343–45

Hoyt CS, Caltrider N. Hemispheric visually-evoked responses in congenital esotropia. *J Pediatr Ophthalmol Strabismus* 1984; **21**: 19–21

Hoyt CS, Jastrebski GB, Marg E. Amblyopia and congenital esotropia visually evoked potential measurements. *Arch Ophthalmol* 1984; **102**: 58–61

Hoyt CS, Mousel DK, Weber AA. Transient supranuclear disturbances of gaze in healthy neonates. *Am J Ophthalmol* 1980; **89**: 708–12

Hubel DN, Wiesel TN. Integrative action in the cat's lateral geniculate body. *J Physiol (London)* 1961; **155**: 385–98

Hubel DN, Wiesel TN. Receptive fields, binocular interaction, and functional architecture in the cat's visual cortex. *J Physiol (London)* 1962; **160**: 106–54

Hubel DN, Wiesel TN. Binocular interaction in striate cortex of kittens reared with artificial squint. *J Neurophysiol* 1965; **28**: 1041–59

Hubel DN, Wiesel TN. The period of susceptibility to the physiological effects of unilateral eye closure in kittens. *J Physiol (London)* 1970; **206**: 419–36

Huber A. Duanes retraction syndrome. Consideration on pathophysiology and aetiology. In: *Strabismus II: Proceedings of the Fourth Meeting of the International Strabismologic Association*. Reinecke RD. (ed.) Grune & Stratton, Orlando 1984; pp. 345–60

Ing MR. Early surgical alignment for congenital esotropia. *Trans Am Ophthalmol Soc* 1981; **79**: 625–63

James R. Combined superior oblique muscle tendon resection and inferior oblique muscle recession for dissociated vertical deviation: A report of 25 cases. *Binocular Vision* 1987; **2**: 137–51

Jampel RS. Representation of the near response on the cerebral cortex of the Macaque. *Am J Ophthalmol* 1959; **48**: 573–81

Jampolsky A. Ocular Deviations. *Int Ophthalmol Clin* 1964; **4**: 567–701

Jay W, Hoyt CS. Abnormal brain stem auditary evoked potentials in Stilling–Turk–Duane retraction syndrome. *Am J Ophthalmol* 1980; **89**: 814–18

Kalina RE. Ophthalmological examination of children of low birth weight. *Am J Ophthalmol* 1969; **67**: 134–6

Keith CG, Kitchen WH. Ocular morbidity in very low birth-weight infants. In: Reinecke RD. (ed.) *Strabismus II: Proceedings of the Fourth Meeting of the International Strabismological Association*. Grune & Stratton, Orlando 1984 pp. 45–53

Knapp P. A and V patterns. In: Dabezier OH, (ed.) Symposium on Strabismus. CV Mosby 1971; St Louis pp. 242–54

Kommerel G, Mehdorn E. Is an optokinetic defect the cause of congenital and latent nystagmus? In: Lennerstrand G, Zee DS, Keller EL. (eds) *Functional Basis of Oculomoticity Disorders*. Pergamon Press; Oxford 1982; 159–167

Kratz KE, Spear PD. Effects of visual deprivation and alterations in binocular competition on responses of striate cortex neurons in the cat. *J Comp Neurol* 1976; **170**: 141–52

Kriss A, Timms C, Elston J, Taylor D. Pattern – and flash – evoked potentials in patients with dissociated vertical deviation. *Doc Ophthalmol* 1988; **69**: 283–291

Kriss A, Timms C, Elston J, Taylor D, Gresty M. Visual-evoked potentials in dissociated vertical deviation – a re-appraisal. *Br J Ophthalmol* 1989; **73**: 265–70

Kushner BJ. Strabismus and amblyopia associated with regressed retinopathy of prematurity. *Arch Ophthalmol* 1982; **100**: 256–61

Kushner BJ. The Role of Ocular torsion on the etiology of A + V patterns. *J Pediatr Ophthalmol Strabismus* 1985; **22**: 171–79

Lang J. Microtropia. *Arch Ophthalmol* 1969; **81**: 758–62

Levy NS, Cassin B, Newman M. Strabismus in children with cerebral palsy. *J Pediatr Ophthalmol* 1976; **13**: 72–74

Lossef S. Ocular findings in Cerebral Palsy. *Am J Ophthalmol* 1962; **54**: 1114–8

Ludwig IH, Parks MM, Getson PR, Kammerman LA. Rate of deterioration in accommodative esotropia correlated to the AC/A relationship. *J Pediatr Ophthalmol Strabismus* 1988; **25**: 8–13

Malp LE, Porter JD. Neural control of vergence eye movements: Activity of abducens and Oculomotor Neurons. *J Neurophysiol* 1984; **52**: 743–61

Margolis S, Pachter BR, Breinin GM. Structural alterations of extraocular muscle associated with Apert's Syndrome. *Br J Ophthalmol* 1977; **61**: 683–9

McKusick VA. *Mendelian Inheritance in Man*. Johns Hopkins University Press, Baltimore & London 1978; pp. 359–60

Miller JE. The electromyography of vergence movements. *Arch Ophthalmol* 1959; **62**: 790–4

Miller NR, Kiel SM, Green WR, Clark AW. Unilateral Duane's

retraction syndrome (type I). *Arch Ophthalmol* 1982; **100**: 1468–72.

Nash AJ, Hegmann JP, Spivey BE. Genetic analysis of vergence measurements in populations with varying incidence of strabismus. *Am J Ophthalmol* 1975; **79**: 978–84

Nashold BS, Seaber JH. Defects of Ocular motility after stereotactic midbrain lesions in Man. *Arch Ophthalmol* 1972; **88**: 245–8

Nixon RB, Helveston EM, Miller K, Archer SM Ellis FD. Incidence of strabismus in neonates. *Am J Ophthalmol* 1985; **100**: 798–801

Palmer P, Dubowitz LMS, Levene MI, Dubowitz V. Developmental and neurological progress of preterm infants with intraventricular haemorrhage and ventricular dilation. *Arch Dis Child* 1982; **57**: 748–53

Parks MM. Abnormal accommodative convergence in squint. *Arch Ophthalmol* 1958: **59**: 364–80

Parks MM. The monofixation syndrome. *Trans Am Ophthalmol Soc* 1969; **67**: 609–15

Parks MM. The overacting inferior oblique muscle. The XXXVI de Schweinitz Lecture. *Am J Ophthalmol* 1974; **77**: 787–97

Parks MM. Dissociated hyperdeviations. In: Duane TD, Jaeger EA. (eds) *Clinical Ophthalmology* Vol. I Harper & Row, Philadelphia 1982; p. 1–4

Pratt-Johnson JA. Central disruption of fusional amplitude. *Br J Ophthalmol* 1973; **57**: 347–50

Pratt-Johnson JA, Barlow JM, Tillson G. Early surgery in intermittent exotropia. *Am J Ophthalmol* 1977; **84**: 689–94

Rabinowitz IM. Visual function in children with hydrocephalus. *Trans Ophthalmol Soc UK* 1974; **104**: 353–65

Rabinowitz IM, Walker JM. Disorders of Ocular Motility in Children with Hydrocephalus. *Transactions of the 4th International Congress of Orthoptics.* Henry Kimpton, London 1975; 279–86

Ramsay J, Taylor D. Congenital crocodile tears: a key to the aetiology of Duane's syndrome. *Br J Ophthalmol* 1980; **64**: 518–22

Reisner SH, Perlman M, Bentovim N, Dubrawski C. Transient lateral rectus muscle paresis in the newborn infant. *J Pediatr* 1971; **78**: 461–65

Rethy I. Development of simultaneous fixation from the divergent anatomic eye position of the neonate. *J Pediatr Ophthalmol Strabismus* 1969; **6**: 92–7

Reynolds JD, Biglan AW, Hiles DA. Congenital Superior Oblique Palsy in Infants. *Arch Ophthalmol* 1984; **102**: 1503–5

Robb RM, Rodier DW. The variable clinical characteristics and course of early infantile esotropia. *J Pediatr Ophthalmol Strabismus* 1987; **24**: 276–82

Rothstein TB, Romano PE, Shoch D. Meningoyelocele. *Am J Ophthalmol* 1974; **77**: 690–3

Ruttum M, Von Noorden GK. Orbital and facial arthrometry in A and V pattern strabismus. In: Reinecke RD, (ed.) *Strabismus II: Proceedings of the 4th Meeting of the International Strabismological Association.* Grune & Stratton, Orlando 1984; 363–9

Simons K, Reinecke RD. Amblyopia screening and stereopsis. In: *Transactions of the New Orleans Academy of Ophthalmology.* St Louis, CV Mosby 1978; 15–50

Sondhi N, Archer SM, Helveston HM. Development of normal ocular alignment. *J Pediatr Ophthalmol Strabismus* 1988; **25**: 210–11

Stanworth A. Defects of ocular movement and fusion after head injury. *Br J Ophthalmol* 1974; **58**: 266–71

Steinberg M, Rendle-Short J. Vestibular dysfunction in young children with minor neurological impairment. *Dev Med Child Neurol* 1977; **19**: 639–51

Stevens PR. Anisometropia and amblyopia. *Br Orthopt J* 1960; **17**: 66–73

Tamler E, Jampolsky A. Is divergence active? An electromyográphic study. *Am J Ophthalmol* 1967; **63**: 452–9

Taylor DM. Is congenital esotropia functionally curable? *J Pediatr Ophthalmol Strabismus* 1974; **2**: 3–35

Taylor DSI, Vaegan, Morris JA, Rogers RG, Warland J. Amblyopia in bilateral infantile and juvenile cataract. *Trans Ophthalmol Soc UK* 1979; **99**: 170–5

Tsutsui J, Fukai S. Human Strabismic Cases Suggestive of asymmetric Projection of the visual pathway. In: Reinecke RD (ed.) *Strabismus Proceedings of the Third Meeting of the International Strabismological Association.* Grune & Stratton, New York 1978; pp. 79–88

Urist MJ. The aetiology of the so-called A and V syndrome. *Am J Ophthalmol* 1958; **46**: 835–44

Urrets-Zavalia A, Solares-Zamora J, Olmos HR. Anthropological studies of the nature of cyclovertical squint. *Br J Ophthalmol* 1961; **45**: 578–96

Van Hof-Van Duin J, Mohn G. Stereopsis and optokinetic nystagmus. In: Lennerstrand G, Zee DS, Keller EL (eds) *Functional Basis of Oculomoticity Disorders.* Pergamon Press; Oxford 1982; pp. 113–9

Van Vliet AGM. On the Central Mechanism of Latent Nystagmus. *Acta Ophthalmol* 1973; **51**: 772–81

Von Noorden GK. Factors involved in the production of amblyopia. *Br J Ophthalmol* 1974; **58**: 158–64

Von Noorden GK. The nystagmus compensation (blockage) syndrome. *Am J Ophthalmol* 1976; **82**: 283–90

Von Noorden GK. Current concepts of infantile esotropia. *Eye* 1988; **2**: 343–358

Von Noorden GK, Avilla CW. Nystagmus Blockage Syndrome Revisited. In: Reinecke RD (ed.) *Strabismus II: Proceedings of the fourth meeting of the International Strabismological Association.* Grune & Stratton, Orlando 1984; pp. 75–82

Von Noorden GK, Brown DJ, Parks M. Associated convergence and accommodative insufficiency. *Doc Ophthalmol* 1973; **34**: 393–403

Von Noorden GK, Dowling JE, Ferguson DC. Experimental amblyopia in monkeys. 1. Behavioural studies of stimulus deprivation amblyopia. *Arch Ophthalmol* 1970; **84**: 206–14.

Van Noorden GK, Wong GM. Surgical results in nystagmus blockage syndrome. *Ophthalmology*, 1986; **93**: 1028–31

Waardenburg PJ. Genetics and Ophthalmology In: *Neuro-ophthalmology* Vol. 2 Blackwell Scientific Publications, Oxford 1963; pp. 1009–36

Waardenburg PJ. Genetics and Ophthalmology. In: *Neuro-Ophthalmology*, Vol. 2 Blackwell Scientific Publications, Oxford 1963; pp. 1009–36

Wiesel TN, Hubel DN. Receptive fields of cells in striate cortex of very young, visually inexperienced kittens. *J Neurophysiol* 1963(a); **26**: 994–1002

Wiesel TN, Hubel DN. Effects of visual deprivation on morphology and physiology of cells in the cat's lateral geniculate body. *J Neurophysiol* 1963(b); **26**: 978−93

Wiesel TN, Hubel DN. Single cell responses in striate cortex of kittens deprived of vision in one eye. *J Neurophysiol* 1963(c); **26**: 1003−17

Wiesel TN, Hubel DN. Extent of recovery from the effects of visual deprivation in kittens. *J Neurophysiol* 1965(a); **28**: 1060−72

Wiesel TN, Hubel DN. Comparison of the effects of unilateral and bilateral eye closure on cortical unit responses in kittens. *J Neurophysiol* 1965(b); **28**: 1029−40

Wiesel TN, Hubel DN. Ordered arrangement of ocular dominance columns in monkeys lacking visual experience. *J Comp Neurol* 1974; **158**: 307−18

Wybar KC, Walker J. Surgical management of strabismus in hydrocephalus. *Trans Ophthalmol Soc UK* 1980; **100**: 475−8

45 Incomitant Strabismus and Cranial Nerve Palsies

JOHN ELSTON

Incomitant strabismus in childhood is rare: no precise epidemiology is available, but it is notable that amongst 149000 new patients presenting with strabismus (adults and children) to an eye hospital, only 126 (0.84%) had one of the commonest varieties of incomitant strabismus, Duane's syndrome (Kirkham 1970). Incomitant strabismus may also present to paediatricians, neurologists and neurosurgeons, making data collection difficult.

In infancy, diagnosis may be difficult because of problems with the examination of the pupil responses and the limited range of eye movement, particularly lateral and upgaze that can readily be elicited. Horizontal eye movement testing may be augmented by the spinning test; the infant is held, with the head supported, facing the examiner who spins around the vertical axis. The eyes deviate against the direction of spinning and saccade back to refixate. Provided the infant has a normal afferent visual and central nervous system, the integrity of the infranuclear ocular motor system can be assessed clinically by comparing the speed and extent of the refixation saccades in each eye. In this way a lateral rectus palsy, for example, can be differentiated from a concomitant convergent squint. In older children, the adoption of a consistent abnormal head posture, and unwillingness to turn the eyes in the direction of the abnormal posture may be the presenting sign of incomitant strabismus. Children who do not move their eyes normally may also be referred as having a sensory visual defect.

Incomitant strabismus is caused by two broad groups of disorders: developmental abnormalities (principally Duane's, Mobius', and Brown's syndromes) and ocular motor palsies.

Developmental abnormalities

Duane's syndrome

Although originally described in the European literature at the end of the 19th century, the disorder is properly named after Duane who described 54 cases in 1905, detailing the consistent ocular features. There is a congenital deficiency of abduction of the eye, associated with variable impairment of adduction, retraction of the globe and narrowing of the palpebral aperture on adduction (Fig. 45.1) and abnormal oblique movements (Duane 1905). The disorder is usually unilateral, in which case it is commoner on the left side (Pfaffenbach et al. 1972) but may be bilateral (15–20% cases) (Cross & Pfaffenbach 1972, Isenberg & Urist 1977). It is commoner in females than males (Pfaffenback et al. 1972) and may be familial (Kirkham 1970) (Fig. 45.2). There is a spectrum of abnormality of eye movement, and some authors have tried to classify the condition into types I, II and III, depen-

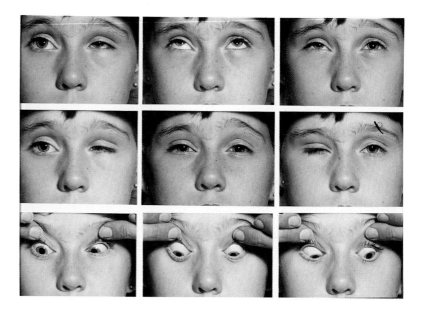

Fig. 45.1 Bilateral typical Duane's syndrome. There is no deviation in the straight ahead position, narrowing of the palpebral fissure in the adducting eye and weak abduction.

dent on the relative limitations of abduction and adduction. Type I has normal adduction, type II normal abduction and reduced adduction, and type III reduced abduction and adduction. Although there is some electrophysiological (electromyography) support for this classification (Huber 1974) it is not very useful clinically since all cases of Duane's syndrome are explicable on a single pathology (see below). The syndrome may be best regarded as typical (as described by Duane) or atypical (having other features such as marked reduction of adduction).

One of the notable features of the condition is the frequently normal development of sensory and motor binocular function despite profoundly abnormal eye movements. Binocularity may only be maintained with an abnormal head posture, usually of head turn towards the side of the lesion. Amblyopia, usually due to anisometropia or astigmatism, occurs in 10% of cases, 25% if the condition is bilateral.

Other systemic developmental abnormalities may be present in cases of Duane's syndrome. The most important are perceptive deafness (10.7%, Kirkham 1970) which may be severe in infancy and lead to a speech defect, and the Klippel–Feil anomaly, an abnormality of the cervical spine leading to a short neck with reduced movements and a low posterior hair line. The triad of Duane's, deafness and Klippel-Feil may be inherited as an autosomal dominant condition (known as Wildervanck's syndrome) with variable penetrance and different features in affected family members (Kirkham 1970). These, or other development anomalies such as auricular malformation, Goldenhar's syndrome, hemivertebra, syndactyly or

other (usually terminal) limb malformations may be present in up to one third of cases (Pfaffenbach *et al.* 1972). It is suggested, that since all these structures develop between the fourth and eighth week of intrauterine life, a teratogenic influence, either genetic or external, may operate at this stage.

The pathophysiology of the condition was a matter of speculation until the development of the technique of extraocular muscle electromyography. A study in 1972 showed normal innervation of the medial rectus, but a wide variation of lateral rectus innervational abnormalities, with co-firing on adduction, reduced activity on attempted abduction, and inappropriate activity on up and downgaze (Scott & Wong 1972). It became clear that retraction (and secondary palpebral aperture narrowing) on adduction was due to co-contraction often in the superior and inferior as well as the lateral rectus, and the abnormal oblique movements (such as elevation in adduction) are also due to a primary innervational anomaly. The results were taken to indicate an absent VIth nerve, with the peripheral IIIrd nerve supplying all the extraocular muscles in an abnormal way; a primary brain stem origin for the abnormality was thought likely. This conclusion had been reached earlier, principally on clinical grounds, by Hoyt and Nachtigaler (1965). Confirmation of the EMG findings was provided by Strachan and Brown (1972), who showed paradoxical innervation of the lateral rectus, and Huber (1974) who was able to distinguish the clinical subtypes of Duane's with EMG and suggest that the features depended on the relative contribution and pattern of IIIrd nerve supply to the lateral rectus, and fibrosis in

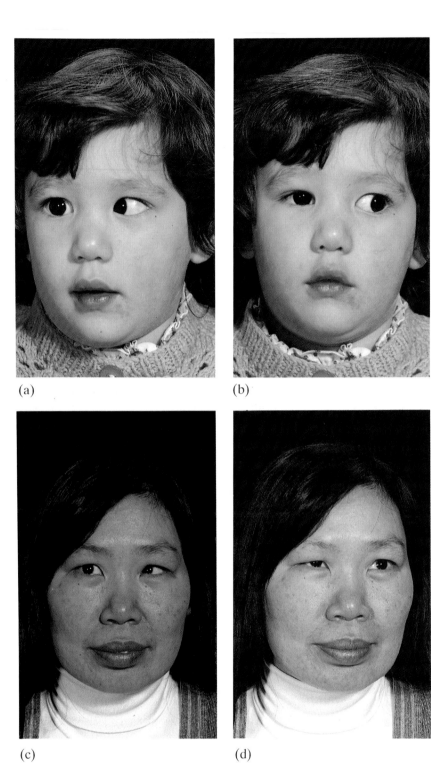

(a)   (b)

(c)   (d)

Fig. 45.2 A typical right Duane's syndrome in a child (a, b) with a similar abnormality in her mother (c, d).

the muscle. There is no doubt that the traction test is positive in Duane's syndrome, and the abnormal oblique movements may also, to some extent, be due to rotation of the globe around its anteroposterior axis dictated by the unyielding muscle.

The first comprehensive report of the postmortem findings, both intracranial and orbital in a case of bilateral Duane's syndrome appeared in 1980 (Hotchkiss *et al.* 1980). Both abducens nuclei and nerves were absent from the brain stem, and the lateral rectus muscles were partly innervated by branches from the oculomotor nerves. An autopsy in a case of unilateral (left) Duane's confirmed these findings, and firmly established the disorder as a developmental neurological abnormality (Miller *et al.* 1982). There may be a more extensive pontine abnormality than an absence of motor neurone cell bodies in the abducens nucleus in some cases. Nine out of 14 patients with Duane's showed increased latency in wave III of the brain stem auditory-evoked potential (Jay & Hoyt 1980) which is generated by the superior olivary complex in the pons. Seventeen out of 18 cases of congenital crocodile tears in the literature also had Duane's syndrome, suggesting more extensive pontine dysgenesis in these cases (Ramsay & Taylor 1980).

A syndrome exactly mimicking Duane's syndrome has occurred in a child with lateral rectus myositis (Timms *et al.* 1989).

A vertical retraction syndrome has been described and suggested to be a related entity. The features are congenital limitation of up or downgaze, with retraction and narrowing of the palpebral aperture on attempting the opposite movement. The superior rectus is more often involved than the inferior rectus and there is a variable esotropia or exotropia. The literature is sparse however, and there are no reports of pathology: some cases described (Pruksacholawit & Ishikawa 1976) may well be partly recovered congenital IIIrd nerve palsies. Other unusual patterns that may be related include an adduction deficit with simultaneous abduction on attempted lateral gaze into the field of action of the apparently paretic muscle (Wagner *et al.* 1987).

MANAGEMENT

The parents of a child with Duane's syndrome need an explanation of the underlying developmental problem, emphasising that although the condition is not progressive, it will not resolve, and it is not possible to create normal eye movements surgically. The developmentally significant associations (see above), particularly deafness, should be excluded. An accurate refraction is required, and anisometropia and amblyopia treated.

The overall plan depends on the primary position alignment, the presence of an abnormal head posture, the severity of the retraction and the pattern of upshoot and downshoot, and accompanying A, V or X pattern (Kraft 1988).

If the child is binocular with the head held straight, no surgical treatment is necessary or possible; if binocular with a noticeable head posture, (turn towards the side of the lesion) then surgery to move the eye in the direction of the head turn may be helpful. Specialized surgical techniques are required, however, since standard strabismus surgery may reduce eye movements even further. A temporal transfer of the superior and inferior rectus to produce some abduction, combined with a small medial rectus recession may be required (Gobin 1974). In cases where retraction on adduction is the chief cosmetic abnormality, it can be reduced by recessing the medial and lateral rectus equally on the affected eye. Similarly up- and downshoots of the eye may be amenable to mechanical stabilization of the position of the extraocular muscles on the globe (Fig. 45.2). In cases with a constant strabismus (usually convergent) surgery will also be required.

Möbius' syndrome

The syndrome of congenital facial diplegia with failure of abduction was first described by Von Graefe in 1880, more completely by Möbius in 1888 (Van Allen & Blodi 1960). The facial palsies are often incomplete (sparing the lower face) and asymmetrical but are an invariable feature. The eyes, which do not close normally but are protected by Bell's phenomenon, are often straight, not convergent (Fig. 45.4), suggesting bilateral horizontal gaze palsies. Forty five out of 61 cases reviewed by Henderson (1939) showed both these signs, whilst 15 had in addition bilateral partial IIIrd nerve palsies. The vertical eye movements are otherwise normal, as are the pupils, the vision, and the optic nerves and fundus. Eighteen of the 61 cases had partial atrophy of the tongue, which characteristically shows longitudinal furrowing and fasciculation (Fig. 45.5). There may also be paralysis of the soft palate. More widespread abnormalities such as corneal anaesthesia (Fig. 45.6) may also occur in Möbius and Möbius-like syndromes (Miller *et al.* 1989).

Other associated developmental anomalies include skeletal malformations — agenesis or dysgenesis of limbs, syndactyly or polydactyly (Rogers *et al.* 1977) — and pectoralis muscle defect. Mental deficiency is relatively rare (10% of Henderson's cases), belying the external appearance.

The condition may be familial (Merz & Wojtowicz 1967) but Baraitser (1977) has shown in a study of the siblings and parents of 15 children diagnosed as Möbius' syndrome that if primary skeletal defects, agenesis of limbs, syndactyly, etc. are included as obligatory in the diagnosis, the risk to subsequent offspring is very low (2%). A number of other con-

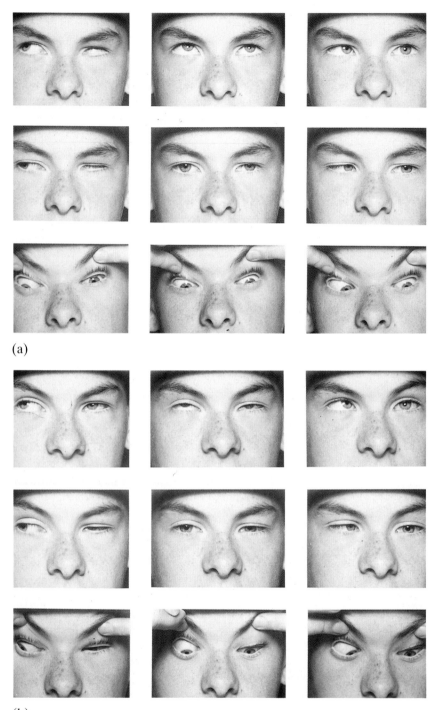

(a)

(b)

Fig. 45.3 (a) Left Duane's with gross upshoot of the left eye on adduction. (b) same patient following splitting and recession of the left lateral rectus.

ditions, however, may present with Möbius-like facies in infancy. These include disorders of the anterior horn cell such as hypoplasia of the involved cranial nerve nuclei (Towfighi *et al.* 1979) brain stem tegmental necrosis (Thakkar *et al.* 1977) and myopathy, for example facio-scapulo-humeral dystrophy (Hanson & Rowland 1971).

In Möbius' syndrome, the facial muscles show no EMG potentials on attempted activity (Merz & Wojtowicz 1967): the lateral rectus may however, show some evidence of co-contraction with the medial rectus on attempted abduction (Van Allen & Blodi 1960; Merz & Wojtowicz 1967). There is some evidence, therefore, for a supranuclear (or possibly

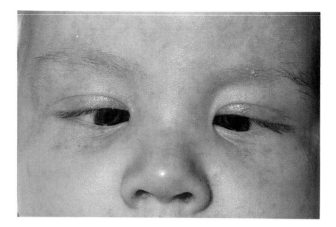

Fig. 45.4 Möbius' syndrome. Marked convergence with bilateral sixth nerve palsy and a seventh nerve palsy evidenced by rather 'expressionless' eyes. Many parents of infants with Möbius syndrome find their child's apparent (but false) lack of response, due to the facial palsy, difficult to accept.

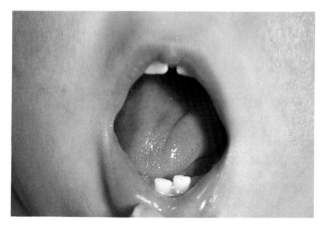

Fig. 45.5 Hypoplasia of the tongue with longitudinal furrowing in Möbius syndrome.

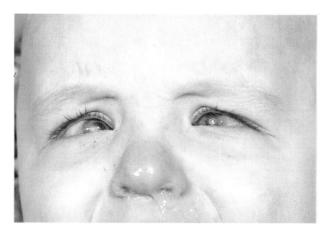

Fig. 45.6 Möbius-like syndrome with anaesthetic corneas from fifth nerve palsy and exposure due to VIIth nerve palsy.

infranuclear) abnormality of horizontal gaze, but postmortem evidence shows that the underlying problem is agenesis of the VIth, VIIth and XIIth cranial nerve nuclei (Towfighi *et al.* 1979). The extraocular muscles themselves are normal, but a traction test is often strongly positive probably due to secondary fibrotic changes.

MANAGEMENT

These children should be under the care of a paediatric neurologist: the ophthalmologist may be needed to identify and treat amblyopia. Surgery may have a role in some cases (Miller *et al.* 1989).

Brown's syndrome

True Brown's syndrome (as opposed to simulated Brown's syndrome) is a developmental abnormality of the superior oblique tendon, whose anterior portion appears to be congenitally short. The result is a failure of elevation of the affected eye, which is complete when the eye is adducted, and lessens progressively with abduction (Fig. 45.7) (Brown 1973). Other features include a positive traction test on attempted passive elevation of the eye in adduction, and a V pattern of eye movement, with exotropia in upgaze. Although overaction of the ipsilateral superior oblique is classically absent, it may be present in one fifth of patients (Sato *et al.* 1987). The palpebral aperture usually widens on adduction. These features serve to differentiate the condition from failure of elevation in adduction due to superior oblique overaction. 10% of all cases are bilateral (Brown 1973), and the condition may be familial (Moore *et al.* 1988). Mirror image Brown's syndrome has been described in twins (Wortham & Crawford 1988).

The trochlear and superior oblique tendon appear to be derived from the same mesenchymal tissue, and develop into seperate entities by differential growth (Sevel 1981). In the embryo, septa extend from the tendon to the trochlea, and the syndrome may be due in some cases to persistence of these septa; in others, anterior tendon development is defective. Some cases improve spontaneously with age, and this may be due to progressive atrophy or disruption of the abnormal septa. The condition may be simulated, usually by trauma to the trochlear, occasionally by inflammatory disease (rheumatoid arthritis), a metastasis (Slavin & Goldstein 1987), or trochlea involvement by tumour (Biiedner *et al.* 1988).

Children with true Brown's syndrome usually pres-

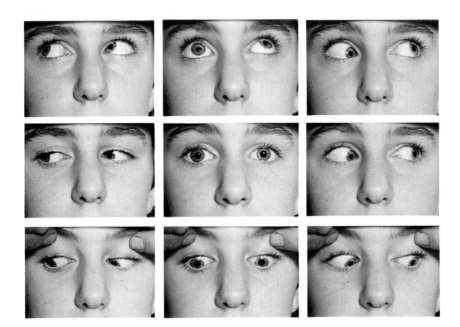

Fig. 45.7 Right Brown's syndrome with poor elevation of the eye in adduction but no residual hypotropia in the primary position.

ent with an abnormal head posture, turning their heads to move the affected eye into abduction, sometimes combined with elevation of the chin, in order to achieve binocularity. Sometimes binocularity has been lost by the time of presentation, in which case the parents notice a vertical strabismus, with overelevation of the normal eye the most prominent feature.

MANAGEMENT

There is an overall tendency for spontaneous improvement (Waddel 1982) and complete resolution may occur, preceded by a period of intermittency between the ages of 7 and 10 often characterized by an audible and palpable 'click' as the tendon passes through the trochlear. In children who are binocular, with no deviation in the primary position and no gross head posture, management can be expectant. Without these features, or in the presence of a marked eye movement defect, with reduced area of binocular single vision a superior oblique tenotomy is required (Scott & Knapp 1972). Because of the frequency of complete superior oblique palsy with inferior oblique overaction following this procedure, some authorities recommend a simultaneous inferior oblique recession (Parks & Sprague 1987). At surgery the diagnosis is confirmed by the forced duction test; to differentiate between oblique and rectus muscle abnormality more completely the test is performed in two stages. Firstly with the eye pushed backwards into the orbit the oblique muscles are tested and secondly pulled outwards the rectus muscles are put to test.

Extraocular muscle fibrosis syndrome

This condition, also known as generalized fibrosis or strabismus fixus is a congenital, often familial developmental abnormality of the extra-ocular muscles and levator. The features are bilateral ptosis and external ophthalmoplegia, affecting vertical movements more than horizontal. The eyes are fixed in downgaze, and a head posture of chin elevation is adopted. Attempting upward movements often produces nystagmoid convergence (Catford 1966; Crawford 1970) whilst the eyes may diverge on attempted downgaze (Fells *et al.* 1984). There is usually an exotropia, and no binocular vision; myopia and astigmatism are common, as is amblyopia. The fibrosis syndrome may be an autosomal dominant condition, or sporadic; patients are otherwise physically and neurologically normal.

Operative findings include a strongly positive traction test (Catford 1966) and the replacement of extraocular muscles by dense fibrous tissue. This tissue may have anomalous insertions on the globe. (Apt & Axelrod 1978). The condition may also occur unilaterally, usually in a limited form, affecting the inferior rectus principally (Fig. 45.8) (Von Noorden 1970).

MANAGEMENT

Refractive error and amblyopia must be identified and

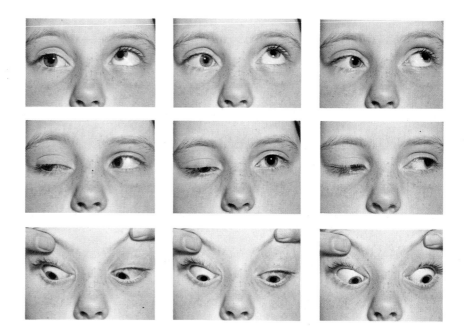

Fig. 45.8 Right inferior rectus fibrosis with right hypotropia especially in upgaze. There is a right pseudoptosis.

treated conventionally. To reduce or overcome the abnormal head posture, a very large recession or a free tenotomy of the affected muscles, possibly combined with post-operative traction sutures, is required. Surgical treatment of the ptosis should be cautious because of the absence of Bell's phenomenon.

Others

Goldenhar's syndrome (oculo-auriculo-vertebral dysplasia with hemifacial microsomia) may be accompanied by congenital ophthalmoplegia. A postmortem study in one case showed agenesis of the IV and VIth nerve nuclei (Aleksic *et al.* 1976).

In the craniofacial dysostoses, individual extraocular muscles, particularly the superior oblique and superior rectus, may be absent, poorly developed or insert anomalously on the globe (Robb & Boger 1983). Rarely, an anomalous muscle insertion may be an isolated abnormality not associated with other orbital pathology (Rosenbaum & Jampolsky 1975; Mather & Saunders 1987).

Acquired oculomotor nerve dysfunction

The oculomotor system consists of supranuclear, internuclear, nuclear and infranuclear components; the latter only will be considered in this section. Infranuclear oculomotor disorders in childhood may be isolated, or associated, either with other symptoms (for example pain or headache), or signs (for example

other cranial nerve palsies). Isolated individual ocular motor (IIIrd, IVth or VIth cranial nerve) disorders will be discussed first.

Children with IIIrd, IVth or VIth cranial nerve palsies may present to ophthalmologists, neurologists, neurosurgeons or paediatricians, so that it is difficult to collect data from a representative group of patients, and the epidemiology is sparse. In an unselected, retrospective study of 1000 cases of all ages (all with acquired palsies), Rush and Younge (1981) found that 90% of the patients were over 19 years at presentation, suggesting that these conditions are rare in childhood.

Presentation

Isolated ocular motor nerve palsies in infancy usually present with the parents' observation of an abnormality of eye or eyelid movement, or pupil size. Older children may complain of double vision, and although this symptom can be the result of the recognition of physiological diplopia, it should always be taken seriously. The distance esotropia of a mild lateral rectus palsy, for example, may be minimal, but early diagnosis is important. Other presentations in childhood include the shutting of one eye, adoption of an abnormal head posture or the observation of abnormal eye movements.

A full history is important; recent infections including exposure to neurotropic viruses, may be of aetiological importance. General symptoms such as headache and fever should be sought, and may determine the urgency of investigation. The drug history may be relevant, for example, tetracycline (Maroon & Mealy 1971) and nalidixic acid (Cohen 1973) may cause intracranial hypertension.

The differential diagnosis includes concomitant strabismus, neuromuscular disease, orbital disease and central nervous system dysfunction. Myasthenia gravis may present in infancy and childhood with ptosis and ophthalmoplegia (Berkovitz *et al.* 1977). Juvenile myasthenia resembles the adult type, and may be associated with thyroid dysfunction. Neonatal myasthenia, due to cross-placental transfer of anti-acetylcholine receptor antibodies from a mother with the disease, is usually transient. Mitochondrial cytopathy may present in childhood with symmetrical ophthalmoplegia and ptosis (Land *et al.* 1981).

Orbital disease in childhood, such as metastatic neuroblastoma, usually presents as a mass lesion with proptosis, but may also mechanically restrict the eye movements. Orbital trauma in older children may produce a 'blow out' fracture with limited eye movements; the prognosis is poor in children, and although surgery to repair the orbital floor defect carried out after the initial swelling has subsided may be indicated, the results are not good (McGarry & Fells 1984).

Central nervous system disease must also be excluded before the diagnosis of peripheral ocular motor palsy is made. For example, skew deviation of any aetiology may mimic a vertical muscle palsy. Monocular elevation paresis (double elevator palsy) may be caused by a unilateral pretectal lesion (Jampel & Fells 1968); in this condition there is no ocular deviation in the primary position or downgaze, no ptosis and normal pupils, but defective upgaze in both adduction and abduction (Metz 1981). Divergence paralysis with raised intracranial pressure produces the signs of a mild bilateral VIth nerve palsy and may be the same condition (Kirkham *et al.* 1972).

Third nerve

CONGENITAL PALSY

This is certainly a rare condition (Victor 1976). Unilateral cases only are described in the literature. The clinical features are ptosis, (Fig. 45.9a-c) and exotropia with variable involvement of IIIrd nerve innervated extraocular muscles producing reduced adduction, elevation and depression (Victor 1976, Miller 1977). The pupil although usually large may be smaller than the normal size, although the smallness has never satisfactorily been explained (Lotufo *et al.* 1983), and

was present in only 2 out of 12 cases in Victor's series, seven having larger pupils (Victor 1976). Amblyopia on the affected side is almost invariable.

Many cases develop signs of abnormal re-innervation (Fig. 45.9 d-f) superimposed on limited normal re-innervation, either oculomotor synkinesis ('misdirection regeneration') or cyclic spasms of oculomotor function. These two disorders appear clinically to be closely related; they both consist of elevation of the lid (and failure of inhibition of the levator on downgaze) and miosis, which either occurs predictably on adduction (oculomotor synkinesis) or unpredictably, but often triggered by attempted adduction (oculomotor spasms). Other precipitants of oculomotor spasms, which are shortlived, lasting seconds to half a minute, are fixing with the affected eye and attempted downgaze. They also occur spontaneously, and in sleep (Loewenfeld & Thompson 1975). The condition, although rare, is probably commoner than was formerly appreciated since Fells & Collin (1979) diagnosed nine cases over a 4-year-period. It may also develop after a IIIrd nerve palsy acquired in the first 2 years of life. The mechanism is obscure, but the clinical features imply a supranuclear abnormality; the close resemblance to oculomotor synkinesis suggests that this, too, is probably due to a similar supranuclear control mechanism based on more sustained neuronal circuitry. Since oculomotor synkinesis in acquired palsy develops following peripheral IIIrd nerve trauma, either in head injury or from tumours or aneurysm, the implication is that congenital IIIrd nerve palsy is due to peripheral trauma. This is supported by associations with birth trauma (Victor 1976), long tract signs (4/10 cases) or generalized developmental delay (2/10 cases) (Balkan & Hoyt 1984). Other, more unusual aetiologies include infarction of the IIIrd nerve nucleus in a child who did not survive (Norman 1974), and nuclear aplasia.

Another, rare variant of a supranuclear disorder involving IIIrd nerve innervated structures is congenital medial rectus palsy with associated divergence of the affected eye on attempted adduction (Wilcox *et al.* 1981; Wagner *et al.* 1987).

Management

Because of the associated neurological abnormalities, all cases should be assessed by a paediatrician. Amblyopia must be treated with patching, which may be combined with the use of low concentration (0.1%) pilocarpine, which, by mediating accomodation, will bring the child into focus for near objects. Surgical

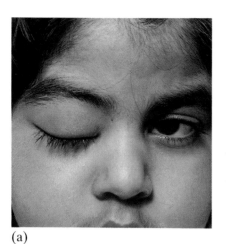

(a)

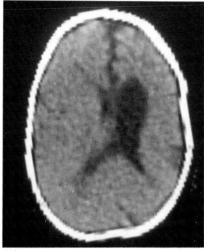

(b)

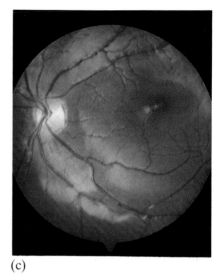

(c)

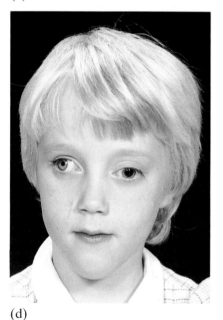

(d)

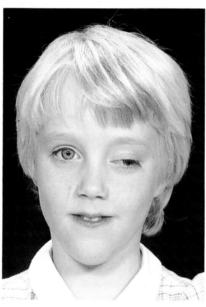

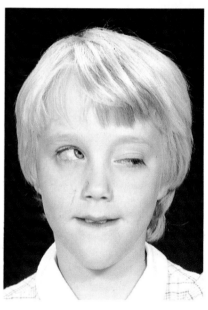

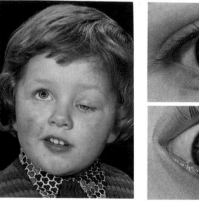

(e)

Fig. 45.9 (a) Right IIIrd nerve palsy, associated with, (b) a porencephalic cyst. The left optic disc (c) shows band atrophy reflecting the left homonymous hemianopia from right optic tract involvement. (d) Third nerve palsy with aberrant regeneration, causing relative lid elevation on adduction. The cause was 'ophthalmoplegic migraine' and after a further episode the aberrant regeneration was abolished. (e) Congenital IIIrd nerve palsy with smaller pupil on the affected side (see text).

treatment will be needed, and if the eye is markedly exotropic, should be carried out early (e.g. during the second year) to allow it to be used during occlusion treatment without a gross head turn. It is important for the parents to appreciate that normal eye movements can never be achieved, but it is usually possible to centre the eye in the orbit in the primary position. The ptosis is not usually severe enough to require nearly treatment to enable patching to be effective. If it does require treatment at a late stage, the lid should be raised cautiously, as Bell's phenomenon may be defective, and corneal exposure may become a problem.

ACQUIRED PALSY

The important consideration in this group is the aetiology; the clinical features vary according to the extent of IIIrd nerve involvement, and the associated symptoms according to the underlying cause. The important differential diagnosis, if the pupil is not involved, is myasthenia gravis which may present in infancy or childhood (Berkovitz *et al.* 1977).

Closed head trauma is a potent cause of IIIrd nerve palsy at all ages, and the commonest single cause (six cases) in Miller's series of 17 acquired childhood cases. Trauma alone may not be a sufficient explanation, however, and if a IIIrd nerve palsy follows minor head injury without loss of consciousness or skull fracture, neuroradiological investigation (CT scan) is indicated. Three patients with parasellar or clivus tumours presented with a IIIrd nerve palsy in such circumstances, the nerve being stretched over the tumours (Eyster *et al.* 1972).

Infection was the next commonest cause in Miller's series (4/17). Thirteen of 147 cases of bacterial meningitis caused by haemophilus influenzae, neisseria meningitidis, and streptococcus pneumonia had IIIrd nerve palsies (a different 13 had VIth nerve palsies), all of which recovered fully on treatment, unlike nerve deafness in meningitis (Dodge & Swartz 1965). Other infectious agents described include varicella (Sharf & Hyams 1972) in which the pupil may be involved, infections mononucleosis (Nellhaus 1966) and tuberculosis.

Tumours may present as an isolated IIIrd nerve palsy; this has been described in craniopharyingioma (Hoff & Patterson 1972) leptomeningeal sarcoma (Miller 1976) and as a complication of enlargement of the third ventricle associated with intracranial tumour (Osher *et al.* 1978). Although intracranial aneurysms can occur in early childhood (Matson 1965; Patel & Richardsons 1971), the earliest ages at which posterior communicating artery aneurysm has caused isolated, pupil involved, IIIrd nerve palsies is 16 and 17 (Miller 1977).

Charcot coined the phrase 'ophthalmoplegic migraine' in 1890, and large numbers of cases were described by Mobius and Ehlers (Alpers & Yaskin 1951). These early cases were diagnosed clinically, however, and it is now clear that the symptoms and signs can result from many causes, so that full neuroradiological investigation is mandatory. The condition presents with pain in or above the eye, sometimes with vomiting, for 24–48 hours; as the pain lessens, the eyelids droops, the eye becomes exotropic and the pupil dilates over the next 24–48 hours. The palsy recovers over the next 3 days to 1 month (Bickerstaff 1964). The condition may be recurrent, either on the same or opposite side; the first attack almost always occurs before the age of 12, and it is commoner in boys. There may be a family history of migraine (it has also been described in siblings) (Van Pelt & Andermann 1964), and the first attack may be in infancy (Fig. 45.9c).

The aetiology is uncertain; carotid angiography following the onset of the palsy has been described as normal (Alpers & Yaskin 1951) or showing narrowing of the intracavernous carotid artery (Walsh & O'Doherty 1960). It has been suggested that the intracavernous vasa nervorum to the IIIrd nerve are in spasm or blocked, that the nerve is compressed by oedema of the intracavernous carotid, or that the increased cerebral volume that may accompany migraine compresses the nerve (Harrington & Flocks 1953). The recognition of the development of oculomotor synkinesis after migrainous ophthalmoplegia (O'Day *et al.* 1980) supports the suggestion of a peripheral (probably microvascular) aetiology.

Despite extensive investigation including arteriography and CT scanning, some cases of acquired IIIrd nerve palsy in childhood remain unexplained (Mizen *et al.* 1985). Characteristically, there is no recovery of function in these cases.

The pattern of recovery in acquired IIIrd nerve palsy depends largely on the cause, and varies from complete, to incomplete with or without oculomotor synkinesis or, if the onset was in infancy, cyclic spasm.

Management

The management begins with patching to prevent or treat amblyopia. Spontaneous recovery must be allowed for before surgery is contemplated, and stable orthoptic measurements for at least 6 months must be obtained. The operation needed will depend on the extent of recovery, and whether or not there is a vertical as well as horizontal component. In cases with oculomotor synkinesis and lid elevation in adduction, the abnormal movements can be used to advantage, by recessing the lateral and resecting the medial rectus of the contralateral (normal) eye. This effectively treats both the horizontal strabismus and the ptosis on the affected side. Unusually large recessions and resections are usually required when surgery is on the affected eye.

Fourth nerve

CONGENITAL PALSY

A congenital or very early onset IVth nerve palsy becomes apparent when the infant is old enough to have developed head control (2–4 months). It is usually unilateral. The characteristic turn and tilt of the head away from the side of the lesion is then adopted in the interests of binocularity. The demonstration of a vertical strabismus when the head is straightened, and elevation of the affected eye when the head is tilted to that side in the Beilschowsky head tilt test (Fig. 45.10) are possible by the age of 6 months (Reynolds *et al*. 1984). The differential diagnosis of torticollis in infancy includes disorders of the sternomastoid and cervical spine, hemianopias and other eye movement disorders such as nystagmus, oculomotor apraxia, and Brown's and Duane's syndromes.

When the child is old enough to allow full eye movement testing, the underaction of the superior oblique and consequent overaction of ipsilateral inferior oblique and contralateral inferior rectus become evident. A large vertical fusion range will be demonstrable. The aetiology is uncertain; some cases may be familial, and there do not seem to be any associated neurological or developmental defects. Patients with Goldenhar's syndrome may have a congenital IVth nerve palsy due to agenesis of the nucleus (Aleksic *et al*. 1976).

Some apparently unilateral cases are in fact bilateral (Reynolds *et al*. 1984). Scott and Kraft (1986) found that a third of their cases were bilateral, but often highly asymmetric, with the lesser affected eye masked by the contralateral hypertropia.

Management

Provided the child remains binocular and does not have a gross head posture, surgical treatment can be delayed until it is possible to assess the visual system fully orthoptically. An ipsilateral inferior oblique recession is the best treatment, but sometimes a superior oblique tuck is also necessary. Bilateral cases need to be detected and treated with bilateral surgery in the first instance (Kushner 1988).

ACQUIRED PALSY

Acquired IVth nerve palsy is usually bilateral; the physical signs, apart from underaction of the superior oblique muscles, consist of a V pattern of eye movement with esotropia, and increasing excyclotorsion in down gaze. Patients therefore adopt a head posture of chin depression to achieve binocularity. The differential diagnosis includes alternating skew deviation, in which a vertical strabismus, with the adducting eye higher, develops on lateral gaze, and the V pattern due to bilateral inferior oblique 'overaction' seen in concomitant strabismus (see above).

The commonest cause is closed head trauma; if there is no history of trauma, full neurological examination and investigation is indicated, since posterior fossa tumours may present this way. Surgical treatment must be deferred until spontaneous recovery has stopped; bilateral advancement of the anterior half of the superior oblique tendons corrects the excyclotorsion and increases depression in adduction, reducing the V pattern. A bilateral palsy is frequently asymmetric.

Sixth nerve

CONGENITAL PALSY

The commonest form of congenital lateral rectus palsy is Duane's syndrome, considered in more detail above. Diagnostic features include familial occurrence and increased frequency in girls than boys, and on the left rather than right side. Transient unilateral lateral rectus palsies in newborn infants were first recognized in 1962 (Benson 1962). Subsequent reports have established that the condition is benign and not associated with either other neurological or developmental abnormalities, or strabismus in childhood. It may be relatively common, but not often detected (Reisner *et al*. 1971) with figures of one in 182 and one in 124 normal neonates quoted (de Grauw *et al*. 1983).

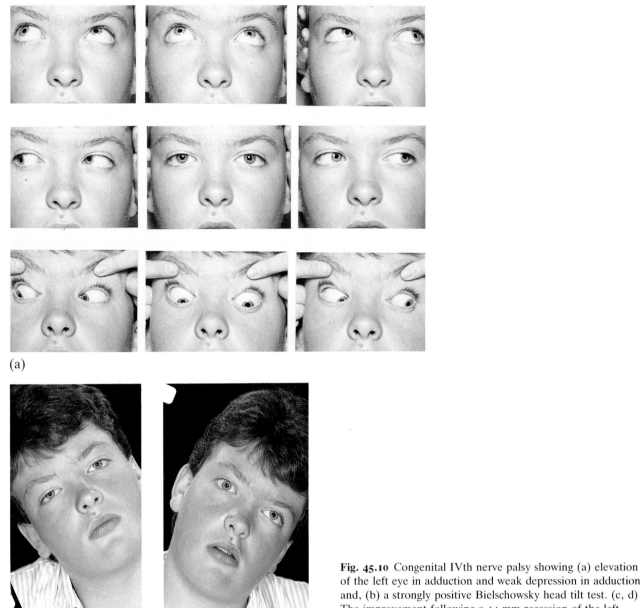

(a)

(b)

Fig. 45.10 Congenital IVth nerve palsy showing (a) elevation of the left eye in adduction and weak depression in adduction and, (b) a strongly positive Bielschowsky head tilt test. (c, d) The improvement following a 14 mm recession of the left inferior oblique.

Curiously, it is commoner on the right side; typically the pregnancy is normal, but the delivery is more likely to have been by forceps than in normal neonates. The full recovery with normal binocularity suggests that it is a peripheral lesion. Normal neonates who show this abnormality should have a full medical and neurological examination, but if this is normal, may not need further investigation, and should be treated expectantly.

ACQUIRED PALSY

Dependent on the age of the child, acquired abduction deficit in childhood will present with a head turn away from the palsied muscle (if unilateral) or double vision (unilateral or bilateral palsies), worse for distance fixation. The child may not complain of double vision, but be seen to shut one eye, for example when watching television. Alternatively, parents may notice the sudden onset of a convergent strabismus. Associated symptoms such as headache, drowsiness, or earache may give important aetiological clues.

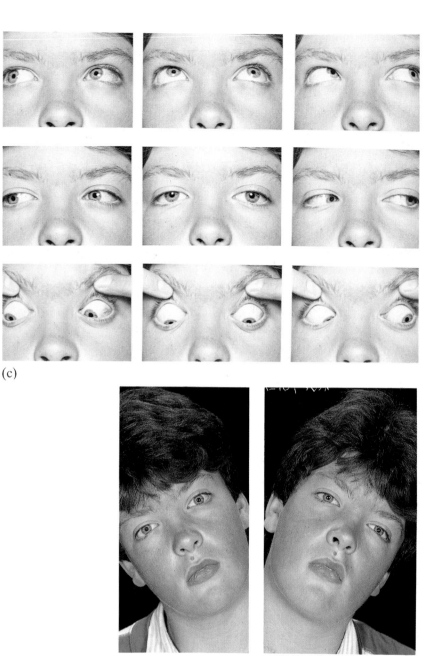

Fig. 45.10 *Cont.*

(c)

(d)

If hydrocephalus is excluded, the commonest single cause appears to be a tumour, (Robertson *et al.* 1970) and amongst tumours, pontine glioma is predominant. Lateral rectus palsy is the commonest presentation of this tumour which occurs at an average age of 6.5 years. Brainstem gliomas are amongst the commonest central nervous system tumours of childhood and adolescence (Panitch & Berg 1970) and may produce unilateral or bilateral VIth nerve palsy, rarely a IIIrd nerve palsy. Benedikt's syndrome (IIIrd nerve palsy with contralateral ataxia and tremor due to destruction of the cerebello-rubro-thalamic tract) or Weber's syndrome (IIIrd nerve palsy with contralateral hemiparesis) may develop. The abduction deficit is usually progressive, and may evolve into a gaze palsy (Bucy & Keplinger 1959). Pyramidal signs and other cranial nerve palsies, most frequently facial palsy, develop thereafter (Bray *et al.* 1958). Thirty five percent of cases develop papilloedema at some stage. By contrast, metastatic neuroblastoma, which may cause an isolated lateral rectus palsy in its early stages, presents in children under the age of three. Other primary intracranial tumours, in the posterior fossa particularly, may present with raised intracranial pressure which produces papilloedema and bilateral abduction deficit. In these cases, as with IIIrd nerve palsy, minor head trauma may precipitate the palsy (Robertson *et al.* 1970). A lateral rectus palsy has been described as the presenting sign in orbital rhabdomyosarcoma (Sananman & Weintraub 1971).

Head injury is the next commonest cause reported (Robertson *et al.* 1970). Brainstem injury may produce associated signs such as VIIth nerve palsy (Fig. 45.11). Benign intracranial hypertension can present in childhood, either in its idiopathic form, or secondary to middle ear disease and cerebral venous sinus thrombosis, or drugs. Those incriminated include tetracycline (Maroon & Mealy 1971), nalidixic acid (Cohen 1973) and steroids (Cohen 1973).

Infection is another relatively common cause, and lateral rectus palsy may occur in bacterial meningitis (Dodge & Swartz 1965) and has been described in varicella (Nemet *et al.* 1974). Vascular causes are unusual in the paediatric age group, although an arterio- venous malformation has been incriminated (Robertson *et al.* 1970) and micro vascular disease in the second decade (Moster *et al.* 1984).

In some cases, no cause may be established, yet full recovery occurs. Such benign VIth nerve palsies in childhood were first recognized in 1967 (Knox *et al.* 1967) when 12 cases, aged 18 months to 15 years at presentation were described. The features are now well established: the palsy is isolated, painless, and resolves spontaneously within 8–12 weeks. Investigation, including CT scanning and CSF examination is normal. The original cases were described as following a viral illness with fever and upper respiratory tract infection, and accompanying peripheral blood lymphocytosis. The condition has also been described following immunization, for example for rubella, rubeola and mumps (Werner *et al.* 1983) or occurring without an identifiable precipitant (Boger *et al.* 1984). It may be recurrent (Bixenman & Von Noorden 1981) usually ipsilaterally (Boger *et al.* 1984) and occur in infants as young as 2 1/2 months. Recovery may be incomplete especially after multiple recurrences, and extraocular muscle surgery may be necessary (Bixenman & Von Noorden 1981). Amblyopia may develop during the period of palsy, and prophylactic patching is advisable (Scharf & Zonis 1975).

The aetiology is obscure, and both microvascular (arteritic) and primary demyelinating pathologies have been proposed (Werner *et al.* 1983). It is a diagnosis of exclusion that is made retrospectively and after a

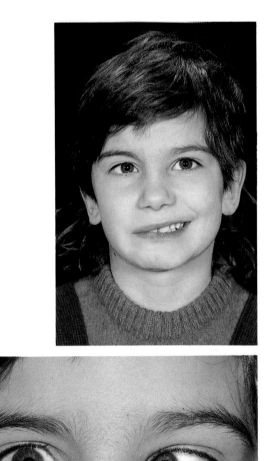

Fig. 45.11 Traumatic right VIth and VIIth nerve palsy.

period of close observation: full neurological examination and investigation are mandatory.

Amongst other causes of VIth nerve palsy in childhood are those that follow lumbar puncture, and in the older age group, those associated with multiple sclerosis and posterior fossa developmental abnormalities (Bixenman & Laguna 1987).

Management

The management depends on the underlying cause; once this is established, the natural history becomes clearer, and the extent of spontaneous recovery more predictable. Patching to prevent amblyopia, or the teaching of a head posture to maintain binocularity may be all that is necessary. If full recovery does not occur, surgery is necessary; if near full abduction returns, with a normal abducting saccadic velocity but a persistent esotropia, binocularity can be regained either by recession of the medial and resection of the lateral rectus, or by an injection of botulinum toxin into the medial rectus. If an injection is used, a short period of exotropia must be expected (Elston & Lee 1985).

In unrecovered lateral rectus palsy, because of the secondary overaction of both the ipsilateral and contralateral medial rectus muscles, a large esotropia is produced, and the treatment objective becomes more limited; the re-establishment of binocularity in the primary position and downgaze. It is necessary to redistribute the forces generated by the extraocular muscles on the affected side, and to provide an adducting vector by a full vertical muscle temporal transfer together with recession of the medial rectus. Botulinum toxin injection of the medial rectus may be helpful in such cases (Fitzsimmons et al. 1988).

COMBINATIONS OF IIIRD, IVTH AND VITH NERVE PALSIES

If isolated ocular motor nerve palsies are rare in childhood, a review of the available literature suggests that combinations of palsies are extremely unusual. The differential diagnosis includes conditions discussed above and considered in more detail later such as myasthenia gravis and mitochondrial cytopathy. Fisher's syndrome of ophthalmoplegia, ataxia and areflexia may occur in childhood, with the youngest reported case at 22 months (Marks et al. 1977). Six of the 8 cases of less than 18 years discussed by these authors had internal as well as external ophthalmoplegia, but relative sparing of the levator is characteristic, and argues against the condition being exclusively a peripheral neuropathy. Increased CSF protein without cells is characteristic, and in children the condition appears to have a benign course with complete recovery.

Combinations of ocular motor palsies are most commonly due to lesions in the cavernous sinus or superior orbital fissure. Clinical differentiation between these two sites is difficult, and they are best regarded together as the sphenocavernous syndrome. This consists of a IIIrd, IVth, and VIth nerve palsy with involvement of the first and, in the cavernous sinus, second division of the Vth (trigeminal) nerve. There may also be involvement of the oculosympathe-

tic nerve, and sometimes an optic neuropathy; proptosis may develop. Apart from double vision, pain is often a prominent symptom. Subtle pupillary signs including sinuous pupil reactions and supersensitivity to 0.1% pilocarpine occur (Slamovits et al. 1987).

The sphenocavernous syndrome has been described in childhood most frequently due to rhabdomyosarcoma (Sananaman & Weintraub 1971; Takahash et al. 1982). Other causes include a primary intrasellar germinoma that evolved into a choriocarcinoma (Guiffre & Lorenzo 1975) and hystiocytosis X (Beller & Kornbleuth 1951). The rarity of ocular motor nerve involvement in this condition, however, has been emphasized (Moore et al. 1985). Burkitt's lymphoma which is rare in developed countries presents at an average age of 11.5 years with abdominal involvement; it has however, been described as causing bilateral total external ophthalmoplegia by extension from the ethmoid sinus (Trese et al. 1980). A craniopharyngioma can rarely invade the cavernous sinus and produce ocular motor palsies (Neetens & Selosse 1977).

The orbital apex syndrome differs from the above in presenting with proptosis, optic neuropathy, and (at least initially) mechanical limitation of eye movement. Other signs, such as oculo sympathetic involvement and conjunctival oedema frequently develop. Secondary neuroblastoma and other metastatic disease (e.g. leukaemia) are the commonest causes in childhood.

Neuromuscular disease and incomitant strabismus in infancy and childhood

A number of neuromuscular disorders, including myopathies, muscular dystrophies, mitochondrial cytopathy and myasthenia gravis may involve the extraocular muscles and levator in infancy and childhood. The differential diagnosis, which may also include the fibrosis syndrome and combinations of IIIrd, IVth, and VIth nerve palsies, may be difficult and depends on the clinical features and family history as well as muscle enzyme studies, electromyography and muscle biopsy.

Amongst congenital myopathies, which produce muscle weakness and hypotonia, congenital fibre type disproportion (CFTD) may rarely be associated with exotropia, ophthalmoplegia and ptosis from birth (Owen et al. 1981). Centronuclear myopathy, a familial cause of generalized muscle weakness, is consistently associated with ptosis and external ophthalmoplegia in the survivors to the second decade (Bradley et al.

1970). Visually insignificant mid cortical cataracts have also been reported in this condition (Hawkes & Absolon 1975).

The eye movements are normal in both congenital and Duchenne muscular dystrophy, although there may be orbicularis oculi weakness in both (Honda & Yoshioka 1978). Myotonic dystrophy, however, may present in infancy or childhood with either ptosis (including eyelid myotonia) or more often reduced eye movements (Dodge et al. 1965). Such cases have been misdiagnosed as Möbius' syndrome; the family history and examination of relatives may be important in making the correct diagnosis.

In the whistling face, or Freeman–Sheldon syndrome, there is a high incidence of strabismus and ptosis; the extraocular muscles are stiff on forced duction testing (O'Keefe et al. 1986). The children have many other features attributable to increased muscle tone including a small mouth which may make anaesthesia hazardous. They are usually of normal intelligence and the inheritance is autosomal dominant.

Mitochondrial cytopathy has diverse neuromuscular and central nervous system manifestations. The onset is in the first or second decade in the majority of cases, characteristically with progressive external ophthalmoplegia and limb weakness on exertion. Ptosis is also a common presenting symptom (Petty et al. 1986). A pigmentary retinopathy is not usually prominent in childhood, but electrodiagnostic studies may be abnormal.

The younger the age at presentation, the more likely the patient is to develop systemic abnormalities such as cardiac conduction defects, generalized hypotonia, cerebellar ataxia, endocrine abnormalities, (e.g. diabetes mellitus) and retinal pigmentation (Mitsumoto et al. 1983). A family history suggesting mitochondrial inheritance may be helpful in making the diagnosis. Muscle biopsy (including extra ocular muscle biopsy) will show ragged red fibres (Ringel et al. 1979).

Myasthenia gravis is rare in the first decade; neonatal myasthenia, due to cross placental transfer of anti-acetylcholine receptor antibodies, occurs in approximately one in seven children of myasthenic mothers, and, recovers spontaneously in 1–12 weeks. Congenital myasthenia has the same clinical characteristics, but occurs in the absence of antibodies and is commoner in boys than girls. It may be inherited as an autosomal recessive trait in some cases. Unlike the juvenile variant (see below) it shows no tendency to remit, and may be due to a different disease process (Simpson 1981).

Juvenile myasthenia, with onset before 17 years, (Fig. 45.12) occurs nearly five times more commonly in girls than boys; the spontaneous remission rate is high (30% by 15 years of follow-up) and higher after thymectomy (Rodrigues et al. 1983).

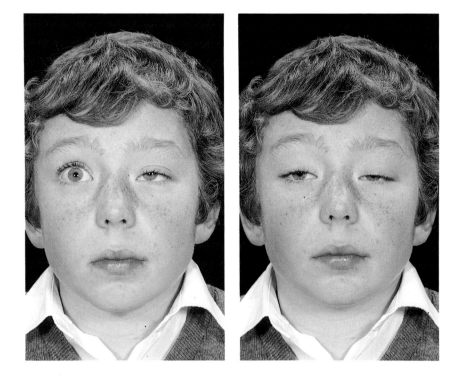

Fig. 45.12 Myasthenia with variable ptosis, squint, and orbicularis weakness. Photographs taken 10 min apart.

Rarely, other diseases may produce an ophthalmoplegia; in a-beta-lipoproteinaemia, for example, mild ptosis, and exotropia may be the presenting signs (Yee *et al.* 1976).

Head trauma and incomitant strabismus

Trauma is a common and largely preventable cause of mortality and morbidity in childhood. Children arc injured in road traffic accidents both as pedestrians and as unrestrained back seat passengers: they may be injured at play (e.g. falling from a tree) or occasionally deliberately by their parents or others responsible for their care. Various types of incomitant strabismus may result.

Closed head injury with or without skull fracture may cause a complete IIIrd nerve palsy; the injury is usually severe, and may be associated with prolonged loss of consciousness and other neurological signs (Elston 1984). Bilateral IVth nerve palsies follow less severe head injuries, often without loss of conciousness, when the head is flexed on the neck. The IVth nerve roots are avulsed from the superior medullary velum. The diagnosis is difficult to make on eye movement testing and frequently missed; measurements of ocular torsion are necessary to distinguish a unilateral from a bilateral IVth nerve palsy. Sixth nerve damage may result directly from trauma, or develop secondary to raised intracranial pressure.

Concomitant strabismus (usually esotropia) may also be precipitated by closed head trauma; any case, however, in which there is an inconsistency between the severity of the reported trauma and the subsequent physical signs should be investigated neuroradiologically. A predisposing lesion may be responsible.

Facial trauma may also cause strabismus. In a blow out fracture, anterior orbital trauma results in a fracture of either the medial wall or orbital floor, with displacement of orbital contents. There is enophthalmos and limitation of eye movement due to trapping of either the extraocular muscles or their associated fascia in the fracture. Extraocular muscle dysfunction may also be due to intramuscular haemorrhage, in which case spontaneous recovery may be expected, or traumatic denervation. Whereas in adults, spontaneous improvement is the rule, in children this is not the case, and early surgery to free trapped tissue is advised, but may not be successful (McGarry & Fells 1984).

References

Aleksic S, Budzilovich G, Choy A *et al.* Congenital ophthalmoplegia in oculoauriculo vertebral dysplasia — hemifacial microsomia (Goldenhar—Gorbin syndrome). *Neurology* 1976; **26**: 638−44

Alpers BJ, Yaskin EH. Pathogenesis of ophthalmoplegic migraine. *Arch Ophthalmol* 1951; **45**: 555−66

Apt L, Axelrod RN. Extra-ocular muscle fibrosis. *Am J Ophthalmol* 1978; **85**: 822−9

Balkan R, Hoyt CS. Associated neurologic abnormalities in congenital third nerve palsies. *Am J Ophthalmol* 1984; **97**: 315−9

Baraitser M. Genetics of Mobius syndrome. *J Med Genetics* 1977; **14**: 415−7

Beller AJ, Kornbleuth W. Eosisophilic granuloma of the orbit. *Br J Ophthalmol* 1951; **35**: 220−5

Berkovitz S, Beklin M, Tenenbaum A. Childhood myasthemia gravis. *J Pediatr Ophthalmol* 1977; **14**: 269−73

Benson PF. Transient unilateral external rectus muscle palsy in newborn infants. *Br Med J* 1962; **1**: 1054−5

Bickerstaff ER. Ophthalmoplegic migraine. *Rev Neurol* 1964; **110**: 582−7

Biedner B, Monos T, Frilling F, Mozeo M, Yassur Y. Acquired Brown's syndrome caused by frontal sinus osteoma. *J Pediatr Ophthalmol Strabismus* 1988; **25**: 226−30

Bixenman WW, Laguna JF. Acquired esotropia as initial manifestation of Arnold-Chiari Malformation. *J Pediatr Ophthalmol Strabismus* 1987; **24**: 83−6

Bixenman WW, Von Noorden GK. Benign recurrent sixth nerve palsy in childhood. *J Pediatr Ophthalmol Strabismus* 1981; **18**: 29−34

Boger WP, Puliafito CA, Magoon EH, Syndnor CF, Knupp JA, Buckley EG. Recurrent isolated sixth nerve palsy in children. *Ann Ophthalmol* 1984; **16**: 237−44

Bradley WG, Price DL, Watanabe CK. Familial centronuclear myopathy. *J Neurol Neurosurg Psychiatry* 1970; **33**: 687−93

Bray PF, Carter S, Taveras JM. Brainstem tumours in children. *Neurology* 1958; **8**: 1−7

Brown HW. True and simulated superior oblique tendon sheath syndromes. *Doc Ophthalmol* 1973; **34**: 123−36

Bucy PC, Keplinger JE. Tumours of the brain stem with special reference to ocular manifestations. *Arch Ophthalmol* 1959; **62**: 541−54

Catford GV. A familial musculo-fascial anomaly. *Trans Ophthalmol Soc UK* 1966; **86**: 19−36

Cohn GA. Pseudotumour cerebri in children secondary to administration of adrenal steroids. *J Neurosurg* 1963; **20**: 784−6

Cohen DN. Intracranial hypertension and papilloedema associated with nalidixic acid therapy. *Am J Ophthalmol* 1973; **76**: 680−2

Crawford JS. Congenital fibrosis syndrome. *Can J Ophthalmol* 1970; **5**: 331−6

Cross HE, Pfaffenback DD. Duane's retraction syndrome and associated congenital abnormalities. *Am J Ophthalmol* 1972; **73**: 442−50

de Grauw AJC, Rotteveel JJ, Cruyserg JRM. Transient sixth cranial nerve paralysis in the newborn infant. *Neuropediatrics* 1983; **14**: 164−5

Dodge PK, Gamsford I, Byers RK, Russell P. Myotonic dystrophy in infancy and childhood. *Paediatrics* 1965; **35**: 3−19

Dodge PK, Swartz MN. Bacterial meningitis — a review of selected aspects. *N Engl J Med* 1965; **272**: 954−60

Duane A. Congenital deficiency of abduction, associated with impairment of adduction, retraction movements, contraction of the palpebral fissure and oblique movements of the eye. *Arch Ophthalmol* 1905; **34**: 133−59

Dulley B, Fells P. Long term follow-up of orbital blow-out fractures with and without surgery. In: Ravalt AP, Lenz M (Eds.) *Orbital Disorder*, Proceedings of the 2nd International Symposium. Karger, Basel 1975; **14**: 467−70

Elston JS. Traumatic third nerve palsy. *Br J Ophthalmol* 1984; **68**: 538−43

Elston JS, Lee JP. Paralytic strabismus: the role of botulinium toxin. *Br J Ophthalmol* 1985; **69**: 891−6

Eyster EP, Hoyt WF, Wilson CB. Oculomotor palsy from minor head trauma. *J Am Med Assoc* 1972; **220**: 1082−6

Fells P, Collin JRO. Cyclic oculomotor palsy. *Trans Ophthalmol Soc UK* 1979; **99**: 192−6

Fells P, Waddell E, Alvarez M. Progressive, exaggerated A-pattern strabismus with presumed fibrosis of extraocular muscles. In: Reinecke RD (ed.) *Strabismus II: Proceedings of the Fourth Meeting of the International Strabismological Association*. Grune & Stratton, Orlando 1984; 335−43

Fitzsimmons R, Lee JP, Elston JS. Treatment of unrecovered VIth nerve palsy with combined botulinium toxin chemodenervation and surgery. *Ophthalmology* 1988; **95**: 1535−42

Gobin MH. Surgical management of Duane's syndrome. *Br J Ophthalmol* 1974; **58**: 301−6

Guiffre R, Lorenzo ND. Evolution of a primary intrasellar germinomatons teratoma into a choriocarcinoma. *J Neurosurg* 1975; **42**: 602−4

Hanson PA, Rowland LP. Mobius syndrome and facio-seapulo-humeral dystrophy. *Arch Neurol* 1971; **24**: 31−9

Harrington DO, Flocks M. Ophthalmoplegic migraine. *Arch Ophthalmol* 1953; **40**: 643−55

Hawkes CH, Absolon MJ. Myotubular myopathy associated with cataract and electrical myotonia. *J Neurol Neurosurg Psychiatry* 1975; **38**: 761−4

Henderson JL. The congenital facial diplegia syndrome: clinical features, pathology and aetiology. *Brain* 1939; **62**: 381−403

Hoff JT, Patterson RH. Craniopharyngiomas in children and adults. *J Neurosurg* 1972; **36**: 299−302

Honda Y, Yoshioka M. Ophthalmological findings of muscular dystrophies: A survey of 53 cases. *J Pediatr Ophthalmol Strabismus* 1978; **15**: 236−8

Hotchkiss MD, Miller NR, Clark AW, Green WR. Bilateral Duane's retraction syndrome: a clinicopathologic case report. *Arch Ophthalmol* 1980; **98**: 870−4

Hoyt WF, Nachtigaller H. Anomalies of ocular motor nerves. *Am J Ophthalmol* 1965; **70**: 443−8

Huber A. Electrophysiology of the retraction syndromes. *Br J Ophthalmol* 1974; **58**: 293−300

Isenberg S, Urist MJ. Clinical observations in 101 consecutive patients with Duane's retraction syndrome. *Am J Ophthalmol* 1977; **84**: 419−25

Jampel RS, Fells P. Monocular elevation palsy caused by a central nervous system lesion. *Arch Ophthalmol* 1968; **80**: 45−57

Jay W, Hoyt CS. Abnormal brain stem auditary evoked potentials in Stilling-Turk-Duane retraction syndrome. *Am J Ophthalmol* 1980; **89**: 814−8

Kirkham TH. Duane's syndrome and familial perceptive deafness. *Br J Ophthalmol* 1969; **53**: 335−9

Kirkham TH. Inheritance of Duane's syndrome. *Br J Ophthalmol* 1970; **54**: 323−9

Kirkham TH, Bird AC, Sanders MD. Divergence paralysis with raised intracranial pressure. *Br J Ophthalmol* 1972; **56**: 776−82

Knox DL, Clark DB, Schuster FF. Benign VI nerve palsies in children. *Pediatrics* 1967; **40**: 560−4

Kraft SP. A surgical approach for Duane's syndrome. *J Pediatr Ophthalmol Strabismus* 1988; **25**: 119−31

Kushner BJ. The diagnosis and treatment of bilateral masked superior oblique palsy. *Am J Ophthalmol* 1988; **105**: 186−95

Land JM, Hockaday JM, Hughes JT, Ross BD. Childhood mitochondrial myopathy with ophthalmoplegia. *J Neurol Sci* 1981; **51**: 371−82

Loewenfeld IE, Thompson HS. Oculomotor palsy with cyclic spasms. A critical review of the literature and a new case. *Surv Ophthalmol* 1975; **20**: 81−124

Lotufo DG, Smith JL, Hopen GR, Pollard F. The pupil in congenital 3rd nerve misdirection syndrome. *J Clin Neuro-Ophthalmol* 1983; **3**: 193−5

Marks HG, Augustyn P, Allen RJ. Fisher's syndrome in children. *Pediatrics* 1977; **60**: 726−9

Maroon JC, Mealy J. Benign intracranial hypertension. *JAMA* 1971; **216**: 1479−80

Matson DD. Intracranial aneurysms in childhood. *J Neurosurg* 1965; **23**: 578−83

Mather TR, Saunders RA. Congenital absence of the superior rectus muscle: A case report. *J Pediatr Ophthalmol Strabismus* 1987; **24**: 291−6

McGarry B, Fells P. Difficulties in the management of orbital blow-out fractures in patients under 20-years-old. In: Ravalt AP, Lenk M (Eds.) *Transaction of the Vth International Orthoptic Congress*, Lips, Lyon 1984; 283−7

Merz M, Wojtowicz S. The Mobius syndrome. *Am J Ophthalmol* 1967; **63**: 837−40

Metz HS. Double elevator palsy. *J Pediatr Ophthalmol Strabismus* 1981; **18**: 31−5

Miller NR. Isolated oculomotor nerve palsy in childhood from leptomeningeal polymorphic sarcoma. *J Pediatr Ophthalmol* 1976; **13**: 211−4

Miller NR. Solitary oculomotor nerve palsy in childhood. *Am J Ophthalmol* 1977; **83**: 106−111

Miller NR, Kiel SM, Green WR, Clark AW. Unilateral Duane's retraction syndrome (type I). *Arch Ophthalmol* 1982; **100**: 1468−72

Miller MT, Ray V, Owens P, Cheu F. Möbius and Möbius-like syndromes. *J Pediatr Ophthalmol Strabismus* 1989; **26**: 176−89

Mitsumoto H, Aprille JR, Wray SH, Nemni R, Bradley WG. Chronic progressive external ophthalmoplegic (CPEO) clinical morphological and biochemical studies. *Neurology (Cleveland)* 1983; **33**: 452−61

Mizen TR, Burde RM, Klingele TG. Cryptogenic Oculomotor nerve palsies in children. *Am J Ophthalmol* 1985; **100**: 65−7

Moore AT, Pritchard J, Taylor D. Histiocytosis X: an ophthalmological review. *Br J Ophthalmol* 1985; **69**: 7−14

Moore AT, Walker J, Taylor D. Familial Brown's syndrome. *J Pediatr Ophthalmol Strabismus* 1988; **25**: 202−4

Moster ML, Savino PJ, Sergott RC, Bosley TM, Schatz NJ. Isolated sixth-nerve palsies in younger adults. *Arch*

Ophthalmol 1984; **102**: 1328–30

Neetens A, Selosse P. Oculomotor anomalies in Sellar and Parasellar pathology. *Ophthalmologica (Basel)* 1977; **175**: 80–104

Nemet P, Ehlich D, Lazar M. Benign abducens palsy in varicella. *Am J Ophthalmol* 1974; **78**: 859

Nellhaus G. Isolated oculomotor nerve palsy in infections mononucleosis. *Neurology* 1966; **16**: 221–4

Norman MG. Unilateral encephalomalacia in cranial nerve nuclei in neonates: report of two cases. *Neurology* 1974; **24**: 424–7

O'Day J, Burston F, King J. Ophthalmolplegic migraine and aberrant regeneration of the oculomotor nerve. *Br J Ophthalmol* 1980; **64**: 534–6

O'Keefe M, Crawford JS, Young JDH, Macrae WG. Ocular abnormalities in the Freeman-Sheldon syndrome. *Am J Ophthalmol* 1986; **102**: 346–9

Osher RH, Corbett JJ, Schatz NJ, Savino PJ, Orr LS. Neuro-ophthalmological complications of enlargement of the third ventricle. *Br J Ophthalmol* 1978; **62**: 536–42

Owen JS, Kline LB, Oh SJ, Miles NE, Benton JW. Ophthalmoplegia and ptosis in congenital fiber type disproportion. *J Pediatr Ophthalmol Strabismus* 1981; **18**: 55–60

Panitch HS, Berg BD. Brain stem tumour of childhood and adolescence. *Am J Dis Child* 1970; **119**: 465–472

Parks MM, Sprague EH. Simultaneous superior oblique tenotomy and inferior oblique recession in Brown's syndrome. *J Am Acad Ophthalmol* 1987; **94**: 1043–7

Patel AN, Richardson AG. Ruptured intracranial aneurysms in the first two decades of life. *J Neurosurg* 1971; **35**: 571–3

Petty RKH, Harding AE, Morgan-Hughes JA. The clinical features of mitochondrial myopathy. *Brain* 1986; **109**: 915–38

Pfaffenbach DD, Cross HE, Kearns TP. Congenital anomalies in Duane's retraction syndrome. *Arch Ophthalmol* 1972; **88**: 635–9

Pruksacholawit K, Ishikawa A. A typical vertical retraction syndrome: a case study. *J Pediatr Ophthalmol* 1976; **13**: 215–20

Ramsay J, Taylor D. Congenital crocodile tears: a key to the aetiology of Duane's syndrome. *Br J Ophthalmol* 1980; **64**: 518–22

Reisner SH, Perlman M, Ben-Tovim N, Dubrawski C. Transient lateral rectus muscle paresis in the newborn infant. *J Pediatr* 1971; **78**: 461–5

Reynolds JD, Biglan AW, Hiles DA. Congenital superior oblique palsy in infants. *Arch Ophthalmol* 1984; **102**: 1503–5

Ringel SP, Wilson WB, Barden MT. Extra-ocular muscle biopsy in chronic progressive external ophthalmoplegia. *Ann Neurol* 1979; **6**: 326–39

Robb RN, Boger WP. Vertical strabismus associated with plagiocephaly. *J Pediatr Ophthalmol Strabismus* 1983; **20**: 58–62

Robertson DM, Hines JD, Rucker CW. Acquired sixth-nerve palsy in children. *Arch Ophthalmol* 1970; **83**: 574–9

Rodriguez M, Gomez MR, Howard FM, Taylor WF. Myasthenia gravis in children: long term follow-up. *Ann Neurol* 1983; **13**: 504–10

Rogers GL, Hatch GF, Gray I. Mobius syndrome and limb abnormalities. *J Pediatr Ophthalmol* 1977; **14**: 134–8

Rosenbaum AL, Jampolsky A. Pseudoparalysis caused by anomalous insertion of superior rectus muscle. *Arch*

Ophthalmol 1975; **93**: 535–7

Rush JA, Younge BR. Paralysis of cranial nerves III, IV and VI. Cause and prognosis in 1,000 cases. *Arch Ophthalmol* 1981; **99**: 76–9

Sananman ML, Weintraub MI. Remitting ophthalmoplegia due to rhabdomyosarcoma. *Arch Ophthalmol* 1971; **86**: 459–61

Sato SE, Ellis FD, Pinchoff BS, Helveston EM, Rummel JH. Superior oblique overaction in patients with true Brown's syndrome. *J Pediatr Ophthalmol Strabismus* 1987; **24**: 282–7

Scharf J, Zonis S. Benign abducers nerve palsy in childhood. *J Pediatr Ophthalmol* 1975; **12**: 165

Scott AB, Knapp P. Surgical treatment of the superior oblique tendon sheath syndrome. *Arch Ophthalmol* 1972; **88**: 282–6

Scott WE, Kraft SP. Classification and treatment of superior oblique palsy. *J Pediatr Ophthalmol Strabismus* 1986; **0**: 265–75

Scott AB, Wong GM. Duane's syndrome: an electromyographic study. *Arch Ophthalmol* 1972; **87**: 140–7

Sevel D. Brown's syndrome — a possible etiology explained embryologically. *J Pediatr Ophthalmol Strabismus* 1981; **18**: 26–31

Sharf B, Hyams S. Oculomotor palsy following varicella. *J Pediatric Ophthalmol* 1972; **9**: 245–7

Simpson JA. Myasthenia gravis and myasthenic syndromes. In: Walton J (ed.) *Disorders of Voluntary Muscle.* Churchill Livingstone, Edinburgh 1981; pp. 585–624

Slamovits TL, Miler NR, Burde RM. Intracranial oculomotor nerve paresis with anisocoria and pupillary parasympathetic hypersensitivity. *Am J Ophthalmol* 1987; **104**: 401–7

Slavin ML, Goodstein S. Acquired Brown's syndrome caused by focal metastasis to the superior oblique muscle. *Am J Ophthalmol* 1987; **103**: 598–9

Strachan IM, Brown BH. Electromyography of extraocular muscles in Duane's syndrome. *Br J Ophthalmol* 1972; **56**: 594–9

Takahash T, Murase TT, Isayama Y, Tamaki N, Fujiwara K, Matsumoto S. Rhabdomyosarcoma presenting as Garcia's syndrome. *Surg Neurol* 1982; **17**: 269–72

Thakkar N, O'Neil W, Duvally J, Liv C, Ambler M. Mobius syndrome due to brain stem tegmental necrosis. *Arch Neurol* 1977; **34**: 124–6

Timms C, Russell-Egitt I, Taylor D. Acquired Duane's syndrome. *Binocular Vision* 1989; **4**: 109–12

Towfighi J, Marks K, Palmer E, Vannucci R. Mobius syndrome: neuropathological observations. *Acta Neuropathol (Berl)* 1979; **48**: 11–17

Trese MT, Krohel GB, Hepler RS, Naeim F. Burkitt's lymphoma with cranial nerve involvement. *Arch Ophthalmol* 1980; **98**: 2015–7

Van Allen MW, Blodi FC. Neurological aspects of the Mobius syndrome. *Neurology* 1960; **10**: 249–59

Van Pelt W, Andermann F. On the early onset of ophthalmo plegic migraine. *Am J Dis Child* 1964; **107**: 628–31

Victor DI. The diagnosis of congenital unilateral third-nerve palsy. *Brain* 1976; **99**: 711–8

Von Noorden GK. Congenital hereditary ptosis with inferior rectus fibrosis. *Arch Ophthalmol* 1970; **83**: 378–80

Waddel E. Brown's syndrome revisited. *Br Orthopt J* 1982; **39**: 17–21

Wagner RS, Caputo AR, Frohman LP. Congenital unilateral adduction deficit with simultaneous abduction: A variant of Duane's Retraction syndrome. *Ophthalmology* 1987; **94**:

1049−54

Walsh JP, O'Doherty DS. A possible explanation of the mechanism of ophthalmoplegic migraine. *Neurology* 1960; **10**: 1079−84

Werner DB, Savino PJ, Schatz NJ. Benign recurrent sixth nerve palsies in childhood. *Arch Ophthalmol* 1983; **101**: 6073−8

Wilcox LM, Gittinger JW, Breinin GM. Congenital adduction palsy and synergistic divergence. *Am J Ophthalmol* 1981; **91**: 1−7

Wortham E, Crawford JS. Brown's syndrome in twins. *Am J Ophthalmol* 1988; **105**: 562−3

Yee RD, Cogan DG, Zee DS. Ophthalmoplegia and disassociated nystagmus in abetalipoproteinaemia. *Arch Ophthalmol* 1976; **94**: 571−5

Appendix — Problems

P1 Clinical Investigations of Bilateral Poor Vision From Birth

DAVID TAYLOR

When the eyes are found to be normal (Table P1.1) it is important to exclude 'pseudo blindness' as in delayed visual development or saccade palsies (the absence of rapid eye movements makes the baby appear blind). Babies with normal fundi can still be blind from such conditions as Leber's amaurosis, cone dysfunction syndromes, cerebral blindness (perinatal anoxia, meningitis, developmental anomalies or hydrocephalus), or high ametropia. The nystagmus may be primary, not due to eye disease, and this itself will give rise to poor vision.

When the fundus is thought to be normal it is most important to exclude the presence of optic nerve hypoplasia by a combination of direct and indirect ophthalmoscopy.

Abnormalities of the pupil reactions are useful in the clinical investigations of bilateral poor vision from birth. A paradoxical pupil (in which the pupil is larger in the light than in the dark) is indicative of retinal disease, whereas sluggishly reacting pupils indicate anterior visual pathway disease. A relative afferent pupil defect suggests there is asymmetrical anterior visual pathway disease.

A paediatric neurological consultation and further

Table P1.1 Common causes of poor vision in infancy with reportedly normal eyes.

	Ophthalmoscopy	Pupils	EEG	Flash ERG	Flash VEP	Pattern VEP	CT/MRI Scan	Slit lamp
DVM	Normal	Normal	Normal	Normal	Normal	Normal	Normal	Normal
Optic nerve hypoplasia	Abnormal but direct ophthalmoscopy essential	Afferent defect	Normal	Normal	Abnormal	Abnormal	Normal or Abnormal or Not usually indicated	Normal
Optic atrophy	Abnormal	Afferent defect	Normal unless associated brain diseases	Normal	Abnormal	Abnormal	Depends on cause	Normal
Cortical blindness	Normal	Normal	Often abnormal	Normal	Usually abnormal	Usually abnormal	Usually abnormal	Normal
Albinism	Abnormal	Normal	Normal	Normal	Cross-over defect		Not usually indicated	Iris transillumination
Cone dystrophy	Normal or abnormal	Normal or paradoxical	Normal	Abnormal	Abnormal	Abnormal	Normal or not usually indicated	Normal
Retinal dystrophy	Usually abnormal	Normal	Normal	Abnormal	Usually normal	Usually normal	Normal	Normal
Leber's amaurosis	Normal	Paradoxical	Normal	Very abnormal or absent	Abnormal	Absent		

investigations such as visually evoked responses, electroretinogram, CT scanning, and biochemistry are carried out where indicated. Invasive tests such as CT scanning should not be used unless positive information, which is going to influence management, is likely to be gained.

Figure P1.1 gives guidelines to follow.

The history of the child's prenatal, perinatal and postnatal development, and the history of the onset of the poor vision or of the age at which it was detected are vital in the clinical investigation of suspected poor vision from birth. A family history, including the presence of consanguinity and some general questions into the child's general developmental milestones, as well as the presence of any systemic abnormalities such as seizures and the medications that the child

may be on for these is most important. The visual assessment of the child is carried out in the usual way.

Examination of the external eyes will reveal the presence of nystagmus or squint and the anterior segment of the eye can be inspected both by the naked eye and with the use of the slit lamp to exclude such conditions as albinism, cataract, corneal abnormalities, etc.

It is vital that every patient is refracted since high ametropia can give rise to poor vision from early in life.

The vitreous should be examined with the ophthalmoscope, direct or indirect, and with the slit lamp and such abnormalities as haemorrhage from non-accidental injury or bleeding disorders as in the leukaemic can be excluded. Retrolental fibroplasia,

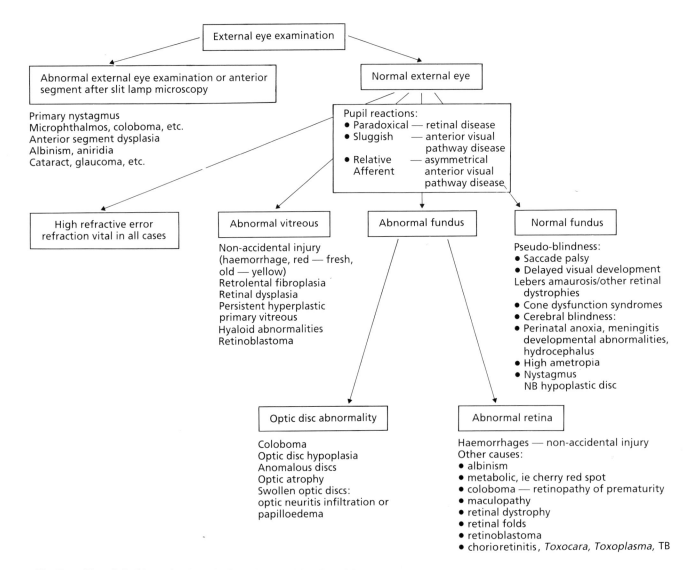

Fig. P1.1 The clinical investigation of bilateral poor vision from birth.

retinal dysplasia, persistent hypoplastic primary vitreous, hyaloid abnormalities and retinoblastoma seedlings may be found on examination.

The fundus should be examined with the pupil dilated with both the direct and indirect ophthalmoscope. Optic disc abnormalities such as coloboma, hypoplasia, anomalous optic disc, optic atrophy or swollen optic discs may reveal the cause of the poor vision. And similarly retinal abnormalities including, coloboma, retinopathy of prematurity, maculopathy, retinal dystrophy, retinal folds, retinoblastoma, retinitis, haemorrhages, albinism, or metabolic disease (for instance cherry red spot) may be diagnosed.

P2 Red Eye in Infancy

SCOTT LAMBERT AND CREIG HOYT

Infant most commonly develop a red eye secondary to an ocular infection or hemorrhage. Infections during infancy can be life-threatening and should be treated promptly.

Causes

Conjunctivitis

The most common cause of a red eye during infancy is conjunctivitis. Conjunctivitis during the first 48 hours may be a toxic reaction to silver nitrate prophylaxis. A purulent discharge during the first week of life is suggestive of gonococcal conjunctivitis. A Gram stain should be immediately performed and if Gram-negative diplococci are seen in the neutrophils, a third-generation cephalosporin should be administered systematically (Holmes *et al.* 1987). Chlamydia conjunctivitis usually occurs during the first 3 weeks of life and is typically bilateral. Prophylaxis with topical erythromycin, or tetracycline may prolong the interval before a child becomes symptomatic from chlamydial conjunctivitis. The diagnosis may be definitively established by immunofluorescent staining of conjunctival scrapings or by identifying intracytoplasmic inclusion bodies in conjunctival epithelial cells. Chlamydial conjunctivitis should be treated with a 2 week course of systemic erythromycin. A variety of other bacterial agents may also cause conjunctivitis in neonates. Conjunctival cultures should be performed and antibiotic treatment initiated based on the results of these cultures.

Keratitis

Keratitis may also cause a red eye in infancy. Keratitis is usually caused by a viral infection in infants, but on occasion can be bacterial. Herpes simplex and adenovirus are the most common causes of viral keratitis during infancy. Vesicles are also usually present on the eyelids or in the periorbital region in infants with a primary herpes simplex infection. Corneal involvement may consist of a punctate or a dendritic keratopathy. Vesicles on the skin may be cultured for herpes simplex. Infants suspected of having an ocular herpes simplex infection should be treated with systemic Acyclovir because of their high risk of developing a disseminated herpes simplex infection (Nahmias & Hagler 1972). Topical antiviral therapy is also recommended.

Adenovirus conjunctivitis

Adenovirus conjunctivitis may also occur during infancy. It is usually bilateral and associated with periorbital edema, a mucoserous discharge and conjunctival chemosis and hyperemia. Follicles do not develop in the conjunctiva of infants. The diagnosis should be made only after carefully excluding other more serious infections.

Endophthalmitis

Endophthalmitis may also occur in infants. It is usually endogenous and requires immediate systemic antibiotics. It may follow surgery for congenital heart defects or result from a systemic infection with an agent such as group B beta streptococcus acquired at birth. Meningitis frequently occurs concurrently. Although an intraocular tap may be necessary on occasion, the responsible pathogen can usually be identified by culturing blood, cerebrospinal fluid, urine or an infected wound (Greenwald *et al.* 1987).

Chorioretinitis

An active toxoplasmosis chorioretinitis may also on occasion be associated with a red eye during infancy. An accompanying vitritis and iridocyclitis is usually present which may obscure the underlying chorioretinitis. Active toxoplasmosis chorioretinitis should be treated with a course of systemic antibiotics (Feldman & Remington 1987) (see Chapter 11).

Haemorrhage

A periocular haemorrhage may also cause a red eye during infancy. Subconjunctival haemorrhages may occur spontaneously, or secondary to trauma or conjunctivitis. If a red eye exists after trauma, a ruptured or perforated globe should be suspected. If necessary, an examination under anaesthesia should be performed to determine the intraocular pressure and to carefully inspect the globe. Subconjunctival haemorrhages may also occur spontaneously or secondary to a valsalva manoeuvre, as in coughing during a Pertussis infection. Subconjunctival haemorrhages are frequent in the neonate due to birth trauma. In the older child non-accidental injury should be considered as a cause.

Other causes

There are several other causes of red eye in infancy:

Uveitis — This can be either primary or secondary to an intraocular tumour or infiltration (see Chapter 23.)

Glaucoma — Red eye occurs sometimes when the intraocular pressure is sudden and severe. The eye may be red, as well as photophobic, the cornea is usually cloudy and the infant usually fractious.

Vascular malformations and shunts — A red eye may be associated with conjunctival vascular malformations or arteriovenous shunts which involve the orbital venous system.

Episcleritis and scleritis — This is very rare in infancy but may occur in autoimmune disease, dry eye and graft versus hosts disease.

Foreign bodies — Foreign bodies should be suspected if there is a localized area of redness and especially if there is localized fluorescein staining. Slit lamp examination may be required and it is important to look under the upper lid.

References

Feldman HA, Remington JS. Toxoplasmosis. In: Behrman RE, Vaughan VC (eds) *Nelson's Textbook of Pediatrics*, 13 edn WB Saunders Philadelphia 1987; pp. 736–736

Greenwald MJ, Wohl LG, Sell CH. Metastatic bacterial endophthalmitis: A contemporary reappraisal. *Surv Ophthalmol* 1986; **2**: 81–101

Holmes KK, Hook EW, Judson FN *et al*. Policy guidelines for the detection, management and control of antibiotic-resistant strains of *Neisseria gonorrhoeae*. *Morbidity Mortality Wkly Report* 1987; **36**: 13–14

Nahmias AJ, Hagler AJ. Ocular manifestations of herpes simplex in the newborn. *Int Ophthalmol Clin* 1972; **12(2)**: 191–213

P3 Sticky Eye in Infancy

SCOTT LAMBERT AND CREIG HOYT

Nasolacrimal duct obstruction

A sticky eye during infancy is usually indicative of congenital dacrostenosis or blepharoconjunctivitis. Mild congenital dacrostenosis may only be associated with epiphora, but a moderate or severe obstruction is generally associated with dacrocystitis and a mucopurulent discharge although the eye will water in between attacks of stickiness. The diagnosis can be confirmed by expressing mucopus from the lacrimal sac. Increasing the hydrostatic pressure in the lacrimal sac by applying digital pressure over the lacrimal sac may hasten the resolution of nasolacrimal duct obstruction (Kushner 1982). Most nasolacrimal duct obstructions resolve spontaneously by 6 months of age (Peterson & Robb 1978). If dacrocystitis persists beyond 6 months of age, the lacrimal system should be probed (Katowitz & Welsh 1987). It may be performed earlier if the conjunctivitis is severe and uncomfortable for the child.

Conjunctivitis

Conjunctivitis may be bacterial, viral or allergic in aetiology. Bacterial conjunctivitis is usually associated with conjunctival papillae and a purulent discharge. When bacterial conjunctivitis is suspected, a Gram stain and cultures should be obtained to exclude a *Neisseria gonorrhoeae* or *N. meningicoccus* infection and to direct antibiotic therapy. Gonococcal conjunctivitis is typically associated with a copious purulent discharge and lid oedema. Gonococcal conjunctivitis should be treated promptly with systemic antibiotics. Untreated gonococcal conjunctivitis can rapidly progress to a corneal perforation. *N. meningococcus* conjunctivitis is also associated with a purulent discharge and places a child at increased risk of meningicoccal meningitis and should be treated promptly with systemic antibiotics as well (Al-Mutlaq *et al.* 1987).

A conjunctival infection with a variety of other bacterial agents including *Streptococcus pneumoccus* and *Haemophilus influenza* may also result in a purulent ocular discharge. A conjunctival infection with *Staphlococcus aureus* usually is accompanied by a mucopurulent discharge and crusting along the margins of the eyelids.

Viral

Viral conjunctivitis is most commonly caused by an adenovirus infection and is usually bilateral and associated with a mucoserous discharge and pre-auricular adenopathy. A punctate keratopathy may also develop which occasionally progress to subepithelial opacities. Antibiotics are ineffective against an adenovirus infection. A herpes simplex blepharoconjunctivitis (type I or type II) may also be associated with a sticky eye. A primary infection is usually accompanied by vesicles on the eyelids. A keratitis may or may not be present. Infants with an ocular herpes simplex infection should be treated with systemic acyclovir. Topical antiviral agents should be used to treat non-neonates with herpes simplex keratitis or blepharoconjunctivitis.

Allergic conjunctivitis

Allergic conjunctivitis may also be associated with a mucopurulent discharge, lid oedema, and conjunctival chemosis and hyperemia. Affected patients usually have intense puritus as well. Gram staining of a conjunctival scraping typically reveals eosinophils. If the allergic reaction is to a topically applied ocular preparation, the adjacent skin will frequently have an eczematoid dermatitis. Treatment should be initiated with cold compresses and topical 4% cromolyn sodium applied 4–6 times a day. Short courses of topical steroids may also be administered.

Parinaud's oculoglandular syndrome

A sticky eye may also be caused by Parinaud's oculo-glandular conjunctivitis. Affected children typically have unilateral conjunctival hyperemia with a watery discharge, a conjunctival granuloma and regional lymphadenopathy. A gram-negative bacillus transmitted by cats has been implicated as the causative agent for the condition known as catscratch disease (Wear *et al.* 1985).

Vernal catarrh

Vernal conjunctivitis may also be associated with a mucoserous discharge but it is rare in infancy. In addition, affected patients usually have severe photophobia. Giant papillae are typically present on the upper tarsal conjunctiva or along the limbus. A punctate epithelial keratitis or a corneal plaque may develop (Buckley 1981). The condition most commonly affects children in warm climates and is associated with seasonal exacerbations.

The diagnosis can be established by identifying eosinophils from the conjunctival scraping of a child with giant papillary conjunctivitis. Topical cromolyn sodium 4% and steroids should be used to treat acute exacerbations. A superficial keratectomy may be necessary if a vernal plaque fails to resolve after treatment with topical cromolyn and steroids (Buckley 1981).

Other causes

Dry eye

A dry eye may be found in dysautonomia (Riley–Day syndrome), or other causes of deficient tear production. The discharge is usually not mucopurulent and is due to the accumulation of mucus in response to the dryness.

Foreign bodies

Foreign bodies that do not excite an acute reaction may cause stickiness by reactive mucopus production.

References

Al-Mutalaq F, Byrne-Rhodes KA, Tabbara KF. *Neisseria meningidis* conjunctivitis in children. *Am J Ophthalmol* 1987; **104**: 280–2

Buckley RJ. Vernal keratopathy and its management. *Trans Ophthalmol Soc UK* 1981; **101**: 234–8

Katowitz JA, Welsh MG. Timing of initial probing and irrigation in congenital nasolacrimal duct obstruction. *Ophthalmol* 1987; **94**: 698–705

Kushner BJ. Congenital nasolacrimal system obstruction. *Arch Ophthalmol* 1982; **100**: 597–600

Peterson RA, Robb RM. The natural course of congenital obstruction of the nasolacrimal duct. *J Pediatr Ophthalmol Strabismus* 1978; **15**: 246–50

Wear DJ, Malty RH, Zimmerman LE, *et al.* Cat scratch disease bacilli in the conjunctiva of patients with Parinaud's oculoglandular syndrome. *Ophthalmology* 1985; **92**: 1282–90

P4 The Odd-looking Eye

JOHN ELSTON

Many parents cannot put into words what they see with their eyes. Nowhere is this more true than with leukocoria when they may be at a loss to describe the glinting reflex they see in certain gaze directions.

The first step is to establish with the parent and if possible the child, the exact complaint. 'Odd-looking eye' may be used to refer to abnormalities of the eye lids, (e.g. a lump) or eye movements, (e.g. incomitant strabismus) as well as the eye itself. The problem is best approached anatomically. The odd-looking eye may have an abnormal colour, iris or pupil, this is determined by investigation including slit lamp examination.

Trauma is always worth bearing in mind as a cause of an odd-looking eye; it may be responsible for traumatic mydriasis, iris prolapse, iris root dialysis or hyphaema.

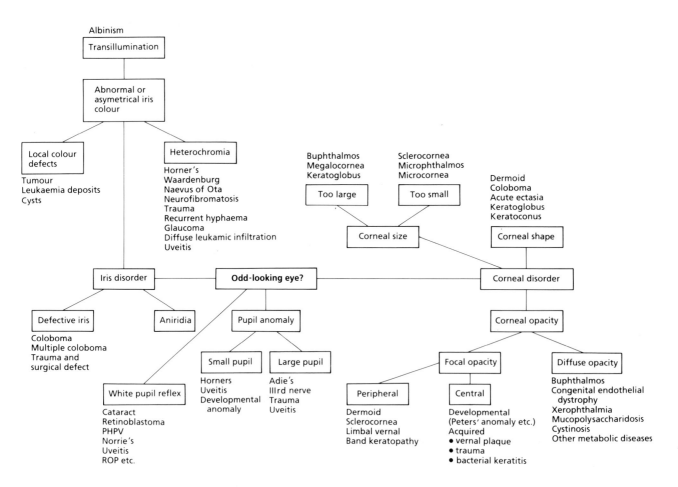

Fig. P4.1 Causes of an odd-looking eye.

P5 The Lump in the Lid

SCOTT LAMBERT AND CREIG HOYT

Rhabdomyosarcoma

Although a variety of disorders can cause lumps in the lids of children, most can be distinguished clinically by their pattern of growth and clinical appearance. The most serious disorder which needs to be considered when evaluating a lump in the lid is a rhabdomyosarcoma. It most commonly occurs in children between 5 and 8 years of age. It may begin as a discrete mass or as a diffuse swelling of the upper eyelid associated with ptosis. Proptosis usually develops soon thereafter as the mass gradually enlarges. If a rhabdomyosarcoma is suspected, a CT scan of the orbit should be performed to look for bony destruction and a non-encapsulated mass. A biopsy is necessary to confirm the diagnosis. Combined radiation therapy and chemotherapy has resulted in a high cure rate for orbital rhabdomyosarcomas (Abrahamson *et al.* 1979).

Other than rhabdomyosarcomas, most other lumps in the lids of children are benign. A careful clinical examination will usually allow these lesions to be distinguished from one another.

Capillary hemangiomas

Capillary hemangiomas frequently involve the eyelids. At birth they are usually clinically insignificant, but during the first 6 months of life they may enlarge. Superficial capillary hemangiomas are often referred to as 'strawberry nevi' and have a reddish coloration. Subcutaneous capillary hemangiomas are manifested clinically as soft, bluish lumps. Capillary hemangiomas should be treated if they cause form-deprivation or anisometropic amblyopia. They may be treated with an intralesional injection of depot steroids or systemic steroids (Kushner 1982). While both are quite effective in hastening the involution of capillary hemangiomas if performed during infancy rebound growth may occur after discontinuing systemic steroids. If a capillary hemangioma is not causing amblyopia treatment is not necessary. Most capillary hemangiomas spontaneously involute later in childhood.

Dermoids

Dermoids are choristomas which primarily arise along the upper orbital rim in the margin of the eyebrow. They are manifested clinically as slow growing, painless, well-encapsulated nodules which may or may not be mobile. They may spontaneously rupture causing a cellulitis. On occasion dermoids have stalks extending through bony canals to the underlying orbital dura. Although their clinical appearance is usually diagnostic, a computed tomographic scan of the orbit is helpful in identifying dermoids with intraorbital extensions prior to surgery. Dermoids should be treated surgically by complete excision.

Chalazion

A chalazion is a lipogranuloma of the eyelids which is manifested clinically as a painless, hard nodule. They are uncommon during infancy, but occur frequently in older children. A *Staphylococcus aureus* blepharitis often occurs concurrently. Warm compresses, cleaning of the lid margins with bland solutions, massage and topical antibiotics frequently hasten their resolution. If conservative therapy proves ineffectual, they may also be treated by surgical drainage or with intralesional depot steroids.

Orbital cysts

Orbital cysts may occur in association with microphthalmia (Weiss *et al.* 1985). The cysts may often be palpated. Both the orbital cyst and the deformed microphthalmic globe should be excised and replaced with a prosthesis for improved cosmesis.

Styes

Styes are commonly treated by the child's paediatrician or general practitioner, so they are often not seen by ophthalmologists. They are painful abscesses of the sebacious glands at the root of the lashes. They can often be cured simply by removing the lash and allowing the abscess to drain. Antibiotic ointment may sometimes be necessary.

Other causes

1 Naevi, basal cell carcinomas and metastatic tumours are all rare in infancy.
2 Molluscum contagiosum, verrucae and simple papilloma.
3 Inflamatory lesions due to Sarcoidosis, fungal infections (especially in immune compromised infants) or foreign bodies.
4 Juvenile Xanthogranuloma
5 Squamous cell carcinoma is rare except in patients with Xeroderma pigmentosa.
6 Cysts are usually developmental, occuring in the upper outer or inner quadrant away from the lid. If they are small and mobile they may be found in the lid itself. Traumatic implantation cysts are rare.
7 Calcifying epithelioma of Malherbe is a pink, hard lump arising in a lid hair follicle.

References

Abrahamson DH, Ellworth RM, Tretter P *et al.* The treatment of orbital rhabdomyosarcoma with irradiation and chemotherapy. *Ophthalmology* 1979; **86**: 1330–5

Kushner BJ. Intralesional corticosteroids injection for infantile adnexal hemangioma. *Am J Ophthalmol* 1982; **93**: 496–506

Weiss A, Martinez C, Greenwald M. Microphthalmos with cyst: clinical presentation and computed tomographic findings. *J Pediatr Ophthalmol Strabismus* 1985; **22**: 6–12

P6 Abnormal Blinking and Eye Closure

DAVID TAYLOR

Many stimuli give rise to blinking: corneal touch, irritation or drying, Vth nerve stimulation especially via the divisions that supply the lids, a flash of light or a loud sound. In addition to the normal 'background' or periodic blinking, the function of which is to spread tears over the eye, the blink rate is normally modified by the state of arousal, excitement and a variety of psychogenic factors.

Normal blink reflex in infancy

Fifth cranial nerve stimulation produces a bilateral contraction of the orbicularis oculi (blink) which has two distinct components (Rushworth 1962); the early response occurring after about 10 ms ipsilaterally, followed by a bilateral late response after about 30 ms. Habituation occurs to the late response in particular. The early response is prolonged in the child under 2 years of age (Clay & Ramseyer 1976). The late response achieves its shortest latency by 6 years and it is not reliably present in the neonate (Kimura *et al.* 1977). The reflex response to bright light, to sound or to corneal stimulation seems to have different components and different latencies to the response to direct Vth nerve stimulation.

The blink rate in infants is much lower than in adults, it may be only one or two blinks per minute.

Insufficient blinking

The integrity of the cornea is vitally dependent on the blink reflex and abnormalities of blinking may rapidly give rise to decompensation with ulceration. In lateral medullary disease (Ongeboer de Visser & Moffie 1979) the reflex may be abnormal, but in high brain stem and thalamic lesions it is retained. Blink reflexes are abnormal in Vth nerve lesions and VIIth nerve lesions, and in neuromuscular junction disease, muscle disease or in structural abnormalities involving the lids. The spontaneous blink rate is markedly decreased in many patients with basal ganglia disease and in some psychiatric states, but it is unusual in these cases for it to cause corneal damage.

Excessive blinking

In investigating excessive lid movements in children the clinician needs to determine whether the child has lid twitches, excessive normal blinking, whether he is 'peering', 'screwing up the eye' or whether he has an abnormality of lid opening.

Lid twitches

LID MYOKYMIA

Small twitches confined to the eyelid are common experiences for adults and not unusual in children. They usually affect the outer aspects of the upper or lower lids and are mildly irritating but of no other significance.

Although said to occur in adults who are chronically tired or who drink too much coffee, in childhood no cause in usually found and the condition improves spontaneously within a few days or weeks.

FACIAL MYOKYMIA

If the myokymia consists of fine, continuous facial and lid contractions that lasts for some weeks and especially if it is associated with intermittent facial contracture a lesion, usually neoplastic, in the dorsal pons should be suspected (Waybright et al. 1979).

Myokymia, usually involving the whole face may also occur in peripheral facial neuropathies and with the Guillain–Barré syndrome.

Excessive blinking

EYE BLINKING TIC

This is much the most common cause of abnormal blinking and it is usually possible to make the diagnosis by history alone. The examination should reveal no abnormality. It disappears in sleep. It occurs most frequently in boys between 6 and 8 years old, and there may be a family history of similar tics.

The onset is often ill-defined and the excessive blinking is bilateral or unilateral usually occurring in groups lasting moments to a few minutes which are not accompanied by discomfort and are often not a great inconvenience to the child. In some cases the blinking occurs when the child is embarrassed or when stressed such as during school lessons and it may be accompanied by head shaking, nostril flaring or pulling faces.

Management consists of ensuring that there is no abnormality on examination and giving strong reassurance. Mostly, the parents are worried that there is an underlying problem and their concern springs from this worry which itself may make the blinking worse. Reassurance that the blinking will not harm the child and that it is a form of habit spasm is usually enough to cause its improvement, even if it takes several weeks or months to do so. Nonetheless there

as a high frequency of behavioural problems in these children and psychiatric assessment is often necessary.

GILLES DE LA TOURETTE SYNDROME

This syndrome often starts in children as a repetitive facial twitch or spasm, often unilateral, that is associated with explosive, stereotyped repetitive actions such as shouting, barking, gesticulation, behavioural disturbances or gaze deviation (Frankel & Cumming 1984). It may be familial (Pollack et al. 1977). In the early years it appears to be a simple eye blinking tic in many cases.

EYE CONDITIONS

Refractive error, poor vision, dry eye, lid disease, corneal disease, subtarsal foreign body, uveitis, conjunctivitis all may cause photophobia and blinking. They can all be excluded by history and examination and the treatment is that appropriate to the condition. The key to the diagnosis is the history. Blinking, or peering may occur in children with a squint, especially a divergent squint and it occurs most frequently in bright sunlight.

LACRIMAL OBSTRUCTION

Anyone who has tried to hold back a tear will know that the attempt is accompanied by excessive blinking, presumably in an attempt to make the blink-tear pump mechanism work more effectively. Any cause of excessive tear production or poor tear drainage, even if not accompanied by actual watering of the eye, may be associated with an increased blink rate.

BLINK – SACCADE SYNKINESIS

Some patients with saccade palsy, in particular congenital oculomotor apraxia, may make blinks at the time that they attempt to look laterally. In some way this appears to help them to generate more normal velocity eye movements, but there is often an accompanying head thrust. Sometimes the parents or doctors notice the blink most.

Peering — refractive errors/media opacities

A gentle half closure of the eyelids classically occurs in myopia or other refractive errors, and sometimes in opacities of the media to achieve a pinhole effect to give better acuity.

Blepharospasm

Blepharospasm is the term applied to 'screwing up' the eye; contracture of all the orbicularis oculi including the brow and some facial muscles. The contractures are much longer than blinks lasting several seconds or longer.

ESSENTIAL BLEPHAROSPASM

This is bilateral blepharospasm with facial spasm that may be associated with other dystonic movements. It is so rare in childhood that an alternative diagnosis should be sought.

HYSTERICAL OR PSYCHOGENIC BLEPHAROSPASM

This occurs in young people; it is bilateral and intermittent. It is rarely disabling, may be prolonged and generally is much more difficult to treat than hysterical blindness. It usually ceases spontaneously after a period of some weeks or months, after the underlying stress factor is relieved.

HEMIFACIAL SPASM

Occasionally this starts in childhood (Shaywitz 1974; Langston & Tharp 1976). The spasms are present during sleep and are usually unilateral. They start with the orbicularis oculi but in moments the whole side of the face is screwed up (Fig. P 6.1). The electromyographic picture is characteristic although usually not associated with brainstem disease. Miller (1985), citing numerous cases from the literature, believes that a large proportion of these patients may have intrinsic or extensive compression of the VIIth nerve as it leaves the brainstem; certainly children with hemifacial spasm should be investigated thoroughly, including CT scan and angiography. There is some controversy as to whether surgery is indicated in the cases where compression by small anomalous blood vessels is thought to be the underlying cause.

DRUG-INDUCED BLEPHAROSPASM

Blepharospasm associated with dystonic movements of the limbs is often drug induced, the most frequent drugs involved being antiemetics, especially phenothiazines, antihistamines and carbamazepine. Drugs which cause dry eye may also cause excessive blinking or blepharospasm. Strychnine poisoning occurs from time to time in country areas where it

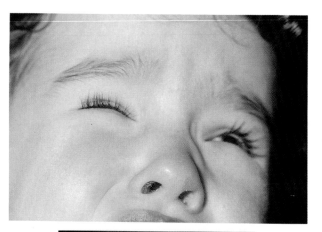

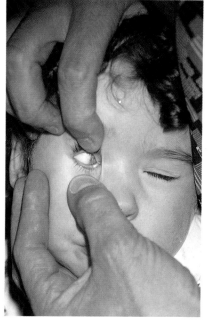

Fig. P6.1 Two-year-old child with intermittent right hemifacial spasm from 1 year. The attacks occurred about 20 times a day, were painful and caused the whole right half of the face to go into spasm. The attacks resolved spontaneously after 13 months and never recurred over 6 years. There were no abnormalities on CT scanning. The eye movements were normal, the Bell's phenomenon was present during the attack and there were no cranial nerve defects during the intervals between attacks.

may be used to poison bait for carnivores; it is usually other farm animals that eat the bait and suffer from tonic seizures when stimulated by touch or sound. The seizures involve face and limb muscles. Human poisoning is usually intentional but rare nowadays.

TETANUS

Risus sardonicus — the spasm of facial muscles

including the lids — is a classic sign of tetanus intoxication.

BLEPHAROSPASM IN EYE DISEASE

Children may screw up the side of the face and the eyelids in response to local pain from uveitis, keratitis, dental or sinus disease, or in conditions causing Vth nerve irritation. Screwing up one eye in sunlight is a frequent symptom in intermittent divergent squint.

HEREDITARY BLEPHAROSPASM

A family with blepharospasm involving the brow was described by Irvine *et al.* (1968).

SEIZURES

During seizure activity in children there are often associated lid and face movements and blepharospasm. These may be unilateral or bilateral and are often associated with a deviation of the eyes. This is most often seen with petit mal epilepsy; the attacks are brief and most usually associated with a 'blank spell' with cessation of speech and other activities for a few seconds although complex movements of the head and face, lips, tensing, or fumbling with the fingers may also occur.

BRAINSTEM LESIONS

The clinical picture with blinking associated with brainstem lesions is very different from the common psychogenic blinking (Figs. P6.2, P6.3). Often the abnormality is unilateral and consists of a spasm of the orbicularis lasting moments associated with forced lateral gaze or elevation of the eye. When they apear to be brought on by lateral gaze the term blepharoclonus has been applied (Keane 1978). The contraction may be accompanied by discomfort and since it may last many months or years the child may spend much time in pain. The pain and the intermittent nature of the problem may make it difficult to see because the child tends to cover his head when he feels the spasm starting. There may be an associated VIIth nerve weakness or other brainstem signs when the spasm is not present.

In adults, rostral brainstem lesions have been described giving rise to bilateral blepharospasm (Jankovic & Patel 1983).

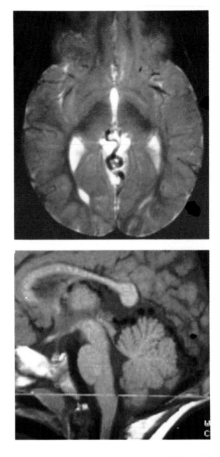

Fig. P6.2 Right-sided facial spasm occurred about every 10 min in this 3-year-old who had anomalous shunt vessels secondary to an occluded sigmoid sinus demonstrated by angiography and MRI scanning. The child had become severely dehydrated at age 1 year and was 'off colour' for 6 months afterwards when the blepharospasm started. The abnormal vessels lie in the cerebellar, cerebellomedullary and pontine cysterns.

Abnormal lid opening

Difficulty in opening the eyes has been described in myotonic dystrophy (Dodge *et al.* 1965) and in the myotonia associated with Schwartz–Jampel syndrome (Schwartz & Jampel 1962). Apraxia of lid opening has been described in adults with cerebrovascular disease or basal ganglia disease. They have an involuntary intermittent inability to open the lids despite elevation of the brow.

Investigation and management

The taking of a detailed history is the surest way to the correct diagnosis and most cases can be diagnosed on history alone, although the examination is also a very important facet in the process.

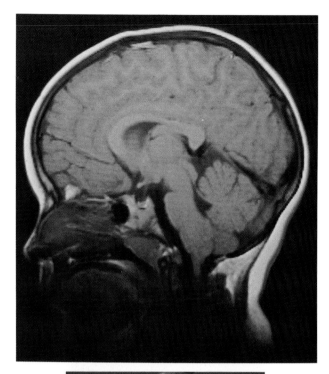

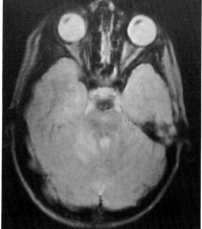

Fig. P6.3 Presumed pontine glioma presenting with unilateral blepharospasm. She presented with attacks of right-sided blepharospasm occurring every few minutes and accompanied by discomfort. CT scans carried out on two occasions were normal and MRI scan done 2 years after the onset demonstrated the tumour. This scan carried out 4 years after the onset showed no change in the size of the tumour.

The following questions may be asked, couched in appropriate language for each patient.

1 Is it the blink or the blink time that seem abnormal?
2 Does it occur in any specific situation or at any time? i.e.

(a) At any time of the day?

(b) In sun or bright light?

(c) In relation to stress, shyness or social situation?

(d) When they are trying to look at something?

(e) In the wind?

(f) In dry air, e.g. in central heating?

3 Is the eye or the lid ever red, sore painful or itching?
4 Is it just a portion of the lid that twitches, the whole lid, the lid and surrounding facial muscles or other parts of the body?
5 Are there any eye movement abnormalities?
6 Is there any associated central nervous system disease?
7 Are there any psychiatric, behavioural or psychological problems?
8 Is there a family history?

By the systematic asking of these questions a diagnosis can usually be reached and confirmed by careful examination and further investigation where necessary. The commonest cause of the complaint of excessive blinking is probably psychogenic blinking; this must be a positive diagnosis as well as diagnosis by exclusion of disease.

References

Clay SA, Ramseyer JC. The orbicularis oculi reflex in infancy and childhood. *Neurology* 1976; **26**: 521–4

Dodge PR, Gamstrop I, Byers RK, Russell R. Myotonic dystrophy in infancy and childhood. *Pediatrics* 1965; **35**: 3–19

Frankel M, Cummings JL. Neuro-ophthalmic abnormalities in Tourette's syndrome: functional and anatomic implications. *Neurology* 1984; **34**: 359–61

Irvine AR, Daroff RB, Sanders MD, Hoyt WF. Familial reflex blepharospasm. *Am J Ophthalmol* 1968; **65**: 889–890

Jankovic J, Patel SC. Blepharospasm associated with brainstem lesions. *Neurology* 1983; **33**: 1237–40

Keane JR. Gaze evoked blepharoclonus. *Ann Neurol* 1978; **3**: 243–5

Kimura J, Bodensteiner J, Yamada T. Electrically elicited blink reflex in normal neonates. *Arch Neurol* 1977; **34**: 246–9

Langston JW, Tharp BR. Infantile hemifacial spasm. *Arch Neurol* 1976; **33**: 302–3

Miller NR. Normal and abnormal eyelid position and movement. In: Eds *Walsh and Hoyt's Clinical Neuro-ophthalmology*, 4th edn. Vol. 2. Williams & Wilkins, Baltimore 1985; pp. 982–6

Ongerboer de Visser BW, Moffie D. Effects of brain stem and thalamic lesions on the corneal reflex; an electrophysiological and anatomical study. *Brain* 1979; **102**: 595–608

Pollack MA, Cohen NL, Friedhoff AJ. Gilles de la Tourette's syndrome: familial occurrence and precipitation by methylphenidate therapy. *Arch Neurol* 1977; **34**: 630–32

Rushworth G. Observations on blink reflex. *J Neurol Neurosurg Psychiatr* 1962; **25**: 93–108

Schwartz O, Jampel RS. Congenital blepharophimosis associated with a unique generalised myopathy. *Arch Ophthalmol* 1962; **68**: 52−60

Shaywitz BA. Hemifacial spasm in childhood treated with carbamazepine. *Arch Neurol* 1974; **31** 13

Waybright EA, Gutman L, Chan SM. Facial myokymia. *Arch Neurol* 1979; **36**: 244−5

P7 Dry Eye and Inappropriate Tearing

DAVID TAYLOR

Signs and symptoms

The child with a dry eye never actually complains that it is 'dry'! He says that it is 'burning'. It may also be irritable, somewhat red, gritty and with a small to moderate amount of discharge. The symptoms are often worse in dry atmospheres such as in a hot department store or in dry weather, and they may first present when the central heating is turned on. Sometimes the parents or the child's doctor will have tried a variety of drops. One clue to the underlying cause being a dry eye is that many different drops make the eye feel better, but only momentarily. The parents should be asked whether he sleeps with his eyes even a tiny bit open at night, and if so, whether the cornea is exposed; this is most important in lid or orbital abnormalities and when corneal abnormalities are found along areas that are likely to be exposed. Excessive blinking or screwing up the eyes is another frequent symptom. An enquiry should be made into the presence of joint, skin, gut and respiratory disease, any previous eye disease or local treatment, especially radiotherapy. Rarely he may complain of photophobia or itching.

Diagnosis

Dry eye in a child is relatively uncommon and this is one of the main reasons why it is underdiagnosed. Having suspected it, diagnosis depends on three main procedures.

EXTERNAL INSPECTION

This includes blink rate and blink effectiveness (is the cornea completely covered by the blink?), the presence of Bell's phenomenon, lid abnormalities, skin lesions and scars around the eyes and elsewhere should be looked for.

SLIT LAMP EXAMINATION

This should include looking at the lids for blepharitis, meibomitis, at the tear film for mucus and debris, signs of instability of the film, focal drying, punctate keratitis shown with rose bengal or fluorescein stain, scarring of the lids and conjunctiva, conjunctival thickening or wrinkling. Mucus filaments and plaques may also be seen.

Slit lamp observations of the tear film should include the tear film break-up time (BUT) (Norn 1969; Baum 1985). If a dry spot appears within ten seconds of a blink this is considered abnormal. A variety of entities other than dry eye may reduce BUT (Baum 1985).

Slit lamp examination may also show the presence of a narrower than normal tear meniscus alongside the lid or the presence of a Dellen, which is a localized area of thinning of the cornea at a persistent dry spot.

SCHIRMER'S TEST

The Schirmer's tear test may be difficult to perform in children but where it is possible it may give useful confirmation of a clinical impression of dryness.

After carefully and reassuringly explaining the procedure to the child, a filter paper strip is placed in the lower fornix laterally, and the length of the filter paper that has been wetted is noted after 5 min. Less than 5 mm is definitely abnormal and most children will wet 15 mm or more. Anaesthetic drops may need to be used but this will reduce the tear production by lessening reflex tearing from corneal stimulation — some ophthalmologists use this as a test of reflex tearing.

Dry eyes from tear mucin deficiency

The very innermost layer of tears is formed from mucin produced in goblet cells of the conjunctiva and is very important in its ability to stabilize the tear film. Its importance in dry eye is not as obvious as it may seem (Thoft 1985) nonetheless in conjunctival and corneal surface disease mucus abnormalities seem to be important (Holly & Lemp 1977). Vitamin A deficiency and trachoma are the commonest causes worldwide but in the Western world the Stevens–Johnson syndrome, burns and, pemphigoid (occasionally seen in older children) are the main causes.

Dry eyes from tear lipid-layer deficiency

The meibomian glands produce a thin oily layer on the surface of the tears which reduces evaporation, and deposits of meibomian secretion at the lid margins prevent entry of skin fatty acids which could disrupt the integrity of the film (Tiffany 1985). Blepharitis, meibomitis and damage to these glands by irradiation may be a contributory factor to dry eye symptoms, and meibomitis and blepharitis should be treated vigorously by massage and cleaning of the lid margins using bland isotonic solutions on a cotton wool ball, or

cotton wool bud, gently but firmly at least twice a day. A short course of an antibiotic/corticosteroid combination ointment, applied in small quantities to the very margin of the lid may help at the beginning of the treatment.

Aqueous tear deficiency — kerato-conjunctivitis sicca (KCS)

The aqueous middle layer of the tear is produced in the lacrimal glands and this is deficient in most dry eye states.

KCS is classically a disease of middle age and it usually develops in the absence of systemic disease. When it occurs with rheumatoid arthritis, systemic lupus erythematosus, sarcoidosis, coeliac disease, Hashimoto's thyroiditis, systemic sclerosis or other autoimmune disease it is known as Sjögren's syndrome.

Defective aqueous tear production also occurs in a variety of other diseases in childhood.

Congenital alacrima

Traditionally, it was thought that neonates produce no tears but Patrick (1974) showed that tears are present from the first day of life and he proposed that the absence of tearing and crying was accounted for by an efficient tear pump.

It is common experience that the parents of some children note that he does not tear when he cries when upset. This, when not accompanied by any external eye abnormality or other symptoms, is of no concern and is presumably due to an abnormality of reflex tear secretion to emotional stimuli. A congenital absence of the lacrimal gland has been proposed but this is difficult to prove. Treatment, in the absence of symptoms or signs other than the absence of emotional tearing itself, is never required. Since damage to the cornea may follow in a minority of these children (Sjögren & Erikson 1950), they should be seen from time to time and especially frequently if there are symptoms (O'Driscoll 1975).

Unilateral cases with corneal dessication and blindness (Morton 1884; Smith et al. 1968) are rare.

A bilateral, hereditary alacrima due to hypoplasia of the lacrimal gland suggested by pharmacological testing and by lacrimal gland biopsy, has been described as an autosomal dominant trait (Mondino & Brown 1976).

Defective reflex tearing

In children with congenital insensitivity to pain or with Vth nerve damage from tumour or trauma, there is, in addition to the neuropathic effects of the anaesthesia, also a defect in reflex tearing which further jeopardizes corneal integrity.

Localized drying

Localized drying can occur because of lagophthalmos, either due to lid abnormalities following excessive ptosis surgery, proptosis, or facial palsy. Following squint surgery where small pieces of conjunctiva may be left standing above the rest, or in conjunctival tumours, around dermoids, etc. small Dellen (localized tiny dimples caused by dessication) may form and, although they are not a problem by themselves, they weaken the cornea's resistance to infection and keratitis may result.

Infective keratitis from drying can be very difficult to treat and needs vigorous treatment directed both toward the infection and the drying.

Familial glucocorticoid deficiency with achalasia of the cardia

In early childhood these children develop hypoglycaemia and changes in skin pigmentation, dysphagia due to achalasia of the cardia, and symptomatic dry eyes (Allgrove et al. 1978).

Ectodermal dysplasia

The ectodermal dysplasias are a group of skin conditions characterized by dry skin with (in the hypohydrotic forms), absence of sweat glands and sebaceous glands, poor hair formation and dental abnormalities. A decrease in tear formation is present in ectodermal dysplasia (Wilson et al. 1973) and also in the related syndrome associated with ectrodactyly and cleft palate, 'EEC' syndrome (Baum & Bull 1974). Eyelid cysts, palmoplantar keratosis, hypodontia and hypotrichosis occur as a possible autosomal recessive trait (Font et al. 1986).

Other ocular abnormalities including lacrimal drainage anomalies (Beckerman 1973) and a macular dystrophy (Ohdo 1983) also occur in association with ectodermal dysplasia. Although they are usually autosomal recessive, the genetics are complicated and requires the help of a geneticist experienced in dermatological problems.

With cranial and facial malformations

Dry eyes have been described with Goldenhar's syndrome (Sugar 1967; Baum & Feingold 1973; Mohandessan & Romano 1978) or with craniosynostosis (Schroder & Dietze 1973). They have also been noted in Duane's syndrome (Pfaffenbach et al. 1972; Ramsay & Taylor 1980).

In multiple endocrine neoplasia type IIb

Along with their Marfanoid habitus and characteristic facies with large lips, multiple mucosal neuromas and café au lait spots, thickened peripheral and corneal nerves and an increased tendency to thyroid, adrenal and parathyroid tumours these young people may have lid neuromas, thick lids, nasal displacement of the lacrimal puncta and decreased tear formation (Spector et al. 1981).

Familial dysautonomia (Riley–Day syndrome)

The Riley–Day syndrome is an autosomal recessive condition almost exclusively occurring in children of Ashkenazi Jewish parentage. The underlying defect is unknown but may involve the gene concerned with nerve growth factor.

Systemic features include emotional lability, paroxysmal hypertension, sweating, cold hands and feet, and a blotchy skin. They tend to drool and have difficulty in swallowing and they lack fungiform papillae on the tongue (Riley et al. 1949; Brunt & McKusick 1970).

As well as a progressive sensory neuropathy (Axelrod et al. 1981) which gives rise to absent deep tendon reflexes, a profound corneal hypoaesthesia, together with lack of tears combines to make corneal ulceration prominent amongst these children's problems (Fig. P7.1). They also have an increased incidence of myopia, exodeviations, anisocoria, ptosis and retinal vascular tortuosity (Dunnington 1954; Goldberg et al. 1968).

There are several syndromes which closely resemble the Riley–Day syndrome; probably the most certain way to establish the diagnosis is by the histopathological changes on sural nerve biopsy (Pearson et al. 1975), but this procedure is not often necessary. Other confirmatory findings include the induction of miosis by 0.1% pilocarpine (Fig. P7.2) or 2.5% methacholine, which indicates denervation hypersensitivity, and the absence of flare after intradermal injection of histamine.

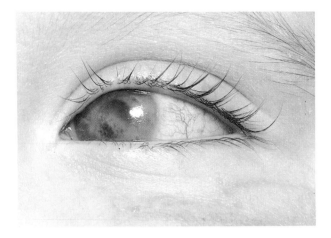

Fig. P7.1 Corneal drying, ulceration, scarring, and vascularization in familial dysautonomia. The combination of anaesthesia and dryness makes keratitis a significant problem for many of these children.

The management of the child as a whole requires conscientious symptomatic and supportive therapy which is the only way to prolong their lives (Axelrod *et al.* 1976), but it is unusual for them to survive beyond 30 years. The care of their eyes require an unusual degree of dedication by their parents and the ophthalmologist, the main treatment being directed towards the dryness.

Sjögren's syndrome

This syndrome is not common in childhood, occurring mainly in adults who have rheumatoid arthritis or other autoimmune disease, together with dryness of the mouth and other mucous membranes, and with dry eye. They may also have bronchitis, pneumonia, pulmonary disease together with the other manifestations of autoimmune disease. It is occasionally seen in children with polyarteritis nodosa, Wegener's granulomatosis or the Churg−Strauss syndrome (asthma, eosinophillia, and fever).

Other syndromes with alacrima

Alacrima has also been described in patients with congenital absence of the lacrimal puncta and aptyalism (Caccamise & Townes 1980) in craniosynostosis (Schroder & Dietze 1973) in the Goldenhaar syndrome and (Romano 1978) where it was also associated with a neuroparalytic keratitis. Alacrima has also been noted after craniofacial surgery in craniofacial dysostoses.

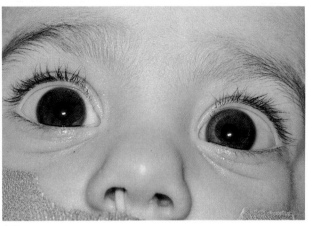

(a)

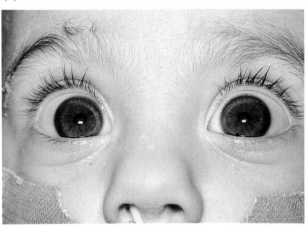

(b)

Fig. P7.2 (a) Familial dysautonomia at the time of instillation of pilocarpine 0.1%. There is no change in pupil size in normal children. (b) Same patient, same lighting conditions 20 min later. The denervation hypersensitivity is indicated by the pupil constriction.

Treatment of dry eyes

Treatment of dry eyes is frequently unrewarding for both doctor and patient. The doctor's treatment is helped by the occurrence of spontaneous relative remissions but the patient is only actively helped by his own or his parents compliance with what is often a demanding but successful regime (Lemp 1987).

Treatment of the cause

Treatment of the cause is only possible in drug induced dry eyes and in xerophthalmia. Biannual vitamin A administration prevents xerophthalmia (Djunaedi *et al.* 1988).

Reduction of tear loss

Avoidance of dry atmospheres, of excessive central heating, the active use of humidification of the main living and sleeping rooms, and of locally increasing humidity by the use of glasses with side arms or of goggles (even swimming goggles) are important methods to reduce the loss of tears by evaporation. Parent's lives may be radically altered even to the extent of having to choose holidays in humid climates. Hydrophilic contact lenses, frequently wetted with preservative-free isotonic drops may help, but are prone to infection (Mackie 1985).

Conservation of tears, first by punctal occlusion with gelatin or silicone rods and later permanently by punctal thermocautery may be helpful (Wright 1985).

Stimulation of tear production, enhancement of the lipid layer of the tear film, osmotic systems, methyl cellulose inserts, and constant infusion apparatuses have all been used with varying success (Wright 1985).

Reduction of the wetted area

Although strongly resisted by parents, a lateral third or half tarsorrhaphy, which can easily be reduced later is an essential part of treatment of severe dry eye states where there is associated corneal hypoaesthesia; it should be performed before irretrievable corneal damage has occurred.

Treatment of excess mucus

It is debatable whether in dry eye mucus is a help or a hindrance to the vitality and comfort of the cornea. Ten percent or 20% acetylcysteine drops may be tried four times daily for those children in whom tacky mucus may be causing corneal epithelial defects.

Treatment of dry, exposed corneas

Taping or padding the lid, unless expertly done can be more harmful than helpful and is best avoided unless it can be carefully controlled. A temporary tarsorrhaphy with butyl-cyanoacrylate glue or suture may help and the use of simple eye ointment (ointment without antibiotic) or if infected, antibiotic eye ointment is a good temporary solution.

Artificial tears

Artificial tears are the mainstay for symptomatic dry eyes. A variety are available from simple saline solution, polyethyline glycol, polyvinyl alcohol, methyl alcohol, and dextrans. An expensive alternative suggestion for severe, acute problems is Healonid. The advantage of the water soluble polymers over saline is mainly in that they have a longer action. It may be that hypo-osmolar solutions are more effective (Gilbard 1985). Although there is probably little to choose between the various forms, most ophthalmologists have their favourite preparations, but it is probably better not to use preparations that have the preservative benzalkonium which unstabilises the tear film. If used frequently, preservative-free drops preferred.

Inappropriate tearing

Eye irritation including subtarsal foreign body

The symptom of a watering eye calls for a thorough search for a subtarsal foreign body, for uveitis, external eye disease and, for a misplaced lash. The commonest source of a persistent watering eye with a foreign body sensation is a subtarsal foreign body. It may be transparent so it can be prudent to sweep the tarsal conjunctiva with a cotton wool bud; one newly appointed British consultant acquired instant fame and fortune in so diagnosing one of our previous Queens who had fruitlessly consulted several greybeards previously!

Crocodile tears

The gastrolacrimal reflex, is also known as 'crocodile tears', from the legend that crocodiles weep before eating their victims. It is usually found in patients following traumatic or inflammatory conditions of the facial nerve, or the greater superficial petrosal nerve, presumably by misdirection of the regrowing secretomotor fibres that subserve salivation.

Congenital crocodile tears are usually associated with Duane's syndrome or what has been described as a VIth nerve palsy (Ramsay & Taylor 1980) and these patients also have other deformities including oxycephaly, facial asymmetry, syndactyly and other limb deformities deafness, and abnormal auricles. This association between Duane's syndrome and crocodile tears is thought to be a discrete lesion in the vicinity of the abducens nucleus with innervation of both the lateral rectus and the salivary gland by oculomotor fibres, the latter abnormally carrying fibres from the salivatory areas in the brainstem (Ramsay & Taylor 1980).

References

Allgrove J, Clayden GS, Grant DB, MaCaulay JC. Familial glucocorticoid deficiency with achalasia of the cardia and deficient tear production. *Lancet* 1978; **8077**: 1284−6

Axelrod FB, Iyer K, Fish I, Pearson J, Sein ME, Speilholz N. Progressive sensory loss in familial dysautonomia. *Pediatrics* 1981; **67**: 517−22

Axelrod F, Mittag TW, Green JP. Familial dysautonomia. *Nature* 1976; **262**: 742

Baum J. Clinical manifestation of dry eye states. *Trans Ophthalmol Soc UK* 1985; **104**: 415−23

Baum J, Bull MJ. Ocular manifestation of the ectrodactyly, ectodermal dysplasia, cleft-palate syndrome. *Am J Ophthalmol* 1974; **78**: 211−6

Baum JL, Feingold M. Ocular aspects of Goldenhar syndrome. *Am J Ophthalmol* 1973; **75**: 250−53

Beckerman BL. Lacrimal anomalies in anhidrotic ectodermal dysplasia. *Am J Ophthalmol* 1973; **75**: 728−80

Brunt PW, McKusick VA. Familial dysautonomia. *Medicine* 1970; **49**: 343−74

Caccamise WC, Townes PL. Congenital absence of the lacrimal punctae associated with alacrima and aptyalism. *Am J Ophthalmol* 1980; **89**: 62−5

Djunaedi E, Sommer A, Pandji A, Taylor HR. Impact of vitamin A supplementation on xerophthalmia. *Arch Ophthalmol* 1988; **106**: 218−23

Dunnington JH. Congenital alacrima in familial autonomic dysfunction. *Arch Ophthalmol* 1954; **52**: 925−31

Font RL, Seabury-Stone M, Schanzor MC, Lewis RA. Apocrine hidrocystomas of the lids, hypodontia, palmar plantar hyperkeratosis, and onychodystrophy. A new variant of ectodermal dysplasia. *Arch Ophthalmol* 1986; **104**: 1811−3

Gilbard JP. Topical therapy for dry eye. *Trans Ophthalmol Soc UK* 1985; **104**: 484−98

Goldberg MF, Payne JW, Brunt PW. Ophthalmologic studies of familial dysautonomia. *Arch Ophthalmol* 1968; **80**: 732−43

Holly FJ, Lemp MA. Tear physiology and dry eyes. *Surv Ophthalmol* 1977; **22**: 69−82

Lemp MA. Recent developments in dry eye management. *Ophthalmology* 1987; **94**: 1299−305

Mackie IA. Contact lenses for dry eyes. *Trans Ophthalmol Soc UK* 1985; **104**: 477−83

Mohandessan MH, Romano PL. Neuroparalytic keratitis in Goldenhar−Gorlin syndrome. *Am J Ophthalmol* 1978; **85**: 111−3

Mondino BJ, Brown SI. Hereditary congenital alacrima. *Arch Ophthalmol* 1976; **94**: 1478−80

Morton AS. Congenital, unilateral absence of lacrimation. *Trans Ophthalmol Soc UK* 1884; **4**: 350−1

Norn MS. Dessication of the precorneal tear film. 1. Corneal wetting time. *Acta Ophthalmol* 1969; **47**: 865−80

O'Driscoll TG. Alacrima. *Trans Ophthal Soc UK* 1975; **95**: 13−14

Ohdo S, Hirayama K, Terawaki T. Association of ectodermal dysplasia ectrodactyly and macular dystrophy. *J Med Genet* 1983; **20**: 52−7

Patrick RK. Lacrimal secretions in full-term and premature babies. *Trans Ophthal Soc UK* 1974; **94**: 283−90

Pearson J, Dancis J, Axelrod F, Grover N. The sural nerve in familial dysautonomia. *J Neuropath Exp Neurol* 1975; **34**: 413−24

Pfaffenbach DD, Cross HE, Kearns TP. Congenital anomalies in Duanes syndrome. *Arch Ophthalmol* 1972; **88**: 635−9

Ramsey J, Taylor D. Congenital crocodile tears: a clue to the aetiology of Duanes syndrome? *Br J Ophthalmol* 1980; **64**: 518−22

Riley CM, Day RL, Greeley DMcL, Langford WS. Central autonomic dysfunction with defective lacrimation. *Pediatrics* 1949; **3**: 468−72

Romano P. Neuroparalytic keratitis in Goldenhar syndrome. *Am J Ophthalmol* 1978; **85**: 111−3

Schroder D, Dietze U. Bilateral congenital absence of tears, keratitis sicca and premature synostosis of all cranial sutures. *Klin Monatsbl Augenheilk* 1973; **163**: 239−41

Sjögren H, Erikson A. Alacrima congenita. *Br J Ophthalmol* 1950; **34**: 691−4

Smith RS, Maddox SF, Collins BE. Congenital alacrima. *Arch Ophthalmol* 1968; **79**: 45−8

Spector B, Klintworth GK, Wells SA. Histologic study of the ocular lesions in multiple endocrine neoplasia syndrome type IIB. *Am J Ophthalmol* 1981; **91**: 201−14

Sugar HS. An unusual example of the oculo-auriculo-vertebral dysplasia syndrome of Goldenhar. *J Pediatr Ophthalmol* 1967; **4**: 9−11

Thoft RA. Relationship of the dry eye to primary ocular surface disease. *Tr Ophthalmol Soc UK* 1985; **104**: 452−7

Tiffany JM. The role of meibomian secretion in the tears. *Trans Ophthalmol Soc UK* 1985; **104**: 396−401

Wilson FM, Grayson M, Pieroni D. Corneal changes in ectodermal dysplasia. *Am J Ophthalmol* 1973; **75**: 17−27

Wright P. Other forms of treatment of dry eyes. *Trans Ophthalmol Soc UK* 1985; **104**: 497−8

P8 Photophobia

SUSAN DAY

Definition

Photophobia is light sensitivity which makes the child uncomfortable in normal lighting conditions. A child may be unable to relate his symptom, and parents may interpret slight closing of the eyes in bright sunlight as light sensitivity. True photophobia in which the child is uncomfortable is an uncommon symptom in infants and children.

Causes

Corneal

Most causes for true photophobia are of corneal origin. Photophobia may be caused either by epithelial disruption, as with a foreign body, or by intrastromal changes, such as with corneal oedema.

The most important cause of corneal photophobia is buphthalmos. Buphthalmos is the hallmark of congenital glaucoma. The corneas are enlarged due to breaks in Descemet's membrane which allow stretching of the cornea in the infantile eye. The cornea further thickens as a result of abnormal Descemet's function, and with this thickening haziness may occur. With extensive changes, actual scar forma-

tion may develop which ultimately may limit clarity of the media.

The baby with congenital glaucoma may be extremely photophobic. Mothers report that their babies keep their eyes closed at all times in outdoor lighting and that only with dim illumination in the home will the eyes open. The child may be erroneously treated for possible nasolacrimal duct obstruction since the photophobia also results in epiphora. The accurate diagnosis, however, must be expediently made, as early treatment can prevent blindness in these infants.

Corneal dystrophies may also create photophobia in the infant period. Congenital hereditary endothelial dystrophy, a rare autosomal recessive condition, may result in corneal clouding in the first few months of life. The photophobia is less striking than with buphthalmos, perhaps since the epithelium is not as disturbed.

Aniridia is a familiar cause of photophobia as a consequence of the abnormal irides and may include a corneal epithelial component of photophobia particularly in the older child. With aniridia, epithelial disruption with pannus formation occurs peripherally in many individuals.

Another cause of corneal photophobia is scarring. This most commonly occurs after trauma in which a corneal or corneal–scleral wound involves the optical axis. Iatrogenic scarring from refractive procedures can also create glare; hopefully this would not be found in children.

Another major cause of corneal photophobia is with disruption of the corneal epithelium, as with keratitis or corneal foreign body. Keratitis commonly occurs in conjunction with common childhood diseases such as chickenpox and measles. It is important to exclude concurrent uveitis in such patients. Herpetic keratitis may occur in children highlighting the need to do a careful fluorescein assessment in any child with keratitis. Congenital herpetic keratitis is particularly important to diagnose as its treatment warrants systemic anti-viral agents to prevent significant central nervous system sequelae. Corneal foreign bodies occur commonly in children, and may be particularly difficult to diagnose due to examination constraints and to lack of a clear cut history. Other epithelial disruptions, as caused by trauma, such as by children's finger nails, may be the cause of photophobia. Cystinosis, a systemic metabolic disorder, results in crystalline-like deposits in the corneal stroma. This tends to be a progressive condition and photophobia may become a feature of the child's symptoms. Several forms of cystinosis occur, with one presenting within the first few years of life and the other remaining clinically silent until the mid-teens. The diagnosis is particularly important to make, as renal malfunction is another hallmark feature of this condition.

Uvea

Abnormalities of the uvea can result in photophobia as well. Two mechanisms are present for this. Firstly, the uveal pigment acts as a filter to incoming light. If the uveal pigment is missing, as with albinism, photophobia may be present. Another uveal abnormality, aniridia, may cause photophobia since the pupillary aperture is large and constant. Uveitis includes photophobia in its triad of symptoms: pain, redness, photophobia. Childhood iritis is most commonly either infectious in aetiology (such as with chickenpox) or traumatic in origin, perhaps in association with corneal abnormalities. One of the more significant forms of iritis is that associated with juvenile rheumatoid arthritis (JRA), which unfortunately does not usually have associated photophobia. This form of childhood iritis must be found in its early stages by routine slit lamp examination of the child with diagnosis of JRA.

Lens

Partial cataract can result in photophobia. This symptom is uncommon in infants with complete cataracts, but may be present in children with partial cataracts. The symptoms of photophobia are important to discuss in patients undergoing chemotherapy, since posterior subcapsular cataracts may occur in association with dry eye in this treatment and since posterior subcapsular cataract are particularly prone to create photophobia. Subluxed and dislocated lenses can also induce photophobia. The diagnosis of Marfan's syndrome, homocystinuria, previous trauma, and Weill–Marchesani syndrome must be considered.

Optic nerve

Although visual loss is by far the most important symptom of optic neuritis, photophobia may be a concurrent symptom. The photophobia is almost paradoxical, as vision may be extremely poor, yet light may be particularly aggravating. Some patients report that fluorescent bulb illumination are particularly bothersome with optic neuritis.

Vitreous

Vitritis as an isolated finding, is not common in infants and children. There is usually an associated chorioretinitis or endophthalmitis. Nevertheless, in children on chemotherapy, possible candida vitritis may be present. Metastatic endophthalmitis may result in a difficult-to-define photophobia. This diagnosis must be entertained in any child who has had previous trauma, including manipulations such as dental work.

Retina

Congenital cone dystrophies may result in a presentation of photophobia in an infant. The infant appears not to have photophobia indoors, but will immediately close the eyes when taken outside. The key feature which distinguishes this condition from other causes of photophobia is relatively poor vision which is hallmarked during infancy by nystagmus. Nystagmus may be very difficult for the parents to notice, and even primary care physicians may have difficulty discerning any abnormality. As the child grows older, vision difficulties become more apparent in addition to the light sensitivity.

Macular oedema may also result in photophobia. This condition may cause light sensitivity in the postoperative aphakic infant and child. These children must have a complete examination, as secondary glaucoma could also cause photophobia.

Central nervous system

The central nervous system rarely can account for photophobia. Children with meningitis and encephalitis may be extremely light sensitive. Such symptoms are common with less serious conditions such as childhood measles. The mechanism for the photophobia is rather curious; the Vth cranial nerve, responsible for much of the sensation in the periorbital region, is also responsible for meningeal innervation. It is possible that the photophobia is a referred symptom. Such children nevertheless must be examined to exclude the possibility of concurrent keratitis or iritis (Huber 1976; Safran *et al.* 1980; Cummings & Gittinger 1981).

Strabismus

The apparent light sensitivity associated with strabismus is far different than the child with a corneal foreign body. Nevertheless, the child with an intermittent exotropia will consistently close one or the other eye when going from indoors to outdoors. This is interpreted as photophobia by the parents. The squinting is felt by some to eliminate diplopia in such a child (Wang & Chryssanthou 1988). It is thought that fusion control is more difficult in brightly illuminated situations; thus an exophoria becomes a manifest tropia.

Other causes

Other causes of photophobia are perhaps more difficult to define. They are important, however, as apparent light sensitivity is a rather common complaint. Children who are very fair skinned seem to be photophobic. Although a complete examination is in order, normal findings provide reassurance to the parent that this will most likely be outgrown. Another interpretation of photophobia is in the child, typically 5–7 years old, who suddenly begins to blink in furious spurts. Very often, no anticipated conjunctivitis, foreign body, allergy, or other pathology is found. It is important to observe during the examination for an apparent on/off switch for the blinking. One can be reassured that this is a benign condition when the blinking seems to be an attention getting device.

EXAMINATION

The examination must be tailored depending on the degree of co-operation, yet complete to exclude all possible conditions. It is best to consider what the most likely diagnoses are given the child's age. In an infant, congenital glaucoma must be the primary diagnosis of exclusion. In the toddler, trauma and possible corneal foreign body must be sought, since a specific history is often lacking. Another cause in this age group is keratitis associated with a childhood illness. In the preschool child, conditions which are also associated with reduced vision must be considered. At this age, objects of interest become smaller and vision good enough to learn the alphabet is a far greater demand than vision required for a 2-year-old to stack blocks. Monochromatism, albinism, and aniridia may often first come to an ophthalmologist's attention at this time. In the school-age child, the attention getting form of photophobia seems prevalent. A further common cause at this age is manifestation of intermittent exotropia.

All aspects of the examination are important, even when the ophthalmologist is accustomed to not performing systematically a complete examination in young age groups. Visual acuity, slit lamp examination, ocular motility, and fundus examination are essential. When all appears to be normal, then electroretinography and visual evoked responses should be requested.

MANAGEMENT

The management of a child with photophobia is highly dependent on the underlying cause. Buphthalmos, of course, requires immediate steps to lower the intraocular pressure. Iritis may need cycloplegic agents and steroids. Herpetic keratitis requires antiviral agents.

Management of the specific symptom of photophobia is rather practical, consisting of the use of tinted glasses, hats which shade the sunlight, change of residence, and avoidance of brighter outdoors illumination. In children with monochromatism, special brown tinted glasses may enhance vision as much as possible, and children with albinism often respond favourably to rose tinted spectacles. Management of children who blink excessively is predominently one of parental education, although occasionally 'magic drops' consisting of artificial tears will help the child. The management of such children certainly requires discussion with the parents, emphasizing the normal aspects of the examination and the high probability that the symptoms will be outgrown.

References

Cummings JL, Gittinger JW. Central dazzle: a thalamic syndrome? *Arch Neurol* 1981; **38**: 372–4

Huber A. *Eye Signs in Brain Tumours*, 3rd edn. CV Mosby Co., St Louis 1976

Safran AB, Kline LB, Glaser JS. Positive visual phenomena in optic nerve disease. In: *Neuro-ophthalmology* JS Glaser (ed). CV Mosby Co. St Louis 1980; **10**: 225–231

Wang M, Chryssanthou G. Monocular eye closure in intermittent exotropia. *Arch Ophthalmol* 1988; **106**: 941–2

P9 The Watering Eye

SUSAN DAY

Signs and symptoms

Tearing in childhood is a common clinical problem, especially within the first year of life.

A child with excessive tearing causes great frustration for the parent. In stores, strangers will ask why the baby is 'crying', the skin becomes excoriated from frequent wiping and rubbing and parents avoid taking the child to windy or dusty places, where the tearing is aggravated. The paediatrician's reassuring words that the child will 'outgrow' the condition often lose their credibility.

Associated symptoms must be elicited to focus on the appropriate diagnosis. Presence of a scratchy sensation will lead the examiner to suspect a foreign body; morning discharge may point to a diagnosis of keratitis or exposure keratopathy. Photophobia is the most ominous associated symptom since congenital glaucoma may present with it. More than one excellent physician has misdiagnosed nasolacrimal duct obstruction or external infection for infantile glaucoma simply by failing to register the complaint of photophobia.

Diagnosis

External inspection

The epiphora may be obvious, with a watery appearance just as if the child had been crying. The skin may be shiny, roughened, or erythematous. More subtle tearing problems may be represented by a larger-than-usual tear meniscus above the lower lid. Secondary bacterial infection may occur with a non-patent nasolacrimal system; dacryocystitis and, more commonly conjunctivitis with purulent discharge may then be the presenting symptom.

Slit lamp examination

The slit lamp examination will help assess for presence or absence of the nasolacrimal punctae. If congenital abnormalities of the punctae are present, involvement of the upper and lower punctae must usually co-exist in order for epiphora to be apparent but the lower punctae are probably also a cause of epiphora when involved alone. An unsuspected foreign body or corneal abrasion may also be detected with the slit lamp. Other evidence of keratitis or corneal abnormality must be sought.

Fluorescein testing

Fluorescein is a valuable method of diagnosing causes of epiphora. Corneal abrasions, keratitis, and other superficial irregularities may be detected because of the bright green staining of epithelial defects when viewed in blue light. Fluorescein can also be used to judge patency of the nasolacrimal system: 5 minutes after instillation, it should be visible either in the nasal cavity or the oropharynx by inspection with a cobalt blue light.

Intraocular pressure

In the baby with excess tearing who also has photophobia, the physician must ensure that glaucoma is not present. Any corneal enlargement, clouding, or breaks in Descemet's membrane (Haab's striae) visible on slit lamp exam suggest this diagnosis. The intraocular pressure must be assessed by an applanation technique, such as with the Perkins hand-held tonometer. Tactile measurements are notoriously inaccurate. Chloral hydrate sedation will allow accurate measurement of the intraocular pressure (Jaafar 1988). If the diagnosis is obvious, then an examination under anesthesia proceeding to surgery is appropriate even though the anaesthesia will have to be modified to measure intraocular pressure (Walton 1979; Quigley 1982; De Luise & Anderson 1983). (See Chapter 25.)

Causes and treatment

Non-patent nasolacrimal system

Epiphora first apparent between 3 and 6 weeks after birth affects approximately 6% of all neonates (Calhoun 1987). In large part, management is by the primary care physician and includes antibiotics to prevent secondary infection and massage to encourage establishment of patency (Peterson and Robb 1978; Nelson *et al.* 1985; Paul 1985). The ophthalmologist may be consulted if there is no resolution by 6–9 months, if there is recurrent infection, or anxious parents. Treatment by the ophthalmologist must include proper medical management including massage and antibiotics where there is clinical infection (Kushner 1982). With persistent epiphora, then probing of the nasolacrimal system is indicated. Some ophthalmologists advocate probing as young as 3 months citing high success rate and ability to perform as an outpatient procedure as its advantages (Baker 1985) whereas others prefer to delay probing, hoping for natural resolution of the problem and opting for general anesthesia and a more controlled environment to encourage better success (Kushner 1982). The technique of probing as well as indications for more extensive surgery are discussed elsewhere (see Chapter 21).

Foreign body

The history of recent trauma accompanied by excess tearing and foreign body sensation usually leads to an obvious suspicion of a corneal or conjunctival foreign body. In preverbal children, the history may be more difficult to obtain. The diagnosis must usually be made with the aid of magnification with either the slit lamp or, in instances of less co-operation, loupes or a +20 lens. When the foreign body is not immediately apparent, the upper lid should always be everted for closer inspection.

Removal of a foreign body requires sufficient co-operation from the patient. If the foreign body is not embedded, removal with an applicator moistened with topical anesthetic may be possible. If not easily dislodged, a dental burr drill or needle must be used. General anesthesia or systemic ketamine and topical anaesthesia with appropriate monitoring is required when co-operation is in doubt, as chloral hydrate sedation will not allow the necessary manipulation.

Keratitis/conjunctivitis

A watery eye is a common symptom in keratitis. The child often has a history of upper respiratory infection. Eye involvement is usually bilateral but may be asymmetrical in its onset or severity. Epidemic keratoconjunctivitis must be accurately diagnosed so that further transmission to schoolmates, neighbours, and family members can be kept at a minimum with proper hygiene. Keratitis related to chickenpox (Marsh 1973), measles (Fedukowicz & Stenson 1985), and mumps (Riffenburgh 1961) must be carefully examined for associated uveitis or optic neuritis. Rarely, watery irritated eyes may be the earliest symptom related to Stevens–Johnson syndrome although the severity of the associated systemic findings pre-empts the eye findings. Such children deserve early assessment and careful following by an ophthalmologist.

Allergic conjunctivitis

Although itching represents the primary symptom of this condition, excess tearing is a prominent feature. The diagnosis is usually easy to make on the basis of seasonal exacerbations, known allergic associations, such as asthma, hay fever or eczema. (See Chapter 15.)

Contact lens-related epiphora

In the older child or the aphakic infant with contact lenses epiphora may result from numerous causes. Improper fitting, change in corneal curvature, build-up of deposits, chips or tears at the edge of the contact lens can all create watery eyes from epithelial irregularities. The upper tarsal plate must be assessed for giant papillary conjunctivitis (GPC) in the long-term contact lens wearer (Allansmith 1977). Treatment may include refitting of lenses, obtaining new lenses, and disodium cromoglycate for patients with GPC (Allansmith & Abelson 1983). In all such patients, especially infant aphakes, care must be taken that no corneal ulcer is present, and parents of contact lens wearing infants are warned to be sure to have the lens removed within a few hours in the event of a red, sticky, watery, or photophobic eye.

Congenital glaucoma

As previously mentioned, epiphora in conjunction with photophobia may herald congenital glaucoma. Buphthalmos and corneal clouding are also usually present. The diagnosis must be made on the basis of clinical findings including documentation of elevated intraocular pressure, and treatment usually surgical; instituted promptly to prevent irreversible optic nerve damage. (See Chapter 25.)

Crocodile tears

One peculiar form of tearing occurs only when the patient salivates, most typically when eating, but also possible when the patient is thinking of a good meal (Golding–Wood 1963). The lesion may be is at the level of the geniculate ganglion of the VIIth cranial nerve but central mechanisms have been postulated. In this region, the preganglion parasympathetic fibers to the lacrimal gland are coursing with similar fibres to the submandibular gland. Presumably, a 'miswiring' is present in this region, resulting in the anomalous tearing with salivation. Most typically this phenomenon occurs after injury or surgery on the ear (Axelsson & Laage-Hellman 1962) or as a sequel to Bell's palsy (McGovern 1940). Congenital crocodile tears has been reported in association with another 'miswiring' phenomenon, Duane's syndrome (Ramsay & Taylor 1980).

References

Allansmith MR, Abelson MB. Ocular allergies. In: Smolin G, Thoft R (eds.) *The Cornea*. Little, Brown & Co., Boston/ Toronto, 1983; pp. 231–43

Allansmith MR, Greiner JV, Henriquez AS *et al.* Giant papillary conjunctivitis in contact lens wearers. *Am J Ophthalmol* 1977; **83**: 697–708

Axelsson A, Laage-Hellman JE. The gusto-lacrimal reflex: the syndrome of crocodile tears. *Acta Otolaryngol* 1962; **54**: 239–42

Baker JD. Treatment of congenital nasolacrimal system obstruction. *J Pediatr Ophthalmol Strabismus* 1985; **22**: 34–5

Calhoun J. Problems of the lacrimal system in children. *Pediatr Clin N Am* 1987; **34**: 1457–65

De Luise VP, Anderson DR. Primary infantile glaucoma. *Surv Ophthalmol* 1983; **28**: 1–19

Fedukowicz HB, Stenson S. *External Infections of the Eye*, 3rd edn. Appleton-Century-Crofts, Norwalk, Connecticut 1985

Golding-Wood PH. Crocodile tears. *Br Med J* 1963; **1**: 1518

Jaafar MS. Care of the infantile glaucoma patient. In: RD Reinecke (ed.) *Ophthalmology Annual* 1988. Raven Press New York; 1988; pp. 15–37

Kushner BJ. Congenital nasolacrimal system obstruction. *Arch Ophthalmol* 1982; **100**: 597–600

Marsh RJ. Herpes zoster keratitis. *Trans Ophthalmol Soc UK* 1973; **93**: 181–90

McGovern FH. Paroxysmal lacrimation during eating following recovery from facial palsy. *Am J Ophthalmol* 1940; **23**: 1388–42

Nelson LB, Calhoun JH, Menduke H. Medical management of congenital nasolacrimal duct obstruction. *Ophthalmology* 1985; **92**: 1187–90

Paul TO. Medical management of congenital nasolacrimal duct obstruction. *J Pediatr Ophthalmol Strabismus* 1985; **22**: 68–70

Peterson RA, Robb RM. The natural course of congenital obstruction of the nasolacrimal duct. *J Pediatric Ophthalmol Strabismus* 1978; **15**: 246–50

Quigley HA. Childhood glaucoma, results with trabeculotomy and study of reversible cupping. *Ophthalmology* 1982; **89**: 219–26

Ramsay J, Taylor DSI. Congenital crocodile tears: a clue to the aetiology of Duane's syndrome. *Brit J Ophthalmol* 1980; **64**: 518–22

Riffenburgh RD. Ocular manifestations of mumps. Special reviews. *Arch Ophthalmol* 1961; **66**: 739–42

Walton DS. Diagnosis and treatment of glaucoma in childhood. In: Chandler PA, Grant WM (eds.) *Glaucoma*. Lea & Feibiger, Philadelphia 1979; pp. 319–290

P10 Proptosis

DAVID TAYLOR

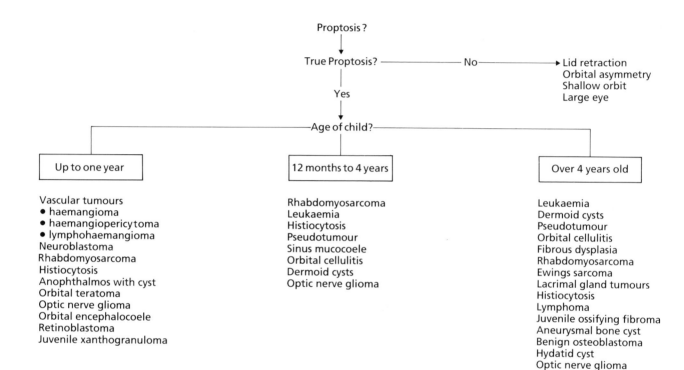

Fig. P10.1 The causes of proptosis vary with the age of the child and there is considerable overlap between the age-groups and between various centres. The table lists causes in approximate order of frequency. Details of each condition should be sought from the text. In making a clinical diagnosis the history and progression of the condition as well as the clinical findings are of vital importance.

P11 Eye Pain

SUSAN DAY

Definition and anatomy

'My eye hurts' is about as simple a definition of this symptom as can be found. Eye pain is a highly subjective complaint, and one which does not always match the physical findings. In a preverbal child, eye rubbing, light sensitivity, excessive blinking, irritability with a red eye may be viewed by the parent as being associated with pain. The older child may complain of eye pain when the underlying cause is anything from a foreign body to an attention-getting device.

In general, the aetiology for eye pain can be better defined on the basis of the quality of the pain. A superficial foreign body sensation implies epithelial irregularities or foreign bodies on the cornea or conjunctiva. A deeper aching pain is complained of with severe intraocular pressure elevation and uveitis. Eye pain more specifically characterized by burning or itching leads one toward concerns about dry eye, allergy, and chemical irritation. Pain induced by bright light classically implies uveitis although photophobia can also occur in patients with retinal and optic nerve disease as well as glaucoma.

Eye pain occurs when pain receptors are stimulated. Over-stimulation of other types of sensory fibres does not cause pain; thus another explanation such as induced ciliary body spasm must be found for the statement that 'light hurts my eyes'. Two fibre systems, myelinated and unmyelinated, transmit pain fibres; the former appears to transmit sharp transient pain sensations, the latter transmits dull aching sensations.

Pain fibres innervating the eye and periorbital structures arise from the trigeminal, or Vth cranial nerve. The first (ophthalmic) division is the most important division responsible for eye pain. It innervates the globe, forehead, lacrimal gland, canaliculi, and lacrimal sac as well as the frontal sinus, upper lid, and side of the nose. Its intracranial source is the Gasserian ganglion, from which it extends through the cavernous sinus. Branching just behind the superior orbital fissure into the lacrimal, frontal and nasociliary nerves, it then enters the superior orbital fissure. An important intracranial branch of the ophthalmic division supplies the meninges. The second major branch (V2), the maxillary nerve, supplies the cheek, lower eyelid, sometimes a small lower segment of the cornea, upper lip, side of the nose, maxillary sinus, roof of mouth, and temporal region; it too arises from the Gasserian ganglion and courses either within or just lateral to the cavernous sinus. It then passes through the inferior orbital fissure after giving rise to dural branches. Although coursing within the orbit, its terminal branches do not include intraorbital structures. The third (V3) division, or mandibular nerve, supplies sensation to other regions of the cheek as well as sensation within the mouth and preauricular area. After rising from the Gasserian ganglion, it passes through the foramen ovale to the infratemporal fossa. Although pain is most commonly generated at the site of the insult, referred pain may occur if the sensory pathway is stimulated in other regions. This phenomenon is particularly important when discussing eye pain, as intracranial stimulation of the dura may result in a sensation of retrobulbar pain.

The cornea represents one of the areas of greatest density of pain nerve endings in the body, with the greatest concentration occurring in the central cornea. There are more fibres horizontally than vertically, corresponding to the exposed area of the interpalpebral fissures.

Non-corneal structures show, in descending order, less sensitivity: eyelids, caruncle, and conjunctiva (Norn 1973).

Other ocular structures can be associated with pain including the uvea, sclera and optic nerve sheaths. Although the precise mechanism for the pain is poorly understood, but it's amelioration, either natural or in response to treatment has led to commonly accepted explanations. The aggravating pain of ciliary body spasm is often relieved with cycloplegic agents. Anti-inflammatory agents can abate pain associated with episcleritis and, less commonly, scleritis. Pain of retrobulbar optic neuritis has been interpreted as nerve sheath inflammation. The retina and optic nerve have no pain fibres in and of themselves.

Eye pain in any given individual may include several components which require therapeutic attention. The child with a corneal foreign body will have a corneal cause for pain as well as possible reflex ciliary body spasm. Therapeutically, the epithelium must be restored by removal of the irritating cause and pressure patching if the epithelial defect is sufficiently large, and cycloplegic agents will help alleviate the ciliary spasm.

Causes

Cornea

The majority of eye pain in children is associated with underlying corneal pathology. Trauma can result in either a corneal abrasion or in a corneal foreign body. The verbal child may report that the eye feels like it has sand in it, or feels scratchy. Commonly, a child's cornea may be scratched by fingernails; this usually occurs rather innocuously, since a toddler's eye is at the height where an adult's hand rests.

Cat scratches to the eye are particularly a worry due to the abundance of aerobic and anaerobic bacteria under the claws. The presence of a localized granuloma, preauricular adenopathy and a positive response to cat-antigen gives rise to the cat scratch disease or

preauricular syndrome of Parinaud (Carithers 1970, 1978). Corneal injury may also be non-accidental, and children's eyes have been burned with cigarettes. Foreign bodies most often occur as a child is playing with toys which can break and become splintered. The symptoms are identical to that of an abrasion. Corneal abrasions and foreign bodies often result in severe photophobia as well as pain. With time a red eye may develop or a corneal infiltrate may ensue.

Infection represents the second most common cause of cornea-induced eye pain. Keratitis typically occurs with epidemic kerato-conjunctivitis but can also be present with other viral causes. Herpetic keratitis, although uncommon in children, must be clearly differentiated from these other causes. Keratitis is a common association of allergic conjunctivitis; a scratchy foreign body symptom thus may accompany this condition. Keratitis may occur in children who wear contact lenses, either acutely due to malfitting contact lenses, or chronically due to changing dimension of the child's cornea or deposit build-up on the lens. A sterile or bacterial ulcer must be ruled out in contact lens wearers. Exposure keratopathy can occur in children with especially prominent eyes and shallow orbits, such as occurs with craniofacial abnormalities. Children with Down's syndrome may fail to sufficiently close their eyes when sleeping, thus resulting in chronic keratopathy. Their symptoms may be aggravated by chronic blepharitis (Shapiro & France 1985). Most corneal dystrophies do not result in pain although some epithelial dystrophies may cause painful photophobia.

Conjunctiva

Isolated conjunctivitis does not cause pain unless there is an associated keratitis or iritis. If pain is present, then episcleritis must be considered as an alternative or associated diagnosis.

One common circumstance in which the conjunctiva is apparently responsible for eye discomfort is in the post-operative strabismus patient. The conjunctival suture often causes a foreign body sensation probably by corneal stimulation. One argument for the cul-de-sac incision is to provide better post-operative comfort since the suture position is away from the immediate peri-limbal position.

Episclera

Inflammation of the episclera can be either nodular, as in the chicken pox lesion, or diffuse. Episcleritis is associated with marked injection and may involve the overlying conjunctiva as well.

Lacrimal gland

Pain secondary to dry eyes is an uncommon occurrence in children. Dry eyes may occur as a side-effect of cancer chemotherapy; these children are often given artificial tears prophylactically. Absent tear production associated with Riley–Day syndrome, although a cause of dry eyes and recurrent corneal ulceration, is devoid of any eye pain since corneal sensation is absent. Lacrimal gland swelling is rare in children though it may occur with parotid gland swelling in mumps. Dacryodenitis occurs rarely in association with a childhood viremia and produces vague discomfort around the eyes. Lacrimal gland infarction associated with sickle cell disease can result in rapid swelling of the gland and mimic acute bacterial cellulitis. Childhood inflammatory orbital disease, with signs and symptoms compatible with orbital pseudotumour, is often associated with pain (Mottow & Jakobiec 1978).

Lacrimal sac

Acute dacryocystitis may occur in infants with a nonpatent nasolacrimal system. The pain is accompanied by swelling in the region of the nasolacranial sac as well as other signs of acute infection.

Glaucoma

The eye pain of congenital glaucoma is also associated with photophobia. Both result from corneal abnormalities as the neonate's cornea is stretched by the high pressure. With breaks in Descemet's membrane, stromal edema and epithelial irregularities develop, leading to pain and photophobia. The child whose pressure is brought under control may continue to have light sensitivity as a consequence of corneal scarring.

Uvea

Since the iris is supplied with pain fibres, iritis is associated with pain which may be augmented by ciliary spasm. The symptom of pain may be difficult to sort out from photophobia: the combination results in an extremely uncomfortable eye. Childhood iritis may occur in association with infection (measles, chickenpox), often in conjunction with keratitis. The iritis of juvenile rheumatoid arthritis is only occasionally painful. Iritis may occur in conjunction with hyphema which is usually traumatic. If not associated with trauma, infiltrative processes such as childhood leukemia or juvenile xanthogranuloma must be considered.

More posterior forms of childhood uveitis include pars planitis and toxocara lesions. These inflammations usually present as visual loss rather than with eye pain. Because the iris and uvea include many pain fibres, this must be considered when doing laser procedures on co-operative children. A laser peripheral iridectomy or retinal photocoagulation may be uncomfortable.

Optic nerve

The retina and optic nerves do not contain pain fibers but the optic nerve sheath does. Eye pain may occur with childhood optic neuritis. As with adult optic neuritis, the pain most commonly is initiated by looking from side to side; this puts the inflamed nerve sheath on stretch, eliciting pain. More chronic distention of the nerve sheath, such as occurs with optic nerve sheath glioma in children, does not elicit pain.

Lids

Acute distention of all or part of the lids results in vague pain. A child with a stye (hordeolum) complains of pain much more consistently than those with chalazion. Preseptal cellulitis results in tremendous stretching of the lid tissue, and pain is one of the hallmark symptoms.

Lids of children with chronic allergy may itch rather than cause true pain. Their skin becomes scaly with the eczematous reaction.

Orbit and CNS

Orbital pain may result from local irritation of pain fibers. Such pain usually implies an acute event, such as a rapidly expanding mass or pseudotumour (Mottow & Jakobiec 1978). The pain, however, may be referred pain from intracranial irritation of the dura. Cavernous sinus inflammation, such as occurs in individuals with Tolosa–Hunt syndrome, causes pain within the orbit, but does not often occur in children (Kline 1982). Rarely brainstem glioma may present with episodic pain, sometimes with facial spasm.

Painful IIIrd nerve palsy

Adults with posterior communicating artery aneurysms may complain that for years before their acute painful IIIrd nerve palsy they had had intermittent eye or orbital pain, but unless they complain of diplopia or have physical signs when they are examined they usually go undiagnosed for years. Ophthalmoplegic migraine, although its name implies an associated headache, is often pain free.

Painful VIth nerve palsy

In childhood the sudden onset of a VIth nerve palsy, the sudden worsening of an existing concomitant squint with the appearance features of incomitance or the onset of a convergent squint worse in the distance, together with facial pain should make one think of petrous apex osteitis secondary to mastoiditis or suppurative otitis media (Gradenigo's syndrome). This was common in pre-antibiotic days but now painful VIth nerve palsy is probably more frequently seen with orbital or retro-orbital disease.

Herpes zoster ophthalmicus (HZO)

Although relatively unusual in children it does occur and it may give rise to severe discomfort in the acute phase. Post-herpetic neuralgia, however, seems to be exceptionally unusual in children. As opposed to adults with HZO, children with this condition have a significant incidence of systemic disease including immune deficiency and leukaemia. Treatment with antiviral agents and steroids may reduce the incidence of post-herpetic neuralgia.

Trigeminal neuralgia

Trigeminal neuralgia is predominantly a disease of old age (Poser 1975) but cases have been described in early childhood (Harris 1943). It may be secondary to pontine tumours or tumours including vascular anomalies which press on the Vth nerve. It has been associated with multiple sclerosis (Harris 1950) but, especially in childhood, this is probably not significant. The pain is severe and paroxysmal lasting seconds but leaving the child shaking and upset for a while afterwards. The fact that it is facial pain causing the problem is not obvious in the smaller child who may not be able to communicate his problem so well. Detailed neuroradiology of the course of the Vth nerve is indicated.

Headache

A child may occasionally talk about eye pain when in fact the complaint is a more generalized headache. The interpretation as 'eye pain' may be an important localizing symptom for a further discussion of childhood headache. (See Problem 16.)

Functional eye pain

The child between 5 and 8 years has learned that complaining about pain leads to parental attention. Occasionally, this complaint may centre around his eyes. The child may really be asking to get glasses, as further questioning may reveal this motive. Siblings of children with bona fide eye problems may have observed the extra commotion and attention given the sibling and hope for equal treatment by complaining of eye pain. Nevertheless, a diagnosis of a functional disorder is purely one of exclusion in any child which usually can be made with ease after listening to and observing the child.

Diagnostic techniques

Since the vast majority of underlying pathology is either corneal or conjunctival in origin, these structures must be carefully examined under magnification.

The slit lamp examination can be performed on children of all ages. Staining the cornea with fluorescein or rose bengal should only be performed after corneal sensation has been assessed. In children who cannot co-operate for a slit lamp, the cobalt blue Wood's light which is normally used for assessing fit of hard contact lenses can be used or a +20 lens with the cobalt blue filter fitted over the indirect ophthalmoscope.

In a non co-operative child, the +20 lens or operating loupes may provide adequate magnification. If one decides that a lid speculum must be used, a topical anaesthetic drop must be used. Application of the drops to the fellow eye may suppress the blink reflex reducing squeezing of the lids. If a lid speculum is not available, a paper clip with the round end bent over will provide lid retraction. When a foreign body is suspected but not seen, double lid eversion must be performed. When metallic foreign bodies are suspected in the setting of a metal-on-metal, e.g. hammer and nail injury, one must consider radiologic studies to exclude foreign bodies situated more deeply in the eyes. It is also important to document the absence of foreign bodies after treatment if any doubt is present.

The slit lamp or magnification with loupes also provides information about the adnexal structures and is particularly important in cases of chronic keratoconjunctivitis.

The diagnosis of congenital glaucoma includes accurate measurement of intraocular pressure. The Perkin's tonometer is particularly helpful, as the pneumotonometer appears to be more affected by corneal scarring. Examinations under sedation may be necessary for accurate intraocular pressure assessment since the pressure is liable to be altered under anaesthesia.

The assessment of possible preseptal cellulitis is aimed at excluding the diagnosis of orbital cellulitis or primary ocular infection. The globe itself must be seen, as lid swelling can occur secondary to endophthalmitis, and as signs of orbital cellulitis are found by examining the globe. A lid speculum is usually required.

The diagnosis of iritis may be particularly difficult to make in children: the slit lamp must be used. Miosis as well as irregularity of the pupil due to synechiae may support the diagnosis of iritis when examination with the slit lamp is difficult. Many direct ophthalmoscopes include a slit aperture which can be used in lieu of a slit lamp if the situation demands.

Neuroradiological studies are required whenever orbital swelling persists or when the quality of retro-orbital pain and presence of associated symptoms suggests intracranial pathology. Orbital abscesses, optic nerve sheath pathology, lacrimal gland swelling are all usually detectable with these studies. A bone scan is rarely indicated when concern about a lacrimal gland infarct in association with sickle cell disease is present. Debate often occurs as to when a neuroradiological study should be performed in cases of presumed periorbital cellulitis. If the child fails to respond to intravenous antibiotics after 36−48 hours, then CT or MRI scanning should be performed to exclude the possibility of orbital mass (such as retinoblastoma, rhabdomyosarcoma, or abscess).

Treatment

The treatment of eye pain depends upon the underlying cause. Corneal abrasions are often left unpatched in children, since the patch itself may be uncomfortable. If the symptoms have persisted for 2 days, then a pressure patch is indicated. The addition of a cycloplegic agent to prevent ciliary spasm may make the patient more comfortable. If the cause of the abrasion is potentially infectious, (such as a cat scratch) then the patient must be followed very carefully to ensure that a corneal ulcer does not develop.

Foreign bodies must be removed. Start simply, as if you were removing an eye lash, pulling the lower lid down and instructing the patient to look around. Then try an applicator moistened with topical anesthetic. If these simple techniques do not work, then the examiner must judge if the child is sufficiently cooperative to have the foreign body removed with more traditional techniques of dental burrs or small gauge needles. When in doubt, sedate the child or arrange anesthesia, as the risk of a more significant scar is not worth the pride of doing it 'the adult way'. Many children can co-operate, however, and it is up to the examiner to set the stage for co-operation. Folk remedies in some middle Eastern countries have relied upon women who remove the foreign body with their tongue; although this treatment has apparently withstood the test of time, its mention here should not be taken as an endorsement!

References

Carithers HA. Cat-scratch disease. *Am J Dis Child* 1970; **119**: 200−3

Carithers HA. Oculoglandular disease of parinaud. *Am J Dis Child* 1978; **132**: 1195−200

Harris W. Trigeminal neuralgia at an exceptionally early age. *Br Med J* 1943; **2**: 39

Harris W. Rare forms of trigeminal neuralgia and their relation to disseminated sclerosis. *Br Med J* 1950; **2**: 1015−9

Kline L. The Tolosa−Hunt syndrome. *Surv Ophthalmol* 1982; **27**: 79−95

Miller N. Anatomy and physiology of the trigeminal nerve. In: Miller N (Ed.) *Walsh and Hoyt's clinical neuro-ophthalmology*, 4th edn. Williams & Wilkins, Baltimore 1985; 999−1043

Mottow LS, Jakobiec FA. Idiopathic inflammatory orbital pseudotumor in childhood. I. Clinical characteristics. *Arch Ophthalmol* 1978; **96**: 1410−17

Norn M. Conjunctival sensitivity in normal eyes. *Acta Ophthalmol* 1973; **51**: 58−66

Poser CM. Facial pain: diagnostic dilemma, therapeutic challenge. *Geriatrics* 1975; **30**: 110−5

Shapiro MB, France TD. The ocular features of Down's syndrome. *Am J Ophthalmol* 1985; **99**: 659−63

P12 Blurred Vision

SUSAN DAY

Signs and symptoms

A young child rarely complains that he is unable to see unless the visual loss is acute and bilateral. Poor vision is usually suspected by the parents, other relatives, or school teachers on the basis of the child's behaviour. Parents may relate that the child sits close to the television, seems disinterested in all objects except those in his hand, or holds a book close to one eye. They may note a turn of the head or squeezing of the eye lids when an effort to see is being made. School teachers may sense a child's difficulty in seeing the blackboard or in reading a book. Difficulty with vision is often perceived as an underlying cause for a child's slow learning or poor reading abilities.

Acute bilateral vision loss is rare. A change in behaviour is noted, such as a child's stumbling around a familiar room. He may complain that the lights should be turned on or, paradoxically, complain bitterly of photophobia. The observant child may even say that colours have become faded.

Associated symptoms, both ocular and systemic, usually point to causes of visual loss other than refractive error. Eye pain or redness, photophobia, and leukocoria may be observed by those close to the child. Headache, failure to thrive, seizure disorders, delayed or premature puberty, all may accompany visual loss in the child. The ophthalmologist needs to inquire about systemic health in every child who presents with visual loss.

Monocular visual loss or 'blurred' vision presents in an entirely different fashion. For chronic underlying causes, strabismus may occur, since there is no fusional drive to 'keep the eyes straight'. A non-seeing eye will usually turn inward if the defect is present from an early age and will turn outward in older individuals, but there are very many exceptions to this classic teaching. When strabismus is associated with poor vision in one eye, the visual loss cannot be attributed to simple amblyopia until other more ominous causes of visual loss have been excluded.

Monocular visual loss often causes failure at a school screening examination. These tests usually assess vision monocularly and may include other tests of binocular function.

Finally, concern about possible blurred vision may be raised in the context of a family history of eye problems.

Diagnosis

Visual acuity

This must be assessed at both distance and near since a discrepancy between the two will possibly suggest a refractive error. When blurred vision is the presenting complaint or when the recorded acuity is less than expected, the ophthalmologist must check the visual acuity himself. Hesitation on the child's part, adopting an abnormal head position, squeezing the eyes shut, all can be seen only by observing not only what the child sees but how the child sees. Record this behaviour in the patient's notes: this provides much more information than a simple fractional notation.

Refraction

See Chapter 8.

Optic nerve function

These include assessment for pupillary responses, colour vision, and visual fields as well as clinical evaluation of the optic nerve appearance. These functions should be checked carefully whenever systemic symptoms demand or whenever acuity cannot be improved to an expected level despite appropriate optical correction. For details of specific examination techniques, see Chapter 7.

Media examination

This includes a search for any preretinal abnormality interfering with vision. The retinoscope provides the quickest way to assess media clarity and should be used before the pupils are dilated. In this way, the impact of ptosis, corneal irregularities, anterior segment abnormalities, lens opacities, and vitreous opacities can be ascertained in the normal non-dilated state. Although the retinoscope will not always pinpoint the location of the abnormality, it will highlight the amount of interference with the optical axis.

Whenever the retinoscopy defines a problem with media clarity other than ptosis a slit lamp examination is mandatory. This will define whether the alteration is corneal, anterior segment, lenticular, or in the vitreous (see Chapter 7). The direct and indirect ophthalmoscope may aid in further definition of posterior media abnormalities.

Fundoscopy

Both the direct and indirect ophthalmoscope should be used whenever the cause for blurred vision remains a puzzle. Details, such as changes in the retinal nerve fiber layer and foveal pigment irregularities are best appreciated with the direct ophthalmoscope, whereas the panoramic view is gained from indirect ophthalmoscopy; both are necessary.

Neurological testing

When the history suggests a neurological cause for blurred vision simple neurological examination such as finger-to-nose testing of cerebellar function or observation of tandem-walking skills is a helpful aid to diagnosis and assessment. Other testing of cranial nerves, motor function and cognitive tasks may be undertaken when appropriate.

Causes and treatment

Refractive error

Blurred vision in association with refractive error reflects not only the type of refractive error but also the accommodation. It is uncommon for children to present with refractive-error blurred vision before 9–12-years-old because of the prevalence of low to moderate hyperopia with excellent accommodation. Change in refractive error toward myopia typically occurs between 10 and 14 years (Brown 1938; Slataper 1950). The increase in myopia is more pronounced before than after puberty and changes are more pronounced in a myopic child than a hyperopic child (Mantyjarvi 1985).

Children with hyperopia in general do not have reduced vision unless the refractive error exceeds 5–6 diopters. Uncommonly, however, bilateral isoametropic amblyopia may be found with hyperopia as low as four diopters. The most common form of presentation of moderate hyperopic refractive errors is as accommodative esotropia rather than blurred vision.

Myopic children typically have blurred distance vision with difficulty seeing the school blackboard, habitual television viewing at a close distance, and peering in an attempt to see. Such a child may try on someone's glasses and note the dramatic improvement in vision. Extremely high myopic refractive errors capable of inducing isoametropic amblyopia may present early as parents become concerned about the child's vision.

Purely astigmatic refractive errors are unusual causes for blurred vision despite the high incidence of astigmatism in the first years of life (Mohindra & Held 1981; Dobson et al. 1984). Gwiazda et al. (1985) were unable to find any differences in visual development in astigmatic infants who were given correction and those who were not given optical correction. Nevertheless, true meriodional amblyopia has been demonstrated (Mitchell et al. 1973) in adults.

Refractive errors are rarely responsible for poor

school performance. Print in school books is usually large, and refractive errors which are significant usually present as difficulty with distance vision (Tongue 1987).

'Failed school examination'

The parents often bring a child for further examination with a note from school expressing concern about a failed vision screening examination. Often the parent will volunteer that there is not any problem with the child's visual behaviour. Occasionally, the parent will be afraid that the child is going blind, has a brain tumour, or has been medically neglected.

Although a child who has failed a screening exam deserves a thorough examination to exclude pathology, the 'yield' is very low. Most commonly, the child's co-operation or understanding of the test may have been limited, and a simple thorough recheck may reveal normal acuity. Secondly, the content of the screening exam may include areas such as 'visual motor integration', 'accommodative facility', and other measurements not in general regarded as important by ophthalmologists. It helps if the ophthalmologist is acquainted with the local screening techniques and participates in their establishment and review (Simon & Metz 1985).

Media opacities

Anything which interferes with a clear image being focussed on the retina may be regarded as a media opacity and the closer it is to the nodal point of the eye, the more significant it is. Thus, a posterior capsular cataract usually has a more devastating effect on vision than an anteriorly placed lens opacity.

The most anterior of media opacities is lid anomalies. Ptosis can occlude the visual axis or induce astigmatism which creates a 'blur'. It most commonly induces amblyopia with unilateral involvement although refractive errors are frequently also present. Capillary hemangiomas also warrant early intervention whenever their presence interferes with the visual axis or induces astigmatism (Nelson et al. 1984; Pasyk et al. 1984).

Acquired corneal clouding or inflammation can induce visual blurring. Keratitis from any cause may reduce acuity in association with irritation and watery discharge. Symptoms due to keratoconus usually present during the second decade as slowly progressive visual loss, perhaps with multiple attempts at correction with glasses or contact lenses (Leibowitz 1984).

Dystrophies presenting within the early years of life can result in recurrent epithelial defects or reduced vision (Waring et al. 1984).

Blurred vision as a consequence of anterior segment inflammation is usually associated with pain, redness, and photophobia, however in Still's disease (juvenile rheumatoid arthritis or JRA) vision may become impaired without any associated symptoms. Iridocyclitis is most commonly found in the pauciarticular form, seronegative for rheumatoid factor, and positive on antinuclear antibody testing. The ocular involvement may even precede arthritic involvement.

In the older child with cataract a blurring of vision may occur, such as with an acquired metabolic or traumatic cataract or in a child who has been on long-term systemic or topical steroids. A unilateral or sometimes bilateral congenital cataract may cause symptoms and present in older children. The child may also report glare when a partial cataract is present.

Vitreous opacities including haemorrhage, vitritis, retinoblastoma seedlings or vitreous cysts are uncommon causes of blurred vision. When the vitreous is too opacificied to allow visualization, other diagnostic tests must be performed such as ultrasound and/or CT scanning of the eyes and orbits.

Retinal vitreous and optic nerve causes

RETINOBLASTOMA

Approximately 5% of children with retinoblastoma have visual difficulties as a presenting feature (Ellsworth 1987). More slowly growing and unilateral tumours may present at a later age and retinoblastoma must be excluded in any child presenting with poor vision or strabismus.

PERSISTENT HYPERPLASTIC PRIMARY VITREOUS (PHPV)

Mild PHPV may cause blurred vision if the refractive error differs significantly from the fellow eye, or if there is progression opacity or secondary glaucoma.

RETINOPATHY OF PREMATURITY (ROP)

Retinopathy of prematurity can create various levels of reduced vision, but fortunately resolves spontaneously in the vast majority of cases. Nevertheless, ROP represents a significant cause of visual loss amongst children (Phelps 1981).

When they are older, premature infants may have blurred vision from myopia (Nissenkorn *et al.* 1983; Gordon & Donzis 1986), or as a consequence of isoametropic amblyopia or of vitreous or retinal detachment.

COATS' DISEASE

Coats' disease is characterized by poor vision, usually unilateral, affecting males more than females, usually within the first decade of life (Ridley *et al.* 1982) (see Chapter 27.5).

RETINAL DYSTROPHIES

The visual disturbances with retinal dystrophies are variable. Family history of early visual loss may be present, and bilaterality is the rule. There may be associated systemic findings. Blurred vision is rarely a complaint in retinitis pigmentosa in the early stages; rather, night-blindness and loss of peripheral visual field occur. These children also tend to have high myopic or hypermetropic refractive errors. (See Chapter 27.3.)

SYSTEMIC DISEASE

Retinal involvement from systemic disease warrants particular consideration since the ocular findings may lead directly to the systemic diagnosis. Blurred vision may also occur as a consequence of side effects of treatment.

Leukaemia, the most common childhood malignancy, can involve the eye in many ways. Most commonly, leukemic retinopathy reflects anaemia, hyperviscosity, and thrombocytopenia. When haemorrhage or leukaemic infiltration directly involves the macula, then vision may be affected. Opportunistic infections such as candidiasis and cytomegalovirus may result in progressive visual loss (Rosenthal 1983).

Juvenile onset diabetes may present within the first year of life, but retinopathy is uncommon in the first decade (Lynn *et al.* 1974; Palmberg *et al.* 1981). Blurred vision may, however, result from myopia induced by rapid shifts in blood glucose levels, or from optic atrophy associated with DIDMOAD (see Chapter 29.).

Metabolic disorders can create blurred vision on a retinal basis, including Batten's disease, mucopolysaccharidoses, mucolipidoses, and other neurometabolic diseases.

Optic nerve

Optic neuropathies can at times present startling examples of acute visual loss. The child may describe the loss more as 'dim' vision than 'blurry' vision. Childhood optic neuritis may follow a viral illness. The ophthalmologist usually sees the patient after a CT scan has been ordered by the paediatrician. Poor pupil responses, poor colour vision, and a central scotoma or constricted visual fields with poor acuity all point to a diagnosis of optic neuritis rather than papilloedema.

Dominant optic atrophy, with its slow deterioration of vision during the first two decades, represents a subtle often misdiagnosed form of decreased vision in children. The key to its diagnosis is to assess other family members and to recognize the classic wedge-shaped area of temporal optic nerve pallor (Hoyt 1980).

In Leber's optic neuropathy the presentation is usually in the second or third decade. Typically, involvement is first in one eye with an interval of days to weeks before the second eye is affected. Central vision is lost, and colours become faded. Although the condition typically affects males, females can also develop Leber's optic neuropathy. Acutely, there is optic disc swelling, but optic atrophy ensues although a variable recovery of vision may occur years later. (See chapter 29.)

Optic atrophy without ocular post-inflammatory or hereditary causes suggests a central nervous system abnormality. Although this usually results in bilateral involvement, unilateral involvement does not exclude this group of disorders.

Congenital optic nerve abnormalities can also be associated with later poor vision especially when the lesion is unilateral and discovered later or as a result of school testing.

Finally, whenever fundus findings suggest a retinal or optic nerve disorder which does not seem to neatly fit into a category, trauma, either accidental or non-accidental must be suspected. Usually suspicion is raised on the basis of an odd sounding history or unusual reaction of the child when interrogation hints at concern about possible trauma. When non-accidental injury is suspected, medical as well as legal issues to protect the child must be addressed.

Central nervous system abnormalities

Blurred or reduced vision can result from involvement of the visual pathways; any prechiasmal lesion will result in optic atrophy. Increased intracranial pressure may cause papilloedema regardless of its location and visual blur may occur intermittently as a consequence of this. Papilloedema does not typically cause visual symptoms but if severe and especially if it is also chronic there may be rapid unilateral or bilateral loss of vision. These 'obscurations' are transient, lasting only seconds, and are posture related. Children usually refer to them as blackouts, greyness or dimming.

A severely atrophic optic nerve will not appear swollen despite increased intracranial pressure since no retinal nerve fibre layer is present to become swollen. A child with a central nervous system mass (especially in the posterior fossa) is often ill, complaining of vomiting and headache. He may also observe diplopia as a consequence of associated cranial nerve palsy although suppression may mask this symptom.

The parachiasmal syndrome of visual defect, growth and other hyperthalamic disturbances represents a particular challenge. The usual causes in children are optic pathway glioma and craniopharyngioma. Various combinations of optic atrophy and papilloedema occur depending on the duration of the process and the tempo of the intracranial disease.

Hydrocephalus is a not uncommon cause of visual loss in children; the usual cause of the visual loss is papilloedema but dilation of the third ventricle results in splaying of the chiasm with subsequent bilateral optic atrophy.

Cortical blindness represents a particularly frustrating diagnosis, since there are so few ophthalmological findings. This term has also been used erroneously when hydrocephalus or midline masses were present. Cortical blindness often follows perinatal anoxia but also occurs with meningitis or encephalitis.

Hysterical/malingering visual loss

See Chapter 33.

References

Brown EVL. Net average yearly changes in refraction of atropinized eyes from birth to beyond middle life. *Arch Ophthalmol* 1938; **19**: 719–34

Dobson V, Fulton AB, Sebris SL. Cycloplegic refraction of infantile and young children: the axis of astigmatism. *Invest Ophthalmol Vis Sci* 1984; **25**: 83–7

Ellsworth RM. Retinoblastoma. In: Duane T (ed.) *Clinical ophthalmology*, Vol. 3, Harper & Row, Philadelphia 1987; pp. 1–19

Gordon RA, Donzis PE. Myopia associated with retinopathy of prematurity. *Ophthalmology* 1986; **93**: 1593–8

Gwiazda J, Mohindra I, Brill S, Held R. Infant astigmatism and meridional amblyopia. *Invest Ophthalmol Vis Sci* 1985; **25**: 1269–76

Hoyt CS. Autosomal dominant optic atrophy: a spectrum of disability. *Ophthalmology* 1980; **87**: 245–51

Leibowitz HM. Keratoconus. In: Leibowitz HM (ed.) *Corneal disorders* WB Saunders, Philadelphia, 1984; pp. 100–20

Lynn JR, Snyder WB, Vaiser A (eds) *Epidemiology of Diabetic Retinopathy*. Grune & Stratton New York, 1974

Mitchell DE, Freeman RD, Millodot M *et al.* Meridional amblyopia: evidence for modification of the visual system by early visual experience. *Vision Res* 1973; **13**: 535–57

Mantyjarvi MI. Changes of refraction in schoolchildren. *Arch Ophthalmol* 1985; **103**: 790–2

Mohindra I, Held R. Refraction in humans from birth to 5 years. In: Fledelius HC, Alsbirk PH, Goldschmidt E (eds) *Documenta Ophthalmologica Proceeding* Series 28, Third International Conference on Myopia, Copenhagen 1980. Dr W Junk NV publishers, The Hague 1981; pp. 19–27

Nelson LB, Melick JE, Harley RD. Intralesional corticosteroid injections for infantile hemangiomas of the eyelid. *Pediatrics* 1984; **74**: 241–5

Nissenkorn I, Kremer I, Ben-Sira I *et al.* Myopia in premature babies with and without retinopathy of prematurity. *Br J Ophthalmol* 1983; **67**: 170–3

Palmberg P, Smith M, Watman S *et al.* The natural history of retinopathy in insulin-dependent juvenile onset diabetes. *Ophthalmology* 1981; **88**: 613–8

Pasyk KA, Dingman RO, Argenta LC, Sandal GS. The management of hemangiomas of the eyelid and orbit. *Head Neck Surg* 1984; **6**: 851–7

Phelps DL. Vision loss due to retinopathy of prematurity (Letter). *Lancet* 1981; **1**: 606

Ridley ME, Shields JA, Brown GC *et al.* Coats' disease: evaluation of management. *Ophthamology* 1982; **89**: 1381–7

Rosenthal AR. Ocular manifestations of leukaemia. *Ophthalmology* 1983; **90**: 899–905

Simon JW, Metz HS. School vision testing (Editorial). *J Pediatr Ophthalmol Strabismus* 1985; **22**: 5

Slataper FJ. Age norms of refraction and vision. *Arch Ophthalmol* 1950; **43**: 466–81

Tongue AC. Refractive errors in children. *Pediatr Clin North Am* 1987; **34**: 1425–37

Waring GO, Rodrigues MM, Laibson PR. Corneal Dystrophies. In: Leibowitz HM (ed.) *Corneal Disorders* WB Saunders Philadelphia, 1984; pp. 57–99

P13 Investigation of Acquired Poor Vision in Childhood

DAVID TAYLOR

In the investigation of suspected poor vision in childhood, taking a detailed history is important to be sure that the disease is really acquired and to detail its onset.

If the onset is acute, a careful examination of the anterior and posterior segments may well reveal the cause. If the anterior and posterior segments are normal on examination the cause of the visual loss may be intracranial such as hydrocephalus, meningitis or encephalitis; the child may have optic neuritis or optic nerve compression. When the examination is completely normal one should always consider hysterical blindness, but not be put off the possibility of there being underlying organic disease by the presence of non-organic symptoms.

If the onset is ill-defined or chronic the abnormality may be discovered by careful examination of the anterior and posterior segments. If these are normal the cause may still be optic nerve compression because optic atrophy takes many weeks to appear. High ametropia must be ruled out by refraction and optic neuritis should be considered if the onset is relatively recent. In a normal child, in whom the visually evoked responses are abnormal, intracranial causes of blindness such as tumours, hydrocephalus, meningitis, encephalitis or leucodystrophies (adrenoleucodystrophy typically presents as blindness in young boys) can be ruled out by appropriate investigations. Hysterical blindness is often chronic in its onset. The figure gives guidelines but should not be thought of as being complete.

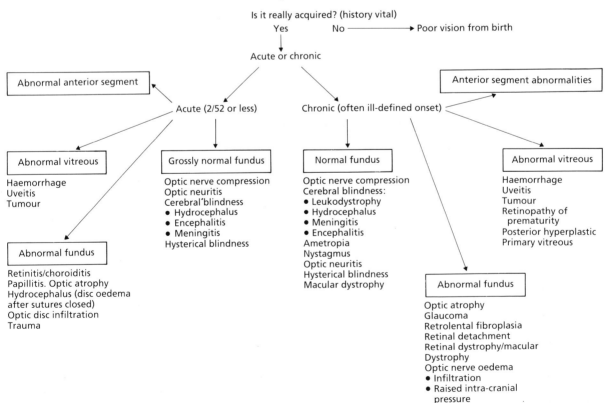

Fig. P13.1 The investigation of bilateral acquired poor vision in childhood.

P14 The Deaf-Blind Child

NICHOLAS CAVANAGH

The association of both ocular and auditory dysfunction is not rare, and apart from congenital rubella, it occurs in many syndromes. It follows from this, that a case can well be made for all deaf children to have full ophthalmological examination, and vice versa. Indeed, Rogers *et al.* (1988) having screened three hundred and sixty hearing impaired students for visual problems, found an overall 43% had either significant refractive errors or pathologic findings (Usher's syndrome contributed about 15% of the pathology). Regenbogen and Godel (1985) found 45% of 150 deaf children had ocular anomalies interfering with good vision.

How might it be best to group and subdivide what would otherwise be an extremely diverse collection of diseases with only ocular and auditory involvement in common? One approach is to consider them under the following headings and refer to the index to locate more details about each condition mentioned.

Diseases associated with the deaf-blind child

1 Conditions with lens problems, e.g.
Congenital rubella;
Congenital toxoplasmosis;
Congenital cytomegalovirus;
Alport's syndrome.
2 Conditions with pigmentary or other retinopathy, e.g.
Usher's syndrome;
Cockayne's syndrome;
Mucopolysaccharidoses;
Alström's disease;
Stickler's disease;
Refsum's disease;
Congenital rubella;
Toxoplasmosis.
3 Conditions with anterior segment changes, e.g.
Mucopolysaccharidoses;
Cogan's syndrome (keratitis and deafness);
Trisomy 8;
Alport's disease;
Congenital rubella.
4 Conditions with optic disc abnormalities, e.g.
DIDMOAD;
Von Recklinghausen's disease;
Trauma;
Friedreich's ataxia;
Spinocerebellar degeneration;
Prematurity;
Meningitis;
Syphilis;
Metachromatic leukodystrophy;
Trisomy 13;
CHARGE association.

A child with the double handicap has more than the sum of the problems of either of the handicaps on their own. He poses an enormous management difficulty. McInnes and Jeffrey (1977) sum up his predicament like this. 'The deaf-blind child is one whose condition of visual and auditory impairment results in multisensory deprivation which renders inadequate the traditional approach to child rearing used to alleviate the handicap of blindness, deafness, and retardation.' Such children depend for their case upon a truly multi-disciplinary approach from a team which would include ophthalmologist, audiologist, ENT surgeon, psychiatrist, geneticist, psychologist, specialist teacher and may also include cardiologist, cardiothoracic surgeon, plastic surgeon, neurosurgeon, etc., all being co-ordinated by a paediatrician, perhaps ideally by a paediatric neurologist. Whilst it is a truism in paediatrics that specialists have to relate to the child both directly and through his parents, in the case of the multisensory deprived child the role of the parents/carers is pivotal both in terms of greater commitment of time to be in direct physical contact with the child than would be the case with the normal child, and also because of the more prolonged dependance of the child on a one to one relationship.

Management of the deaf-blind child

The role of the ophthalmologist is, in the first place, to assist in establishing the diagnosis, since this will permit more accurate genetic and prognostic advice, specific treatment when available, and better overall management. Later, he may be involved in the provision of treatment for some remediable conditions such as cataract, corneal defects, glaucoma or refractive errors. This commitment should be on-going.

Parents of newly diagnosed children often wish to be put in contact with other similarly affected families. In the UK a National Deaf-Blind and -Rubella Association has been formed, and this has established a National Advisory Service with a team of advising teachers to assist the deaf-blind child and his family.

Detailed description of the aims and practice of management of the deaf-blind child is beyond the scope of this brief section and the reader is referred to McInnes and Telfrey (1982) or *Multiply Handicapped Children* (1986) by R. Wyman, 1986. However some general comments can be made. Deaf-blind children may be initially hypo or hyper-reactive and nearly all show a dislike of being touched. An attempt has to be made to overcome this by contact with the child on a one to one basis through activities he enjoys such as eating, toileting, etc., employing whatever residual hearing and vision there is. Initially the aim has to be

to encourage the child to tolerate, accept and co-operate passively with the parent or carer who should either stand behind, but in contact with the child or seat him between his knees.

This phase has the dual effect of allowing the parent to understand and assess the child's abilities and level of function and thus enable him to formulate later programmes that fit those abilities. Through co-active, co-operative and reactive stages the child can be led gradually to the point when he can be encouraged to formulate objectives and solve them himself, rather than be simply manipulated. With the ability to use information to solve problems, formal education can begin. Intervention must aim to provide help that covers all areas of development including gross and fine vision, social and emotional, language and concepts, perception and life styles, as well as specific visual and auditory problems. It is important not to mislabel these children as retarded on the grounds of delayed development.

References

McInnes JM, Telfrey JA. The deaf−blind child. In: Freeman JR, Scott E (eds) *Visual Impairment in Children and Adolescents*. Grune & Stratton 1977; pp. 337−64

McInnes JM, Telfrey JA. *Deaf−blind Infants and Children*. Open University Press, Milton Keynes 1982

Regenbogen L, Godel V. Ocular deficiencies in deaf children. *J Pediatr Ophthalmol Strabismus* 1985; **22**: 231−3

Rogers GL, Pillman RD, Brenner DL, Leguire LO. Screening of school aged hearing impaired chilren. *J Paediatr Ophthalmol Strabismus* 1988; **25**: 230−2

Wyman R. *Multiply Handicapped Children*. 1986 Souvenir Press (Human Horzers Series), London

P15 Optic Atrophy in Infancy

DAVID TAYLOR

Presentation and diagnosis

Small children with optic atrophy do not have any pathognomic mode of presentation connected with the optic atrophy itself. The history is vital and particular attention should be paid to any family history of poor vision, consanguinity of the parents, the progress of the pregnancy and any suspicion of lack of weight gain as well as any immediately prenatal problem. The most important time in a child's life for acquiring non refractive visual defects is in the perinatal period, particularly if the baby is premature and of low birth weight. The parents of these children should be questioned in detail about their baby's early life; whether the child had to be in an incubator, have added oxygen, be ventilated or any difficulty in breathing. Episodes of bradycardia or apnoea must be noted, also whether the child had to be resuscitated, or the parents warned by the neonatologist that survival was in jeopardy.

If the onset was in postnatal life the mode of onset and progression of the visual defect should be detailed as well as possible, including the parent's opinion on the child's vision. Many observant parents will make relevant observations about vision and even about the state of the pupils, the presence of nystagmus, squint or structural abnormalities of the eye. Their observations should be noted because they will be useful in determining progression; because no objective measurements can be made this does not reduce the value of the clinical observations.

An assessment of the child's vision should be made together with the state of his pupil reactions, which if reacting sluggishly to light or showing a relative afferent pupil defect, will suggest anterior visual pathway disease. In older children an acquired defect of colour vision may help in identifying optic nerve disease, especially if asymmetrical.

The careful examination of the fundus with both direct and indirect ophthalmoscope is mandatory to the diagnosis of optic atrophy. The optic disc itself will appear pale with fewer than normal vessels on the surface. The pallor may be diffuse or segmental, and it is most important to pay attention to the presence of nerve fibre layer atrophy which will show as an enhancement of the normal reflex from the retinal vessels which normally do not stand up greatly above the internal limiting membrane. In optic atrophy where the nerve fibre layer has atrophied the vessels stand out, if the optic atrophy is severe the vessels stand out like cords seen in the light reflected in parallax from the internal limiting membrane as it passes over the vessels.

The differential diagnosis on fundoscopy is between optic atrophy and optic disc hypoplasia or other congenital anomalies, or glaucoma and here it is most important that the optic disc is examined by direct ophthalmoscopy. Structural abnormalities of the optic disc may also be mistaken if the outline of the disc is not grossly abnormal and similarly glaucoma may be missed if the cupping of the optic disc is not noticed during a hasty examination. It is most important to pay very close attention to the state of the optic disc in order not to mistake the normal appearance of an infant's disc when the visual defect may be due to some other cause, for instance delayed visual development.

It is not possible to establish a cause in every case (Repka & Miller 1988) and in published series the cause varies enormously from centre to centre; the tertiary referral teaching centre will see cases biased by a close association with neurology, neurosurgery or metabolic departments, whilst developmental centres will see mainly cerebral palsy cases.

Causes

Fig. P15.1 gives guidelines for diagnosis, details can be acquired from the text.

Optic atrophy occurs in late prenatal or early postnatal life. Early onset damage to the anterior visual system results in a hypoplastic disc or an anomalous optic disc, and in postnatal life optic atrophy is an indication that the damage is anterior to the lateral geniculate body. When the optic atrophy is definitely unilateral the cause is anterior to the chiasm and when it is definitely bilateral it is either due to bilateral disease or disease involving pathways posterior to the chiasm. It is possible that later pre-natal brain damage may, by transynaptic degeneration give rise to optic atrophy without hypoplasia, but there is little clear evidence for this. Prenatal causes of optic atrophy include the hereditary optic neuropathies and metabolic causes. If there is a history of prenatal or perinatal problems this may well be the cause, especially if the degree of anoxia was severe; the clues to this being in the history.

One should be cautious about attributing optic atrophy to a relatively mild perinatal insult and it is rare for optic atrophy caused by perinatal problems to not be associated with other cerebral damage. Postnatal causes include tumours invading or encroaching on the visual pathways. Clues to this in the diagnosis may be in the history of progression of the visual defect, and associated eye movement disorder or the presence of systemic disease such as neurofibromatosis. There may be a clear history of trauma or meningitis and a careful history should be taken of any drug ingestion.

Hydrocephalus may also result in optic atrophy, but it is an extremely unusual presenting symptom. Optic atrophy in hydrocephalus may be difficult to assess even in later life as acuity may be preserved much later than other aspects of vision. Babies with lactic acidosis (i.e. in Leigh's disease, mitochondrial cytopathy, pyruvate decarboxylase or cytochrome oxidase deficiency) have a high incidence of optic atrophy, sometime profound (Hayasaki *et al.* 1986). Other optic neuropathies and many of the hereditary optic neuropathies present later in childhood.

Investigations

Structural eye disease must be excluded and even if the retina appears normal it is as well to carry out an

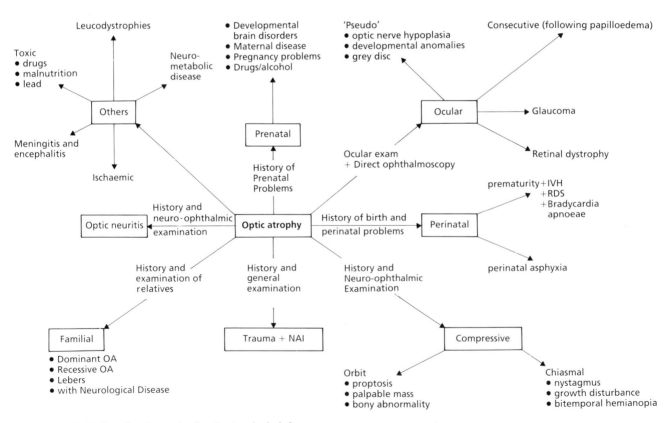

Fig. P15.1 Guidelines for diagnosis of optic atrophy in infancy.

electroretinogram. The integrity of the visual pathways may also be assessed by visually evoked cortical responses. A CT or MRI scan may be indicated, but a CT scan should be avoided wherever possible, due to the (small) risks of X-ray scanning in young children. Systemic investigations are carried out where appropriate.

Prognosis

The prognosis depends on the diagnosis and the natural history of that condition. Much caution should be used in giving a prognosis to parents whose child has recently suffered optic atrophy from an acute cause such as tumour or hydrocephalus, since very dramatic recovery can take place up to 2 or occasionally more years after the onset of the visual loss. As a general rule it is better to be optimistic than pessimistic and this should especially be so if there is still some response to a flash stimulus on the visually evoked cortical responses; every paediatric ophthalmologist has seen examples of remarkable late recovery in vision with optic atrophy or cerebral disorders in infancy.

The uncertainty about the prognosis, however should not inhibit the ophthalmologist from registering the visual handicap with the appropriate authority, although reassessment should be suggested periodically.

References

Hayasaka S, Yamaguchio K, Mizuro K, Miyabayashi S, Narisawa K, Tada K. Ocular findings in childhood lactic acidosis. *Arch Ophthalmol* 1986; **104**: 1656–8

Repka MX, Miller NR. Optic atrophy in children. *Am J Ophthalmol* 1988; **106**: 191–4

P16 Headaches

DAVID TAYLOR

Headache in childhood is common (Hockaday 1983). The incidence varies but in all studies headache occurs in over half of all children but is not necessarily reported to their doctor (Hockaday 1983).

Certain principles are important:
1 The shorter the history the greater the reason for concern.
2 The younger the child the more likely it is that the headache is organic (Hockaday 1983).
3 The history is usually the clue to the diagnosis: most cases are diagnosed on history alone.
4 Important historical detail (i.e. trauma) may be missing.
5 Every headache that interferes with the child's ordinary activity must be regarded seriously unless it is shown to follow a pattern acceptable as migraine.

It is possible to subdivide most headaches into one of four groups (Lance 1978).
1 Acute single episodes (minutes or hours):
  (a) Intracranial disease: meningitis; encephalitis; subarachnoid haemorrhage; and trauma.
  (b) Arterial hypertension.
  (c) Systemic infections with fever.
  (d) Sinusitis and mastoiditis.
  (e) Uveitis or glaucoma.
2 Acute recurrent episodes:
  (a) Migraine and migraine-like syndromes.
  (b) Raised intracranial pressure — intermittent hydrocephalus.
  (c) Subarachnoid haemorrhage.
3 Subacute (days or weeks):
  (a) Intracranial tumour, abscess, or subdural haematoma
  (b) Benign intracranial hypertension.
4 Chronic:
  (a) Stress
  (b) Eyestrain
  (c) Temporomandibular joint and dental problems.
  (d) Psychological or psychiatric states.

There are numerous areas where the above guidelines overlap. For instance, intracranial tumour may present as a chronic headache or stress headaches may present to the doctor with only a short history, but the important point is that a detailed history will correctly classify virtually all headaches.

Stress headaches

Stress headaches are the commonest of childhood headaches, and as modern treatments for stomach ulcer pain decimate the role-models for stomach-ache among children's relatives, the symptom of headache becomes a more frequent excuse for missing days at school.

The mechanism producing the pain may be increased muscle tension, hence the term 'tension' headache, and this is borne out by the occurence of ache and pain in groups of muscles that are caused to contract in a sustained manner. Tension was thought to induce relative ischaemia by vasoconstriction (Wolff 1963), though not all the evidence for this has been corroborated.

The headaches have usually occurred for some months by the time the child is seen by an ophthalmologist and they are usually bifrontal or bitemporal only rarely are they occipital in childhood. They are unusual below 6 years of age. Headaches are frequent in other family members, in particular in the mother. They do not have the migraine accompaniments of visual or other prodromal symptoms and vomiting, although they may feel ill at ease or unwell enough to make them want to lie down.

The headaches occur daily or a few times a week but they are not often clearly related to any particular factor (such as school, working, exercise, etc). Occasionally they are clearly related to the 'causative' factor, e.g. they only occur at school, in church or at the weekly scout meeting.

The underlying stress factors which give rise to the tension is often much more difficult to identify than in hysterical visual defects. The parents should be asked to search for appropriate factors such as teasing at school, poor performance or being 'understretched' at school, or sibling rivalry. Attempts need to be made to modify their life to get around the stress. Analgesics such as paracetamol are helpful but should only be used occasionally. Only rarely is further treatment such as relaxation therapy or psychiatric or psychological help needed. Probably the most important treatment, after exclusion of organic disease, is explanation and reassurance of parent and child.

Hypertension

Although rare in childhood, hypertension is a significant cause of serious disability, e.g. blindness and neurological complications (Hulse *et al.* 1979; Trompeter *et al.* 1982).

One of the main problems is failure of doctors who see a child with neurological problems in the early stages (e.g. facial palsy, convulsions, and altered levels of consciousness), to take the blood pressure. Many hospitals do not even have paediatric sphigmomanometer cuffs! The delay in diagnosis significantly increases the permanent sequelae of the hypertension. The cause is usually renal or renovascular disease with reflux nephropathy and chronic glomerulonephritis being the most common.

Although headache is rarely caused by hyperten-

sion, it is the most common symptom of childhood hypertension, it is usually severe and generalized, it may wake the child or be present on waking and be made worse by stooping or lifting heavy objects. Hypertensive retinopathy or papilloedema is often present (Trompeter *et al.* 1982) on the first examination.

The visual defect may occur from hypertensive damage to the retina, optic nerve and choriod (Hayreh 1986d) and from cortical blindness. Optic nerve infarction occurs as a sudden event when the systemic blood pressure has dropped in a patient in whom ophthalmic and cerebral arterial blood vessels have constricted by autoregulation to compensate for the high blood pressure. The sudden drop in blood pressure causes flow in the constricted vessels to cease, even though the blood pressure may be 'normal' (Hulse *et al.* 1979; Hayreh *et al.* 1986a)

Retinal (Hayreh 1986b) and, more commonly, choroidal (Hayreh 1986c) damage are less frequent causes of permanent visual sequelae, but may cause focal defects.

Hemianopias (Hulse *et al.* 1979) and cortical blindness may result from hypertensive encephalopathy and stroke.

Altered intracranial pressure

Raised intracranial pressure (ICP)

Headache is very frequent in patients with raised ICP and increases in severity and frequency as the ICP rises.

Intermittent at first if the ICP rise is transient, the headaches may become constant and be exacerbated from time to time presumably as the ICP varies. The older child is often manifestly distressed by the pain and may describe it as 'bursting' or 'blowing up'. With sudden rises in ICP, as in posterior fossa tumours, there may be vomiting, sometimes 'projectile'. For example, he vomits with a suddenness and force that is disastrous for the house furnishings and his parents' clothes. The vomiting often improves the headache. Younger children just go 'off colour' or babies become disgruntled and unhappy. Raised ICP in infants can be felt by tenseness of the open fontanelle and the 'expert parent' may know how to recognize the association between tense fontanelle and the child going off-colour.

A major difficulty in paediatric neuroophthalmology is headaches which occur in children with treated hydrocephalus. Many of these resolve themselves simply into those caused by RICP from a blocked shunt or other obvious headache syndrome but there remains a group in whom no cause is found; the shunt is functioning, the scan shows no changes suggestive of currently raised ICP, there is no intellectual deterioration and no papilloedema. Undoubtedly a number of these have stress headaches, perhaps exacerbated by parental worries about the child, but in some there is no stress factor identifiable and can only be managed by reassurance, analgesics, and close monitoring. Occasionally intracranial pressure monitoring may help (Minns 1977).

The headache is usually generalized but in some instances overlies the area of an abscess or tumour. Pituitary tumours may have a point headache at the vertex; it is instructive to ask the child to point with one finger to where the ache is.

Classic observations on the localization and significance of headache were made by Northfield (1938) and Wolff (1963), the localization of the headache is probably less significant than the other aspects.

Benign intracranial hypertension

Benign intracranial hypertension (BIH, pseudotumour cerebri) is not uncommon in childhood. It can occur without obvious precipitating cause (Grant 1971). Causes may include: withdrawal of steroids, vitamin A intoxication, tetracycline ingestion, lateral sinus thrombosis (often after dehydration in infancy or head trauma, even minor), hyperviscosity, as in polycythaemia and thrombocytosis, and systemic lupus erythematosus (Grant 1971; Carlow & Glasser: 1974; Weisberg & Chutorian 1977; Orcutt et al. 1984). Probably the most common cause is withdrawal of the steroids used in the treatment of leukaemia, eczema, or autoimmune disease. Grant (1971) found an equal sex incidence in children.

The headaches are often frontal and severe but rarely associated with vomiting. The children are often unwell during an attack. Transient visual loss, lasting never more than two or three seconds may occur in severe papilloedema of any cause. They are known as obscurations and are often posture-related, most frequently the child loses vision on standing up. Many children, perhaps because the vision loss is so transient do not describe 'loss of vision' but 'blurriness, blacking, mistiness' or other terms.

The papilloedema is usually bilateral and roughly symmetrical. But it may be highly asymmetrical or even unilateral when there is an anomaly of the optic nerve or its dural sheath, (Sedgwick & Burde 1983),

when there is direct involvement of one optic nerve or when there is profound unilateral optic atrophy with insufficient nerve fibres remaining to form papilloedema.

Visual loss is not often associated with BIH in childhood, but Baker et al. (1985) made it quite clear that severe visual loss can occur especially when the papilloedema is severe, when dural venous sinus thrombosis is the cause, and when there are retinal nerve fibre layer haemorrhages.

Diagnosis is essentially one of exclusion, made much easier by scanning. Middle ear disease, drug ingestion, previous dehydration, trauma and hyperviscosity of the blood can be excluded by appropriate historical questions and examination.

Treatment of the headache of BIH is treatment of the condition. The number of different modes of treatment implies that none is clearly superior. These include Diamox, steroids, repeated lumbar punctures, glycerol ingestion and of course withdrawal of any precipitating factor. Most cases show spontaneous improvement but for those in whom the headaches do not improve and are disabling, if there is a consequent or threatened neurological deficit or threatened visual loss, a variety of surgical procedures may be indicated including ventriculo-peritoneal shunting, bitemporal decompression and optic nerve sheath decompression. In the latter procedure (Galbraith & Sullivan 1973) a slit is made in the optic nerve sheath usually from the nasal side and has a low morbidity in adults and children (Billson & Hudson 1975; Tompkins & Spalton 1984; Hupp et al. 1985). Various techniques have been used including multiple slits (Sergott et al, 1988) and fenestration via a lateral orbitotomy (Corbett et al. 1988). The procedure may improve vision even after patients have failed to improve following one or more lumbarperitoneal shunting procedures (Sergott et al. 1987). The optic nerve subarachnoid space is patent postoperatively (Brourman et al. 1988) and the mechanism of its action is probably by causing decompression of the optic nerve and the intracranial contents by filtration of CSF through the slit or fenestration (Keltner 1988).

Low intracranial pressure

Lumbar puncture headaches seem to be much less frequent in children who do not suffer the days of severe bursting headache of some adults who have had lumbar punctures. Some, however complain of headache and may be 'grizzly' for a few hours.

Eye and oculomotor disease

Eye disease especially uveitis, glaucoma, and corneal disease gives rise to eye pain; chronic eye pain is often also referred to areas around the eye and may result in symptoms of headache.

Parents, teachers and others frequently suspect that refractive error or eye muscle 'imbalance' cause headache, but only occasionally are they right.

The headaches usually are related to school or reading and are very rarely present on waking. They are most often frontal or around the eyes and they are present almost every day, often not being present on weekends or holidays.

The causes can be divided into those from refractive errors, latent strabismus convergence insufficiency, and accommodation defects. Refractive errors usually cause headaches or 'eyestrain' by making the child peer at objects through narrow palpebral fissures in a pin hole effect. It is probably the prolonged muscular contraction that causes the symptoms.

Latent strabismus usually does not cause headache or eyestrain, even with large angle deviations; occasionally however when the latent deviation is barely controlled, symptoms may develop.

Eyestrain is more frequent when there is convergence insufficiency. The symptoms are usually directly related to reading and the child complains that he cannot read or that concentration is difficult. Diagnosis is simply made by getting the child to look at a near detailed (accomodative) target and observing the eye position or asking him to tell you when he sees double; considerable exhortation should be used after the initial test to see how hard he is trying! Treatment is by near point exercises.

Accomodation defects result in reading difficulty similar to presbyopia. Nearly all are psychogenic and respond well to reassurance, relief of stress factors when these can be identified, and near-point exercises. Organic causes of accomodation defects include Adie's pupil, pharmacological blockade by atropine like drugs, incipient nerve palsies. Not many clinicians will correctly diagnose at the first visit the child or young person who presents with symptoms of defective accommodation secondary to a Sylvian aqueduct syndrome but they do occur!

Bone and sinus disease

Sinus disease and osteomyelitis related to it is not uncommon in older children but the severity and frequency are less since the advent of antibiotics. The pain is usually localized over the affected sinus or in the case of the ethmoids it is usually felt 'between the eyes'. It is often severe and intermittent, worse on bending or coughing and often better on lying down. There may be tenderness on pressing or tapping on the affected area. The diagnosis can be confirmed by radiology but often the help of an otorhinolaryngologist is required.

Headache with intracranial disease

Meningism

Irritation of the meninges (meningism) causes headache and a stiff neck which increases and becomes painful on flexing. The cause can be infectious meningitis when fever is also present or blood in the CSF following subarachnoid haemorrhage from aneurysm, arteriovenous malformation, or trauma. Local tenderness or ache may occur if the meningeal disease is localized. Minor trauma giving rise to meningism from subarachnoid haemorrhage should make one suspicious of an arteriovenous malformation.

Trauma

The headaches that occur soon after head trauma are usually related to meningism, sinus diseases or direct skull, or muscle trauma, but headaches frequently continue for several months after the trauma. This post-traumatic headache is less frequent in children than in adults and usually has a better prognosis, but is more frequently associated with temper tantrums, lack of concentration, and behaviour disorder (Dillon & Leopold 1961).

Migraine

Migraine is an important cause of headache in children and is frequently associated with visual or ocular symptoms (Bille 1962).

Migraine is paroxysmal, occurring in attacks lasting hours or days, every few weeks or months. The child is free of symptoms in the intervals between attacks.

A variety of premonitory symptoms preceed the attacks by a matter of hours and include dizziness, nausea, excitability, depression; children however are often unaware of them until asked directly. Classically, visual symptoms occur next but are not often of the typical 'fortification spectrum' type complained of by adults. Scotomata, scintillating spots or hemianopias are frequent and transient and the headache follows within the hour. Usually the headache is very severe, unilateral and of a boring quality. There may be associated symptoms of sensory or motor disturbances in the head or limbs and dysphasia. Photophobia is severe in some children and many like to lie down in a darkened quiet room. The headache passes off in hours but can last days and leaves many patients feeling weak and shaky for a while.

Some authors make a distinction between classic and common migraine (Spector 1984); the classic form being associated with the premonitory visual symptoms.

Many cases have typical or partial attacks and the diagnosis in these cases in particular rests on the history alone, Scintillating scotomas, hemianopia, central scotoma, altitudinal hemianopia, diplopia, and the other symptoms may occur without headache (Wiley 1979; O'Connor & Tredici 1981).

Migraine is probably related to calibre changes in meningeal vessels that penetrate the outer cortex (Blau 1978) and although it has been reported to resolve after the removal of brain arteriovenous malformation (Troost et al. 1979) this is distinctly unusual. If the history is typical and if there is a family history, further investigations are not usually necessary. That the visual symptoms are usually cortical is attested to by their occurence in people without eyes (Peatfield & Rose 1981).

Episodic mydriasis may occur in childhood migraine during the headache (Woods et al. 1984).

Complicated migraine

HEMIPLEGIC

In this form the migraine attacks are accompanied by a hemiplegia or hemisensory attack. The attacks may alternate from side to side (Hosking et al. 1978) and it may familial (Zifkin et al. 1980).

OPHTHALMOPLEGIC

This condition usually has its onset in childhood with the sudden onset of a unilateral IIIrd nerve palsy usually involving the pupil (Friedmann et al. 1962). Pain or headache is not always present (Durkan et al. 1971). The IIIrd nerve palsy usually resolves at least partially, only to recur after an interval of up to a few years. The mechanism is obscure, but is probably peripheral. Anomalous reinnervation may occur and then be obliterated by a further attack. The diagnosis should only be made after careful exclusion of other causes by scanning and arteriography. There may be a family history of migraine.

Fourth and VIth nerve pareses are even less frequent.

BASILAR

This is presumed to be due to transient abnormalities of the vertebrobasilar vascular system (Bickerstaff 1961). Symptoms include vertigo, hemianopias, ataxia, and occipital headache. It is important to establish the absence of hypertension and neurological signs or symptoms between attacks.

RETINAL, CHOROIDAL AND OPTIC NERVE

These are diagnosed by the history of the visual defects. They are monocular transient visual defects including altitudinal hemianopias, central or arcuate scotomas or total visual loss. Permanent visual loss has occurred in some cases, attributed to a variety of mechanisms (Spector 1984). It is usually diagnosed in adults only.

CLUSTER HEADACHES (Raeder's syndrome, Horton's cephalalgia, migrainous neuralgia, etc.)

These excruciating, recurrent facial headaches sometimes with sympathetic nervous system signs are found in middle-aged adults, but occasionally can be dated back to late childhood.

Other causes of headache

Hypoglycaemia causes irritability and headache in some children (Hockaday 1982).

Fever of any cause may be associated with headache and many of the exanthematas especially measles, cause eye pain on lateral gaze.

Nerve entrapment may occur in children with bone disorders such as fibrous dysplasia, mucopolysaccharidoses or histiocytosis X.

Arthritis of the temporomandibular joint or at the craniocervical junction are rare but may occur in children predisposed to 'wear and tear' arthritis by injury, developmental defects or metabolic disease, e.g. ochronosis.

Investigation

The diagnosis is made by the history, the examination

either confirms it or excludes any associated abnormalities such as hypertension or central nervous system signs. A small proportion of patients will require further investigation by plain X-rays, CT scanning or MRI scanning, especially those in whom raised ICP intracranial tumour or sinus disease is suspected.

References

Baker RS, Carter D, Hendrick EB, Buncic JR. Visual loss in pseudotumour cerebri of childhood. *Arch Ophthamol* 1985; **103**: 1681−6

Bickerstaff ER. Basilar artery migraine. *Lancet* 1961; **1**: 15−17

Bille B. Migraine in School children. *Acta Paediat Scand* (Suppl.): 1962; **51** 00−00

Billson FA, Hudson FA. Surgical treatment of chronic papilloedema in children. *Br J Ophthalmol* 1975; **59**: 92−5

Blau JN. Migraine: a vasomotor instability of the meningeal circulation. *Lancet* 1978; **11**: 1136−9

Brourman ND, Spoor TC, Ramocki JM. Optic nerve sheath decompression for pseudotumor cerebri. *Arch Ophthalmol* 1988; **106**: 1378−83

Carlow TJ, Glaser JS. Pseudotumor cerebri syndrome in systemic lupus erythematosus. *JAMA* 1974; **228**: 197−200

Corbett JJ, Nerad JA, Tse DT, Anderson RL. Results of optic nerve sheath fenestration for pseudotumor cerebri. *Arch Ophthalmol* 1988; **106**: 1391−7

Dillon H, Leopold RL. Children and the postconcussion syndrome. *J Am Med Ass* 1961; **175**: 86−91

Durkan GP, Troost BT, Slamovits S, Spoor TC, Kennerdell JS. Recurrent painless oculomotor palsy in children. A variant of ophthalmoplegic migraine? *Headache* 1971; **21**: 281−4

Friedman AP, Harter DH, Meritt HH. Ophthalmoplegic migraine. *Arch Neurol* 1962; **7**: 320−31

Galbraith JEK, Sullivan JH. Decompression of the perioptic meninges for relief of papilledema. *Am J Ophthalmol* 1973; **76**: 687−92

Grant DN. Benign intracranial hypertension: a review of 79 cases in infancy and childhood. *Arch Dis Child* 1971; **46**: 651−5

Hayreh SS, Servais GE, Virdi PS. Fundus lesions in malignant hypertension IV. Focal intraretinal periarteriolar transudates. *Ophthalmology* 1986a; **93**: 60−74

Hayreh SS, Servais GE, Virdi PS. Fundus lesions in malignant hypertension V. Hypertensive optic neuropathy. *Ophthalmology* 1986b; **93**: 74−8

Hayreh SS, Servais GE, Virdi PS. Fundus lesions in malignant hypertension VI. Hypertensive choroidopathy. *J Am Acad Ophthalmology* 1986d; **93**: 1383−400

Hayreh SS, Servais GE, Virdi PS, Marcus ML, Rojas P, Woolson RF. Fundus lesions in malignant hypertension III.

Arterial blood pressure, biochemical and fundus changes. *Ophthalmology* 1986d; **93**: 45−60

Hockaday JM. Headache in children. *Br J Hosp Med* 1983; **27**: 383−92

Hosking GP, Cavanagh NPC, Wilson J. Alternating hemiplegia: complicated migraine of infancy. *Arch Dis Child* 1978; **53**: 656−00

Hulse JA, Taylor DSI, Dillon MJ. Blindness and paraplegia in severe childhood hypertension. *Lancet* 1979; **11** 553−6

Hupp SL, Glaser JS, Frazier-Byrne S. Optic nerve sheath decompression Review of 17 cases. *Arch Ophthalmology* 1987; **105**: 386−9

Keltner J. Optic nerve sheath decompression. *Arch Ophthalmol* 1988; **106**: 1365−9

Lance JW. Outpatient problems headache. *Br J Hosp Med* 1978; **19**: 377−9

Minns RA. Clinical application of ventricular pressure monitoring in children. *Z Kinderchir* 1977; **22**: 430−43

Northfield DW. Some observations on headache. *Brain* 1938; **61**: 133−62

O'Connor PS, Tredici TJ. Acephalgic migraine, fifteen years experience. *Am Acad Ophthalmol* 1981; **88**: 999−1002

Orcutt J, Page NGR, Sanders MD. Factors affecting visual loss in benign intracranial hypertension. *Ophthalmology* 1984; **91**: 1303−13

Peatfield RC, Rose F C. Migrainous visual symptoms in a woman without eyes. *Arch Neurol* 1981; **38**: 466−6

Sedwick LA, Burde RM. Unilateral and asymmetric optic disc swelling with intracranial abnormalities. *Am J Ophthalmol* 1983; **6**: 484−7

Sergott RC, Savino PJ, Bosley TM. Modified optic nerve sheath decompression provides long-term visual improvement for pseudotumor cerebri. *Arch Ophthalmol* 1988; **106**: 1384−90

Spector RH. Migraine. *Surv Ophthalmol* 1984; **29**: 193−207

Tomkins CM, Spalton DJ. Benign intracranial hypertension treated by optic nerve sheath decompression. *J R Soc Med* 1984; **77**: 141−3

Troost BT, Mark LE, Maroon JC. Resolution of classic migraine after removal of an occipital lobe arteriovenous malformation. *Ann Neurol* 1979; **5**: 199−201

Trompeter RS, Smith RL, Hoare RD, Neville BGR, Chandler C. Neurological complications of arterial hypertension. *Arch Dis Child* 1982; **57**: 913−7

Weisberg LA, Chutorian AM. Pseudotumor cerebri of childhood. *Am J Dis Child* 1977; **131**: 1243−8

Wiley RG. The scintillating scotoma without headache. *Ann Ophthalmol* 1979; **11**: 581−5

Wolff HG. *Headache, and other related pain.* Oxford University Press, New York 1963

Woods D, O'Connor PO, Fleming R. Episodic unilateral mydriasis and migraine. *Am J Ophthalmol* 1984; **98**: 229−35

Zifkin B, Andermann E, Andermann F, Kirkham T. An autosomal dominant syndrome of hemiplegic migraine, nystagmus, and tremor. *Ann Neurol* 1980; **8**: 329−31

P17 Peculiar Visual Images

DAVID TAYLOR

Children probably have visual experiences that are not 'usual' much more frequently than is realized. They have difficulty in describing them, preferring to call their vision blurred or fuzzy or just 'funny' to giving a more accurate description which they have difficulty in expressing. Their parents, quite understandably, often do not report the symptoms because they have difficulty in understanding them. Ophthalmologists rarely ask children whether they have odd visual images because of a mistaken fear of being misunderstood.

Dysmetropsia

Changes in the size or shape of an object.

Micropsia

A sensation that objects are smaller than they should be is a common experience in childhood and it is usually not based on any organic disease unless associated with other symptoms. Micropsia with metamorphopsia, hallucinations or visual defects is always organic.

Most of the children I have seen with this condition have been between 7 and 15 years, of either sex and it has been an isolated complaint. Often they have been reading in bed in the evening and have noticed a progressive diminution in the size of their book; looking up they see familiar surroundings clearly but greatly diminished in size; if they walk around they have a peculiar sensation that they are in a Lilliputian land. The sensation frightens only the most timid. It lasts a few minutes and usually goes more quickly than it comes. Sometimes the disappearance is instantaneous whereas the onset is so gradual that it is difficult to say when it began. There is no adequate explanation of the cause but it could be related to a 'mismatch' between accommodation and convergence because when divergence is induced by mirrors or prisms in the absence of a change in accommodation or change in image size, an increase in the perceived size of the image is experienced. The reverse occurs when convergence is induced. The symptoms usually disappear in a few months and reassurance is the only treatment.

Micropsia also occurs with retinal macular disease, particularly with macular oedema or any disease in which the retinal elements are abnormally separated including dystrophies and neuroretinitis. In retinal micropsia there is usually an uncorrectable acuity defect, only a minimal colour defect and the child notices blurred or distorted central vision especially if the disorder is bilateral (Fig. P17.1).

Micropsia may be noticed at the first wearing of myopic spectacles or contact lenses for hypermetropia, and it may be prolonged if the lenses are too strong.

Cerebral abnormalities have been reported as causing micropsia including migraine, cortical defects

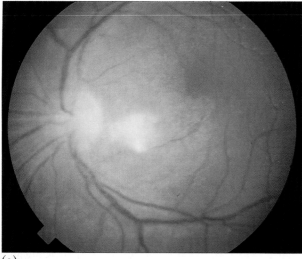

(a)

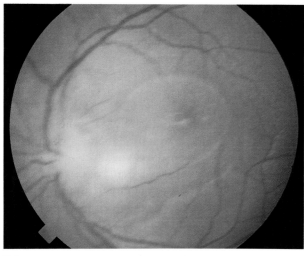

(b)

Fig. P17.1 (a) Neuroretinitis with micropsia. This 9 year-old girl complained of dullness of the vision in both eyes, and smallness of objects with distortion on the right. The white area temporal to the optic disc represents retinal nerve fibre swelling and vascular leakage. The retinal oedema extends to the fovea. (b) As the retinal oedema increased and extended across the macula the acuity dropped to 6/36 and the micropsia disappeared.

and a chiasmal tumour (Bender & Savitsky 1943) which gave rise to a nasal/temporal field size difference. Hallucinations also occurred with Lilliputian images (Savitsky & Tarachov 1941) in a child with scarlet fever.

The key to the diagnosis, therefore, is the history and examination of the child: with isolated micropsia and no abnormality on examination there is no need for further investigation.

Macropsia

Macropsia is much rarer than micropsia. It may occurs with retinal diseases where the foveal cones are pushed together or with cortical disease. Rarely it is found as a non-organic or benign disorder in the same way that micropsia occurs.

Metamorphopsia

Distortion of central vision, which the child reports as 'lines are bent', 'objects appear broken up' or, in younger children that things are blurred or that they just can not see properly, occurs only with organic disease, usually of the anterior visual system. It is accompanied by clinical or neurophysiological evidence of central visual disorders. Metamorphopsia also occurs with brain abnormalities but it is usually accompanied by hallucinations or with visual field defects or both.

Erythropsia and 'coloured clouds'

A sensation that everything is red (erythropsia) is sometimes noted by patients, including children, for a few days or weeks after cataract surgery, it does not seem to have any significance and usually does not trouble the child very much.

'Coloured clouds' are a sensation reported by some children and adults when lying in a sleepy state in oblique sunlight or bright light. They see whorls of multicoloured lights, predominantly red and blue which swirl in their vision when the lids are closed; it is normal and is probably an entoptic phenomenon.

Entoptic phenomena

Entoptic phenomena are visual observations of normal phenomena within the eye that are made in unusual viewing conditions. Examples include the viewing of retinal vessels by rubbing the eye with a light through closed lids, or seeing spots moving when looking at a bright clear blue sky or an open field of snow (Scheerer's phenomenon).

Phosphenes and photopsias

Phosphenes are transient tiny spots of light seen in an otherwise intact field of vision which usually occur because of retinal stimulation. There are many examples of phosphenes including:

1 The bright lights seen when the eye is rubbed through closed lids.

2 Bright lights may occur as a result of retinal traction in vitreous disease. When associated with seeing spots these are an indication for careful ophthalmoscopy since they are the cardinal symptoms of a retinal tear.

3 'Moores's lightning streaks' are larger blue or white lights that meander in the vision for a second or so especially when the lights are dimmed. Their origin is unknown and they seem to be harmless.

4 Flick phosphenes are eye movement-related spots of light caused by retinal traction.

5 Transient flashes of light may be seen in retinal embolic disease.

Photopsias are larger, longer lasting, visual phenomena that may also be related to movement. Davis *et al.* (1976) described their occurrence in patients with optic neuropathies, the relationship to movement presumably being due to traction on the optic nerve. Rarely a patient with an optic neuropathy may complain of seeing a bright light or a flash of light when stimulated by sound (Page *et al.* 1982; Jacobs *et al.* 1987). Thus many of the transient flashes of light seen by children can be of serious significance and should never be dismissed as being 'invented'.

Complaints about poor vision in special lighting conditions should never be dismissed. They may be a form of photophobia (see Appendix, Problem 8), due to an optic neuropathy causing altered visual perception or due to a cerebral defect.

Monocular diplopia

Monocular diplopia in children, requires especially careful questioning to determine its true nature. It is most often due to small axial cataracts or corneal disease, cataracts where one part of the lens has a higher refractive index than another, or occasionally due to retinal disease or simple refractive errors (Coffeen and Guyton 1988). Careful questioning may also reveal more than two images, each of varying sharpness.

An interesting example of monocular diplopia occurs when, in a child who has anomalous retinal correspondence associated with squint, the eyes are re-aligned surgically; he sees two images with the eye that was squinting before surgery. It fades gradually over weeks or months as one or other image predominates depending on the success of the re-alignment. With both eyes open there can be a bin-

ocular triplopia. Diplopia may occur with brain disease (Safran *et al.* 1981) when either eye is viewing and is very rare. In many cases no cause can be found and the underlying problem may be hysterical (see Chapter 33).

Hallucinations

Hallucinations, being entirely personal subjective phenomena, are impossible for the clinician to verify, so their definition by Esquirol as 'false sensory impressions not due to disease of the sense organs' makes a positive diagnosis impossible. There is, however, no totally satisfactory definition of these images which the patient thinks are real, but which arise within the mind in the absence of sense organ stimulation.

Pseudohallucinations are described as hallucinations where the subject realizes they are not 'real' images. Illusions are misinterpretations of actual images.

Social deprivation

Children deprived, intentionally or otherwise, of social contact may develop elaborate visual and auditory images of imaginary friends or animals that can last hours and are usually enjoyed by the child, who is preoccupied by them (Bender 1954). They are probably extensions of the normal imaginary companions that many children have (Bender & Vogel 1941).

Sensory deprivation and visual loss

Persons who have been isolated for prolonged periods, especially in conditions of total sensory deprivation may develop elaborate visual and other sensory hallucinations which are often quite pleasant.

Hallucinations occur quite frequently in visual loss, this is a common experience for cataract surgeons in an elderly population and is enhanced by the patient's nervousness and exposure to drugs especially alcohol (and its withdrawal) and premedication drugs.

Patients with sudden cortical visual loss have formed hallucinations that usually, but not always, occur in the area of defective visual field (Lance 1976). These hallucinations are 'irritative' phenomena that are similar to those that occur after encephalitis (Mize 1980) or with epilepsy. However they occur in any part of the visual field. Patients with eye disease may develop hallucinations that diminish in their clarity, frequency and duration as the blindness progresses (White 1980). When vivid, pleasant hallucinations occur in the elderly with preserved intellectual functions and eye disease, they are known as the Charles Bonnet syndrome (Damas-Mora *et al.* 1982). I have seen a child with adrenoleukodystrophy with cortical blindness and optic atrophy who had vivid and pleasant hallucinations of animals.

Visual phenomena with localized brain disease

Hallucinations should not be thought of as arising from disease of any particular part of the brain, but some phenomena are more common with disease of certain areas of the brain (Gittinger *et al.* 1982). Disease of the posterior visual pathways and particularly the occipital cortex usually gives rise to unformed crude, repetitive hallucinations. These are usually 'irritative' i.e. due to an epileptic form of discharge as opposed to the hallucinating due to anterior visual pathways disease which 'releases' the brain from vision which normally suppresses unwanted discharges (Cogan 1973).

Temporal lobe lesions are said to give rise to formed and detailed visual and olfactory hallucinations. In one case, that of an elderly man with a stroke the hallucinations were exclusively provoked by watching TV (Safran *et al.* 1981).

The evidence for midbrain disorders giving rise to hallucinations is less clear. L'Hermitte (1922) and Van Bogaert (1927) described cases with pathological confirmation. Van Bogaert coined the term Peduncular Hallucinosis because he believed that involvement of the cerebral peduncles was a vital feature. The name is so euphonic that it has remained. The hallucinations are remarkably vivid (Geller & Bellur 1987), like a film in many cases, coloured and occasionally accompanied by unformed sound.

Hypnagogic and hypnopompic

Hallucinations on going to sleep (hypnagogic) or waking (hypnopompic) are quite common in adults. They are often pleasant and have the frustrating quality that when they are concentrated upon they disappear. Although said to be common, occurring in perhaps one fifth of a population of physicians (Lessell 1975), I have found them so rarely in children that I am reluctant to ask.

Drugs

Barbiturates, valium, and alcohol withdrawal after chronic intoxication may all be associated with hallucinations. Chronic abuse is very rare in childhood, but must be remembered with the withdrawal of barbiturates in epileptic children.

Atropine, cyclopentolate and some other cycloplegic drugs are potent causes of visual hallucinations which occur as part of an organic psychosis with confusion and signs of intoxication (hot, red-faced, dilated pupils, tachycardia).

Ketamine, widely used for examinations under anaesthesia, produces visual and frightening hallucinations especially if the child is wakened roughly.

LSD and mescalin cause hallucinations that may occur long after the taking of the drug but usually within the first 6 hours, starting shortly after ingestion. Micropsia, macropsia, palinopsia and remarkable formed visual hallucinations that are not stereotyped also occur (Lessell 1975).

Psychoneuroses and psychiatric disease

Hallucinations, particularly auditory, occur in about 15% of children with behaviour problems (Bender 1954). Powerful, auditory and visual hallucinations, often religious or persecutory and frightening are characteristic of schizophrenia which may have its onset in later childhood. They are true hallucinations, believed by the patient. In adolescent psychoses, hallucinations occur in 75% of children and are most frequently auditory or auditory and visual (Garralda & Ainsworth 1987).

Children with conductor emotional disorders who also suffered from hallucinations, were older than similar children without hallucinations. They also had lower IQs and were more frequently admitted to hospital for the disorder. The hallucinating children were more likely to be depressed, to have a family history of mood changes and to have more symptoms suggestive of cognitive perceptual disorder (Garralda 1984a). When followed to adulthood the association with hallucinations did not carry an increased risk for psychoses, depressive illness, organic brain disease, or other psychiatric disorder (Garralda 1984b).

Palinopsia (visual perseveration in time)

Palinopsia is when there is a 'flashback' of part of a visual scene that was experienced seconds, minutes, or hours previously. Part or the whole of the visual field may be affected by the palinopsic image and there may also be auditory perseveration (Lessell 1975). It occurs in evolving lesions of different types, usually in defective areas of the visual fields. There is almost invariably a visual field defect and the right parietal lobe is most frequently affected (Bender *et al.* 1968).

Occipital epilepsy

Benign occipital epilepsy of childhood is a condition which may be familial and gives rise to unformed visual experiences of transient loss of vision that occur in brief attacks up to several times a day. Electro-encephalography shows epileptiform discharges over the occipital region that are abolished by eye opening. Symptoms may be improved by antiepileptic drugs (Nagendran *et al.* 1989).

References

Bender L. Hallucinations in children. In: *A Dynamic Psychopathology of Childhood*. C Thomas, Springfield, Ill 1954

Bender MB, Feldman M, Sobin AJ. Palinopsia. *Brain* 1968: **91**: 321−38.

Bender MB, Savitsky N. Micropsia and teleopsia limited to the temporal fields of vision. *Arch Ophthalmol* 1943; **29**: 904−8

Bender L, Vogel BF. Imaginary companions of children. *Am J Orthopsychiatry* 1941; **11**: 56−65

Cogan DG. Visual hallucinations as a release phenomena. *Alb von Graefes Arch Klin exp Ophthalmol* 1973; **188**: 139−50

Coffeen O, Guyton DL. Monocular diplopia accompanying ordinary refractive errors. *Am J Ophthalmol* 1988; **105**: 451−60

Damas-Mora J, Skelton-Robinson M, Jenner FA. The Charles Bonnet syndrome in perspective. *Psychol Med* 1982; **12**: 251−61

Davis FA, Bergen D, Schauf C, McDonald WI, Deutsch W. Movement phosphenes in optic neuritis: a new clinical sign.

Neurology 1976; **26**: 1100−04

Garralda ME. Hallucinations in children with conduct and emotional disorders. The clinical phenomenon. *Psychol Med* 1984A; **14**: 589−96

Garralda ME. Hallucinations in children with conduct and emotional disorders. The follow-up study. *Psychol Med* 1984b; **14**: 597−604

Garralda ME, Ainsworth P. Psychoses in adolescence. In: Coleman J (Ed.) *Working with Troubled Adolescents*. Academic Press, London 1987; 169−86

Geller T. Bellur SN. MRI Confirmation of mesencephalic infarction during life. *Ann Neurol* 1985; **21**: 602−03

Gittinger WW, Miller NR, Keltner JL, Burde RM. Sugarplum fairies. Visual hallucinations. *Surv Ophthalmol* 1982; **27**: 42−8

Jacobs L, Karpic A, Bozian D, Gothgen S. Auditory−visual synesthesia. *Arch Neurol* 1987; **38**: 211−16

L'Hermitte J. Syndrome de la Calotte du pédoncule Cérébral. Les Troubles Psycho-Sensoric dans les lésions du mésocephale. *Rev Neurol* 1922; **2**: 1359−65

Lance JW. Simple formed hallucinations confined to the area of a specific visual field defect. *Brain* 1976; **99**: 719−34

Lessell S. In: *Glaser JS, Smith JL Neuro-ophthalmology*, vol. 8. Glaser JS, Smith JL (eds) CV Mosby, St Louis 1975; pp. 27−44

Mize K. Visual hallucinations following viral encephalitis; a self report. *Neuropsychologica* 1980; **18**: 193−202

Nagandran K, Prior PF, Rossiter M. Benign occipital epilepsy of childhood: a family study. *J R Soc Med* 1989; **82**: 684−5

Page NGR, Bolger JP, Sanders MD. Auditory evoked phosphenes in optic nerve disease. *J Neurol Neurosurg Psychiatr* 1982; **45**: 7−12

Safran AB, Kline LB, Glaser JS, Daroff RB. Television induced formed visual hallucinations and cerebral diplopia. *Brit J Ophthalmol* 1981; **65**: 707−11

Savitsky N, Tarachov S. Lilliputian hallucinations during convalescence from scarlet fever in a child. *J Nerv Ment Dis* 1941; **93**: 310−12

Van Bogaert L. L'hallucinose pédonculaire. *Rev Neurol* 1927; **47**: 608−17

White NJ. Complex visual hallucinations in partial blindness due to eye disease. *B J Psychiatr* 1980; **136**: 284−6

P18 The Child Who Fails at School

NICHOLAS CAVANAGH

The ophthalmologist is usually unwillingly dragged into a child's educational problems but nonetheless it is important that he understands the variety of reasons why a child may have come to see him. The psychologist is the expert in this area and all children with significant learning problems will need assessment by one as early as possible.

Some indications of the extent and nature of the problem will have been provided by the school with comments and reports. These will need to be supplemented by a history from the parents and child, and sometimes it is helpful to see them separately. The history should cover early development, social circumstances, behaviour of the child and the family's perception of the problems.

Causes of failure

These include adverse social circumstances, emotional disturbance, mental retardation, progressive degenerative disease of the CNS, ocular and/or auditory handicap, specific disability, and educational.

Intellectual

The commonest reason is that the child is moderately or severely mentally handicapped. Alternatively the child may have been normal mentally and then regressed with time because of a degenerative disease of the brain. Conditions causing regression are often associated with visual failure.

Specific learning disability

A child may be of normal intelligence but have a specific disability. One such example is dyslexia, but another might be a specific problem of memory whether of long or short term memory or of auditory or of visual memory. Other examples include perceptual problems or specific language disabilities. Many specific disabilities are compounded by attentional deficits, dyspraxia, or behavioural problems (see Chapter 36).

Social and emotional

Social and/or emotional causes of school failure may be mainly due to the child and his family, or in part due to an adverse interaction between the child and his teacher in school. Causes in the former category include the child having a 'difficult' personality, poverty, poor parenting, abuse, bereavement, mixing with the 'wrong' crowd, drug taking, truancy, etc. Examples in the latter category might include child-teacher personality conflict or poor social integration of the child with his peers due to cultural or racial differences.

Educational reasons

The school or its teachers may be at fault or the syllabus inappropriate, boring or too advanced for the child. Not all children respond well to all teaching methods and school-based factors in educational failure should be sought.

Hearing defects

Clearly serious hearing defects will have significant implications for learning. Less severe defects may go unrecognized longer and have deteriorating effects for that reason. Hearing loss may fluctuate and therefore underly erratic achievements. It is postulated that hearing impairment during the sensitive years of speech acquisition may have lasting repercussions upon language abilities.

Sight and oculomotor defects

Although there is a significant proportion of dyslexics who have a variety of minor visual and oculomotor anomalies, (see Chapter 36) it is not proven that these are the cause of the problem and exercises, etc. alone without remedial teaching are unlikely to cause significant improvement. Uncorrected refractive errors, convergence insufficiency, poor vision from any cause and some oculomotor disturbances may occasionally be implicated in educational failure.

The ophthalmologist's role

The ophthalmologist has a simple role. He has to exclude significant eye disease, refractive error or oculomotor dysfunction. Some ophthalmologists may take a greater interest in dyslexia and give their opinion as to the need for occlusion treatment, etc. (see Chapter 36). Their role as wise counsel and guide to the appropriate investigation and management of the child who fails at school should not be overlooked.

P19 Abnormal Pupil Appearance in Infancy

DAVID TAYLOR

Parents often have difficulty in expressing their observations regarding abnormalities of their child's pupils. They may be encouraged to be specific as to whether the pupil is large, small, or abnormally shaped or sited, but when the abnormality is actually due to the iris or the appearance of the pupil reflex it may be more difficult for the parent to find the appropriate words.

Their vagueness should not be dismissed, because it is rarely a symptom, without foundation. Examination, including slit lamp microscopy and fundoscopy, usually reveals the cause. The figure below gives guidelines on the causes, the details of which should be sought in the text (Fig. P19.1 and Chapter 37).

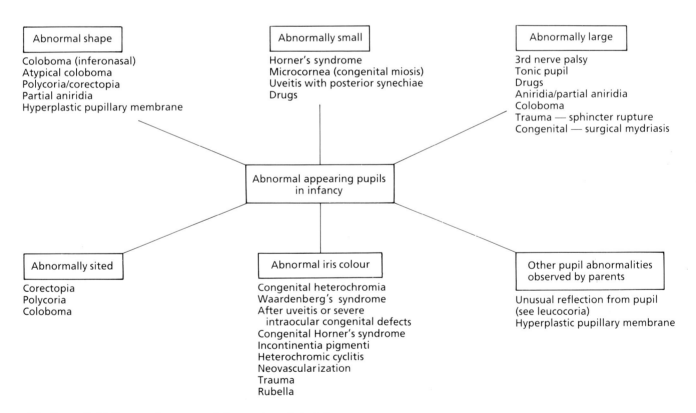

Fig. P19.1 Guidelines on the causes of abnormal pupils in infancy.

P20 Clinical Investigation of Anisocoria

DAVID TAYLOR

When anisocoria is found in a child a simple stage by stage routine can be followed as outlined in Figure P20.1. This is designed to be a guide only.

Pharmacological testing may occasionally be helpful, but most cases can be diagnosed clinically by their size in different lighting conditions and by their neurological accompaniments.

Slit lamp examination will reveal developmental abnormalities and sinuous reactions.

The pupil reactions to a bright light and to a near stimulus are noted. The pupil sizes in the dark and in bright light are recorded and preferably photographed. Physiological anisocoria is common in minor degrees; it is usually equal in light and dark and the reactions are normal.

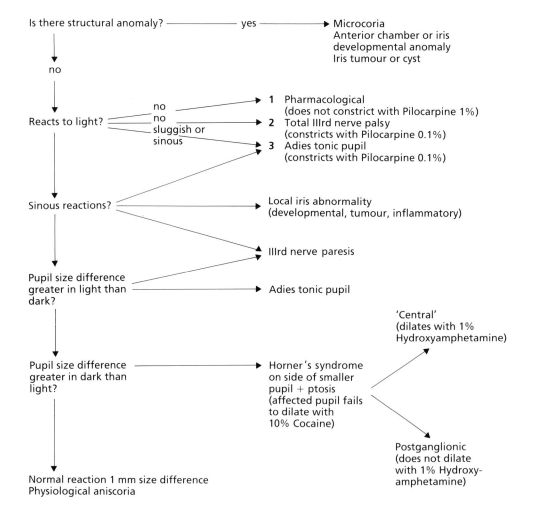

Fig. P20.1 A guide to the routine investigation of anisocoria.

P21 Wobbly Eyes in Infancy

DAVID TAYLOR

It is surprising how few parents notice nystagmus. Their attention is more frequently drawn to the associated squint or poor vision. The history of the nystagmus is important, both prenatal factors such as drug ingestion or a difficult delivery and of postnatal factors such as the mode of onset, associated systemic and ocular illnesses, drugs, and the history of the vision itself.

Some information can be gleaned from the directional characteristics of nystagmus. Nystagmus may be purely vertical, horizontal, or rotary which are characteristics of certain disorders, or they may have specific characteristics (i.e. monocular, see-saw, etc.) which have anatomical or pathogenetic significance (Fig. P21.1)

If the nystagmus is not specific in its characteristics it may help to follow the guidelines of Fig. P21.2. They are not complete but may be helpful in systematically reaching a diagnosis.

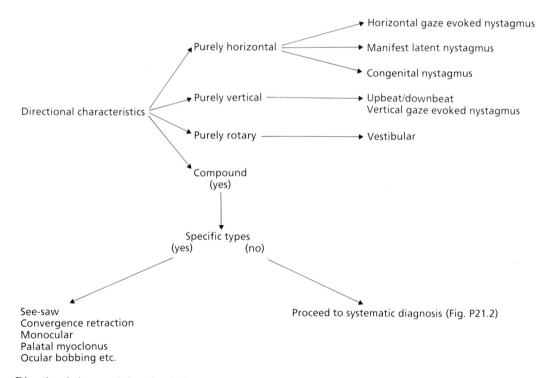

Fig. P21.1 Directional characteristics of wobbly eyes in infancy.

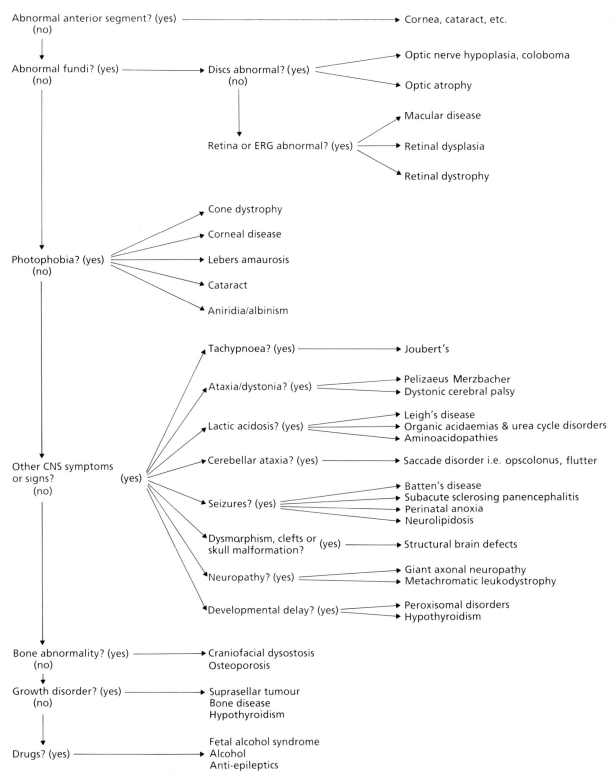

Fig. P21.2 Systematic diagnosis of wobbly eyes in infancy.

Index

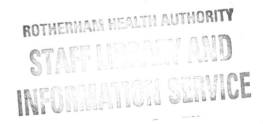